Canine Medicine and Therapeutics

Canine Medicine and Therapeutics

Second edition

edited by

E. A. Chandler BVetMed, FRCVS
J. B. Sutton JP, MRCVS
D. J. Thompson BA, MVB, MRCVS

for the

British Small Animal
Veterinary Association

BLACKWELL
SCIENTIFIC PUBLICATIONS
OXFORD   LONDON   EDINBURGH
BOSTON   PALO ALTO   MELBOURNE

First published 1979
Second edition 1984
Reprinted 1986

Spanish edition 1984

Printed and bound in Great Britain by
Butler & Tanner Ltd
Frome and London

DISTRIBUTORS

USA
   Blackwell Mosby Book Distributors
   11830 Westline Industrial Drive
   St Louis, Missouri 63141

Canada
   The C V Mosby Company
   5240 Finch Avenue East,
   Scarborough, Ontario

Australia
   Blackwell Scientific Publications
      (Australia) Pty Ltd
   107 Barry Street,
   Carlton, Victoria 3053

British Library
Cataloguing in Publication Data

Canine medicine and therapeutics—2nd edn.
   1. Dogs—Diseases
   I. Chandler, E. A.
636.7′0896   SF991

ISBN 0-632-01069-X

Contents

Contributors

W. E. Allen PhD, MVB, MRCVS
Royal Veterinary College Field Station, Hawkshead Lane, North Mymms, Hatfield, Herts AL9 7TA

B. G. Bagnall MA, PhD, DrMedVet, MVSc, MRCVS Smith Kline Animal Health Products, Apple Brook Research Center, 1600 Paoli Pike, West Chester, Pennsylvania 19380, USA.

J. Barker BVetMed, MRCVS
Eastfield Veterinary Clinic, Station Road, North Thoresby, Grimsby

K. C. Barnett MA, PhD, BSc, FRCVS DVOphthal
Animal Health Trust Small Animals Centre. Lanwades Park, Kennett, near Newmarket, Suffolk CB8 7PN

P. G. C. Bedford PhD, BVetMed, FRCVS DVOphthal
Royal Veterinary Field College Station, Hawkshead House, North Mymms, near Hatfield, Herts

D. Bennett BSc, BVet Med, MRCVS
The Veterinary Hospital, University of Liverpool, Crown Street, Liverpool L7 7EX

W. P. Beresford-Jones MA, PhD, MRCVS
Sandbanks, Maidstone Road, Seal, near Sevenoaks, Kent TN15 0EH

B. M. Bush PhD, BVSc, FRCVS
Beaumont Animals Hospital, Royal Veterinary College, Royal College Street, London NW1 0TU

J. R. Campbell PhD, BVMS, FRCVS
Royal Dick School of Veterinary Studies, Summerhall, Edinburgh

Mrs M. L. Clarke FRCVS 'Wheelwrights', 82 Strand Street, Sandwich, Kent CT13 9HX

H. J. C. Cornwell PhD, BVMS, MRCVS
Department of Pathology, Veterinary School, Bearsden Road, Glasgow G61 1QH

R. Curtis PhD, MSc, BVSc, DTVM, FRCVS
Animal Health Trust Small Animals Centre, Lanwades Park, Kennett, near Newmarket, Suffolk CB8 7PN

P. G. G. Darke PhD, BVSc, MRCVS, DVR
Royal Dick School of Veterinary Studies, Summerhall, Edinburgh

A. T. B. Edney BA, BVetMed, MRCVS
Pedigree Petfoods, Division of MARS LT., Animal Studies Centre, Freeby Lane, Waltham-on-the-Wolds, Melton Mowbray, Leicestershire LE14 4RT

I. R. Griffiths PhD, BVMS, FRCVS
Department of Veterinary Surgery, Veterinary Hospital, Bearsden, Glasgow G61 1QH

R. E. W. Halliwell MA, PhD, VetMB, MRCVS
College of Veterinary Medicine, Department of Medical Sciences, Box J126 JHMHC, University of Florida, Gainesville 32610, USA

J. W. Harvey PhD, DVM
College of Veterinary Medicine, Department of Medical Sciences, Box J126 JHMHC, University of Florida, Gainesville 32610, USA

D. E. Jacobs PhD, BVMS, MRCVS
Royal Veterinary College, Royal College Street, London NW1 0TU

D. J. Meyer DVM
College of Veterinary Medicine, Department of Medical Sciences, Box J 126 JHMHC, University of Florida, Gainesville 32610, USA

D. E. Noakes PhD BVetMed, MRCVS
Royal Veterinary College Field Station, Hawkshead Lane, North Mymms, Hatfield, Herts AL9 7TA

D. B. Murdoch BVMS, DVR, MRCVS
Parkside Veterinary Surgery, 2 Sefton Road, New Ferry, Wirral, Merseyside L62 5AT

J. P. Renton PhD, MRCVS
Department of Veterinary Surgery, University of Glasgow Veterinary School, Bearsden Road, Glasgow · G61 1QH

V. L. Voith DVM, PhD
Director, Animal Behaviour Clinic, University of Pennsylvania, School of Veterinary Medicine, 3800 Spruce Street, Philadelphia, PA 19104, USA

A. E. Waterman BVSc, DVA, PhD, MRCVS
Department of Veterinary Surgery, University of Bristol, Langford House, Langford, Bristol BS18 7DU

L. L. Werner DVM
Director, Clinical Immunology Laboratory, College of Veterinary Medicine, Box J126 JHMHC, University of Florida, Gainesville 32610, USA.

CONTRIBUTORS TO FIRST EDITION

We are grateful to the following original authors of the first edition, who have not contributed directly to the second edition:

R. K. Archer MA, PhD, ScD, FRCVS
J. E. Cox BSc, BVetMed, MRCVS
J. O. Joshua FRCVS
N. G. Wright PhD, BVMS, DVM, MRCPath, MRCVS

Preface to first edition

Canine Medicine and Therapeutics has been produced by the British Small Animal Veterinary Association as an authoritative text on a subject in which even the most experienced veterinary surgeon will confess to have some deficiencies.

The concept that the BSAVA should organise a multi-author book on canine medicine, was developed by the Association's Publications Committee and is a radical departure from their smaller manuals of instruction. To produce the book, an editorial board was formed of past Presidents of the BSAVA with publishing experience and in addition two serving Officers of the Association. The 22 contributors were selected with great care and represent expert knowledge in the subjects allocated.

The book is primarily intended for the practising veterinary surgeon and aims to instruct and update in all spheres of medicine. The final year student should also find *Canine Medicine and Therapeutics* an invaluable and refreshingly clear account of all medical problems in the dog.

Although each chapter gives comprehensive cover of the subject, including notes on anatomy and physiology where applicable, the authors have been guided by the editorial board to produce an essentially practical book on medicine. Word and illustration limits were also imposed on the authors on the grounds of economy and speed of production. In this way a concise volume on canine medicine has been produced in a very short time. For those requiring further reading a bibliography is also included with each chapter with further notes on the value of references.

The BSAVA is most grateful to the authors for their hard work and cooperation and the assistance of Blackwell Scientific Publications at all stages of production.

E. A. Chandler
J. B. Sutton

April 1979

Preface to second edition

The British Small Animal Veterinary Association welcomes with the second edition of Canine Medicine and Therapeutics seven new authors, who add more experience, knowledge and two new chapters to its already well recognised text.

While the layout and style of the book remains unchanged and ideally suited to the veterinary surgeon in practice and the student in clinical years, a good amount of new knowledge and material has been added. There are more references, more illustrations, both black and white and colour, and the size of the book has been increased generally. Most chapters have been re-written but in varying amounts, reflecting varying increases in available information.

The success of the first edition was entirely due to the expertise of the original authors and the hard work of the editorial team. The second edition has been a considerable challenge for the BSAVA and it is with justificable pride that it is now introduced.

E. A. Chandler
J. B. Sutton
D. J. Thompson

1
Cardiovascular System

P. G. G. DARKE

The canine species has considerable cardiovascular reserves, but many domesticated dogs are not sufficiently extended for signs of cardiovascular insufficiency to be immediately apparent. Cardiac *disease* can be present for a long time before signs of cardiac *failure* are noticed. However, the presence of cardiac disease is readily detected and recognition of stages of the development of cardiac failure, following compensation and decompensation, is necessary for decisions on therapy and management.

There is good collateral circulation in most canine tissues, and thrombosis or atherosclerotic disease is uncommon. When cardiac output is well within normal demands, the heart rate and rhythm in dogs are notably influenced by vagal tone. Regular slowing of the heart rate under this influence (and acceleration) is found in many normal animals and recognised as 'sinus arrhythmia'.

Table 1.1 shows the overall incidence of cardiac disease in dogs presented to an American clinic (Detweiler & Patterson 1965). Of 4831 dogs presented at the clinic, 545 had evidence of cardiac disease. Of this series, 71 dogs (13.0%) were in congestive cardiac failure.

CONGENITAL CARDIOVASCULAR DISEASE

Congenital malformations involving the cardiovascular system may cause serious disease. Table 1.2 shows the incidence of congenital lesions in a survey of 290 dogs (Patterson 1971).

There is evidence that certain congenital malformations, in particular patent ductus arteriosus, may not be as common in Britain, yet atrioventricular dysplasias may be more frequently encountered.

Patent ductus arteriosus

The ductus normally seals within days of birth, as part of adjustments made by the circulation following pul-

Table 1.1 The incidence and type of cardiac disease in 4831 dogs (Detweiler & Patterson 1965).

	Number of cases	Per cent of cardiac disorders
Congenital disorders	27	(5.0)
Acquired disorders	518	(95.0)
Chronic valvular disease	297	54.5
Myocardial disease	68	12.4
Chronic valvular and myocardial disease	94	17.2
Others	59	10.8

Table 1.2 The incidence of congenital lesions in a survey of 290 dogs (Patterson 1971).

		Per cent of total
Patent ductus arteriosus	82	25.2
Pulmonic stenosis	57	17.6
Aortic stenosis	40	12.3
Persistent right aortic arch	23	7.1
Ventricular septal defect	20	6.1
Systemic venous anomalies	13	4.0
Atrial septal defects	12	3.7
Tetralogy of Fallot	11	3.4
Mitral insufficiency	9	2.8
Incompletely diagnosed	42	12.9
Others	16	4.9
	325	

(Some dogs had more than one defect)

monary inflation. Persistence of patency leads to shunting of part of the outflow from the left side of the heart to the right-sided (pulmonary) circulation during both systole and diastole. This leads to increased demands of left-sided cardiac output and overloading of the lungs. Cardiac insufficiency, pulmonary congestion and oedema, or congestive cardiac failure can develop within weeks or months of birth, and clinical signs are related to these phenomena.

Clinical examination of an affected animal usually yields certain · clear diagnostic features. Mucous membranes appear normal in the majority of cases but, in a few cases where pulmonary hypertension becomes severe, a reversal of shunting may occur so that output from the right side of the heart enters the aorta. This will produce cyanosis. The pulse is usually rapid and can be characteristically jerky, due to a very rapid rise and fall in strength.

Auscultation may reveal congestion of the lungs and a harsh systolic murmur which is generally audible over most of the cardiac area and accompanied by a diastolic murmur, which is usually maximal over the base of the heart on the left side. The waxing and waning of this continuous sound is usually described as a 'machinery' murmur. Occasionally the murmur is loudest at the thoracic inlet and if pulmonary hypertension develops the diastolic component can disappear. Radiography reveals evidence of pulmonary congestion and elevation of the trachea following cardiomegaly. It is sometimes possible to identify enlargement of the aortic arch and pulmonary vessels. Deep Q waves and abnormally tall R waves are frequently found on ECG, especially in leads II and III. Confirmation of the presence of patent ductus arteriosus requires cardiac catheterization and angiography, with the catheter tip in the aortic arch.

The long-term survival of dogs with uncorrected patent ductus arteriosus is poor. Thoracotomy and surgical closure of the defect by double ligation with silk is *relatively* simple and successful in cases where the ductus is a clearly defined vessel and in the absence of further defects which can accompany this lesion. Surgery should be undertaken as soon as possible after diagnosis, as the outcome is likely to be less successful if the dog's maturity is awaited. In the presence of congestive cardiac failure, surgery should be preceded by medical therapy to allow improved cardiac function.

Pulmonic stenosis

Malformation of cusps of the pulmonic valve is the most common form of this deformity, although narrowing may occur above or below the valve. As a dog grows with the lesion, relative obstruction of the right ventricular outflow develops. Clinical signs may initially be absent, but the growth of some dogs is stunted. Exercise intolerance and marked dyspnoea are often early signs of cardiac insufficiency and, following right-sided cardiac failure, venous congestion, ascites and hepatomegaly develop. The latter may be obvious at the time of clinical examination, but in

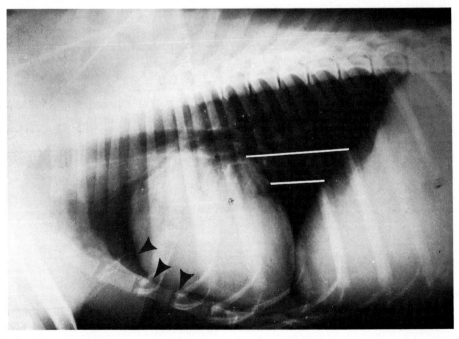

Fig. 1.1 Lateral view of the thorax of a young Labrador with a harsh systolic murmur of congenital pulmonic stenosis. Right ventricular enlargement is present (black arrows). Additionally, the caudal vena cava is enlarged (white lines) and ascites is indicated by the loss of hepatic outline.

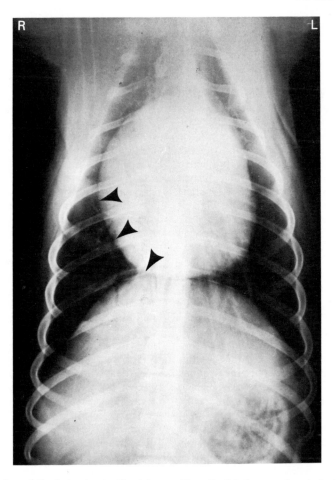

Fig. 1.2 Dorsoventral view of the Labrador in Fig. 1.1. Right ventricular enlargement is indicated by the rounded silhouette (black arrows) and displacement of the cardiac apex to the left.

compensated cases clinical findings can be restricted to the presence of a harsh systolic murmur, usually maximal well forward on the right (occasionally left) side of the thorax, near the sternum.

The right ventricular portion of the cardiac shadow on lateral radiographs appears to be rounded and the cardiac apex may be displaced slightly caudally or dorsally (Figs. 1.1, 1.2). In addition, a post-stenotic bulging of the pulmonary artery may be seen. There is frequently marked negativity of the QRS complex on ECG, with large S waves in all three conventional limb leads. Confirmation of the defect requires cardiac catherization. Right-sided angiography usually demonstrates marked hypertrophy of the right ventricular wall and post-stenotic dilatation of the pulmonary artery. Systolic pressure in the right ventricle is at least double the normal value of 30 mmHg. The possibility of the simultaneous occurrence of other lesions

(e.g. septal defects) should be considered. Surgical relief of the stenosis by dilation with forceps introduced through the right ventricular wall or by section under a patch graft has been successful in some cases. Treatment of right-sided or congestive cardiac failure can help in many cases.

Aortic stenosis

This deformity is most commonly found as a fibrous bar or ring below the valve (sub-aortic stenosis). In many cases no signs of dysfunction are noticed, although fainting (syncope) is not uncommon and left-sided or congestive cardiac failure can develop. The most obvious clinical finding is generally the presence of a harsh systolic murmur centred over the aortic region at the heart base. The murmur may radiate up the aortic arch. Radiographic evidence is often limited to signs of left-sided cardiac enlargement, although bulging of a post-stenotic dilatation of the aortic arch may be seen. Electrocardiographic findings are frequently unremarkable, but dysrhythmias are sometimes recorded. Left-sided cardiac catheterization is required to demonstrate abnormally high left ventricular systolic pressure relative to the aortic pressure. The stenosis and post-stenotic dilatation may be apparent with angiography. Surgical correction requires cardiac by-pass and is not normally considered. A guarded prognosis should be made in untreated cases as, although many affected dogs do not show signs of cardiac failure, sudden death is quite common and the development of dysrhythmias may complicate the management of those dogs with congestive cardiac failure. Propranolol may reduce this risk.

Atrial and ventricular septal defects

Either atrial or ventricular septal defects ('hole in the heart') can be found in combination with other abnormalities and often their presence is identified only in the investigation of other lesions. This applies particularly to an atrial defect, which may be found at one of several sites. While the primary defect gives rise to shunting of blood from the left to the right atrium, and this produces a murmur and a degree of right ventricular overload, clinical signs may be minimal. Similarly, ventricular septal defects occur frequently in combination with pulmonic stenosis and as part of the tetralogy of Fallot. The defect is usually high in the septum, where it can contribute to right ventricular overload. There is a systolic cardiac murmur which is usually harsh, and most audible well forward on the right side of the thorax, but which may be heard also on the left side. Any clinical signs of cardiac insufficiency due to a simple defect are usually related either to pulmonary congestion or to right-sided cardiac failure. In uncomplicated cases of either type of defect, there can be radiographic evidence of this congestion and right-sided cardiac enlargement. However, the ECG is often within normal limits. While a ventricular defect can be detected following cardiac catheterization for angiography (with contrast material in the left ventricle), blood pressure studies and blood gas analysis, catheterization of the left atrium for identification of an atrial defect is not easily achieved. Surgical correction of either defect requires cardiac by-pass and medical treatment is only required if signs of right-sided or congestive cardiac failure develop.

Tetralogy of Fallot

This defect is essentially due to an embryonic failure of the division of the aortic trunk to meet the interventricular septum, so that the aortic arch receives some of the outflow from the right ventricle. There is effective stenosis of the outflow from the right ventricle to the pulmonary artery. The tetralogy includes pulmonic stenosis, ventricular septal defect, dextroposed aorta and right ventricular hypertrophy, which develops in response to the increased outflow resistance. There is consequent shunting of deoxygenated blood into the peripheral circulation (right-to-left shunt). The age at which clinical signs are first appreciated depends in part on the degree of over-riding of the aorta. The affected animal is generally stunted and exercise intolerance with dyspnoea and fatigue or syncope are common findings. Mucous membranes are often deeply coloured and cyanosis readily occurs. There is generally a harsh systolic murmur, but the site and intensity are variable. Radiolucency of the lungs due to undercirculation is often a prominent radiographic finding and right-sided cardiac enlargement may be apparent. Right ventricular cardiac catheterization will indicate raised intraventricular pressure and angiography will demonstrate the right-to-left shunt. Peripheral blood gas analysis will usually reveal reduced oxygen tension, and polycythaemia may be detected haematologically. Surgical correction is difficult, requiring cardiac by-pass, and the prognosis is poor, even with attempted medical management.

Congenital mitral or tricuspid insufficiency

Incompetence of the left or right atrioventricular valve due to dysplasia has been found in a number of young dogs. This causes a systolic murmur and cardiac insufficiency similar to the findings in ageing dogs with acquired fibrosis (endocardiosis) of these valves. Diagnosis can be confirmed angiographically and treatment and management are similar to those required for older dogs with valvular incompetence.

Persistent right aortic arch

An abnormality in the development of the aortic arch can result in the dorsal aorta passing to the right of the trachea and oesophagus. In these circumstances, a vascular ring causes occlusion of the oesophagus, as the ligamentum arteriosum passes above the oesophagus to reach the pulmonary artery. This gives rise to no signs of cardiac dysfunction, but the occlusion of the oesophagus causes persistent regurgitation of solid food from the time that it is first offered. The condition is confirmed by radiography following a barium meal. The stricture should be sectioned surgically to relieve the problem. Other similar vascular rings are occasionally found.

Pericardiodiaphragmatic hernia (peritoneopericardial diaphragmatic hernia)

This is an occasional finding in dogs, where failure of the diaphragm to close the abdomen from the thorax, together with incomplete formation of the mediastinum and the pericardial sac, permits the abdominal cavity to communicate with the pericardial sac. Abdominal contents (usually mesentery, intestine or both) can pass into the pericardial sac. This may cause no clinical signs, but digestive upsets, dyspnoea or right-sided cardiac failure can develop. Cardiac sounds are usually muffled and intestinal sounds may be heard in the cardiac region. Radiographic signs include a greatly enlarged, smooth cardiac silhouette with, in some cases, the presence of gas-filled loops of intestines within the pericardial sac. This is confirmed with radiology following barium meal. Surgical correction via the abdomen is readily achieved, but medical treatment for right-sided cardiac failure should be instituted before surgery is attempted if signs of cardiac failure are present.

Portosystemic anastomoses

Various forms of anastomoses between the hepatic portal vein and other vessels, usually the caudal vena cava, are found either as congenital lesions or secondary to hepatic cirrhosis. Such anastomoses cause shunting of portal venous blood away from the liver, so that nutrients are poorly metabolised and the liver tends to atrophy. Poor physical development, poor appetite and numerous neurological signs can be seen as the dog grows. These include depression, ataxia, circling, wandering, seizures, blindness and head-pressing. The neurological disturbance is associated with hyperammonaemia, due to the failure of conversion of ammonia to urea by the liver. Other signs include polydipsia, salivation, vomiting and ascites. Diagnosis is aided by biochemical findings of low plasma urea and high ammonia levels, together with abnormal retention of bromsulphalein (BSP) and the presence of heavy deposits of ammonium biurate crystals in the urine (Chapter 14). Confirmation re-

quires portal angiography, with contrast material being introduced into the spleen or mesenteric artery. Surgical correction is usually unsuccessful since the circulation and liver cannot readily adapt to sudden changes.

Arteriovenous fistulae

Direct communication between an artery and a vein, by-passing a capillary bed, is unlikely to cause serious signs if the connection is small, but significantly large fistulae are found in dogs. These anomalies may be congenital or acquired. Signs are related to alterations in blood flow in the region of the body that is affected, causing, for example, excessive venous filling with tissue swelling and oedema, or ischaemia with ulceration and gangrenous necrosis of a limb extremity. In addition, with a large defect, increased venous return and consequent overload of the right side of the heart can result in pulmonary congestion or oedema and right-sided cardiac failure. In many cases, a sac-like aneurysm develops, and a thrill or murmur may be detected locally. Angiography aids the diagnosis. In appropriate cases, surgical correction can be undertaken.

Others

Many other congenital defects have been described in individual cases. Not all cases of congenital heart disease are readily diagnosed, even with sophisticated aids to diagnosis. A specific diagnosis may be of no practical consequence, as correction usually requires expensive equipment (for cardiac by-pass) with well-trained ancillary staff, which are not readily available to the profession. Cardiac failure that results from congenital lesions must be treated as it arises.

Hereditary considerations

It has been demonstrated that patent ductus arteriosus in Poodles, pulmonic stenosis in Beagles, and persistent right aortic arch in German Shepherd Dogs in the USA (Patterson 1971) and subaortic stenosis in Boxers in Britain are hereditary in certain lines of dog. In addition, patent ductus arteriosus in Pomeranians and Collies, pulmonic stenosis in Bulldogs, Chihuahuas and Fox Terriers, tetralogy of Fallot in Keeshonds, sub-aortic stenosis in German Shepherd Dogs and Newfoundlands, and persistent right aortic arch in Irish Setters, occur significantly more commonly in these breeds in the USA than the overall breed incidence would indicate, which suggests that certain lines in these breeds may carry a hereditary factor for these congenital malformations. Such considerations warrant attention when cardiovascular anomalies are diagnosed in Britain.

ACQUIRED CARDIAC DISORDERS

Organic lesions

Valvular and endocardial disorders

Valvular fibrosis (endocardiosis)
Fibrosis of the atrioventricular valves is a progressive change which probably starts early in life and which very commonly causes valvular incompetence. The incidence and severity of lesions increases with age but the precise cause is unknown. Cardiovascular compensation for valvular incompetence may be followed by cardiac failure as the valvular leakage increases. The left atrioventricular (mitral) valve is generally more severely affected than the right atrioventricular valve. Stages in the development of cardiac dysfunction following progressive mitral incompetence have been defined by Ettinger and Suter (1970) (see p. 10). Signs of cardiac dysfunction may not develop for months or years following mitral incompetence, as the heart and circulation can compensate adequately by myocardial hypertrophy, an increase in heart rate and peripheral vasoconstriction. Valvular incompetence is found most commonly in small breeds of dog, especially chondrodystrophoid types. The effect of valvular insufficiency is compounded by subsequent dilatation of the cardiac chambers and the atrioventricular annular ring. Degeneration of chordae tendineae and myocardial necrosis and fibrosis also frequently accompany valvular insufficiency, the latter associated with arteriosclerosis of small intramural coronary vessels. This process frequently provokes dysrhythmias in the advanced stages of valvular insufficiency.

Mitral incompetence is marked by a systolic murmur of increasing duration and intensity. It is initially audible most clearly over the fifth intercostal space. The murmur may be appreciated in a dog as young as 5 or 6 years of age, and it is frequently encountered in dogs from 8 years onwards. Any murmur detected before 5 years of age should arouse suspicions of the presence of a congenital lesion, especially if signs of cardiac failure are present.

Incompetence of the right atrioventricular (tricuspid) valve occurs less commonly as a primary disorder than in combination with mitral incompetence. Clinical signs are related only to severe decompensation following valvular insufficiency, when right-sided cardiac failure develops. The maximum intensity of the systolic murmur of tricuspid incompetence is usually at about the fourth intercostal space on the right side of the thorax.

Fibrosis of the aortic and pulmonic valves occurs to a limited extent, but it is rarely sufficient to cause significant dysfunction.

Treatment. Atrioventricular valve replacement requires cardiac by-pass, beyond conventional resources. Stages in the development of congestive cardiac failure must be treated as they arise (p. 20).

Bacterial endocarditis
Blood-borne infection affecting heart valves of dogs may arise from any septic focus, such as infected bite wounds, dental, prostatic or uterine infections, or bronchopneumonia. Vegetative lesions develop most frequently on the left atrioventricular or aortic valves. Organisms that may be found include Streptococci, Staphylococci, *Escherichia coli*, *Erysipelothrix rhusiopathiae* and *Pseudomonas pyocyanea*. Signs of endocarditis in dogs refer to sepsis and fever (anorexia, lethargy, joint pain) rather than cardiac failure (see p. 14).

Rupture of chordae tendineae may result from fibrosis that occurs simultaneously with endocardiosis. This causes the rapid development of congestive cardiac failure and cannot readily be diagnosed *in vivo*.

Intracardiac neoplasms are a rare finding in ageing dogs. Signs can be associated with congestive cardiac failure and diagnosis requires angiography or echocardiography.

Most valvular disease in the dog results in incompetence, producing systolic cardiac murmurs that are usually maximal over the valve concerned. Murmurs can be auscultated or recorded by phonocardiography. Harsh stenotic murmurs arise occasionally from valvular vegetations of endocarditis and from endocardial neoplasms. Murmurs of endocarditis often change character rapidly from day to day, and may have a diastolic component.

Myocardial disorders
A number of disease processes affect myocardial function, the specialised conduction tissues and cardiac rhythm. Myocardial disease is more common than is recognised by many clinicians.

Myocarditis
This is usually found in conjunction with generalised infections or inflammatory disease, including parvovirus in very young pups.

Fibrosis
Resulting from inflammation, infarction, ischaemia or cardiac dilatation, this can contribute to loss of myocardial function in cardiac failure, and can act as an ectopic focus for tachydysrhythmias.

Neoplasia
Lymphosarcoma and carcinomata occasionally metastasise and haemangiosarcoma can develop in the myocardium. Myocardial neoplasia can cause pericardial effusion and signs of right-sided cardiac failure (p. 12). Chemodectomas ('heart base' tumours) arise in the aortic body and congestive cardiac failure and pleural effusions can develop. Neoplasms can cause conduction disturbances and bradydysrhythmias (p. 15).

Idiopathic cardiomyopathy
Myocardial failure of unknown aetiology occurs commonly in large and giant breeds of dog, resulting in the rapid development of right-sided or congestive cardiac failure. Atrial fibrillation is commonly associated with this disorder.

Infarction
Embolic spread of septic or neoplastic material can cause fatal dysrhythmias ('cardiac arrest'), but small areas of myocardium are affected by intramural coronary arteriosclerosis, which frequently accompanies endocardiosis.
    Atherosclerosis of the coronary arteries is rare in dogs.

Myocardial rupture
This may result from fibrosis. It causes pericardial effusion ('tamponade') and acute cardiac failure. Myocardial contusion is a common sequel to road accidents, which can result in temporary dysrhythmias.

Metabolic and endocrine disorders
Myocardial function is influenced by certain endocrine and electrolyte disturbances. The effect of hyperkalaemia, following adrenocortical insufficiency, is notable: there is hypovolaemia, bradycardia and slowed impulse conduction, and, with persistence of this disease, myocardial atrophy occurs. Hypokalaemia or upsets in calcium balance also have profound effects on myocardial function. Thyroid, parathyroid and adrenal dysfunction can all be significant. Hypoxia causes decreased myocardial contractility and an increased sensitivity to dysrhythmias.

Toxaemic disease
Toxaemias, including uraemia, pyometra and gastric dilatation/torsion can either provoke ectopic pacemaker activity (producing premature atrial or ventricular beats) or interfere with impulse conduction (causing heart blocks). In addition, myocardial contractility may be depressed so that cardiac output will fall.
    Certain drugs, notably anaesthetics and cardiac glycosides also affect the myocardium.

Effect
Many myocardial disorders provoke *dysrhythmias*, due either to myocardial irritability, activating ectopic pacemakers (tachydysrhythmias, see p. 16) or to disturbances in impulse conduction (causing bradydysrhythmias, see p. 15). If caused by functional disturbances these dysrhythmias can develop in the absence of detectable organic lesions. ECG will confirm dysrhythmias and conduction disturbances and may demonstrate further signs of myocardial dysfunction (disturbances of the S–T segment, negativity of T wave and bundle branch blocks) which can signify hypoxia or disease of the myocardium. However, the type of dysrhythmia or ECG disturbance does not necessarily indicate the nature of the aetiology or the severity of the disorder.

Significance
Myocardial disease and dysrhythmias tend to cause a decrease in cardiac output and may result in congestive cardiac failure, weakness or syncope.

Treatment
If a specific cause can be detected (e.g. sepsis) then appropriate therapy (e.g. antibiotics) may be effective. Therapy for dysrhythmias may be essential when they are severe. The value of positive inotropic drugs (e.g. digoxin or dobutamine) in myocardial dysfunction is debatable.

Pericardial disorders
Several forms of effusion are found:

Haemorrhage
Haemorrhage may be:

1 Neoplastic (e.g. from haemangiosarcoma of the myocardium).
2 Due to rupture of the myocardium (e.g. in road

accident trauma). Spontaneous left atrial rupture has been reported in dogs, usually in association with mitral incompetence.

3 Idiopathic (spontaneous): probably the most common cause in larger breeds of dog (Gibbs *et al* 1982).

4 Due to coagulopathy (see Chapter 11).

Transudation
Can occur with generalised oedematous disorders (hypoproteinaemia, congestive cardiac failure or neoplastic obstruction of circulation).

Exudation (pericarditis)
Can be due to tuberculosis (now rare) or penetrating wounds or foreign bodies (uncommon).

Fibrinous pericarditis
(Inflammatory or secondary to other disease, e.g. autoimmune disease or uraemia).

Significance
Pericardial effusions tend to cause reduction in right ventricular filling, reduced cardiac output and signs of right-sided, then congestive, cardiac failure. These signs often develop very rapidly ('tamponade'). Accumulation of large quantities of pericardial effusion usually causes muffling of heart sounds, which can be inaudible in severe cases, and the pulse may be weak. Confirmation of pericardial distension requires fluoroscopic radiography or echocardiography. However, radiographic signs suggesting pericardial effusion include a globular appearance of the heart in the absence of gross elevation of the trachea, often with a notably sharp outline to the heart. Unfortunately, details of the cardiac outline are often obscured by the pleural effusion of heart failure.

In acute right-sided or congestive cardiac failure associated with pericardial effusion, pericardiocentesis is recommended for therapy and investigation (p. 23). Diuretic therapy (p. 22) is usually desirable to relieve the effects of congestive cardiac failure.

Vascular disorders
Massive atherosclerosis and thrombosis of the coronary arteries, common in man, is very rare in dogs. However, a number of vascular disorders are encountered:

Thrombosis
Thrombosis of arteries and veins may develop as a result of vascular damage (autoimmune or parasitic), in association with infection or amyloidosis, or for no clear reason. Affected sites include:

1 The aorta at the bifurcation of the iliac arteries, where occlusion causes sudden weakness and hypothermia of the hindquarters, with pain, a degree of hyperaesthesia, and loss of the femoral pulse.

2 Pulmonary arteries, causing acute and non-specific signs, including tachypnoea, lethargy and tachycardia. A weak pulse and pale mucous membranes are also commonly found. Diagnosis requires contrast radiography (angiography).

3 A variety of organs affected by thromboembolic spread, including the kidneys, lungs, intestinal tract or central nervous system, causing infarction.

Embolic spread of septic or neoplastic material
Dissemination of these lesions to tissues similar to those affected by thrombosis may occur. This is especially common with endocarditis.

Arteriosclerosis
Arteriosclerosis of small intramural coronary vessels is a common finding in ageing dogs, frequently associated with mitral incompetence. Small areas of myocardial fibrosis result, which can act as ectopic pacemakers.

Polyarteritis
Polyarteritis (periarteritis nodosa) is an inflammatory disorder affecting small arteries, and is probably the result of autoimmune disease. Haemorrhage may develop in a number of organs (Chapter 10) and pyrexia, stiffness, leucocytosis and renal (glomerular) damage may be found (Chapter 10). Vasculitis can also develop in response to certain infections (especially hepatitis virus).

Disseminated intravascular coagulation
This is a relatively common disorder in association with shock, toxaemia or neoplasia (Chapter 11).

Cerebrovascular accident ('stroke')
There is considerable doubt as to whether in dogs there is a direct counterpart of this phenomenon, so commonly encountered in man. Many clinicians recognise a disorder involving an upset in balance that occurs suddenly in aged dogs, which probably results from a disturbance of the vestibular system: vasospasm, encephalitis and otitis media have been implicated, but obvious pathological lesions may be absent from many cases. Recovery is usual within a few days, even in the absence of treatment.

Neoplasia
1 'Heart base' tumours arise from chemoreceptor tissue (chemodectomas) or ectopic thyroid tissue in

the region of the aortic body in ageing dogs, with a marked preponderance reported in Boxers and Boston Terriers. Affected dogs may show no clinical signs until either the tumour is sufficiently large to occlude venous return to the heart, causing hydrothorax or oedema, or it invades the myocardium, causing haemorrhage into the pericardial sac. In either circumstance, congestive cardiac failure can develop. Carotid body tumours also occur.

2 Haemangiosarcoma develops in a number of tissues in ageing dogs, with German Shepherd Dogs being commonly affected. Splenic, hepatic, cardiac and pulmonary tissues are frequently involved. Recurrent haemorrhage into body cavities, including the pericardial sac, is found in some cases.

Parasitic infections

Heartworm disease. Due to the nematode *Dirofilaria immitis*, heartworm disease may be encountered in dogs imported from tropical or subtropical regions, including Africa, Asia, Australia, the central Americas and eastern seaboard of the USA. The parasite is transmitted in larval form by mosquitoes. The larvae develop in the dog's tissues before migrating into the circulation, when they are carried to the right side of the heart and the pulmonary vessels. The immature worms develop over a period of 2–3 months, causing arteritis of pulmonary vessels which may produce fibrosis and pulmonary hypertension. The resulting clinical signs are coughing, dyspnoea and exercise intolerance. Right-sided cardiac enlargement and failure can ensue. The most reliable diagnostic test is the detection of larvae (microfilariae) in stained blood smears. Signs of right-sided cardiac enlargement may be detected radiographically and electrocardiographically, and gross distension of pulmonary arteries may be evident on radiographs.

Treatment for congestive cardiac failure may be necessary (p. 21). In areas where Dirofilaria is endemic, prophylaxis is necessary, but in imported dogs, where adult worms may be encountered, thiacertarsamide sodium (0.22 ml/kg BID i.v. for 2 days) is usually effective, although toxicity can occur at this dose rate. Alternatively, levamisole (10 mg/kg BID for 2 weeks) can be used (Carlisle 1980).

Angiostrongylus vasorum is an intravascular nematode that may be found especially in Greyhounds imported from Eire. It causes vasculitis that affects particularly the pulmonary arteries and arterioles, resulting in pulmonary thrombosis and sometimes consolidation. Occasionally, haemorrhage or oedema can occur in peripheral soft tissues. Angiostrongylus is diagnosed by detecting larvae in faeces. These may be seen even in direct smears of faeces, but faecal flotation is otherwise necessary. Pulmonary tissue and vascular changes on radiographs are not very specific. Treatment with levamisole (7.5 mg/kg orally for 5 days) is usually effective.

Functional cardiac disturbances

A number of dysrhythmias can be caused by idiopathic disturbance to the vagus, pacemaker or impulse conduction (p. 15). Vagal hyperactivity can be induced by disorders of the central nervous system, by reflex stimulation from carotid sinus pressure, or by excessive glycoside administration.

1 Sinus arrhythmia, which is usually a reassuring sign of normal cardiac function in dogs, can be accentuated by excessive vagal tone.
2 Sinus arrest, which can be a form of excessive sinus arrhythmia, producing long pauses alternating with groups of beats. This disorder occurs most commonly in small and brachycephalic breeds of dog.
3 Sinoatrial and atrioventricular blocks.
4 Sinus bradycardia, which implies that the resting heart rate is less than 70 per minute, but the sinus node is still the pacemaker. This reduced heart rate can result from excessive vagal action and it can occur in normal dogs or with glycoside toxicity.

CLINICAL SYNDROMES RESULTING FROM CARDIOVASCULAR DISORDERS

Clinical signs will appear only when there is failure of compensation by the circulation. Compensation for failure of cardiac output to meet tissue requirements is stimulated mainly by baroceptors, but it also involves the kidneys. A normal heart can multiply its output and the following mechanisms operate:

1 Vasoconstriction, stimulated by the sympathetic nervous system and angiotensin, occurs in cutaneous, renal, alimentary and splenic tissues, and increases the circulating volume.
2 Tachycardia, as a result of sympathetic stimulation and vagal inhibition, increases cardiac output, at the progressive cost of stroke volume (due to reduced ventricular filling).
3 Increased myocardial contractility, stimulated by catecholamines and increased venous return.
4 Retention of sodium and water by the kidneys, in

response to aldosterone, stimulated by the renin–angiotensin mechanism. This increases the circulating volume.

5   Increased stroke volume, initially resulting from the increased ventricular filling pressure that is caused by increased circulating volume and elevated central venous pressure.

However, these mechanisms can be inappropriately regulated, causing volume overload (1, 4 and 5), pressure overload (1 and 3) and excessive tachycardia (2), with the result that the myocardium becomes over-stretched. Myocardial hypoxia and inefficiency then cause a further fall in cardiac output. Volume overload results in tissue congestion and oedema, which may primarily affect one or other side of the circulation in the early stages.

Readily detectable signs of compensation for cardiac failure include tachycardia, enlargement of cardiac chambers and loss of sinus arrhythmia. Signs of failure include congestion of the pulmonary circulation if the left side of the heart is mainly affected, or congestion of the systemic circulation including liver and spleen, often with ascites, in right-sided cardiac failure. However, neither side of the circulation is isolated and failure of one side usually influences the other.

Left-sided cardiac failure

Left-sided cardiac failure can be caused by:

1   Congenital cardiac disorders (e.g. sub-aortic stenosis or mitral dysplasia)
2   Mitral valve incompetence due to endocardiosis.
3   Myocardial failure (see p. 7).

Signs of left-sided failure relate to pulmonary congestion with interstitial and/or alveolar oedema, and to decreased cardiac output. Stages in the development of clinical signs following mitral incompetence have been defined by Ettinger and Suter (1970). These are as follows:

Stage I. Normal activity does not produce undue fatigue, dyspnoea or coughing.

Stage II. The dog is comfortable at rest, but ordinary physical activity causes fatigue, dyspnoea or coughing.

Stage III. The dog is comfortable at rest, but minimal exercise may produce fatigue, dyspnoea or coughing.

Stage IV. Congestive cardiac failure: dyspnoea and coughing are present even when the dog is at rest. Signs are exaggerated by any physical activity.

As the development of left-sided cardiac failure following mitral incompetence is usually progressive over a period of many months or years, and because this disease is by far the most commonly encountered cause of cardiac failure, the diagnosis of the stages of progression of this disease is described in more detail.

Stage I is represented merely by the presence of a systolic murmur (grade I/V) as an incidental finding, indicating mitral incompetence. The heart rate remains within the normal range, and sinus arrhythmia will usually be present. The pulse will be normal in character and rhythm, and there will be little evidence of cardiomegaly with either clinical or radiographic examinations.

Stage II is marked by some exercise intolerance and breathlessness, but a client's complaint is most likely to be their dog's coughing. Although Ettinger and Suter (1970) suggest that this is usually provoked by exercise, the cough is frequently first noticed by the client at night. The heart rate is likely to remain elevated after exercise, although it may return to normal when the dog is at rest. Increased respiratory sounds may be present in the thorax, and evidence of left-sided or generalised cardiac enlargement, together with pulmonary venous congestion, may be detected on thoracic radiographs (Figs. 1.3, 1.4).

Stage III is marked by laboured respirations and very poor exercise tolerance, in addition to coughing, which is often paroxysmal and followed by attempts to regurgitate. The heart rate becomes elevated even at rest, and dysrhythmias, particularly premature (ectopic) beats, may be detected. There is usually an increase in respiratory sounds, the systolic cardiac murmur becomes loud and prolonged, and the cardiac sounds are audible over a larger area than usual. Generalised cardiomegaly is detected radiographically and left-sided cardiac enlargement may be pronounced. Pulmonary venous congestion or hilar oedema is marked, and evidence of systemic venous congestion may be seen: enlargement of the caudal vena cava and the liver is often noted.

Stage IV concerns dogs with congestive cardiac failure which results from decompensation. Dyspnoea, orthopnoea and coughing occur even at rest and the abdomen can be enlarged by ascites and hepatomegaly. Mucous membranes may be slightly pale, and the pulse is sometimes rapid and jerky, but it tends to

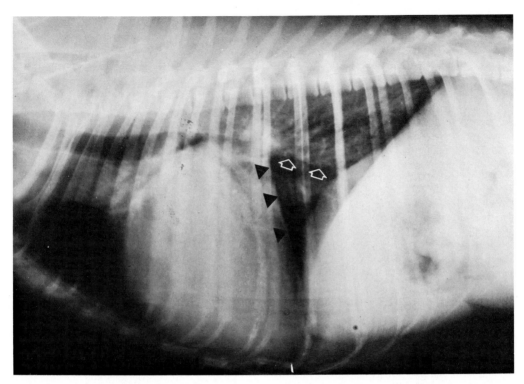

Fig. 1.3 Lateral view of the thorax of an 11-year-old miniature poodle with persistent coughing, resulting from left-sided cardiac failure, following mitral incompetence. Marked elevation of the trachea, upward tilting of the caudal vena cava and straightening of the caudal border of the heart (indicated by black arrows) represent left atrial enlargement. There is diffuse alveolar and interstitial density in the dorsal region of the diaphragmatic lung lobe (white arrows), representing pulmonary congestion and oedema.

become weak and irregular with advanced disease. Respiratory râles are audible over much of the thorax. In some cases, heart sounds can be muffled by the presence of pleural effusion, but a holosystolic murmur of Grade IV–V/V often obliterates the first and second sounds and it may be audible beyond the normal area of auscultation of heart sounds. Radiography will demonstrate widespread pulmonary congestion and oedema, possibly hydrothorax, and gross left-sided or general cardiomegaly. The caudal vena cava may appear to be large and hepatomegaly can often be detected. Cardiac dysrhythmias, including atrial and ventricular ectopic beats are commonly detected by auscultation and ECG, and atrial fibrillation is encountered in large dogs.

Dogs in this stage of decompensation are at risk of sudden death, but many dogs with mitral incompetence will not reach this limit for some years.

A problem is posed by the fact that the most prominent sign of Stages II and III is coughing, and by the frequency with which a murmur of mitral incompetence is detected in ageing dogs. The cough of left-sided cardiac failure resembles that of other chronic respiratory disorders in ageing dogs, particularly chronic bronchitis, which may be present in animals at Stage I of left-sided cardiac failure, where a murmur is an incidental finding. Differentiation of the features of Stages I from those of II and III is therefore important.

Acute decompensation

Acute decompensation following left-sided cardiac failure causes marked signs of pulmonary oedema: severe dyspnoea can develop within a few hours. This can be accompanied by respiratory noise (bubblings), coughing and cyanosis. Respiratory sounds (râles) in the thorax may be so pronounced that cardiac sounds are almost inaudible. Gross tachycardia, with weak pulse and dysrhythmias are common findings. Radiographs demonstrate an alveolar pattern that is much more widespread than in slowly-developing left-sided cardiac failure.

The differential diagnoses of coughing and dys-

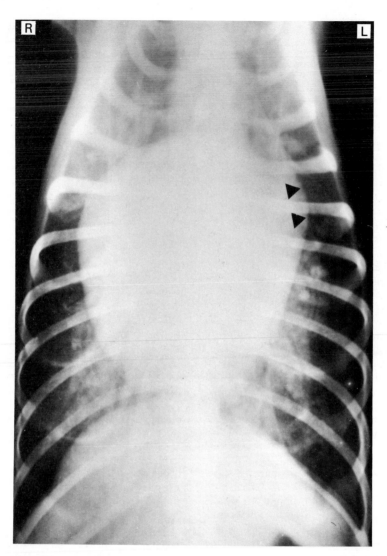

Fig. 1.4 Dorso-ventral view of the thorax of a dog with left-sided cardiac failure. There is generalised cardiac enlargement, but the left atrium is notably enlarged (black arrows). Pulmonary oedema is present in the diaphragmatic lobes.

pnoea, both prominent signs of cardiac failure, are discussed in Chapter 2 but the combination of dyspnoea and tachycardia poses problems in differential diagnosis. Potential causes of dyspnoea with tachycardia include: left-sided cardiac failure; heatstroke; pulmonary oedema (primary); pneumonias; and intrapulmonary or pleural haemorrhage.

Right-sided cardiac failure

Right-sided cardiac failure can be caused by:

1 Congenital cardiac disorders such as pulmonic stenosis, tricuspid dysplasia or tetralogy of Fallot, and ventricular septal defects or patent ductus arteriosus if pulmonary hypertension develops.
2 Tricuspid incompetence due to endocardiosis.
3 Pericardial effusions.
4 Extensive and severe respiratory disease, causing pulmonary hypertension (cor pulmonale).
5 Myocardial failure.
6 Left-sided cardiac failure—due to increased total blood volume and pulmonary hypertension.
7 Dirofilaria—in imported dogs.

Signs of right-sided failure are caused mainly by systemic venous congestion. Abdominal enlargement and breathlessness are prominent when the disease is advanced, but clinical examination may reveal a number of features at earlier stages. Hepatomegaly and splenomegaly may be detected, and venous engorgement can be identified in some cases. Abdominal enlargement develops as a result of the formation of ascites, which is often accompanied by hydrothorax. Subcutaneous oedema is not a common finding in dogs in cardiac failure.

Pressure of ascites and hepatomegaly on the diaphragm will contribute to breathlessness, and tachypnoea is enhanced by the formation of hydrothorax. The effusions into body cavities are modified transudates, typically straw-, orange- or pink-coloured and slightly opaque. There is a moderate (20–30 g/l) protein content, and typically a specific gravity of 1.018–1.020. The effusion is similar to that found with certain neoplasms in body cavities or following hepatic cirrhosis (cf. Chapter 14).

Right-sided cardiac failure generally leads to congestive failure if the disorder is progressive. Digestive upsets are a feature of some cases, and probably contribute, together with hepatic dysfunction, to the loss of bodily condition that occurs.

Congestive cardiac failure

This can develop as a primary disorder, especially if sudden in onset. Frequently, it is a sequel to either left or right-sided cardiac failure, as failure of one side of the circulation influences the other.

Causes of congestive cardiac failure as a syndrome include:

1 Progression from right- or left-sided cardiac failure.
2 Myocardial failure, especially cardiomyopathy in giant breeds.
3 Congenital disorders (especially patent ductus arteriosus).
4 Severe brady- or tachydysrhythmias.

Signs of failure include:

1 Dyspnoea (due to pulmonary congestion and/or oedema).
2 Tachypnoea (due to hydrothorax).
3 Coughing (due to pulmonary congestion and/or oedema).
4 Fatigue, especially with any exercise or excitement.

5 Abdominal enlargement (due to ascites and hepatomegaly).
6 Inappetence, depression and weight loss.
7 Congested mucous membranes or pallor (occasionally cyanosis), with sluggish capillary refill.

Clinical findings can include:

1 Tachycardia (or bradydysrhythmia) and a weak pulse (indicating myocardial failure).
2 Cardiac murmurs (usually systolic) due to:
(a) valvular fibrosis
(b) congenital lesions
(c) gross cardiac dilatation
(d) (endocarditis—uncommon).
3 Dysrhythmias due to:
(a) myocardial disease or failure
(b) conduction disturbance.
4 Muffling of heart sounds (pericardial or pleural effusions).
5 Cardiomegaly, pulmonary congestion or oedema, pleural or abdominal effusions (physical or radiographic findings).
6 ECG changes:
(a) prolongation and/or splitting of QRS complex (ventricular enlargement); prolonged or enlarged P wave (left or right atrial enlargement).
(b) dysrhythmias:
 (i) premature atrial beats
 (ii) premature ventricular beats
 (iii) paroxysmal tachycardias
 (iv) atrial fibrillation
 (v) total atrioventricular block
(c) reduced voltages (pleural or pericardial effusion).
7 Elevated transaminase, alkaline phosphatase and urea levels can be found, and leucocytosis is common.

Congestive cardiac failure (decompensation) may be precipitated in a dog previously compensating for cardiac disease by a number of stressful situations:

1 Infections, toxaemias (bite wounds, pyometra, renal failure).
2 Discontinuation of cardiac therapy.
3 Excessive excitement or exercise.
4 Excessive heat or humidity.
5 Trauma, surgery, anaemia.
6 Intravenous fluid therapy or high sodium intake.
7 Pregnancy.

Fainting episodes (syncope) or collapse at exercise ('heart attack')

There are many potential causes of collapse in dogs, particularly acute disorders affecting the central nervous system. It should be emphasized that cardiological causes rarely include massive coronary artery occlusion. The variety of differential diagnoses quoted here merely exemplifies the large number of causes.

Cardiological causes

1 Severe low-output cardiac disease, e.g. acquired mitral incompetence or congenital aortic stenosis.
2 Bradydysrhythmias: atrioventricular block (multiple missed beats or total block); sinoatrial block (multiple missed beats); sinoatrial arrest; sinus bradycardia.
3 Tachydysrhythmias: paroxysmal atrial or ventricular tachycardia (or fibrillation).

Bradydysrhythmias can be associated with excessive vagal tone (p. 15). Signs of collapse due to cardiac insufficiency tend to be seen with excitement or exercise. There may be sudden flaccid collapse and equally rapid recovery, or generalized weakness and lethargy. Few prodromal or postictal signs are usually noted.

Vascular causes

1 Congenital or aquired arteriovenous fistulae (pulmonary, hepatic or peripheral tissues).
2 Pulmonary artery obstruction (thrombosis, Angiostrongylus or Dirofilaria).
3 Vascular occlusion (especially thoracic neoplasms).
4 Aortic thrombosis (causes weakness not syncope).
5 ('stroke'?).

Some of these disorders may cause cyanosis, an uncommon finding in cardiac disease other than with congenital right-to-left shunts or pulmonary oedema.

Central nervous system disorders

1 Epilepsy—this is an excitatory disorder with, in most cases, tachypnoea, salivation, tonic and clonic spasm, urination or defaecation, postictal bewilderment and sometimes hunger and thirst (cf Chapter 5). The disorder occurs most often at rest or on waking. There are often prodromal signs.
2 Narcolepsy (a functional disturbance: spontaneous falling into deep sleep).
3 Other causes of cerebral hypoxia: anaemia, haemorrhage, haemoglobinopathy; vascular disease.
4 Metabolic dysfunction or toxaemia: hypoglycaemia (e.g. due to an islet cell tumour of the pancreas, hepatic failure or physical exhaustion); hypocalcaemia (eclampsia); hypoadrenocorticalism; hepatic failure (portocaval shunts, cirrhosis, neoplasia); uraemia.

With these disorders, collapse or weakness may be intermittent. The animal may also be otherwise unwell.

5 CNS lesions: encephalitis (viral); congenital disorders; otitis media; trauma.
6 Poisoning (e.g. barbiturates).

Respiratory disease

This occurs especially as upper airway obstruction in brachycephalic breeds, and includes stenotic nares, elongated soft palate, laryngeal collapse, tracheal collapse, laryngeal paralysis ('roarer') and neoplastic obstruction of the respiratory tract. Dyspnoea with noise and cyanosis can be prominent features of collapse in these disorders (Chapter 2).

Idiopathic collapse

Collapse can occur at exercise in a number of sporting breeds, including Labradors, Pointers and Springer Spaniels. No clear cause has been determined, despite extensive investigation. Claims that hypoglycaemia may be a cause appear to be unsubstantiated. It is important that clients be reassured that recurrent collapse is not necessarily fatal or distressing to the dog.

Hindlimb weakness

Exercise intolerance that includes ataxia and hindlimb weakness, without loss of consciousness, can also be a sign of cardiac insufficiency. Alternative causes include aortic thrombosis and spinal, orthopaedic or neuromuscular disorders, in which the animal usually remains conscious: congenital spinal disorders ('wobblers', vertebral malformations); trauma (spinal or bilateral fractures or hip luxation); acquired spinal disorders (prolapsed intervertebral disc, neoplasia, CDRM); neuromuscular disorders (myasthenia gravis, cramp, polymyositis, azoturia, botulism, myotonia); peripheral nerve disease (neoplasia, polyneuritis, brachial plexus neuritis, louping-ill, trauma).

Full investigation of these disorders includes a detailed history, thorough clinical, cardiological and neurological examination and biochemical tests.

Endocarditis

Cases usually present with vague signs of fever. Clinical signs are related more to the effects of infection than to incompetence or stenosis of cardiac valves. Some or all of the following may be found:

1 Persistent or recurrent pyrexia with lethargy, anorexia, weight loss.
2 Intermittent lameness and tenderness in joints.
3 Pale mucous membranes.
4 Signs referable to the kidneys, lungs, joints, myocardium or the central nervous system, if there has been embolic spread to these systems.

Systolic murmurs are common, and not readily differentiated from other causes, but occasionally a diastolic murmur, otherwise a rare finding in the dog, is detected. The nature of a murmur often changes rapidly in endocarditis. Haematology indicates leucocytosis and anaemia in most cases. Serum globulin levels are usually raised, and repeated blood samples for culture may identify the causal organism. However, the recent use of antibiotics will prevent successful culture. Radiography and electrocardiography are not usually helpful aids to diagnosis of endocarditis (but associated dysrhythmias of myocarditis are common).

CARDIAC RHYTHM AND DYSRHYTHMIAS

All cardiac tissue has intrinsic rhythmicity. The sinus node is the dominant pacemaker, but sites in conduction tissue (the atrioventricular node, bundles of His and the Purkinje system) can act as substitute pacemakers (producing 'escape' beats) if there is no stimulus from the normal pacemaker. Additionally, myocardial lesions (p. 7) can act as irritant foci, producing ectopic pacemakers, tachycardias or fibrillation, which will interfere with normal cardiac activation if sufficiently premature.

Diagnosis of a dysrhythmia does not necessarily indicate the underlying pathological lesion or aetiology, and dysrhythmias *per se* may or may not contribute significantly to cardiac failure. However, they often indicate underlying myocardial disease that may itself cause loss of myocardial contractility. Although definitive diagnosis requires an ECG, auscultation provides an indication of most dysrhythmias.

Sinus arrhythmia, a regular, phasic increase and decrease in heart rate, producing 'groups' of beats usually synchronous with respirations, is very common in normal dogs. It is usually abolished in tachycardia (e.g. in cardiac failure), but it can be accentuated in ventilatory dyspnoeas and in brachycephalic breeds.

Bradydysrhythmias and conduction disturbances

Conduction disturbances can be caused by excessive vagal tone (functional) or by myocardial lesions (abscesses, fibrosis or neoplasia). Bradydysrhythmias can also be found with myocardial depression (with toxaemias, electrolyte disturbances or glycoside toxicity). In some cases there is no clear aetiology.

Disturbances include sinus bradycardia or arrest, sino-atrial or atrioventricular blocks and intraventricular conduction disturbances (e.g. bundle branch blocks).

Clinical features

Sinus arrest (or pause):
This is a form of accentuated sinus arrhythmia, in which long pauses occur between groups of beats. These may be synchronous with respirations. This is common in brachycephalic breeds, but it may be significant if prolonged, causing syncope.

'Missed' or dropped beats
Absence of one or more beats in a normal sequence is of limited significance unless frequent. It may indicate sino-atrial or atrioventricular block.

Bradycardia
With a heart rate less than 70 per minute, if the rhythm is notably regular, it may indicate complete heart block (total atrioventricular block), with a slow and usually regular, ventricular 'escape' rhythm. This may be serious, as neoplasia, sepsis or toxaemias can be the cause and this dysrhythmia can cause syncope or congestive cardiac failure. If any indication of sinus arrhythmia is present, the bradycardia may be vagally induced. Severe bradycardia can be caused by hyperkalaemia (hypoadrenocorticalism or toxaemias).

Significance
Syncope, exercise intolerance or lethargy can result from bradydysrhythmias if sufficiently severe. Gross bradycardias can contribute to congestive cardiac failure.

Treatment
The principles include reversal of any excessive vagal activity and stimulation of the ventricular rate if necessary.

1 Any glycoside therapy should be withdrawn or reduced.
2 The dog should be checked for evidence of other generalised disease (toxaemia or endocrine disturbance).

3 Atropine may be used to block vagal activity, 0.5–2.0 mg can be administered subcutaneously or intravenously. If this is effective, the drug may be given orally (Eumydrin; Winthrop). However, other visceral effects of atropine may not be desirable for long-term use.

4 Isoprenaline, a beta-adrenergic stimulant, can increase the heart rate in sinus arrest, sinus bradycardia or blocks, at an oral dose of 15–30 mg T I D. However, sudden death has been reported with this drug in dogs, possibly due to ventricular fibrillation.

5 Severe bradydysrhythmias causing syncope or congestive cardiac failure will respond to stimulation with an artificial pacemaker. These are usually installed to increase the ventricular rate in animals that are suitably young or that are unlikely to have serious myocardial disease. Second-hand pacemakers are suitable for use in dogs, if re-sterilized according to manufacturers' recommendations. A pacing lead is passed via the jugular vein into the right ventricle under local anaesthesia. A temporary external pacemaker is then required to control the ventricular rate while the dog is anaesthetized and the permanent pacemaker is placed subcutaneously in an area susceptible to minimal trauma. The life of modern batteries is usually several years. The ideal pacing rate is probably 90–100 beats per minute in dogs.

Tachydysrhthmias

Irritant foci (ectopic pacemakers) can be stimulated by most myocardial diseases (p. 7). Irritation and excitability are exacerbated by hypoxia, acidosis or catecholamines, which are features of anaesthesia and toxaemias. Disturbances include atrial or ventricular ectopic beats, fibrillation or tachycardias.

Clinical features

1 *Premature beats* (ectopic atrial or ventricular beats) are heard as premature and louder beats (a 'tripping' in tachycardia). Any murmur may be altered and there may be a pulse deficit for the beat. These are a common finding in congestive cardiac failure, but occasional premature beats can be heard in normal dogs.

2 *Atrial fibrillation* (or flutter) is heard as a true arrhythmia—a 'chaotically' random rhythm with variation in intensity of cardiac sounds and of any murmur. Usually there is a pulse deficit, with variations in strength. This is a serious dysrhythmia, found especially in large or giant breeds of dog with cardiomyopathy.

3 *Paroxysmal tachycardias* (atrial or ventricular) are heard as a continuous tachycardia, or in intermittent bursts, with a regular rhythm. The pulse is usually weak. This dysrhythmia usually represents severe myocardial disease which can cause weakness or syncope. Congestive cardiac failure often ensues.

Treatment

The basic principle is to reduce myocardial irritability, suppressing ectopic pacemaker activity, the liability to develop fibrillation, and the heart rate. Most effective agents also tend to reduce myocardial contractility, which may or may not be desirable. Most agents are contraindicated in bradydysrhythmias as, by reducing contractility, they can exacerbate congestive cardiac failure.

1 Lignocaine (2% solution without adrenaline) can be very successful in reducing ventricular tachycardia, ventricular fibrillation or multiple ventricular ectopic beats, but it has to be administered intravenously and it is very rapidly excreted. It is of value, therefore, mainly for acute tachydysrhythmias. The usual dose is 2–5 mg/kg i.v. as a single bolus, or 20–120 μg/kg per minute in an intravenous drip. The cardiac rhythm should be monitored by E C G: overdosage with lignocaine can cause convulsions or bradydysrhythmias.

2 Quinidine sulphate and procainamide decrease myofibril excitability and prolong the refractory period. This suppresses ectopic beats and paroxysmal tachycardias (especially of ventricular origin), and can occasionally reverse atrial fibrillation in dogs. Toxic effects include depression, anorexia, gastrointestinal disturbances and incoordination. These are exacerbated by glycoside therapy. The dose for quinidine is 6–10 mg/kg every 4–8 hours orally.

3 Beta-adrenergic blockade (e.g. propranolol) reduces myocardial contractility, conduction velocity and response to catecholamines. Propranolol has also a direct effect against tachydysrhythmias. Atrial tachycardias, and ventricular ectopic beats and tachycardias can be reduced, and the heart may be protected against ventricular fibrillation. This drug is especially useful for reducing the ventricular rate in atrial fibrillation. The normal dose of propranolol is 0.5–2.0 mg/kg T I D orally.

4 Newer antidysrhythmic drugs include disopyramide, which has similar applications to quinidine but which appears to be more effective and less toxic. The dose rate is currently related to that recommended in man (50–200 mg orally T I D or more frequently in dogs).

5 Cardiac glycosides, especially digoxin can be of value in atrial tachycardias (although beta-blockade may be more effective) and in reducing the ventricular rate in atrial fibrillation, especially in combination with beta-blockade, if this is not fully effective. For dosage and application, see p. 21.

6. Calcium antagonists (verapamil, nifedipine) have anti-tachydysrhythmic effects, but they have not yet found much favour in this application in dogs.

7 D.C. shock can be effective in converting ventricular fibrillation (one form of 'cardiac arrest') to normal contractions in dogs, and it can reverse atrial fibrillation in a few dogs, especially with the aid of quinidine. However, since the majority of cases are not converted, and it is probably myocardial disease rather than the atrial fibrillation that contributes to cardiac failure, this technique is not usually worth serious consideration.

It is only severe tachydysrhythmias (tachycardias, multiple ventricular ectopic beats and possibly atrial fibrillation) that require therapy. While other dysrhythmias may represent myocardial damage, the dysrhythmia *per se* may not be very prejudicial to cardiac output. However, agents such as beta-adrenergic blockers may have a long-term 'protective' effect on the myocardium.

INVESTIGATION OF CARDIOVASCULAR DISORDERS

History

Signs such as syncope, dyspnoea or ascites that develop suddenly may readily suggest cardiovascular insufficiency, but signs of cardiac failure such as exercise intolerance and coughing often develop insidiously.

Careful questioning is required to establish the pattern of disease and to elicit such minor details as the development of exercise intolerance.

Examination

Careful clinical examination, especially auscultation, is essential for the assessment of cardiac failure.

Observations

1 Subcutaneous oedema resulting from cardiac failure is uncommon in dogs. It is more often associated with hypoproteinaemia.

2 Ascites causes the classically pear-shaped abdomen in right-sided or congestive cardiac failure.

3 Dyspnoea or tachypnoea are common findings in congestive cardiac failure and if acute pulmonary oedema is involved, frothing at the mouth can be seen.

4 The colour of mucous membranes is often normal, but:

(a) Pallor may be observed in cardiac failure or cardiogenic shock.

(b) Cyanosis is a feature of congenital disorders with right-to-left shunts but it may also be noted in cases where pulmonary oedema develops. It is otherwise uncommon.

(c) Congestion of the mucous membranes may be noted in the presence of right-sided or congestive cardiac failure, with sluggish capillary refill.

5 Jugular pulsation is not readily appreciated in dogs, but it can be seen in right-sided cardiac failure.

Palpation

1 Precordium: a strong impulse beat may be appreciated in the presence of cardiomegaly and a thrill is sometimes felt in the presence of the vibration of a severe murmur (e.g. of congenital disease).

2 Pulse: character, rate and rhythm. These phenomena are not always readily determined in obese or uncooperative patients. A pulse deficit can exist with dysrhythmias such as atrial fibrillation or premature ventricular beats, where individual contractions may be insufficiently productive to create a palpable pulse wave. The character of the pulse is influenced not only by cardiovascular function but also by fever, pain and anaemia. Variations in intensity of the pulse can be appreciated in dysrhythmias.

3 Abdomen: hepatomegaly can be palpated in the presence of venous congestion.

Percussion

1 The area of cardiac dullness may be increased with cardiomegaly or pericardial effusion.

2 The presence of pleural fluid can be detected as ventral dullness in right-sided cardiac failure (see Chapter 2).

3 A fluid wave can be appreciated in the abdomen with ascites of right-sided or congestive cardiac failure.

Auscultation

Attention should be paid to:

1 The intensity of cardiac sounds, which can be increased with fever, anaemia or cardiac enlargement, but which is decreased in the presence of a pleural or pericardial effusion.

2 The area over which cardiac sounds are heard. This is increased by cardiac enlargement in congestive cardiac failure. Cardiac sounds can be displaced or muffled by neoplasms.

3 The rate: this should be compared with the pulse rate. The range for normal dogs is 70–140 beats per minute. The heart rate usually becomes progressively elevated in cardiac failure.

4 The rhythm: a regular irregularity (usually consistent with respirations) is normal in the dog (sinus arrhythmia). Many dysrhythmias can be identified with careful auscultation (p. 15):

(a)   Ectopic beats (premature and loud and usually followed by a compensatory pause).

(b)   Atrial fibrillation—'chaotic' rhythm, totally random, with variation in intensity of sounds and a pulse deficit.

(c)   Missed beats, representing partial heart block.

5 Abnormal sounds: most murmurs in the dog are systolic, due to congenital lesions or acquired valvular incompetence, but:

(a)   Murmurs may represent changes in viscosity of blood (anaemia, hypoproteinaemia),

(b)   A characteristic 'machinery' murmur, waxing and waning throughout systole and diastole, is heard with patent ductus arteriosus.

(c)   Diastolic murmurs can be heard with endocarditis. The site at which a murmur is loudest often indicates the origin of the sound.

(d)   Pulmonary râles can be heard in the presence of left-sided or congestive cardiac failure.

A stethoscope is the most important instrument in the diagnosis of cardiological disorders. The entire cardiac area must be auscultated for murmurs and for a sufficient length of time to identify any occasional dysrhythmia.

Further investigation

Radiology

This is a very valuable aid in the diagnosis of cardiac disorders. However, assessment remains subjective in view of the variations in chest shape and size between different breeds.

Clear radiographs, if possible taken at maximal inspiration, are essential for detailed examination. Lateral and preferably, dorsoventral rather than ventrodorsal, exposures should be made. Radiographs should be examined for the following features:

1 Enlargement of the entire cardiac outline: the normal craniocaudal length is approximately 2.5–3.5 intercostal spaces, increased by cardiac enlargement; the trachea normally lies at an acute angle to the vertebral column, being displaced dorsally by enlargement; the normal heart appears flattened laterally in dorsoventral projections and it does not usually occupy more than two-thirds of the width of the thorax. Progressive cardiac enlargement is a notable feature of the development of congestive cardiac failure. A very rounded cardiac silhouette may suggest pericardial effusion.

2 Enlargement of individual cardiac chambers (indicating primarily left- or right-sided disease).

3 Pulmonary congestion or oedema, especially in the perihilar region in left-sided cardiac failure. Conversely, hypovascularity can occur in the presence of right-to-left shunts or hypovolaemia.

4 Enlargement of the liver and the caudal vena cava, evidence of venous congestion, right-sided or congestive cardiac failure.

5 Pleural and abdominal effusions in right-sided or congestive cardiac failure.

Cardiac catheterization and the use of contrast media (angiography) is essential for confirmation of the presence of many congenital and acquired cardiovascular lesions. The results of angiography are most readily interpreted from cineradiography, from videotape recordings, from an image intensifier or from films recorded by a rapid cassette changer.

Electrocardiography

ECGs record only myocardial events. Minimal information on valvular or congenital diseases is provided. The technique may be performed with a dog standing or lying on its right side, but it is important that the patient be insulated from the ground, and as relaxed as possible. Einthoven's triangle, employing leads attached to the limbs, is still most frequently employed, and most electrocardiographs are constructed to record this lead system.

Information that may be derived from ECGs includes:

1 Heart rate.

2 Heart rhythm:

(a)   the activity of normal or ectopic pacemakers is determined. Tachydysrhythmias (p. 16) are readily diagnosed.

(b)   the conduction of the cardiac activation impulse is identified and bradydysrhythmias and conduction disturbances should be apparent.

3 Waveform:

(a)   changes in myocardial function due to hypoxia, electrolyte, endocrine or acid-base imbalance can be identified.

(b) alterations can represent changes in the cardiac electric field, due to cardiac chamber enlargement. In particular:

(i) tall P waves (P pulmonale) may be found with right atrial enlargement.

(ii) notched and prolonged P waves (P mitrale) may represent left atrial enlargement.

(iii) large positive voltage and prolongation of QRS complex may occur with left ventricular enlargement.

(iv) negativity of QRS complex, especially in leads I and II can represent right ventricular hypertrophy, particularly with congenital lesions such as pulmonic stenosis and tetralogy of Fallot.

However, in many cases where gross chamber enlargement exists, the ECG remains within normal limits.

Phonocardiography

Recording the pattern of heart sounds synchronously with an ECG aids the identification of a murmur, its pitch and position in the cardiac cycle. Ejection murmurs, typical of congenital stenotic lesions, tend to be diamond-shaped (crescendo–decrescendo). Murmurs tend to occupy an increasing proportion of the systolic interval with increasing valvular incompetence.

The third heart sound (S_3—ventricular filling) is often found in atrial dilatation and overload following mitral incompetence.

Cardiac catheterization

Catheters are passed either through the femoral artery and the aortic valve to the left ventricle or through the jugular vein and the right atrium to the right ventricle, in a technique that is essential for verifying the presence of cardiac lesions, especially congenital disorders. The technique is required for various advanced diagnostic procedures:

1 Angiography, necessary to confirm the presence of congenital shunts and strictures.
2 Direct blood pressure measurement, valuable in the diagnosis of stenotic and shunting congenital disorders.
3 Blood gas analysis (oxygen and carbon dioxide partial pressures and pH), particularly useful for the identification of shunts through congenital lesions.
4 Cardiac output studies and the identification of circulatory overload in congestive cardiac failure.

Cardiac catheters are best placed with the aid of image intensification (fluoroscopy).

Echocardiography

Echocardiography uses an ultrasonic beam and scanner with a display screen to visualise echoes from boundaries between intracardiac structures. Bone and lung interfere with the signal, but in man, the depth of myocardium and septum (increased in hypertrophy), the size of cardiac chambers (increased in dilatation), the size and the contents of the pericardium (effusions) can be assessed, and valves, their lesions and function, and even congenital lesions such as septal defects can be seen.

Echocardiography has been applied successfully to dogs, but variations in chest shape and size between breeds limit the value and interpretation of results except in very skilled hands. Undoubtedly, this technique offers great potential for non-invasive assessment of cardiac function in dogs. However, good equipment is currently very expensive.

MANAGEMENT AND TREATMENT OF CARDIAC DISEASE AND FAILURE

Congenital lesions

The finding of a cardiac murmur in a dog under 2 years of age strongly suggests the presence of a congenital lesion. A murmur may be encountered in one of three ways:

1 Detected incidentally, with no overt signs of cardiovascular dysfunction.
2 Associated with stunting, breathlessness, exercise intolerance or syncope.
3 Associated with congestive cardiac failure.

The overall prognosis is poor for dogs with congenital cardiac lesions:

1 Sudden death, or at least syncopal attacks, may occur with sub-aortic stenosis.
2 Poor growth, severe exercise intolerance and death within the first two years of life are likely with tetralogy of Fallot.
3 Congestive cardiac failure is likely to develop within the first few years of life with patent ductus arteriosus and pulmonic stenosis, and it may develop with other lesions.
4 Conversely, atrial or ventricular septal defects may cause minimal disturbance to circulation.

When a murmur indicating the presence of some congenital lesion is first detected in a puppy, certain decisions should be made:

1 Whether the dog should be returned by the owner to the breeder in view of the overall prognosis.
2 Whether further investigation should be undertaken to determine the cause and to define more closely the prognosis and whether management is possible: this may require specialised equipment to achieve a clear diagnosis.
3 Whether surgical correction may be possible or advisable:
(a)   surgery is relatively simple for patent ductus arteriosus.
(b)   crude dilation of a stenosed pulmonic valve via a right ventricular wall puncture is possible.
(c)   most other commonly encountered congenital lesions have been repaired successfully in dogs, but repair requires sophisticated surgery and cardiac bypass.
4 The client should, alternatively, be warned of the prognosis and the possible development of congestive cardiac failure that may require management and therapy.

Progressive left-sided cardiac failure
(following mitral incompetence)

When a murmur representing mitral incompetence has been detected in a dog, the stage of development indicates the level of necessary treatment (p.10). It is important that dogs be checked regularly for signs of progression and to monitor the response to treatment.

Stage 1. No therapy is necessary, therapeutic procedures such as elective surgery may be undertaken safely. If the dog is obese, it should be strictly dieted. A salt-free diet should be considered and the client should be warned to restrict the dog's exercise if tiredness is noted.
Stage II. The dog's exercise should be limited to that which causes no distress, and obesity should not be tolerated. The dog's sodium intake should be reduced to a minimum. Xanthine derivatives are often beneficial for relief of coughing.
Stage III. Exercise should be kept to a minimum, with no prolonged walks, or hill- or stair-climbing. The remaining provisions for Stage II should be maintained. Diuresis is instituted as necessary for coughing.
Stage IV. In congestive cardiac failure, further to

Stages II and III, intensive diuresis and complete rest are essential. Cage rest is strongly advised, but a quiet home environment may be less stressful. Sedation is worth consideration in excitable dogs, barbiturates or opiates are more suitable in circulatory failure than phenothiazine derivatives such as acetylpromazine. Digitalization is beneficial in some cases, but vasodilator therapy may be most useful. Antidysrhythmic drugs may be required if dysrhythmias are severe.

Congestive cardiac failure

The prognosis for dogs with congestive cardiac failure depends on the cause, the response to treatment and the degree of disease in other organs. Prognosis is guarded in the presence of congenital or myocardial disease, but it may be reasonable with pericardial effusions and valvular incompetence. The response to treatment may be assessed:

1 Clinically, by:
(a)   loss of retained congestive fluids (this can be measured by a reduction of weight), abdominal size and respiratory signs.
(b)   improvement in the dog's activity, alertness and body condition.
(c)   reduction of tachycardia.
(d)   reduction in dysrhythmias.
2 Radiographically, by:
(a)   reduction in cardiac size
(b)   reduced pulmonary congestion and oedema
(c)   reduced retention of body fluids
(d)   reduction in size of the caudal vena cava and the liver.

Unfortunately, apparently identical cases frequently do not respond equally well to similar treatment. Poor response to treatment may indicate:

1   Inadequate therapy
2   Myocardial failure (myopathy, cardiac dilatation, dysrhythmias)
3   Neoplasia (heart base tumour, haemangiosarcoma, endocardial tumour)
4   Cardiac crises—ruptured chordae tendineae, atrial rupture
5   Heart worm (imported dogs)
6   Primary respiratory disease
7   Other organ or system failure (e.g. renal or hepatic failure)

Further radiography assists the assessment of progress. ECGs will demonstrate dysrhythmias.

Traditional approach

Drugs were employed to attempt to encourage the heart to work more efficiently, with relief of clinical signs.

1 Cardiac glycosides were used to increase myocardial contractility, to control tachycardia and to prolong diastole (and therefore improve ventricular filling and coronary perfusion), possibly at the cost of increased myocardial oxygen consumption.
2 Xanthine derivatives were employed to increase myocardial contractility, to cause bronchodilation and to induce diuresis.

Modern approach

Many drugs now employed aim to relieve the workload and inappropriate responses of the heart and circulation to cardiac failure (p. 10).
Therapeutic aims are as follows:

1 To counteract sodium and water retention (with diuretics and possibly spironolactone or captopril).
2 To cause arteriolar vasodilation (with hydralazine, captopril or prazosin), reducing excessive back pressure (afterload) on the ventricular outflow, thus increasing cardiac output, reducing valvular incompetence and myocardial stretching, and improving tissue perfusion.
3 To encourage venous capillary dilatation (with prazosin, frusemide or captopril), reducing volume overload (preload) and tissue oedema.
4 To reduce myocardial contractility and energy and oxygen consumption (with beta-adrenergic blockade or calcium antagonists).
5 To reduce the heart rate (with beta-adrenergic blockade or glycosides).
6 To reduce myocardial irritability and dysrhythmias (with beta-adrenergic blockade or calcium antagonists).

Additionally, traditional management (rest and salt-free diets) remain valuable adjuncts to therapy.

Details of therapy for cardiac failure

Digitalization

Cardiac glycosides have been employed for at least two centuries. They are still widely used, but may readily be misused; inadequate dosage is usually ineffective, while prolonged or excessive administration can result in toxicity, the signs of which may not be instantly recognised. The benefits of digitalization include an increase in myocardial contractility, which

assists cardiac output. By vagal stimulation the cardiac pacemaker is slowed, there is depression of the atrioventricular node and an increase in ventricular conduction time. Thus, the diastolic interval is prolonged, which aids ventricular filling.

However, the increased myocardial contractility occurs at the expense of increased energy consumption. The vagal stimulation can produce excessive bradycardia or atrioventricular blocks and permits an increase in the incidence of ventricular ectopic pacemakers. In addition, glycosides increase the irritability of the ventricular myocardium, so that ectopic ventricular beats, paroxysmal ventricular tachycardia and ventricular fibrillation occur more readily with digitalization. Toxic effects are exacerbated by low plasma potassium levels. Indications for digitalization include congestive cardiac failure and atrial fibrillation. Contraindications include heart blocks, multiple ventricular ectopic beats or paroxysmal ventricular tachycardia. If signs of toxicity develop, the drug should be withdrawn for at least 24 hours.

Techniques for digitalization. The preparation of choice is digoxin, which is absorbed and excreted more rapidly in dogs than digitoxin. It is important to use a refined product with reliable potency such as Lanoxin.
Techniques include:

1 Rapid digitalization, which should be performed with the dog under close supervision, preferably with cage rest. A *total loading dose* of 0.05–0.20 mg/kg bodyweight is calculated, to be given orally in divided doses over 48 hours. The doses should be administered, for example, 8-hourly until signs of effective digitalization (slowed heart rate, increased intervals on an ECG) are perceived. The drug should then be withdrawn for at least 24 hours, and daily administration resumed at one-quarter to one-tenth of the dose required for digitalization, in divided doses.
2 Slow digitalization, which can be achieved with an intelligent client's cooperation with the dog being treated as an outpatient. The initial dose rate should be 0.02 mg/kg bodyweight daily in divided doses for a period of 1 week. If the effect has been inadequate, the level may be raised slightly during subsequent weeks. Again, administration should cease for at least 24 hours if signs of toxicity develop, and a lower dose re-introduced.

The quantity of glycosides required for digitalization cannot be predicted, but if facilities exist, measurement of plasma digoxin indicates that a level of 2 μg/l is ideal. Every case must be treated as though a clinical experiment. It is very important that a client be warned of signs of toxicity (depression, anorexia, vomiting).

Diuresis

Modern diuretic agents, such as frusemide and the thiazides, are very potent. They inhibit the tubular resorption of sodium and, therefore, the water that accompanies the sodium (saluresis). The response to therapy is rapid and these agents are effective even when the cardiac output is impaired. Frusemide has an additional benefit in provoking venodilation. In congestive failure, all detectable retained fluid, such as ascites, can disappear within 4–5 days with intensive treatment, even without additional cardiac therapy. Diuresis can be used in conjunction with most cardiac drugs. Care should be taken over their use in uraemic patients, as cardiac output may be reduced.

It is advisable to weigh a dog before administration is started, and to monitor the loss of weight that should result from diuresis. For intensive therapy with frusemide an oral dose of 5 mg/kg bodyweight may be employed three times daily for 5–7 days. In acute cardiac failure, the drug can be administered intravenously. For less intensive therapy, half this dose should be employed, and for maintenance 1 mg/kg bodyweight once daily may suffice. This dose can be adjusted by the client according to the dog's progress. With intensive diuresis, it is important to determine that urine *is* being excreted.

Significant loss of potassium can occur with sustained intensive diuresis, but it is probably of little concern at maintenance levels in dogs. Oral supplementation with potassium chloride can avoid this problem, but this agent can easily be overdosed and may irritate the gastrointestinal tract. Therapy with a potassium-sparing mineralocorticoid antagonist such as spironolactone (10–50 mg three times daily, orally) in combination with diuretics is worth consideration. This drug is, itself, a mild diuretic, but it is expensive and can also be overdosed.

Xanthine derivatives

These drugs (e.g. aminophylline, etamphylline or theophylline) are bronchodilating agents with limited myocardial stimulant and diuretic effects. Their value lies mainly in improved respiratory function for a dog that is coughing (Stages II–III of cardiac failure) and for this purpose they may be employed in combination with diuretics. These drugs can be irritant to the stomach, and should be withdrawn if vomiting occurs. Their effect is not very prolonged and it is important that treatment be administered several times daily.

Modern cardiovascular agents

Arteriolar vasodilators. These can reduce back-pressure (afterload) on the heart, reducing valvular incompetence, increasing cardiac output, improving tissue perfusion and reducing cardiac dilatation and myocardial tension. However, they are expensive, they can cause syncope and they may cause tachycardia (especially hydralazine at high dose rates).

Prazosin (Hypovase; Pfizer) at 0.02–0.05 mg/kg TID orally and hydralazine at 0.5–2.0 mg/kg BID orally are the agents most often employed in dogs.

Venodilators. These can reduce volume overload (preload) and reduce tissue oedema. However, they can reduce ventricular filling and cardiac output excessively. Prazosin (as above) and frusemide (mainly a diuretic) have been employed in dogs.

Beta-adrenergic blockers. These agents reduce the heart rate, myocardial contractility, myocardial oxygen consumption and also suppress tachydysrhythmias. *But* they can exacerbate congestive cardiac failure by reducing myocardial contractility. They are of particular value in atrial fibrillation, especially with cardiomyopathy in large and giant breeds of dog. The drug usually employed in dogs is propranolol (Inderal; ICI) at 1–5 mg/kg TID orally.

Angiotensin inhibitors (angiotensin-converting enzyme inhibitors). These drugs are general peripheral vasodilators and aldosterone inhibitors. By reducing sodium and water retention and peripheral resistance, they are of great potential value in congestive cardiac failure, but they are relatively expensive. Captopril has been used successfully at 0.1–2.0 mg/kg TID orally.

Calcium antagonists. These drugs tend to reduce myocardial contractility and oxygen consumption, cause peripheral and coronary vasodilatation and reduce ectopic tachydysrhythmias. However the loss of contractility may not be desirable in congestive cardiac failure. Verapamil and nifedipine are most well known but they have not been widely employed in dogs.

Low sodium diets

Essentially, all routinely-prepared commercial foods, for example canned and dried products, biscuits, meal and even domestic bread, contain added salt. Obviously, some prepared meats such as ham and sausages also have high levels of salt. In addition, eggs, milk and milk products, and fish contain significant quantities of sodium. Because sodium retention occurs with cardiac failure, and an adult dog's nutritional requirement for sodium is minimal, it is worth trying to avoid these foods for a dog in the later stages of cardiac failure.

A suggestion is to cook food (meat, chicken, potatoes, rice or pasta) for the dog without adding salt. In addition, some breakfast cereals contain no salt, most fruit and vegetables contain little sodium, and salt-free savourings can be bought from chemists.

Commercial salt-free canine diets have been available, but they do not appear to be well accepted by dogs. Palatability can be improved by salt-free savourings or frying. It is very important to ensure that a dog with heart failure is encouraged to eat food, but that obesity is avoided.

Paracentesis
Paracentesis of fluid that has accumulated in the thorax is desirable to relieve respiratory distress. Paracentesis of ascites is usually necessary only to assess the nature of the fluid and to relieve pressure from the diaphragm. Removal of large quantities of modified transudate deprives the animal of vital protein. If response to diuretic therapy is good, fluid will be rapidly withdrawn without paracentesis.

If the presence of pericardial effusion is suspected, paracentesis of the pericardium may be required. The skin is prepared aseptically and local anaesthetic is introduced subcutaneously and into the intercostal space. Following this, a plastic cannula and stylet (19 gauge × 2–3 inches is suitable) with three-way tap attached, is introduced into the fifth intercostal space two thirds of the way down the left side of the thorax. The pericardium can usually be felt scratching the tip of the needle. It is penetrated and the stylet is withdrawn. If the needle is introduced too far, the myocardium may be felt moving on the end of the needle, and if an ECG is being recorded, ectopic ventricular beats are likely to be seen.

A sample of fluid is withdrawn and examined visually. Portions should be placed in EDTA (for cytology), heparin (for proteins) and sterile (for culture) bottles. If the fluid appears haemorrhagic, no more should be withdrawn until it has been checked for clotting. Blood of insidious haemopericardium is usually deep red ('port wine') in colour and it does not usually clot. On the other hand, inadvertent puncture of a major vessel of the heart will produce bright normally-clotting blood. In this case, the cannula should be withdrawn and the animal monitored and treated for shock. As much pericardial effusion as possible should be removed to relieve pressure on ventricular filling. Purulent or transudative effusions are usually recognisable by their appearance. Clinical improvement following adequate drainage is usually very rapid, but recurrence may occur.

Endocarditis

It is essential that, once an organism has been cultured and its sensitivity to antibiotics has been determined, suitable agents are used at high dose rates, sufficiently frequently and for an adequate length of time (e.g. 3–4 times daily for 1 month). Treatment is expensive, and failure is common, partly as a result of embolic spread to other vital tissues. Supportive therapy, with a high protein diet, anabolic steroids and vitamin preparations is important.

Other surgical procedures

Repair of a pericardiodiaphragmatic hernia and removal of adult heartworms from the right ventricle are beyond the scope of discussion in this book. Removal of an aortic thrombus is of doubtful value, as collateral circulation is usually adequate to sustain the dog's activity. It is more important to concentrate on reducing the risk of further thrombosis with agents such as heparin. However, the use of such agents requires close monitoring of the coagulation time.

REFERENCES

BECKETT S.D., BRANCH C.B. & ROBERTSON B.T. (1978) Syncopal attacks and sudden death in dogs: mechanisms and etiologies. *J. Am. Anim. Hosp. Assoc.* **14**, 378. (An outline of some of the many disorders that can cause collapse).

BOHN F.K., PATTERSON D.F. & PYLE R.L. (1971) Atrial fibrillation in dogs. *Br. Vet. J.* **127**, 485. (A philosophical account of 55 cases. An over-pessimistic prognosis is probably given by this series of cases).

BONAGURA J.D., MYER C.W. & PENSINGER R.R. (1982) Angiocardiography. *Vet. Clinics N.Am.* **12** (2), 239. (A well-illustrated review of findings with a number of cardiac disorders in dogs and cats).

BUCHANAN J.W. & PATTERSON D.F. (1965) Selective angiography and angiocardiography in dogs with congenital cardiovascular disease. *J. Am. Vet. Rad. Soc.* **6**, 21. (Description of techniques used in this procedure).

CARLISLE C.H. (1980) Heartworm disease in dogs with particular reference to protocol for treatment. In *The Veterinary Annual*, 20th edn, C.S.G. Grunsell & F.W.G. Hill, Bristol, Scientechnica. (A comprehensive account, including clinical features, diagnosis and treatment).

DARKE P.G.G. (1974) The interpretation of electrocardiograms in small animals. *J. Small Anim. Pract.* **15**, 537. (A review of the basic concepts of this technique, with illustrations of the common dysrhythmias).

DETWEILER D.K. & KNIGHT D.H. (1977) Congestive heart failure in dogs: therapeutic concepts. *J. Am. Vet. Med. Assoc.* **171**, 106. (Details of pathophysiology and the traditional treatment of congestive heart failure, including techniques for digitalisation).

DETWEILER D.K. & PATTERSON D.F. (1965) The prevalence and types of cardiovascular disease in dogs. *Ann. N.Y. Acad. Sci.* **127**, 481. (A classical, comprehensive article surveying the incidence, diagnosis and treatment of congenital and acquired cardiovascular disorders).

DETWEILER D.K. & PATTERSON D.F. (1967) Abnormal heart sounds and murmurs of the dog. *J. Small Anim. Pract.* **8**, 193. (A straightforward guide to murmurs and their origins).

ETTINGER S.J. (1983) *Textbook of Veterinary Internal Medicine*, 2nd edn, Section IX: Diseases of the Cardiovascular system. W.B. Saunders, Philadelphia. (A large section in this standard textbook, bringing Ettinger & Suter (1970) more up to date).

ETTINGER S.J. & SUTER P.F. (1970) *Canine Cardiology*. W.B. Saunders, Philadelphia. (*The* comprehensive textbook on this subject, although a new edition is overdue).

EYSTER G.E., EYSTER J.T., CORDS G.B. & JOHNSTON J. (1976) Patent ductus arteriosus in the dog: characteristics of occurrence and results of surgery in one hundred consecutive cases. *J. Am. Vet. Med. Assoc.* **168**, 435. (A large survey, describing the results of surgery and demonstrating that early correction is important).

FISHER E.W. (1967) Cardiac failure. *J. Small Anim. Pract.* **8**, 137. (A clear and concise account of the generation of congestive cardiac failure).

GIBBS C., GASKELL C.J., DARKE P.G.G. & WOTTON P.R. (1982) Idiopathic pericardial haemorrhage in dogs: a report of 14 cases. *J. Small Anim. Pract.* **23**, 483. (Clinical findings, therapy and outcome are described in detail).

HAMLIN R.L. (1977) New ideas in the management of heart failure in dogs. *J. Am. Vet. Med. Assoc.* **171**, 114. (Reassessment of the therapeutic approach to heart failure that avoids the toxic and non-beneficial effects of glycosides).

HAMLIN R.L. & KITTLESON M.D. (1982) Clinical experience with hydralazine for treatment of otherwise intractable cough in dogs with apparent left-sided heart failure. *J. Am. Vet. Med. Assoc.* **180**, 1327. (Successful use of an arterial vasodilator in dogs with heart failure no longer responsive to traditional therapy).

HAYES H.M. (1975) A hypothesis for the aetiology of canine chemoreceptor system neoplasms, based upon an epidemiological study of 73 cases among hospital patients. *J.* *Small Anim. Pract.* **16**, 337. (73 cases of 'heart base' and carotid body tumours and a theory for their occurrence in Boxers and Boston Terriers).

HILWIG R.W. (1976) Cardiac arrhythmias in the dog: detection and treatment. *J. Am. Vet. Med. Assoc.* **169**, 789. (A fairly straightforward and clear description of dysrhythmias and some therapeutic possibilities).

KLEINE L.J., Zook B.C. & Munson T.O. (1970) Primary cardiac haemangiosarcomas in dogs. *J. Am. Vet. Med. Assoc.* **157**, 326. (An account of 31 cases of haemangiosarcoma—mainly in German Shepherd Dogs—arising in the heart).

LIU S-K., Maron B.J. & Tilley L.P. (1979) Canine hypertrophic cardiomyopathy. *J. Am. Vet. Med. Assoc.* **174**, 708. (Clinical features of one form of idiopathic cardiomyopathy).

LOMBARD C.W., Tilley L.P. & YOSHIOKA M. (1981) Pacemaker implantation in the dog: Survey and literature review. *J. Am. Anim. Hosp. Assoc.* **17**, 751. (Summarises in some detail 22 cases, with a mainly successful outcome).

McINTOSH J.J. (1981) The use of vasodilators in treatment of congestive heart failure in dogs: a review. *J. Am. Anim. Hosp. Assoc.* **17**, 255. (A clear description of these modern drugs and their application).

MURDOCH D.B. & BAKER J.R. (1977) Bacterial endocarditis in the dog. *J. Small Anim. Pract.* **18**, 687. (A good review of this disease, with a presentation of three further cases).

MYER C.W. & Bonagura J.D. (1982) Survey radiography of the heart. *Vet. Clin. N.Am.* **12** (2), 213. (A detailed review of cardiac radiology with a comprehensive description of changes with numerous different disorders).

PATTERSON D.F. (1971) Canine congenital heart disease: epidemiology and aetiological hypotheses. *J. Small Anim. Pract.* **12**, 263. (A very extensive review of published reports (mainly American), with breed incidence.)

PENSINGER R.R. (1971) Congestive heart failure in dogs. *J. Am. Vet. Med. Assoc.* **158**, 447. (A clear account of the development and traditional management of congestive heart failure).

TILLEY L.P. (1979) *Essentials of Canine and Feline Electrocardiography*. C.V. Mosby, St. Louis, Philadelphia. (An excellent comprehensive and readable guide to the recording and interpretation of small animal ECGs).

WYBURN R.S. & Lawson D.D. (1967) Simple radiography as an aid to the diagnosis of heart disease in the dog. *J. Small Anim. Pract.* **8**, 163. (A helpful guide to the simple use of radiography for cardiological diagnosis).

2
The Respiratory System

P. G. G. DARKE

INTRODUCTION

Difficulty can be experienced in achieving definitive diagnoses of respiratory disorders, owing to the small size and restlessness of some dogs, and the relative inaccessibility of intrathoracic structures.

The respiratory system is the main site not only for gaseous exchange, but also for heat dissipation in this species. Additionally, the nasal chambers operate as an air filter, which may be a factor in the relatively high incidence of nasal tumours in dolichocephalic breeds.

There is a wide range of thoracic configuration in dogs, the deep and narrow thorax of a Great Dane contrasting, for example, with the shallow, broad thorax of a Bulldog. Similarly, the airway of a Greyhound is exceptionally clear, whereas the activity of a Bulldog, Pekingese or Yorkshire Terrier may be restricted by respiratory tract obstruction. Hyperthermia is a considerable threat to small breeds with narrow airways and with poor respiratory reserves, particularly if obese.

Pathological disorders of the respiratory system are here divided into those affecting the airway, the lungs and the pleural cavity, respectively. The approach to investigation of respiratory disease depends on the presenting clinical signs (e.g. coughing, dyspnoea), which are considered separately. The respiratory system is in intimate association with the heart and circulation and disease of one system frequently affects the other.

PATHOLOGICAL DISORDERS

Airway

The trachea and upper divisions of bronchi will be considered together. Nasal and laryngeal disorders are considered in Chapter 3.

Inflammation
This may result from the action of infectious agents (viral, bacterial or parasitic), secondary bacterial infection, chemical or mechanical irritants (smoke, dust, pollutants) or inhaled regurgitated or mis-swallowed material. The principal clinical sign is coughing and this can readily become self-perpetuating.

Primary infections
It has been demonstrated that the virus of canine distemper, adenoviruses, reovirus, parainfluenza virus and herpesvirus are found as primary pathogens in Britain. Further agents may yet be identified. Viral infection may be followed by bacterial invasion and multiplication of organisms that are normally commensal: this invasion frequently modifies the course of disease. Experimental infection has proved that the bacterium *Bordetella bronchiseptica* can also be a primary pathogen.

The main route of infection is by inhalation. The usual response to infection is tracheobronchitis, but the upper respiratory tract, in particular the larynx and tonsils, is often involved.

Respiratory infection can occur in dogs of all ages, and dogs with systemic immunity to adenovirus may not be protected against the respiratory challenge of this virus. Canine distemper infection in a young animal normally results in systemic illness and it causes development of further clinical signs (Chapter 13).

Kennel cough is a term often loosely assigned to any acute coughing of uncertain origin in dogs. The disorder is frequently encountered in dogs that are temporarily confined together at, for example, pet shops or boarding kennels. Most commonly, acute coughing is the only major sign of kennel cough in an otherwise apparently healthy dog. The cough is usually dry, hacking and paroxysmal and it is often followed by retching. The client may be erroneously concerned about the possibility of a bone in the dog's throat. In uncomplicated cases, the signs subside in a few days even without therapy. Clinical findings are usually minimal, but coughing can be stimulated by tracheal palpation, and harsh vesicular or bronchial sounds may be detected in the thorax. Laboratory and radiographic findings are usually unremarkable in an un-complicated case. Treatment can usually be restricted to proprietary anti-tussive agents. Antibiotics are unlikely to be effective in simple cases, but they may protect against complications if the dog is unwell or if the cough is persistent.

Secondary infections

More widespread clinical signs are encountered in some cases: mild malaise with pyrexia, serous ocular and nasal discharges and tachypnoea can occur. Occasionally, secondary bacterial infection can cause bronchopneumonia. The dog may be systemically ill, with depression, anorexia and pyrexia. The cough may be moist, and bubbling or squeaking sounds may be heard in the thorax. This degree of infection requires treatment with broad-spectrum antibiotics for at least a week.

Other irritants

Acute coughing can be precipitated by the inhalation of irritants such as smoke, industrial chemicals, irritants or dust, or of regurgitated or mis-swallowed ingesta.

Chronic bronchitis

Chronic bronchitis can result from infection or from continued exposure to irritants which induce chronic reactive changes in the mucosa. These include hyperplasia, excessive mucus production, and mucus stasis, following the slowing of ciliary activity. Clinically, a cough develops which is variable, but often harsh, unproductive and paroxysmal, and it may be noticed particularly after overnight rest. The disorder affects adult and ageing dogs most commonly, and is possibly most severe in dogs of small breeds. Chronic bronchitis frequently coincides with valvular insufficiency in ageing animals and requires differentiation from heart failure (p. 11).

The dog's physical condition is normally good in an uncomplicated case and many affected dogs are obese. Auscultated respiratory sounds are usually normal but there may be crackling or wheezing. The results of routine laboratory examinations are usually unrewarding. Swabs from tonsils or sputum for bacteriology tend to give misleading results, but tracheal or bronchial washings are more valuable. Radiography can demonstrate bronchial wall thickening in some cases, but the degree is not directly related to the severity of clinical signs. Bronchoscopy may reveal strands or plugs of mucus in the lower airway, and roughening and thickening of the mucosa are often evident. These findings are not specific, but they allow the exclusion of possible differential diagnoses (p. 41).

Relief may be obtained with mucolytic (e.g. bromhexine) and anti-tussive drugs, or where all else fails, with corticosteroids, but the long-term results of therapy are often unrewarding. Removal of the animal from any dry, smoky, dusty or polluted atmosphere is essential for recovery, and daily artificial air humidification (e.g. in a shower room) can help to loosen mucous secretions. Recurrence of clinical signs following an improvement is common and clients should be advised of this. The mucosal changes are usually not completely reversible, but although chronic bronchitis can lead to bronchopneumonia, bronchiectasis or emphysema, these complications have not been commonly demonstrated in dogs.

Parasitic infection

Filaroides osleri is probably transferred from dam to offspring via sputum or faeces. The overall incidence is not high, but in certain localities or kennels, the disorder is encountered reasonably commonly. Infection causes tracheobronchitis and the formation of reactive nodules containing the parasite in the lining of the airway. Affected dogs are usually under 5 years of age, but clinical signs are noted mainly at 6–18 months of age. While some dogs with nodules in the airway show no signs of infection, most have a persistent, harsh, paroxysmal cough that is unresponsive to routine treatment. A few dogs lose weight and some develop dyspnoea and expiratory noise (wheeze), due to partial airway obstruction.

Physical findings are generally unremarkable. Larvae will be identified in the faeces of some, but not all infected dogs when examined by the Baermann technique. A diagnosis is most readily made by bronchoscopy, with which nodules can be seen at the bifurcation of the trachea. Confirmation is by finding larvae or eggs in microscopic examination of nodules, sputum or tracheal washings removed from the airway. Nodules are often too small for radiographic detection.

Treatment requires the use of an anthelmintic: levamisole administered orally at a daily dose rate of 7.5 mg/kg body weight for at least two weeks, has proved to be effective, and albendazole may be alternative therapy (25 mg/kg body weight orally for five days). A determined attempt should be made to trace and examine other in-contact dogs and if possible, the dam. They should receive similar treatment if evidence of infection is present.

A second course of treatment has proved necessary in some cases and surgical removal of nodules should be considered if respiratory distress is prominent. Secondary bacterial infection may require treatment with antibiotics in a few cases.

Trauma

Occasionally, the trachea may be damaged by dog bites or choke chains. Dog bites can cause serious tissue swelling, introduce infection and cause subcutaneous emphysema. Local damage may require surgical attention. Damage to the trachea by choke chains can produce local haemorrhage and coughing, even if the damage is not great.

Tracheal collapse

Tracheal collapse can occur as a result of congenital malformation or hypoplasia of the trachea, but the disorder is more commonly encountered as a dorsoventral flattening of the trachea that first becomes evident in middle-aged or ageing miniature and toy breeds (especially Yorkshire Terriers). The flattening is most marked at the thoracic inlet. Affected dogs usually develop dyspnoea with pronounced respiratory noise, stimulated by exercise or excitement. Dyspnoea is frequently activated by a paroxysm of wheezy coughing. Distortion of the trachea can be palpated cranial to the thoracic inlet in some dogs.

Marked narrowing of the trachea on one or other side of the thoracic inlet is detected on plain radiographs in only a few cases, as it is unusual to expose at the time of collapse. It is very important that radiographs be recorded with the head and neck extended to demonstrate the defect clearly, but fluoroscopy is usually necessary for confirmation. With bronchoscopy, the dorsoventral narrowing of the airway is clearly seen, and secondary tracheitis may be present.

The results of surgical treatment have not been convincingly reliable. Relief may be obtained with sedation and by avoiding heat, severe exercise and excitement. Obese dogs should be rigorously dieted. Antitussive therapy (p. 43) and corticosteroids can help relieve secondary inflammation and severe coughing. However, euthanasia may be requested as persistence of the coughing and dyspnoea cause distress to both dog and client. Client education about the persistence of the problem is essential, since medical treatment is at most palliative.

Foreign bodies

These are not commonly inhaled by dogs. When inhalation occurs, foreign bodies can cause acute upper airway obstruction with choking and cyanosis, but sufficiently small objects (twigs, hair or grass seeds) can lodge in bronchi. They initially cause acute coughing and sometimes haemoptysis, but the cough persists if the object is not dislodged and expectorated. Pulmonary lobar collapse or infection can follow. Clinical findings may be minimal in uncomplicated cases and many foreign bodies are non-radiopaque. Bronchos-

copy is the most reliable technique for their detection and removal (using forceps). Trans-thoracic surgery is required if simple removal is not successful.

Tumours

Invasion of the airway by primary neoplasms is uncommon, bronchogenic carcinoma being most frequently recorded. Chronic unproductive coughing is a typical sign, occasionally with haemoptysis. If the lesion is sufficiently large, respiratory noise may be apparent, due to airway obstruction. There may be radiographic evidence of a lesion if sufficiently large (>5 mm), but bronchoscopy or cytology of tracheobronchial washings is necessary for confirmation of diagnosis. Primary tracheal tumours are rare.

Tumours surrounding the airway can cause signs of respiratory dysfunction. Pressure from thyroid neoplasms, gross lymphomegaly, local abscesses and even gross cardiomegaly can affect respirations. Dyspnoea is the most prominent sign, often first noticed with the demands of excitement or exercise, and accompanied by respiratory noise. Coughing, usually dry and unproductive, may develop as a result of concurrent tracheitis, and retching or regurgitation are common, due to oesophageal obstruction. Tumours in the neck region may be palpated but thoracic radiography is often required for the identification of tumours affecting the lower airway. Exploratory surgery, with the removal of the lesion or material for biopsy, may be required to establish a definitive diagnosis and prognosis.

Allergy

Although bronchial asthma has been induced experimentally in dogs, the naturally-occurring form of this disease appears to be rare. However, pulmonary infiltration with eosinophilia may have an allergic basis (p. 34).

Lungs

Infections

Viral

Viral infections may cause pneumonia with focal oedema. Secondary bacterial invasion is a common sequel in the absence of antibacterial therapy.

Bacterial

Bordetella bronchiseptica is occasionally a primary pathogen, but many secondary agents such as Pasteurella spp., haemolytic Streptococci, Pseudomonas spp. and *Escherichia coli* invade the lower airway to cause bronchopneumonia. This invasion can be a sequel to viral infection, fluid inhalation, haemorrhage, oedema, or partial obstruction of the airway. Food or fluids can be inhaled following regurgitation with oesophageal or pharyngeal disorders or incompetent oral therapy. Pulmonary necrosis, oedema and infection can result (inhalation pneumonia).

Clinical signs of pneumonia include coughing, often soft in character, with tachypnoea and pyrexia. Radiography usually reveals diffuse, alveolar opacity or consolidation, often affecting ventral regions of the lungs (Figs. 2.1, 2.2). Viral infections may be self-limiting, but bacterial involvement requires frequent therapy with broad-spectrum antibiotics for at least two weeks.

Tuberculosis is now rarely encountered in dogs in the UK. It may be seen as a granulomatous reaction in pulmonary tissue, often with few initial clinical signs other than loss of condition.

Granulomatous reaction can also result from infection by Actinomyces spp. or Nocardia spp. These agents are commonly also associated with pleurisy. Radiographic findings are variable, with diffuse and even miliary distribution of lesions, but bronchial lymph node enlargement and pleural effusions can be seen. In view of the public health risk, euthanasia is advised for confirmed cases of tuberculosis.

Pulmonary abscesses are not commonly found in dogs, although localised infection and abscessation can follow penetration of the oesophagus by a foreign body such as a bone, the thoracic wall by trauma or the trachea by a foreign body (e.g. grass seed).

Other infections
Toxocara larvae may cause pneumonia during their passage through pulmonary tissue in puppies during their first weeks of life. Dyspnoea and coughing are

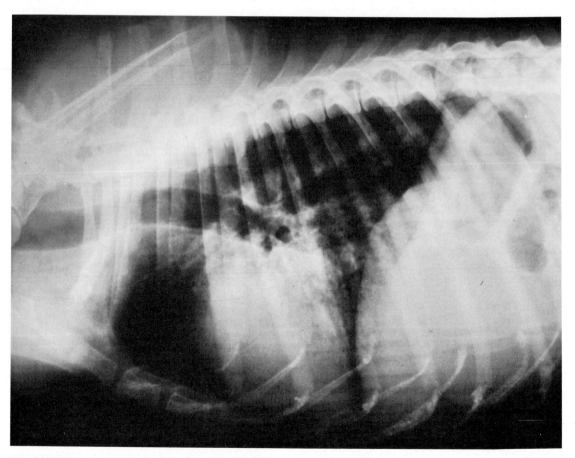

Figs. 2.1 & 2.2 Radiographs of the thorax of an 11-year-old Shetland Sheepdog with malabsorption and a cough following oral misdosing. Ill-defined blotchy densities in the lower left cardiac and diaphragmatic lung lobes indicate an alveolar pattern. At post-mortem examination, inhalation pneumonia was confirmed.

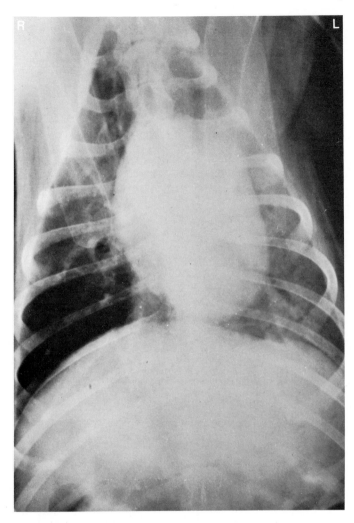

Fig. 2.2

clinical signs, and secondary bacterial infection can occur. Therapy should be directed towards the latter, since agents active against nematode larvae are not yet licensed for use in the UK.

Toxoplasma gondii and fungi have been reported to be associated with pneumonia in dogs, but rarely in the UK.

Pneumonia and consolidation may be a sequel to infection with *Angiostrongylus vasorum*, a parasite causing vasculitis in a number of tissues (Chapter 17).

Neoplasia
Primary pulmonary neoplasia is uncommon, usually involving a local spread by adenocarcinoma (Figs. 2.3, 2.4) in aged dogs.

Secondary neoplasia is very common following metastatic haematogenous or lymphatic spread from mammary or osseous neoplasms (Fig. 2.5), carcinoma of the tonsils, thyroid or abdominal organs (Fig. 2.6), or malignant melanoma. The predilection of many of these neoplasms for spread to the lungs is an indication for routine thoracic survey radiography.

Haemangiosarcoma or lymphosarcoma can also invade pulmonary interstitial tissue.

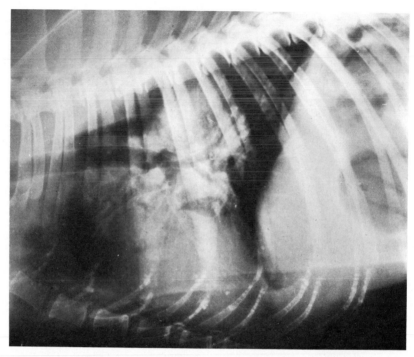

Fig. 2.3 (lateral) & **Fig. 2.4** (ventrodorsal) views of the thorax of an 11-year-old Labrador with a persistent cough, showing an area of homogenous density in the upper right cardiac lung lobe. This was confirmed as adenocarcinoma at post-mortem examination.

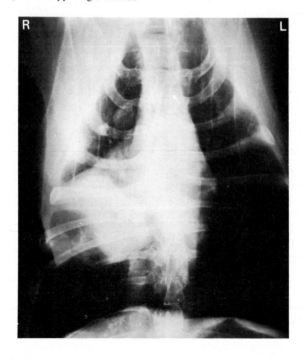

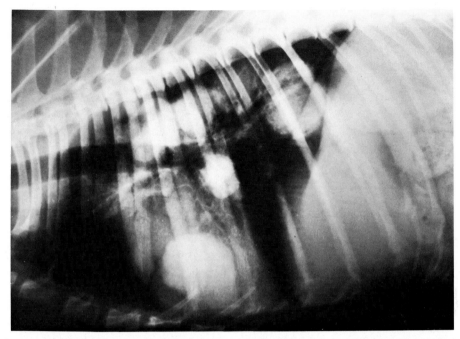

Fig. 2.5 Lateral view of the thorax of a Miniature Poodle with prominent 'golfball' metastases from a mammary neoplasm. Such lesions may not be visible unless at least 4 mm in diameter.

Clinical findings in neoplasia

Metastatic pulmonary neoplasia does not commonly cause coughing in dogs, but coughing is the most consistent sign of primary neoplasia. Other signs frequently include non-specific weight loss and lethargy. When infiltration of pulmonary tissue has become extensive, tachypnoea develops, noticed initially following stress or exercise, but later continuously. Occasionally there is marked reluctance to move, associated with thoracic pain, and lethargy, anorexia, pyrexia and debility can develop following secondary infection. Clinical examination or history should reveal the primary site of a neoplasm that has metastasised. Loss of thoracic resonance can sometimes be appreciated by percussion, and heart sounds may be muffled, despite the loss of body fat.

Radiography is of prime importance in establishing a diagnosis and if there is any doubt about the findings, the examination should be repeated within a few weeks. Typical findings are solitary masses (primary neoplasia), multiple nodules or diffuse interstitial infiltration (secondary neoplasia). The absence of visible masses does not rule out the presence of metastases, which may be too small for radiographic identification if less than about 5 mm in diameter or on less-than-perfect films. Bronchoscopy is not very rewarding in most cases. Occasionally there may be recurrent attacks of acute lethargy and tachypnoea following haemorrhage from an ulcerated neoplasm such as haemangiosarcoma. In these circumstances pallor of the mucous membranes, with tachycardia and radiographic evidence of pleural effusion are common. Haematology indicates anaemia consistent with acute haemorrhage and the presence of the haemorrhage may be confirmed by paracentesis. The haemorrhagic fluid usually fails to clot.

In a few cases, a presenting sign is lameness, with tender, swollen limbs resulting from so-called hypertrophic pulmonary osteoarthropathy (HPOA). This is due to sub-periosteal haemorrhage and new bone formation, apparently in response to reflex activity via the vagus nerve, which is stimulated by extensive pulmonary disease or pleural or mediastinal masses.

Specific diagnosis of a pulmonary mass may be made only by needle biopsy or by exploratory thoracotomy. Even primary tumours, which might be excised, are usually malignant and the results of therapy are not very rewarding.

Other alveolar disorders

Pulmonary oedema

Pulmonary oedema is potentially a life-threatening and yet therapeutically responsive disorder in dogs.

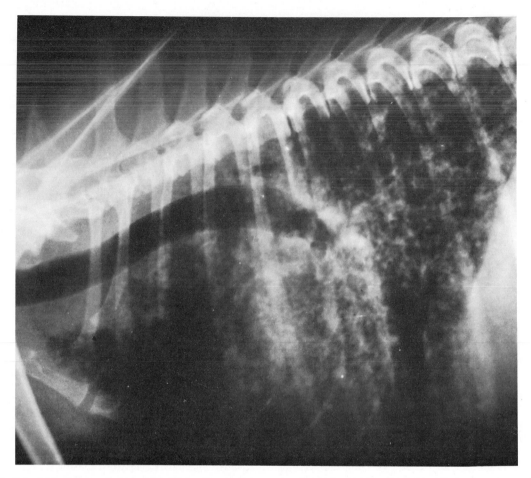

Fig. 2.6 Lateral view of a crossbred bitch with marked dyspnoea. A 'miliary' interstitial pattern is seen throughout the lung field. This is a much less common manifestation of metastases than in Fig. 3. A hepatic carcinoma was the primary source of neoplasia.

The most common cause is left-sided cardiac failure, due, for example, to valvular insufficiency, congenital lesions or myocardial failure (Chapter 1). Pulmonary oedema results much less commonly from the inhalation of toxic fumes from fires, ingestion of poisons such as organophosphates, ANTU or paraquat, and bee stings or snake bites. Anaphylaxis, electrocution, lymphatic obstruction, neurological and immunological disturbances are among other disorders that can cause oedema directly or indirectly. Hypoproteinaemia, anaemia or pulmonary damage can exacerbate alveolar and interstitial oedema.

Severe pulmonary oedema produces respiratory distress varying from tachypnoea to severe dyspnoea with air hunger (sternal recumbency, neck extended, mouth open and lips drawn back) and wheezy or bubbling respiratory noise. Attempts to cough may produce frothy mucus which is sometimes pink-coloured. The cough is usually soft in character and respirations are noisy. There is often restlessness and coughing at night with pulmonary oedema following left-sided cardiac failure. Cyanosis of mucous membranes can occur in severe cases and widespread râles can be detected by auscultation. Cardiac sounds may be dominated by respiratory sounds, but tachycardia, with dysrhythmias or murmurs may be heard if the cause is cardiac failure. The rectal temperature often falls with severe dyspnoea.

Radiographic examination (with careful handling of the patient) is usually rewarding. In the presence of alveolar oedema, widespread disseminated mottling and blotchy opacities are seen, often throughout the lung field. The pattern may be most dense in the hilar region following cardiac failure (Figs. 1.3, 1.4). In these circumstances, evidence of cardiomegaly with marked left atrial and ventricular enlargement is likely to be noted. The pattern in interstitial oedema is more hazy. Whatever the cause, serial radiographs should be recorded, as there may be rapid changes associated with progressive deterioration, or improvement following therapy. Differentiation of oedema from acute pneumonia or intrapulmonary haemorrhage, and the assessment of possible cardiac failure, may not be simple.

Frusemide or thiazide diuretics (intravenously in the first instance) are usually the most effective therapy. Bronchodilating agents such as the xanthine derivatives (theophylline, etamphylline) are also indicated. Sedation is often beneficial, and oxygen therapy may be attempted, but handling a dog to administer oxygen can cause further distress. Cardiac glycosides or vasodilators may be indicated in cardiac failure (Chapter 1), and corticosteroids in the case of shock or allergy. The use of antibiotics should be considered in order to prevent the development of bronchopneumonia.

Intrapulmonary haemorrhage

This can be caused by ulceration of a neoplasm, trauma to the airway, pulmonary contusion or, commonly, coagulopathy (Chapter 11). In rural areas, coagulopathy is frequently due to warfarin poisoning. Signs, usually of sudden onset, include lethargy and shallow, rapid respirations, with dyspnoea if severe. A soft cough, which may result in haemoptysis, is a common feature. Examination of the animal may reveal further sites of haemorrhage or trauma, and pale mucous membranes. With most coagulopathies the clotting time will be prolonged, but further detailed laboratory examination will be needed to identify the clotting factor concerned (Chapter 11). Routine haematology is likely to reveal regenerative anaemia.

Radiography will identify localised areas of mottled or floccular opacity, which may be restricted to the ventral regions of isolated lung lobes. Sometimes, evidence of concurrent intrapleural haemorrhage will be detected. Therapeutically, little can be done to remove the material from the lungs, but the re-establishment of normal coagulation is an urgent priority, with administration of vitamin K1 for warfarin poisoning or the transfusion of fresh blood or plasma to supply clotting factors. The dog should be rested and it is wise to administer broad-spectrum antibiotics for 5–7 days to suppress secondary bacterial infection. Uncomplicated intrapulmonary haemorrhage often resolves remarkably rapidly without therapy but there is a potential risk of pulmonary collapse or fibrosis.

Miscellaneous disorders

Emphysema

Vesicular emphysema is occasionally encountered in dogs, somtimes as a result of airway obstruction or chronic bronchitis, but often of uncertain aetiology. The significance of emphysema in dogs is uncertain, but signs are usually related to the predisposing cause, and a marked expiratory effort can be seen in advanced cases. Crackling sounds may be detected by auscultation of peripheral lung areas. Classically, the presence of abnormal radiolucency in the peripheral lung field is an indication of this disorder on radiographs, but in the presence of changes associated with chronic bronchitis, identification is not clear. Treatment must be aimed at reversing the predisposing cause or at relief of coughing.

Paraquat poisoning

Paraquat poisoning is caused in dogs by the consumption of the concentrated form of this herbicide, either directly or through malicious baiting of materials such as carcasses. The poison causes necrosis of alimentary mucosae and widespread damage to internal body tissues, resulting in renal failure and severe lung disease. Principally, there is fibroblastic infiltration and epithelial necrosis in alveoli and bronchioles, together with widespread alveolar haemorrhage and oedema. This causes progressive loss of capacity for gaseous exchange. Following initial vomiting, tachypnoea develops into severe dyspnoea and air hunger over a few days. The body temperature tends to fall and the heart rate rises late in the disorder, when cyanosis may be noted. Clinical findings are otherwise minimal, though ulceration of the buccal mucosa is often seen.

In most cases, a rising level of plasma urea and the results of urinalysis will be consistent with acute renal failure (Chapter 15). In many cases, remarkably few abnormalities will be detected radiographically unless intra-alveolar haemorrhage and oedema have been severe, when diffuse increased pulmonary density may be detected. In a few cases, mediastinal or subcutaneous emphysema follows the severe dyspnoea. A positive diagnosis can be made from chemical tests on the urine in the early stages, but frequently the poisoning can only be suspected from circumstances, as paraquat is rapidly excreted. Very little response to therapy can be achieved in rapidly developing cases and the condition warrants euthanasia on humane grounds.

Pulmonary thromboemboli

Pulmonary thromboemboli and infarction are encountered occasionally, often with no clearly recognisable clinical signs, unless the lesion is very large. Pulmonary thrombosis can result from trauma elsewhere in the body, infection with bacteria or parasites (Angiostrongylus spp. or, in imported dogs, Dirofilaria spp.; Chapter 17) and it has been associated with renal amyloidosis. Clinical signs include sudden lethargy and depression, dyspnoea, tachycardia and weak pulse. Therapy is mainly supportive if a definitive diagnosis can be achieved: radiographic signs include a localised diffuse alveolar opacity similar to other alveolar diseases. The prognosis is poor.

Acquired collapse
Acquired collapse of a lung lobe can be a sequel to partial obstruction of a bronchus by neoplasms, bronchial secretions or foreign bodies. Lobar collapse may also result from pressure of pleural effusions, pneumothorax, or abdominal contents passing through a rupture of the diaphragm. Specific clinical signs are minimal but the disorder will be detected radiographically by a shift of tissues towards the collapsed lobe, and increased density of the affected lobe. The possible causes should be considered and treatment directed accordingly. Lobar collapse occasionally leads to torsion of an affected lung lobe and pleural effusion.

Eosinophilic 'pneumonia'
Eosinophilic pneumonia (pulmonary infiltration with eosinophilia) occurs occasionally in dogs. The cause is uncertain, although in some cases the response indicates an allergic phenomenon. The clinical signs vary from coughing to dyspnoea and may be acute in onset or persistent. Radiographs may reveal a diffuse alveolar/interstitial pattern similar to that of bronchopneumonia, and persistent eosinophilia is detected with routine haematology or airway washings. Response to corticosteroid therapy may be dramatic.

Other lesions
Lung cysts, blebs and bullae (congenital or acquired) are occasionally encountered. They are usually airfilled and may communicate with an airway or they may be independent. Generally they cause no clinical signs unless very large, when they interfere with lung expansion, causing breathlessness at exercise. They are detected as thin-walled structures without normal vascularisation or bronchi on radiographs. Occasionally, air-filled cysts may rupture, causing pneumothorax. This may necessitate surgical attention; small cysts usually require no therapy.

Pleural cavity

Trauma
Road accidents and dog fights can cause rib fractures and intercostal tears which give rise, directly or by trauma to lung lobes or associated structures, to pneumothorax, intrapleural haemorrhage or exudative pleurisy, any of which may cause tachypnoea. In addition, there will be localised swelling and pain and extensive damage to the thoracic wall, so that the integrity of this structure is destroyed. Subcutaneous emphysema will often be detected when such cases are examined clinically.

Percussion may demonstrate the presence of air or fluid in the thorax by increased or decreased resonance, respectively. Radiography is an important aid to diagnosis for proof of rib fractures and for the detection of pneumothorax or pleural effusions.

Pneumothorax
Pneumothorax allows lungs to retract and undergo partial or total collapse. It can be caused by penetration of the thoracic wall, pulmonary tissues, the airway or the oesophagus, and rarely it occurs spontaneously. The disorder is usually bilateral. Signs include tachypnoea, especially if the dog is stressed, with reluctance to move freely or lie down normally. There may be cyanosis in severe cases. Increased resonance is often easily detected by thoracic percussion. Vesicular sounds are absent from affected regions of the thorax.

Radiography is required to confirm the diagnosis, with signs of elevation of the cardiac shadow from the sternum, areas of increased lucency in the peripheral regions of the thorax with absence of the vascularity that would indicate normal pulmonary tissue, and partial collapse of lung lobes (Fig. 2.7). In the absence of shock or severe respiratory distress, the dog should be rested and sedated. In more severe cases, aspiration should be undertaken in a fashion similar to the paracentesis of fluids (p. 36), using a three-way tap in the upper region of the thorax, mid-way along its length. One withdrawal of air followed by rest and sedation may be sufficient in many cases, but recurrence may require the use of an under-water air trap or exploratory thoracotomy for the repair of a leaking wound.

Ruptured diaphragm
Ruptured diaphragm is a serious sequel to road accident trauma. Clinical signs referable to 'diaphragmatic hernia' may not become evident to the owner for several days or weeks after an accident, because, firstly, the lack of respiratory reserve may not become evident until the animal becomes more active, second a rupture may suddenly enlarge, and third, a pleural

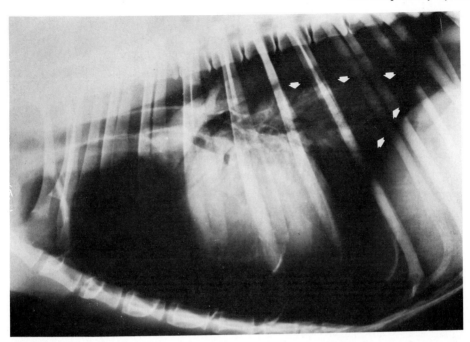

Fig. 2.7   Lateral view of the thorax of a two-year-old Terrier with a fractured pelvis and dyspnoea following a 50-foot fall. Gross pleural lucency is seen, together with elevation of the heart from the sternum and collapse of lung lobes. (The outline of diaphragmatic lobes is indicated with arrows). There is also pneumomediastinum: the azygos vein is seen.

effusion can develop slowly. In an acute case with a large rupture, there may be considerable respiratory distress, cyanosis and shock. Tachypnoea and reluctance to lie down may be signs of less severe damage. Chest movements may be accentuated, and severe dyspnoea can develop. The commonly-described empty abdomen is by no means always evident.

Thoracic percussion often reveals lack of resonance and there may be unilateral muffling and apparent displacement of heart sounds. Occasionally, increased resonance will be appreciated with percussion if, for example, the stomach passes through the hernia. The presence of audible borborygmi in the thorax is a variable finding and not always distinct. Loss of continuity of the line of the diaphragm on radiographs should always arouse suspicions of a rupture (Fig. 2.8). A detailed study of the radiographs, with additional information following the oral administration of barium to outline the position of components of the digestive tract, is often necessary to ascertain the presence of a rupture of the diaphragm and the viscera that have passed through the rupture. Care should be exercised in handling a dyspnoeic animal.

Occasionally, only small components of tissue such as a lobe of the liver may protrude through a rupture, giving rise to pleural effusion and local adhesions. The effusion should be withdrawn by paracentesis to assess its nature and to allow clearer radiography. Surgical repair of ruptured diaphragm requires very careful management of gaseous anaesthesia.

Pleural effusions

The presence of an effusion causes similar clinical signs, whatever the nature of the effusion. Diffusion of small quantities of serous fluids through the pleural cavity is a normal phenomenon. Accumulation of fluids results from excess production, failure of absorption, or the escape of abnormal fluids into the cavity.

Clinical signs generally refer to the loss of thoracic capacity for expansion of lungs and this will often be insidious and progressive in onset. Tachypnoea is a cardinal sign, usually with shallow respirations, which is noticed first after exercise or stress and later even at rest, although it can be masked by a reduction in the dog's activity. As respirations become embarrassed even at rest, the dog tends to adopt a position that assists ventilation (instead of lateral recumbency, a sitting position or a position lying on the sternum is adopted, often with elbows abducted).

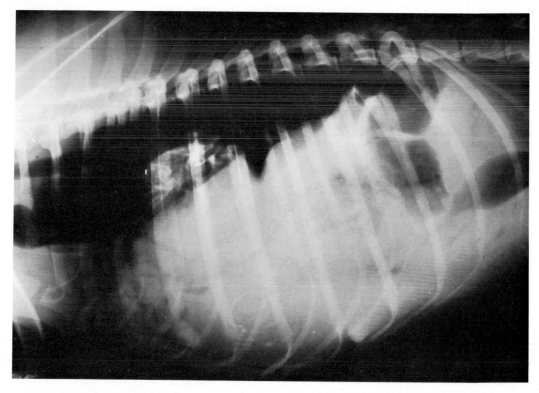

Fig. 2.8 Lateral view of the thorax of a two-year-old Collie with ruptured diaphragm. Lung lobes are collapsed, there is loss of cardiac and diaphragmatic outlines, and dense structures are present in the thorax.

Careful percussion of the thorax will often reveal a marked distinction between lack of resonance in the ventral thorax, due to the presence of fluid, and increased resonance over the upper thorax where the lungs 'float' on the fluid. Muffling of heart sounds may be total, so that the heart rate may be appreciated only by palpation of the pulse, or with electrocardiography.

Great care should be taken in handling a patient for radiology if more than mild tachypnoea is present. Marked tachypnoea indicates minimal respiratory reserve and since it is dangerous to place an affected dog in dorsal recumbency, a dorso-ventral exposure is the position of choice. A lateral view may be all that is necessary to confirm the presence of intrapleural fluid and a standing lateral exposure can be useful (Fig. 2.11). This avoids excessive handling and allows the clear demonstration of a fluid line in the thorax in most cases. Further radiography should be delayed until sufficient fluid has been withdrawn to permit safe handling of the animal and the recording of clearer intrathoracic detail. Radiographic evidence of the presence of pleural effusion includes general homogeneous opacity in the lower thorax, with clear outlining of the radiolucent borders of lung lobes by interlobular fissure lines appearing between lung lobes and the thoracic wall, especially at the extremities of the thorax (Figs. 2.9, 2.10).

Paracentesis of the thorax is relatively simple, although in some cases 'pocketing' of fluid can occur in the presence of adhesions, preventing easy withdrawal. Following aseptic preparation of the site and the infiltration of subcutaneous, intercostal and pleural tissues with local anaesthetic, a needle (19G × 19 mm is suitable) with a three-way tap or syringe attached is introduced with sterile precautions into the 7th or 8th intercostal space, two-thirds of the way down the thorax. The needle should be directed along the inside wall of the thorax, rather than straight into the cavity. Better drainage is achieved, with less risk to intrathoracic tissues, by the use of a sterile plastic cannula, particularly if it is punctured with a number of holes before sterilisation. A skin incision to allow the introduction of this type of cannula should be made to one side of the thoracic puncture to avoid fistulation after paracentesis.

Samples of fluid should be taken into tubes contain-

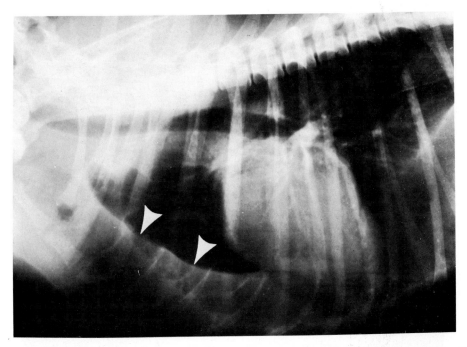

Fig. 2.9 Lateral view of the thorax of a whippet with pleural effusion (chyle). Some loss of outline of normal struc- tures (heart, diaphragm) is apparent, together with pleural opacity causing reduced lung size (indicated by arrows).

ing EDTA and heparin and into sterile tubes for cy- tology, bacteriology and biochemistry respectively. However, the appearance of the fluid can be a very useful guide to diagnosis if it is not contaminated by blood. Care should be taken in handling purulent effusions, as in a few cases (e.g. tuberculosis) they can be infectious to man. Effusions are often categorised as transudates or exudates, according to protein and cellular content, but this division is somewhat arbi- trary and may be of little clinical relevance.

True transudates

True transudates are capillary filtrates with a protein content of less than 30 g/l and a specific gravity less than 1.018. Transudates are translucent or only slightly opaque and colourless, and they contain few cells. They are rarely found in dogs other than in hypoproteinaemic disorders. The most common cause of hypoproteinaemia is protein-losing nephropathy, usually due to widespread glomerulonephritis or amy- loidosis (Chapter 15). True transudates also occur with protein-losing enteropathies, of which lymphan- giectasis is the only recorded cause in dogs (Chapter 14). Pleural transudation is rarely a sequel to starva- tion, malabsorption, or hepatic failure in dogs.

In the presence of true transudation, plasma protein levels will be low, with albumin less than 20 g/l. Glom- erulonephritis or amyloidosis will be marked by heavy proteinuria. Therapy must be aimed at the replace- ment of plasma protein by transfusion of plasma in severe cases, the feeding of a high quality protein diet and the use of anabolic steroids. Attention should be paid to the underlying renal disease (Chapter 15). Protein-losing enteropathy will usually be associated with chronic diarrhoea and progressive weight loss. There may be laboratory evidence of malabsorption. The prognosis is guarded.

Modified transudates

Many pleural effusions may be described as *modified transudates*, typically straw-coloured or pink, and slightly opaque. The protein (approximately 30 g/l) and cellular content and the specific gravity (approxi- mately 1.018) are higher than those of a true transu- date, which may result in part from a reaction of the pleura to long-standing transudation. Right-sided or congestive cardiac failure (Chapter 1), tumours or ad- hesions causing obstruction to venous or lymphatic flow, and abdominal tissues protruding through a rup- tured diaphragm are potential causes.

Following the removal of as much fluid as possible, radiographs should be examined for evidence of car-

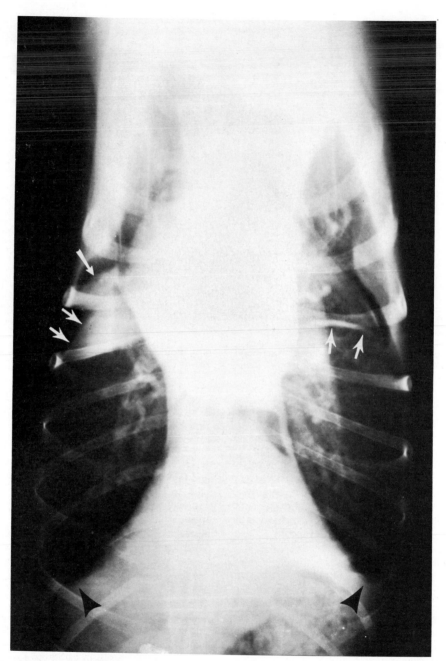

Fig. 2.10 Ventro-dorsal view of a dog with pleural effusion. Marked interlobular fissure lines are seen (white arrows) and there is rounding of the costophrenic angles (black arrows). The cardiac and diaphragmatic silhouettes are often more masked than in this view, where the fluid appears to be localized.

diomegaly, neoplasia or ruptured diaphragm. Fluid should also be removed to relieve respiratory distress. Thoracotomy may be indicated for confirmation of the presence of a neoplasm, but few lesions in this region are amenable to surgery. Cardiac failure should be treated rigorously as necessary (Chapter 1). Repeated thoracentesis for removal of fluids is not an ideal therapeutic approach, for protein contained in the fluid will be replaced by further losses from plasma.

Despite knowledge of these potential causes, unexplained hydrothorax is occasionally encountered, and repeated removal of fluid may be necessary, if only to relieve respiratory distress.

Haemothorax

This can be caused by trauma to the thorax or thoracic tissues, rupture of a neoplasm (especially haemangiosarcoma), tearing of an adhesion or some coagulopathy. If the haemorrhage is at all insidious, the effused blood will only partially clot. Clinical signs include sudden lethargy, tachycardia, tachypnoea and pallor of the mucous membranes. Tachypnoea results from anaemia in addition to the loss of thoracic capacity. The onset of signs is usually sudden, but haemorrhage may be self-limiting and fairly rapid improvement in the dog's condition can be seen. Recurrent episodes of gradual remission and acute relapse are common. With coagulopathies, other sites of haemorrhage may be evident and the clotting or bleeding times may be prolonged. The anaemia is usually regenerative, whatever the cause.

Other effusions, including purulent exudate, may contain large numbers of erythrocytes. Similarly, contamination of samples by inadvertent minor trauma during paracentesis is quite common. Treatment of acute haemothorax must include the removal of sufficient blood to allow improved breathing and the use of intravenous fluid therapy to correct hypovolaemia. Blood transfusions should be reserved for very severe blood loss or for the supply of clotting factors by the use of fresh blood or plasma in coagulopathies. Vitamin K1 must be administered in warfarin poisoning: the action of this agent will be apparent within a few hours. Attempted removal of all blood from the thoracic cavity is unnecessary as materials are readily recycled, but there is a risk of fibrinous adhesions and permanent lung collapse if removal is not attempted. Recurrence or persistence of haemorrhage is an indication for thoracotomy to establish a diagnosis or to permit haemostasis.

Pyothorax

The presence of purulent material in the thorax indicates exudative pleurisy. The exudate is dense, occasionally granular and often foul-smelling, varying in colour from yellow through green to brown. An affected dog not only develops tachypnoea, but it is also rapidly debilitated by toxaemia. Lethargy, anorexia and weight loss are common signs. Often the mucous membranes become rather pale and there is pyrexia in the early stages, but this is a variable finding in chronic cases. Generalised lymphomegaly may be found. The effusion is highly cellular, containing polymorphonuclear neutrophils, debris and (usually) bacteria (which can be identified with Gram's stain). The protein and fibrin content is usually high. Routine haematology will indicate marked leucocytosis, often with anaemia.

The source of the infection is seldom established. Certain infections, including nocardiosis and tuberculosis are probably due to primary invasion. Infectious agents may be introduced by haematogenous spread, injury to the thoracic wall, or damage to the oesophagus or respiratory tissue by foreign bodies. Micro-organisms include Streptococci, Staphylococci, Proteus spp., *Escherichia coli*, or Pasteurellae. Infections may involve more than one agent, but in a number of cases it is impossible to identify a causal organism.

The effusion may be 'pocketed' by adhesions and removal by paracentesis may not be very successful, even when repeated in a number of sites. Parenteral antibiotic therapy with agents appropriate to the sensitivity of the infective organisms is required more than once daily for many weeks together with supportive treatment for debility. If no bacterial agent is identified, broad-spectrum antibiotics should be employed. Lavage of the thorax with saline and antibiotics can be attempted and the use of proteolytic agents such as streptokinase (Varidase; Lederle) can be considered, to facilitate the breakdown of adhesions. However, these procedures can be painful, and proteolysis is usually unnecessary. The introduction of an indwelling catheter obviates the need for repeated puncture of the thoracic wall. Thoracotomy may be indicated for very persistent cases, following careful anaesthesia, to break down adhesions and to attempt to identify the source of infection. The overall prognosis must be very guarded, as treatment will be expensive and tedious, and success is by no means guaranteed: even if the infection is cleared, pulmonary function may be restricted.

Chylothorax

This is an occasional finding, with few diagnostic signs other than those related to pleural effusions, and with loss of condition in long-standing cases. The onset is usually gradual and there may be simultaneous peritoneal effusion. The chyle is characteristically milky-white and opaque although it is sometimes blood-tinged. The fluid stains readily for fats and large numbers of lymphocytes will be identified by microscopic examination. The cause may be neoplastic or traumatic rupture, erosion or obstruction of a lym-

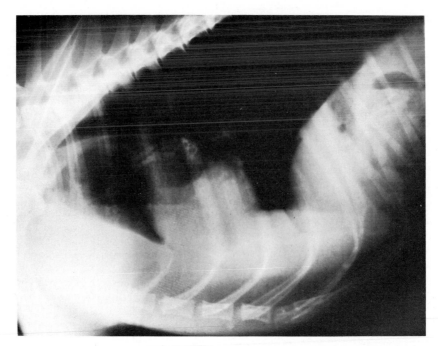

Fig. 2.11 'Standing lateral' view of the thorax of the dog in Fig. 2.9, using a horizontal X-Ray beam. A horizontal fluid line is often well demonstrated by this position in cases of doubt over the presence of pleural effusion.

phatic duct, but in a number of cases the origin is indeterminate even at post-mortem examination.

Plain radiography will usually not reveal the cause, even after removal of effusion, but if lymphangiography is carried out using contrast material, the point of leakage can be detected in some cases. Unfortunately, the picture is often confused by the large number of lymphatic structures revealed by this technique, and the lack of experience of most investigators. The effusion should be removed to relieve respiratory embarrassment. Occasionally there will be no recurrence following paracentesis, but repeated effusion is an indication for exploratory thoracotomy with a view to ligating a leaking lymphatic vessel or the lymphatic duct. It is wise to restrict the intake of fats (with the exception of medium chain triglycerides such as coconut oil, which are not absorbed into the lymphatic system) to reduce the production of chyle. Attention should be paid to the maintenance of high levels of protein and carbohydrates in the diet.

Neoplastic effusions

Few primary neoplasms affect the pleural cavity *per se* other than mesothelioma, which usually gives rise to a sanguineous effusion in which large numbers of mesothelial cells can be detected microscopically. Generalised neoplasms can also cause effusions. These include carcinomata, for which cytology can sometimes be rewarding, and haemangiosarcoma, from which haemothorax develops. Other neoplasms create effusions which are modified transudates in character, through pressure on venous and lymphatic vessels. These include the 'heart base' (aortic body) tumour and lymphosarcoma. Most effusion-producing neoplasms are malignant, but in the absence of cytological evidence of malignancy, detection and confirmation of a diffuse neoplasm may be very difficult. Repeat radiographs should be examined carefully for evidence of neoplasia following withdrawal of effusions in ageing dogs.

Mediastinum

Technically, mediastinal structures are extrapleural, in direct contact with tissues of the neck. Being also in close contact with the pleura and pulmonary tissues, the mediastinum is affected by many of the same generalised disorders. Mediastinal tumours include thymic and aortic body ('heart base') neoplasms and bronchogenic carcinoma, but lymphomegaly, granulomas and abscesses are also found. In general, these produce clinical signs related to:

1 Pressure on the airway, causing dyspnoea, coughing and/or respiratory noise
2 Pressure on the oesophagus, causing regurgitation, retching or dysphagia
3 Loss of thoracic capacity causing tachypnoea, or
4 Pressure on venous and lymphatic vessels, producing pleural effusions or oedema of the head, neck or forelimbs.

Horner's syndrome (Chapter 5) is occasionally encountered in cases where the sympathetic nerve chain is affected by pressure in the cranial region of the thorax. There is an association between thymomas in the dog and myasthenia gravis.

Escape of air from bronchi, the trachea or the oesophagus following trauma or even severe respiratory distress can cause pneumomediastinum (Fig. 2.7). This usually also gives rise to subcutaneous emphysema of the head and neck, but it is not generally serious unless associated with pneumothorax.

Radiology is an important aid in the diagnosis of mediastinal diseases, which rarely cause specific clinical signs. Displacement of the oesophagus, trachea or heart by mediastinal masses may be clear on radiographs. The use of a small quantity of barium to identify the position of the oesophagus is valuable. Further investigation of a mediastinal lesion is likely to require thoracotomy.

Congenital pericardiodiaphragmatic hernia, in which the abdominal cavity connects directly with the pericardial sac, is occasionally encountered. Abdominal contents such as mesentery or intestines·may surround the heart. Clinical signs, if they occur, may include digestive upsets, dyspnoea or right-sided cardiac failure. Muffling of heart sounds is generally apparent with auscultation, but radiography is required for definitive diagnosis.

DIFFERENTIAL DIAGNOSIS AND MANAGEMENT OF COUGHING

Aetiology of coughing

Coughing is stimulated by irritation or inflammation of the mucosa of the airway at sites between the pharynx and larger bronchioles, the larynx being particularly sensitive. The sensory pathway of irritation is mainly the vagus nerve, but motor control of coughing is via more complicated pathways and the mechanism includes closure of the larynx, and action of the intercostal muscles and the diaphragm. The stimulus may be chemical, physical, viral or bacterial irritation, the excessive production or stasis of mucus, or the presence of material such as oedematous or purulent exudate arising from the lungs.

Coughing helps remove material, but continued unproductive coughing may be disadvantageous as materials can be disseminated into unaffected parts of the lung. Coughing can also result in emphysema, pneumothorax, or pneumomediastinum and the effort is debilitating to the dog. In addition, continued coughing annoys owners.

Differential diagnosis of coughing

Acute coughing

Kennel cough (viral/bacterial); airway irritation (smoke, dust, chemicals); foreign body inhalation; pulmonary oedema; intrapulmonary haemorrhage (trauma, coagulopathies); inhalation pneumonia; allergic (eosinophilic) pneumonia.

Persistent coughing

Chronic bronchitis/bronchiectasis; left-sided cardiac failure (pulmonary oedema or congestion); tracheal collapse; parasitic infection (Filaroides); foreign body; bronchopneumonia; pressure on airway by tumours, enlarged lymph nodes, abscesses or enlarged heart; airway neoplasia; (pleurisy).

Investigation of coughing

History

History that may suggest a diagnosis:

Age
1 Young animals may have congenital lesions (e.g. tracheal hypoplasia), and Filaroides and other respiratory infections are prevalent in young dogs.
2 Older dogs are more likely to develop chronic bronchitis, left-sided cardiac failure or neoplasia.

Breed
1 Ageing Boxers are frequently affected by neoplasia.
2 Yorkshire Terriers and toy breeds are liable to tracheal collapse.
3 Ageing West Highland white Terriers often present with coughing and marked crepitant sounds in the thorax, suggesting emphysema.
4 Many Irish Setters develop regurgitation (e.g. with megaloesophagus) accompanied by inhalation pneumonia.
5 Small breeds appear to be predisposed to chronic bronchitis and to left-sided cardiac failure due to acquired mitral incompetence.

6 Brachycephalic breeds frequently develop upper airway obstruction and inflammation.

Weight loss
Weight loss may indicate severe or generalised systemic disease (neoplasia, chronic bronchopneumonia or regurgitation and inhalation).

Speed of onset
Coughing due to inhalation and infections develops suddenly, but other disorders develop more insidiously and progressively.

Environment
Known exposure to boiler dust or cigarette smoke may indicate chronic bronchitis. Recurrent seasonal disease might suggest pulmonary infiltration with eosinophilia. Recent kennelling or purchase from a pet shop suggests infection, but this likelihood might be reduced by respiratory vaccines.

Exercise tolerance
Exercise tolerance is reduced in cardiac failure, neoplasia or airway obstruction.

Nature of the cough
The nature of a cough is not as certain an indication of a cause as might be imagined, but:

1 A honking or wheezing cough suggests airway obstruction or tracheal collapse, while a loud, harsh dry cough suggests airway irritation (including infection) and a soft, moist cough, especially if accompanied by nasal discharge, can represent alveolar disease (bronchopneumonia or pulmonary haemorrhage).
2 Chronic bronchitis or left-sided cardiac failure often provokes coughing at night or on waking, while coughing due to airway obstruction tends to be provoked by exercise.

Clinical findings
Unfortunately, neither history nor the clinical examination yields a definitive diagnosis in many cases of coughing. However, the following points should be borne in mind. There is usually weight loss following neoplasia or bronchopneumonia. The rectal temperature can be elevated with bronchopneumonia and some acute respiratory infections. There may be pallor of the mucous membranes with intrapulmonary haemorrhage, and cyanosis with respiratory obstruction or severe interstitial or alveolar disease. Lymphomegaly is not commonly found. The pharynx and tonsils should be examined for disease. Tracheal deformity may be palpated in tracheal collapse and peri-

tracheal masses may be felt in the neck. Tracheal manipulation will often reveal the character of a cough, through provocation.

There are usually moist râles present with pulmonary oedema or bronchopneumonia, dry rhonchi in nonproductive chronic bronchitis and crackling sounds may be auscultated in the presence of emphysema. Cardiac murmurs associated with valvular insufficiency are common in ageing dogs, but the area over which the heart is heard is increased, the heart rate is usually elevated and dysrhythmias are often present in cardiac failure (Chapter 1). In chronic bronchitis, in the presence of *compensated* cardiac disease, the heart rate is likely to be normal and accentuated sinus arrhythmia, usually synchronous with respirations, may be present. Auscultation is not specifically rewarding in many other coughing dogs.

Laboratory aids to diagnosis
These are not particularly helpful in the investigation of coughing. Apart from bronchopneumonia, where marked leucocytosis is usual and eosinophilia can occur, and intrapulmonary haemorrhage, where regenerative anaemia may be anticipated, there are rarely significant haematological or biochemical abnormalities. Faecal examination by the Baermann technique is diagnostic in some cases of filaroidiasis, and sputum from these cases will usually contain larvae.

Radiology
In the majority of coughing dogs, this does not provide diagnostic information, as many airway irritations produce no significant radiographic changes. However, it is a valuable aid in eliminating the possibility of some lower airway and pulmonary disorders, including neoplasia, bronchopneumonia and evidence of left-sided cardiac failure or megaloesophagus. It is important to make radiographic exposures at the time of maximal inspiration to identify the fine detail of pathological changes against the contrast of air-filled lungs. This is best achieved in an anaesthetised dog by using positive pressure inflation of the lungs, if there is no contraindication for anaesthesia. In addition, this allows exposures to be made with a minimum of movement. Short exposures at high kilovoltages are important for good results. A grid should be used with depth of tissue greater than 14 cm.

Bronchoscopy
Bronchoscopy is an important additional aid for the thorough investigation of coughing due to airway lesions or obstruction. It enables a clinician to observe the airway, obtain tissue biopsies or samples of secre-

tions for cytology, bacteriology and parasitology and to remove lesions or foreign bodies. The ideal instrument for this purpose is a flexible fibre-optic bronchoscope, with lighting and biopsy channels, but its cost restricts availability. Useful information can be gained, particularly in larger dogs, with rigid tube endoscopes when these are equipped with distal lighting.

Bronchoscopy should be undertaken only when the risk of anaesthesia is not considered to be significant. It is not advised in the presence of dyspnoea or cardiac failure. Premedication with phenothiazine derivatives such as acetylpromazine should be employed. It is debatable whether atropine should be used: although this drug will suppress some cardiac dysrhythmias and bronchoconstriction resulting from vagal stimulation, it may add to the stasis of mucus in the airway that occurs with bronchitis. Deep anaesthesia or muscular relaxants are required to permit laryngeal relaxation for bronchoscopy. While relaxation can be achieved with short-acting barbiturates, gaseous anaesthesia will allow inflation of lungs for radiology and it safeguards the supply of oxygen.

The endotracheal tube is withdrawn under deep anaesthesia, the dog is placed on its sternum and the pharynx and larynx are examined thoroughly. The larynx can be sprayed with local analgesic, and then the sterilised and lubricated bronchoscope is introduced gently into the airway. This is examined in detail and any distortion is noted: the instrument is then passed, if size permits, into each mainstem bronchus in turn, to observe the mucosa and bronchial contents.

In exudative pulmonary disorders (e.g. bronchopneumonia) mucopurulent material may be seen emerging from particular bronchi. This is also a region where small foreign bodies can lodge, where tumours can develop, and where the mucosa may become roughened and thick strands or plugs of mucus may be found in chronic bronchitis. The nodules of parasitic bronchitis are usually found at the tracheal bifurcation. In acute tracheobronchitis (kennel cough) the mucosa of the trachea is usually hyperaemic and purulent material may be present, whereas normal mucosa is pink in colour and small blood vessels and tracheal rings are easily identified.

A foreign body should be removed carefully with crocodile forceps and any lesion or abnormal tissue should be taken for histological examination. Swabs for bacteriology can be introduced through a tubular endoscope with crocodile forceps, and after withdrawal of the endoscope, mucopurulent material can be sampled. It is possible to take samples of material from the lower airway for cytology by washing with 5–10 ml of sterile saline and withdrawing it through a sterile tube. The significance of the results of cytology

of bronchial washings in dogs is poorly documented. Potentially, neoplastic cells may be detected and predominance of certain cell types may be helpful in diagnosis. A technique for obtaining washings by tracheal puncture in unanaesthetised dogs has been described (Creighton & Wilkins 1974), but valuable bronchoscopic findings are missed by this technique.

Therapy for coughing

Should be directed towards:

1　Avoidance of sources of irritation:
(a)　dry, smoky or dusty atmospheres,
(b)　sudden temperature changes,
(c)　collars (shoulder harnesses are better),
(d)　obesity (overweight dogs should be strictly dieted),
(e)　heavy exercise.

2　Loosening of materials in the airway, which can be assisted:
(a)　with mucolytic agents such as bromhexine or carbocisteine,
(b)　with expectorants—ammonium chloride, balsams,
(c)　by placing the dog in an atmosphere humidified by steam several times daily—for example, a shower room,
(d)　by use of a nebulizer that introduces very fine aerosol water droplets through a face mask.

3　Reduction of irritation:
(a)　antihistamines? (often incorporated in proprietory medicines). Sodium cromoglycate may be effective in the few truly allergic cases in dogs.
(b)　local demulcents (glycerine, syrup, honey)
(c)　corticosteroids may assist in some cases of acute and severe airway inflammation (kennel cough) and chronic bronchitis, but they should be used with caution.

4　Suppression of coughing, especially in cases where paroxysmal coughing is *unproductive* and distressing, using:
(a)　cough centre depressants (opiates: dextromethorphan, codeine).
(b)　sedatives (barbiturates) and tranquillisers (phenothiazine derivatives: acetylpromazine, chlorpromazine).
Many commercial anti-tussive preparations contain a mixture of two or more of these agents.

5 Bronchodilation—using:

(a) adrenergics: e.g. orciprenaline, terbutaline, iso-etharine, phenylephrine, ephedrine or salbutamol.

(b) xanthine derivatives: aminophylline, etamiphylline, theophylline.

6 Elimination of infection with antibacterial therapy:

(a) in the presence of acute respiratory disease when bronchopneumonia may develop: severe tracheobronchitis; inhalation pneumonia; viral pneumonia; pulmonary trauma; intrapulmonary haemorrhage or oedema.

(b) in the presence of bronchopneumonia: if possible, a bronchial washing or a sample of sputum should be gained for bacteriological culture and antibiotic sensivity testing.

(c) if the character of respiratory disease changes so that generalised illness develops or purulent sputum is produced.

In the absence of sensitivity test results, broad-spectrum antibacterial agents should be employed (ampicillin, tetracyclines or potentiated sulphonamides) more than once daily for at least a week. In the absence of resolution of bronchopneumonia, therapy should be maintained for much longer. The use of antibiotics for uncomplicated kennel cough is generally unnecessary. This is supported by evidence that these agents penetrate the upper respiratory tract very poorly. There is evidence that the penetration of the airway by tetracyclines is facilitated by bromhexine.

DIFFERENTIAL DIAGNOSIS OF TACHYPNOEA AND DYSPNOEA

Physiological or association with generalised disease
(often open-mouthed panting)
Hyperthermia (heat stroke)
Excitement/fright/nervousness
Pain, fever
Shock, acidosis
Anaemia/hypoxia
Parturition, eclampsia
CNS disorders (encephalitis/trauma)
Endocrine disorders (phaeochromocytoma/hyperthyroidism?)

Airway obstruction (usually also coughing and respiratory noise)
Foreign body, neoplasm, trauma

Laryngeal paralysis/collapse/oedema
Soft palate overlength or oedema
Laryngeal or tracheal trauma or haemorrhage
Tracheal collapse
Peritracheal masses: tumours (thyroid, lymphatic, thymic, heart base), abscesses, gross cardiomegaly
Filaroidiasis
Cardiac enlargement

Loss of thoracic capacity for pulmonary expansion
Effusions—haemorrhagic, purulent, chylous, transudative, neoplastic
Ruptured diaphragm (or congenital pericardiodiaphragmatic hernia)
Pneumothorax
Mediastinal or pleural neoplasms
Gross cardiomegaly
Intra-abdominal masses, ascites, gastric dilatation
Oesophageal dilatation

Loss of pulmonary capacity for gaseous exchange
Bronchopneumonia
Interstititial pneumonia
Pulmonary oedema
Metastatic neoplasia
Pulmonary haemorrhage
Paraquat poisoning
Pulmonary emphysema
Lung lobe torsion
(Pulmonary thrombosis)

Investigation of dyspnoeas

Changes in the character of respirations often do not become obvious to a client until respiratory disease is widespread and well advanced, for there is considerable functional reserve capacity in a normal dog, and if the disease is insidious in onset, the dog may adapt its behaviour to compensate by becoming less active. For this reason, the history is not always very revealing. However, road accidents (causing intra-pulmonary haemorrhage, ruptured diaphragm, pneumothorax or haemothorax), access to poisons (paraquat, warfarin), old age (neoplasia?) and progression (pleural effusion) may each indicate a cause.

Observations
During physical examination the dog should be handled with care as struggling can cause sudden death. The character of respirations should be noted:

1 Tachypnoea (an increase in respiratory rate), often shallow in character, occurs in restrictive pulmonary disease (where the elastic recoil is reduced), in disorders where there is loss of thoracic capacity for pulmonary expansion or in the presence of interstitial or alveolar disease. Tachypnoea can also be physiological, in which case breathing is usually open-mouthed.

2 Dyspnoea—a disturbance in respiration (laboured, difficult, painful)—is most marked with airway obstructions, when cyanosis and respiratory noise may be evident:

(a) Stridor (inspiration noise) indicates an upper airway obstruction.

(b) 'Asthmatic' wheeze at the end of expiration indicates lower airway obstruction.

(c) Orthopnoea (sternal recumbency, elbows abducted) suggests pleural effusion and/or cardiac failure.

Clinical findings

The mucous membranes may be normal, cyanosed (indicating airway obstruction or failure of gaseous exchange) or pale (in the presence of intrapulmonary or intrathoracic haemorrhage, or pyothorax). Percussion can be helpful: increased resonance can be detected in pneumothorax, decreased resonance may be appreciated in the presence of widespread pulmonary consolidation or neoplasia, and a distinct line may be identified between the ventral dullness and increased dorsal resonance in the presence of pleural effusions. Pulmonary râles are audible with auscultation in the presence of pulmonary oedema or bronchopneumonia. Cardiac sounds are muffled by pleural effusions and may be displaced by intrapleural masses. Cardiac murmurs, tachycardia and dysrhythmias may be associated with cardiac failure when it causes pulmonary oedema.

Investigation

Routine haematology may reveal marked leucocytosis following bronchopneumonia and exudative pleurisy, or anaemia resulting from intrapulmonary or intrathoracic haemorrhage. The level of plasma urea usually rises rapidly following paraquat poisoning. The results of biochemical tests are otherwise usually unrewarding. Pleural effusions should be examined cytologically, biochemically and bacteriologically.

Radiology is of great importance in the diagnosis of respiratory distress. The presence of pleural effusions or masses, rupture of the diaphragm and traumatic injury to ribs can be detected. Radiographic examination is essential for confirmation of the presence of generalised alveolar disease or metastatic pulmonary infiltration and it is an important aid to the diagnosis of cardiac enlargement. Radiography is almost the sole means of detecting mediastinal disorders. In many circumstances, it is difficult to obtain clear radiographs in the presence of pleural effusions or respiratory distress. The ideal of obtaining inspiratory films for clear contrast is not always readily achieved, and penetration with high kilovoltage levels and short exposures is essential.

Paracentesis of the thorax is an essential procedure in the presence of an effusion, to relieve dyspnoea and to establish a diagnosis, by analysis of the fluid and by repeating radiography. Biopsy of pulmonary lesions may be the sole means of confirming a diagnosis indicated by radiography. Biopsy can be achieved at thoracotomy, when the removal of a solitary mass may be considered or by transthoracic needle puncture. Using a Menghini or Trucut (Travenol) biopsy needle, large or widespread lesions can be sampled. Biopsy samples should be preserved in formol saline for histopathological examination. Respiratory function tests are not fully developed for use in dogs. In man, considerable reliance is placed on the patient's cooperation for these tests, which provide valuable diagnostic information.

MANAGEMENT OF ACUTE RESPIRATORY DISTRESS

It should be stressed that any dog with respiratory distress should be handled with great care as there may be very little reserve of respiratory capacity. Major details of history should be determined rapidly, including the possibility of trauma, access to poisons or electric shock, the rapidity of onset and the degree of deterioration. The general condition of the dog should be evaluated as quickly as possible—the level of consciousness, the colour of mucous membranes, the capillary refill time, the character of respirations and the rate, rhythm and character of cardiac sounds and pulse are of prime concern.

Rapid or deep chest movements do not necessarily mean that air is being passed or gases utilised. The respiratory failure may be ventilatory (airway obstruction) or hypoxic (gas transfer in lungs). Immediate therapeutic considerations may outweigh further diagnosis at this point. Priorities should include:

1 Establishment of a patent airway. If the dog is unconscious or severely incapacitated, immediate tracheal intubation may be indicated. If an upper airway problem exists, tracheotomy should be considered.

It is important to ensure that passage of air is taking place at the nose, mouth or tube. This may be assessed by listening closely, by the appearance of condensation on a mirror or by the movement of a fine piece of cotton wool. The removal of material blocking an airway is not readily achieved by aspiration in dogs without intubation or tracheotomy.

2 Administration of oxygen by mask, if handling does not distress the patient. Oxygen may be given through an endotracheal tube or tracheotomy tube, or by enrichment of the atmosphere in some form of oxygen tent, particularly if the dog is cyanosed or pale. This will not resolve problems associated with poor gaseous exchange, in which high carbon dioxide levels and respiratory acidosis occur.

3 As soon as steps have been taken to encourage gaseous exchange and oxygen supply, attention should be paid to circulatory function. If cardiac function appears to be normal, but there is evidence of shock or hypovolaemia, fluid (Ringer's lactate or saline with bicarbonate) should be administered intravenously. Bradycardia, heart block or poor blood pressure may be counteracted by the use of isoprenaline (Saventrine).

If cardiac function appears to be poor, and there is evidence of pulmonary oedema, diuretics and xanthine derivatives (aminophylline, etamphylline or theophylline) should be administered intravenously.

Sedation should be considered, as the distress of severe dyspnoea increases the respiratory requirement. Acetylpromazine or chlorpromazine may be used in the absence of circulatory failure. Opiates should be used only with caution owing to depression of the respiratory centre. When the dog's distress has been relieved sufficiently, further assessment should be carried out to make a diagnosis. Radiology is of particular importance and this should be undertaken before thoracentesis.

The perfect management of a patient with severe respiratory distress requires extensive facilities, including positive pressure ventilation, oxygen humidification, and the assessment of arterial and venous blood pressures, blood gases and acid–base levels, and cardiac function. In addition, intensive nursing and continuous observation are required. The full range of these facilities is rarely available in general practice, but the successful treatment of acute respiratory distress with routine equipment can be very satisfying.

REFERENCES

AMIS T.C. (1974) Tracheal collapse in the dog. *Aust. Vet J.* **50**, 285. (A clear, concise account of 15 cases).

BARBER D.L. & HILL B.L. (1976) Traumatically induced bullous lung lesions in the dog: a radiographic report of three cases. *J. Am. Vet. Med. Assoc.* **169**, 1085. (A report, review and discussion of aetiology and clinical findings with lung cysts and bullae).

BEMIS D.A. & APPEL M.J.G. (1977) Aerosol, parenteral and oral antibiotic treatment of *Bordetella bronchiseptica* infections in dogs. *J. Am. Vet. Med. Assoc.* **170**, 1082. (Experimental results demonstrating that oral or parenteral antibiotic treatment is ineffective for this infection).

BIRCHARD S.J., CANTWELL H.D. & BRIGHT R.M. (1982) Lymphangiography and ligation of the canine thoracic duct: A study in normal dogs and three dogs with chylothorax. *J. Am. Anim. Hosp. Assoc.* **18**, 769. (An excellent review of the aetiology of chylothorax with details of successful ligation of the thoracic duct in three cases).

BRODEY R.S. (1971) Hypertrophic osteoarthropathy in the dog: a clinicopathological survey of 60 cases. *J. Am. Vet. Med. Assoc.* **159**, 1242. (A definitive account of many cases of 'HPOA').

BRODEY R.S. & CRAIG P.H. (1965) Primary pulmonary neoplasms in the dog: a review of 29 cases. *J. Am. Vet. Med. Assoc.* **147**, 1628. (A detailed account of clinical and pathological findings).

CREIGHTON S.R. & WILKINS R.J. (1974) Transtracheal aspiration biopsy: technique and cytologic examination. *J. Am. Anim. Hosp. Assoc.* **10**, 219. (A simple technique for obtaining lower airway samples without requiring anaesthesia or visualisation).

DARKE P.G.G. (1976) Use of levamisole in the treatment of parasitic bronchitis in the dog. *Vet. Rec.* **99**, 293. (Successful treatment of filaroidiasis in eight dogs).

DARKE P.G.G., GIBBS C., KELLY D.F., MORGAN D.G., PEARSON H. & WEAVER B.M.Q. (1977). Acute respiratory distress in the dog associated with paraquat poisoning. *Vet. Rec.* **100**, 275. (Account of 10 cases, none of which survived).

DONE S.H. (1970) Some aspects of pathology of the lower respiratory tract of the dog: a review. *J. Small Anim. Pract.* **11**, 655. (A dated review of some pathological findings).

DONE S.H., CLAYTON JONES D.G. & PRICE E.K. (1970) Tracheal collapse in the dog: a review of the literature and report of two new cases. *J. Small Anim. Pract.* **11**, 743. (Described by the title).

ETTINGER S.J. (1983) *Textbook of Veterinary Internal Medicine* (2nd Edn) Section VIII: Diseases of the Respiratory System. W.B. Saunders, Philadelphia. (Very comprehensive text, covering the whole subject in depth).

GIBBS C. (1973) Radiological features of intrathoracic neoplasia in the dog and cat. In *The Veterinary Annual*, 14th Edn, eds. C.S.G. Grunsell & F.W.G. Hill. J. Wright, Bristol. (Concise illustrated account of the radiographic appearance of pulmonary and pleural neoplasms in dogs and cats).

HALL L.W. (1964) The accident case—V. The diagnosis of thoracic injuries. *J. Small Anim. Pract.* **5**, 35. (Short article on traumatic lesions; good radiographic illustrations).

HARVEY C.E. & O'BRIEN J.A. (1972) Management of respiratory emergencies in small animals. *Vet. Clin. N. Am.* **2** (2), 243. (A clear account of practical aspects of handling respiratory failure).

HOBSON H.P. (1976) Total ring prosthesis for surgical correction of collapsed trachea. *J. Am. Anim. Hosp. Assoc.* **12**, 822. (Description of surgery using plastic syringe cases to give partial relief of tracheal obstruction. The author reports 'success in 50–60 cases').

LORD P.F., GREINER T.P., GREENE R.W. & DE HOFF W.D. (1973) Lung lobe torsion in the dog. *J. Am. Anim. Hosp. Assoc.* **9**, 473. (A detailed account of 14 cases, with radiographs).

LORD P.F., SUTER P.F., CHAN K.F., APPLEFORD M. & ROOT C.R. (1972) Pleural, extrapleural and pulmonary lesions in small animals: a radiological approach to differential diagnosis. *J. Am. Vet. Rad. Soc.* **13**, (2), 4. (A description of the radiographic appearance of small pleural and pulmonary lesions, and experimentally-produced pleural effusion).

PERMAN V. & OSBORNE C. (1974) Laboratory evaluation of abnormal body fluids. *Vet. Clin. N. Am.* **4** (2), 255.

REIF J.S. (1969) Solitary pulmonary lesions in small animals. *J. Am. Vet. Med. Assoc.* **155**, 717. (Differential diagnosis of the radiographic finding of single pulmonary lesions).

RONDEBUSH P., GREEN R.A. & DIGILIO K.M. (1981) Percutaneous fine-needle aspiration biopsy of the lung in disseminated pulmonary disease. *J. Am. Anim. Hosp. Assoc.* **17**, 109. (A description of one technique for lung biopsy, the only method of confirming a diagnosis in diffuse lung disease or with solitary lesions).

RUBIN G.J., NEAL T.M. & BOJRAB M.J. (1973) Surgical reconstruction of collapsed tracheal rings. *J. Small Anim. Pract.* **14**, 607. (Clear radiographs are used to demonstrate this disorder and a technique for repair is described).

SUTER P.F., CARRIG C.B., O'BRIEN T.R. & KOLLER D. (1974) Radiographic recognition of primary and metastatic pulmonary neoplasms of dogs and cats. *J. Am. Vet. Rad. Soc.* **15** (2), 3. (A very thorough review of pulmonary neoplasia and its radiographic appearance).

SUTER P.F. & CHAN K.F. (1968) Disseminated pulmonary disease in small animals: a radiographic approach to diagnosis. *J. Am. Vet. Rad. Soc.* **9**, 67. (The radiographic appearance of diffuse alveolar, interstitial and bronchovascular pulmonary diseases is described in detail).

SUTER P.F. & LORD P.F. (1974) Radiographic differentiation of disseminated pulmonary parenchymal disease in dogs and cats. *Vet. Clin. N. Am.* **4** (4), 687. (A clear account of the differential diagnosis of this type of disease).

THORDAL-CHRISTENSEN A. & CLIFFORD D.H. (1953) Actinomycosis (nocardiosis) in a dog with a brief review of this disease. *Am. J. Vet. Res.* **14**, 298. (An old review of all types of nocardiosis, including pleural and pulmonary infections).

VENKER-VAN HAAGEN A.J. (1979) Bronchoscopy of the normal and abnormal canine. *J. Am. Anim. Hosp. Assoc.* **15**, 397. (A beautifully illustrated and diagrammed article giving full details of bronchoscopy).

WALKER R.G. (1959) Traumatic pneumothorax in small animals. *Vet. Rec.* **71**, 859. (Differential diagnosis and management are discussed in detail).

WALKER R.G. (1968) Pulmonary complications in suspected warfarin poisoning in the dog. *Vet. Rec.* **83**, 148. (A brief account of the diagnosis of the respiratory complications of this disease).

WALKER R.G. & HALL L.W. (1963) Rupture of the diaphragm: report of 32 cases in dogs and cats. *Vet. Rec.* **77**, 830. (A detailed report of clinical findings and surgical repair).

WHEELDON E.B., PIRIE H.M., FISHER E.W. & LEE R. (1974) Chronic bronchitis in the dog. *Vet. Rec.* **94**, 466. (Clinical and pathological details of a limited number of cases).

WILSON G.P., NEWTON C.D. & BURT J.K. (1973) A review of 116 diaphragmatic hernias in dogs and cats. *J. Am. Vet. Med. Assoc.* **159**, 1142. (A fairly brief review of findings in a large number of cases, including the results of surgical treatment).

3

Ear, Nose, Throat and Mouth

P. G. C. BEDFORD

DISEASES OF THE EAR

Inflammatory disease of the ear is one of the most common conditions encountered in canine practice, to which the vast selection of remedial products currently available to the practitioner bears witness. However, despite the therapeutic barrage possible, it can still prove difficult to treat ear disease effectively. As with other disease problems only the identification of cause amongst the various manifestations of pathological response will offer the best chance of cure. Treatment applied along symptomatic lines only can be of no permanent value, and may indeed allow an acute reversible condition to slide into one of irreversible chronicity. Superficial disease of the ear is usually heralded quite simply by otorrhoea and discomfort, but the associated aetiology is complex and an awareness of this complexity together with the differential diagnoses is therefore essential in producing the cure. Thus, the use of anti-inflammatory drugs may lead to a temporary improvement, but as long as the cause remains unidentified and untreated, the disease will recur once this therapeutic restraint has been removed. Similarly, the indiscriminate use of antibiotic preparations that are of no specific value in terms of cause can predispose the disease site to the added complication of fungal infection, and the use of inflammatory acaricidal preparations in the absence of ear mites is nothing less than bad medicine. Shotgun therapy is no substitute for the identification of cause and the application of specific therapy. In theory, at least, effective treatment should not be difficult for the various causes of disease are well known, and a specific approach for each cause exists. The problem lies in diagnosis, either due to an absence of specificity through lack of effort which, to some extent, may have been conditioned by the range of remedial products available, or due to the fact that at the time of examination the cause may be masked by secondary complications. Thus the initiatory grass seed may be hidden by the presence of a copious discharge, and the

presence of that discharge, together with the multiplying bacterial and fungal residents of the normal ear, will be contributory to the total pathogenic response.

Aetiopathogenesis of ear disease

The ear has three distinct yet intimately connected anatomical regions: the external ear (auris externa) which consists of the pinna and the external auditory canal; the middle ear (auris media) which consists of the tympanic membrane and a large tympanic cavity containing the three auditory ossicles; and the internal ear (auris interna) which consists of the spiral cochlea and the semi-circular canals. The external and middle ears function in the collection and transmission of sound, whilst the internal ear is associated with the functions of hearing and balance. Traditionally, a separate disease entity is ascribed to each region, namely otitis externa, otitis media and otitis interna. Otitis externa is by far the most common disease of these three, and indeed otitis media and interna usually occur as extensions of chronic external ear disease. The presenting clinical features of otitis externa and media are the same, namely otorrhoea and the various manifestations of aural discomfort, and indeed in long-standing otitis externa, rupture of the tympanic membrane and involvement of the middle ear practically always occur. It is only in an otitis interna that a loss of balance and possible deafness are observed clinically.

Otitis externa

The possible factors that are involved in the initiation of otitis externa are several. They range from problems inherent to the structure of the ear itself to concomitant skin disease, but irrespective of the cause the ensuing pathological process is the same (Fig. 3.1). Inflammation of the integument is seen as hyperaemia

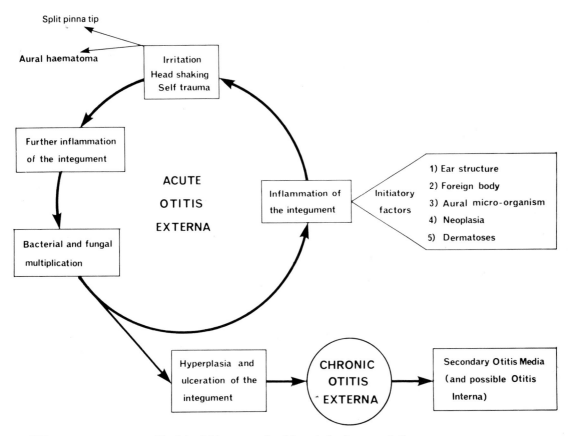

Fig. 3.1 Otitis externa: the vicious circle of cause and effect.

and oedematous swelling, and head shaking and self trauma further exacerbate this response. The ceruminous discharge which is constantly present increases in those ears in which there is subsequent bacterial and/or fungal involvement. If the disease process remains unrelieved, the resultant vicious circle of inflammation and tissue change ultimately produces an irreversible chronic state which is invariably further complicated by an otitis media.

The structure of the ear is perhaps the most important factor to be considered in the initiation of inflammation within the external auditory canal. The lining integument of the canal contains a large number of alveolar glands and it continuously produces ear wax, a sticky mixture of sebaceous material and cerumen which coats the integument as a protective barrier. A build-up of wax leads to inflammation within the integument, but normally the wax production is balanced by its continuous loss from the ear. The evaporation of moisture from the wax is an essential feature in this vital process, and adequate ventilation

of the external auditory canal is necessary to allow the drying out to occur. The hanging flap type of pinna of the Cocker Spaniel or the Basset Hound not surprisingly denies adequate ventilation of the canal, and as such contributes to the accumulation of ear wax and tissue debris. Similarly, the narrow lumen of the canal in the Miniature Poodle with its tight rugal folds retains ear wax most readily, and there are those breeds like the German Shepherd Dog and the Dachshund in which the benefit of an adequate canal lumen is offset by excessive normal wax production. Some hair is normally present in the external auditory canal in most breeds, but an excessive quantity directly contributes to the build-up of ear wax and prevents adequate drainage and ventilation. Ear conformation apparently plays another part in the aetiology of otitis externa in that different microorganisms appear to be associated with these structural variations. Thus the Miniature Poodle appears to be predisposed to either pure fungal infection or mixed fungal and Gram-positive bacterial infections, whilst in those breeds with the pendulous pinna it is the Gram-negative bacteria that most commonly occur in otitis externa (Pugh *et al* 1974).

Although the ear mite *Otodectes cynotis* is undoubtedly the most common cause of otitis externa in the cat, it is of less overall significance in the dog (Frazer 1965; Pugh *et al* 1974). The clinical picture of otocariasis varies between the two species in that it tends to be only in the kitten that severe signs of disease are seen, whilst the adult cat appears to tolerate even a heavy infestation extremely well. Indeed many treated feline patients seem to be resistant to reinfestation (Joshua 1965). However, in a dog of any age the presence of the mite is always attended by an acute reaction characterised by much head shaking, traumatic ear scratching and an initially dry discharge.

It should be remembered that the integumental lining of the external auditory canal is an extension of the body skin and that the only practical difference is the added presence of the ceruminous tubular glands deep in the connective tissue. As such, otitis externa can be an extension of concomitant skin disease or allergy (Frazer 1965; Pugh *et al* 1974). Foreign body irritation of the integument is an important cause of otitis externa, and the ubiquitous grass seed should be identified and removed at the primary consultation. The involvement of soap, pet ear preparations and even water as potential causes of disease will be revealed by good history taking. Neoplastic growth involving the external ear is relatively uncommon in the dog, but its presence can be a source of irritation, and inflammation of the integument can occur as the result of inadequate canal drainage and ventilation. Inflammatory polyps and tubular gland adenomas, which may be identified by a blue bubble appearance, can fill the external auditory canal, while mast cell tumours and squamous cell carcinomas can involve both the pinna and the canal. Rarely, the tympanic bulla may be involved in adnexal tumour formation.

It may be that the several bacteria and fungal organisms which are involved in otitis externa can act in an initiatory capacity, but as all these organisms with the exception of the Gram-negative bacteria exist as commensals in the normal ear, it is far more likely that it is as secondary agents they exert their pathogenic effect (Frazer *et al* 1970). There is no doubt that the bacteria and fungi do multiply in the presence of the inflammation (Marshall *et al* 1974). Staphylococci appear to be the commonest bacteria in both the normal and the diseased canine ear, but in disease they are seldom found in pure culture. Staphylococcal and streptococcal bacteria appear early in the disease process. The Gram-negative bacteria *Pseudomonas* spp., *E. coli* and *Proteus* spp. exert their pathogenic effect

as secondary contaminants introduced as the result of self trauma. They are involved in the most severe and long-standing cases of otitis externa, and *Pseudomonas aeruginosa* is commonly involved in otitis media. Of the fungal organisms that can be isolated from the canine ear, the yeast *Pityrosporum canis* is perhaps the most significant. It is often present in the normal ear, and in disease it is usually the commonest microorganism isolated. Again, it is most unlikely that it acts as an initiator of disease, but it is likely that its multiplication in an inflammatory environment contributes to the overall inflammatory response. It is commonly isolated in association with staphylococcal organisms, but it can be found in pure culture and in this respect it is likely that long-term antibiotic therapy may contribute to its dominance.

Otitis media

Disease of the middle ear occurs more commonly in dogs than may at first be realised, and in any long-standing otorrhoea its involvement should always be suspected, if not assumed. The clinical signs of otitis media are precisely the same as those of external ear disease, namely constant discharge and discomfort, but in addition involvement of the temperomandibular joint is a remote but possible complication.

Although an ascending otitis media via the Eustachian tube is possible (Lane 1976), most middle ear disease occurs as the predictable extension of external ear disease in which the barrier of the tympanic membrane has perforated. The tympanic membrane or myringa is a thin composite structure of epithelium and connective tissue which is subject to the same inflammatory and ulcerative processes as the integument lining the external auditory canal. The majority of perforations occur in the central area of the pars tensa, and subsequent healing is only possible in the absence of infection: in most long-standing cases of otitis media, myringal remnants are hard to detect and any post-cure closure is by granulation tissue. Once the myringa has perforated, the disease process spreads medially to involve the mucoperiosteal lining of the tympanum, and eventually the whole of the tympanic bulla becomes filled with pus. Some organisation may occur within the tympanum, and destruction of bone or new bone formation will proceed in the wall of the bulla.

Otitis interna

Disease of the inner ear or labyrinthitis is uncommon in the dog, and when it does occur it is usually as the extension of an otitis media. Therefore, clinical signs of middle and outer ear disease are apparent, together with abnormalities in posture and movement.

Deafness may occur through an involvement of the organ of Corti, or may be simply associated with occlusion of the external auditory canal and changes within the tympanic bulla in long-standing disease. However, acquired deafness is uncommon in the dog. (Congenital deafness can be associated with albinism in animals, and a congenital degeneration of the organ of Corti in which the tectorial membrane is displaced, distorted or replaced by a coagulum, the cochlear nerve and the spiral ganglion cells are degenerated and the scala media may be collapsed, occurs in Collies, Dalmations, Cocker Spaniels and Bull Terriers.)

Diagnosis

Otitis externa

The presenting clinical signs of otitis externa are otorrhoea, irritation as witnessed by head shaking and ear rubbing or scratching, and discomfort or pain. Violent flapping of the pinna can result in the splitting of its tip and haematoma formation. Facial wounding or traumatic dermatitis below the level of the tragus may be present as the result of self trauma. The patient may tilt its head towards the affected side, and if the ear is extremely painful, depression and possible inappetence will have been noticed by the owner. In this context a complete anamnesis is of value in investigating the initiating cause, and a complete physical examination will reveal the possibility of concomitant skin disease. The submandibular lymph nodes may be enlarged. Diagnosis of the initiating cause demands a thorough examination of the ear, and although time and numbers must always dictate the length of the possible diagnostic procedure to some extent, it is true to say that in some patients satisfactory diagnosis will only take a few minutes, and, in others, examination under general anaesthesia will be essential. A common approach is to apply therapy symptomatically for a week as a screening procedure, and to pick up the unimproved condition for further investigation at the time of the second consultation. Despite the pressures of practice, this cannot be regarded as the ideal, and every effort should be made to isolate the cause at the primary examination. The diagnostic procedure involves the following considerations:

1 The anamnesis
2 The clinical signs
3 A complete physical examination
4 The examination of the ear which may involve cleaning of the canal, and anaesthetic restraint:
(a) The appearance of the integument
(b) The discharge: colour: microbiological examination
(c) Auriscopic examination
(d) Examination of the myringa
(e) Radiography of the middle ear

The integument will be hyperaemic and possibly oedematous in the acute condition, but hypertrophied or hyperplastic with stenosis or occlusion of the external auditory canal in the chronic state. The colour of the discharge may be a guide to the type of microorganism which can be present. Pure *Pityrosporum canis* and mixed *P. canis*/staphylococcal infections may be indicated by a dark brown to black discharge, predominantly staphylococcal or streptococcal infections may be indicated by a dark yellow to light brown discharge, whilst the Gram-negative bacteria may be characterised by a pale yellow discharge (Frazer *et al* 1961, 1970; Pugh *et al* 1974). Of course, specific identification of the type of microorganism present requires swab-taking for subsequent laboratory diagnosis. Swabs must be carefully procured: they must be taken before any cleansing procedure, and the skin and surrounding hair must not be touched. But even assuming that the swabs are carefully taken and transported quickly to the laboratory, the final report may be difficult to interpret. The relative importance of the microorganisms isolated can be very difficult to decide unless the bacteriological examination is at least semi-quantitative and a suitable range of microorganisms is looked for. Specific antibiotic therapy may then be used.

A complete examination of the external auditory canal requires the use of the auriscope. The ear mite is pinhead-sized, and appears white in the light of the auriscope, It is negatively phototropic, and its rapid escape movements are readily discernible. Mites exist in dry ears only, and will vacate a canal in which the discharge is wet. In a number of cases the external auditory canal will require cleansing, and, possibly, the use of general anaesthesia in the recalcitrant patient with a painful ear will be necessary. Foreign body identification and extraction, and the diagnosis of integumental ulceration, invariably necessitate anaesthesia, and it is an essential procedure for examination of the myringa. The length and shape of the external auditory canal with its bend at the division of the horizontal and vertical portions necessitate the use of a long aural speculum. This examination is uncomfortable even in the normal ear. Adequate cleansing of the horizonatal part of the canal is difficult unless a Spreull needle is employed. Gentle lavage with a 0.5% cetrimide solution is advocated, but even so a diseased myringa can easily be perforated if care is not taken.

Cetrimide is perhaps the least ototoxic antiseptic agent thus utilised, and in the event of accidental myringotomy, provided that infected debris is not flushed into the middle ear and a normal saline wash is used to counter the irritant effect of the cetrimide, subsequent otitis media rarely occurs and the myringal puncture wound will heal rapidly. Once the distal external auditory canal has been adequately cleaned, the normal myringa will be seen as a whitish sheet of tissue, sloping away from the speculum ventrally. Perforations usually occur in the central area, but in long-standing cases, identification of the myringa can be difficult and remnant tissue only may be present. In many patients, the lumen width of the canal will not permit sight of the myringa, and in these cases palpation of the structure using the Spreull needle or a blunt probe is a useful procedure (Fig. 3.2). The probe can be balanced

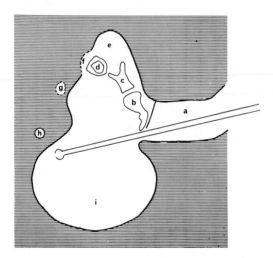

Fig. 3.2 The tympanic bulla, demonstrating the use of the Spreull needle in both diagnosis and bulla lavage; (a) external auditory canal; (b) malleus; (c) incus; (d) stapes; together (b), (c) and (d) make up the ear ossicles. (e) Epitympanic recess; (f) foramen ovale; (g) foramen rotundum; (h) Eustachian tube; (i) tympanic bulla (hypotympanicum).

on the intact structure, but it will pass through a perforation to rest on the medial wall of the tympanum. Tapping the probe against the bony wall of the bulla confirms its position. Where perforation has occurred an otitis media will be present, and radiography of the bulla can be helpful in the prognosis.

Otitis media

The presenting clinical signs of otitis media are the same as those of external ear disease. The anamnesis will usually reveal a long duration otorrhoea, and

indeed there will have been no remission of discharge even following drainage surgery to the external auditory canal. There is persistent, relatively gentle head shaking, and the affected ear may be tilted downwards. The patient may be lethargic, rarely febrile, but occasionally inappetent and there may be obvious pain on palpation of the ear. The diagnostic procedure involves the following considerations:

1 The anamnesis
2 The clinical signs
3 A complete physical examination
4 The examination of the ear under a general anaesthetic:
(a) the external ear
(b) microbiological examination
(c) examination of the myringa
(d) the patency of the Eustachian tube
5 Radiography of the middle ear
6 Exploratory surgery of the bulla

The patient should be examined under a general anaesthetic and the myringa either inspected visually or palpated using a blunt probe (Fig. 3.2). The probe should be directed ventrally to avoid damage to the round and oval foramina in the event of a perforation being present. In the majority of cases, the myringa will be perforated or unidentifiable, but in an early ascending otitis media it will be intact and will distend laterally into the lumen of the distal external auditory canal. In the occasional patient visualisation and palpation of the myringa may be impossible due to stenosis and distortion of the canal and here radiography of the canal using a contrast material (Lipiodol) can be useful. Approximately 4 ml are instilled into the previously cleaned canal with the dog in lateral recumbency, and in the event of myringal perforation the contrast material will enter the tympanum after a few minutes. However, this technique is not entirely reliable, for the presence of any exudate or granulation tissue in the distal canal area will impede medial movement of the contrast material. The patency of the Eustachian tube may be tested quite simply, but initially and usually, it requires adequate washing out of the tympanum. With a cuffed endotracheal tube in place, saline solution containing a fluorescein marker is introduced into the tympanum via a Spreull needle. The saline will drain into the nasopharynx if the Eustachian tube is patent, and it may be seen at the contralateral nostril. Contrast material can also be used to demonstrate the patency of the Eustachian tube radiographically. Similarly, air can be gently pumped into the middle ear using an insufflator, and a whistling noise in the nasopharynx may

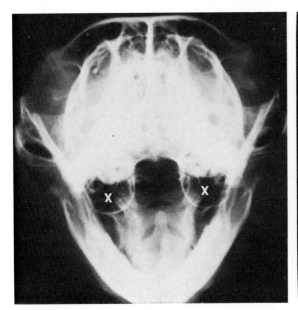

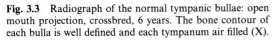

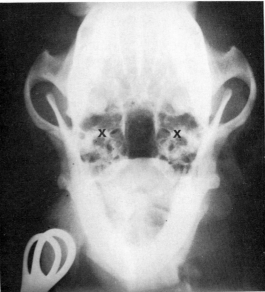

Fig. 3.3 Radiograph of the normal tympanic bullae: open mouth projection, crossbred, 6 years. The bone contour of each bulla is well defined and each tympanum air filled (X).

Fig. 3.4 Radiograph of diseased tympanic bullae in otitis media: open mouth projection, Poodle, 8 years. Bilateral bone change is present within each bulla (X).

be heard if the Eustachian tube is patent. Radiography of the tympanic bulla is of value in an assessment of otitis media (Figs. 3.3, 3.4). Lateral and open mouth views are particularly valuable in demonstrating changes in and around the bulla. Both destructive and proliferative changes in the wall of the bulla can be visualised, whilst granulation tissue and discharge material will obscure the air space. On occasion surgical exploration of the bulla can further the diagnosis in terms of foreign body material and neoplasia.

Microbiological examination of the discharge represents a most vital step in the diagnostic and subsequent therapeutic measures. Staphylococci, streptococci, *Clostridium welchii* and *P. canis* may all be isolated with regularity, but it is the common presence of *Pseudomonas* spp. that represents the most difficult aspect of the medical treatment of otitis media.

Otitis interna

Inflammatory disease of the inner ear is demonstrated by obvious neurological signs in addition to the clinical signs of otitis media. Nystagmus may be seen, extreme lateral flexion of the cervical and thoracic spine may occur, and the patient usually circles or falls to the affected side when attempting to walk. Further diagnostic criteria are not necessary and not usually sought after. However, the caloric test of vestibular function is worthy of brief mention. Caloric stimula-

tion of the endolymph within the vestibular apparatus is easily achieved by irrigating the external auditory canal with hot or cold water. Warm water stimulation of the endolymph results in nystagmus with a beat to the same side, whereas with cold water stimulation the nystagmus beat is to the opposite side. If the vestibular apparatus is non-functional then nystagmus does not occur.

Deafness, when present, is a readily noticeable diagnostic feature.

Treatment

The success of therapy employed in the treatment of canine ear disease depends in the first instance on the identification and correction of the initiating cause and thus the prevention of the complications related to secondary tissue change. The complex aetiological picture may render the application of specific therapy difficult, and the progression of an acute condition into one of chronicity is the result of incomplete diagnosis and inadequate therapy.

Otitis externa

Medical therapy is inappropriate should the cause of disease be the inadequate ventilation and drainage of the external auditory canal. Resection of the lateral wall of the canal should be completed before associated secondary tissue changes further complicate the disease process. Foreign body material and excess hair should be removed, and otocariasis treated by using a suitable acaricide such as benzyl benzoate. Such agents are effective only against the adult parasite and therapy should make allowance for the 3-week life cycle involved. It should always be remembered that the cat acts as a reservoir of infestation for the dog. Secondary and contaminant infection requires the use of specific antibiotic and antifungal therapy based on a laboratory diagnosis, and there is always a place for the use of topical, and in some instances systemic, corticosteroid therapy to control inflammation and oedema. Adequate cleansing of the ear can be a necessary adjunct to diagnosis and the effectiveness of subsequent therapy. Wax and debris accumulation will potentiate the disease process, and its physical presence will impede the activity of local therapeutic agents. Ceruminolytics are most helpful in this respect, for overzealous cleansing of the ear can be harmful. Local anaesthetic preparations may be used if pain is present; their usage, however, should not be simply a symptomatic one but only in the presence of a specific diagnosis.

The use of medical therapy in chronic ear disease can have no permanent therapeutic value. Adequate ventilation and drainage of the external auditory canal is impaired or destroyed by hyperplastic tissue changes, and recurrence will always be the order of the day. The surgery of lateral canal wall resection, or partial or complete ablation of the canal will be required if cure is to be effected. Verrucose overgrowth of the integument lining the pinna may occur in chronic otitis externa, and it represents a constant source of irritation and discomfort. Corticosteroid applications can offer no permanent relief, and treatment is by the removal of the swellings using electrocautery.

Otitis media

Attention must be paid to the concurrent external ear disease, and in many instances corrective external auditory canal surgery will have been attempted. Complete ablation of the canal in the presence of an otitis media will result in a chronic fistulisation of the operation site. Often it is only when canal surgery has been attempted to control the otorrhoea that the tympanic bulla is suspected of being involved in the production of discharge. Most cases of otitis media do respond to the relatively simple techniques of bulla irrigation, and as an adjunct to this medical approach resection of the lateral wall of the canal should be completed initially. This exposes the horizontal canal, facilitating access

to the middle ear for the subsequent lavage procedure whilst allowing ventilation and drainage to take place. Myringotomy is necessary in the presence of an ascending otitis media, and a blunt probe is used for the perforation, being pushed through the ventral half of the myringa. The tympanic bulla is irrigated via a Spreull needle under general anaesthesia every third day using a 0.5% cetrimide solution, or sterile normal saline, until the washings are clear of debris. Bleeding may occur during this process, but it is of no concern. Cetrimide is used for its excellent cleansing activity, but it should be subsequently washed out of the bulla using sterile normal saline, for not only will its retained presence act as a tissue irritant, but the possible ototoxic effect and the added disadvantage that *Pseudomonas* will actually flourish in its presence must both be considered. The tympanum is then finally drained using suction and infused with a mixture of the indicated antibiotic, usually polymyxin B, and a corticosteroid. The technique is repeated a maximum of five times, after which refractory cases should be considered for bulla osteotomy. Systemic broad-spectrum antibiotic and corticosteroid therapy is pursued throughout the course of treatment.

Otitis interna

Irrigation of the middle ear and bulla osteotomy can be of real value in the treatment of otitis interna. However, when there are marked tissue changes in the bulla, such as the filling of the tympanum with granulation or osseous tissue, treatment will require a vestibular osteotomy. Parenterally administered corticosteroids and broad-spectrum antibiotics should accompany the irrigation procedure and any surgical technique. The recovery time is long, and although complete balance can be restored, the head tilt may persist permanently.

DISEASES OF THE NOSE

The structure and function of the nasal cavity are such that air drawn in at the nostrils is warmed, filtered free of particulate matter and bacteria, and moistened almost to saturation point en route to the lungs. The nasal cavity is simply a bony shell which is divided longitudinally in the midline by a bone and cartilaginous septum into two separate chambers. The size and disposition of the nasal chamber varies considerably between the brachycephalic and dolichocephalic breeds. Each chamber is functionally subdivided into a series of air-conducting passages by the intricate structural, almost meshwork, arrangement of the turbinate bones (Fig. 3.5). Thus, a current of inspired air

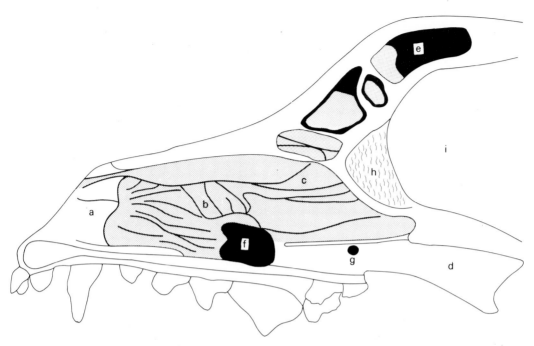

Fig. 3.5 The right nasal chamber and the paranasal sinuses; (a) rhinarium and external naris; (b) maxilloturbinate structure; (c) ethomoturbinate structure; (d) choana (internal naris); (e) frontal sinus; (f) maxillary sinus; (g) sphenoidal sinus; (h) cribriform plate; (i) cranial cavity.

is effectively broken up and warmed, whilst its filtration and humidification are accomplished by the ciliated mucus-secreting epithelium lining these passageways. The paranasal sinuses are atavistic extensions of the nasal cavity (Fig. 3.5). The sphenoidal sinus is of no clinical significance, whilst the maxillary sinus is simply a lateral diverticulum of the nasal chamber and is technically not a true sinus. The frontal sinus is separated from the nasal chamber and its anterior and posterior compartments drain into the ethmoturbinate structure. Olfactory function in the dog is highly developed, and it is within the deeper recesses of the ethmoturbinates that the olfactory neuroepithelium lies. Thus anorexia may be related to a loss of olfactory function when nasal disease is present, and the removal of nasal discharge in the inappetent patient constitutes sound nursing advice.

Nasal breathing is normal for the resting animal, but mouth breathing is necessary in a high environmental temperature and with physical activity. It also occurs where a disease process severely obstructs the normal nasal passage of air. Obstruction is related to either a disruption of the normal anatomy by chronic inflammatory change and neoplasia, or else it is the presence of copious discharge which is responsible. Sneezing and snorting are reflex actions to clear the airway, whilst gagging and coughing reflect the nasopharyngeal drainage of discharge in nasal disease.

Diagnosis

Anamnesis

The anamnesis usually relates either to the appearance of rhinorrhoea or the onset of dyspnoea manifested by sneezing, snorting, gagging or coughing and mouth breathing. Factors of age and incident related to the onset of the clinical signs, the duration of those signs, the degree of dyspnoea, the characteristics of the nasal discharge, facial deformity and possible pain are determined at this time. The initial response of the nasal mucosa to challenge in most cases is an increase in the amount of serous discharge produced, and this together with sporadic or persistent sneezing is the common feature in early nasal disease. In chronic disease, sneezing tends to occur less commonly, whilst the discharge produced is thicker, much more mucoid and, with infection and tissue breakdown, often purulent. Paroxysms of sneezing can result in epistaxis, and tissue breakdown may be indicated by blood-tinged discharge or rank haemorrhage (Fig. 3.6). Nasal discharge may not be noticed too readily if the

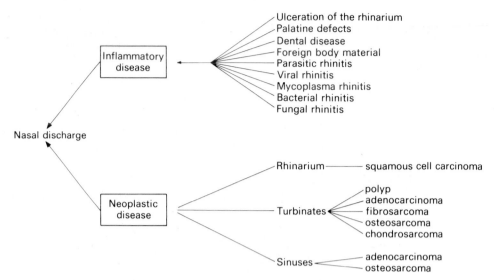

Fig. 3.6   The differential diagnosis of nasal discharge.

patient is a nostril licker, and noisy respiration can be related to soft palate, laryngeal and tracheal deformities, as well as nasal obstruction.

Clinical examination
A complete physical examination is routine, and it should include temperature, pulse, the pattern of respiration, an assessment of pulmonary function and any indication of systemic disease. Attention is paid to the oral cavity, the oropharynx and any facial deformity or palpable asymmetry related to the nasal cavity. Pain over the frontal, nasal or maxillary bones is significant, and a softness of tissue in these areas would denote advanced endonasal tumour. An epiphora can occur simply as the result of nasal irritation, but it also occurs with blockage of the nasolacrimal duct by invasive tumour. The external nares are checked for patency, movement during respiration, ulceration, tumour formation and the presence of nasal discharge. Rhinarial and nasal airway patency may both be simply assessed by holding a strand of cotton wool to each nostril in turn to demonstrate air movement. Sinus percussion is valueless. Nasal discharge material is taken for subsequent microbiological evaluation, and blood samples may be indicated for haematological and serological examinations.

Further examination of the patient requires general anaesthesia, and tracheal intubation is essential to prevent the possible inhalation of nasal discharge and facilitate irrigation of the nasal chambers. Examination of the oral cavity includes inspection of the teeth, inspection of the tonsils and oropharynx, and inspec-

tion and palpation of the hard and soft palates. The nasopharynx is examined by drawing the soft palate forward and then by using a warmed illuminated dental mirror. Anterior rhinoscopy in the small dog may prove impossible, but in most dogs the anterior nasal turbinates may be visualised using a long auriscope cone. A copious discharge can complicate the examination, but it is possible to locate and remove foreign body material using alligator forceps, occasionally identify neoplasms and even diagnose a rhinomycosis. Irrigation of the nasal chamber is achieved by packing off the nasopharynx and flushing warm water or saline into the nose via a length of lubricated polythene tubing (a dog catheter is suitable). The wash can dislodge foreign bodies and, by clearing the discharge, helps with differential diagnosis in the next part of the examination, radiography of the nasal cavity.

A complete radiographic examination is an essential part of the diagnostic procedure, and lateral, ventrodorsal, occlusal and frontal sinus projections are required. A lateral thoracic projection should be included as routine if endonasal neoplasia is suspected, even though metastasis would appear to be extremely rare. A lateral projection of the nasal cavity allows visualization of the superimposed nasal chambers and frontal sinuses (Fig. 3.7), a ventrodorsal open mouth projection demonstrated the nasal chambers and the posterior limits of the ethmoturbinate mass in particular (Fig. 3.8), the occlusal projection is for the nasal chambers only (Fig. 3.9), whilst the frontal sinus projection (anteroposterior) excludes the nasal chambers (Fig. 3.10). The practitioner will find that the occlusal

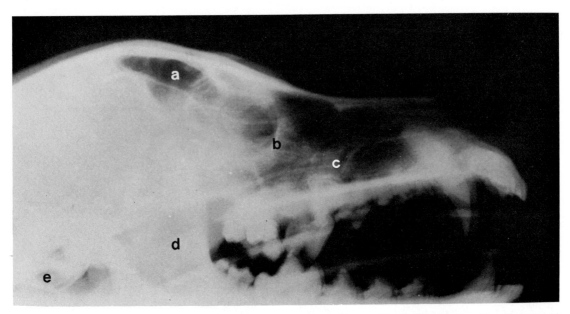

Fig. 3.7 Radiograph of the normal nasal cavity: lateral projection, crossbred, 6 years; (a) frontal sinuses; (b) ethmoturbinates; (c) maxilloturbinates; (d) soft palate; (e) tympanic bullae.

projection using non-screen film will usually prove the most valuable, clearly demonstrating the turbinate structures and usefully contrasting the diseased nasal chamber with the normal side in the patient with a unilateral discharge. Placing the film inside the oral cavity avoids the superimposition of the mandible over the nasal cavity, and allows the nasal chambers to be seen clearly and in entirety. The interpretation of nasal cavity radiographs relies upon the contrasts seen within the trabecular pattern of the ethmoturbinate mass and the appearance of the air spaces within the rest of the cavity. Nasal discharge and hypertrophic and neoplastic tissue changes obliterate air space, whilst increased areas of negative contrast are indicative of the tissue destruction that occurs with both neoplasia and in aspergillosis.

Exploratory rhinotomy

There are occasions when a specific diagnosis is not possible without surgical invasion of the nasal cavity. Radiographically early tumour formation without marked invasive and destructive changes can be difficult to differentiate from hyperplastic rhinitis, whilst the aetiology of a chronic rhinitis may remain obscure. Direct visualisation of the intranasal structures together with the removal of biopsy material necessitates rhinotomy. The nasopharynx is packed off and the nasal chamber thoroughly irrigated. The skin is opened to one side of the midline from the posterior

limit of the rhinarium to the posterior limit of the frontal sinuses, and as wide as possible length of nasal, maxillary and frontal bone removed to expose the nasal chamber and the anterior frontal sinus (Figs. 3.11, 3.12). The piece of bone is lifted so that the nasal septum remains intact, and the width of this bone flap should be sufficient to allow adequate examination of the intranasal structures and the manipulation of the biopsy instrument. Haemorrhage is heavy only if radical turbinectomy is attempted and then the nasal chamber should be packed off using ribbon bandage which is removed some 5 days after surgery. The wound is closed routinely using subcutaneous and skin sutures. A subcutaneous emphysema may occur over the site of the bone resection within 24 hours of surgery, but though spectacular it is of no serious or permanent consequence.

The nostrils

Stenosis of the nostrils

Distortion or collapse of the external nares occasionally occurs as the result of severe wounding or extensive ulceration with necrosis of the nasal cartilages. Congenital stenosis of the airway through the nostrils is a common anatomical defect in brachycephalic breeds. Here the defect may or may not contribute to the brachycephalic 'airway obstruction syndrome'

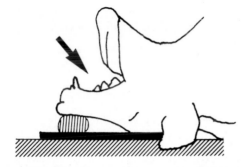
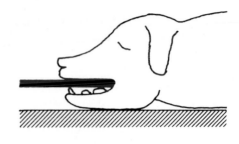

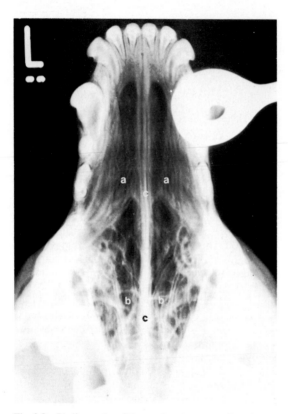
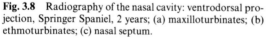

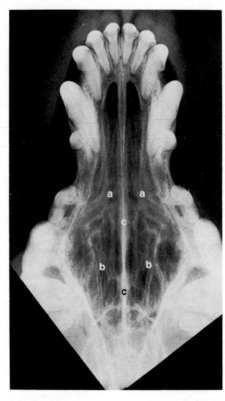

Fig. 3.8 Radiography of the nasal cavity: ventrodorsal projection, Springer Spaniel, 2 years; (a) maxilloturbinates; (b) ethmoturbinates; (c) nasal septum.

Fig. 3.9 Radiography of the nasal cavity: occlusal projection, crossbred, 6 years; (a) maxilloturbinates; (b) ethmoturbinates; (c) nasal septum.

which involves the entire nasal–pharyngeal–laryngeal region. The shortened upper jaw compresses the nasal chambers and the nasopharynx into a much shorter space than normal, and a resultant increased inspiratory effort can pull the pharyngeal wall, the laryngeal saccules and the arytenoid cartilages into the airway, to further interfere with air flow. The movement of an

overlong soft palate (overlong relative to that of the dolichocephalic) into the anterior laryngeal airway during inspiration is an additional and major cause of dyspnoea in the brachycephalic dog, and the result of so much anatomical distortion is the commonplace noisy snuffling type of respiration which may be associated with severe airway obstruction, particularly

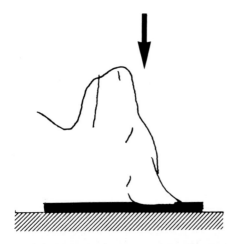

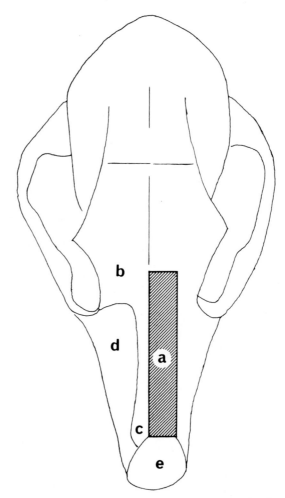

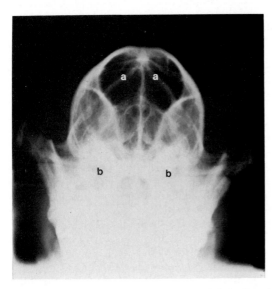

Fig. 3.10 Radiography of the frontal sinuses: Labrador, 4 years; (a) frontal sinuses; (b) tympanic bullae.

Fig. 3.11 The dorsal aspect of the skull, demonstrating the site of exploratory rhinotomy; (a) the site of rhinotomy; (b) the frontal bone; (c) the nasal bone; (d) the maxillary bone; (e) the rhinarium.

in later life. In addition and particularly in the Bulldog breed, glosso-epiglottic mucosal displacement and tracheal hypoplasia may be present to add to the overall problem (Bedford 1982, 1983).

Stenosis of the nares in the brachycephalic is due to an overbending of the wing of the dorsal parietal nasal cartilage, causing the rhinarial tissue on its medial aspect to be held against the philtrum. The subject is thus denied the facility of nasal inspiration, either completely or in part, and resorts to mouth breathing. The defect should be corrected as early as possible, and is easily and effectively treated either by wedge resection of the tissue around the medial aspect of the wing of the dorsal parietal cartilage, or else by excision

of an ellipse of tissue from the dorsolateral junction of skin and rhinarium. The wound is sutured to pull the nostril open.

Idiopathic ulceration (pemphigus vulgaris)
Ulceration of the external nares may be due to excoriation resulting from the persistent licking of nasal discharge, but an intractable ulcerative condition of autoimmune origin is seen occasionally, particularly in the German Shepherd Dog of any age. The condition is usually bilateral, resulting in crusting of the nostrils, chronic persistent sneezing, rhinorrhoea and even sporadic epistaxis. If untreated extensive erosion of the alar cartilages can occur, and this can lead to

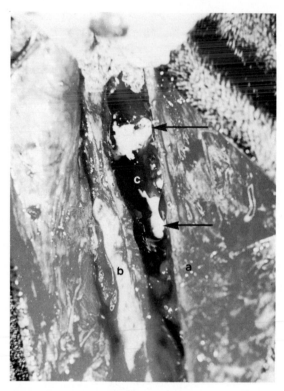

Fig. 3.12 Exploratory rhinotomy demonstrating the presence of *Aspergillus* colonies (arrows) on the ethmoturbinate structure. (a) Left nasal bone; (b) right maxilla; (c) rhinotomy exposing the ethmoturbinate structure.

distortion or even collapse of the nostrils. Secondary bacterial contamination may be present, and Gram-negative organisms are a common finding. Diagnosis rests upon the histopathological findings and the demonstration of auto-antibodies and complement by immunofluorescence. As with other manifestations of bullous autoimmune skin disease, treatment can be difficult. Cryotherapy and radiotherapy have proved useful where the involvement is extensive but high steroid doses (2–4 mg/kg bodyweight prednisolone) offers perhaps the most effective means of control. Ascorbic acid is a helpful adjunct to steroid therapy.

Foreign bodies and trauma
The lodgement of foreign body material within the nostril is unusual, the ubiquitous grass awn normally finding its way into the nasal chamber. Persistent sneezing and nasal discharge are the presenting clinical signs. Wounds of the nostril usually heal well, but stenosis of the airway can occur where the damage is extensive.

Neoplasia
Squamous cell carcinoma of the nostril is locally malignant, and surgical excision is followed by rapid recurrence of the neoplasm, usually within 2–3 months. However, excellent results have been achieved with radiotherapy, and the lesion is eminently suitable for cryosurgery.

The nasal cavity

Foreign body rhinitis
The presence of an endonasal foreign body represents an uncommon cause of rhinitis in the dog, but the diagnosis is always probable in the patient that presents with a sudden onset of violent and persistent sneezing. The grass awn is seasonal, and its presence is obviously related to a walk in the country or a romp in the garden. With time the violent sneezing and head shaking give way to a less outwardly distressing chronic nasal discharge. Secondary infection with both bacteria and fungal organisms is a feature of the chronic foreign body presence, and the resulting discharge will be purulent. Anterior rhinoscopy is easily accomplished under a general anaesthetic using a long wide-bore auriscope speculum, and the retrieval of foreign body material lodged in the anterior nasal cavity is often possible without resorting to major surgery. In the chronic case, swabs for microbiological examinations should always be taken for the established secondary infection will require specific therapy. Occasionally a needle may be chewed through the palatine bone (Fig. 3.13) or the soft palate, or, rarely, during swallowing, bone or a piece of wood may pass from the nasopharynx forward through the choanae to lodge in the posterior nasal chamber (Fig. 3.14). With foreign bodies lodged in the posterior nasal chamber discharge may be lost from the nostril, but the lesion will be one of a posterior rhinitis primarily and gagging and retching will be part of the presenting clinical picture.

Rhinitis related to dental disease
Periapical abscessation associated with severe periodontal disease, caries or dental fractures is rarely a cause of nasal discharge. Loss of the canine tooth, particularly in the Daschshund, may result in a low grade nasal discharge due to oronasal fistulation.

Rhinitis due to palatine defects
The presence of food material in the nasal cavity, which has gained entrance via a defect in either the hard or soft palate, will produce a rhinitis. A secondary bacterial involvement will result in a purulent

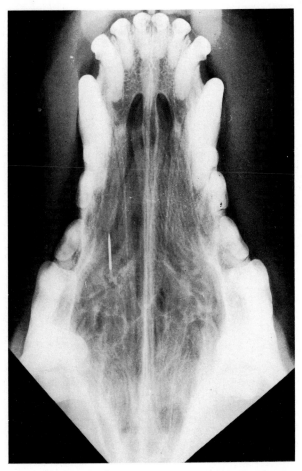

Fig. 3.13 Radiograph of the nasal cavity demonstrating the presence of a needle in the left nasal chamber. Occlusal projection, Springer Spaniel, 2 years.

nasal discharge. Congenital hypoplasia of the soft palate is primarily associated with a posterior rhinitis, and though most of the discharge is usually swallowed, sneezing and nasal discharge at the external nares are the presenting clinical signs. The simple procedure of feeding and drinking at head height can prove most effective in the presence of a minor lesion, but palatoplasty is essential where the defect is extensive. Rhinitis and nasal discharge also accompany congenital and traumatic defects of the hard palate: a small traumatic defect may close by granulation, but surgery involving bridging of the defect using mucoperiosteal flaps is necessary to close the larger traumatic and congenital defects. The indicated antibiotic and a corticosteroid are used to treat the rhinitis.

Parasitic rhinitis

Two intranasal parasites have been recorded in the dog. The nasal mite, *Pneumonyssus caninum* is seen in the United States, Australia and South Africa, whilst the occurrence of the pentastomic 'tongue worm', *Linguatula serrata*, in the UK is apparently extremely rare. Whereas the effects of nasal mite infestation are generally not serious, being confined to occasional mucous discharge, sneezing and head shaking, the presence of *L. serrata* usually results in a severe rhinitis in which sporadic coughing and sneezing occur, and an often blood-stained nasal discharge is seen. The host is often severely ill and a positive diagnosis, which depends upon the demonstration of eggs in the nasal discharge, is difficult. Exploratory rhinotomy often proves to be an essential diagnostic procedure, and as

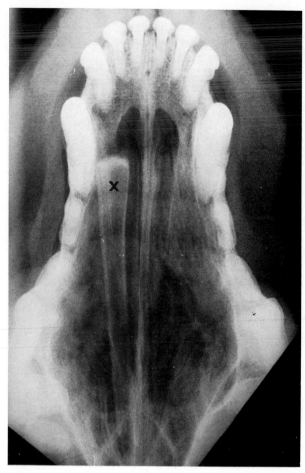

Fig. 3.14 Radiograph of the nasal cavity demonstrating the presence of a chicken bone (x) in the left nasal chamber. Occlusal projection, Cocker Spaniel, 5 years.

effective medical treatment is not possible, the parasite is physically removed at the time of surgery to effect the cure.

Viral rhinitis

Recent research into the aetiology of canine upper respiratory tract disease has demonstrated the important role of several viruses in the initiation of acute rhinitis (Wilkins & Helland 1973; Wright *et al* 1974) (see also Chapter 2). Canine adenovirus, specifically CAV Toronto A26/61, is considered to be a primary pathogen in laryngotracheitis, whilst herpesvirus is known to cause a range of infections in the dog, including neonatal disease, tracheobronchitis or 'kennel cough', vesicular lesions on the genitalia of both dogs and bitches, and encephalitis. A parainfluenza virus with antigenic properties similar to Simian SV5 virus

has also been incriminated as a primary cause of canine upper respiratory tract disease, and the severe rhinitis which occurs in canine distemper is well recognised. In many cases of viral rhinitis, the organism in fact is responsible only for a mild or subclinical infection; but it is this local challenge which predisposes the patient to secondary bacterial disease, which in turn exacerbates and prolongs the initial condition, often producing severe secondary complications. Thus, the logical step to control the infection is the initiation of bacteriological sensitivity tests and the specific use of the indicated antibiotic therapy. Uncontrolled infection produces irreversible hyperplastic changes within the nasal epithelium, and nasal discharge will thus persist as a function of mucus hypersecretion.

The occurrence of a specific rhinitis syndrome in the

Irish Wolfhound breed is attributed to primary herpesvirus infection with a secondary bacterial involvement (Wilkinson 1969). The disease is seen in very young dogs, most being affected at birth. Initially, there is a watery bilateral discharge, noisy respiration and episodic sneezing. The discharge becomes catarrhal, then purulent and it may be blood-tinged due to erosion of the nasal mucosa. There may be early spontaneous resolution, but with chronic hyperplastic change there is persistence of the nasal discharge, and a cough indicates pulmonary involvement. Severely affected patients are subject to growth retardation and recurrent periods of acute rhinitis. Specific medical therapy is not possible, and symptomatic treatment is of temporary value only. The prognosis is related to the extent of the pulmonary involvement, but marked improvement has been obtained following radical turbinectomy procedures. It has been suggested than a hereditary factor may be involved in the aetiology of the condition, and that dormant herpesvirus within the genital tract of the bitch is inhaled with uterine or vaginal fluids by the puppy during whelping. Several bacteria, particularly *Bordetella bronchiseptica* and *Pasteurella multocida*, are then involved as secondary pathogens.

Bacterial rhinitis

A number of bacteria and mycoplasmas may be isolated from nasal discharge material, but it is difficult to be certain of their precise role in rhinitis. Undoubtedly some organisms are of no significance, being merely present as contaminants, but others do exert a pathogenic effect, and specific antibiotic therapy is of value where this is so. It is possible that some bacteria may be responsible for actually initiating an acute rhinitis, and this is probably the case with *Bordetella bronchiseptica*, and possibly *Pasteurella multocida*. At one time *B. bronchiseptica* was considered to be the casual agent of canine distemper because of the frequency at which it was isolated from the respiratory tract of infected dogs. Subsequently it has been regarded as being a secondary invader following primary viral infection, but recent experimental work has shown that it will produce infectious respiratory disease in its own right (Thompson *et al* 1976). Other bacterial organisms require some predisposing lesion or challenge to create an environment in which they can multiply to exert their pathogenic effect as secondary invaders. Antibiotic therapy must be selected on the basis of sensitivity tests, and in acute rhinitis a cure may be effected. The use of broad-spectrum antibiotics without such sensitivity testing is likely to be less effective. The treatment of chronic rhinitis in which hyperplastic and hypertropic changes have led to the hypersecretion of mucus and distortion or occlusion of the turbinate airways (Fig. 3.15) requires a somewhat different approach. Bacterial isolation and specific antibiotic therapy may clear the infection, but dyspnoea, inadequate drainage and the recurrence of infection will only be prevented by radical turbinectomy. Routine cultural examinations should be maintained throughout a convalescent period of approximately 6 weeks following such surgery to prevent infection of the operation site.

Fungal rhinitis

Nasal mycosis is a relatively common condition particularly in the young patient, and the routine examination of nasal discharge material should always include fungal identification procedures. The importance of *Aspergillus fumigatus* cannot be stressed too much, for the rapid destruction of turbinate material can only be prevented by early diagnosis and specific therapy. It is of interest to speculate whether the organism is of primary aetiological significance, or whether it acts as a secondary pathogen following a previous challenge. Its spores are commonplace, and logically rhinomycosis should also be as ubiquitous if the organism is a primary pathogen. Primary fungal disease in man is recognised as the result of defective cell-mediated immunity, for example, mucocutaneous candidiasis due to a specific T-cell deficiency. It is possible that canine rhinomycosis occurs as the result of a similar defect. However, there is invariably an accompanying bacterial infection with aspergillosis, and it is therefore possible that the fungus is only of importance as a secondary pathogen. Indeed, it is even possible that Aspergillus may act in both ways and this would explain in part the variation in response that there is to medical therapy.

Aspergillosis is seen most commonly in the dolichocephalic animal under 4 years of age. The infection initially involves the caudal region of the ventral maxilloturbinates, and subsequently extends anteriorly. A copious unilateral or bilateral mucopurulent discharge is present, and it may be flecked with blood, indicating the aggressive nature of the infection. Occasionally there is epistaxis, and the patient may also exhibit pain and facial distortion; rarely is the animal systemically ill. Various diagnostic techniques may be employed: the organism may not always be present in material subjected to direct smear and cultural examination, and the skin sensitivity test has proved most unreliable. However, the serological double diffusion test is of value, apparently only reading positive in the presence of a clinical infection, and radiology can be of specific diagnostic value, for turbinate destruction without increased soft tissue shadow is seen as areas

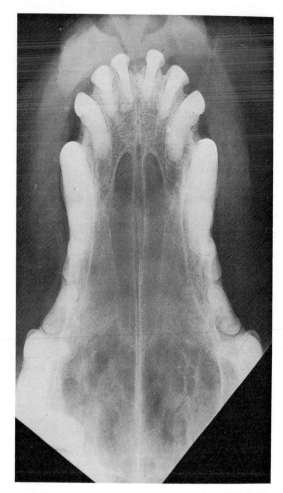

Fig. 3.15 Chronic rhinitis: Cocker Spaniel, 4 years. Occlusal view prior to irrigation.

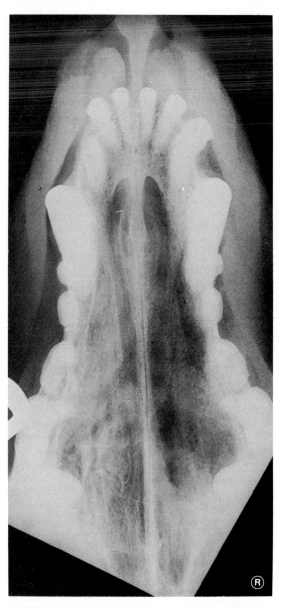

Fig. 3.16 Aspergillosis in right nasal chamber: German Shepherd Dog; 3 years.

of negative contrast on the occlusal films (Fig. 3.16). This appearance is pathognomonic for the disease. Diagnosis may depend upon exploratory rhinotomy when the aspergillus colonies may be identified on the turbinate mass by their whitish 'mould-like' appearance (see Fig. 3.12), or as the result of biopsy when histological examination demonstrates the branching septate hyphae of the fungus and the 'sunburst' appearance of its conidiophores (Fig. 3.17). When considering the differential diagnosis of nasal discharge in the dog it should be remembered that on occasion aspergillosis can accompany endonasal neoplasia. Initially therefore the serological and radiographical results may appear to be at odds with one another, but exploratory rhinotomy will confirm the findings.

The treatment of aspergillosis involves some discussion of the possible health hazard, and a guarded prognosis should always be given. In early disease or where little radiographic change is demonstrable, systemic and local antifungal therapy should be employed initially. The prolonged use of such drugs as nystatin, amphotericin B, thiabendazole and clotrinazole has been advocated but the failure of this

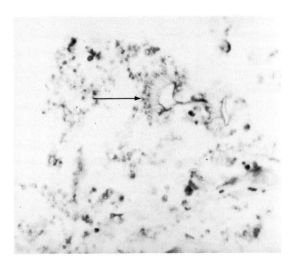

Fig. 3.17 *Aspergillus fumigatus* demonstrating the 'sunburst' appearance of the conidiophores (arrow).

medical therapy or the radiographic presence of considerable turbinate necrosis dictates that radical turbinectomy must be employed. Indeed, whilst a medical cure is possible, turbinectomy plus medical therapy is the most likely treatment to effect that cure. Postoperatively, Lugol's iodine (1%) is flushed through the nasal cavity and frontal sinus via an indwelling polythene tube for 5 days, and systemic thiabendazole is given at a dose rate of 20 mg/kg per day for up to 6 weeks. There is always nasal discharge following surgery, and routine bacteriological and fungal examinations maintained throughout the recovery period will dictate the use of any additional therapy.

Endonasal neoplasia
Endonasal malignant neoplasia is the most common cause of nasal discharge in the older dolichocephalic patient, and it should be remembered that such neoplasia is also an occasional finding in the young animal. The usual site of tumour development is the ethmoturbinate region (Fig. 3.18), and facial and palatine distortion are seen with tumours of long duration. Commonly, it is the adenocarcinoma, the fibrosarcoma, the osteosarcoma and the chondrosarcoma that occur, and the clinical picture is one of dyspnoea with unilateral, sometimes bilateral, mucopurulent discharge and bouts of heavy epistaxis and violent sneezing. Occlusion of the nasal cavity by the tumour mass can result in the swallowing of discharge, and erosion of the nasolacrimal duct will produce an 'ocular' discharge. Pain can accompany long-standing neoplasia, but metastasis appears to be extremely rare.

The prognosis is grave due to the ineffectiveness of cytotoxic therapy, the problems of radiotherapy and the rapid recurrence within 3–4 months of surgery.

The surgical management of turbinate neoplasia is therefore not advocated, but exploratory rhinotomy does have a part to play in the procedure of differential diagnosis. Occasionally benign fibrous polyps, which may enlarge to fill the nasal chamber, extend into the nasopharynx or protrude from the nostril. They are confirmed by their gross appearance and by histology. Their presence is occasionally accompanied by blood-staining of the associated discharge due to a pressure-induced destruction of the anterior ethmoturbinate tissues. They occur in chronic hyperplastic rhinitis and their removal relieves the associated dyspnoea. The prognosis is good, but they should be differentiated from an aggressive type of fibrous tissue neoplasm in which rapid recurrence follows excisional surgery. The radiographical differential diagnosis between early tumour and hyperplastic rhinitis can also be difficult and here exploratory rhinotomy can be of value. A positive radiographical diagnosis of tumour is only possible where there is obvious bone destruction, the loss of air shadow and, in the more advanced

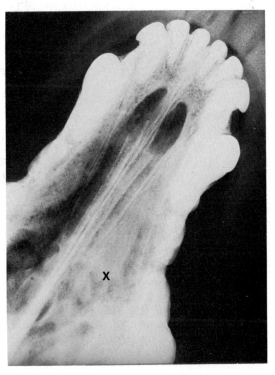

Fig. 3.18 Development of a tumour (x) in the ethmoturbinate region, Crossbred, 8 years.

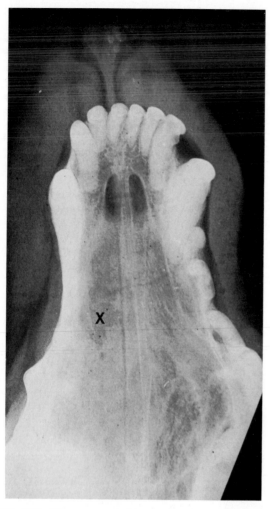

Fig. 3.19 The appearance of tumour invasion together with the concurrent bone destruction of the right maxilla (X), Labrador cross, 10 years.

case, the breakdown of the nasal septum and tumour invasion of the centrolateral turbinates (Fig. 3.19).

The paranasal sinuses

Primary conditions of the paranasal sinuses are of rare occurrence and disease involving these structures is usually an extension of that affecting adjacent tissues. The maxillary 'sinus' is a lateral outpouching of the nasal chamber at the level of the carnassial tooth and it is in free communication with the middle and ventral nasal meati. Congenital sinus cysts are extremely rare,

but this structure may be involved as a complication of carnassial tooth-root abscessation. However, the frontal sinus is a definitive structure, its size and disposition varying considerably between the breeds. It is a mucous membrane-lined compartment which communicates with the nasal chamber via a narrow drainage ostium between the ethmoturbinate scrolls. Primary sinus neoplasia is seen but more commonly tumour presence within the sinus is the result of an invasive turbinate-based growth. Although a 'sinusitis' as an extension of a rhinitis is a theoretical possibility, the condition which is often so described is, in fact, a retention mucocele due to impaired drainage through a blocked ostium and diseased turbinate mass. Turbinectomy restores drainage to the sinus, and it is this sinus discharge which presents as nasal discharge for a considerable time following surgery. Frontal sinus aspergillosis occurs commonly in rhinomycosis and the sinus must be opened at rhinotomy to facilitate inspection and debridement, and to allow the post-operative instillation of the iodine solution.

DISEASES OF THE MOUTH

The mouth has several parts to play: it functions in the prehension and mastication of foods, drinking, gustation, swallowing, digestion, heat exchange, grooming and respiration during exercise. It consists of the lips and the buccal cavity, the latter comprising the vestibule of the mouth and the oral cavity proper. The lips form a mobile external opening to the buccal cavity, and consist of skin, muscle, connective tissue and mucous membrane. The vestibule is the space between the teeth and the cheeks which communicates with the oral cavity proper by way of the interdental spaces. The parotid and zygomatic salivary ducts open into the posterior dorsal part of the vestibule via small raised papillae in the cheek at the level of the upper carnassial teeth. The oral cavity proper is formed by the hard and soft palates dorsally, the dental arcades and gums laterally and anteriorly, and the tongue and the sublingual mucosa ventrally; it opens into the oropharynx posteriorly. The hard palate is formed by the palatine processes of the palatine, maxillary and incisive bones on each side and its oral surface is thrown up into transverse ridges covered by stratfield squamous epithelium. The dog has 28 deciduous teeth, and its 42 tooth permanent dentition (3142/3143) is present at approximately 6-7 months of age. The molar teeth have no deciduous representation and the third molar is the last to erupt. The largest tooth is the upper fourth premolar, the carnassial tooth, and it is usually this one that is involved in facial sinus production. The gums, or gingivae, are composed of dense fibrous connective tissue which is covered by a highly vascularised mucosa. The tongue is composed of muscles which originate from the hyoid apparatus; it is a multipurpose organ which is utilised in the imbibition of fluids, the prehension and mastication of foodstuffs, swallowing, grooming and gustation. The submandibular and the multilobular sublingual salivary glands open anteriorly under its body at the base of the frenulum linguae on the sublingual caruncle, and the dorsum of the tongue posteriorly bears several papillae which house the taste buds and assist in grooming and feeding.

Diagnosis

Oral disease is indicated by an anamnesis of inappetence or anorexia, quidding, halitosis, rubbing or pawing of the lips and excessive salivation. A complete physical examination of the patient is routine, and haematological and serological examinations can be necessary for the oral lesions may be indicative of a systemic disease. Particular attention is paid to an associated lymphadenopathy or any other palpable swelling in the head region. Adequate initial inspection of the mouth is possible in most patients without resorting to anaesthetic restraint and the lips, teeth, gingivae, tongue, hard and soft palates, the oropharynx and the palatine tonsils should be examined. Severe pain on opening the mouth is most likely to be associated with the presence of tonsillar carcinoma, eosinophilic myositis or craniomandibular osteopathy. Halitosis is associated with the local problems of stomatitis and periodontal disease, accompanies gastrointestinal and respiratory disease, and occurs in uraemia and severe diabetes. The excess saliva produced is initially thin, clear and seromucous, but with chronicity it will become tenacious and pungent: blood may be present in ulcerative conditions and purulent material can be seen in severe periodontal disease. The non-pigmented buccal mucosa is normally pink and smooth, and the capillary refill time is short. Further inspection involving detailed examination and palpation, radiography and biopsy procedures requires a general anaesthetic. Radiography is invaluable in demonstrating the presence of foreign bodies, the investigation of space-occupying lesions and neoplastic growth, and can be useful in determining the extent of a dental problem. Bacterial and fungal examinations are of limited value, for a wide variety of these micro-organisms can be cultured from the normal mouth (Snow *et al* 1969).

The lips

Developmental abnormalities
Fissures of the upper lip (harelip or primary palate clefts) occur occasionally in the dog, usually in association with cleft of the secondary palate. The fissure may be either central through the philtrum, unilateral or bilateral, and it can involve the dental arcade and even extend into the incisive foramen, but in the absence of an accompanying palatine defect a fissure does not present as a clinical problem.

Trauma
Lip trauma occurs as the result of chewing sharp and abrasive objects, road traffic accidents and dog fights, and the biting of electric wires. Any surgical reconstruction should be immediate, and skin grafting may be necessary when tissue is missing or has subsequently sloughed following a severe electrical burn.

Cheilitis and lip-fold dermatitis
Inflammation of the lips occurs as the result of lip trauma, erosion of the buccal mucosa due to the presence of dental tartar or malpositioned teeth, and as part of a specific skin disease. This latter category includes contact dermatitis, demodectic mange, dermatomycosis, pemphigus vulgaris and, in the young patient, pustular dermatitis associated with staphylococcal infection. The clinical signs of cheilitis include self trauma, wetness and loss of lip hair and oral malodour. Treatment requires attention to the specific cause and the alleviation of the secondary inflammation.

Lip-fold dermatitis or labial dermatitis, is cheilitis in which there is chronic inflammation and ulceration of the lower lip fold. It is commonly seen in the Spaniel breeds, but any individual with a deep furrowed lip fold can be affected. It is normally bilaterally present, and the long-standing condition may involve the labial commissures. It occurs as the result of saliva running into the lip fold and being retained there by the lip hair: the initial inflammatory response is subsequently complicated by the establishment of chronic bacterial infection. The presenting clinical signs include the constant drooling of saliva, self trauma, oral malodour and brown staining of lip hair. Treatment requires repeated antibacterial washes and corticosteroid cream application. Removal of the hair in and around the lip folds is a useful adjunct to medical therapy, but cure for the chronic condition necessitates the surgical ablation of the lip folds.

Neoplasia
The external lip surface is subject to the same neoplastic

involvement as the rest of the body skin; non-malignant papillomas, adenomas, carcinomas and malignant melanomas are the most common. The mucosal surface is one of the sites involved in infectious oral papillomatosis in the young dog, whilst squamous cell carcinoma is the commonest malignancy seen here in the older patient.

The buccal cavity

Developmental abnormalities

Developmental abnormalities of the buccal cavity include inferior and superior prognathism, cleft hard palate (secondary palate), and various dental anomalies associated with the permanent dentition. Severe prognathism can occasionally result in a dental interlock which can interfere with normal jaw growth. Maxillary micrognathism has been selectively bred for in several breeds, and the resultant obstructive dyspnoea produced is a tribute to the wisdom of mankind. In cleft hard palate the lateral palatine processes fail to develop sufficiently to unite in the midline, and the resultant degree of oronasal communication varies considerably. In severe cases the inability to produce a vacuum between the tongue and the palate by sucking prohibits effective nursing, and supplemental nourishment is a necessary life support. Pharyngostomy intubation (see p. 74) is of real value, for surgical correction using sliding mucoperiosteal flaps must be delayed until the patient is at least 2 months, but ideally 5 months, of age.

The dental anomalies which occur are rarely anodontia, more commonly oligodontia involving the incisors, premolars and last molars, supernumerary teeth which result in abnormal dental and gingival contours predisposing to food retention and early periodontal disease, and commonly the retention of deciduous teeth, which can produce occlusal defects and abnormal attrition of the permanent dentition.

Foreign bodies and trauma

Acute oral foreign bodies are common, and the patient usually presents in severe distress, drooling saliva and pawing the mouth. The chronic presence of foreign body material is associated with stomatitis, dysphagia, halitosis and less self-trauma. Pieces of wood and bone can be jammed across the hard palate, and their removal can be complicated by interdental space fixation. Bone can be wedged between the upper and lower arcades, and fish hooks, needles and pins can cause complication by their penetration of the buccal tissues.

Traumatic damage is usually related to road traffic accidents, dog fights and electrical and caustic burns. Radiography is of value should damage to deep tissues

and bone be suspected. Wounds of the tongue should be sutured with non-absorbable material to prevent the shape distortions that can occur with healing by secondary intention. The general therapeutic principles are those of antibiosis, penicillin being the drug of choice for the majority of oral infections, surgical repair and attention to nutrition.

Inflammatory disease

Stomatitis is generalised inflammation of the mouth, and it is either a primary disease process or occurs as a secondary feature to a systemic problem. Gingivitis is a localised inflammation of the gums, and glossitis is inflammation of the tongue.

Primary glossititis is frequently of traumatic origin; dental tartar erosion, foreign body penetration, chemical and electrical burns and insect stings are the usual causes. Treatment involves the removal of the cause and the use of corticosteroids to control any associated swelling. A gangrenous glossitis characterised by sloughing of the anterior third of the tongue may be related to strangulation, but chronic nephritis and leptospirosis should be considered within the differential diagnosis. The condition is painful, and the presenting clinical signs are those of anorexia, excess salivation and halitosis. Adequate treatment is difficult, and consists of antibiosis, corticosteroids and vitamin A and C therapy. The end result is usually a considerable slough of the anterior tongue with subsequent impaired fluid intake. In the German Shepherd Dog lesions of calinosis circumscripta can involve any area of the tongue, but are most commonly seen on the anterior margins (Fig. 3.20). They would appear to be of no serious consequence, but their removal necessitates surgery. Primary gingivitis occurs as the result of dental tartar accumulation, bacterial infection and alveolar periostitis. The gingivae initially become hyperaemic, they may bleed easily and with chronicity there is ulceration, exudation and recession of gum tissue tooth root material. Treatment involves the removal of dental tartar and antibiotic therapy, usually with penicillin.

Bacteriological examinations are of limited value, but can be helpful with the resistant case. Prophylaxis represents the most useful approach, and routine dental treatment on a biannual basis should reduce the incidence of the disease. Secondary gingivitis occurs in chronic debilitating diseases such as nephritis with subclinical uraemia, infectious diseases such as canine distemper and leptospirosis, avitaminosis C, and heavy metal poisoning like lead and copper in which a classical 'blue line' of haemorrhage at the gingival margin is specifically diagnostic.

Primary stomatitis is usually the extension of severe

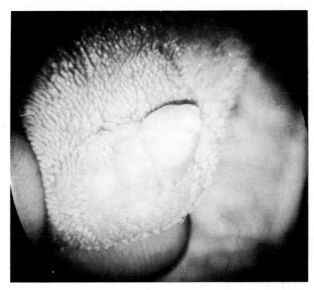

Fig. 3.20   A lesion of calcinosis circumscripta involving the tip of the tongue, German Shepherd Dog, 18 months.

gingivitis and periodontal disease, but chemical, thermal or mechanical trauma can be the cause. Vincent's stomatitis is a severe and usually recurrent infection produced by a combination of spirochaete and fusiform bacilli. Initially, the gingival margin is involved, but there is rapid extension of the infection towards the root apex and considerable concurrent loss of tissue. Treatment is most often unrewarding, but penicillin therapy for up to 3 weeks may be effective when given in conjunction with oral hygiene. Extensive debridement and tooth removal has also been advocated, but the results are often poor. Mycotic stomatitis due primarily to *Candida albicans* with secondary bacterial infection presents as a most painful condition due to extensive ulceration of the mucosal surface. The prognosis is generally good, and treatment consists of topical nystatin applied 4 times daily over a period of approximately 2 weeks. Systemic antibiosis is usefully employed to control the bacterial secondaries, and corticosteroid therapy used judiciously can be of value in controlling pain. The vitamin supplementation of a high protein diet appears to be a useful aid to tissue repair. A similar type of necrotising stomatitis is also seen in which there are recurrent episodes of extensive ulceration of the buccal mucosa. Mycotic and bacterial infections are involved, and the possible inclusion of herpesvirus in the aetiology should be allowed for in the therapeutic regimen employed.

Stomatitis also occurs in the systemic disease conditions of chronic nephritis, diabetes and heavy metal poisoning. Treatment involves attention to the specific cause, systemic antibiosis to control secondary infection, oral hygiene, and the use of atropine sulphate to reduce salivation. One important differential diagnosis of oral pain is eosinophilic myositis, an idiopathic myopathy involving the muscles of mastication (see Chapter 6, p. 162). Pain, muscle swelling and, occasionally, exophthalmos accompany dullness and anorexia in the acute disease, whereas the chronic form is characterised by progressive atrophy of the muscles of mastication. A viral aetiology is suspected, and dramatic response can be obtained using corticosteroid therapy.

Dental disease
Retention of the deciduous canine teeth, and the incisor teeth to a lesser extent, occurs with some frequency in the toy and brachycephalic breeds, and is due to the failure of root resorption. Enamel hypoplasia due to defective calcification during development prior to eruption is usually attributed to concurrent canine distemper infection, but it can also be associated with nutritional deficiency and severe parasitism. Such teeth stain readily and tend to be involved more often in periodontal disease. Staining of developing teeth will occur with prolonged tetracycline therapy.

Fracture of the teeth is usually associated with mandibular and maxillary fracture consequent to road traffic accidents, or the catching of hard objects. If the pulp cavity is not exposed or damaged, the tooth should be left *in situ*, but pulp exposure is acutely painful and extraction is usually required. Pulp

necrosis following pulp exposure can result in periapical abscessation. Dental attrition is due to the wearing
away of enamel and dentine, a condition which particularly affects the canine teeth of the stone-carrying or
wire-chewing dog. Facial sinus (malar abscess, carnassial abscess) is the result of periapical abscessation of
the roots of the upper fourth premolar tooth, either
due to severe periodontal disease and alveolar plate
necrosis or tooth fracture. It presents as either a soft
fluctuating swelling or a draining sinus below the medial canthus of the eye, the usual patient being the
middle-aged dolichocephalic. Extraction of the carnassial tooth and maxillary debridement are necessary
to provide adequate drainage, and systemic antibiosis
is mandatory.

Periodontal or paradontal disease (alveolar periostitis) is the commonest dental disease of dogs, its incidence increasing with age in all breeds. It is an inflammatory condition of the periodontal membrane of
complex aetiology, but usually related to the accumulation of dental tartar and the extension of a marginal
gingivitis. Bacterial infection gains access to the alveo-
lus, and the destruction of the periodontal ligament
leads to a loosening of the tooth and its possible eventual loss. The clinical features are halitosis, inappetence, dental tartar, gingivitis and gingival ulceration,
pus in the gingival sulcus and loose teeth. The treatment of the early case necessitates scaling of the teeth,
possible gingivectomy and systemic antibiosis: in the
advanced case extensive tooth extraction may be
necessary to control the condition.

Dental calculus or tartar is mineralised bacterial
plaque, the mineral component being mainly calcium
hydroxyapatite, derived from the saliva. Calculus
formation is greatest in sites adjacent to the salivary
duct openings, and the precipitation of hydroxypatite
acts as a nidus for the crystallisation of inorganic salts.
Bacteria act upon salivary urea to release ammonia,
and this raises the oral pH to initiate the precipitation
of the calcium salts on the plaque. Calculus lies supra-
gingivally initially, but with time subgingival tartar
builds up to propagate the gingivitis and eventually
produces the alveolar sepsis. The routine cleaning and
scaling of teeth is essential, but it must be remembered
that once the periodontal ligament has been damaged,
treatment can only slow down the process of periodontal disease. There is experimental evidence to show
that grinding masticatory work is essential for the
health of the periodontium (King 1947); the shearing
forces cleanse the teeth and remove plaque and calculus. In many miniature breeds of dog the diet is such
that dental work is minimal, and consequently periodontal disease enjoys its high incidence.

Dental caries is a disease of the calcified tissues of
the teeth in which the inorganic part is demineralised
and the destruction of the remaining organic portion
is brought about by the bacterial fermentation of
carbohydrates. Its incidence in the dog is low due to
the anatomical form of the teeth, with few fissures to
trap food, bacteria and debris, whilst the salivary alkaline pH and high urea level neutralise the oral acids
to prevent enamel breakdown. Caries most commonly
affects the first maxillary molar tooth, and occasionally involves the second maxillary molar and the first
and second mandibular molars. The associated clinical
signs range from nothing to a painful pulp exposure
and infection which necessitate tooth extraction.

Salivary gland disease

Sialadenitis is due to penetration wounding, blunt
trauma, invading foreign body and, rarely, obstructive
sialolith formation; this latter is an uncommon condition in the dog usually involving the parotid duct
when it occurs. The gland is swollen, a purulent discharge may be seen escaping from the duct intraorally
or through an externally draining fistula, and there is
pain when the mouth is opened. Treatment involves
the early use of antibiosis and hot fomentations;
abscess formation necessitates surgical drainage. A
zygomatic sialadenitis is most unusual, but will present
with the same clinical picture as retrobular abscessation with exophthalmos and pain.

Salivary mucocoeles are the non-painful, fluid-filled
swellings seen usually in young dogs that arise beneath
the tongue, in the posterior intermandibular space
(cervical) and occasionally within the pharynx as a
result of saliva leaking from either gland or duct. A
bilateral involvement is possible, and the cause of this
apparently spontaneous leakage remains unknown.
The submandibular and sublingual glands have both
been implicated, but most of the evidence suggests
that it is the anterior portion of the sublingual gland
that is responsible. The sublingual swelling, or ranula
(Fig. 3.21) lies alongside the frenulum linguae, and
can interfere with eating and drinking. The cervical
mucocoele is the most common and it can enlarge to
massive proportions but is rarely a clinical problem
(Fig. 3.22), whilst pharyngeal mucocoele can obstruct
respiration and interfere with deglutition. Diagnosis is
on the presenting clinical features, and sialography
(Fig. 3.23) can be of value in deciding the site of origin
of the cervical mucocoele (Glenn 1966, 1972). Aspiration is of temporary remedial value only, and excision of
the submandibular/sublingual salivary gland complex
is required to effect the cure (Spreull & Head 1967).

Neoplasia of the salivary glands is uncommon. The

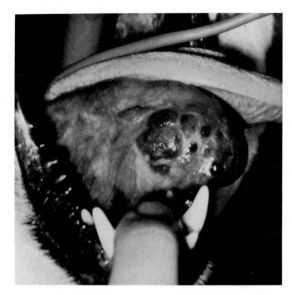

Fig. 3.21 A sublingual salivary mucocoele: German Shephe. Dog cross, 3 years.

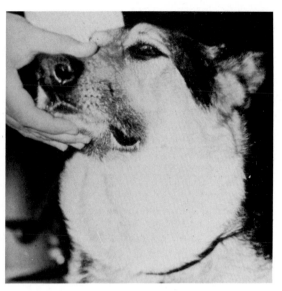

Fig. 3.22 A cervical salivary mucocoele: German Shepherd Dog, 2 years.

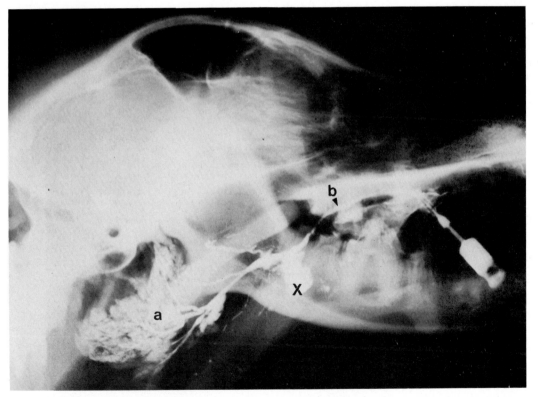

Fig. 3.23 An example of diagnostic sialography. The technique was useful here in confirming the unusual parotid origin of a small cervical salivary mucocoele (X). Leakage from the parotid duct was the result of a grass awn migration: (a) parotid gland; (b) parotid duct.

mandibular and parotid glands are the ones usually affected and the slow-growing adenocarcinoma is the tumour usually involved. Treatment by excision is possible in the absence of metastasis to the regional lymph nodes.

Neoplasia

In the young dog the benign 'warts' of infectious oral papillomatosis develop with varying degree on the buccal and pharyngeal mucosa, and on the tongue. The disease is self-limiting, lasting some 6–12 weeks, but therapy may prove necessary if the involvement is an extensive one. Papillomas can physically interfere with mastication, and halitosis indicates a secondary bacterial stomatitis due to food retention. Autogenous wart vaccines and sodium bismuth tartrate may be of value, whilst simple scissor excision represents the most expedient measure. A benign fibrous tissue gingival tumour occurs commonly in the brachycephalic breeds, particularly the Boxer and the Bulldog, and is known as epulis or periodontal fibrous hyperplasia (Fig. 3.24). Several tumours are usually present, each being cauliflower-like in appearance, firm to the touch and apparently non-painful. Their appearance is attributed to chronic inflammation and they originate from the periodontal membrane: both jaws can be affected, but it is commonly the upper jaw at the level

of the premolar and molar teeth. There can be an associated halitosis, but clinical problems occur only if they interfere with mastication. Treatment, when necessary, consists of excision using electrocautery and the occasional removal of an involved tooth; however, recurrence is the rule. Oral lesions of transmissible venereal cell tumour result from licking the primary lesion but spontaneous regression of these cauliflower-like friable tumours usually occurs without the necessity of surgical or cytotoxic therapy.

The incidence of malignant neoplasia in the mouth is high (Dorn *et al* 1968; Brodey 1970), and it is gingival tissue which is most commonly involved. The three most common oral tumours are the fibrosarcoma, malignant melanoma and squamous cell carcinoma. The fibrosarcoma is seen in the younger dog, and despite its uncommon metastasis, the prognosis remains poor due to its extensive invasiveness and lack of response to radiotherapy. The malignant melanoma also carries a poor prognosis and is particularly common in the Chow and Great Dane: it is a rapidly-growing invasive tumour with metastasis involving the regional lymph nodes and the lungs. However, oral squamous cell carcinoma carries a good prognosis for, unlike its tonsillar counterpart, it is late to invade and metastasise, and is extremely radiosensitive. Differential diagnosis of these tumours is vital, and involves biopsy, exfoliative cytology, and thoracic radiology, particularly if malignant melanoma or

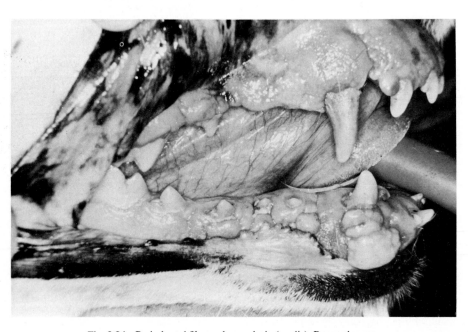

Fig. 3.24 Periodontal fibrous hyperplasia (epulis): Boxer, 4 years.

squamous cell carcinoma are suspected. Chemotherapy is of uncertain value currently, but radiation therapy is advocated for squamous cell carcinoma: 3000–5000 rad should be effective given over a 2 week period. However, the presence of regional lymphadenopathy always indicates a poor prognosis even though the chest radiographs are normal.

DISEASES OF THE THROAT

Description of the disease conditions which affect this complex anatomical structure will be discussed under the two broad headings of 'the pharynx' and 'the larynx'. The region covered extends from the choanae of the nasal cavity and the posterior limits of the oral cavity caudally to the cranial oesophageal opening and the anterior trachea.

THE PHARYNX

The pharynx is the muscular tube which connects the oral and nasal cavities to the oesophagus and larynx; it is common, therefore, to both the respiratory and alimentary systems (Fig. 3.25). The anterior part is divided by the soft palate (secondary palate) into a dorsal nasopharynx and a ventral oropharynx. The nasopharynx functions in respiration, conducting air from the nasal cavity to the free edge of the soft palate

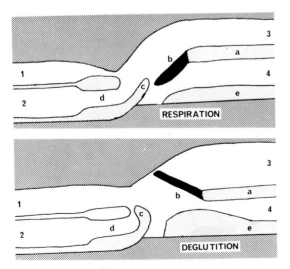

Fig. 3.25 Diagrammatic representation of the structures of the canine throat region: (1) oesophagus; (2) trachea; (3) nasopharynx; (4) oropharynx; (a) hard palate; (b) soft palate; (c) epiglottis; (d) laryngeal airway; (e) tongue.

in the resting animal. Its lateral walls bear the internal openings of the Eustachian tubes, and, during deglutition, its lumen is functionally obliterated by the upward displacement of the soft palate. The oropharynx functions in both respiration and deglutition, being involved in mouth breathing and the conduction of food to the oesophagus. During deglutition the shape of its lumen changes due to the posterior movement of the root of the tongue and the displacements of the epiglottis, larynx and soft palate. Its lateral walls, or fauces, bear the paired palatine tonsils; each tonsil is an elongated, elliptical lymph node situated just caudal to the palatoglossal fold within its own sinus or crypt formed from folds in the pharyngeal wall. They are easily visible in the dog, and it should be remembered that in the young animal it is normal for the tonsil to stand out from its crypt. In addition to the palatine tonsil, diffuse lymphoid tissue in the root of the tongue is referred to as lingual tonsil, whilst the lymphoid tissue in the nasopharynx is referred to as pharyngeal tonsil or adenoid. The canine soft palate is a particularly long and highly mobile caudal extension of the hard palate. In the dolichocephalic it arises at the level of the last upper molar tooth, and at rest its free border is just in contact with the anterior ventral epiglottis. In the brachycephalic breeds the free border extends more caudally into the pharynx because of the shortness of the upper jaw, and this relative overlength can result in severe glottic obstruction.

Diagnosis

The signs of pharyngeal disease are variously inappetence, dysphagia, excessive dyspnoea, retching, gagging and coughing. A physical examination will reveal signs of systemic disease, regional lymphadenopathy or associated upper cervical masses, abnormalities of the mucosa which is normally pink, smooth and shiny, tonsillar abnormality, the presence of discharge, and defects of the soft palate. More detailed investigation will necessitate the use of a general anaesthetic at which time radiography to delineate possible foreign body presence or tumour formation will be possible (Lee 1974). Microbiological examinations are of limited value for a wide variety of bacterial and fungal organisms can normally be cultured. Prominence of the palatine tonsils can be misleading, but true enlargement may be due to neoplasia: often the colour is a better guide to possible disease involvement. The facility of fluoroscopy and barium swallow studies are of considerable value in the differential diagnosis of dysphagia of inapparent related cause.

Disease conditions

Foreign body induced disease

The presence of needles, pins or splinters of wood lodged in either the piriform fossa, the subepiglottic space, the nasopharynx or a tonsillar crypt will initiate an acute irritation and pharyngitis. Cure is simply effected by the prompt removal of the cause, and the use of systemic antibiotic and steroid therapy. Penetration of the pharyngeal wall and the subsequent migration of foreign body material may result in retropharyngeal abscess formation. Treatment necessitates surgical drainage of the abscess and systemic antibiosis: in such cases the foreign body may never be found.

Infection

Primary pharyngitis is not common in the dog, and infection usually occurs as part of concurrent nasal or systemic diseases, or as the result of foreign body presence.

Tonsillitis on the other hand is a commonly diagnosed condition. It occurs occasionally as a primary disease problem in young dogs, usually involving the smaller breeds, and exhibiting a recurrent pattern up to puberty. The presenting features are those of pyrexia, inappetence, coughing, retching and possible malaise but the therapeutic response to broad spectrum antibiosis is usually relatively prompt. Glycerine and thymol preparations can afford some relief, but mild analgesia may be necessary in the occasional severe case. However, the common appearance of tonsillitis amongst all age groups and breeds is as a secondary response to primary disease elsewhere. It will be seen in alimentary tract disease characterised by persistent vomiting, or it will commonly accompany chronic dental conditions. Secondary tonsillitis occurs with the respiratory tract disorders of rhinitis and bronchitis, and those patients with chronic anal conditions can be similarly affected. Treatment is aimed at rectifying the cause, and only then, with the persistence of gagging, choking and coughing, should tonsillectomy be advocated.

Occasionally normal tonsils, due to their relative oversize in a small oropharynx, will contribute to an obstructive dyspnoea, and here tonsillectomy is of distinct value.

Soft palate problems

Dyspnoea related to the soft palate is due to either the glottic obstruction produced by its relative overlength in the brachycephalic, or the rhinitis which accompanies the congenital insufficiency of this structure.

Several factors contribute to the respiratory obstruction that occurs commonly in the brachycephalic, The net result is either the production of the classical snuffling respiration with no interference in physical activity, or severe obstruction during inspiration which can lead to cyanosis and collapse. This second is usually a progression of the first, and is due to chronic structural deformation with reduced patency of the upper airway. Panting in hot weather is a common cause of crisis in such patients, the rapidly-induced pharyngeal and laryngeal oedema adding to the overall insufficiency of the airway with serious consequence. Here the use of steroid therapy to reduce the oedema, and sedation to reduce the necessity for mouth breathing prove invaluable first-aid measures, but permanent relief necessitates the relief of the underlying dyspnoea. Specific reference has been made to the role of the soft palate in this syndrome, in that it is the mismatch of soft palate length relative to the reduced pharynx size which results in the palate being sucked into the glottis during inspiration and logically the excision of excess palatine tissue represents both prophylaxis and cure. However, other stenosing features may be present, and displacement of the glosso-epiglottic mucosa, eversion of the laryngeal ventricles and actual collapse of the epiglottis and the arytenoid cartilages may all be present and require surgical attention.

The congenital hypoplastic condition of the soft palate characterised by unilateral or bilateral absence of tissue (Fig. 3.26), or the cleft which is associated with a hard palate defect/or a harelip (Fig. 3.27) either leads to an aspiration pneumonia and death of the suckling puppy, or its presence is indicated at weaning by a chronic rhinitis and nasal regurgitation. Surgical correction of the defect is necessary, but providing the condition is stabilised using a simple feeding regimen and indicated antibiotic/corticosteroid therapy, palatoplasty may be left until the patient is ideally 5 months old. Wound breakdown is a common occurrence with such surgery, and pharyngostomy intubation (Fig. 3.28) (Bohning et al 1970) is usefully employed during the convalescent stage. Rubber or polythene tubing with an external diameter of approximately 8 mm is introduced through the pharyngeal wall at the piriform fossa, and passed into the stomach until the distal end lies some 4 cm beyond the cardia. The patient is fed suitably sized liquidised meals 4-8 times a day for a 10-day postoperative period; the maximum size of each meal should be approximately 100 ml for the largest patient.

A unique and most dramatic condition which presumably involves the soft palate in some way is seen occasionally in most breeds, but particularly so in the Bull Terrier. The condition is characterised by 20-60

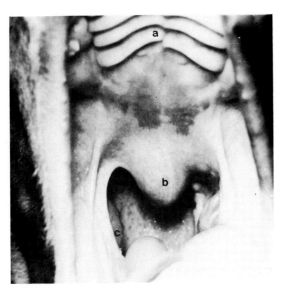

Fig. 3.26 Soft palate hypoplasia in an 8-month-old Weimaraner. (a) Hard palate; (b) 'uvula' formation of the hypoplastic soft palate; (c) right tonsil.

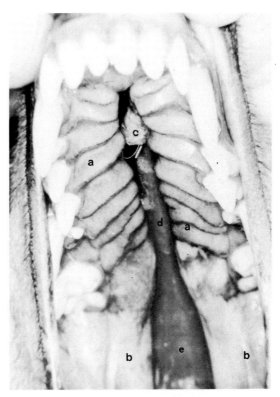

Fig. 3.27 Cleft involving both the hard and soft palates in a 4-month-old Jack Russell Terrier. (a) Hard palate; (b) soft palate; (c) foreign body material within the nasal cavity; (d) nasal cavity; (e) nasopharynx.

second periods of noisy forced inspiratory effort and expiratory flapping of the lips. Despite the alarming appearance of the patient, collapse and cyanosis are not seen and the dog returns to normal immediately. This condition may be due to either a nasopharyngeal spasm, failure of the epiglottis to disengage from the glottis after deglution, or glottic entrapment of the soft palate. Treatment is not necessary, but the dyspnoea may be relieved by either pulling the dog's tongue forward where possible or by rapidly and sharply compressing its chest.

Pharyngeal paralysis
Dysphagia is due either to the discomfort associated with local problems of pharyngitis, tonsillitis, neoplasia, temporomandibular disease, craniomandibular osteopathy and eosinophilic myositis, to cricopharyngeal achalasia or to a pharyngeal paralysis. Lesions of the glossopharyngeal, vagus and trigeminal nerves, of unknown aetiology, result in the insidious onset of a disease condition characterised by the dropping of the lower jaw, the drooling of saliva, nasal regurgitation and an associated rhinitis, and the inability to swallow food and water. In the majority of cases the paralysis is temporary and recovery is complete. In these patients life is maintained by the utilisation of pharyngostomy intubation; the important differential diagnosis is cricopharyngeal achalasia.

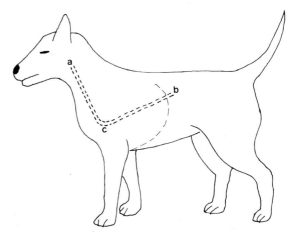

Fig. 3.28 Pharyngostomy intubation. The length of the tubing used equals the distance from the piriform fossa (a), to the tenth chondrocostal junction (b), via the acromion process (c).

Neoplasia

Tonsillar squamous cell carcinoma in the older patient is the commonest pharyngeal neoplasm, the presenting clinical features being dysphagia or anorexia, palpable mandibular lymphadenopathy and severe pain. The tonsil may be enlarged, either firm and scirrhous or softer and friable, bleeding to the touch, and its often apparent unilateral involvement may be found to be bilateral post mortem. The tonsil drains to the medial retropharyneal lymph node, and metastasis is initially found here. In fact, the diseased tonsil may not be enlarged at all, but pain and dysphagia are due to the retropharyngeal metastases, these tumours being so large that they effect a ventral displacement of the pharynx and larynx. Treatment of the primary lesion is not possible due to the presence of those metastases, and frequent pulmonary spread.

Occasionally lymphosarcoma can involve the palatine tonsils and the retropharyngeal lymph nodes. The tonsils appear bilaterally enlarged with smooth surfaces. Again, treatment other than the suppressive effect of steroid therapy is not possible due to the disseminative nature of the disease.

Very occasionally pharyngeal airway obstruction is seen, due to non-neoplastic cystic swellings arising from the tonsillar crypts (Fig. 3.29). Relief is effected by their surgical excision.

Cricopharyngeal achalasia

The differential diagnosis of dysphagia in the absence of obvious predisposing clinical disease in the young dog, in particular the Cocker Spaniel, includes a consideration of failure of the upper oesophageal sphincter to relax. Swallowing is impossible, and the oral and nasal return of food, rhinitis and nasal discharge, and tonsillitis will respond to the corrective surgery of cricopharyngeal myotomy (see also Chapter 14).

THE LARYNX

The larynx is a complex, valve-like musculocartilaginous tube situated immediately posterior to the root of the tongue and the soft palate which provides connection between the oropharynx and the trachea. It is suspended from the temporal bone by the hyoid apparatus, and its cartilaginous framework consists of the epiglottis, the paired arytenoid cartilages and a shield-shape cricoid cartilage (Figs. 3.30, 3.31). The framework is united and supported by several muscles, ligaments and membranes. The paired dorsal cricoarytenoid muscles are its only muscles of abduction, and the motor nerve supply to all the laryngeal musculature except the cricothyroid is via the paired recurrent laryngeal nerves. Sensory nerve supply is via the cran-

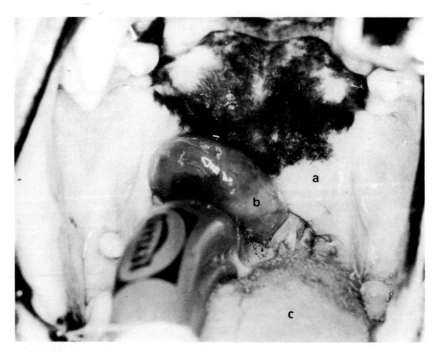

Fig. 3.29   A tonsillar cyst (right): Labrador, 4 years. (a) Soft palate; (b) cyst; (c) tongue.

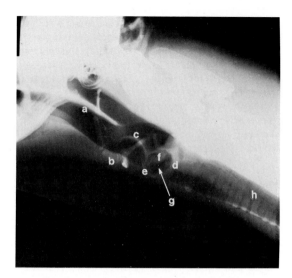

Fig. 3.30 Lateral radiograph of the pharynx and larynx: Greyhound, 6 years. (a) Soft palate; (b) hyoid apparatus; (c) epiglottis; (d) cricoid cartilage; (e) thyroid cartilage; (f) arytenoid cartilage; (g) lateral ventricle; (h) trachea.

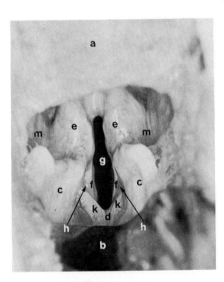

Fig. 3.31 The rostral features of the larynx: the view in to the glottis is obtained using a laryngoscope to displace the apex of the epiglottis ventrally: (a) soft palate; (b) laryngoscope blade; (c) epiglottal cartilage; (d) vestibule; (e) arytenoid cartilages; (f) vocal folds; (g) rima glottidis; (h) lateral ventricles; (k) vestibular folds; (m) piriform fossae.

ial and recurrent laryngeal nerves. The aryepiglottic folds and the lateral ventricles are well developed, and in this species the glottis is valvular. Disease involving the laryngeal musculature or its nerve supply leads to altered or lost voice, degrees of airway obstruction even to the extent of asphyxiation, or foreign body aspiration.

The larynx functions in deglutition, in respiration and in phonation. Voice is produced on expiration, an air current being driven through the narrowed rima glottidis with the larynx in adduction. Voice change is an early indication of laryngeal disease, but this important sign may often pass unnoticed. In respiration the larynx provides communication between the pharynx and the trachea, the glottis being actively abducted during inspiration and passively reduced during expiration. Its function in deglutition is to prevent the aspiration of food material and saliva: the 'valve cap' of the epiglottis is displaced posteriorly by caudal movement of the root of the tongue to deny entrance to the glottis (see Fig. 3.25), whilst the rima glottidis closes by the adduction of the paired arytenoid cartilages, and the vocal folds.

Diagnosis

Disease of the larynx is an important cause of obstructive dyspnoea, and its diagnosis should be considered whenever the patient presents in stridor. Voice change may not be noticed, but noisy respiration, cough, reduced exercise tolerance, episodes of cyanosis and even asphyxiation are significant diagnostic pointers. Superficial examination of the patient will describe the type and extent of the dyspnoea, reveal a possible traumatic origin and delineate cervical lymphadenopathy and swelling. Satisfactory examination of the larynx itself demands a general anaesthetic: arytenoid deformity is usually obvious at this stage, and with the tongue pulled forwards and the epiglottis depressed by the laryngoscope the glottis may be inspected (Fig. 3.31). A light plane of anaesthesia is required to observe the movement of the arytenoid cartilages. These movements should be correlated with respiration, and in laryngeal paralysis absence of arytenoid movement during inspiration results in non-dilation of the rima glottidis, and indeed the vocal cord(s) may be seen to be actually drawn in to the midline. During expiration the rima glottidis may 'enlarge' due to the same passive vocal cord movement. Radiographic examination of the larynx is not an essential diagnostic procedure, but it can prove helpful in identifying fractures, foreign bodies and neoplasia, and demonstrating displacement due to, or involvement with, cervical space-occupying lesions.

Disease conditions

Trauma

The position which the larynx occupies in the neck is a relatively well-protected one, but traumatic damage related to compression or puncture wounding is possible as the result of a road traffic accident or a dog fight. Choke chain restriction injury can result in fracture of the hyoid apparatus, and the laryngeal cartilages may be involved. Fracture of the latter is an extremely rare occurrence, but it is more likely to be seen in the older patient in which cartilage has lost its elasticity and may be calcified. Dislocation of the arytenoid–cricoid articulation and separation of the laryngeal–tracheal junction will result in severe airway obstruction. The treatment of traumatic damage involves the restoration of the airway, and indeed tracheotomy may be necessary. Steroid therapy should be employed to control inflammation and oedema, and open wounding necessitates the use of antibiotics. The possibility of laryngeal paralysis due to nerve damage where severe trauma has occurred should be considered in the prognosis given.

Iatrogenic laryngeal mucous membrane damage can result from attempted intubation when the glottic reflex is still present, or the tube used is too large and non-lubricated. The resultant 'tube cough' is due to inflammation, oedema and even erosion of the mucous membrane, particularly at the level of the glottis. Laryngeal oedema induced by panting occurs in the brachycephalic breeds and obese animals, the patient presenting with a stridor of sudden onset and possible cyanosis. Treatment involves the restoration of an adequate airway, sedation in a cool environment in the case of heat stroke, and the use of steroids.

Infection

Acute laryngitis is usually part of a generalised respiratory infection, and several epitheliotropic viruses and bacteria are involved in the aetiology. Chronic proliferative laryngitis is rare and is characterised by granulomatous tissue change involving the arytenoid cartilages and the aryepiglottic folds, which results in stenosis of the airway and dyspnoea.

Laryngeal paralysis

Inability to dilate the rima glottidis during inspiration due to laryngeal paralysis is an important differential diagnosis in the investigation of the dyspnoeic patient.

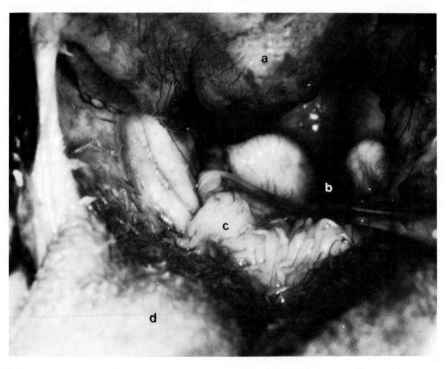

Fig. 3.32 Displacement of the glosso-epiglottic mucosa in respiratory dyspnoea: Bulldog, 2 years. (a) Resected soft palate; (b) laryngeal vestibule; (c) displacing glosso-epiglottic mucosa being held in the vestibule by forceps; (d) dorsum of the tongue.

Accidental or surgical trauma involving the recurrent laryngeal nerve, or a neuropraxia related to abscess formation, lymphadenopathy and neoplasia can result in a unilateral paralysis of the larynx. Phonation may be affected, but such a paralysis may be of little clinical significance except in the racing dog. Congenital laryngeal paralysis (Venker-van Haagen 1980) is an unusual entity, but it has been recorded with certainty in the Siberian Husky and the Bouvier. The paralysis may be either unilateral or bilateral, this latter particularly resulting in a muted bark, stridor, reduced exercise tolerance and even cyanosis and collapse. The most common type of laryngeal paralysis, however, is that which occurs in the older patient within the larger breeds and has been attributed to a neurogenic atrophy of the laryngeal musculature (O'Brien *et al* 1973). In the U K this disease is seen particularly in the Labrador, the Setter and the Springer Spaniel breeds, and is characterized by a stridor of several months duration which eventually progresses to obstructive dyspnoea and collapse on exertion. The paralysis is usually bilateral. Treatment may involve steroid therapy in the early stages to reduce laryngeal oedema, but restoration of the airway by partial laryngectomy or arytenoid cartilage lateralization is essential to prevent severe obstruction.

Displacement of the glosso-epiglotic mucosa

In brachycephalic and Chow-chow patients with chronic inspiratory dyspnoea, a displacement of the glosso-epiglottic mucosa or the ventral part of the aryepiglottic fold can occur as a function of the increased inspiratory effort (Bedford 1983). The tissue is lifted into the laryngeal aditus, and further reduces the patency of the anterior laryngeal airway (Fig. 3.32). Entrapment of the epiglottis is temporary, the mucosa returning to its normal position on expiration. The condition is considered to be part of the process of laryngeal collapse, and treatment is by the surgical excision of the displacing tissue.

Laryngeal collapse

Collapse of the larynx with resultant stenosis of the airway accompanies chronic, severe obstructive dyspnoea, and is seen most commonly in the brachycephalic airway obstruction syndrome. The reduced nasal airway, possible stenotic nostrils, relative soft palate overlength, and compression of the pharynx by the root of the tongue result in an obstructive dyspnoea, and laboured inspiration produces collapsing forces in the pharynx and larynx. Induced oedematous

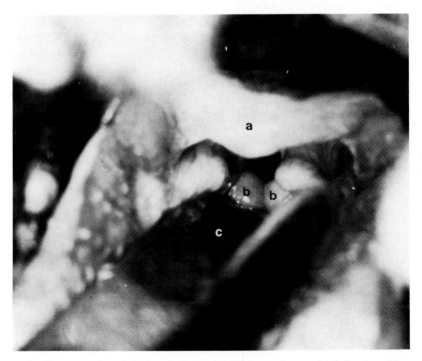

Fig. 3.33 Laryngeal collapse: eversion of the laryngeal saccules: Pekingese, 5 years. (a) Soft palate; (b) everted saccules; (c) laryngoscope blade.

swelling further contributes to the dyspnoea, and eventually eversion of the lateral ventricles, inversion of the corniculate and cuneiform processes of the arytenoids together with scrolling of the epiglottis can occur. The canine lateral ventricles are large structures, and the inspiratory 'suck' turns their oedematous mucous membrane linings inside out (Fig. 3.33). They appear as balls of tissue in the lumen of the glottis, obscuring the vocal cords and narrowing the airway, and subsequent fibrosis results in their permanent presence. Medial and rostral collapse of the arytenoids, epiglottic scrolling and the aryepiglottic folds results in severe, potentially fatal glottic airway obstruction (Fig. 3.34).

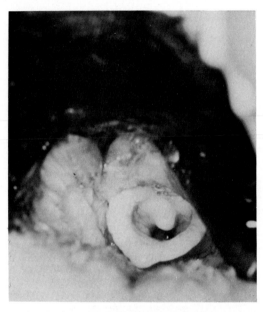

Fig. 3.34 Laryngeal collapse: medial and rostral displacement of the arytenoid cartilages and epiglotic scrolling to produce severe airway obstruction: Pug, 7 years.

The treatment of laryngeal collapse involves the surgery of ventriculectomy, partial laryngectomy and correction of the other predisposing factors involved in the syndrome. However, tracheal fenestration may prove necessary.

Neoplasia
Laryngeal polyps arising from the vocal cord(s) are occasionally seen, but rarely cause dyspnoea; however, chondromas and granulomas following penetration wounds or radical surgery can attain a size which may cause serious airway obstruction. Primary malignancies of the larynx are rare, but adenocarcinomas,

osteosarcomas, mast cell tumours and chondrosarcomas can occur (Wheeldon *et al* 1982). Thyroid adenocarcinomas, lymphosarcomas and heart base tumours may affect laryngeal function by recurrent laryngeal neuropraxia.

REFERENCES

The ear
FRAZER G. (1965) Aetiology of otitis externa in the dog. *J. Small Anim. Pract.* **6**, 445.
FRAZER G., GREGOR W. W., Mackenzie C. P., Spreull J. S. A. & Withers A. R. (1970) Canine ear disease. *J. Small Anim. Pract.* **10**, 725.
FRAZER G., WITHERS A. R. & SPREULL J. S. A. (1961) Otitis externa in the dog. *J. Small Anim. Pract.* **2**, 32.
JOSHUA J. O. (1965) *The Clinical Aspects of Some Diseases of Cats*. Heinemann, London.
LANE G. J. (1976) Canine middle ear disease. In *Veterinary Annual*, 16th edn. John Wright, Bristol.
MARSHALL M. J., HARRIS A. M. & HORNE J. M. (1974) The bacteriological and clinical assessment of a new preparation of the treatment of otitis externa in dogs and cats. *J. Small Anim. Pract.* **15**, 401.
PUGH K. E., EVANS J. M. & HENDY P. G. (1974) Otitis externa in the dog and cat: an evaluation of a new treatment. *J. Small Anim. Pract.* **15**, 387.

The nose
BEDFORD P. G. C. (1978). The differential diagnosis of nasal discharge in the dog. In *Veterinary Annual*, 18th edn, John Wright, Bristol.
BEDFORD P. G. C. (1982) Tracheal hypoplasia in the English Bulldog. *Vet. Rec.* **111**, 58.
BEDFORD P. G. C. (1983) Displacement of the glosso-epiglottic mucosa in canine asphyxiate disease. *J. Small Anim. Pract.* **24**, 199.
THOMPSON H., McCANDLISH A. P. & WRIGHT N. G. (1976) Experimental respiratory disease in dogs due to *Bordetalla bronchiseptica*. *Res. Vet. Sci.* **20**, 16.
WILKINS R. J. & HELLAND D. R. (1973) Antibacterial sensitivities of bacteria isolated from dogs with tracheobronchitis. *J. Am. Vet. Med. Assoc.* **162**, 47.
WILKINSON G. T. (1969) Some observations on the Irish Wolfhound rhinitis syndrome. *J. Small Anim. Pract.* **10**, 5.
WRIGHT N. G., THOMPSON H., CORNWALL H. J. C. & TAYLOR D. (1974) Canine respiratory virus infections. *J. Small Anim. Pract.* **15**, 27.

The mouth
BRODEY R. S. (1970) The biological behaviour of canine oral and pharyngeal neoplasms. *J. Small Anim. Pract.* **11**, 45.
DORN C. R., TAYLOR D. N., SCHNEIDER R., HIBBARD H. H. & KLAUBER M. R. (1968) Survey of animal neoplasms in Alameda and Contra Costa Counties, California. II. Cancer morbidity in dogs and cats from Alameda County. *J. Nat. Cancer Inst.* **40**, 307.
GLEN J. B. (1966) Salivary cysts in the dog: Identification of sub-lingual duct defects by sialography. *Vet. Rec.* **78**, 488.

GLEN J. B. (1972) Canine salivary mucocoeles. Results of sialographic examination and surgical treatment of fifty cases. *J. Small Anim. Pract.* **13,** 515.

KING J. D. (1947) Experimental investigations of paradontal disease. IV. Gnawing of sugar-cane in the treatment of non-ulcerated gingival disease in man. *Br. Dent. J.* **82,** 61.

SNOW H. D., DONOVAN M. L., WASHINGTON J. O. & FONKALSRUD E. W. (1969) Canine respiratory disease in an animal facility. *Arch. Surg.* **99,** 126.

SPREULL J. S. A. & HEAD K. W. (1967) Cervical salivary cysts in the dog. *J. Small Anim. Pract.* **8,** 17.

The throat

BOHNING R. H., DEHOFF W. D., McELHINNEY A. & HOFSTRA P. C. (1970) Pharyngostomy for maintenance of the anoretic animal. *J. Am. Vet. Med. Assoc.* **156,** 611.

LEE R. (1974) Radiographic examination of localised and diffuse tissue swellings in the mandibular and pharyngeal area. *Vet. Clinics N. Am.* **4,** 723.

O'BRIEN J. A., HARVEY C. E., KELLY A. M. & TUCKER J. A. (1973) Neurogenic atrophy of the laryngeal muscles of the dog. *J. Small Anim. Pract.* **14,** 521.

VENKER-VAN HAAGEN A. J. (1980) Investigations on the pathogenesis of hereditary laryngeal paralysis in the Bouvier. Thesis, Utrecht University.

WHEELDON E. B., SUTER P. F. & JENKIN T. (1982) Neoplasia of the larynx of the dog. *J. Am. Vet. Med. Assoc.* **180,** 642.

4

The Eye

R. CURTIS AND K. C. BARNETT

CLINICAL EXAMINATION

In any clinical examination it is essential that a routine is established in order that important clinical signs are not overlooked. The eye, because of its peculiar visual accessibility, may show a variety of concurrent signs and frequently secondary signs may mask the primary lesion. Identification of the primary cause is essential for the correct choice of treatment. It is obligatory to obtain as full a history as possible, giving particular attention to the sequence of events in time. Since some ocular conditions are manifestations or consequences of systemic disease, the health status of the patient must be established, with such additional clinical examination as is deemed necessary. It is unwise to allow the history given by the owner to prejudice the manner in which the eye is examined initially.

The room in which ocular examinations are conducted should be well lit but also capable of being blacked out, preferably with a small pilot light to provide minimal background illumination.

Restraint is rarely a problem, but the practitioner should always be prepared to tranquilise, or even anaesthetise, a patient if adequate examination is otherwise not possible. Local (topical) anaesthesia frequently facilitates examination in certain cases.

Preliminary examination and ophthalmoscopy

Before the eyes are examined in detail the head should be observed in full light from the front for any gross anatomical defects or abnormalities of the adnexa or globe and to detect subtle differences between the eyes less obvious on closer inspection: for example disparity in the size of the globes, palpebral apertures and pupils (anisocoria). Some neuro-ophthalmological signs such as ptosis, nystagmus, strabismus and Horner's syndrome may be obvious at this stage (see Chapter 5). After cleaning away any ocular discharge the structures of the eye are examined methodically, and in sequence, commencing with the eyelids and working backwards to the retina.

A useful preliminary appraisal of the eye, and especially the lens, may be made by distant direct ophthalmoscopy. With the direct ophthalmoscope set at '0' and held at a distance of about 0.6 m from the patient, lens opacities may be clearly seen against the tapetal reflex.

The anterior structures of the eye, including the lens, are best examined initially with a focal light source or pencil beam, preferably in conjunction with a monocular or binocular loupe. The direct ophthalmoscope is also suitable and both methods may be supple- by slit-lamp biomicroscopy, if available.

Routine examination of the vitreous body and fundus may be accomplished by direct or indirect ophthalmoscopy. In the UK the direct ophthalmoscope is still widely used, but in the USA it has been largely supplanted by the binocular indirect ophthalmoscope. Essentially the choice is one of individual preference.

The conventional direct ophthalmoscope produces a real, erect and greatly magnified image, but only a small area of the fundus is visible at one time. Settings (lenses) of the direct ophthalmoscope appropriate to various structures within the eye are shown in Fig. 4.1. Many practitioners prefer to commence by examining the retina (a slight negative setting is usual), working forward with lenses of increasing dioptre.

In indirect ophthalmoscopy the light source and the eye of the examiner are positioned at a distance from the patient's eye and a convex lens is interposed to produce an inverted image of low magnification but wide field (approximately 40° with a 20 dioptre lens). In its simplest form indirect ophthalmoscopy can be carried out with nothing more than a pen torch and a lens of appropriate strength. The instrument most commonly used is the binocular indirect ophthalmoscope which has the following advantages over the direct ophthalmoscope:

1 The patient is usually less apprehensive.
2 A comparison of the two eyes may be made more readily.

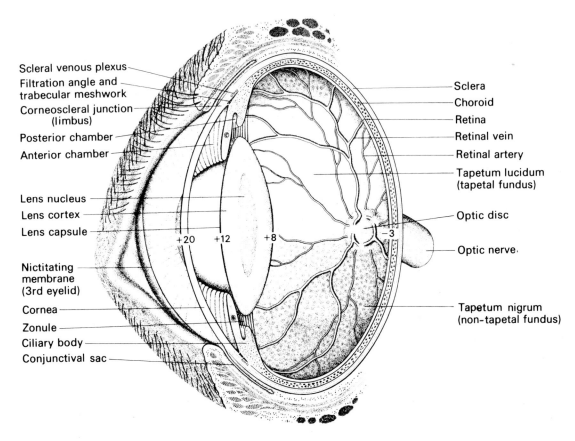

Fig. 4.1 Diagrammatic section of the canine eye. The figures indicate lens settings (in dioptres) of the direct ophthalmoscope appropriate to certain structures within the eye.

3 The area of fundus visible is larger and the periphery more accessible.
4 The fundus is usually clearer when diffuse lenticular opacities are present.
5 Stereopsis, or three-dimensional effect, is achieved.

An instrument with considerable potential in veterinary ophthalmology is the monocular indirect ophthalmoscope (American Optical Company) which

combines most of the desirable features of the direct and binocular indirect ophthalmoscopes. It is hand-held and produces an erect image of wide field. It is the simplest of all ophthalmoscopes to use.

If it is considered necessary to examine the peripheries of either the lens or the retina it is essential that the pupil be dilated. Tropicamide (Mydriacyl) is a suitable mydratic and preferred to atropine.

Pupillary light reflex (PLR)

An appreciation of pupil size and mobility is an important part of the routine examination. In a darkened room the pupil should contract briskly when a beam of light is directed into the eye. Both eyes should always be tested, and if the responses are dissimilar an attempt should be made to deduce which eye is abnormal. To fully appreciate the PLR the contralateral eye

Table 4.1 Comparison of direct and indirect ophthalmoscopes.

	Direct	Binocular Indirect	Monocular Indirect
Image	Erect	Inverted	Erect
Magnification (approx)	×15	×3	×4
Field (disc diameters)	2	10	7
Stereopsis	No	Yes	No

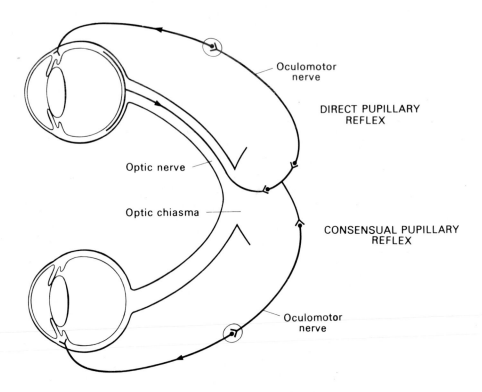

Fig. 4.2   Direct and consensual pupillary light reflexes.

should be covered.

When one eye only is stimulated the pupil of the other should constrict (the consensual PLR—Fig. 4.2). A positive response establishes the integrity of the afferent pathway (optic nerve) on the side stimulated and the efferent pathway (oculomotor nerve) on the opposite side.

It should be remembered that the PLR is not a test of vision, merely of the integrity of nervous pathways.

Examination of the eyelids

Special care should be taken to locate supernumerary or ectopic cilia, for which a loupe and strong illumination are essential. Thorough examination of the palpebral conjunctiva and inspection behind the third eyelid (e.g. for foreign bodies) is best performed with forceps and under topical anaesthesia (e.g. 0.5% proparacaine hydrochloride (Ophthaine)).

Lacrimal apparatus

Hyposecretion and hypersecretion may be measured with the Schirmer Tear Test. Wetting of more than 10 mm on test paper in 1 minute indicates adequate tear production; less than 5 mm or more than 25 mm indicate hyposecretion or hypersecretion respectively.

Patency of the nasolacrimal duct may be established either by instilling fluorescein into the conjunctival sac or by infusing saline into one (preferably the upper) of the puncta situated within the lid margins near the medial canthus; dye or saline should appear in the nostril if the duct is patent.

In any case of hypersecretion and blepharospasm, even in adult dogs, a special search should be made for supernumerary or ectopic cilia using a loupe and a focal light source.

Corneal integrity

Fluorescein-impregnated papers, because of their sterility and ease of use, are preferable to drops for the demonstration of corneal ulcers and abrasions. Rose bengal is useful for demonstrating desiccated tissue (e.g. in keratoconjunctivitis sicca) which stains bright red.

Slit-lamp biomicroscopy

The slit-lamp biomicroscope is of considerable value in determining the depth and extent of lesions of the cornea, lens and sometimes the vitreous body. Full-field illumination also provides a large and greatly magnified image of the cornea, anterior chamber and lens which is unrivalled. Hand-held models are available.

Tonometry

Tonometry is the measurement or assessment of intra-ocular pressure (IOP).

Digital tonometry, in which ocular tension is assessed by applying the tips of the index or second fingers to the globe over the closed upper lid, is fairly satisfactory in identifying differences in pressure between the two eyes but requires experience for absolute changes in pressure to be appreciated. The most frequently used instrument for measuring IOP in veterinary practice is the Schiøtz tonometer. This inexpensive but useful instrument consists essentially of a footplate, incorporating a protruding and weighted plunger, and a recording scale; the footplate is applied vertically to the cornea and the length of the plunger allowed to protrude, being dependent on the indentibility of the cornea, is registered as a deflection on the scale; the intraocular pressure is then determined from calibration tables, which have now been determined for the dog and are quoted in recent textbooks on veterinary ophthalmology.

Applanation tonometers, of which there are several types, depend on the principle that the force required to flatten a given area of cornea is proportional to the IOP. The most accurate and convenient (and the most expensive) tonometer is the Mackay–Marg electronic tonometer; this instrument incorporates a transducer probe, the function of which is based on the applanation principle. Besides accuracy it has the advantage that it may be used with the eye in its normal position. The normal IOP in the dog lies between 15 and 30 mm Hg.

Gonioscopy

The diagnosis of primary glaucoma in the dog cannot be considered complete without examination of the iridocorneal, or filtration, angle. Because this structure cannot be seen with the ophthalmoscope alone, a special highly convex contact lens (goniolens) is required. The lens is inserted into the eye following topical anaesthesia. Several types of goniolens are available, of which perhaps the most suitable for canine work is the Barkan gonioscopic lens.

Electroretinography

The electroretinogram (ERG) is a graphic record of the changes in electrical potential which occur when the retina is stimulated by light. Such potentials are detectable at the cornea by means of a contact lens electrode and, after amplification, are usually displayed on an oscilloscope screen, from which a photographic record may be obtained. Although it is possible to obtain an ERG in a conscious dog, satisfactory results are usually best obtained with the patient anaesthetised.

The normal canine ERG comprises a negative 'a' wave (arising in the photoreceptor layer) followed by a positive 'b' wave (arising from the inner nuclear layer and Müller cells). During dark adaptation the latencies and amplitudes of these waves change as the predominantly cone (photopic) response becomes a predominantly rod (scotopic) response. Responses to repeated light stimuli (flicker) also afford a means of distinguishing rod and cone function.

The method has considerable, and largely unexploited, potential in the early diagnosis of progressive retinal atrophy, and is also useful in the assessment of retinal function when opacities of the ocular media preclude satisfactory ophthalmoscopy of the fundus (e.g. prior to cataract extraction).

THE EYELIDS

The eyelids are mobile folds of skin which enclose muscular and glandular tissues and a poorly developed fibrous tarsal plate. They are lined by conjunctiva (palpebral) which is continuous with the bulbar conjunctiva at the fornix. The orbicularis oculi muscle (VIIth cranial nerve) closes the eye and the upper lid is raised by the levator palpebrae muscle (IIIrd cranial nerve). Eyelashes (cilia) and associated sebaceous glands are present in the upper lid, but are poorly developed in the lower lid. The Meibomian (tarsal) glands open at the lid margins. The third eyelid (membrana nictitans) is well developed and consists of a cartilaginous plate and lymphatic tissue and is covered by conjunctiva. The position of the third eyelid is dependent on the position of the globe and on changes in the retrobulbar mass; it has no motor nerve supply.

Blepharospasm

This is an important and common ocular sign indicating pain, particularly in the conjunctiva or cornea, but sometimes more deep-seated. It presents as a constant or frequent blinking of a narrowed palpebral fissure due to the contraction of the orbicularis oculi muscle. It may indicate the presence of a foreign body under the upper, lower or third eyelid but it is also a clinical sign of many other eye diseases.

Blepharitis

Inflammation of the eyelid (blepharitis) is usually secondary to conjunctivitis. Treatment should include attention to the primary condition, careful cleaning of the lids and application of an antibiotic ointment.

Periorbital dermatitis

The skin of the eyelids is particularly prone to various skin diseases including ringworm and both demodectic and sarcoptic mange. An ulcerative condition of the eyelid margin, sometimes referred to as 'mucocutaneous disease', is occasionally seen, particularly in the German Shepherd Dog. Sometimes other mucocutaneous junctions are involved (e.g. lips, anus, vulva); the aetiology is unknown. Pyoderma of the eyelids is due to a staphylococcal infection which also commonly affects the muzzle and chin. This condition may be treated with systemic antibiotics.

Chemosis

Chemosis (conjunctival oedema) may be due to injury, infection or, more commonly, allergy (e.g. to insect bites). Bilateral chemosis is sometimes seen in puppies as a reaction to certain foods.

Hordeolum

The term hordeolum refers to an acute localised pyogenic infection at the lid margin (stye) involving either the sebaceous gland of a cilia follicle (external hordeolum) or a meibomian gland (internal hordeolum), the latter being the more common. Topical anti-biotic therapy, the application of heat and possibly surgical incision are indicated.

Chalazion

A chronic inflammation of a meibomian gland, usually presenting as a firm, discrete nodule over which the skin is mobile. Care should be taken to distinguish it from a neoplasm. The mass should be removed surgically by incision and curettage or total excision.

Ptosis

Drooping of the upper lid (ptosis), with narrowing of the palpebral fissure, may be due to a lesion of the oculomotor nerve or involvement of the sympathetic innervation of the eye in Horner's syndrome (see Chapter 5).

Lagophthalmos

Inability to close the eyelids is seen in some exophthalmic breeds, particularly the Pekingese. In certain cases the condition may be improved by the application of artificial tears; tarsorrhaphy or shortening the palpebral fissure at the lateral canthus may also be considered.

Entropion

Inturning of the upper or lower eyelid, or both. It may or may not involve the lateral canthus and may be unilateral or bilateral. The cause is commonly hereditary and the condition is first seen from a few weeks to several months of age. Certain breeds are particularly affected. It is occasionally associated with injury or with enophthalmos. Treatment is surgical, but in young dogs, provided the cornea is not significantly affected, it may be advantageous to delay surgery until maturity (Plate 4.1).

Ectropion

Eversion of the lower lid, with exposure of conjunctiva, is usually due to too long an eyelid. The condition is seen particularly in certain breeds but is less common than entropion. It is occasionally associated with injury or gross swelling of the lid. Treatment is surgical (Plate 4.2).

Distichiasis

The presence of an abnormal row of eyelashes (distichiasis) is probably the most common hereditary eye abnormality in the dog. The cilia emerge from, or just posterior to, the orifices of the meibomian glands. The condition is often congenital.

Epilation affords temporary relief only. Electrolysis, applied correctly and successfully, destroys the follicles but is a tedious procedure if cilia are numerous. Various surgical techniques are available for the removal of the cilia-bearing tissue but cicatrisation can cause subsequent problems (Plate 4.3).

Ectopic cilia

Single or small tufts of supernumerary eyelashes may sometimes arise from the palpebral conjunctiva, usually of the upper lid, causing epiphora, blepharospasm and frequently focal corneal ulceration. Occasionally the problem does not arise until several years of age. Simple excision of the offending follicle is effective (Plate 4.4).

Eyelid neoplasms

According to one study (Krehbiel J.D. & Langham R.F. (1975) *Am. J. Vet. Res.* **36,** 115) the most common tumours of the eyelids are, in order: sebaceous adenomas, squamous papillomas, sebaceous adenocarcimonas, benign melanomas and malignant melanomas; squamous cell carcinomas are relatively uncommon. The majority of the eyelid tumours are benign and even those that are histologically malignant, even if locally infiltrative, tend not to metastasise. As elsewhere around the eye there may sometimes be difficulty in distinguishing proliferative nodular lesions from true neoplasms. In general, eyelid tumours should always be removed surgically. An exception is the papillomatous lesion of possible viral origin encountered in young dogs which may regress spontaneously.

Nictitating membrane (third eyelid)

Apparent prominence of the third eyelid may be due to lack of pigment in the free border. True prominence may be associated with any painful eye disease which causes a degree of enophthalmos; it also occurs as an anatomical feature in certain breeds. Unilateral prominence occurs in Horner's syndrome. Prominence associated with exophthalmos suggests a retrobulbar abscess or neoplasm. Inflammatory conditions include follicular conjunctivitis. A plasma cell infiltration has been recorded in the German Shepherd Dog. Hypertrophy and prolapse of the nictitans gland both occur and may require surgical removal of the gland. Neoplasia of the third eyelid is uncommon, but of the tumours occurring the squamous cell carcinoma is the most frequent. Excision of the third eyelid frequently leads to other ocular disease and should only be undertaken in cases of proven malignancy.

THE EYEBALL

Abnormalities of size and position

Microphthalmos
In microphthalmos the eye is congenitally small with variation from a small pigmented cyst in the orbit to an anatomically and functionally normal eye slightly smaller than usual. Often other eye anomalies are present, particularly cataract and nystagmus. Severe microphthalmos, together with blindness and deafness, occurs in a proportion of puppies when both parents carry the blue merle gene.

Enophthalmos
In enophthalmos the eye is sunken, which is normal to some degree in the Collie breeds. It is sometimes present in young dogs, in particular the Flat-Coated and other Retrievers. Enophthalmos leads to prominence of the third eyelid and is found in cases of microphthalmos, Horner's syndrome and, especially, painful conditions of the anterior segment which cause retraction of the globe, for example distichiasis and corneal ulceration. Enophthalmos may also be associated with atrophy of the orbital pad of fat in debilitating diseases.

Exophthalmos or proptosis
These are terms used to describe prominence of an eyeball of normal size. Exophthalmos is normal to a degree in the brachycephalic breeds and in these dogs the third eyelid is retracted. Exophthalmos, together with prominence of the third eyelid, is due to a space-occupying retrobulbar lesion which may be an abscess, orbital neoplasia or, rarely, haemorrhage. A retrobulbar abscess is usually due to a foreign body and is unilateral, sudden in onset and accompanied by pain

and heat. Exophthalmos due to a tumour may lead to deviation of the eye as well as prominence. Exophthalmos can also occur in eosinophilic myositis when one or both eyes are affected.

An exophthalmic eye often appears larger due to the wider palbebral aperture; similarly, when the two pupils are of different size, the eye with the more dilated pupil may appear large.

Hydrophthalmos

An enlarged globe due to stretching of the ocular tunics following chronic glaucoma is termed hydrophthalmos or buphthalmos. The condition is irreversible and is accompanied by blindness. In many instances a high intraocular pressure is maintained and the condition is painful, necessitating enucleation of the globe. If left untreated the final outcome is phthisis bulbi.

Phthisis bulbi

In this condition the eye is small and shrunken due to atrophy of the globe caused by severe inflammation, often following prolonged glaucoma. Both microphthalmos and phthisis bulbi may lead to secondary entropion.

Strabismus or squint

Deviation of the visual axis arises through an imbalance of the extraocular muscles; one or both eyes may be affected with optical axes in any direction. The condition may be congenital or associated with a cranial nerve lesion. Lateral deviation of the globe often follows the replacement of a prolapsed eyeball.

Nystagmus

Nystagmus denotes involuntary oscillation of one or both eyeballs, intermittent or continuous, with variable direction and excursion. The condition may be congenital in puppies with severe visual defects such as dense corneal opacities, partial cataract or retinal abnormality. It is sometimes seen in dogs which have been blind for prolonged periods. Acquired nystagmus may be associated with otitis media, brain tumour, cerebellar disease, trauma or senility (Chapter 5).

The red eye

An inflamed eye with perilimbal (pericorneal) hyperaemia may be encountered in several conditions and often presents a diagnostic challenge. The most important causes of a red eye are conjunctivitis, anterior uveitis (q.v.) and glaucoma (q.v.) (Table 4.2). The nature of the hyperaemia is an important diagnostic criterion. In conjunctivitis the superficial (conjunctival) vessels are hyperaemic whilst in anterior uveitis and glaucoma the deeper episcleral (ciliary) vessels (which are not normally readily visible) are engorged. The conjunctival vessels are mobile over the globe whereas the ciliary vessels do not move with the conjunctiva. Hyperaemic conjunctival vessels, but not ciliary vessels, can be blanched with 0.001% epinephrine or 0.12% phenylephrine. In anterior uveitis and glaucoma the conjunctiva itself rarely appears reddened (although it is possible for all three conditions to occur together) whereas in conjunctivitis the redness may extend across the fornices to the palpebral conjunctiva.

Table 4.2　The red eye: differential diagnosis of conjunctivitis, anterior uveitis and glaucoma.

	Conjunctivitis	Anterior uveitis	Glaucoma
Superficial perilimbal hyperaemia	+	−	−
Deep perilimbal hyperaemia	−	+	+
Elevated IOP	−	−	+
Pupil	Normal	Constricted	Dilated
Pupillary light reflex	Normal	Reduced	Reduced
Pain	±	+	+
Discharge	Possibly mucopurulent	Watery	Watery
Other	−	Dull iris Aqueous flare Hypopyon	?Gonioscopic changes ?Corneal oedema

In all cases presenting with a red eye the interior of the eye should be examined and digital, or preferably instrumental, tonometry performed.

Other causes of or factors contributing to a red eye include corneal ulceration, keratitis, keratoconjunctivitis sicca, episcleritis and retrobulbar lesions, including abscesses, foreign bodies and neoplasms.

Conjunctivitis

The bulbar conjunctiva covers the anterior aspect of the globe as far as the corneal limbus; the palpebral conjunctiva lines the inner surface of the eyelids and both surfaces of the third eyelid.

Clinical signs of conjunctivitis are congestion of the blood vessels, ocular discharge varying from serous to mucopurulent, blepharospasm and slight irritation which may lead to self-inflicted damage. Conjunctivitis may be acute or chronic with subsequent hypertrophy and may be unilateral or bilateral. Causal agents include bacteria, viruses, fungi and allergens; it may also be associated with foreign bodies, wind, trauma and ectropion.

Treatment. Cleanliness together with antibiotic drops or ointment with or without corticosteroids, administered topically or subconjunctivally but not systemically. Steroids and antihistamines are indicated in allergic conjunctivitis. Bacteriology is of limited value.

Follicular conjunctivitis

Hyperplasia of the subepithelial lymphoid follicles as a result of non-specific irritation and usually affecting the palpebral conjunctiva and the external surface of the third eyelid. It is best treated by bursting the small follicles by rubbing with a copper sulphate crystal or with cotton wool on mosquito forceps, followed by the application of an antibiotic ointment.

Bilateral conjunctivitis

This occurs in distemper and other systemic pyrexias; it may also be a primary condition.

Subconjunctival haemorrhage

This commonly follows trauma and treatment is unnecessary.

Chemosis or conjunctival oedema

This is usually due to allergy, trauma or the presence of a foreign body. Chemosis following trauma to the head can lead to severe drying of the cornea, possibly resulting in loss of the eye.

The wet eye

Lacrimation with a subsequent rust-coloured tear streak, wetting of the hair on the cheek and possibly dermatitis is due to overproduction of tears. Inadequate drainage of tears is called epiphora. The fluorescein test (one drop of fluorescein in the eye and examination of the nostril a few minutes later for evidence of a green stain) is not always reliable as a test for lacrimal duct patency, and if negative it should not be assumed that the duct is absent or blocked. Irrigation via a nasolacrimal duct cannula, under local or general anaesthesia, together with probing with a dilator, would be the next step in an investigation.

Overproduction of tears occurs in all eye diseases where there is irritation. Common causes include the presence of supernumerary eyelashes or ectopic cilia, nasal folds, entropion, foreign bodies, conjunctivitis, corneal ulcers, glaucoma and hypertrophy of the glands of the third eyelid.

Inadequate drainage is due to either congenital or acquired closure of the puncta or canaliculi, or both. It can also occur in cases of ectropion where the puncta are not in contact with the tear film. An infection of the lacrimal sac and duct (dacryocystitis) is often accompanied by a persistent, and usually unilateral, purulent conjunctivitis. Dacryocystitis or blockage of the canaliculus by mucus in cases of catarrhal conjunctivitis may both lead to epiphora.

Treatment. Surgical, including irrigation of the nasolactimal duct system.

The dry eye

Keratoconjunctivitis sicca

This condition is due to impaired tear secretion and can be unilateral or bilateral. There are many possible causes, but in the majority of cases the cause is unknown. The clinical signs include a tacky and profuse mucoid ocular discharge, a thickened and red conjunctiva, vascularisation, ulceration, pigmentation and opacity of the cornea, loss of lid mobility, a narrowed palpebral fissure and dry nostrils. Severe corneal changes can sometimes lead to eventual blindness. There is considerable variation in the degree of severity, but all cases have a diminished Schirmer Tear Test result. Rose Bengal (1%) may be used to stain devitalised corneal epithelial cells (Plate 4.5).

Treatment. Medical therapy is based upon the frequent application of an artificial tear preparation to preserve the tear film. Preparations including hydroxy-propyl methylcellulose (hypromellose) (Isoptoplain) or polyvinyl alcohol (PVA) (Liquifilm) are particularly suitable. The most common reason for failure is insufficient frequency of application, and an initial rate of application of at least ten times per day is a reasonable guideline. If deemed necessary topical antibiotics and corticosteroids may be given. Pilocarpine drops given orally are sometimes used to stimulate lacrimal gland secretion (for details see specialist texts). Severe cases may be treated surgically by parotid duct transposition; the results are usually effective, but overproduction of tears may present a real problem to the owner.

THE CORNEA

The cornea is an avascular structure comprising several layers, with the collagenous substantia propia, or stroma, occupying most of the thickness. This is bounded anteriorly by stratified squamous epithelium, which is continuous with the bulbar conjunctiva, and posteriorly by a single cell layer, the endothelium (mesothelium). Beneath the endothelium is a tough elastic layer known as Descemet's membrane. Both limiting membranes, but particularly the endothelium, contribute to a delicate pump mechanism which maintains the cornea in a state of deturgescence compatible with transparency. Impairment of this mechanism, for example following endothelial damage or a rise in intraocular pressure, leads to corneal oedema and thus corneal opacity.

The anterior surface of the cornea is kept moist by the tear film. The corneal reflex, or reflection of light from an instrument or any other light source, should normally be sharp and regular and is most useful for revealing alterations or irregularities of the surface. Sensitivity of the cornea (Vth cranial nerve) may be tested with a wisp of cotton wool to evoke a blink reflex.

Keratitis

Inflammations of the cornea are common in the dog and of varying types. Aetiology includes bacterial, viral and fungal infections, trauma, foreign bodies, impaired tear secretion, glaucoma, and anterior luxation of the lens. Certain breeds of dog exhibit specific types of keratitis and certain types of dog, especially brachycephalic breeds, are more prone to keratitis than others. Keratitis may affect part or all of the cornea, and may be unilateral or bilateral. Presenting signs include corneal opacity, vascularisation and pigmentation; blepharospasm, lacrimation and photophobia may be present.

Infections involving the corneal stroma may be treated with subconjunctival and systemic antibiotics in addition to topical preparations. Because anterior uveitis may also be present topical atropine may be indicated. Chronic keratitis results in fibrosis and pigmentation.

Vascular keratitis

Both superficial and deep (interstitial) types occur. In the superficial form new blood vessels extend from the bulbar conjunctiva and branch in a treelike form (vascular arborisation) on the cornea. In the deep form neovascularisation appears as straight brushlike vessels in the corneal stroma and is often accompanied by oedema. Photophobia may accompany the blepharospasm and lacrimation may occur with superficial keratitis.

Treatment. An attempt should be made to identify the cause. Corticosteroids are indicated to control excessive vascularisation and both steroids and atropine may be useful for associated anterior uveitis.

Pigmentary keratitis

Pigmentary changes are usually secondary to vascular keratitis, with the pigment being carried via the blood vessels from the pigmented limbus. They are superficial and sometimes bilateral, but the two eyes may not be equally affected. Occasionally cases of deep pigmentation are encountered, particularly in the West Highland White Terrier and Pug. When the pigmentation does not appear to be secondary to neovascularisation it may be uveal in origin.

Chronic superficial keratitis or pannus

Pannus is a progressive and bilateral, but not necessarily symmetrical, condition in which the cornea undergoes subepithelial neovascularisation, granulation and pigmentation extending from the limbus. It is seen typically in the German Shepherd Dog and crossbreeds of this breed, and sometimes in the Collie breeds. Onset occurs in middle age (usually 3–7 years). The cause is unknown but autoimmune phenomena, initiated or exacerbated by environmental factors, are suspected.

The lower temporal quadrant is most frequently

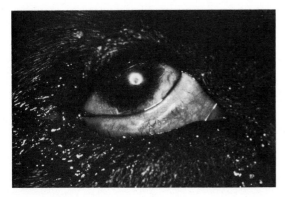

Plate 4.1 Entropion of the lower lid in a German Short-haired Pointer.

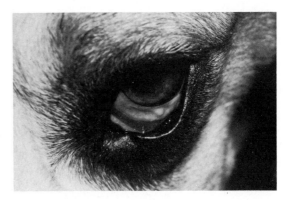

Plate 4.2 Ectropion in a Beagle.

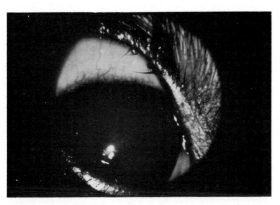

Plate 4.3 Distichiasis, with secondary corneal ulceration, in a Shetland Sheepdog.

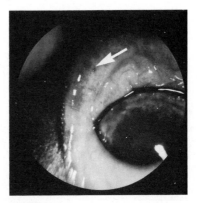

Plate 4.4 An ectopic cilium arising from the base of a meibomian gland and penetrating the palpebral conjunctiva.

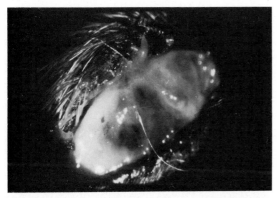

Plate 4.5 Keratoconjunctivitis sicca in a West Highland White Terrier. The thick tacky discharge is characteristic.

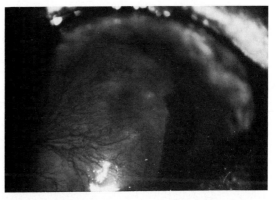

Plate 4.6 Corneal pannus (chronic superficial keratitis) in a German Shepherd Dog.

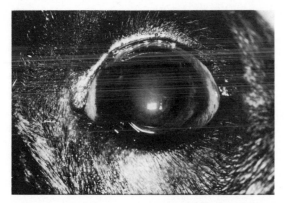

Plate 4.7 Indolent ulcer (recurrent epithelial erosion) in an 8-year-old Boxer.

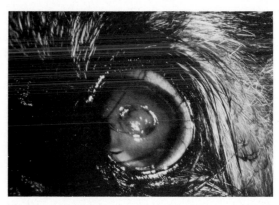

Plate 4.8 Deep corneal ulcer with hypopyon and corneal oedema in a Pekingese.

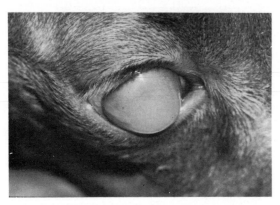

Plate 4.9 Corneal oedema (blue-eye) and keratoglobus in a Weimaraner following vaccination with attenuated CAV-1.

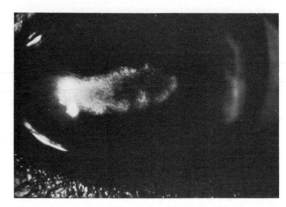

Plate 4.10 Corneal lipidosis in a Cavalier King Charles Spaniel. The corneal lesion is subepithelial and unaccompanied by inflammatory changes.

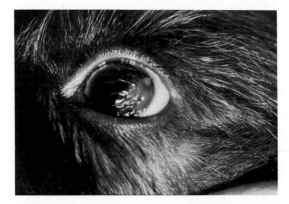

Plate 4.11 Corneal dermoid in a crossbred. The skin-like tissue is limited almost entirely to the cornea.

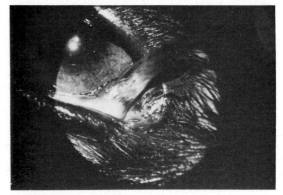

Plate 4.12 Conjunctival dermoid in a German Shepherd Dog. The cornea is unaffected but note the deformity of the outer canthus.

affected, but the condition may ultimately involve the whole cornea, corneal opacity and pigmentation rendering the eye blind. Occasionally the third eyelid is involved (Plate 4.6).

Treatment. The condition may be controlled, but not cured, by topical or subconjunctival steroid therapy. The authors' preference is for topical fluocinolone (Synalar) lotion given six times daily initially and reducing gradually over a period of six weeks, by which time most moderate lesions have resolved. Ultimately, however, further steroid therapy will be required. Heavy depositions of pigment can often be treated successfully by superficial keratectomy.

Corneal ulceration

Corneal ulceration implies loss of epithelium (superficial ulceration, corneal erosion) or epithelium together with stroma (deep ulceration).

The causes are many and include trauma (especially resulting from distichiasis, ectopic cilia, entropion, conjunctival lithiasis, etc.), infectious agents and degenerative, and therefore predisposing, conditions of the cornea; also chemical and thermal burns. Accompanying signs of ulceration are redness, pain, blepharospasm, photophobia and lacrimation. Diagnosis is confirmed by the ability to stain with fluorescein, which may be rendered more obvious under Wood's lamp (Plates 4.7, 4.8).

Treatment. It is important to identify and remove the cause, if possible. Particular attention should be given to locating ectopic cilia, which are frequently overlooked. Antibiotic eye ointment and chemical cauterisation should be applied when necessary. For cautery, phenol is preferred to iodine or silver nitrate. Washing and lubrication is important for burns. The indolent ulcer, seen particularly in the Boxer and Pembroke Corgi, should be cauterised and all loosely adherent epithelium removed from the edge of the ulcer. Topical atropine drops should be administered in all cases when iritis is present. Suturing of the third eyelid across the cornea is an extremely valuable procedure for the deep ulcer, or the ulcer which fails to respond to topical therapy.

Collagenase ulcers

Rapid degeneration (melting) of the cornea with deep ulceration can result from the liberation of collagenase from *Pseudomonas* spp. and also from the corneal tissues themselves. Initially reported in the USA, the condition has recently been encountered in the UK. Treatment should include antibiotics active against *Pseudomonas*, anticollagenases such as EDTA or acetylcysteine and the application of a third eyelid flap.

Descemetocoele

A deep corneal ulcer where corneal erosion has led to exposure of Descemet's membrane (which does not stain with fluorescein). The danger of corneal perforation is significant and treatment should include the application of a third eyelid flap or other precautionary measures.

Corneal oedema associated with canine adenovirus type 1

Corneal oedema ('blue eye') is seen in a proportion of dogs recovering from infectious canine hepatitis (canine adenovirus type 1 infection; see also Chapter 13) but nowadays it is seen more frequently 10-14 days after vaccination with live attenuated virus. This phenomenon, essentially a manifestation of keratouveitis, results from an antigen–antibody reaction within the eye. It is usually unilateral and transient, with the cornea clearing completely without treatment within a few days. Prolonged or severe cases may lead to a bullous keratopathy with small vesicles of fluid appearing in the corneal epithelium. Sometimes the corneal oedema fails to disperse due to extensive damage to the corneal endothelial cells. Corneas which have not cleared within approximately two weeks are unlikely to resolve completely. Glaucoma may develop in a proportion of cases which fail to resolve (Plate 4.9).

Treatment. Topical therapy with atropine and corticosteroids is directed primarily at the anterior uveitis. If secondary glaucoma develops both atropine and steroids should be discontinued, being contraindicated when the intraocular pressure is raised. Hypertonic saline and glycerine applied topically may be useful in some cases to clear the corneal oedema, but are usually of little value.

Other causes of diffuse corneal oedema

Diffuse corneal oedema may occur as a result of an increase in intraocular pressure and in severe cases of anterior uveitis.

Corneal oedema is sometimes encountered in the Chihuahua and some brachycephalic breeds and is probably due to an endothelial dystrophy.

Corneal degenerations and infiltrations

Subepithelial deposition of lipid (corneal lipidosis; Plate 10) produces a well-demarcated round or oval opacity at or near the centre of the cornea; this is usually bilateral. There are no other signs. Treatment is unnecessary and medical treatment is of no avail.

Other corneal opacities may be due to the deposition of cholesterol and calcification of the corneal stroma, with the epithelium sometimes involved. Such lesions may be central or peripheral in position and unilateral or bilateral. Vascularisation occurs in a few cases and may be associated with other corneal disease or certain systemic disorders.

Treatment. Superficial keratectomy is possible in these conditions.

Corneal dermoid

This is a congenital, fleshy, usually pigmented, hairy area on the cornea or, more rarely, the conjunctiva (Plates 4.11, 4.12).

Treatment. Surgical removal.

Differential diagnosis of corneal signs

Corneal vascularisation
Superficial and interstitial keratitis
Pannus
Keratoconjunctivitis sicca
Corneal response to foreign bodies, injury, eyelid tumours, supernumerary eyelashes, nasal folds, entropion and other forms of irritation
Healing of deep or persistent corneal ulcer
Glaucoma

Corneal pigmentation
Pannus
Keratoconjunctivitis sicca
Other forms of chronic keratitis

Corneal opacity
Scar formation
Corneal ulcer (stains with fluorescein)
Corneal oedema
Corneal lipidosis (does not stain with fluorescein)
Corneal degenerations and infiltrations
Small and large opacities due to persistent pupillary membranes
Posterior corneal opacity due to a anteriorly luxated lens
Keratic precipitates and hypopyon

THE ANTERIOR CHAMBER

The anterior chamber is a fluid-filled space between the cornea and the iris (the posterior chamber lies between the iris and lens). Both chambers are occupied by aqueous fluid which is produced by the ciliary body and drains, via the iridocorneal angle, into the scleral venous plexus. The aqueous fluid is derived from plasma, but the composition is modified at the blood–aqueous barrier of the ciliary body. The aqueous fluid is responsible for the intraocular pressure (IOP).

The posterior chamber is of little clinical significance and will not be considered further.

Uveal exudation

Slight changes in uveal permeability affect the chemical composition of the aqueous fluid, notably by increasing its protein content. Significant uveal disturbance allows leakage of higher molecular weight proteins such as fibrinogen and fibrinous strands may appear in the aqueous fluid or at the pupillary margin. The increased protein content may be detectable in a light beam as 'aqueous flare'. Severe uveal disturbance leads to inflammatory cell effusion. Cells dispersed throughout the aqueous fluid are seen with the ophthalmoscope as a multitude of points of light. Cells may precipitate in the lower iridocorneal angle to form a compact mass (hypopyon) which, in severe cases, may fill half the anterior chamber. A small hypopyon is best viewed from the dorsal limbus. Inflammatory cells and cellular debris may adhere to the endothelial surface of the cornea, forming keratic precipitates (KPs). Adherence is facilitated when corneal function is impaired and the presence of KPs suggest the possibility of primary corneal disease.

Although inflammatory cells in the anterior chamber may suggest primary uveitis, their presence is often secondary to a problem elsewhere, for example keratitis or degeneration of the lens. Transudate or exudate in the anterior chamber is usually sterile, resulting from toxicity rather than infection (Plates 4.13, 4.14).

Treatment. Provided that the primary cause is transient or can be relieved, even severe hypopyon can disperse rapidly and no attempt should be made to drain off cellular material. Corticosteroids are the most effective empirical treatment, but concurrent eye disease, particularly corneal ulceration, may preclude their use.

Hyphaema

The presence of blood in the anterior chamber (hyphaema) can arise from a variety of causes, including trauma to the eye or head, penetrating foreign bodies, intraocular neoplasms, glaucoma, Collie eye anomaly, purpura and infectious canine hepatitis. In most instances bleeding is from vessels of the anterior uvea. When diagnosing hyphaema it is important to:

1 Establish that blood is in the anterior chamber and not in the vitreous body.
2 Examine the other eye for abnormalities suggestive of a congenital cause.

Hyphaema is not in itself of great consequence as removal of erythrocytes by phagocytosis is efficient. An extensive blood clot, by impeding aqueous outflow, can cause glaucoma but this is rare. Persistent hyphaema suggests serious ocular disease and should receive a poor prognosis.

Treatment. The primary cause, if determined, should be treated (e.g. uveitis with corticosteroids, glaucoma with miotics or carbonic anhydrase inhibitors). Pilocarpine may be used to constrict the pupil to hasten dispersal and the patient should be kept quiet. Under normal circumstances no attempt should be made to remove blood by paracentesis. Vitamin K, which can lead to prothrombin deficiency, should not be given unless there is specific evidence of a coagulation defect.

Foreign bodies

These have already been considered, being of major importance in association with the cornea. However, penetrating lesions of the cornea, even if treated surgically, occasionally leave fragments of foreign body, or pyogenic foci, within the anterior chamber. If the eye is quiescent foreign bodies are best left *in situ*. Slit-lamp biomicroscopy is a useful aid to their detection.

Luxated lens

A lens which has luxated anteriorly will usually be clearly visible within the anterior chamber, yet it is surprising how frequently the condition is misdiagnosed, presumably because the corneal opacity resulting from contact with the lens suggests a primary keratitis. A focal light source should reveal the lens equator or, if the pupil is dilated, an aphakic crescent between the equator and the iris. Fluorescence under Wood's lamp offers useful confirmation.

Neoplasms

Neoplasms seen within the anterior chamber are not common in the dog, but when they occur they are almost always associated with the uveal tract. Hence care should be taken to distinguish them from iritis. They may be primary or secondary. Amongst the most frequent are melanomas (malignant or benign) (Plate 4.15), adenomas and adenocarcinomas, lymphosarcomas and haemangiomas. Neoplasms of mammary origin are the commonest secondary tumour.

A bilateral condition suggests lymphosarcoma, or another secondary tumour, and primary foci should be sought with attention to lymph nodes and mammary glands. However, ocular manifestations can be a first sign of lymphosarcoma. In spite of the impracticability of biopsy, a provisional diagnosis is necessary for a decision on whether or not to enucleate the eye. Melanomas and adenomas, and adenocarcinomas of the ciliary body, are locally invasive and prone to metastasis; in either case the globe is best enucleated.

Pigmented iris cysts are occasionally found floating in the anterior chamber or attached to the pupil margin. These are of no clinical significance.

Persistent pupillary membranes

Persistent pupillary membranes are strands of tissue present in the anterior chamber which represent incomplete atrophy of fetal mesodermal tissue. Usually they link iris with cornea and may cause local corneal opacity at the point of insertion; sometimes they may attach to the lens, with associated capsular cataract, or traverse the pupil. In young puppies these tissues can be expected to atrophy completely by a few weeks of age and no treatment is necessary. In the Basenji and some other breeds the condition is inherited and is permanent.

THE ANTERIOR UVEA

The anterior uvea comprises the iris and ciliary body. They are considered together because a condition affecting one usually involves the other. Anterior uveitis is synonymous with iridocyclitis. Posterior uveitis (choroiditis) is considered later (see p. 104).

Anterior uveitis

An eye experiencing an acute iridocyclitis exhibits photophobia, pain, blepharospasm and lacrimation, and may present as a red eye. The iris is typically thickened and the surface rough in texture and dull. The pupil is constricted (a pathognomonic sign, with Horner's syndrome the exception) and iris mobility is reduced or lost. Fibrinous strands may be present in the pupil and the aqueous fluid may exhibit flare, hypopyon and sometimes hyphaema. Cells and cellular debris may adhere to the cornea and to the anterior lens capsule.

Close attention should be paid to the perilimbal hyperaemia which is deep rather than superficial and is sometimes referred to as 'ciliary flush'. This is typical of glaucoma also but affords a useful distinction from conjunctivitis, where the hyperaemia is more superficial. Uveitis is accompanied by a fall in intraocular pressure, often to the extent that the eye feels soft.

Consequences of uveitis include adhesions between iris and lens (posterior synechiae) and between iris and cornea (peripheral anterior synechiae). Blockage of the iridocorneal angle and trabecular meshwork with inflammatory debris, and the formation of anterior synechiae (Plate 4.16), can both precipitate an attack of glaucoma; so too can posterior synechiae when pupillary block occurs (iris bombé). Following an episode of uveitis the colour of the iris may darken significantly and remain as a permanent reminder, even in an otherwise wholly recovered eye.

Many forms of anterior uveitis are recurrent.

Pathogenesis

Whilst the clinical sign of anterior uveitis are distinctive and readily recognised they are rarely specific for any one cause. Indeed it is probably true to say that in the majority of cases the cause cannot be established. Uveitis can exist at the histological level without being clinically apparent.

There is little doubt that in many instances of uveitis immunological factors are involved. The presence of an antigen in the eye will lead to the sensitisation of specific lymphoid cells within the uveal tract and of others which arise exogenously. Depending on the nature and duration of the antigenic stimulus both local antibody (from plasma cells) and/or cell-mediated hypersensitivity reactions may proceed within the uvea. In many respects the uvea behaves as a lymph node and some cases of uveitis may be manifestations of lymphoid cell proliferation which in a lymph node would be regarded as functional rather than pathological. As a result of such phenomena the eye can remain sensitised to further antigenic stimulation and may reinflame sometimes months or even years later. In addition, the uveal tissues, or rather their products following cell lysis, can act as autoantigens capable of participating in both humoral and cell-mediated reactions in the same way as microbial antigens. The antigen–antibody reaction, especially through leucocytic chemotaxis, and the release of cytolytic lysosomal enzymes, can bring about uveal cell death and hence augmentation of the reaction. Thus, toxic agents including the cytolytic products of neoplasms and microbial agents, microbes themselves and autoantigens, such as released lens protein, can all initiate and compound a vicious circle which can manifest as a recurrent or chronic phenomenon depending on the nature and duration of the stimulus. Circulating immune complexes can also initiate the cycle.

Specific causes of uveitis

Microbial causes. There are apparently no specific bacterial causes of uveitis apart from infections resulting from penetrating wounds or from generalised systemic infections (e.g. leptospirosis). The toxins produced by *Pseudomonas aeruginosa* in deep keratitis can cause anterior uveitis. Infection with canine adenovirus type 1, the cause of infectious canine hepatitis, commonly produces a mild anterior uveitis after approximately one week as a result of virus invading susceptible tissue of the eye. A proportion of such eyes will subsequently experience a local viral antigen–antibody reaction which can initiate a corneal oedema (blue eye) and a massive, but usually transient, anterior uveitis. Approximately 10 per cent of affected eyes will exhibit complications such as persistent corneal oedema and vascularisation, hypopyon and sometimes glaucoma.

Other possible viral causes of anterior uveitis include canine distemper virus and canine herpesvirus.

Uveitis may sometimes be encountered in certain fungal conditions such as cryptococcosis, blastomycosis and histoplasmosis and the parasite *Toxoplasma gondii* may also be implicated.

In a number of these infections anterior uveitis may result from hypersensitivity reactions rather than from direct infection of the eye.

Other causes. Lens-induced (phacoanaphylactic) uveitis can result from the escape of lenticular material into the eye; this may occur following trauma, spontaneous rupture of the capsule, leakage from mature cataracts, or following extracapsular cataract extraction.

Neoplasia, both primary and secondary, can initiate uveitis.

Treatment

Corticosteroids constitute the most effective treatment

for anterior uveitis and may be administered as drops or ointment, or injected subconjunctivally. Treatment should be continued at least until final resolution has been achieved. Where for some reason corticosteroids are specifically contraindicated, for example when severe corneal ulceration is present, other non-steroidal anti-inflammatory drugs (e.g. indomethasin or phenylbutazone) may be considered.

Atropine sulphate (usually as a 1% or 2% solution) is of value for relieving pain and preventing the development of synechiae and subsequent glaucoma. Because atropine is far less effective as a mydriatic in the inflamed eye, compared with the normal eye, the frequency of application must be increased according to severity and should be consistent with maintaining a dilated pupil.

THE LENS

The lens of the dog is relatively large, measuring 10–12 mm in diameter and 7–8 mm in axial thickness. It is situated immediately behind, and in contact with, the iris, which is displaced forward slightly towards the pupillary margin. The lens occupies a depression in the face of the vitreous body known as the patellar fossa and it is partly adherent to the vitreous on its posterior aspect. The fibres of the suspensory ligament of the lens, or zonule, arise from the pars plana and pars plicata (ciliary processes) of the ciliary body and insert at the lens equator. Changes in size or shape of the lens, through resorption or tumescence, will alter the depth of the anterior chamber.

The lens consists of an outer capsule, thicker anteriorly than posteriorly, an outer cortex and an inner nucleus. Immediately beneath the anterior capsule is the lens epithelium, which is responsible for the active transport of ions and amino acids and for protein synthesis. At the lens equator epithelial cells elongate to form the secondary lens fibres; the manner in which these fibres are laid down results in the formation of anterior and posterior suture lines. The energy source for the lens is glucose which, like other metabolites, is derived from the aqueous fluid.

The lens is viewed through the pupil, with mydriasis being essential for complete examination. The suture lines may appear as opaque lines in certain lights (erect Y anteriorly, inverted Y posteriorly) and their prominence varies considerably from one dog to another. Occasionally in puppies dark opacities, sometimes arrowhead-shaped, occur around the suture lines but these often disappear in the adult. In young puppies, shortly after the eyes are open, it is usual to see remnants of the pupillary membrane resembling a spider's web in the pupil; these remnants are only temporary and disappear by a few weeks of age. In the adult dog it is common to see a short thread of hyaloid artery attached to the posterior aspect of the lens close to the point where the suture lines meet; movement of this faintly opaque remnant occurs in the vitreous with eye movement. The older dog exhibits senile nuclear sclerosis of the lens, a normal age change due to compression of lens fibres and fluid loss. It does not interfere with vision although it may appear as an opacity or opalescence of the centre of the lens in direct light. It should not be confused with cataract and is readily distinguished, using distant direct ophthalmoscopy, by viewing the lens in light reflected from the tapetal fundus.

Cataract

The term cataract denotes any opacity of the lens, including its capsule. Cataract may be classified as primary (no other eye changes apparent) or secondary (associated with a disease of other parts of the eye); in addition, cataracts may arise in association with many systemic disturbances.* Cataract is very common in the dog, but in many cases the aetiology is unknown. Cataracts may be bilateral or unilateral, partial or total, symmetrical or non-symmetrical, progressive or non-progressive, permanent or temporary, congenital or occurring at any time in later life. Temporary cataract is rare in the dog but lens resorption in young dogs with cataract is not uncommon. The position of the opacity may be useful in prognosis: for example, cortical cataracts often progress, whereas capsular cataracts do not.

Some cataracts are inherited. Primary hereditary cataracts are not apparently associated with other ocular disease and are often referred to collectively as 'hereditary cataract'. Cataracts may also be secondary to other inherited ocular disease, e.g. progressive retinal atrophy (q.v.).

Congenital cataract

Congenital cataracts usually result from infectious or toxic insults to the fetus during pregnancy, most of which are not amenable to investigation. In such cases all or at least several puppies in a litter are affected, although the severity may vary from one individual to another. Usually both eyes are affected. Commonly,

---

* In the opinion of the authors it is preferable to restrict the term 'secondary' to events occurring within the eye.

other ocular signs such as persistent pupillary membranes, microphthalmos, nystagmus, iris anomalies and retinal folds may be present. Only in rare instances are congenital cataracts inherited.

Persistent pupillary membranes are sometimes attached to the lens capsule and may be associated with focal cataracts (Plate 4.17). Sometimes a persistent hyaloid artery may have an associated opacity on the posterior capsule and, rarely, intralenticular haemorrhage and lens opacity may accompany a persistent hyaloid artery containing blood.

Primary hereditary cataract

Most forms of primary hereditary cataract are inherited in a simple Mendelian manner (usually recessive) and are thus amenable to some degree of control by judicious breeding. It is important to remember that, on the basis of ophthalmological examination, most hereditary cataracts are not congenital. However, generally speaking, they tend to arise in early life, most being detectable by one year of age. Such cataracts are not usually accompanied by other ocular signs, an important distinction from congenital cataracts.

A remarkable feature of primary hereditary cataract is its marked breed specificity. For each susceptible breed the age of onset, distribution of opacities within the lens, the rate of progression and the extent to which the lesions are bilaterally symmetrical are often characteristic. The ophthalmoscopic appearance of a cataract can thus be of diagnostic value, although the diagnosis of hereditary cataract in one individual alone should only be made with great caution.

Congenital forms of hereditary cataract appear to be limited to the Miniature Schnauzer. Whilst in the remaining breeds the first signs of cataract are seen in early life; in the American Cocker Spaniel and the Golden Retriever cataracts may not appear until middle age. In the Miniature Schnauzer, Staffordshire Bull Terrier and the Boston Terrier bilateral symmetry is always obvious, but in the American Cocker Spaniel and the Golden Retriever asymmetry is commonly observed; in the latter breeds there are also progressive and non-progressive forms. In the Golden Retriever a non-progressive posterior polar cataract and a progressive form of cataract, both of which may occur in the same individual, are probably both expressions of the same dominant gene. Features of primary hereditary cataract in susceptible breeds in the UK are shown in Table 4.3.

Outside the UK, hereditary cataracts have been reported in the Chesapeake Bay Retriever, the Standard Poodle and the West Highland White Terrier (Plates 4.18, 4.19).

Secondary cataracts

Cataract associated with anterior uveitis. Cataract can sometimes follow severe inflammation of the iris or anterior uvea. Accompanying signs include aqueous flare, miosis, lowered intraocular pressure, ciliary infection, photophobia, posterior synechiae and change in colour of the iris.

Cataract associated with glaucoma

Cataract secondary to retinal disease. Cataract often accompanies retinal disease, including detachment, and is frequently encountered in advanced cases of generalised progressive retinal atrophy and sometimes in association with central progressive retinal atrophy. Many cataracts which present in the Miniature Poodle and Cocker Spaniel are secondary to a hereditary retinopathy. In such cases confirmation of retinal dys-

Table 4.3   Primary hereditary cataract.

Breed	Mode of inheritance	Approx. earliest age diagnosed	Approx. age limit for onset*	Remarks
Afghan Hound	Recessive	1 year	3 years	Bilateral, usually asymmetric
American Cocker Spaniel	Recessive (?)	6 months	5 years	Bilateral, asymmetric
Boston Terrier	Recessive	2 months	18 months	Bilateral, symmetric
German Shepherd Dog	Recessive (?)	2 months	3 years	Bilateral, asymmetric
Golden Retriever and Labrador Retriever	Dominant	9 months	6 years	Not necessarily bilateral or symmetric; often polar, sometimes total
Miniature Schnauzer	Recessive	3 months	3 years	Bilateral, symmetric
Old English Sheepdog	Recessive (?)	6 months	5 years	Complicated
Staffordshire Bull Terrier	Recessive	3 months	18 months	Bilateral, symmetric
Welsh Springer Spaniel	Recessive	2 months	3 years	Bilateral, usually symmetric

* Ages for final certification under the BVA/Kennel Club Eye Examination Scheme.

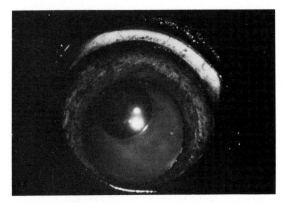

Plate 4.13 Pigmented uveal cyst free in the anterior chamber in a Labrador Retriever.

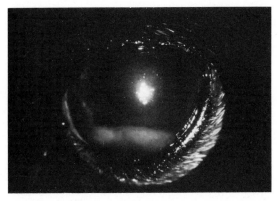

Plate 4.14 Hypopyon resulting from acute anterior uveitis.

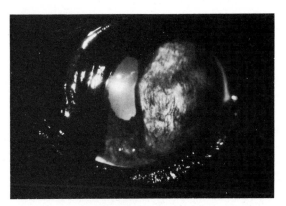

Plate 4.15 Malignant melanoma of the anterior uvea in an Afghan Hound.

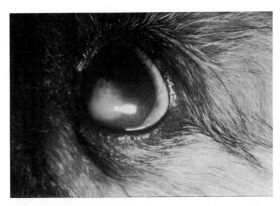

Plate 4.16 Focal corneal scar and anterior synechiae with distortion of the pupil in a Pekingese.

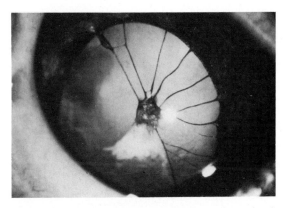

Plate 4.17 Persistent pupillary membranes and associated congenital cataract in an Old English Sheepdog.

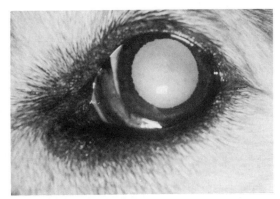

Plate 4.18 Hereditary cataract in a Golden Retriever. The lens opacity is total and illustrates the progressive form of the cataract in this breed.

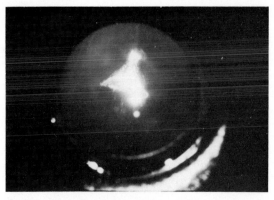

Plate 4.19 Hereditary cataract in a Golden Retriever. In this form the opacity is focal and situated at the posterior pole of the lens.

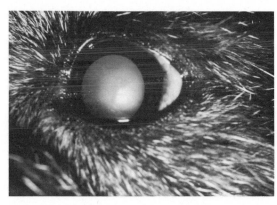

Plate 4.20 Diabetic cataract in an 8-year-old crossbred bitch.

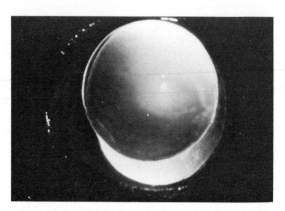

Plate 4.21 Primary lens luxation in a Jack Russell Terrier. The displaced lens is clearly visible in the anterior chamber.

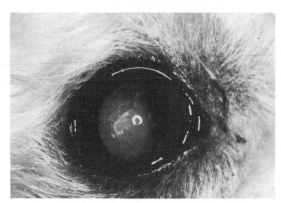

Plate 4.22 Lens luxation secondary to cataract formation in a 12-year-old Poodle with progressive retinal atrophy.

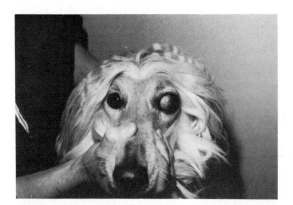

Plate 4.23 Unilateral hydrophthalmos in an Afghan Hound following a blue-eye reaction.

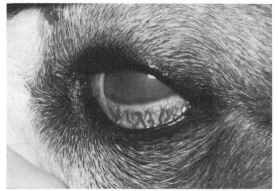

Plate 4.24 Primary glaucoma in a Beagle showing typical congestion of the episcleral vessels and an advancing corneal vascular fringe.

function (e.g. by electroretinography) can be valuable in forestalling unnecessary cataract surgery.

Traumatic cataract
Trauma to the globe, either penetrating or non-penetrating, can lead to cataract formation if there is accompanying damage to the lens capsule. Direct penetration of the anterior lens capsule by a thorn or shotgun pellet invariably leads to cortical damage. The release of lens-specific proteins through a traumatised capsule may initiate a lens-induced (phacoanaphylactic) uveitis or endophthalmitis. Where the degree of inflammation cannot be controlled medically, it may be advisable to remove the traumatised lens.

Diabetic cataract
Cataractous changes commonly accompany diabetes mellitus in the dog. The cataracts tend to be bilaterally symmetrical, rapid in onset and progressive, becoming total within weeks or sometimes even days. Pupillary light reflexes usually remain brisk. Other systemic signs are present (Plate 4.20).

Toxic cataract
A number of toxic chemicals are known to cause cataract, but they are seldom implicated in veterinary practice. Chlorpromazine derivatives are known to be cataractogenic following prolonged use. Various forms of irradiation are also cataractogenic.

Treatment of cataract

Primary cataract. Surgical extraction of the lens should be considered; however, little is to be gained in unilateral cases. The pupillary light reflex, or the electroretinogram, is useful to assess retinal function in bilateral cases.

Secondary cataract. The primary condition should be treated wherever possible. Various medical treatments have been described over the years, but none has survived the test of time.

Leukocoria

Leukocoria is defined as a white pupil.
Cataract is the commonest cause of this clinical sign but retinal detachment, particularly exudative, and retinal dysplasia may present as an opacity in the pupil. Collections of brown pigment granules on the anterior lens capsule, usually about the centre, are often seen in the dog and are remnants of the pupillary membrane. They could be confused with cataract when the lens is viewed against the tapetal reflex in reflected light.

Lens luxation

Lens luxation is not a common condition in the dog, but its occurrence frequently necessitates immediate surgical intervention in order to prevent the development of secondary glaucoma and loss of vision. Unfortunately, many cases still pass unrecognised, being treated as inflammations of the anterior segment.

The term luxation denotes total displacement or dislocation of the lens from its normal position; it implies rupture of the zonule, or suspensory apparatus of the lens, the fibres of which arise from the pars plana and ciliary processes and insert at the lens equator. Subluxation describes an intermediate stage in which there is partial breakdown of the zonule but the lens, although slightly mobile, remains in its grossly normal position. Lens dislocations may result from many causes, which may be classified as congenital, primary, secondary or traumatic. Primary luxations, in which there is no apparent antecedent ocular disease, are the more numerous (at least in the UK); dislocations secondary to other ocular disease are not uncommon but those which are congenital or due to trauma alone are relatively rare.

Primary lens luxation
In the UK spontaneous displacement of the lens in the adult dog has been a clinical problem for many years and the terrier breeds are particularly prone to this condition. It arises in middle age (usually 3–7 years) and either sex may be affected. It is encountered most frequently in the Jack Russell Terrier, but is also seen in the Tibetan Terrier, the Sealyham, the Miniature Bull Terrier, and the Fox Terriers, and isolated cases occur in other Terrier breeds. In the Tibetan Terrier the condition is inherited as an autosomal recessive gene, and this mode of inheritance may well be applicable to other affected breeds.

It has now been established that the cause of primary lens luxation is an inherent weakness of the zonule which, although evident microscopically at an early age, only becomes clinically apparent in adulthood. The essential lesion is always bilateral (Plate 4.21).

Clinical signs
In practice, lens luxation seldom becomes apparent to an owner until the lens has fully dislocated, even though subtle clinical changes may have been apparent in the eye for many weeks or months. Most

luxations are anterior, but sometimes the lens passes posteriorly and ventrally into the vitreous body; it should be remembered also that the lens is often capable of migrating back and forth through the pupil. An anteriorly luxated lens is usually accompanied by a well-demarcated sub-central corneal opacity (which should not be confused with a primary keratitis) and the outline of the lens is clearly visible in the beam of a pen torch. The presence of an aphakic crescent, more obvious if the pupil is dilated, is pathognomonic of a posterior luxation, or of advanced subluxation. If a luxated lens remains in the anterior chamber the development of secondary glaucoma is almost inevitable; if this happens it may be difficult to determine whether lens luxation or glaucoma is the primary condition.

Examination of the contralateral eye in an apparently unilateral case of lens luxation almost always reveals evidence of subluxation. Typically the iris exhibits iridodonesis (trembling resulting from movement of the globe due to lack of support by the lens), deepening of the anterior chamber and the presence of small grey floccular bodies within the pupil which represent masses of vitreous prolapsed into the anterior chamber as a result of zonular rupture. Subluxation is rarely accompanied by other ocular signs, but tonometry will often reveal a moderately elevated intraocular pressure. A subluxated lens will almost invariably luxate, but the interval between luxations in the two eyes can be many months and sometimes as great as two years.

If either luxation or subluxation is diagnosed in one eye only the other eye must be examined at frequent intervals, preferably with tonometry. The owners should be warned that the second lens will ultimately luxate and instructed on what action to take when this happens.

Treatment
An anteriorly luxated lens must be removed surgically regardless of whether or not glaucoma is present. Pre-operative treatment for glaucoma is a wise precaution and renders the operation itself less hazardous. Lendectomy is also indicated in all cases of subluxation and pupil block (a possible consequence of subluxation or luxation, when the lens is held in the pupillary aperture by contraction of the iris). The use of miotics to retain a luxated lens behind the iris has, in the authors' experience, been unsuccessful.

Management of the posteriorly luxated lens is more problematical. Because of the dangers of retinal detachment, the practical difficulty in extracting a lens from the vitreous, and the fact that in this position the lens is not particularly troublesome, a decision not to operate may be justified. There is, however, a commitment to frequent re-examination of the eye and the owner should be warned that if the lens moves spontaneously into the anterior chamber immediate surgery is necessary.

Secondary lens luxation
Dislocation of the lens may result from ocular conditions such as glaucoma, cataract and uveitis.

In glaucoma the immediate cause appears to be increased tension within the zonule as a result of enlargement of the globe, rather than a direct effect of pressure on the zonular tissue. Secondary lens dislocations have been reported in breeds susceptible to primary glaucoma, notably the American Cocker Spaniel, the Basset Hound and the Beagle. It should be remembered that the Terrier breeds may themselves by susceptible to primary glaucoma and very occasionally secondary rather than primary luxations may be encountered (Plate 4.22).

GLAUCOMA

The term glaucoma does not denote a specific disease entity, but rather embraces an array of ocular conditions which have in common a raised intraocular pressure (IOP) incompatible with the functional integrity of the eye. Glaucoma is a cause of blindness in the dog and is clinically important not only on account of loss of vision, but also because of the severe pain which may accompany it; the latter, being difficult to assess clinically, is often underestimated.

The intraocular pressure is attributable to the aqueous fluid; this is secreted by the ciliary body, flows through the pupil into the anterior chamber and exits via the iridocorneal angle and trabecular meshwork, ultimately draining into the vessels of the scleral venous plexus. The IOP is thus dependent upon both the rate of production and the rate of clearance of aqueous fluid, but in the dog almost all types of glaucoma arise through impairment of drainage rather than hypersecretion. The IOP in the normal (normotensive) canine eye lies between 15 and 30 mm Hg.

One of the earliest effects of glaucoma is degeneration of the retinal neuroepithelium and optic disc, with accompanying irreversible vision loss. Sustained pressure leads to degeneration and atrophy of other structures, especially the uveal tract. A further possible sequel is frank enlargement of the globe (hydrophthalmos; Plate 4.23), an irreversible change which is accompanied by total loss of vision.

Since in the dog there are no subjective symptoms of impaired vision, so important in the early diagnosis of glaucoma in man, cases are likely to be presented only when relatively advanced. Prompt recognition of the condition is therefore of the utmost importance.

The canine glaucomas may be classified as congenital, primary and secondary. In congenital glaucoma there is usually an abnormality of the iridocorneal angle (goniodysgenesis); this may be true also of some 'primary' glaucomas, even though the onset of a pathological rise in pressure does not occur until adulthood.

Clinical signs and diagnosis

Insofar as they reflect an elevation in IOP, the clinical signs of glaucoma are similar regardless of the underlying cause. However, much depends on the absolute pressures attained, on their duration and, to some extent, on the age of the dog.

Acute glaucoma is typically a painful condition and is usually accompanied by marked blepharospasm, photophobia and lacrimation. Congestion of the episcleral vessels is a constant feature and in particular the prominence of subconjunctival vessels running at right angles to the limbus is characteristic. Congestion of the conjunctival vessels and chemosis may or may not be present. Diffuse clouding of the cornea may be seen when the elevation in IOP is moderate to high, but some individual dogs appear able to sustain high IOP's without undue loss of corneal transparency. Degenerative changes within the cornea may induce vascularisation which frequently presents as a regular brushlike fringe of vessels advancing from the limbus (glaucomatous pannus).

Pupillary dilation and suppression of the pupillary light reflex are always present in acute glaucoma due to inhibition of the sphincter iridis muscle and damage to the nervous pathways. With sustained pressure the uveal tract begins to atrophy and on gonioscopy synechiae may be seen to transverse the iridocorneal angle. Evidence of retinal degeneration (attenuation of the retinal vessels and patchy areas of tapetal hyper-reflectivity) and, in some long-standing cases, cupping or atrophy of the optic disc may be evident on ophthalmoscopic examination.

A sustained high intraocular pressure will ultimately lead to stretching of the collagenous outer tunic of the globe comprising the sclera and cornea. This may be manifest as tears in Descemet's membrane (evident as white linear streaks against the blueness of the oedematous cornea), thinning of the sclera (scleral ectasia), especially at the equator of the globe, and eventually frank enlargement of the globe (buphthalmos, hydrophthalmus). In the very young animal a small degree of stretching is reversible, but in the adult such a change is irreversible and is associated with permanent blindness. Stretching of the ocular tunics can result in dislocation of the lens. A hydrophthalmic eye eventually becomes hypotensive and shrinks, the condition being known as phthisis bulbi.

Both instrumental tonometry and gonioscopy are aids which should be utilised in any practice with a concern for ophthalmological cases. Digital tonometry (palpation of the globe over the closed upper lid) can be useful on occasions, but even with experience can result in false interpretations; some recourse to instrumentation is therefore necessary. In view of the high cost of applanation instruments the choice is virtually restricted to the Schiøtz tonometer, which utilises the indentation principle. Calibration tables are now available for the use of this instrument in the dog; by comparison, the human calibration tables underestimate the true canine IOP by several mm Hg.

Provocative tests to detect predisposition to glaucoma have been described, but it is doubtful whether they are yet relevant in general practice.

Primary glaucoma

In these forms of glaucoma there is no evidence of concurrent intraocular disease to account for the rise in pressure. Two types are recognised in the dog: open angle glaucoma and narrow or closed angle glaucoma (angle-closure glaucoma). The latter is the more common (Plate 4.24).

Open-angle glaucoma

This condition has been investigated extensively in the Beagle, but instances have been recorded in other breeds. In the Beagle it occurs as an autosomal recessive trait and becomes apparent between 6 and 18 months of age, with gradual progression to blindness by about 4 years if left untreated. During this time the globe slowly enlarges, producing tears in Descemet's membrane and subluxation of the lens. There is no obvious defect of the iridocorneal angle until secondary changes supervene. Primary open-angle glaucoma in the Miniature Poodle occurs much later in life (8 years plus).

Narrow or closed angle glaucoma (angle-closure glaucoma)

Angle-closure glaucoma has been recorded in many breeds, including the American Cocker Spaniel, the English Cocker Spaniel, the Basset Hound, the Miniature Poodle, the Smooth and Wire-haired Fox Terriers and the Sealyham. In the American Cocker Spaniel the condition is familial, but a precise mode of inheritance has not been established. It is typically an acute condition with a rapid elevation in IOP leading to irreversible damage if not treated promptly; however, this stage is probably a culmination of a series of earlier sub-clinical and self-limiting attacks. The essential defect appears to be a narrowing of the iridocorneal angle. During an attack the angle may close completely, predisposing to the formation of anterior peripheral synechiae which contribute to the maintenance of a high IOP.

In the Basset Hound the condition appears to be associated with sheets of mesodermal tissue bridging the iridocorneal angle. It is sometimes classified as congenital rather than primary; however, clinical manifestations are not usually apparent until after one year of age.

Secondary glaucoma

Glaucoma may be secondary to a number of conditions of the eye of which the most important is lens luxation. This possibility should immediately be investigated if an individual of appropriate breed and age is presented with glaucoma. Other lens-induced glaucomas may be associated with intumescence (swelling) and hypermaturation (phacolysis) of the cataractous lens. Inflammatory conditions, principally anterior uveitis, which result in the formation of peripheral anterior synechiae, iris bombé or angle blockage, are not uncommon; of these, secondary glaucoma following 'blue eye' affords a good example. Intraocular

haemorrhage, foreign bodies and neoplasia are also possible causes of secondary glaucoma.

Treatment

The medical treatment of glaucoma depends so much on the individual case that it is difficult to lay down precise guidelines. Examples of therapeutic agents used in the treatment of canine glaucoma are listed in Table 4.4. In many instances ultimate control can be achieved only by surgical procedures, but it should be the aim initially to control the problem by medical means. If, following an attack of glaucoma, the iridocorneal angle fails to open after therapy with miotics the eye may be a candidate for surgical intervention.

Surgical procedures found to be of value in the dog include cyclodiathermy and cyclocryotherapy (which reduce aqueous production through partial destruction of the ciliary body), cyclodialysis (the re-opening of the closed ciliary cleft), iridencleisis (exteriorisation of iridal tissue into the subconjunctival tissues), and a combination of corneal trephination and peripheral iridectomy.

Miotics. Probably the most useful group of agents available. They act principally by opening the iridocorneal angle and increasing aqueous outflow and are administered topically. Demecarium bromide (Tosmilen) is more effective and has longer action than pilocarpine or eserine. In most situations their use should be supplemented by one of the carbonic anhydrase inhibitors.

Table 4.4 Some therapeutic agents used in the treatment of canine glaucoma.

1 *Miotics*—constrict pupil and increase rate of aqueous outflow.
    examples: Pilocarpine (1–2%) t.i.d.
               Eserine (0.25–1%) q.i.d.
               Demecarium bromide (Tosmilen) (0.25–0.5%) s.i.d.
               Phospholidine iodine (0.25%) s.i.d.

2 *Carbonic anhydrase inhibitors*—decrease rate of aqueous formation.
    examples: Acetazolamide (Diamox) 10–25 mg/kg b.i.d.
               Dichlorphenamide (Daranide) 5–10 mg/kg b.i.d.

3 *Adrenergics*—stimulate alpha- and beta-receptors.
        (alpha-receptors increase aqueous outflow; beta-receptors decrease aqueous formation)
    example: Epinephrine (1–2%)

4 *Hyperosmotics*—increase osmotic pressure of blood, thereby drawing fluids from eye.
    examples: Glycerol—oral 1–2 ml/kg
               Mannitol—i.v. 1–2 gm/kg

Carbonic anhydrous inhibitors. This group includes the diuretics acetazolamide (Diamox) and dichlorphenamide (Daranide) which achieve their effect by reducing the rate of production of aqueous fluid by approximately 50%. Acetazolamide may be given intravenously as well as orally. These drugs are suitable for long-term therapy although possible side-effects such as vomiting and diarrhoea may be encountered. They are a useful adjunct to topical miotic therapy.

Sympathomimetics. Epinephrine reduces intraocular pressure both by improving aqueous outflow and reducing aqueous fluid production. It is less effective than drugs of either of the above groups and can be irritant.

Osmotic agents. Oral glycerine and intravenous mannitol have a fairly rapid, although transient, effect and can be useful in acute congestive glaucoma if other measures fail.

THE VITREOUS BODY

The vitreous body, or simply 'vitreous', is an avascular and transparent gel occupying the posterior cavity of the eye; anteriorly it is in contact with the posterior surface of the lens, the zonule and the ciliary body and posteriorly it is intimately related to the surface of the retina. The vitreous contains approximately 98% water and is essentially a network of collagen fibres with hyaluronic acid occupying the spaces between. The peripheral (cortical) areas of the vitreous are relatively more dense and the anterior surface, which is adherent to the lens capsule towards the equator and to the posterior pars plana of the ciliary body, is sometimes referred to as the anterior hyaloid membrane. Loss of vitreal support can lead to detachment of the retina or luxation of the lens.

During embryonic development hyaloid blood vessels extend from the site of the future optic disc to the posterior surface of the lens. The hyaloid vasculature of the 'primary' vitreous atrophies in late gestation, but remnants may persist up to approximately four weeks after birth.

The following conditions of the vitreous body may be encountered.

Persistence of the hyaloid vasculature
Vestiges of the hyaloid vasculature may remain in a variety of forms into adulthood. Not uncommonly a short length of hyaloid vessel attached to the posterior lens surface may be seen wafting in the anterior vitreous.

Persistent hyperplastic primary vitreous (PHPV)
PHPV and persistent hyperplastic tunica vasculosa lentis (PHTVL) have been recorded in many breeds, but have recently been reported as a specific heritable condition in the Doberman Pinscher. Accompanying posterior lens opacities and retrolental fibrovascular proliferation and pigmentation may significantly affect vision.

Posterior lenticonus
An infrequent congenital anomaly in which the posterior polar surface of the lens forms a conical projection into the vitreous. The cause is unknown.

Asteroid hyalosis
In this condition numerous small round white bodies composed of calcium salts and attached to the vitreal filaments are scattered throughout the vitreous. They are refractile and move only slightly with movement of the globe. The condition is common in the older dog, is often unilateral and is not necessarily accompanied by obvious ocular disease. Vision is not significantly affected.

Synchisis scintillans
The appearance of crystal-like bodies composed of cholesterol, which move freely in a degenerate and fluid vitreous, often accompanies retinal disease.

Vitreous syneresis
This term denotes liquifaction of the vitreous which is sometimes encountered in the old dog. Retinal detachment is a possible consequence.

Vitreous haemorrhage
This may occur in cases of retinitis, retinal dysplasia (q.v.), other retinal detachments, Collie eye anomaly and a number of systemic conditions such as hypertension and hypercholesterolaemia. It may also result from trauma or penetrating injuries, for example gunshot wounds. The residues remaining may appear as greyish-white masses.

THE CHOROID

The choroid, or posterior uvea, is a highly vascular and deeply pigmented structure lying between the retina and the sclera. Its innermost layer is a capillary network (choriocapillaris) which serves to nourish the outer layers of the retina. Between this and the large choroidal vessels, and occupying the dorsal half of the choroid, lies the tapetum cellulosum. The choroid is not normally visible on ophthalmoscopic examination unless there is thinning or degeneration of the overlying retina or lack of retinal pigment.

Congenital defects of the choroid and retina usually occur together; choroidal hypoplasia, as part of the Collie eye anomaly syndrome, is considered below. Choroiditis may be part of a generalised uveal inflammation or it may be associated with retinal disease (chorioretinitis or retinochoroiditis, depending on which layer is primarily affected). *Toxoplasma gondii* is a cause of primary choroiditis and chorioretinitis.

THE RETINA

The retina is a thin, transparent membrane in contact with the choroid and extending anteriorly to the posterior extremity of the ciliary body (ora ciliaris retinae). It is a multilayered structure consisting largely of several types of neurone and their synapses. The light-sensitive receptors, the rods and cones, comprise the outermost layer of the 'sensory' retina. Rods account for approximately 95% of the total receptors. Situated between the photoreceptors and the choroid is a single cell layer, the pigment epithelium, which is concerned both with phagocytosis of spent photoreceptor material and various biochemical processes relating to photostimulation. The pigment epithelium is pigmented in the non-tapetal region but not over the tapetum itself. Ophthalmoscopically, the fundus can thus be divided into tapetal and non-tapetal regions.

The tapetal fundus. The normal tapetal fundus is triangular or semilunar in shape and situated above the optic disc. It is surrounded by non-tapetal fundus. In the adult the tapetal fundus may assume a variety of colours, including orange, green and yellow. However, in the young puppy it is violet or blue before assuming the adult colour by about four months of age. Sometimes tapetal colour can be linked to coat colour (e.g. an orange tapetum in the Irish Setter). Pigment may occasionally be present in the pigment epithelium over the tapetum and this must be carefully distinguished from pathological pigmentation. Occasionally a tapetum may be absent and this occurs commonly in Dalmatians. Atrophy, or thinning, of the retina leads to an increase in tapetal reflectivity.

The non-tapetal fundus. The non-tapetal fundus is dark-brown to black, the pigmentation obscuring the choroidal vasculature. However, lack of pigment in the pigment epithelium may occur, especially in sub-albinotic animals such as the merled Collie. In this case the choroidal vessels are clearly visible radiating (approximately) from the optic disc; such a fundus is described as 'tigroid'. A light coloured iris is usually associated with incomplete pigmentation of the non-tapetal fundus.

Clinical examination

The presence of retinal disease will usually be detected when behavioural changes suggestive of deterioration of vision are reported by the owner, or during inspection for other ocular disease or for purposes of certification. Retinal disease *per se* rarely gives rise to specific clinical signs other than dilatation of the pupil and impairment of the pupillary light reflex.

In examining the retina with a direct or indirect ophthalmoscope it is important to dilate the pupil to observe the more peripheral areas. The fundus should be searched for focal lesions, abnormalities of vasculature, changes in reflectivity (usually arising through thinning of the retina over the tapetum), appearance of the choroidal vasculature, pigmentary changes, and changes in the optic disc. It should, in most instances, be possible to distinguish between diseases of hereditary origin, which are usually bilateral and more or less symmetrical, and infectious or inflammatory conditions, which usually are not.

Accurate ophthalmoscopic diagnosis of retinal disease is dependent on a thorough knowledge of the normal canine fundus and full appreciation of variations in vascularity, colour and pigmentation can be gained only by experience. Some typical variations are illustrated in Plate 4.25.

Congenital conditions

Retinal dysplasia

Retinal dysplasia is a congenital malformation characterised by the formation of folds or rosettes in the layers of the neuroepithelium. In severe cases, retinal detachment can occur. The condition can be either

Plate 4.25
1. Normal fundus.
2. Normal fundus (note difference in colour of tapetum lucidum and tortuosity of retinal blood vessels, also position and edge of the optic disc).
3. Generalised progressive retinal atrophy.
4. Central progressive retinal atrophy.
5. Collie eye anomaly showing chorioretinal dysplasia and colobomas of the optic disc.
6. Total retinal detachment.
7. Chorioretinitis or retinal necrosis.

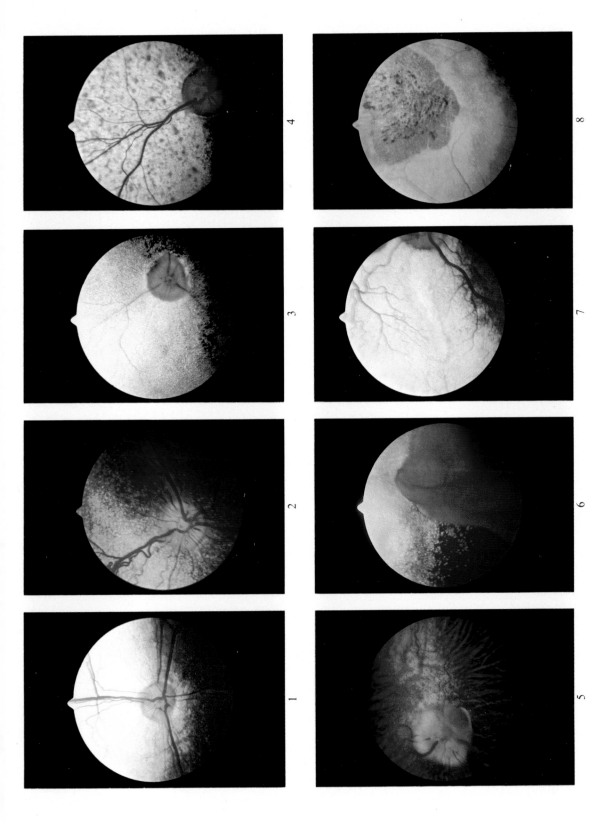

acquired, arising from one of several possible insults during pregnancy or neonatally (e.g. canine herpesvirus, canine parvovirus), or inherited. The former category is rare in the dog, but inherited forms of retinal dysplasia have recently assumed considerable clinical importance.

The ocular signs of inherited retinal dysplasia in the dog vary according to breed. In the Cocker Spaniel and the Beagle the fundus changes are of the multifocal type, with numerous vermiform foci (folds) evident over the tapetal, and to a lesser extent, non-tapetal areas. In severe cases other ocular signs such as microphthalmia and nystagmus may be present. The retinal lesions alone, however, appear not to have any effect on vision. In the English Springer Spaniel a more severe form of multifocal retinal dysplasia has been reported in which accompanying cataractous changes and retinal detachment sometimes occur. In this breed a visual defect does occur depending on the severity of the condition.

In the Bedlington Terrier and the Sealyham Terrier retinal dysplasia presents as an infundibular total retinal detachment, with the retina attaching to the posterior lens capsule; in such cases leukocoria is a presenting sign. Microphthalmia and intraocular haemorrhage may also occur and blindness is typical. Retinal dysplasia with total retinal detachment is also encountered in the Labrador Retriever. In this breed two further types of retinal dysplasia have been described, a multifocal form somewhat similar to that seen in the Cocker Spaniel and a severe form associated with skeletal abnormalities. It has been suggested that these forms may be genetically similar.

Retinal dysplasia is transmitted as a recessive gene in the Bedlington Terrier and the Labrador Retriever, and probably also in the remaining breeds. Dogs with retinal dysplasia should not be bred from and both their parents must at least be carriers.

Collie eye anomaly

Collie eye anomaly (CEA) was first reported in the USA in 1953. It is an inherited congenital defect of the canine fundus which is almost limited to the Rough and Smooth Collies and the Shetland Sheepdog, although a similar condition has been recorded in other breeds. It is encountered in many parts of the world, but especially in Rough Collies in the USA where an incidence of 85–90% has been reported. In the UK it is common in the Shetland Sheepdog, fairly common in the Rough and Smooth Collie, and has recently been reported in the Border Collie, where the incidence is low.

This complex and imperfectly understood condition comprises a variety of seemingly unrelated defects which include choroidal hypoplasia (chorioretinal dysplasia), tortuosity of the retinal vessels and the presence of colobomas, amongst others. The lesions do not progress although secondary changes such as retinal detachment and intraocular haemorrhage may occur. The lesions are not necessarily bilaterally symmetrical. The condition can be mild with no effect on vision or severe enough to cause total blindness, but in the large majority of cases there is no apparent effect on vision. It is now accepted that collie eye anomaly, or at least its main component, choroidal hypoplasia, is inherited as an autosomal recessive gene. Earlier suggestions that other features may be inherited independently have not been substantiated.

Ophthalmoscopic changes

Choroidal hypoplasia is a frequent and pathognomonic finding in CEA, the area of abnormal choroidal vasculature being situated lateral to the optic disc and approximately at the junction of the tapetal and non-tapetal regions. The choroidal vessels appear larger and fewer than in the normal eye and their form and distribution is often bizarre. The vessels are visible because of an accompanying and characteristic lack of pigment in the overlying retinal pigment epithelium. The choroidal pigmentation is also lacking, permitting the whiteness of the sclera to show between the vessels. Whilst the size of the affected area may vary considerably, its general position is constant. Problems of interpretation are sometimes encountered in eyes in which the retinal pigment epithelium is lacking pigment, i.e. subalbinotic or albinotic fundi (for example in the blue merle Collie), and diagnosis must therefore rest on the form of the choroidal vessels; experience is of great importance here. The term choroidal hypoplasia is now considered preferable to chorioretinal dysplasia.

The fundi of a small proportion of puppies with choroidal hypoplasia may in later life appear ophthalmoscopically normal, presumably because an increase in pigment in the retinal pigment epithelium obscures the defective choroidal vasculature. Such individuals have been referred to as 'go-normals'.

Excessive tortuosity of the retinal vessels is an invariable feature in CEA. However, when observed in isolation tortuosity must be interpreted with caution as it is sometimes a feature of normal Collie eyes. Colobomata may be found in about one-quarter of affected eyes. They may appear as single or multiple excavations of the optic disc, or may be situated elsewhere in the fundus, sometimes up to several disc diameters away from the optic disc. Retinal detachments occur in approximately 10% of cases but are rare in dogs over one year of age. Other ocular findings may include retinal haemorrhage (CEA is always to be considered in the differential diagnosis of hyphaemia and the contralateral eye must be examined), the presence of retinal folds, microphthalmia and mineralisation of the central corneal stroma.

Control
Collie eye anomaly is attributable to a recessive gene and in accordance with general principles affected dogs, their parents and their progeny should not be bred from. Contrary to popular supposition, there is no justification in breeding from mildly affected animals in the belief that they are less likely to pass on the condition. As yet there is no way of identifying the carrier state other than by test-mating, which is a perfectly justifiable and useful procedure. The practice of examining puppies at around seven weeks of age should be encouraged, not only to prevent the sale of puppies to owners who might later breed from them indiscriminately but also to identify the 'go-normal' puppies which would escape detection at a later date.

Inherited retinopathies

The canine retina is subject to a number of inherited abnormalities which include progressive retinal atrophy (PRA) and hemeralopia (day-blindness).

PRA is not a single disease entity but rather a collection of aetiologically distinct conditions which, clinically and ophthalmoscopically, can be grouped into two fairly well-defined types, generalised and central (CPRA). In both, the main pathological change is degeneration of the neuroepithelium leading to loss of layer organisation. They are progressive, often to total blindness, and both eyes are affected to approximately the same extent. They are not accompanied by systemic or other neurological signs and are painless. Generally speaking only one form of PRA occurs in a single breed, exceptions being the Cardigan Corgi and the English Springer Spaniel, which may show both.

It is becoming customary to refer to the generalised form of progressive retinal atrophy as 'PRA' and the central form as 'CPRA'. Some authors, for example, Slatter (1981), prefer to classify PRA, CPRA and hemeralopia as types I, II and III, respectively.

Generalised progressive retinal atrophy (PRA)
PRA was first described in the Gordon Setter in 1911 and has since been recorded in many breeds throughout the world, in all of which it appears to be inherited as an autosomal recessive gene. Recent research, utilising techniques such as electroretinography and electron microscopy, has shown that the initial events occurring in the photoreceptor layer may differ markedly from one breed to another. For example, in the Irish Setter abnormalities of both rods and cones (rod-cone dysplasia) is evident histologically by 2–3 weeks of age, whilst in the Toy and Miniature Poodles the photoreceptors appear to function normally initially and only later degenerate, the rods faster than the cones (rod-cone degeneration). In the Norwegian Elkhound the rod receptors are abnormal (rod dysplasia) and only later do the cones degenerate. The basic defects have yet to be defined in most other breeds. Whilst the onset of clinical signs is clearly related to the type of change occurring in the receptor layer, ophthalmoscopically the condition is remarkably similar in different breeds.

Clinical signs
Almost invariably the first sign of PRA is night blindness. The dog may have difficulty in finding its way about when taken for an evening walk, or it may be apprehensive about being left in darkness. Since the peripheral retina appears to be affected first, vision tends to be better directly in front than to the sides; for example, a ball rolled towards the dog will be seen, but not an object passing across the field of view. Distant vision may be better than near vision and stationary objects may be difficult to see. Vision deteriorates progressively, culminating in total blindness.

The age at which the condition may be diagnosed ophthalmoscopically varies from several weeks to several years (Table 4.5) but is fairly specific for any one breed. In the Irish Setter clinical signs are observed within a few weeks of age and blindness is total by about one year; at the other extreme the condition in the Poodle may not be obvious until 2–5 years of age. The variability of onset in the Poodle suggests the possibility of a complex of several genetically distinct conditions.

Ophthalmoscopy
The first ophthalmoscopic sign is increased reflectivity (hyper-reflectivity) of the peripheral tapetal fundus due to thinning of the retina and possibly also changes in the tapetum itself. The non-tapetal fundus appears paler than normal, sometimes appearing mottled as the residual spots of pigment become prominent against the lighter background. Progressive loss of pigment may also enable the choroidal vessels to be visualised in the later stages. The most obvious change, however, is attenuation of the retinal vessels. Initially the finer vessels atrophy and disappear and later the larger vessels become progressively attenuated. In the final stages the vessels of the optic disc themselves may become obliterated and the disc itself appear white

Table 4.5 Progressive retinal atrophy.

Type	Breed affected	Mode of inheritance	Approx. earliest age diagnosed	Age for final certification*
Generalised	Cairn Terrier	Simple autosomal recessive	3 months	5 years
	Cocker Spaniel		1 year	5 years
	Elkhound		1 year	3 years
	Miniature Long-haired Dachshund		3 months	3 years
	Poodle (Miniature & Toy)		2 years	5 years
	Irish Setter		3 months	3 years
	Tibetan Terrier		9 months	3 years
Generalised or central	Cardigan Corgi	—	3 months	3 years
	English Springer Spaniel	—	1 year	5 years
Central	Briard	Recessive (?)	1–1½ years	5 years
	Border Collie	Dominant with incomplete penetrance (?)	2 years	3 years
	Collie (Rough & Smooth)	—	1 year	3 years
	Shetland Sheepdog	—	1–1½ years	3 years
	Golden Retriever	—	1½ years	6 years
	Labrador Retriever	Dominant with incomplete penetrance	1½ years	4 years

* Under joint BVA/KC Scheme

and enlarged with an irregular periphery. The pupillary light reflex is progressively lost and the pupils become dilated. In many advanced cases secondary cataractous changes occur in the lens, but their onset and rate of progression may be very variable.

It is of diagnostic significance that PRA is always bilateral and progressive, with both eyes being affected to a similar extent.

Electroretinography

Electroretinography has been a powerful research tool in differentiating the inherited retinopathies in different breeds. Changes in the electroretinogram appear much earlier than the earliest ophthalmoscopic signs; for example, abnormalities of the ERG have been recorded in the Irish Setter and the Poodle as early as 3 and 10 weeks, respectively. However, partly because of difficulties in standardising the technique and the apparent wide variation in the ERG from one individual to another, the full potential of the method in the early diagnosis of PRA in the field has yet to be realised.

Control

Several countries now have control schemes based on clinical examinations and certification of freedom from the condition. In the UK the joint scheme administered by the Kennel Club and the British Veter-

inary Association provides for final certification at, or after, the age beyond which PRA is unlikely to develop (Table 4.5), with intermediate (temporary) certification of dogs below this age.

Central progressive retinal atrophy

The essential retinal change in central PRA is hypertrophy and migration of pigment epithelial cells. Subsequent degeneration of photoreceptors and loss of retinal architecture tends to be more severe in the central rather than the peripheral retina.

Just as the pathology of central PRA differs from that of generalised PRA so the signs apparent to the owner will vary. Affected dogs have better vision in dull light than in sunlight; they also tend to have better peripheral vision and can see moving objects passing across the visual field, but are unable to recognise even quite large objects placed directly in front of them. Sometimes they may tend to walk past the owner without seeing him until almost level, or if called from a distance they approach in an arc. If spoken to they appear not to look directly at the speaker and the eyes may appear prominent and the expression anxious. The condition does not progress to complete blindness with the same inevitability as generalised PRA and total blindness is not common.

Breeds affected include the Labrador Retriever,

the Golden Retriever, the Collie breeds, the English Springer Spaniel and the Briard. It has been postulated that in the Labrador Retriever the mode of inheritance is dominant with variable penetrance. However, the recent decline in incidence of the condition in the USA, which cannot be satisfactorily explained in genetic terms alone, suggests the implication of environmental factors. The condition may have an autosomal recessive mode of inheritance in the Briard.

Ophthalmoscopy
Pigmentary changes commence slightly above and temporal to the optic disc (area centralis) and extend rapidly until the whole of the tapetal fundus is covered with numerous brownish-black spots of pigment, which often occur adjacent to blood vessels or may link to form a network. In the Rough Collie the annular form of the spots is characteristic. With time the spots may coalesce to leave a few isolated dark areas. Increased tapetal reflectivity and atrophy of the retinal vessels also occur, but rather later than in generalised PRA. There are no obvious changes in the non-tapetal fundus or the optic disc.

Control
The control schemes implemented for central PRA are the same as those for generalised PRA. The International Sheepdog Society has a scheme which includes compulsory examination of all Border Collies entered at the National Sheep Dog Trials. Neither affected animals nor their progeny are admitted to the stud book and both parents of an affected dog must be examined and cleared before their progeny can be admitted. By this means the incidence of PRA in this breed was reduced from above 12% to less than 2% over the period 1965–1975.

Hemeralopia
Hemeralopia (day blindness) has been reported in the Alaskan Malamute and also the Miniature Poodle. Affected individuals are blind in bright light, but visual in dim light. Onset usually occurs within the first six months of life. The basic defect is a degeneration of the cone photoreceptors (detectable with electroretinography), but ophthalmoscopically the retina appears normal. Hemeralopia is inherited as an autosomal recessive trait.

Other retinopathies

Inflammatory retinopathies
Inflammation of the retina usually arises from, or is associated with, inflammatory changes in the choroid, hence the term chorioretinitis. The possible causes are many and include bacteria, viruses, fungi, parasites and neoplasia; often the cause cannot be established. Retinal lesions may take a variety of forms but they are usually not progressive and, if bilateral, are rarely symmetrical. Canine distemper virus and *Toxoplasma gondii* are fairly common causes of retinal disease. They can occur together.

Canine distemper virus can cause ganglion cell death, producing multiple focal greyish lesions with peripheral hyper-reflectivity. However, blindness in distemper is usually attributable to central nervous rather than ocular involvement.

Chorioretinitis and anterior uveitis are common findings in ocular toxoplasmosis. Retinal atrophy secondary to chorioretinitis and focal hyper-reflective lesions of the tapetal fundus may be evident. Sulphonamides and pyrimethamine have been used with variable success in the treatment of toxoplasmosis and corticosteroids may be beneficial in treating the ocular lesions.

Diabetic retinopathy
Retinopathy occurs in diabetes mellitus but is often obscured, ophthalmoscopically, by the rapidly developing cataract which is commonly seen in this condition. Exudative retinopathy occurs in the dog, as in man, but the proliferative form apparently does not.

Hypertensive retinopathy
Focal retinal haemorrhage, retinal oedema, subretinal exudation and retinal detachment may be associated with hypertension or severe chronic renal disease. However, similar serous detachments are sometimes seen in otherwise apparently healthy dogs. Hypertensive retinopathy has also been reported in cases of hypothyroidism.

Other retinopathies
There are many other causes of retinal disease. Toxic or drug-induced retinopathies are characterised by bilateral symmetry. Retinal haemorrhages occur in the various canine bleeding disorders, systemic lupus erythematosus and the hyperviscosity syndrome.

Retinal detachment

Detachment of the retina may be congenital, idiopathic or secondary to other ocular diseases such as Collie eye anomaly, lens luxation, progressive retinal atrophy and degeneration of the vitreous body. Where detachment is complete there is usually a history of sudden loss of vision and the pupillary light reflex is almost absent or lost. Ophthalmoscopically, the retina is seen as mobile clothlike folds hanging from the optic papilla. There is no treatment.

Incomplete retinal detachment may result from subretinal oedema or haemorrhage; for possible treatment a specialist text should be consulted.

The optic disc

The appearance of the optic disc can be of diagnostic value in several ocular conditions. Congenital abnormalities, best exemplified by Collie eye anomaly, include coloboma, or pitting, and optic nerve hypoplasia. Pitting, or cupping, of the optic disc also occurs in glaucoma and the 'disappearance' of retinal vessels over the crater rim is characteristic. Oedema of the optic disc (papilloedema) may be secondary to retinitis or chorioretinitis, or may result from a rise in intracranial pressure.

Optic neuritis, usually a manifestation of infectious systemic disease, can result in blindness. In acute cases the optic disc is hyperaemic and oedematous and focal haemorrhages may be present.

Therapeutics

Table 4.6 gives a basic list of therapeutic agents and their uses.

FURTHER READING

Ophthalmic texts in the English language

AGUIRRE G. (ed.) (1973) *The Veterinary Clinics of North America*. **3**. W. B. Saunders, Philadelphia.

BISTNER S. I., AGUIRRE G. & BATIK G. (1977) *Atlas of Veterinary Ophthalmic Surgery*. W. B. Saunders. Philadelphia.

BLOGG J. R. (1975) *The Eye in Veterinary Practice*. V.S. Supplies, North Melbourne.

BLOGG J. R. (1980) *The Eye in Veterinary Practice I*. Extraocular disease. W. B. Saunders, Philadelphia.

GELATT K. N. (ed.) (1981) *Veterinary Ophthalmology*. Lea & Febiger, Philadelphia.

GRAHAM-JONES O. (ed.) (1966) *Aspects of Comparative Ophthalmology*. Pergamon, Oxford.

HOGAN M. J., ALVARADO J. A. & WEDDELL J. (1971) *Histology of the Human Eye*. W. B. Saunders, Philadelphia.

JENSEN H. E. (1971) *Stereoscopic Atlas of Clinical Ophthalmology of Domestic Animals*. C. V. Mosby, St. Louis.

MAGRANE W. G. (1977) *Canine Ophthalmology*, 3rd Edn. Lea & Febiger, Philadelphia.

PRINCE J. H., DIESEM C. D., EGLITIS I. & RUSKELL G. L. (1960) *The Anatomy and Histology of the Eye and Orbit in Domestic Animals*. C. C. Thomas, Springfield, Illinois.

RUBIN L. F. (1974) *Atlas of Veterinary Ophthalmoscopy*. Lea & Febiger, Philadelphia.

SAUNDERS L. Z. & RUBIN L. F. (1975) *Ophthalmic Pathology of Animals*. S. Karger, Basle.

SLATTER D. H. (1981) *Fundamentals of Veterinary Ophthalmology*. W. B. Saunders, Philadelphia.

SMYTHE R. H. (1958) *Veterinary Ophthalmology*, 2nd Edn. Bailliere Tindall & Cox, London.

Table 4.6 Ocular therapeutics. This basic list of drugs used by the authors is not intended to be exhaustive and in most instances acceptable alternatives are available.

Drug	Principle action	Indication
Atropine (1%)	Mydriasis	Anterior uveitis
Tropicamide (1%)	Mydriasis (short duration)	Pupil dilatation for examination
Phenol liq.	Chemical cauterisation	Corneal ulceration
Fluorescein (2% sol. or strips)	Diagnostic stain	Corneal ulceration
Proparacaine HCl (0.5%)	Topical anaesthesia	Keratoconjunctivitis sicca
Hypromellose (1%)	Artificial tears	Keratoconjunctivitis sicca
Acetylcysteine (20%)	Mucolysis	Keratoconjunctivitis sicca
Demecarium bromide (0.5%)	Miosis	Glaucoma
Dichlorphenamide (50 mg tabs)	Reduces aqueous formation	Glaucoma

Corticosteroids
1. High potency (topical): fluocinolone acetonide (0.025%), betamethasone valerate (0.05%)
2. Medium potency (topical): betamethasone sodium phosphate
3. Low potency (topical): hydrocortisone
4. Subconjunctival (long acting): methylprednisolone acetate
5. Systemic: many preparations available

Antibiotics
1. Topical: ointments containing penicillin or neomycin are useful for the initial treatment of superficial infections but the ultimate choice should depend on the results of sensitivity tests.
2. Systemic: the systemic use of antibiotics for eye infections depends on such factors as penetration of blood-aqueous barrier, duration of effective levels, secretion in tears, etc. Although not to be used indiscriminately, chloramphenicol has certain advantages.

STARTUP, F. G. (1969) *Diseases of the Canine Eye.* Bailliere Tindall, London.

Texts containing useful chapters on the eye
CATCOTT E. J. (ed.) (1979) *Canine Medicine*, 4th Edn. American Veterinary Publications, Illinois.

ETTINGER S. J. (in press) *Textbook of Veterinary Internal Medicine*, Vol. I. 2nd edn. Saunders, Philadelphia.
KIRK R. W. (ed.) (1980) *Current Veterinary Therapy VII* Small Animal Practice. W. B. Saunders, Philadelphia.

5

The Nervous System

JOHN BARKER

THE CLINICAL EXAMINATION OF THE NERVOUS SYSTEM

Of all the techniques available to the clinician, the most useful and the most neglected is that of detailed, orderly clinical examination. What follows is not intended to be exhaustive, but should at least provide the examiner with sufficient facts for reasoned assessment of the case.

Detailed history taking

Include litter histories, vaccination details, previous medical or surgical problems, and incontact health, considered in relation to the onset of the presenting condition.

Record details of the owner's subjective analysis, noting initial signs, rate of onset, rate of progression, remission, response to attempts at therapy, and development of other later signs.

Objective examination

Results should be recorded and graded; examinations should be easily repeatable and serial examinations should be comparable.

1 Stance and demeanour of the animal at rest and moving in straight line away from and towards the examiner, turning, ascending and descending stairs, and negotiating a simple obstacle course (of chairs, for example).

2 Neurological examination should be carried out in a room with uniform artificial light familiar to the examiner. The sequence of examination:

Tapetal reflex. Compare pupil size using a direct ophthalmoscope set at 'O' to obtain tapetal glow.

Pupillary light reflex. Using a *bright* pentorch to observe the direct light reflex in one eye for a count of five, move the light across to the other eye and observe direct response in that, and repeat several times, noting degree of contraction, maintenance of contraction, and comparing the response of each eye. Assessment

of consensual response is made at the same time. Covering the eye not under direct examination should also be employed to demonstrate afferent lesions.

Nystagmus. Observe for head tilt, and then examine the eyes with the head held level for spontaneous nystagmus. The head should then be passively moved up and down and to either side to observe the normal vestibular nystagmus of each eye. Observation of squints, ptosis, asymmetry etc. is made at the same time. If spontaneous nystagmus is present, assessment should be repeated with the animal in left and right lateral recumbency and on its back, and the eyeball movements should be palpated through closed lids.

Menace reflex. With the eye not under examination covered, the blink response to flicking the fingers at the eye (without making contact) should be readily elicited.

Corneal reflex. Contact with the eye induces a blink. The same response can also be used to assess the integrity of facial sensation (trigeminal nerve) by observing the slight blinking that occurs as the skin is stimulated with a blunt needle.

Other cranial nerves. Obviously, facial nerve and trigeminal motor integrity can be assessed as the head is handled. The mouth should be opened fully, and the tongue observed for normal movement, abnormal muscle fasciculation or atrophy. Gag reflex should then be determined, and normal jaw closure observed.

With the room in darkness, and allowing time for the animal to become dark-adapted, tapetal reflex should be re-assessed with a dimmed ophthalmoscope to ascertain that full and equal pupillary dilatation has occurred. Spontaneous nystagmus is sometimes visible at this point as the animal has difficulty fixating the dim light. Detailed examination of each optic disc and tapetal and non-tapetal fundus is then undertaken and pupillary light reflexes are re-assessed. Eyeball tremor may be noted here. Normal lighting is then restored.

Tonic neck response. Is obtained by extending the head and neck upwards. Cervical pain or spasm can be assessed simultaneously.

Conscious proprioception. The fore and hind limbs are assessed as in Fig. 5.1. Abnormal talon wear is noted as the feet are handled.

Hemistanding. The fore and hind limbs of one side are lifted and the animal is made to bear weight on the others.

Hemiwalking. If the hemistanding is achieved with ease, the animal is made to hemiwalk forward one step on each limb. Even very slight paresis will preclude this.

Placing and hopping reactions. Each limb is tested in turn, with observation of normal extensor thrust being made as each foot is brought down to the floor surface with the body suspended.

Spinal reflexes. These are best assessed as a group. Panniculus reflex is obtained by pressing with a blunt probe rostrally from the lower lumbar region lateral to the dorsal spines on either side. The animal can then be laid on one side with head and neck in line with the trunk, and muscle tone ascertained by passive flexion of the limbs. Tendon reflexes (biceps, triceps and patellar) are then tested by briskly tapping the appropriate tendon with a small patellar hammer, and finally withdrawal reflex and awareness are checked by pinching the interdigital web, observing the limb flexion and the conscious central response (lifting head, crying etc.). If no central response occurs, stronger stimulation should be applied. These tests are then repeated with the animal in the opposite lateral recumbency and laid on its back. Anal reflex, tail movements etc. are assessed at this time. The ability of the animal to right itself is then observed. If this is abnormal, and the size of the patient allows, it should then be suspended by the pelvis, and trunk orientation noted.

Having carried out this examination, the clinician should be in possession of most of the relevant clinical signs shown by the patient. Interpretation is then directed to lateralising and localising the lesion(s) to one gross area of the nervous system (or excluding it altogether), e.g. brain, cord and/or peripheral nerve, and thence to more specific localities, without as yet attempting an aetiological diagnosis, which, even with specialised techniques, may simply be impossible. Some clinical signs occur together with such frequency, even when arising from different aetiologies,

that they may be considered as separate entities or syndromes, and are worthy of detailed consideration.

The vestibular syndrome

Animals suffering from vestibular signs may display a combination of the following clinical signs:

1 *Head tilt* to the side of the lesion
2 *Spontaneous nystagmus* with a slow phase to the affected side
3 *Lower limb tone on the affected side*
4 *Tendency to circle* to the affected side
5 *Facial paralysis* and/or other cranial nerve signs
6 *Sympathetic paralysis* of the ipsilateral eye (Horner's Syndrome)

Detailed examination may also reveal abnormalities of normal vestibular nystagmus with squints developing as head position changes, changes in the direction of spontaneous nystagmus with head position, slight paresis or enhanced spinal reflexes, etc. which may be valuable in determining the position of the lesion within the vestibular system, and hence the prognosis.

Peripheral vestibular lesion (inner ear, vestibular nerve). Well-defined vestibular syndrome with horizontal or slightly rotatory nystagmus *not* varying in direction with head position, well-defined ipsilateral facial paralysis, defined low ipsilateral limb tone.

Central vestibular lesion (brainstem or diffuse pathology). Confusing clinical signs tending to obfuscate the vestibular signs, e.g. paresis, proprioceptive losses, ataxia, with nystagmus changing in direction with head position, involvement of several cranial nerves, cerebellar signs (q.v.).

Bilateral vestibular lesions. May be confusing as no or variable head tilt, nystagmus etc. may occur. Suspending such cases by the pelvis may reveal marked deviation of the trunk ventrally.

CSF sampling, and radiography of the petrous temporal bones may be useful adjuncts to clinical examination.

Clinical presentations
1 *Congenital*. Several reports exist of litters of young (up to six weeks) puppies affected to a greater or lesser extent, but usually with marked head tilt. Clinically the condition appears peripheral, but no post mortem lesion has been found. Providing the animals are feeding

normally, compensation and recovery occur with time.

2 *Otitis interna.* There is usually a history of otitis media with pain and slight head tilt followed by acute onset of vestibular signs, often accompanied by facial paralysis or Horner's syndrome. Radiography may confirm. In a number of cases there is no apparent otitis media or other predisposing pathology, simply the acute onset of peripheral vestibular signs. Treatment with long-term (4–6 weeks) or broadspectrum antibiotics is indicated; if otitis media is present, surgical drainage may be required. Recovery is usually fair, but slight head tilt and persisting facial paralysis are common sequelae. Exposure keratitis in the non-blinking eye does not appear to pose a problem in this species, the dog simply retracting the eye, and 'flicking' the third eyelid over the cornea.

3 *Spontaneous syndrome in old dogs.* Quite frequently, old animals are presented with a history of acute onset of well-defined peripheral signs, often with distress and vomiting (so called 'stroke'). Recovery is usually good, providing the owner can be persuaded to maintain the dog for a few days. Slight head tilt may persist, and re-occurences (often milder) may be seen. Treatment has no effect on the clinical course of the recovery.

4 *Central infections.* Vestibular signs frequently occur in the clinical manifestations of encephalitis (q.v.).

The cerebellar syndrome

The primary function of the cerebellum is the co-ordination of muscle during movement and maintenance of posture at rest. Disease is therefore manifested as:

1 *Ataxia* (muscular inco-ordination) which may be so severe that the dog may be unable to stand without repeatedly lurching and falling in any direction. Milder cases adopt a wide-based stance to retain their equilibrium.

2 *Dysmetria.* Limb movement is delayed in onset, and then 'undamped', leading to a grossly inco-ordinated goosestepping gait.

3 *Tremor* of the head and limbs may be very marked, particularly if a titbit is proffered and the dog is invited to approach and attempt to take it accurately from the fingers. Milder cases may show only slight eyeball tremor on ophthalmoscopic examination.

4 *Menace reflex* may be bilaterally or ipsilaterally absent in cerebellar lesions.

5 *Central vestibular signs* (q.v.) may occur.

Clinical presentations

1 *Congenital.* Hypoplasia of the cerebellum is usually seen in young pups as ataxia and marked tremor as they begin to walk. The condition is non-progressive. Herpes viral infections have been implicated in some cases.

2 *Central infections.* Inflammatory disease of the central nervous system frequently involves the cerebellum, and affected animals show the cerebellar syndrome grossly complicated by other neurological deficits (see below).

3 *Inherited conditions.* Animals with storage diseases, or more specific abiotrophy of the cerebellar Purkinje cells, are usually normal at birth, but develop progressive clinical signs after a few weeks. These conditions are rare.

ESSENTIAL CLINICAL KNOWLEDGE

Pathways for senses, reflexes, movement and syndromes

1 Limb position sense: 'conscious proprioception'

Abnormality. Ataxia, knuckling of foot over on to dorsum, poor reflex stepping, swaying (Fig. 5.1).

Route. Muscle receptors→'A' myelinated fibres→dorsal columns of cord→medial lemniscus→thalamus→internal capsule→sensory cortex.

Significant in peripheral neuropathy, and cord lesions.

2 Touch and pressure

Abnormality. Self explanatory, non-visual placing.

Route. Skin receptors→'B' myelinated fibres→scattered in cord→as for limb position sense.

3 Pain

Abnormality. Self explanatory.

Route. Nerve endings→'C' non-myelinated fibres→diffuse, bilateral chiefly in dorsolateral pathways→thalamus→sensory cortex.

Significant in peripheral neuropathy, extensive cord lesions.

4 Hearing

Ear→VIII nerve→lateral lemniscus→thalamus→internal capsule→temporal cortex→'hearing'.

Also→caudal colliculus of midbrain auditory reflexes, 'startle' response. Much crossing over occurs in

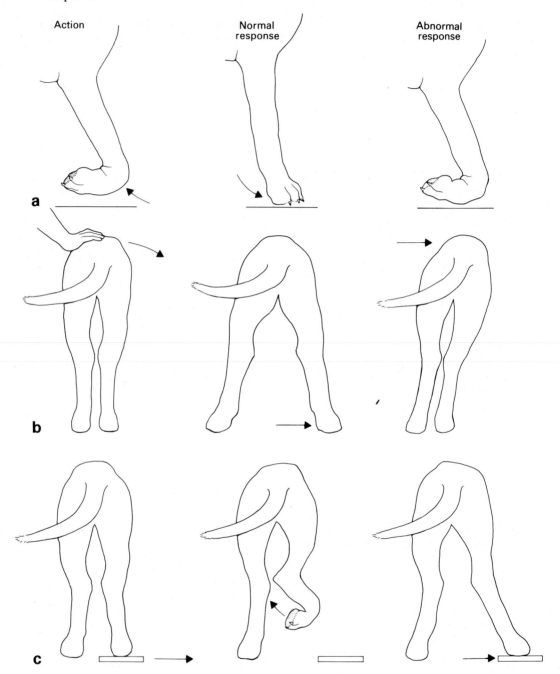

Fig. 5.1 Tests for assessing conscious proprioception: (a) knuckling; (b) sway reaction; (c) reflex stepping.

auditory system, therefore lesions cause bilateral dim-inution.

5 Vision and eye reflexes

Eye→II nerve→optic chiasm (crossing over)→optic tracts→thalamus→internal capsule→occipital cortex→'vision'.

Also→rostral colliculus→III nerve→pupils for pupillary light reflex.

In more detail:

a Pupillary light reflex

Route. As above.

Stimulus. Illuminate one eye.

Result. Bilateral pupillary constriction, in the eye stimulated—'direct' light reflex, in the contralateral eye—'indirect' or 'consensual' light reflex.

b Corneal reflex

Route. Receptors in cornea→V nerve afferent→medulla→VII nerve efferent→orbicularis oculi muscle→'blink'.

Stimulus. Light touch or 'blowing' on cornea.

Result. Direct and consensual. If afferent pathway damaged, blink occurs in affected eye only on stimulation of opposite eye. If efferent pathway is damaged blink cannot occur in affected eye, but consensual is intact.

c Menace reflex

Route. The afferent arm of this reflex is as for 'vision'. The efferent arm however descends in the internal capsule→pons (crossing over)→middle cerebellar peduncle→cerebellar cortex→cerebellar efferent→VII nerve efferent→orbicularis oculi muscle→'blink'. Stronger stimulation causes the recruitment of other cranial nerve nuclei or cervical cord efferents via medial longitudinal fasciculus.

Stimulus. 'Flicking' fingers at the eye under test, other eye covered, without touching or stimulating corneal reflex.

Result. As for corneal reflex. Diffuse cerebellar damage may cause bilateral loss due to efferent arm lesion, unilateral cerebellar damage may cause ipsilateral loss.

d Fixation reflex

Stimulus. Moving object or change in pattern in peripheral visual field.

Response. Turning of head and eyes to bring movement central in visual field.

Requires intact vision and rostral colliculi.

e Horner's syndrome (Fig. 5.2)

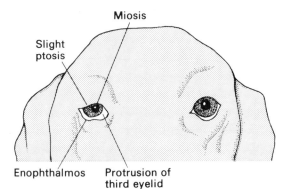

Labels: Miosis; Slight ptosis; Enophthalmos; Protrusion of third eyelid

Fig. 5.2 Horner's syndrome in the dog.

Route. Medulla→cervical cord→sympathetic outflow at T1–2 (majority of fibres to pupil) T3–4→vagosympathetic trunk up neck→the dilator of the pupil; muscle fibres in upper lid and around the orbit; blood vessels of head.

Lesions in cervical cord, or at outflow, or in fibres ascending the neck give rise to unilateral miosis, ptosis, enophthalmos, conjunctival flare.

6 Thalamus

Mass of separate nuclei acting as relay centre for all senses except olfaction. Significant in 'old dog encephalitis'.

7 Internal capsule

All fibres projecting to and from the cortex. Significant in: strokes in man; tumours in the dog; distemper in the dog.

8 Cortex

Depth of 2 mm grey matter divided into lobes named after the overlying bones: frontal, parietal, occipital and temporal; or after their function: motor, sensory, visual, auditory, association etc.

Disease, or dysfunction, of areas leads to specific characteristic clinical signs. Significant in encephalitis, tumours, trauma, epilepsy, hydrocephalus.

9 Limbic system (plus **hypothalamus**): *'emotion and appetites'*

Limbic system
- Pyriform lobe of temporal cortex
- Amygdala
- Hippocampus

→ Fear, Aggression, Emotion

10 Hypothalamus

Pituitary: endocrine functions. Thirst, appetite. Rage. Sexual behaviour: mating, oestral behaviour. Temperature control. Water balance. Sympathetic control. Significant in rabies, pituitary tumours, seizures.

11 Reticular formation: 'arousal'

Mesh of small neurons in midbrain and anterior medulla. Ascending: arousal, consciousness, sleep system.

Significant in consciousness, concussion, drugs, seizures.

12 Descending pathways: 'movement'

a Corticospinal or pyramidal tracts. Long fibres from the motor cortex crossing in hindbrain and descending to cord level but forming a multisynaptic route to the lower motor neurons in the dog. Damage causes 'weakness': hypotonia, hypokinesia and dysmetria (in man causes hemiparesis).

b Extrapyramidal system—less direct route. Cortex-basal ganglia→descending reticular formation→motor nuclei of V, IX, X, XI.→spinal tracts→lower motor neurons especially gamma (tone).

Significance in lesions at any level, but particularly cord.

SPECIALISED DIAGNOSTIC PROCEDURES

Before indulging in some of the more invasive techniques which can be applied to neurological cases, the clinician should pause and consider whether their use might not be more detrimental to the animal under his care than his remaining in some ignorance as to the exact cause or site of the neurological deficit.

The following points should be remembered:
1 Specialised techniques are no substitute for neurological examination, merely adjuncts to it.
2 The results from such examinations require interpretation: it is pointless to be competent in the mechanics of the investigation if the endproduct is meaningless.
3 The endproduct of the investigation must positively benefit the patient (e.g. by allowing surgical intervention or the establishment of an accurate diagnosis or prognosis).
4 There must be minimal risk to the animal from the technique itself. Obviously, non-invasive techniques are to be preferred to invasive if they can yield adequate data. Many investigations require the use of general anaesthesia, often in critically ill animals and this in itself may carry some risk. Animals with raised intracranial pressure should be induced with circumspection, using minimal premedication and ultrashort-acting barbiturates in very low dosage, and maintained on nitrous oxide/oxygen (avoiding halothane which may critically increase intracranial pressure).

Muscle relaxants are often indicated in the positioning of animals for cervical spine radiography and so on, but caution is needed in the physical manipulation of such unconscious, relaxed neurological cases if their recovery from anaesthesia is not to be marred by a deterioration in their clinical condition caused by injudicious and careless handling.

Radiography

Plain films of skull and spine
Non-invasive technique requiring general anaesthesia.

Familiarity with normal radiographic appearance of skull and spine is essential; it often helps to have films of normal animals available for comparison.
1 Raised intracranial pressure: thinning of cranial bones; 'copper beaten' appearance of cranial vault due to gyral pressure; diffuse 'ground glass' appearance of cranial contents due to excess CSF; open suture lines and fontanelles.
2 Local skull changes: fractures, especially in domed-skull breeds; enlargement of foramina (e.g. in cranial nerve schwannomas, carcinoma in the cavernous sinus); opacities of tympanic bullae and petrous temporal bones in otitis media.
3 Spinal column: changes are discussed in spinal cord section.

Contrast techniques
1 Angiography ⎱ Medium in vascular system.
2 Venography ⎰
3 Ventriculography: Medium in ventricles.
4 Myelography: Medium in subarachnoid space of cord.

There are many descriptions of contrast radiographic techniques applied to neurological disease in the dog, but all require general anaesthesia, some are very invasive, some require specialised equipment and some pose great difficulty in interpretation. The following section is biased heavily towards clinical veterinary practice and is therefore not comprehensive.

Angiography
Numerous listed techniques can be found in the literature. Angiography is invasive but it is not likely to cause brain shift or herniation. Theoretically, this is the procedure of choice in brain neoplasia or space-occupying lesions, but there are technical difficulties due to carotid circulation peculiarities in the dog; the need for seriographic equipment and the interpretation of the plates rule out its common application.

Venography
Cavernous sinus venography of the dog is a relatively simple and neglected technique. It is invasive, but much less so than angiography, and can be used to display masses in the orbit, the ventral floor of the cranium and the veins.

Under general anaesthesia, a cannula is inserted into the angularis oculi vein at the medial canthus of the eye and 5–10 ml of meglumine iothalamate (Conray 60) is injected steadily during manual compression of the jugular veins. Exposure is made on completion of the injection.

There are two main problems with this technique.

Firstly, it must be repeated for bilateral comparison, and secondly, interpretation can be difficult.

Posterior spinal sinus venography is possible by introducing contrast media into the saphenous vein during compression of the posterior vena cava by tight abdominal strapping. The value of the technique is limited by its lack of localisation: any lumbar lesion occluding the sinuses causes a total lack of filling along their length.

Ventriculography

This technique involves the introduction of contrast media into the lateral ventricles via a small hole in the cranial vault. It is invasive, but, in general, surprisingly safe and can be used when required in occult hydrocephalus and in demonstrating masses adjacent to and distorting the ventricles. The animal is anaesthetised and a small skin and muscle incision is made midway between the lateral canthus of the eye and the external occipital protuberance.

In young animals, a 22G needle can be introduced directly through the suture line or fontanelle; in older animals a hole is drilled using a bone pin in a Jacob's chuck. The needle is introduced vertically downwards until CFS wells up and can be withdrawn from it. Contrast medium is then introduced. Various types are advocated, including air (5–15 ml), iodo-phenylun-decyclate (Myodil) (1–3 ml) or meglumine iothalamate (Conray 60) (1–3 ml diluted 1:1 with Hartmann's solution). The latter seems the most useful.

Myelography

This is an invasive, but potentially very useful technique in demonstrating sites of cord compression which are not obvious in plain films but which may be amenable to surgery. It involves the introduction of contrast media into the subarachnoid space at the cisterna magna or in the lumbar region (L4–5 or L5–6), the latter involving the insertion of the needle through the cord into the ventral space. Only the former will be considered here, as it is relatively simple. The animal is anaesthetised and cisternal puncture is carried out as for CSF collection (see below). CSF is withdrawn (and undergoes routine analysis, particularly if myelitis is suspected), and is replaced by contrast medium. Here the choice is limited between the oily Myodil, which is immiscible with CSF and has few effects on the meninges, but which flocculates badly and gives interpretation problems, and the use of water-soluble media which are irritant to the meninges and may cause convulsions but which give excellent radiographs. Generally the oily media seem perfectly adequate, especially if introduced smoothly, although they may be superseded by the new, but expensive water-soluble compounds such as metrizamide (Amipaque). Following introduction of contrast, the animal's head is elevated and the x-ray table is inclined, to allow caudal flow of medium along the subarachnoid space, radiographs being taken at intervals along the spine to demonstrate any narrowing or hold-up.

Cerebrospinal fluid analysis

CFS analysis is either a primary investigation or is carried out secondarily to ventriculography or myelography. If the former, it is withdrawn by direct needle puncture of the subarachnoid space at the cisterna magna under general anaesthesia—an invasive technique of some risk. In patients with head trauma, or raised intracranial pressure of any cause, it should be avoided. Withdrawal of fluid at this site increases the pressure gradient between the cranial cavity and the cisterna magna, which may allow caudal shifting of the cranial contents (i.e. tentorial herniation or 'coning' of the cerebellum with dire consequences for the dog).

Cisternal puncture

Under general anaesthesia, and aseptic technique, a 22G needle $1\frac{1}{2}$–$2\frac{1}{2}$ inches long (depending on the size of the subject) is inserted slowly in the dorsal midline between the dorsal notch of the foramen magnum rostrally and the edge of the dorsal arch of the atlas (CI) caudally, with the occipitoatlantal joint flexed. The 'landmarks' for this are in the midline, halfway between the palpable external occipital protuberance of the skull and a transverse line joining the palpable lateral wings of CI, with the dog's head firmly flexed at 90° to its spine (Fig. 5.3). A small 'dimple' in the overlying musculature is usually palpable at the correct spot. If the needle is correctly aligned, slow insertion will result in a distinct loss of resistance as the point enters the subarachnoid space, and clear CSF will well up from the hub. If the needle is incorrectly positioned in the sagittal plane, its point will strike bone, whereupon it should be completely removed and correctly reinserted; if the insertion is to one side, a vertebral sinus may be entered, causing the withdrawal of blood, or blood-contaminated CSF, whereupon the procedure, if primarily intended to yield CSF for analysis, should be abandoned. Various 'correction factors' are published which are intended to compensate for blood contamination of CSF altering its protein and cellular constituents; their value is illusory.

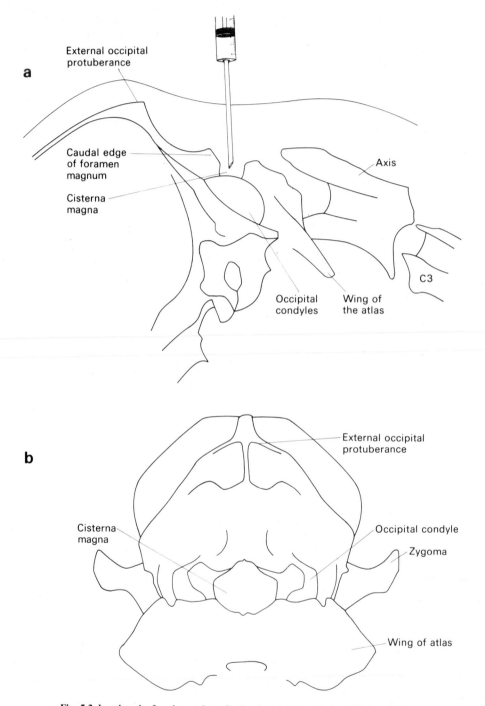

Fig. 5.3 Landmarks for cisternal tap in the dog; (a) lateral view; (b) dorsal view.

CSF Pressure

Measurement of CSF pressure using a simple spinal manometer attached to the inserted needle is advocated in the investigation of, for example, hydrocephalus or intracranial masses. The risks to such patients of cisternal tap are high and CSF pressure, although measured in mm of CSF, is somewhat mercurial, varying as it does with premedication, anaesthetic agents, hyperventilation, jugular pressure, respiration, body position and so on. Intraventricular pressure monitoring might well be of more value particularly in assessing response to treatment of brain oedema.

CSF Laboratory examination

Emphasis is placed on the clinical pathological examination of cerebrospinal fluid in cases of suspected central nervous system (CNS) disease; adequate and experienced laboratory back-up is essential if maximal value is to be obtained from the whole manipulation. Recent attention has been directed to levels of enzymes such as creatinine phosphokinase (CPK) in cerebrospinal fluid. Normally, CPK does not cross the 'blood-brain barrier' and, if present in CSF, is CNS derived. Levels in intracranial neoplasia cases appear to reflect the biological activity of the mass (i.e. the degree of cellular damage it is producing); levels in epilepsy cases may correlate with the subsequent response to therapy. However, at practice level the main analyses are directed at the detection of inflammatory disease.

Cytological examination of CSF should be carried out within 1 hour on fluid collected into plain sterile containers. Normal CSF has a few small lymphocytes and levels of total cell count of 1–8 per mm^3 are obtained. Differential cell counts may be difficult if cell numbers are below 500 per mm^3, and concentration by centrifugation may be needed. Lymphocytic or mononuclear cell increases occur in viral infections, neutrophil increases in bacterial meningitis or abscessation; occasionally tumour cells may be detected.

Otherwise the physical appearance of the sample should be considered. Thus xanthochromia (yellow) may indicate old CNS haemorrhage, frank blood may occur in trauma, and turbidity from high cell numbers may be seen in bacterial infections. Probably the single most valuable test a practitioner can carry out is to estimate CSF globulin using Pandy's reagent (10% aqueous solution of carbolic acid): 2–3 drops of CSF are added to 1 ml of the reagent. Normal CSF shows only slight haze, but CSF with increased globulin causes obvious white turbidity. Increased cellularity and globulin occur in inflammatory conditions, increased globulin alone may occur in oedema.

Electroencephalography

This technique, which is largely non-invasive, involves the recording of the microvolt (μV) potentials arising from the cortical neurons, and the relating of changes in this activity to specific diseases of the animal's brain or to the localising of brain pathology to affected areas. The procedure developed from the wide use of the EEG as an ancillary aid to diagnosis in man, and it is of small wonder that the clinical information revealed in the dog is so paltry, in proportion to the seductive sophistication of the electronics used to record it, when one considers the anatomical differences in the two species. The human cranium is thin, domed, largely unmuscled and encloses a large area of accessible cortex; the canine cranium is small in area, usually massive in thickness and in overlying musculature, and, above all, encloses a small area of inaccessible cortex largely devoted to non-cooperative behaviour. In order to circumvent these difficulties and record cortical activity, it is usually necessary to resort to general anaesthesia, both to allow adequate restraint for recording and to eliminate artifacts arising from movement and muscle potentials which are usually thousands of times greater in amplitude than the cortical signals. By so doing, one modifies the cortical activity of the patient, which one is attempting to observe. However, judicious use of selected sedatives and anaesthetics and the adoption of standardised electrode types, placements and combinations, frequently allows the recording and detection of abnormal cortical activity and its objective evaluation over a period of time; against this should be placed the largely non-specific nature of the changes observed which, without good clinical evaluation of the case, may be valueless in obtaining a diagnosis.

A selection of EEG traces are shown in Fig. 5.4.

THE BRAIN

Clinical approach to suspected brain pathology

If the dog has suffered impaired consciousness, even if only briefly after trauma, hospitalise it and give repeated neurological examinations. It cannot be overstressed that 'unconsciousness' is no reason for failing to adequately assess a neurological case; by simple clinical examination a great deal of valuable information can be rapidly determined and deterioration

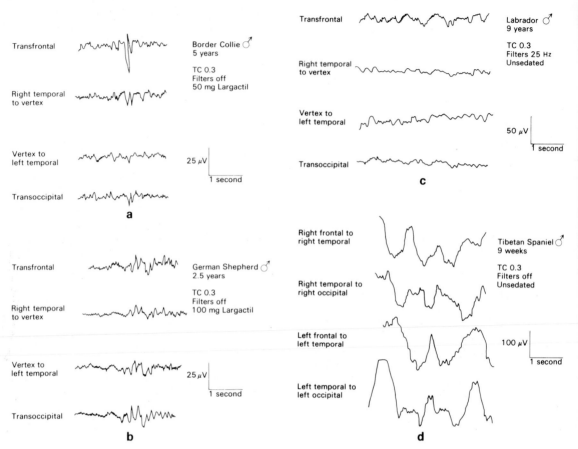

Fig. 5.4 (a) Focal spiking in acquired epilepsy; (b) paroxysmal spiking in generalised epilepsy; (c) diffuse slowing in ODE; (d) hydrocephalus.

Table 5.1   Clinical signs of impairment of consciousness

Level of impairment	Clinical signs
Apathy	Arouse easily; only slight and subtle changes
Drowsiness or torpor	Blunted alertness to normal stimuli
Stupor	Arouse only on vigorous stimulation and immediately relapse when stimulation ceases
Coma	Unresponsive
Death	

can be the more speedily noted (Table 5.1). Raised intracranial pressure may show as impaired consciousness, with or without focal signs, papilloedema (engorgement of the blood vessels of the optic disc), signs of tentorial herniation, progressive rostrocaudal appearance of cranial nerve, vestibular, cerebellar and medulla signs, neck stiffness or onset of extensor rigidity.

During examination, contributing conditions and differential clues can be obtained. For example, pyrexia may indicate infection; hypothermia may indicate brain stem damage; palpation of the skull may reveal recent, or past, trauma, open fontanelles and suture lines; neck rigidity may result from meningitis or cerebellar 'coning': the optic fundus may show papilloedema, optic neuritis, retinitis, haemorrhage, diabetic retinopathy and so on; limb movements and tremors may result from status epilepticus or cerebellar damage. Two clinical warnings are important:

1 Longstanding brain pathology, particularly if space occupying, may give rise to *sudden onset* of marked clinical signs as herniation occurs.

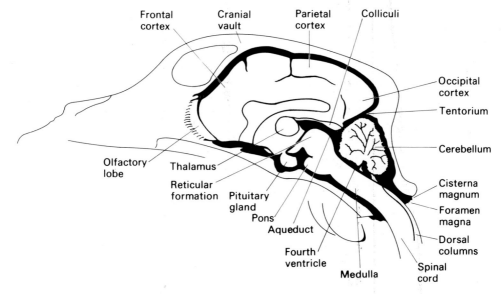

Fig. 5.5 Normal skull-brain relationship in the dog.

2 The animal which has suffered an unobserved epileptiform fit may be presented in postictal confusion, often with ataxia, blindness, stupor, polyphagia or incontinence.

When presented with an acute case, often following trauma, with rapid deterioration, and loss of consciousness it is important to maintain adequate oxygenation. The brain can carry enough glucose for up to 90 minutes of low activity but it cannot store oxygen at all—asphyxia, respiratory depression or even reduced blood flow in surgical hypotension rapidly cause irreversible brain damage. Thus oxygen, with

positive pressure respiration if needed, should be given and adequate steps taken to ensure effective blood circulation before any further procedures are carried out. Incidentally, the unconscious animal which shows signs of hypovolaemic shock will almost certainly have injuries other than to the brain; *a blow to the head does not cause shock*. If indicated, appropriate isotonic fluids and blood can be given, but care should be taken to avoid water loading when brain oedema may be present.

Osmotic diuretics such as mannitol (20%) solution (3 g/kg body weight intravenously), or oral glycerine, may be used to stabilise the brain oedema case long

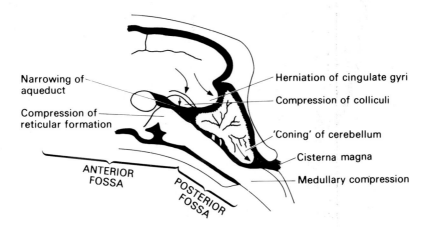

Fig. 5.6 The effects of raised intracranial pressure on skull-brain relationships.

enough for further investigation to be carried out, but any improvement resulting from their use should not be viewed in a false glow of achievement—rapid rebound and deterioration is very common.

Steroids used in very large doses (e.g. dexamethasone 1.1 mg/kg body weight repeated 3-hourly) are effective if extensive structural damage is not present. If in doubt at the time of admission of the animal, steroids should be given anyway, as the earlier they are administered the more effective they are.

Once stability of the patient has been obtained, then more specialised procedures such as EEG and radiography can be applied to obtain more definitive diagnosis.

In acute head injury cases, complications may frequently occur:

Depressed fractures should be elevated and any foreign body or bone fragments should be removed promptly when the patient is stable, with appropriate parenteral antibiotics if the fractures are compound. Clinicians should resist the temptation to apply local medication in open cranial injuries.

Seizures occurring acutely after injury carry a better long-term prognosis than those of late onset some months after injury. Direct cranial nerve damage may occur, but the long-term resolution is generally good.

Subdural haemorrhage in dogs after injury appears uncommon, but such a case might be expected to show progressive deterioration after initial recovery.

Currently, radical exploratory surgery appears to be in vogue in both man and dog but its efficiency or effects seem impossible to assess. Thus patients which are rapidly deteriorating, undergo immediate 'burr hole' surgery bilaterally to expose and decompress the brain; the initial hole is enlarged if bulging of the brain occurs, the dura is opened and the lateral ventricles are tapped to physically extract CSF and thus lower ventricular pressure.

Chronic or long-term cases such as animals with brain tumours, old dog encephalitis, or hydrocephalus, may benefit greatly from steroids, especially in combination with carbonic anhydrase inhibiting diuretics, such as acetazolamide, both drugs being given in normal therapeutic dose levels.

Brain tumours

As discussed in more general terms elsewhere, expanding tumour masses give rise to focal signs and more general dysfunction related to increased intracranial pressure. Focally, the brain is compressed or infiltrated by the mass, local blood supply is compromised and a peritumour zone of cerebral oedema is created which increases the neurological deficit. Many masses metastasise rapidly, both directly and by 'seeding' into the CSF, and the clinical picture is thus rendered more obscure. Once a critical size is achieved a generalised increase in intracranial pressure occurs, often sudden in onset and following ventricular obstruction. This pressure increase is relieved only by herniation of cranial contents caudally. Presented dogs may show headache (manifested by head pressing and pawing, and arising from displacement of the meninges) and personality changes, particularly profound dullness and depression (torpor), sometimes alternating with mania, and shortened attention span. They frequently fail to respond when called, or to recognise familiar human contacts, and are incapable of spontaneous initiation of activity, such as 'asking' to go for walks, or for food. In general, the affected animal loses acquired habits and individuality and tends towards a state of canine dementia, which is very distressing to the attendant owner. Conversely, seizures may be the initial presenting sign often with a significant focal onset or focal residua. Papilloedema, visual field defects (often described by the owner as 'blindness in one eye') blindness or amaurosis may occur. Sensory deficits in touch, pain and proprioception, or motor abnormalities such as 'forced walking', circling to the affected side, or contralateral hemiplegia may occur. Vasomotor or autonomic signs such as bradycardia, and hyperthermia may occur from hypothalamic involvement. Posterior fossa tumours may cause cerebellar or vestibular signs and the onset of cerebellar coning may be marked by vomiting, deep slow respirations, and neck pain. Occasionally, the developing mass may be 'silent' but produce false localising signs by compressing opposite or remote structures, for example contralateral vestibular signs, or focal psychomotor seizures arising from frontal masses indirectly affecting the temporal lobe with its very low seizure threshold.

Diagnosis

Based upon breed and age, detailed clinical neurological examination and history (of previous malignant primaries or developing clinical signs). More specialised techniques such as plain film skull radiographs, venography and ventriculography may be very valuable. Electroencephalography may be disappointing: some brachycephalics have such massive skull and temporal muscle development that signal attenuation does not allow recording of cortical impulses from even anaesthetised and paralysed dogs; or the offending mass may be in the base of the brain or the posterior fossa. CSF collection is dangerous from the cisterna magna: the resulting fall in pressure may be sufficient to allow gross herniation of the compressed brain through the foramen magnum.

Classification of nervous system tumours is complex and often controversial; only aspects of diagnostic or prognostic value will be discussed here.

Tumours may be primary or secondary. The latter may arise by local invasion through the skull or its foramina, or more commonly, by haematogenous spread from remote sites, particularly the mammary glands in the bitch. Most metastases of the brain involve the grey matter of the cerebellum, the hippocampus, the basal ganglia and the meninges, and are frequently multiple. Primary tumours involve various cell types.

Meningiomas are the most frequent of all intracranial tumours. They are solitary and often involve the base of the brain of the dog, where surgical intervention is difficult. They occur most often in dolichocephalic breeds, in individuals aged between 7 and 14 years.

Conversely, oligodendrogliomas and astrocytomas are commonest in brachycephalic breeds, especially the Boxer, Boston Terrier and the Bulldog, in individuals aged 5-11 years. Oligodendrogliomas occur typically in the frontal and temporal lobes bordering the ventricles, or breaking through into them. Astrocytomas are more typically found in the pyriform cortex. Pituitary adenomas may give rise to local signs of aggression and visual abnormalities and general signs of canine Cushing's syndrome or diabetes insipidus. Expansion of the sella by the developing mass is seen radiographically in man, but does not appear to occur in the dog.

Treatment

Extra-axial masses on the dorsal surface of the cortex may be excisable, but only isolated reports occur in the literature. More usually, conservative therapy directed at control of seizures (see p. 126) and of brain oedema (see p. 119) is indicated, with often very useful remissions being obtained. The removal of the peritumour oedema represents in real terms a marked reduction in the size of the advancing 'sphere of influence' of the mass, with corresponding improvement in the dog's neurological state. The use of chemotherapy in dogs is as yet ill defined; radiotherapy similarly awaits evaluation.

Hydrocephalus

This condition is characterised by dilation of the cerebral ventricles with a rise in cerebrospinal fluid volume, usually caused by obstruction to the CSF circulation. In young dogs this may be followed by gross skull enlargement. Hydrocephalus may be active (pro-

gressive and associated with raised intracranial pressure), or arrested (no progressive ventricular enlargement occurs and intracranial pressure is normal at the time of examination).

Pathogenesis

1 Obstruction is the commonest cause of hydrocephalus, resulting in increase in intraventricular static and pulsatile pressure proximal to the blockage, causing compression of white matter with loss of protein and lipid and increased uptake of sodium and water. The cause may be neoplastic, especially in gliomas adjacent to or breaking through into the ventricles, congenital, or related to postinflammatory or posttraumatic damage.
2 Excessive production is theoretically possible in tumours of the choroid plexus ('plexus papillomas').
3 Defective absorption at the arachnoid villae associated with subarachnoid haemorrhage, meningitis or increase in CSF viscosity.

Clinically it is characterised by a wide and often bizarre array of signs usually in young dogs, especially Chihuahuas, Yorkshire Terriers and other 'Toy' breeds. Affected puppies may have open fontanelles but most significantly show disproportionate rate of head growth, seizures, downward and outward strabismus and retardation in comparison with normal animals of the same age. Because of the relatively late completion of myelination in the puppy's brain (at 6 months of age) affected pups may be neurologically normal at birth but progressively lag behind as brain development proceeds. Older animals often display the clinical signs of the primary condition giving rise to a secondary hydrocephalus but it is often remarkable how advanced hydrocephalus can be in adult dogs without clinical evidence. Adult dogs show signs of raised intracranial pressure, dementia and brain herniation but diagnosis often depends on radiography of the skull especially ventriculography. EEG examination is a useful non-invasive technique; CSF pressure measurements appear somewhat valueless in the dog.

Treatment

Hydrocephalus is primarily a surgical condition and the logical treatment is to shunt the obstructed CSF from the lateral ventricles to the right atrium of the heart via a one-way valve system. Surgically, this technique is simple and will probably become more widely used.

Medical treatment of hydrocephalus is aimed at reducing CSF production and oedema and is discussed on p. 119.

Epilepsy

Epilepsy is a disease characterised by paroxysmal and abnormal electrical discharge in the brain, leading to the overt signs we call 'seizures', 'fits' or 'convulsions'. It is a condition of some importance in the dog, as it has a relatively high incidence, and an almost uniquely distressing effect upon the animal's human contacts. Understanding can only be attained if the clinician appreciates the underlying pathophysiology common to all seizures, and avoids the pitfall of equating lists of aetiologies with gains in comprehension. In the following section, the use of the term 'epilepsy' is extended from the narrow veterinary convention delineating convulsions of idiopathic (i.e. unknown) aetiology, to cover any disorder characterised by seizures, in the hope that readers will therefore adopt a common approach to all 'fitting' dogs whatever the cause.

Pathophysiology

Certain key areas of the brain, specifically the reticular formation, the limbic system and the motor cortex, are known to have low thresholds for paroxysmal discharge and hence have a tendency to respond to insult, of metabolic or physical nature, by the production of seizures. Thus epilepsy tends to occur in response to metabolic imbalance, toxins and drugs, or in response to space-occupying masses, or in scar formation following trauma, acting as foci for the production of abnormal discharge which spreads throughout the brain either centrifugally or by normal physiological pathways.

The production and propagation of this seizure discharge depends upon the convulsive threshold of the brain area in which it arises and, also, of the individual as a whole. Thus if the insult to the brain is sufficiently gross to exceed the convulsive threshold, any animal may respond with an overt clinical attack. In some individuals this threshold is high and they will thus rarely respond to even the grossest brain pathology by convulsing; others have a low threshold, and comparatively insignificant or covert insults will result in epilepsy. Animals which have suffered a clinical attack, may subsequently have a lowered threshold and may even continue to have attacks when the initiating cause has been removed or successfully treated. Particular groups such as male animals or the young may show especial susceptibility, and, in adequately studied breeds with a recognised epilepsy problem, a larger than average proportion of the general population appear to fall in the low threshold category, although they may remain clinically normal and undetected. There is no evidence for the often quoted simple autosomal recessive inheritance of epilepsy in the dog, in which the postulates appear to be that homozygosity for the offending gene will in itself precipitate seizures, and that heterozygosity (the 'carrier' state) will be manifested as abnormal EEG activity. Recent reconsideration of the original data has shown that a threshold trait, inherited in a complex manner is a far more acceptable, if less simple, hypothesis.

Clinical approach to an epileptic case

The clinician should attempt to achieve a clear mental image of the seizure suffered by the animal, as he will only rarely be present during an attack. Initial signs of apprehension, behaviour changes, local or unilateral motor activity suggest focal origin to the discharge; such signs may be transient, they may occur alone, or may be engulfed by the more profound signs of a generalised attack as the discharge spreads throughout the brain. In the later attacks of a series, they may be lost altogether. Such attacks, or those of toxic or metabolic origin, are usually generalised and sudden in onset with no prodromal signs; the animal collapses without warning into symmetrical tonic extensor spasms, often whilst drowsy or on awakening. Recovery is often prolonged, with ataxia, central blindness, incontinence and focal paresis, frequently followed by increased thirst and appetite. In a major series of seizures or in status epilepticus, recovery may be incomplete before another attack starts, and, even if control is achieved, the animal may be in a state of dementia for days or even weeks.

In many patients a combination of factors may be needed to precipitate attacks.

1 A genetically determined predisposition, or an age- or sex-modified factor.
2 A general metabolic disturbance lowering threshold (e.g. hypoglycaemia, renal failure or water loading during oestrus).
3 A focal, acquired brain lesion from encephalitis, scarring or space-occupying masses.
4 A 'triggering' factor (e.g. sleep or emotional stress).

Detailed clinical neurological examination, with indicated clinical pathology, radiology and so on *must* be carried out to delineate any of the above factors operating in a particular case.

Electroencephalography of clinical epileptic patients may be of great value in determining the type and origin of the attacks, but it must be carried out under controlled conditions and often involves the use of provocative techniques to expose abnormal discharge between overt seizures. Recording from conscious individuals for brief periods is not of value, mainly because of technical difficulties in recording.

Treatment

Treat the cause if found.

Anticonvulsant therapy is aimed at increasing convulsive threshold and its short-term use is to be deprecated. Usually one drug of choice is used, at least initially, and any alteration of dosage, or withdrawal or introduction of additional medication is carried out slowly. Clinicians and owners should be well aware that complete control of seizures in some animals is impossible and partial success may need to be accepted.

A variety of anticonvulsant drugs are available, but recent research has shown that major differences in the way in which these compounds are absorbed from the gut, are protein-bound in the blood and are metabolised and/or excreted in the dog, compared to man, casts serious doubts over their presumed efficacy in this species. Individual variation in pharmacokinetics poses additional problems, and explains, to some degree, the disappointing therapeutic results.

On the basis of this, the barbiturate and barbiturate-based anticonvulsants such as primidone appear to be most likely to give consistent results. Oral dosage (2-4 mg/kg/day for phenobarbitone, 10 mg/kg/day for primidone) should be monitored by blood assay for phenobarbitone levels (with both compounds, as the parent primidone rapidly disappears from the blood within days of the onset of therapy) in an attempt to achieve therapeutic blood levels. Marked variation in individual sensitivity to these compounds can only be detected and corrected for by this means. As the barbiturates may be hepatotoxic, monitoring of liver enzymes before treatment starts and at intervals during it is obviously indicated.

Other anticonvulsants used chronically in man, such as benzodiazepines, valproic acid and phenytoin, do not appear to achieve therapeutic blood levels when given orally in recommended dose, and again are best monitored by regular blood assay, either when used alone, or in combination with a barbiturate.

Adjuvant therapy

Drugs aimed at specific triggering factors in epilepsy may be of great value in preventing an overt attack. For example many bitches may have seizures precipitated by the water loading that occurs during oestrus; the use of oral acetazolamide in addition to routine anticonvulsants at high risk times in these animals may prevent clinical attacks occurring. Castration or the use of hormones in male epileptics have some proponents.

Status epilepticus

This is continual seizure activity of whatever cause without respite between attacks. Encephalitis, toxins such as strychnine, organophosphates or metaldehyde and metabolic disturbances such as hypocalcaemia or uraemia; all may induce status and *all should be approached in the same manner as 'idiopathic' status.*

This is an emergency and the convulsions should be controlled before specific therapy is attempted.

Intravenous administration of diazepam (2.5-10.0 mg) or clonazepam (0.5-2.0 mg) is the best initial approach. If the animal is not adequately controlled by these drugs, then general anaesthesia (GA) using a minimal induction dose of an ultra-short-acting barbiturate followed by maintenance with an inhalation anaesthetic is indicated. The use of intravenous pento-barbitone sodium in such cases is to be avoided; the 'excitement phase' of recovery from this drug is in reality an expression of its dose-related convulsant activity and is also to be avoided. During the general anaesthesia, additional dosage of parenteral anticonvulsants, including phenytoin sodium, may be given together with fluids and supportive therapy, and specific treatment can be initiated whilst the clinician has total control over the animal's functions. On monitored recovery from the GA, long-term anticonvulsant therapy should be commenced and continued indefinitely or until the clinician is satisfied that the initiating cause has been adequately treated or removed.

Narcolepsy

Narcolepsy is a disease of acute onset in young animals, which has been reported as inherited in the Doberman, and possibly inherited in the Labrador and the Miniature Poodle.

Clinical attacks are precipitated by excitement, feeding or a novel situation, and are either complete, the dog lying flaccidly in any position, or partial, involving only the hindlimbs. Attacks can be aborted by the attendant handling or arousing the animal. Frequency of attacks varies from one or two attacks every few weeks to many per day, depending on the individual.

Diagnosis is based on the clinical signs, EEG study of sleep patterns and on pharmacological provocation with physostigmine (0.03-0.08 mg/kg given i.v.), or suppression with atropine sulphate (0.1 mg/kg given i.v.). Treatment is with methylphenidate at 0.25 mg/kg orally, adjusting the dose to reduce cataplectic attacks to an acceptable level.

Syncope or fainting

The clinician may be given a history which does not allow him to differentiate between the animal which has suffered a seizure and the animal which has fainted or suffered a 'drop attack'.

'Fainting' is a transient loss of consciousness caused by a fall in cerebral blood flow below a critical level, usually due to changes in general systemic blood flow.

'Drop attacks' usually result from direct interruption of arterial supply to the brain.

Fainting occurs in vasodepression in man, when peripheral resistance falls rapidly; in Stokes-Adams's attacks with asystole and tachycardia in Boxers; in transient cerebral ischaemia in coughing attacks or during micturition; or in failure in the supply of blood-borne components such as oxygen or glucose. If the faint is brief, the animal may stagger or 'flop' down with relaxed limbs, but if longer than five seconds, then neurological signs of convulsive movements, extensor rigidity, and pupil dilatation may occur. Recovery from the brief attack is rapid and complete; if neurological signs occur then recovery may be confused and prolonged.

The commonest cause of syncope in the dog appears to be organic heart disease, either due to reduced stroke volume from the affected myocardium or from the valvular lesions. These are usually effort related; in the early stages due to blood shunting to peripheral muscles on exercise, or, later, associated with transient asystoles and reduced coronary flow. Cough syncope may occur in these animals due to direct squeezing of cerebral vessels or to the concussive effect of the CSF pressure rise.

Infectious disease of the central nervous system

Infectious agents are arguably the commonest cause of CNS disorders in the dog. In this species, the overwhelming majority of cases will be viral in origin, bacterial invasion of the CNS occurring sporadically from penetrating wounds, etc.

Canine distemper virus remains a major problem of dogs in the United Kingdom, and its clinical manifestations are protean. A spectrum of conditions exists, graded from syndromes where the virus can be isolated with ease in a fully virulent form, through those where CD antigen can be demonstrated, but not isolated, to those where the role of CD virus is largely speculative.

Classic canine distemper

This is a disease of young, unvaccinated dogs of any breed. Onset of clinical signs is usually quite acute, often preceded by systemic signs of pyrexia, cough, vomiting or diarrhoea.

Objectively, the animal may be torpid or manic, and may have ill-defined generalised seizures, tremor, ataxia, blindness and so-called choreiform movements of head, neck or limbs. Retinitis with scattered areas of tapetal hyper-reflectivity is frequently present.

CSF may show increased cell counts, EEG traces reveal extensive cortical damage, but more specifically, conjunctival smears give positive fluorescent antibody tests for CD antigen. Therapy is largely non-specific, directed to control of secondary infection (including Toxoplasmosis), and supportive measures such as primidone to control seizures, steroids in acute limited dosage to reduce brain oedema, high level 'B' group vitamins, etc.

Chronic canine distemper

This disease is not uncommon, but carries a low index of suspicion amongst clinicians. Mature dogs of any breed, frequently fully vaccinated, can be affected.

Onset of clinical signs is insidious, with no systemic signs. Owners report hindlimb ataxia and weakness with variable progression, often over many months. Objective neurological signs are referable to the cerebellum and brainstem and the dog's personality is intact. Tremor, central vestibular signs and loss of menace reflexes may occur, and the hindlimb weakness may progress slowly to quadriplegia. Retinal lesions may be present. Conjunctival smears may be positive for CD antigen. There is no treatment.

Old dog encephalitis

Confusion is possible between this condition and space-occupying pathology. Affected animals are frequently diagnosed as having 'brain tumours'. Mature dogs, often fully vaccinated, are affected.

Onset of signs is insidious, with no systemic problem. Owners are distressed by the dog's personality change, as many animals appear withdrawn and unresponsive. They may refuse to settle down and rise and pace incessantly. They appear blind, although their attention span is limited and assessment may be difficult. Retinal lesions sometimes occur. The time course is usually months, but animals are commonly put-down as the normal bond with the owners breaks down.

CSF is usually normal. EEG reveals a diffuse cortical depression. There is no treatment.

Polioencephalomalacia (Cerebrocortical necrosis)

There is no age, sex or breed predisposition.

The condition is seen as an acute onset of generalised seizures followed by a short clinical course of personality change, head tilt, blindness and facial twitching and myoclonic jerking. Menace defects are frequently seen and animals may become hemiparetic.

CD antigen has been demonstrated in some cases of this syndrome. Response to therapy is disappointing.

Granulomatous meningoencephalitis

Mostly affects mature animals of any breed. Onset is acute and the course is progressive.

Clinical signs are truly protean, but correlate well with the underlying pathology. Dogs may be grossly ataxic, incoordinated or paretic, may show central vestibular syndrome, facial paralysis, etc., or may have generalised convulsions, depending on the major site of the lesions. Cervical pain is not unusual, and animals can be febrile — leading to a diagnosis of 'meningitis' and attempts at therapy with antibiotics.

The pathology of this condition underlies the complex clinical picture. There is meningitis and perivascular cuffing, and, more significantly, white matter lesions of cerebrum, cerebellum, brain stem, cervical cord, etc., related to blood vessels. Orderly clinical examination should reveal the multifocal nature of the condition, with brain stem signs predominating, and may lead to misdiagnosis as classical canine distemper, even though animals may be vaccinated and mature.

The aetiology of this condition is unknown. Temporary, partial, but useful, remission of clinical signs may follow dosage with high level parenteral steroids; on occasions the response is dramatic.

Reticulosis

Considerable confusion exists over the relationship of granulomatous meningoencephalitis and disseminated reticulosis, and over the gradation from inflammatory reticulosis into neoplastic reticulosis, and over the classification of reticulosis and intracranial lymphosarcomata. Given the current state of canine clinical neurology, this may be largely academic. Disseminated reticulosis is clinically and pathologically related to granulomatous meningoencephalitis, q.v. Discrete focal reticulosis occurs in mature animals, with a possible breed predilection in Terriers and Miniature Poodles. Onset may be acute or insidious, but established clinical signs are those of lateral or focal space-occupying pathology. Animals may also show acute onset blindness sometimes with marked optic neuritis. The response to this condition to high level steroids (2 mg/kg daily) may be very gratifying, with rapid resolution of blindness and other clinical signs.

Aujeskie's disease

Animals may be of any age or sex, but high incidence is associated with pig contact, either directly or *via* the feeding of pig offal, e.g. Hound packs, etc. Onset is acute and the clinical course extremely short. Most animals will die or be destroyed within 48 hours of the onset of signs.

Clinical signs include pyrexia, dullness, emesis, diarrhoea, tachypnoea, crying, hyperaesthesia and seizures. Pruritus and self-mutilation may occur, but are inconstant findings.

Diagnosis is made by virus isolation from fresh brain tissue, and on histological findings.

Parainfluenza virus encephalitis

Isolation of a parainfluenza virus from a dog with posterior paresis has been reported. The virus is normally associated with infectious tracheobronchitis.

Toxoplasmosis

The true role of the protozoan in canine encephalitis is obscure. The organism appears largely opportunist, becoming clinically significant in animals immunosupressed by, for example, CD virus infection. Paired serial blood samples for rising titres against Toxoplasma are indicated,

Cryptococcosis

The saprophytic yeast, *Cryptococcus neoformans*, has been recorded in the UK as causing limb weakness, head tremor and neck pain. Diagnosis was only possible at post mortem.

Metabolic disorders

1 *Hepatoencephalopathy*. Neurological signs arising from hepatic dysfunction are not uncommon. Young animals which are failing to grow, or are losing condition, show drug intolerance (especially to barbiturates or phenothiazine tranquillisers), polydipsia, polyuria, diarrhoea, pyrexia and a plethora of neurological signs such as hysteria, viciousness, central blindness, circling or pacing, and generalised seizures, and in which signs are intermittent with total recovery should arouse suspicion. Careful history-taking will often reveal an association with feeding, especially of high protein food, and converse improvement with starvation. Older animals with hepatic problems, intestinal haemorrhage, etc. may also show hepatoencephalopathy, but in a less defined manner. Diagnosis is confirmed by demonstration of increase in blood ammonia, presence of ammonium biurate crystals in urine sediment, and less specifically, by impaired bromosulphthalein clearance and low blood urea. Ammonia tolerance testing using oral ammonium

chloride can also be employed. In young animals, investigation for possible portosystemic shunts is required. Control of the syndrome is based on low protein diets, and the use of gut-active antibiotics (such as neomycin) and acidifiers to decrease ammonia absorption from the gut.

2 *Uraemic Encephalopathy.* Acute renal failure may give rise to a syndrome characterised by behaviour changes, tremors, facial twitching, head nodding and generalised seizures, sometimes triggered by handling around the head. Affected animals do not show the consciousness changes seen in hepatic syndrome.

3 *Hypoglycaemia.* Functional islet cell tumours in the dog may give rise to episodic weakness, twitching, ataxia or generalised convulsions, associated with exercise or time-locked to feeding. Initial signs may be sporadic and precipitated by stress or abnormal amounts of exercise. Owners may report the condition as poor exercise tolerance or transient collapse. Serial blood glucose determination during exercise or a standard glucose tolerance test may be of value, but determination of fasting glucose/insulin ratio confirms. Terminal cases develop a polioencephalomalacia characterised by continuous seizures and myoclonus, with terminal coma. There are reports of surgical removal of the neoplasm, but hepatic metastases are common in this species, and oral diazoxide (Eudemine) is useful in long-term control.

SPINAL CORD

Spinal cord dysfunction arises from compression of the cord by surrounding structures, or from primary conditions of the cord itself. The results of compression upon the tissues of the cord may well be mediated by its effects upon the blood vessels supplying them; thus slowly developing lesions, such as tumours in the vertebral canal, or malformations of the vertebra themselves, may give rise primarily to venous occlusion and stasis, and white matter degeneration, whereas rapidly compressive or explosive-onset lesions may cause oedema, frank haemorrhage and acute vascular spasm affecting cord segment grey matter, and distant signs arising from failure to the damaged white matter which leads to failure to transmit impulses adequately; removal of distortion, within a limited time period, results in restoration of normal function.

Lesions can thus give rise to local signs from the affected cord segment grey matter, and distant signs arising from failure of the damaged white matter to allow through transmission of normal activity.

Local signs (lower motor neuron signs)
These include defects of sensation, muscle paralysis with neurogenic atrophy, diminished spinal reflex activity (absent jerks, low muscle tone) showing a nerve root pattern of distribution with specific local signs at particular longitudinal levels of the cord.

Table 5.2 Cord segments affected and the local signs

Local sign	Cord segments
Horner's syndrome	Cervical
Forelimb signs	C6–T1
Diaphragm paralysis	C5,6,7
Panniculus reflex (skin twitch) abnormalities	
Segmental input	T1–L3
Motor fibres	C8, T1–2
Segmental intercostal paralysis	Thoracic
Hindlimb signs	L4, 5, 6, 7–S1, 2, 3
Atonic bladder (overflow)	S1, 2, 3

The clinician should be aware that, due to differential embryonic growth, cord segments do not necessarily correspond anatomically with vertebral levels, and hence with spinal nerves, since these are usually identified by the number of the vertebra immediately rostral to the exit of the nerve from the vertebral column. Thus the nerve roots emerging from the cord may traverse a variable distance caudally, within the vertebral canal, before fusing and emerging as a spinal nerve through the intervertebral foramen. The clinical significance of this can be seen especially in the lumbar region, where sacral segments 1, 2 and 3 are within vertebral segment L5, and the last coccygeal cord segment is located at vertebral level L6–7. Thus a compressive lesion posterior to this vertebral level can no longer affect cord tissue, but must involve the descending nerve roots alone and give rise to a lower motor neuron type of injury.

Figs 5.7–5.11 illustrate this point, and allow comparison of radiographic findings with clinical signs.

Distant signs (upper motor neuron signs)
Below the level of the damaged cord, deficits in the areas subserved by the white matter of the affected segments may be observed as:

1 Local enhanced reflex activity (increased or undamped reverberatory jerks, increased muscle tone).

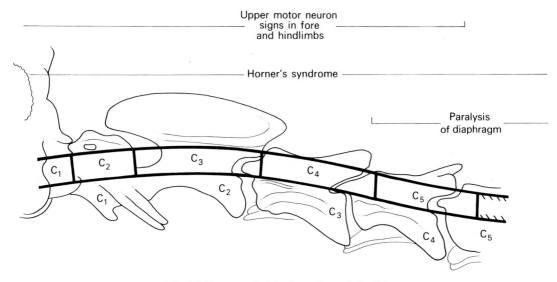

Fig. 5.7 Upper cervical cord-vertebrae relationships.

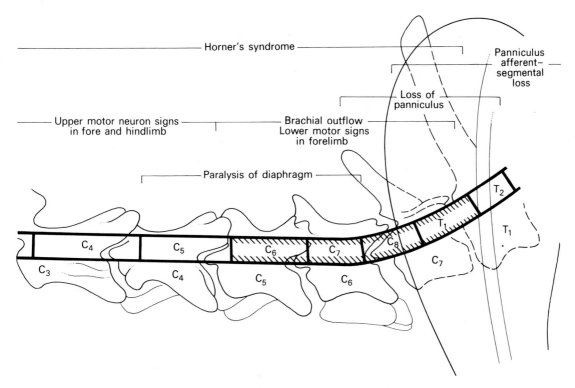

Fig. 5.8 Lower cervical cord-vertebrae relationships.

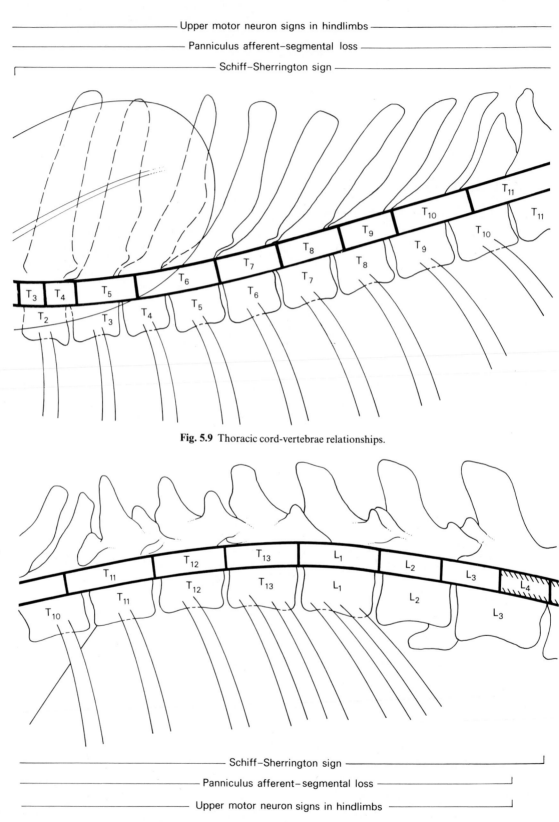

Fig. 5.9 Thoracic cord-vertebrae relationships.

Fig. 5.10 Thoraco-lumbar junction cord-vertebrae relationships.

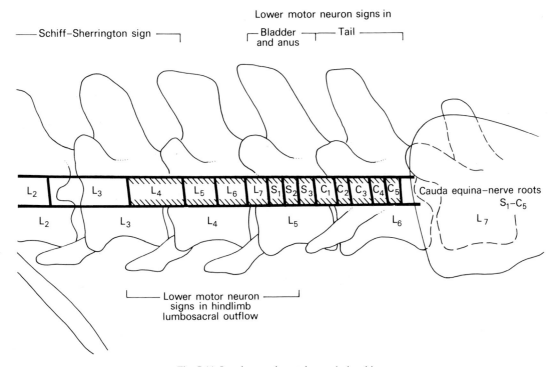

Fig. 5.11 Lumbar cord–vertebrae relationships.

2 Weakness, paresis and loss of voluntary motor control, with disuse atrophy.

3 Defects in postural reflexes dependent upon higher centres (poor limb and joint position sense).

4 Loss of bladder control with appearance of an 'automatic' bladder.

5 Loss of conscious response to pain (a poor prognostic sign, indicating wide transverse distribution of damage at affected segment).

6 Appearance of abnormal local reflexes such as the crossed extensor response (withdrawal of stimulated limb and simultaneous extension of the opposite limb) and the mass response (gross reaction of body posterior to cord lesion to any stimulus) both carrying a poor prognosis, indicating functional cord transection.

7 Schiff–Sherrington response: hyperactivity *above* the level of the cord lesion, usually seen as extensor rigidity of the forelimbs in thoracolumbar transection.

Severity of clinical signs

This depends on the following:
1 Speed of onset of the lesion.
2 Its transverse and longitudinal extent.
3 The normal functional role of the affected segments.
4 The cause.

Clinical examination of a case of cord damage should be aimed at localising the level of the lesion based upon information as set out in Tables 5.1 and 5.2.

However, further investigation may be needed (e.g. plain film radiography). These films should be taken in two planes, with accurate alignment of spine parallel to plate; views under traction (cervical) or in extension or flexion may also be required. They should be examined paying particular attention to the following:

1 The number, shape, density and alignment of vertebra.
2 The size and shape of intervertebral foramina.
3 The width and shape of the vertebral canal.
4 The disc spaces.
5 Soft tissue shadows, or calcification.

Plain films are usually sufficient but if they are not, or if more detailed localisation is needed (e.g. prior to surgery), a myelogram may be needed. CSF removed at this time should undergo routine analysis.

In general, presented cases of spinal cord disease tend to fall into three categories based on management:

Table 5.3 General guide to cord damage at different levels (signs may be unilateral or bilateral)

---

1 High cervical
Ataxia, especially hindlimbs
Poor limb position sense (hind and fore)
Poor reflex stepping (hind and fore)
Increased spinal reflexes (hind and fore)
Horner's syndrome
Paresis

2 Low cervical
Panniculus may be absent
Decreased spinal reflexes (fore)
Paralysis and atrophy (fore)
Horner's syndrome
Ataxia (hind)
Poor position sense (hind)
Increased spinal reflexes (hind)
Paresis

3 Thoracolumbar
Normal forelimbs
Panniculus segmentally absent
Upper motor neuron or lower motor neuron (hind)
Automatic bladder may develop

4 Lumbosacral cord
Lower motor neuron (hind)
Retention of urine with overflow
Paralysis of anus, tail

5 TL cord transection
Extensor rigidity forelegs
Upper motor neuron (hind)
Automatic bladder may develop
Abnormal reflexes may develop (e.g. mass response, crossed extensor in hind, spinal reflex walking)

6 Ascending spinal syndrome
Progresses from TL signs:
Extensor rigidity forelegs
Lower motor neuron signs in hindlegs, anus, tail
Retention with overflow
Paradoxical respiration. Intercostal muscles progressively paralysed and chest falls on inspiration as diaphragm descends

1 Those requiring conservative treatment: usually localised pain, with no other signs and little history. Confinement at home and mild analgesia. Allow time to assess any changes.
2 Those requiring hospitalisation primarily for treatment or for further detailed investigation.
3 Those requiring immediate admission for emergency treatment (e.g. acute or rapidly progressing cord disease or bladder involvement).

Category 3 cases pose an immediate clinical challenge and include cases of acute trauma to the spinal cord usually as the result of a road traffic accident giving rise to a vertebral fracture, dislocation or traumatic disc protrusion. Clinical signs vary with the localisation of the lesion and the severity of the cord damage; the prognosis given to the owner at the time of presentation will however depend solely upon these signs and initial neurological examination should be thorough; radiographic evidence of trauma is of little prognostic value: animals with virtually none may have sustained functional cord transection; animals with gross disarray of the spine on x-ray may have minimal neurological dysfunction.

Prolapsed Intervertebral Discs (PID)

The major clinical problem of PID in the dog lies not in establishing a diagnosis, but in assessing the proper course of treatment and possible prognosis in each individual case; the following section will be biased accordingly. Prolapse of the intervertebral disc occurs in mainly middle-aged animals particularly, but not solely, following chondroid degeneration of the central nucleus in breeds such as the Dachshund and Pekingese. Loss of plasticity of the nucleus, coupled with degeneration of the retaining annulus, subjects the disc to increasing mechanical stress and leads eventually to annular rupture. If the annulus is ruptured partially, the disc bulges and protrudes beyond its normal extent: if completely ruptured, then extrusion of degenerate nuclear material through the annular ring occurs. Unfortunately, since the nucleus is dorsally eccentric, dorsal bulging or extrusion of material is generally the rule, with consequent involvement of the overlying cord and nerve roots. Severity of neurological signs follows the rationale set out previously.

Diagnosis

History is often of minor overexertion or accident prior to onset of signs, which may develop over a period of days or weeks, overnight (the animal displaying a vague discomfort or even mild pyrexia the previous day) or very acutely. Clinical signs are of nerve root or cord compression. Plain film spinal radiography provides accurate diagnosis. The significant features are narrowing of the affected intervertebral space, with perhaps extruded nuclear material visible in the vertebral canal, the predilection sites being C2-3, C6-7, T12-13 and thoracolumbar (TL) junction. T11-12 is normally markedly narrow in the dog and lumbosacral (LS) junction very wide. Calcified nuclear material in a normal width disc is not significant as a localising feature, but may affect the long-term prognosis for future recurrence.

Prognosis and treatment
No sufficiently controlled data exist to favour either surgical or conservative treatment as a standard approach. Each case must be assessed on its merits by the examining clinician.

Cervical protrusions
Pain is usually the predominant clinical sign. Surgical treatment by the fenestration of the affected disc would appear to be the treatment of choice. In certain cases dorsal decompressive laminectomy or ventral decompression through 'slotting' of the vertebral body gives more rapid relief. Prognosis is generally good.

Thoracolumbar protrusions
The treatment and prognosis must be broadly based on certain critical clinical signs of cord damage.

Group A. Animals with pain and minimal other signs can be treated by confinement at home, with mild analgesics, for a minimum period of 4 days.

Group B. Animals with neurological signs, but bladder control intact and pain sensation in hindlimbs intact, should be hospitalised for further investigation and cage confinement. Conservative treatment with rest, analgesics and steroids should be continued until improvement is marked. Nursing care should be directed at the avoidance of decubital ulcers in paraplegic cases.

Group C. Animals with signs as in group B, but with loss of bladder control and intact pain sensation in hindlimbs, may benefit from surgical decompression of the cord if presented early or if deteriorating from milder degrees of cord dysfunction. Otherwise treat conservatively as for group B, with the addition of catheterisation, regular checks for cystitis and antibiotic therapy if indicated.

Group D. Animals with signs as in group C but total loss of pain sensation or animals with the ascending spinal syndrome carry a very poor prognosis.

Neoplasia affecting the spinal cord
Clinical signs of intraspinal neoplasms vary depending upon their position along the cord, and upon the intimacy of their contact with it. Tumours may produce the same clinical signs as any compressive lesion, but the neurological impairment is distinguished by being progressive without remission. Pain is a constant feature.

Intramedullary tumours such as gliomas are very destructive to cord tissue and this may be reflected in the severity of clinical signs; conversely, epidural lymphosarcoma may cause very rapid deterioration. Local pain is most common with epidural masses, possibly because of nerve root involvement. Perineural fibroblastomas arising in this situation characteristically produce local, lower motor neuron-type dysfunction, distributed according to the nerve roots involved, and signs of local, slowly developing compression of the cord. Meningiomas of the cord are perhaps the most interesting types of tumour in that they appear relatively common, and may be amenable to surgical removal.

Clinical diagnosis of cord tumours must be based essentially upon the clinical signs as discussed briefly above, and upon radiography of the spine. The latter, in addition to excluding other sources of cord problems, may reveal enlargement of intervertebral foramina in nerve root tumours, or actual invasion of the vertebral bone itself in malignant sarcoma. Myelography is theoretically valuable to display blockage of the subarachnoid space by the developing lesion but distinction of intramedullary masses, which distend the cord substance, from extramedullary masses, which displace it, may be difficult, although of great prognostic value. The level of subarachnoid obstruction seen in the myelogram may not correspond well with the most favourable level for surgical removal of the mass. CSF analysis at the time of myelography should permit the exclusion of acute infectious myelitis from the differential diagnosis.

Fractures and dislocations

The majority of spinal fractures or dislocations occur around the thoracolumbar junction with clinical signs similar to those of a prolapsed intervertebral disc in this region and vary from local pain and hyper-reflexia in the hindlegs to paraplegia, extensor rigidity of the forelimbs and paradoxical respiration as described under the ascending spinal syndrome.

Treatment should be directed at restoration of cord function and will be discussed with prolapsed intervertebral discs.

The following localised dislocations and fractures may also occur:

Fractured odontoid
This occurs most frequently in animals such as Greyhounds or Whippets somersaulting at speed. The main clinical sign is acute pain and spasm with minimal neurological defects. Radiography under general anaesthetic is required for diagnosis. Treatment comprises confinement and some analgesia.

Atlantoaxial dislocation

This occurs spontaneously in young individuals of Toy breeds with absent or reduced odontoids. The axis dislocates dorsally into the caudal atlas, causing acute neck pain, minimal cord signs and occasional 'drop' attacks. Treatment is surgical and involves exposing the dorsal spine of the axis and passing a wire suture through this, and around the dorsal arch of the atlas, drawing the two together.

Fractures/dislocations of lower lumbar vertebra and sacrum

These commonly result from road traffic accidents in animals hit from behind, and carry a poor prognosis in many cases due to the paresis of hindlegs, bladder and anus resulting from trauma to the extensive nerve roots in the vertebral canal of the dog at this level.

Vertebral deformations

Deformations of the vertebra in the dog are relatively frequent in specific breeds and types, and initial diagnosis tends to be based more on this knowledge than on specificity of clinical signs.

Hemivertebra

A congenital and possibly inherited condition of the small and the brachycephalic breeds, particularly those with 'screw tails'. There is a high incidence in the French and English Bulldog, the Boston Terrier and the Pug, although cases in the Pekingese and West Highland White are not infrequent.

Affected animals are usually asymptomatic or may show signs of thoracic cord compression, with hindlimb ataxia and weakness predominating. The usual age at onset of clinical signs is a few months, often following a minor accident. On examination, lateral deviation and dorsal spinal curvature may be obvious, and low thoracic pain may be displayed by palpation. Definitive diagnosis is by radiography in two planes when the grossly deformed vertebral body will be obvious, usually a single segment in T7–9 region.

Logical treatment would appear to be immediate decompression of the cord in clinically affected animals, but further growth, and hence deformation, precludes a satisfactory outcome.

Lumbosacral stenosis

This condition is characterised by intermittent hindlimb lameness, weakness, with muscle atrophy, urinary and faecal incontinence (i.e. LMN signs), together with pruritus and self-mutilation of hindlegs, tail, perineum, anus and external genitalia. Lumbosacral pain on handling is a constant sign. Plain radiography reveals stenosis of the spinal canal in the lumbosacral region. Reported cases have proved refractory to attempts at conservative treatment, but have responded well to decompressive surgery.

Discospondylitis

This condition occurs most frequently in large, male dogs.

Clinical signs vary with progression; animals are initially pyrexic and anorexic, and may appear depressed. Cord signs develop later, with spinal pain and stiffness and focal neurological defects.

Diagnosis is confirmed radiographically by demonstration of bone lysis and sclerosis, and spondylosis. Various bacteria have been isolated from cases of discospondylitis by blood and urine culture, with *Staphalococcus aureus* predominating. Treatment is by cord decompression in severe cases, with systemic antibiosis for up to six weeks.

PERIPHERAL NERVOUS SYSTEM

The reductionist concept of the 'peripheral nervous system' allows the convenient grouping of a number of clinical entities. It is generally taken to comprise all the cranial nerves except I and II from their points of exit from the brain stem, the segmental nerve roots, the dorsal root ganglia, the autonomic ganglia, mixed spinal nerves, the brachial and lumbosacral plexuses and peripheral nerves themselves.

As well as the various cell types of the ganglia, the system includes fibres which are myelinated (enwrapped in a sheath of Schwann cell cytoplasm) or non-myelinated (protected merely in invaginations of Remak cell) membranes. These fibre types transmit impulses concerned with different sensory modalities and with motor function, and peripheral nerves contain an admixture of them.

In general, the larger the fibre, the more vulnerable it is to trauma to the nerve or nerve root in which it is carried, and the more susceptible it is to demyelinating

Table 5.4 Fibre types and their functions

Fibre type	Function
Myelinated	
'A' large, fast conducting	Motor proprioception (position sense)
'B'	Touch pressure
Non-myelinated	
'C' small, slow conducting	Pain
	Temperature

disease. Thus increasing degrees of nerve damage may produce initially proprioceptive and motor defects alone, followed by loss of touch and pressure sensation and eventually loss of pain response. Similarly, demyelination selectively 'takes out' A and B fibres but leaves pain and temperature sensation intact. These points are of importance when examining cases of suspected peripheral nervous system dysfunction or when assessing the degree of damage in order to arrive at a prognosis.

Differentiation of levels
When faced with a case of suspected peripheral nervous system involvement, the clinician may have great difficulty in discovering the true level of the lesion. Table 5.5 is an attempt to aid in this.

Table 5.5 Differentiation of levels

Level	Signs
Lesion of central nervous system ('upper motor neuron')	Muscle weakness without marked atrophy Enhanced tendon reflexes
Lesion of peripheral nervous system ('lower motor neuron')	Muscle weakness with neurogenic atrophy on muscle biopsy Diminished or altered tendon reflexes Nerve conduction and electromyographic changes Nerve biopsy changes
Lesion of muscle	Increased levels of CPK and transaminases in serum Electromyographic changes Changes seen in muscle biopsy

Nerve biopsy techniques are the best method of accurately discovering the presence of fibre damage and its degree and type, but they require an experienced and knowledgeable neuropathological back-up service to achieve worthwhile results.

Clinically, in veterinary neurology the following points are significant:

1 Peripheral nervous system damage may occur as part of other neurological disease processes but signs of its dysfunction may be masked (e.g. Krabbe's disease
2 The most frequent cause of pathology of the peripheral nervous system in the dog is physical injury.

Physical injury

This occurs from traumatic episodes giving rise to traction, compression, contusion of the nerves or their involvement in lacerations and fractures, or from iatrogenic causes such as plaster casts, tourniquets, intramuscular injections or surgical interferences.

Common manifestations

Forelimb

Brachial plexus paresis. So-called 'radial paralysis' results from traumatic avulsion of the dorsal and, especially, the ventral nerve roots from the spinal cord usually in road traffic accidents. Clinically the pattern of sensory and motor loss in the affected forelimb reflects the nerve root origin of the condition, and does not conform to peripheral nerve fields. There may be ipsilateral loss (motor) of the panniculus reflex with the consensual remaining intact, and Horner's syndrome (see Table 5.2). The latter is especially significant in betraying the nerve root origin of the forelimb paresis, since sympathetic fibres leave the spinal nerve immediately as it emerges through the intervertebral foramen and are spared in lesions distal to that point.

Motor and sensory areas lost vary greatly, from one or two muscle groups with normal sensation, to loss of all groups with gross sensory defects. Muscles have lower motor neuron type paresis and undergo neurogenic atrophy. Nerve biopsy may reveal normal peripheral nerve; electromyography reveals wide distribution of fibre damage, which is supported by muscle histology. In man, myelography reveals diverticula of subarachnoid space through the intervertebral foramina.

Prognosis: some limited recovery of limb function may occur in partial paresis, but total functional recovery is rare.

Treatment: Providing the animal can support the foot clear of the ground and does not mutilate the damaged limb, conservative treatment is best, with contractures avoided by passive physiotherapy by the owner. In the majority of cases, the lesions are too extensive to allow successful use of muscle relocation techniques to restore limb function. Amputation should be considered.

True radial paralysis. This appears very uncommon in isolation from brachial plexus paresis, unless as a complication of trauma or surgical interference to the elbow; the dog cannot extend the paw at first, but compensates well with time.

Hindlimb

Sciatic nerve injury. This commonly occurs proximally with injuries to the pelvis, particularly fracture of the iliac wing, the femoral neck or the acetabulum, following dorsal surgical approach to the hip joint for femoral head excision or during surgery for perineal hernia repair.

Clinically the animal has a 'floppy' gait with ataxia and passive movement of the hock, but can extend and flex the hip normally. The caudal lateral aspect of the thigh is desensitised, with normal sensation medially. The demarcation between normal and desensitised skin areas in the foot occurs in the interdigital space between the second and third digits.

The prognosis depends upon the degree of damage.

Cranial nerve injuries
These are relatively uncommon except as complications of skull fractures; inflammatory processes around the head may however involve cranial nerves, and are included here.

Oculomotor III; trochlear IV; abducens VI. These nerves are motor to the extrinsic eye muscles and levator of the upper lid. They may be damaged in orbital trauma with clinical signs of strabismus (squint) or drooping of the upper lid (ptosis).

The III rd nerve is of great significance in assessing intracranial pathology.

Trigeminal V. This nerve is sensory to the head including cornea and motor to the muscles of mastication. The mandibular division may be involved in a transient paresis of the lower jaw seen in animals with a history of habitually carrying large objects in their mouths. Treatment involves supporting the lower jaw with a bandage or elastic material to allow effective swallowing of liquids; recovery usually occurs within 2–3 weeks. Similar signs are seen in animals with rabies.

The V th nerve may also be involved in inflammatory processes around the head, by extension of tumours of the parynx through the cavernous sinus; the paresis and atrophy resulting from involvement of its motor division must be differentiated from true myopathies of muscles of mastication by muscle biopsy.

Facial nerve VII. This nerve is motor to muscles of facial expression. Involvement of this nerve in inflammatory conditions of the middle ear may give rise initially to hemifacial spasm. As partial closure of the eye and drawing back of the labial commissure on the affected side is so noticeable the unwary may suspect a facial paralysis on the normal, relaxed side.

True facial paralysis results in absent blink or corneal response ipsilaterally, wide palpebral aperture, drooping of the labial commissure, with drooling of saliva and difficulty in prehension of food.

Acoustic nerve VIII. See vestibular syndrome.

Vagus X. Neurogenic atrophy of laryngeal muscles of the dog is a progressive condition of large breeds manifesting itself as a rough bark, or respiratory stridor, followed by obstructive dyspnoea, glottic obstruction and collapse on exertion. Diagnosis is by direct examination of the vocal cords under light anaesthesia to discern the characteristic lack of abduction on vigorous inspiration. Biopsy of the laryngeal muscles reveals neurogenic atrophy but the site of the nerve lesion is unknown.

Peripheral polyneuropathies

Diseases of the peripheral nervous system apart from direct injuries appear to be uncommon, or rather, are diagnosed infrequently in the dog. In man, multiple neuropathy can arise from the following aetiologies: malnutrition or deficiency disease, malignancy, necrotic arteritis, peripheral vascular spasm, uraemia, diabetes mellitus, amyloidosis, as a result of ingestion of drugs and poisons, in disorders of immune response in infections and inborn errors of metabolism.

In animals, relatively few cases of peripheral neuropathy involving only one or two of the above aetiological groups have been reported.

The pathology of polyneuropathies involves damage of two main types to the fibres of the peripheral nerve: demyelination from Schwann cell involvement, and axonal degeneration, occurring together, but to varying degrees.

As previously discussed, the various fibre types (A, B, C) differ in presence or absence of a myelin sheath, in size, in conduction velocities and in the type of information they carry, and they thus differ in their susceptibility to the pathological process; the clinical signs vary accordingly. Demyelinating disease is particularly likely to take out 'A' fibres selectively.

Affected dogs are usually presented with ataxia and weakness of the hindlegs, with poor proprioception and, because of the nature of the fibres conducting the reflex, depression of the knee jerks. Pain sensation is often intact. Clinical diagnosis is often impossible and requires specialised techniques.

Investigation of suspected peripheral polyneuropathy involved electromyography and nerve conduction velocity measurement and the taking and examination of actual biopsies at various sites along the peripheral nerve to study the nature of the pathology, the fibre types involved and the axial location of the lesions.

Acute idiopathic polyneuropathy

The salient feature of this condition (which may in fact be several as yet indistinguishable polyneuropathies) is that animals will gradually recover if maintained for sufficient time.

Clinically there is progressive weakness and diminished spinal reflexes in all limbs, often progressing to tetraplegia. The onset is usually acute and deterioration may occur for up to three weeks before spontaneous recovery begins. The hindlimbs are affected early, and the dog will show weakness and ataxia, with diminished tone and tendon reflexes.

Distal denervating disease

There is no breed or age incidence, but affected animals are usually female. The rate of onset varies, but may progress to tetraplegia and weakness of neck and head muscles. Muscle atrophy may be marked, and limb tone and reflexes diminished. Pain sensation is entirely intact. There is no involvement of bladder or anus.

Recovery is good, and complete in 4–6 weeks.

BREED-RELATED SYNDROMES

A number of neurological conditions share clinical aspects to such an extent that clinicians may despair of distinguishing them. In this situation, the breed-specificity of many syndromes becomes of diagnostic significance. What follows is a list, alphabetical by breed, of some such conditions.

Myelomalacia in Afghan Hounds

This is reported in the literature as ataxia and progressive, fatal paralysis in young Afghan Hounds with a short course of 2–6 weeks. The vertebral white matter of cord appeared to have undergone ischaemic or anoxic damage.

Airedale Terrier cerebellar hypoplasia

Affected puppies show the classical cerebellar signs as described elsewhere.

Basset Hound ataxia

Onset occurs in young male animals under 6 months of age. Clinical signs are those of gradually progressive, pain-free high cord damage, with hindleg ataxia

and poor position sense often the presenting signs. Radiographic examination of the high cervical vertebra reveals narrowing of the vertebral canal especially at C2–3. Steroids and cage rest produce some clinical improvement. Surgical decompression may be indicated, but the condition is believed to be inherited.

Spontaneous subarachnoid haemorrhage in Beagles

This is a condition of acute neck pain and pyrexia seen typically in young Beagles. Affected animals show grossly elevated neutrophil counts and globulin increase in blood samples, and frank or degraded blood on CSF tap. The clinical state of the animal improves dramatically if parenteral steroids are given, but recurrence may be sudden and without warning. It is believed to result from a necrotic polyarteritis of unknown cause.

Progressive axonopathy in the Boxer

An inherited disease of young animals (mostly of 3–6 months of age), with hindlimb ataxia, marked hypotonia, normal flexor response and pain sensation, but striking loss of patellar reflexes. There is no muscle atrophy. Some cases may not progress, but most deteriorate steadily.

Brittany Spaniel hereditary spinal muscular atrophy

Onset is in puppies of 2–8 months old, which develop a curious progressive weakness of proximal muscle groups, i.e. trunk and limb girdles. There may also be involvement of tongue and facial muscles. Muscle atrophy is present, and marked hindlimb tremor may occur. There is no treatment.

Familiar ataxia in the Bull Mastiff

A recently emerged condition in pups of six weeks old and upwards, of either sex, and showing as ataxia, loss of menace reflexes, bizarre centre visual defects and poor proprioception.

Cairn Terrier's storage disease

Globoid cell leucodystrophy has been reported in this breed (and West Highland White Terriers) from 3 months of age onwards. Pups show ataxia, blindness nystagmus, tremor and hindlimb weakness. Abnormal material accumulates in white matter of cerebrum, cerebellum, cord and peripheral nerve—in the latter it is demonstrable by biopsy.

'Fly catching' in the Cavalier King Charles Spaniel

These animals are generally between 8 and 18 months of age and display a bizarre behavioural procedure which involves the fixation, pursuit and catching of imaginary flies, often followed by biting at the hindquarters. The cause is unknown; oral diazepam appears to give some control. A psuedo fly catching syndrome may occur in animals with vitreous 'floaters', which they may discern against a patterned background and pursue vigorously.

Great Danes, Doberman Pinschers ataxia

These breeds typify the condition, which has, however, been reported in other large breeds. The age of onset varies greatly, but the majority of spontaneously arising cases are young; older animals appear more likely to show clinical signs following a particular incident. Signs are again those of high cord damage, with hindleg ataxia the initial sign. Plain film radiography reveals deformation and displacement of vertebral bodies, which tend to be wedge-shaped with corresponding narrowing of the anterior vertebral canal overlying them; in some cases myelography may be indicated to demonstrate this feature, and flexed neck views may be required to show maximal displacement. In the Great Dane, C7 is the most usually affected vertebra; in the Doberman Pinscher, the lesion may be higher. In many cases the occlusion of the vertebral canal is minimal and it is obvious that a considerable gradation occurs between the normal and grossly abnormal vertebral body in these breeds; clinical signs in the presented case may bear little relation in severity to the radiographic findings.

Fox Hound ataxia

Affected animals are adults of either sex, with midthoracic cord damage showing as ataxia with panniculus deficits. Aetiology is unknown, but a similar condition has been reported in Harriers and Beagles.

German Shepherd myelopathy

A common condition in clinical practice, usually starting in animals of five years of age and upward, and characterised by progression from subtle loss of proprioception in one hindlimb to severe posterior ataxia. There is some variation in the rate of progression, and temporary stasis may occur. There is no effective therapy, and the aetiology remains obscure, although there is evidence of immune-mediated disease in these animals.

German Shepherd giant axonal neuropathy

Condition occurs in young animals (14–15 months of age), and is seen as hindleg arreflexia, muscle atrophy and loss of pain sensation with diagnostically significant mega-oesophagus.

German Short-Haired Pointer gangliosidosis

A storage disease of 9–12-month-old animals characterised by impaired vision, convulsions and ataxia.

'Swimmers' in the Irish Setter (hereditary quadriplegia and amblyopia)

These puppies are recognised from their normal littermates by their inability to stand, and their 'swimming' propulsion on their bellies. They appear blind, have nystagmus and marked tremor. The disease is inherited as a fully penetrant autosomal recessive and the lesion is cerebellar, involving Purkinje cell degeneration.

Ataxia in Jack Russell Terriers

Ataxia was reported in Smooth-Haired Fox Terriers when the breed was most popular and declined with that popularity; as the Jack Russell Terrier has increased in numbers a similar entity has now come to light. These animals are under 6 months of age at onset, and display a swaying or prancing hindleg gait with occasional collapse to one side. The genetics of the condition are unknown; the neuropathology is confined to some peripheral neuropathy, focal cord demyelination and degeneration of the superior olivary nucleus and the lateral lemniscus.

Ataxia or abiotrophy in the Kerry Blue Terrier

This is a progressive disorder starting at 9–10 weeks of age with stiffness and incoordination of the hindlegs with a wide-based stance, gradual foreleg involvement and eventual cerebellar signs of intention head tremor when the pups eat or drink, and show marked hypermetria and dysmetria. By 5–6 months of age, the animals, although still strong, cannot coordinate sufficiently to stand and walk. There may be difficulty in distinguishing the clinical signs from those of canine distemper encephalitis, but the disease is breed specific and inherited as an autosomal recessive. The main lesion, as the clinician should suspect, is in the cerebellum, involving the Purkinje cells.

Cerebellar degeneration in the Rough Collie

Affected puppies show marked gait abnormalities and cerebellar syndrome at 4–8 weeks of age.

'Scottie cramp'

These animals are usually under 18 months of age at onset and appear normal at rest. On physical exercise or excitement they indulge in hyperkinetic episodes of abduction of the forelegs, back arching and overflexion of the hindlegs. The forelegs may appear so stiff that forward progression ceases; a sudden onset when running may lead to somersaulting. Attacks can be precipitated by amphetamines or alleviated by phenothiazine ataractics or diazepam. The condition is reported as being inherited on a single autosomal recessive basis; and an apparently identical syndrome has been reported in Dalmatians and Cavaliers. There is no known pathology and the level of the lesion is unknown.

Spinal dysraphism in Weimaraners

Spinal dysraphism is a progressive condition occurring in young Weimaraner puppies at 4–6 weeks of age and characterised by a 'hopping' gait and abnormal proprioception in the hindlimbs. It is believed to be inherited.

FURTHER READING

General interest

Chrisman C. L. (1980) (ed.) *The Veterinary Clinics of North America* **10.** (1) Symposium on Advances in Veterinary Neurology. W.B. Saunders, Philadelphia, London, Toronto.

de Lahunta A. (1977) *Veterinary Neuroanatomy and Clinical Neurology.* W.B. Saunders, Philadelphia, London, Toronto.

Hoerlein B.F. (1978) *Canine Neurology.* 3rd Edn. W.B. Saunders, Philadelphia, London, Toronto.

Jenkins T.W. (1972) *Functional Mammalian Neuroanatomy.* Lea and Febiger, Philadelphia.

Clinical examination

Foster S.J. (1968) Practical Neurological Examination of the Dog. *J. small Anim. Pract.* **9,** 295.

Scagliotti R.H. (1980) In *The Veterinary Clinics of North America: Small Animal Practice* **10.** (2) 417 Current Concepts in Veterinary Neuro-ophthalmology. W.B. Saunders, Philadelphia.

Wright J.A. (1978) Evaluation of CSF in the Dog. *Vet. Rec.* **103,** 48.

Wright J.A. (1980) CSF estimation in the diagnosis of CNS damage in the dog. *Vet. Rec.* **106,** 54.

Wright J.A. & Clayton-Jones D.G. (1981) Metrizamide myelography in 68 dogs. *J. small Anim. Pract.* **22,** 415.

Brain

Braund K.G., Crawley R.R. & Speakman C. (1981) Hippocampal necrosis associated with canine distemper virus infection. *Vet. Rec.* **109,** 122.

Cordy D.R. (1979) Canine Granulomatous Meningoencephalomyelitis. *Vet. Path.* **16,** 325.

Gore R. *et al* (1977) Aujeszky's disease in a pack of hounds. *Vet. Rec.* **101,** 93.

Imagawa D.T. *et al* (1980) Isolation of canine distemper virus from dogs with chronic neurological diseases. *Proc. Soc. Exp. Biol. & Med.* **164,** 355.

Koestner A. (1975) Distemper-associated demyelinating encephalomyelitis. *Am. J. Path.* **78,** 361.

Lincoln S.D. *et al* (1971) Aetiologic studies of Old Dog Encephalitis. *Vet. Path.* **8,** 1.

Lincoln S.D. *et al* (1973) Studies of ODE. *Vet. Path.* **10,** 124.

Lisiak J.A. & Vandervelde M. (1979) Polioencephalomalacia associated with canine distemper virus infection. *Vet. Path.* **16,** 650.

Lisiak J.A. & Vandervelde M. (1979) Polioencephalomalacia in the dog. *Vet. Path.* **16,** 661.

Luginbuhl H., Fankhauser R. & McGrath J.T. (1968) Spontaneous neoplasms of the nervous system in animals. *Progress in Neurological Surgery* **2,** 85.

Sims M.H. & Redding R.W. (1975) The use of dexamethasone in the prevention of cerebral oedema in dogs. *J.A.A.H.A.* **11,** 439.

Vandevelde M., Kristensen B. & Greene C.E. (1978) Primary reticulosis of the CNS in the dog. *Vet. Path.* **15,** 673.

Metabolic disorders

Hill F.W.G. *et al* (1974) Functional islet cell tumour in the dog. *J. small Anim. Pract.* **15,** 119.

Maddison J.E. (1981) Portosystemic encephalopathy in two young dogs. *J. small Anim. Pract.* **22,** 731.

Meyer D.J. (1978) Recognition and diagnosis of canine hepatic encephalopathy in small animal practice. *Florida Vet. J.* **7,** 20.

Strombeck D.R., Weiser M.G. & Kaneko J.J. (1975) Hyperammonaemia and hepatic encephalopathy in the dog. *J.A.V.M.A.* **166,** 1105.

Wolf A.M. (1980) Canine uraemic encephalopathy. *J.A.A.H.A.* **16,** 735.

Spinal cord

Bennett D., Carmichael S. & Griffiths I.R. (1981) Discospondylitis in dogs. *J. small Anim. Pract.* **22,** 539.

Bojrab M.J. (1971) Disc Disease. *Vet. Rec.* **89,** 37.

Griffiths I.R. (1972) Some aspects of the pathology and pathogenesis of the myelopathy caused by disc protrusions in the dog. *J. Neurol. Neurosurg. & Psychiat.* **XXXV,** 403.

Griffiths I.R. (1972) Some aspects of the pathogenesis and diagnosis of lumbar disc protrusion in the dog. *J. small Anim. Pract.* **13,** 439.

Griffiths I.R. (1972) The extensive myelopathy of intervertebral disc protrusions in dogs ('the ascending syndrome'). *J. small Anim. Pract.* **13,** 425.

Kornegay J.N. & Barber D.L. (1980) Discospondylitis in dogs. *J.A.V.M.A.* **177,** 337.

Osterholm J.L. (1974) The pathophysiological response to spinal cord injury. *J. Neurosurg.* **40,** 5.

Tarvin G. & Prata D. (1980) Lumbosacral stenosis in dogs. *J.A.V.M.A.* **177,** 154.

Wright J.A., Bell D.A. & Clayton-Jones D.G. (1979) The clinical and radiological features associated with spinal tumours in 30 dogs. *J. small Anim. Pract.* **20,** 461.

Peripheral nerves

Griffiths I.R. *et al* (1973) Neuromuscular disease in dogs. *J. small Anim. Pract.* **14,** 533.

Griffiths I.R., Duncan I.D. & Swallow J.S. (1977) Peripheral polyneuropathies in dogs. *J. small Anim. Pract.* **18,** 101.

Worthman R.P. (1957) Demonstration of specific nerve paralyses in the dog. *J.A.V.M.A.* **131,** 179.

6
Bones and Muscles

J. R. CAMPBELL AND I. R. GRIFFITHS

INTRODUCTION

Diseases of the locomotor system are primarily associated with lameness or abnormality in gait. A great many of these diseases are traumatic or developmental in origin, without any true pathological abnormality of the tissue elements prior to the onset of the condition, and in many instances treatment of such affections is surgical. Such entities will not be dealt with in this chapter.

Nevertheless, the locomotor system is subject to a variety of pathological changes either of a primary nature or secondary to other diseases or abnormalities. Often the true aetiology is obscure. In order to understand the pathology of the condition a knowledge of the normal anatomy and physiology of the particular structures and their responses to stimuli of various kinds is essential. Each type of structure (i.e. bones, joints, muscles) will therefore be taken separately and these aspects discussed prior to a more detailed consideration of specific disease conditions.

BONE DISEASE

As well as providing support for soft tissues and transmission of force from muscles by leverage, bones also act as a reservoir of certain elements and cell types necessary for the proper function of many systems of the body. In order that the chemical constituents of this reservoir may be available to the organism, bones are capable of being resorbed and simultaneously rebuilt. This process goes on constantly throughout life. Many manifestations of bone disease are due to imbalance between the rate of removal and the rate of reapposition of bone.

Anatomy and physiology of bone

There are two main types of bone; the tubular long bones of the appendicular skeleton and the spine; and the flat bones, primarily the skull, pelvis and scapula though various bone processes such as the spinous processes of vertebrae have features similar to flat bones. The difference in these bones is mainly in relation to their development. Tubular bones develop from a cartilaginous fetal model and ossification occurs initially by endochondral ossification, which continues at the epiphyseal plate throughout the growth period. Flat bones develop directly from sheets of osteogenic cells on a fibrous membrane (intramembranous ossification) without the development of cartilage as an intermediate stage. Increase in the diameter of long bones is also brought about by intramembranous bone formation in the inner layers of the periosteum.

Although these differences apply primarily during bone formation, the flat bones may at a later stage show reactions to stimuli which are at variance with the reaction of tubular bones in similar circumstances and this may be traceable to their different origins.

The long bones consist of a tubular shaft or diaphysis which widens at the ends to form the metaphyses. The articular end of the bone, the epiphysis, arises from a separate centre of ossification and is joined to the metaphysis by the growth cartilage plate. The non-articulating surfaces of bone are covered by a fibrous coat, the periosteum, which in youth may be easily divided into an outer fibrous part and an inner cellular part. Later in life the periosteum becomes thinner and more fibrous. The inner surfaces of the bone shaft and the trabeculae of cancellous bone within the medullary cavity are covered by a thin membrane called the endosteum. Similarly, the surfaces of the flat bones are covered with periosteum and endosteum, but growth plates occur in areas not necessarily associated with articulating epiphysis (e.g. the tuber sacrale and tuber ischii of the pelvis). Such non-articular centres of ossification are sometimes called apophyses and similar non-articular centres occur in some areas in the long bones (e.g. tibial tuberosity).

Bone tissue consists of layers or lamellae of interlacing collagen fibres on which calcium hydroxyapatite is deposited. Such mineralisation is thought to result from the seeding effect of the structure of collagen fibrils, in association with local variations in the pH and mineral levels brought about by activity of the bone cells in the region. The cells concerned in bone production are all derived from mesenchymal cells in the periosteum, endosteum and possibly vascular endothelium (Trueta 1963). Active bone-forming cells on the surface of the bone cortex or trabeculae are called osteoblasts; those contained within the bone lattice, which retain connection with one another and with the source of nutrients by means of cell processes

ly
ti
ti
c
v

t
t

te
l-
t-
a-
he
is-
ce.
nd
so

but
teal
lace
ady

d by
new
rs of
The
es of
ident
parts
Frost

blood
d with
most
aemo-
n their

respective stem cells. Later, in many of the bones, these precursors become quiescent and the medullary cavity becomes largely filled with fat.

Reactions of bone

Skeletal tissue, because of its structure, exhibits limited reaction to disease. In general, the change involves either increased or reduced osteoblastic and/or osteoclastic activity. It is the upset in the balance of these which leads to recognisable changes.

Bone formation can arise through activation of osteoblasts in periostem and endosteum but it is possible also that more primitive mesenchymal elements may differentiate to form chondroblasts or osteoblasts in certain circumstances.

Bone lysis is primarily mediated through the formation of multinucleated osteoclasts which appear at the surface of cortex or trabeculae. However, osteocytes can produce osteolysis around themselves within the matrix of the bone and this may be a more important proportion of osteolysis than has been realised. Osteolysis is achieved by removal of both mineral and organic fractions of bone at the same time.

In addition, the regular deposition of collagen in differently orientated layers may be interfered with, so that the collagen fibrils retain no pattern and are aligned indiscriminately. This type of structure is called 'woven bone' and is deposited in healing fractures and other pathological situations.

Many of the factors which affect these activities are known but their precise mode of action is not clearly understood. Thus vitamin D is known to promote mineralisation, and alkaline phosphatase is produced in greater amounts in areas where mineralisation is taking place, but their exact role in this process is still a matter for conjecture.

Parathyroid hormone promotes resorption of the bone as does reduction in pH. It has been suggested that parathormone acts by blocking the Krebs cycle and causing local increase in acidity, affecting the bone to a greater extent than elsewhere and promoting resorption because of this change in milieu. Calcitonin has been shown to prevent resorption but its mode of action is obscure.

The rate of blood flow in an area must affect the oxygenation and therefore the pH of the tissues, but there are conflicting claims about the effect of increase in blood flow and it is possible that in the absence of any pathological process increased blood flow promotes bone formation, but otherwise it may stimulate bone resorption. However, it may be that in such pathological situations there is localised thrombosis and reduced blood flow associated with hyperaemia of the surrounding area.

Other factors such as corticosteroids, oestrogens and other hormones affect bone deposition and resorption. It has been stated that these effects are produced by modifications of the remodelling process to change the number, rate of activity and duration of active osteons.

Bone tissue reacts to the stresses and strains to which it is subjected; increased compressive forces cause an increase in bone deposition in response. It may be that there is a piezo-electric effect produced by the compression of the bone salt crystals. Whether these suggested electrical changes stimulate the osteoblasts and osteocytes directly or via an effect on blood flow is still a matter for study.

The formation of the organic fraction of bone is dependent on a supply of normal nutrients and reduced bone formation will result from inanition, malabsorption or malnutrition. However, certain vitamins and trace elements may affect the elaboration of organic matrix (e.g. vitamins D and A). Thus porotic or hypertrophic changes may ensue.

DEFINITIONS

Osteopenia. Reduction in the amount of bone.

Osteomalacia. Reduction in the mineralisation of organic matrix.

Osteoporosis. This term has given rise to confusion as it has been used with two distinct meanings:

1 Reduction in the amount of new bone tissue being formed, but with normal rate of resorption.
2 Reduction in the amount and density of bone tissue present.

The term is used in the latter manner to describe the appearance of the bone when the cortices are reduced in thickness and the canals are enlarged either as a result of 1, or as a result of excessive bone resorption. In this sense it is synonymous with osteopenia and is much more commonly used in this descriptive sense.

Osteodystrophia-fibrosa. Increased resorption of bone coupled with deposition of fibrous tissue within the skeleton.

Bone atrophy. Increased resorption following disuse of a limb.

Hypertrophy. Increased deposition of bone.

Osteopetrosis; osteosclerosis. Abnormal denseness of bone.

Exostosis. Local deposit of new bone projecting beyond the normal limits of the skeleton.

Osteophyte. Similar to above but more commonly applied to exostosis near joints.

SPECIFIC DISEASE OF BONE

METABOLIC DISEASE

Rickets and osteomalacia

The distinction between these two names is purely on the basis of the age of the animal. Osteomalacia indicates the failure of mineralisation of newly-formed osteoid tissue. Rickets is the name given when an osteomalacic condition occurs in the young animal and affects the endochondral ossification which continues during growth.

Aetiology
Rickets and osteomalacia occur as a result of depressed mineral concentrations in the blood. Hypocalcaemia can result from dietary insufficiency of calcium or reduced absorption from the gut due to excess phosphate, excess phytate, the presence of beryllium in the ingesta or due to alimentary upset. Hypophosphataemia is much less common in the dog and cat due to the relatively high levels of phosphate in meat and cereals, but can occur in animals on special diets.

Vitamin D promotes the absorption of minerals, particularly calcium, from the gut. It may also directly enhance mineralisation of cartilage and osteoid, although this may be produced simply by its effect on blood mineral levels. The vitamin is produced in the skin or ingested in the food but is altered in the liver to 25-hydroxy vitamin D and then in the kidney to the active form 1,25-dihydroxy vitamin D. Parathyroid hormone increases the formulation of 1,25-dihydroxy vitamin D in the kidney. It has been shown that dogs which have an adequate calcium and phosphorus intake in their diet do not require provision of vitamin D. However the vitamin can prevent the development of rachitic or osteomalacic changes by its effect of increasing the blood calcium concentration, although if the mineral deficiency in the diet is severe other bone defects may be produced because of the bone resorption which vitamin D then causes.

There is also an enterohepatic circulation of vitamin D, the vitamin being excreted in the bile then up to 85% being reabsorbed unless other compounds in the gut or alimentary disease inhibit this.

Pathology

Although there may be some impairment or abnormality of the formation of the organic component of the skeleton, the major abnormality which is present in this dystrophy is failure of normal mineralisation of the formed osteoid. In the young animal there is also failure of mineralisation of the cartilaginous matrix around the hypertrophic cartilage cells in the epiphyseal growth plates. This seems to allow continued survival of these cells, instead of degeneration, and blood vessels from the metaphysis fail to penetrate the cartilaginous mass causing irregularity and increase in thickness of the epiphyseal plate. Throughout the skeleton the bone trabeculae are found to be surrounded by a layer of unmineralised tissue (osteoid) with the osteoblasts still active on the surface. The resulting weakness of these trabeculae causes a disruption of the bone architecture, particularly in the spongiosa of the metaphysis, with the trabeculae appearing contorted and misshapen.

Biochemical estimations on the plasma of affected animals reveals reduction of calcium below 2.2 mmol/l or inorganic phosphate below 1.2 mmol/l. In addition a marked rise in alkaline phosphatase beyond 100 iu is likely to be present.

Clinical signs and diagnosis

The signs depend on the severity of the bone changes. However, hypocalcaemia will also affect muscle activity and neurological efficiency and such effects will complicate the picture. The bones become deformed to some degree. Often the major change is at the epyphysis and metaphysis which become enlarged due to the compression and lateral displacement of unmineralised osteoid and cartilage. Such change is most easily seen at the distal ends of the radius and ulna or may be appreciated by palpation at the costochondral junction although such enlargements are not pathognomonic of rickets. Weakness of the bone shaft may lead to bending of the bones giving a bow-legged appearance, again most noticeable in the forelimbs (Fig. 6.1), or even collapse fractures of the bones. In such an event pain and disinclination to walk may be evident.

Laxity of muscles and ligaments may give a flat-footed, plantigrade appearance or occasionally, in association with some degree of bow-leggedness, knuckling over on the outside toes.

In severe hypocalcaemia increased excitability, muscle tremors, convulsions or coma may be seen, but such neurological disturbances are very uncommon in the dog.

In addition to the clinical signs diagnosis depends on radiological examination. Anteroposterior views of both forelimbs from paw to midradius should be taken and also views elsewhere in the skeleton if collapse fractures are suspected. Widening of the epiphyseal growth plates is pathognomonic of the disease (Fig. 6.1b). Because of some variations in the mineral intake the growth plates do not usually appear regular or completely uncalcified, but areas which are wider and vary in density can be seen, as well as lateral spreading of the growth plate with lateral peaks of mineralisation giving a cupping effect to the metaphysis. Bone density throughout the skeleton will be reduced and thinning and lamellation of the cortices may be evident. Bending of the long bone shafts may be seen on the radiographs. In severe rickets, because of parathyroid stimulation as a result of hypocalcaemia, a more marked porosis of the bones is apparent and folding, compression or complete fractures may be seen. Delayed formation and eruption of teeth will occur in severe cases.

Treatment and prevention

These are both dependent on the provision of an adequate intake of minerals and vitamin D and the elimination of any competing dietary constituent or of concomitant alimentary disease.

The mineral requirement varies from breed to breed but provision of 0.25–1.00% of the diet on a net weight basis, of both calcium and phosphorus is necessary (a ratio of approximately 1:1); the quantity may occasionally be increased to the upper limit for very large or giant dogs which have suffered mineral-deprivation. For most common breeds, 0.3% of each is adequate.

Vitamin D, while not absolutely necessary, will promote mineral transport and deposition and should be given at a rate of 10 iu/kg body weight per day. Vitamin D supplied in the diet or parenterally is, however, much less effective than an equivalent amount formed in the skin by ultraviolet irradiation.

Once the very rapid period of growth is over (i.e. the first 4–5 months of life), rickets is virtually impossible to produce even experimentally and any additives can be reduced gradually. Most proprietary dog foods now contain adequate minerals for skeletal development. Where extra is required it can be given in the form of sterilised bone meal or flour (25% calcium) or calcium phosphate (4% calcium). These compounds also contain phosphorus but since the calcium content is double the phosphorus content the calcium-phosphorus ratio of the minerals in the animal's ingesta is

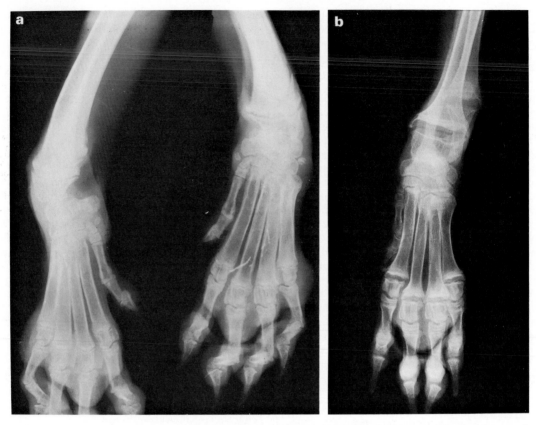

Fig. 6.1 (a) Bowing of the radius and ulna of both forelegs due to a previous rachitic episode. (b) Rickets: the enlargement of the growth plate can be seen at the distal end of the radius and ulna and of the metacarpals. There is generalised loss of bone density.

brought nearer to the optimal 1:1. Calcium supplementation without phosphorus may be supplied in the form of calcium lactate, or calcium borogluconate but the calcium content of these compounds is only 12% and 9% respectively, so correspondingly larger amounts are required. Certain foods contain increased amounts of calcium (e.g. cheese, fish processed with bones). Milk has a satisfactory calcium and phosphate content and ratio but not enough to compensate for gross deficiency in other dietary constituents.

In determining the amount of supplement required it is desirable to estimate the actual mineral content of the diet and calculate the amount of calcium or phosphorus necessary to bring this up to the minimum level. Table 6.1 gives the mineral contents of a number of common foodstuffs and the method of calculating the required supplementation.

Hyperparathyroidism
The parathyroid gland is stimulated to produce hormone primarily by reduction in the concentration of calcium in the blood. Such hypocalcaemia may not be detectable on biochemical estimations of the plasma as the 'feedback system' is very efficient, and increase in parathormone will cause increase in calcium to restore the normal circulating levels very quickly. Mobilisation of calcium by parathormone is brought about by activation of osteoclasts in the bones to produce resorption. Absorption from the gut may also be promoted. Increase in the plasma concentration of inorganic phosphate may produce some direct stimulation of the parathyroid gland but this is thought to be minimal and excess phosphorus probably acts primarily by reducing the plasma calcium level in accordance with the Law of Mass Action.

Primary hyperparathyroidism. This results from hypersecretion of the parathyroid gland as a result of a local glandular abnormality such as adenoma. The appearance of the bones is similar to that seen in

Table 6.1 Mineral content of common foodstuffs calculated on a wet weight basis (after McCance & Widdowson 1946)

	Grams of mineral per 100 g foodstuff	
	Ca	P
Lean meat	0.008	0.280
Fresh milk	0.120	0.095
Egg (whole)	0.056	0.218
Liver	0.008	0.313
Sardines (tinned)	0.409	0.683
Pilchards (tinned)	0.231	0.296
Cheese (cheddar)	0.810	0.545
Brown bread	0.063	0.160
White bread	0.060	0.098

To calculate the amount of supplement required calculate the total daily intake of food and the mineral content:

Dietary constituent	Ca (g)	P (g)
Meat (2 lb = 950 g)	0.076	2.60
Eggs (2 = 120 g)	0.066	0.20
Bread (2 lb)	0.608	1.50
Milk (1 pt = 540 g)	0.650	0.48
Total 2660 g	1.400	4.78
Required (0.3% in diet)	7.900	7.90
Supplement required	6.5	

Amount of bone meal (400 mg Ca/g) required as supplement = 16 g

secondary hyperparathyroidism but diagnosis is more difficult and will be discussed later (see p. 222). It is rare in small animals.

Secondary hyperparathyroidism. This can occur as a result of two separate syndromes: nutritional and renal.

Nutritional secondary hyperparathyroidism (juvenile osteoporosis)

Aetiology
This disease is primarily due to the provision of a diet which is grossly deficient in calcium but contains a much greater amount of phosphorus. Adequate or excess vitamin D will increase the progress and severity of the disease. Because of the calcium deficiency there is a tendency for hypocalcaemia to develop. Parathyroid stimulation results and is able to promote such wide-spread bone resorption that the plasma calcium levels are maintained within normal limits, so preventing rickets. Provision of vitamin D will have a similar effect in the prevention of rickets because vitamin D will promote bone resorption in circumstances where calcium mobilisation from the gut is precluded due to, for example, inadequate concentra-

tion in the ingesta. Provision of vitamin D supplements will therefore exacerbate any bone resorption which is occurring and will prevent any development of concomitant rachitic change. The degree of stimulation of the parathyroid is similar to that seen in rickets but some other, possibly dietary, factor appears to be involved in the causation of rickets, perhaps by inhibiting vitamin D absorption or reabsorption.

Pathology
The changes affect the whole skeleton. There is dramatically increased bone resorption with loss of intramedullary trabeculae, thinning of cortices, increase in number and size of Haversian canals but no change in the rate of bone growth. The effect of this is that the available mineral is continually redistributed through an ever-increasing volume of skeletal structure which as a result becomes weaker and more poorly developed (Fig. 6.2).

On examination of the bones the thin, often rudimentary, cortices are apparent and large numbers of osteoclasts are evident. There may be increase in fibrous tissue in some areas of the bone, particularly on the external surfaces at the metaphysis. Biochemical estimations carried out on the plasma reveal normal calcium levels and normal or increased phosphorus levels. There may also be some increase in alkaline phosphatase.

Clinical signs and diagnosis
Affected animals may be presented with a variety of signs including localised lameness, abnormal gait due to laxity of ligaments similar to rickets, inability or reluctance to stand and walk, widespread bone pain and pathological fractures of the long bones. Occasionally neurological signs are present as a result of collapse fractures of the vertebrae which cause spinal cord pressure. In these cases prognostication is complicated by neurological damage which has already occurred or which may ensue prior to the establishment of more normal bone structure.

Radiography of the skeleton reveals extremely poor bone density, often with very little difference between skeleton and soft tissue, lamellation of the cortices due to the gross increase in size of the Haversian canals or in very severe cases only thin 'pencil line' cortices. The extreme fragility of such bones means that pathological fractures are common, and may take the form of compression (Fig. 6.3a), folding (Fig. 6.3b), or complete fractures. Because of these changes the condition sometimes has been mistakenly diagnosed as osteogenesis imperfecta.

In most cases the growth plates appear normal

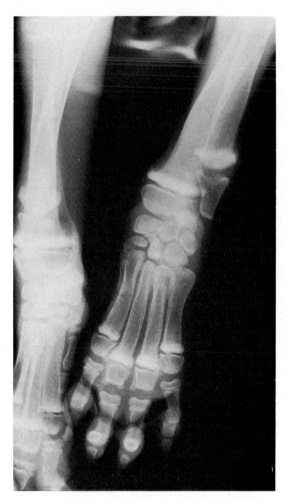

Fig. 6.2 Osteoporosis: radiograph showing lamellation of the cortices, reduced metaphyseal trabeculation with a few coarse trabeculae evident and generalised reduction in bone density except at the primary spongiosa.

although in some there is evidence of a degree of rachitic change. This is most easily seen in the distal epiphysis of the ulna where the peak of the metaphysis appears truncated as a result of failure of ossification at the centre of the growth plate. The metaphysis may show lipping, with the projection pointing away from the epiphysis to form a mushroom shape at the end of the shaft (Fig. 6.3a). There is often an area of radio-lucency at the edge of the metaphysis just on the diaphyseal side of this lip. The area of primary calcification often shows up as a dense white zone in comparison with the surrounding radiolucent bone.

Treatment and prevention

This depends on correction of the mineral deficiency and calculations of dietary requirements should be carried out as in the case of rickets. The most common dietary problem is the feeding of large amounts of meat, which contains very little calcium and much greater amounts of phosphorus. The bones will remain fragile for some weeks after correction of imbalance so no strenuous or boisterous activity must be allowed in the interim or further fractures with deformity may occur. In the case of severe widespread skeletal de-formity euthanasia should be advised.

Regulation of the vitamin D intake is also necessary with reduction of excessive doses where these have been given. Vitamin D can be administered in a num-ber of different forms (e.g. in prepared diets, in mineral supplements, in vitamin supplements); all these sources must be monitored.

In both rickets and nutritional hyperparathyroid-ism, injections of minerals and vitamins are probably less satisfactory than oral administration and should not be used except as an initial booster. Hypocal-caemic porosis is unlikely to occur in older animals as it has been shown that adult dogs can accommodate to a very low calcium intake. However, widespread bone weakness with collapse of the pelvis and compression of vertebrae is occasionally seen in breed-ing bitches which have been maintained for a long time on mineral-deficient diet. Presumably this is due to hyperparathyroidism during pregnancy to mobilise enough calcium for the developing fetal skeletons.

Primary hyperparathyroidism does not produce such dramatic changes and blood estimations are not often helpful because the calcium and phosphorus concentrations in the plasma are maintained within normal limits by excretion of excess in the faeces and urine. Diagnosis of this entity therefore entails den-sometric measurements of the skeletal change, mineral balance studies, or surgical exploration for parathy-roid abnormalities, all of which are expensive and time consuming and may give equivocal results. Estimation of parathormone levels can be carried out but requires very sophisticated laboratory techniques which pre-clude its general use.

Renal hyperparathyroidism ('rubber jaw') (see also Chapters 8 and 15).

Aetiology

Renal dysfunction results in failure of excretion of phosphate with a consequent increase in the plasma concentration of inorganic phosphate. This produces a compensatory reduction in plasma calcium with sti-mulation of the parathyroid gland. Bone resorption is

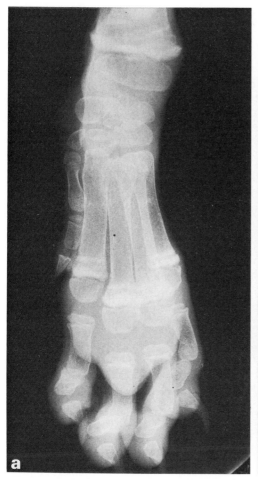
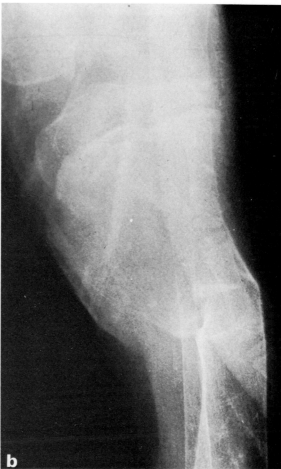

Fig. 6.3 Osteoporosis: (a) typical appearance of a pup with, in addition, areas of increased density in the metaphyses due to collapse and overriding of weakened trabeculae; (b) the appearance of the folding factures which occur in nutritional secondary hyperparathyroidism.

produced but the phosphate released exacerbates the condition and increases the parathyroid stimulation. Calcium phosphate is excreted in the gut but if the renal dysfunction persists, increasing plasma levels of phosphate are produced and more parathormone is released. In renal failure the half life of parathormone is greatly prolonged. Bone resorption occurs at an accelerated rate and the bone is replaced by fibrous tissue.

Clinical signs and diagnosis
Although the whole skeleton is affected, the bones which show the greatest change are those in the head. The reasons for this are not known. In adult dogs the mandible becomes demineralised and soft. The canine teeth can be 'sprung' towards one another at the tips, and fractures of the jaw may occur. The condition is accompanied by signs of renal insufficiency such as polydipsia, but in occasional cases a fracture of the jaw as a result of minimal trauma may precede overt evidence of renal disease.

Radiology of the skull reveals reduced density of the mandible with loss of the alveolar bone plates so that the teeth, which retain their normal density, appear unsupported in the poorly mineralised bone (Fig. 6.4). Resorption of the bone of the terminal phalanges has also been reported but is much more difficult to detect.

In pups with congenital renal abnormalities the other bones of the skull are also affected so that there

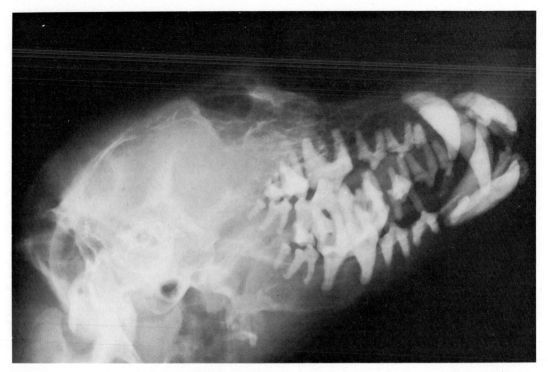

Fig. 6.4 Renal hyperparathyroidism; the reduced density of the mandible and the lack of lamina dura surrounding the tooth roots.

is swelling of the head and abnormal eruption of the teeth. (Brodey *et al* 1961.)

Renal hyperparathyroidism is sometimes mistakenly confused with renal rickets. However, this latter condition is a result of a failure of elaboration of vitamin D in the kidneys and, in humans, gives rise to osteomalacic change in the bones. In 'rubber jaw' there may be some failure of normal activity of vitamin D but no specific clinical abnormality is detectable as a result of such failure.

Treatment and prevention
These are unrewarding in renal osteodystrophy as most cases are associated with chronic irreversible change. Bone changes do not become clinically evident in more acute nephritic syndromes.

Specific treatment would be renal transplantation but this is a rare procedure in animals. Otherwise treatment can only be of a palliative nature, consisting of an increase in the dietary content of calcium.

However, such treatment will not ameliorate the other effects of chronic renal failure.

Prevention of chronic renal disease by vaccination and prompt treatment of acute nephritis are the only prophylactic measures available.

Hypertrophic osteodystrophy

Four forms of hypertrophic osteodystrophy are recognised although the aetiology of three is still a matter of conjecture and controversy.

1 Barlow's disease or infantile scurvy, so called because of its resemblance clinically and radiographically to the condition of this name in the human infant.
2 Hypertrophic osteodystrophy of giant dogs.
3 Hypervitaminosis A.
4 Hypertrophic osteoarthropathy.

Barlow's disease (Moeller–Barlow's disease)
The condition is named after the authors of the first published description of the disease in the human. Scurvy is a disease which is seen in man, primates and guinea pigs but dogs and cats are able to synthesise the vitamin and are not dependent on dietary supplies.

Aetiology
In view of their independence of external sources of ascorbic acid, the aetiology of the condition in dogs remains obscure. Many assays of the vitamin C status

of affected animals have been carried out but specific vitamin C deficiency has never been demonstrated. Blood and urine vitamin C assays carried out in Glasgow have suggested that some affected pups may be producing and excreting more vitamin C than normal animals of the same age. This may suggest some interference with the utilisation of vitamin C and this hypothesis is supported by the fact that the administration of large doses of ascorbic acid often produces dramatic improvement in affected animals. Other suggestions as to aetiology include the excess intake of minerals and vitamins, especially vitamins A and D, hypercalcitoninism or other hormonal imbalance but these theories have not been substantiated.

Pathology

In hypovitaminosis C, the elaboration of connective tissue is interfered with and in the young animal the most severe signs are due to abnormality of the bones and blood vessels. Haemorrhages occur and often these are seen subperiosteally principally at the metaphyseal areas since these are the areas of greatest muscle and ligament attachment to the periosteum. Movement of the periosteum as a result of these stresses causes rupture of the small subperiosteal vessels, due to fragility of the walls as a result of vitamin C deprivation. Subperiosteal haematomas form, which cause swelling of the region. Later these organise and are invaded by osseous tissue so that collars of new bone are formed around the metaphysis, particularly the radius and ulna, the femur and the tibia, although other limb bones are affected to some degree.

The developing bone is also involved in that the developing osteoid is not properly formed and fails to mineralise normally. This results in a degree of porosis throughout the skeleton, but also specific disruptive changes in the region of the primary and secondary spongiosa in the metaphysis. The epiphyseal growth plate matures and calcifies normally, but the absence of normal amounts of new bone laid down on the calcified trabeculae leads to weakening in this area of the bone with collapse of trabeculae and disruption of fragile vessels causing intra-osseous haemorrhage.

Clinical signs and diagnosis

Puppies of between 2 and 6 months of age are affected and the clinical signs are primarily associated with the changes occurring in the metaphyseal area. There is pain and swelling in these regions which, with careful examination, can be differentiated from pain and swelling of the joints. Often pyrexia is present and may reach levels of 105–106°F (40–41°C). The cause of pyrexia is not known but it has been suggested that it may be due to absorption of degradation products from haematomata or simply due to the acute pain suffered by the animal. The pup is unwilling to move or walk and may cry out in pain when approached or touched. There is a degree of dullness but appetite is not reduced, except during pyrexic periods. The condition is most commonly seen in medium-to-large size dogs (e.g. Boxer, Doberman Pinscher, Afghan Hound) but occasionally occurs in smaller breeds.

Diagnosis is dependent on careful clinical evaluation and exclusion of other causes of pyrexia and can

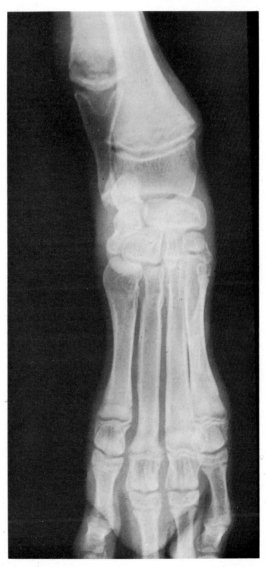

Fig. 6.5 Barlow's disease. Disruption in the metaphyseal area, but normal appearance of the cartilaginous growth plate.

be confirmed by radiography. The metaphyseal areas of the long bones present a characteristic picture. In the early stages the primary changes are seen within the metaphysis. The epiphyseal growth plate appears of normal width and the normally calcified cartilage shows up as a dense white band in comparison with the surrounding abnormal bone (the white line of Frankael). In addition, however, the area of spongiosa in the metaphysis continuous with the growth plate shows areas of increased and reduced density and general disruption (the trummerfeldzone) as a result of poor bone formation, trabecular collapse and haemorrhage (Fig. 6.5). The skeleton in general may show a reduction in density and a 'ground glass' appearance, but this is often difficult to judge in young growing pups.

Soft tissue swelling may be evident around the metaphysis and later in the course of the disease there may be development of spicules of new bone in the sub-periosteal haematomata external to the bone cortex (Fig. 6.6a); these enlarge, coalesce and form an external collar round the bone which then becomes continuous with the cortex, and a residual thickened bone extremity may result (Fig. 6.6b).

Treatment and prevention

Although the changes seen in pups closely resemble those found in human infantile scurvy, and treatment by administration of large amounts of ascorbic acid (0.5–1.00 g/day) often produces dramatic remission of pain (sometimes within 24 hours), return to normal temperature and reduction of swelling of the limbs, there is disagreement about this therapy, some authors claiming that vitamin C is likely to promote hypertrophic bone formation. Should the pain persist, treatment with steroids and analgesics should be given for

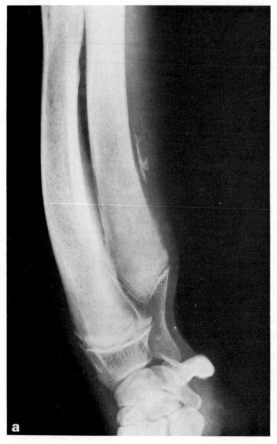
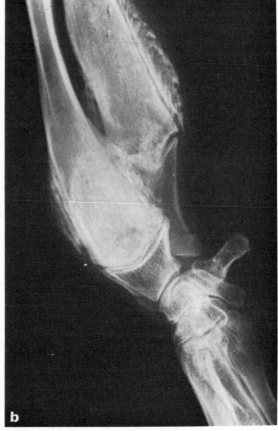

Fig. 6.6 Barlow's disease: (a) a healing lesion in the metaphysis with mineralisation occurring in the subperiosteal area; (b) a more advanced lesion with marked new bone formation and enlargement of the metaphyses, but still disruption in the area of the secondary spongiosa.

a week while the vitamin C administration is continued. It is probably advisable to make sure that excessive amounts of other supplements are not being given in the diet. If extracortical ossification has occurred, swelling of some degree will persist.

It has been stated that the condition resolves in the same way whether it is treated or not and independently of the drugs used (Grøndalen 1976). However, the dramatic response of many cases to administration of vitamin C has convinced the present authors that this should be the treatment of choice. Administration should be continued for several weeks and may be necessary for longer. Once the pup reaches 6–7 months of age no further attacks are likely. If relapse does occur, vitamin C administration often proves unhelpful and prognosis is bad. At present no prophylactic measures are available.

Hypertrophic osteodystrophy in giant dogs

A similar condition is seen in pups in such breeds as Great Dane, St Bernard and Pyrenean Mountain Dog. Where a 'trummerfeldzone' is present aetiology is probably similar. However, in some cases in these large breeds, only the development of extracortical new bone around the metaphysis is evident, and is associated with clinical swelling of the limbs, pain and lameness. These animals are often receiving large mineral and vitamin supplements. Sometimes radiographic examination of the limbs reveals, in addition to the hypertrophic new bone, a triangular projection of non-mineralised epiphyseal growth plate up the centre of the metaphysis, particularly in the ulna. This feature can often be seen in pups of large breeds with no other evidence of bone disease and its significance is not known.

Treatment in these cases is to reduce mineral and vitamin intake to satisfactory levels.

Hypervitaminosis A

Aetiology

This condition is due to the prolonged feeding of a diet containing a large amount of liver. The liver is the main storage organ for many vitamins, including vitamin A, so large amounts will be ingested over a long period.

Pathology

Vitamin A in excessive amounts causes suppression of osteoblastic activity, but high intake over a long period is associated with the development of exostoses in the region of ligament and tendon attachments. The reasons for this are unknown, as reduced osteoblastic activity and increased osteoclasis may be occurring

elsewhere in the skeleton. Hypervitaminosis A is rare in the dog, although it can be produced experimentally.

Diagnosis is dependent on the recognition of exostoses, clinically or radiographically, and confirmation of the dietary regime responsible for the condition.

Hypertrophic osteoarthropathy (pulmonary hypertrophic osteoarthropathy, Marie's disease)
This condition is characterised by swelling of the limbs due to periosteal proliferation mainly of the long bones, particularly the more distal bones of the limbs.

Aetiology

The precise reason for the widespread periosteal proliferation in this condition is not known. It is usually, though not invariably, associated with a chronic intrathoracic lesion, either neoplastic or inflammatory, and it is thought to be due to:

1 Reduced arterial oxygen tension or hypercarbia as a result of impairment of pulmonary function.
2 Formation of intrapulmonary vascular shunts causing reduced Pao_2 or preventing breakdown of vasoactive substances.
3 Some toxic or hormonal factor.
4 Change in vascular perfusion pattern of the limbs as a result of involvement of the autonomic nervous system in the thorax.

This latter theory has been supported by evidence that section of intrathoracic sympathetic fibres results in resolution of the periosteal changes, but usually such improvement is only temporary. Occurrence of a few cases of Marie's disease associated with intra-abdominal abnormalities (Brodey 1971) throws doubts on all these hypotheses.

Pathology

The changes which occur in the skeleton are mainly seen on the radius and ulna, the tibia and the metacarpal and metatarsal bones. The humerus and femur can also be involved, but less commonly the scapula and pelvic bones. There is overgrowth of highly vascular connective tissue with marked new periosteal bone formation which, in the early stages, may be smooth but later produces a very irregular 'palisade' appearance on the surface of the affected bones (Fig. 6.7). The soft tissues overlying these areas are swollen.

Clinical signs and diagnosis

The presenting clinical signs are usually those of chronic pulmonary disease though occasionally an animal is presented with limb swelling and lameness

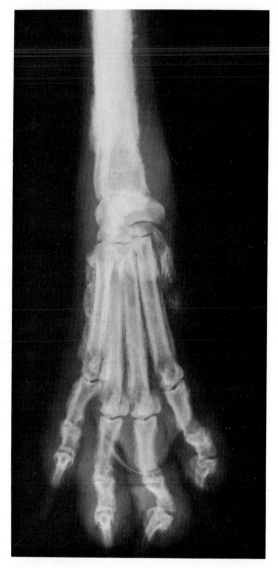

Fig. 6.7 Pulmonary hypertrophic osteoarthropathy (Marie's disease); periosteal new bone forming palisades on the radius, ulna, metacarpals and phalanges.

as the primary complaint. The limbs are hot, oedematous and tender and the animal is unwilling to walk and has a stiff gait. The whole length of the bone is affected down to the joint but not the bone under the articular cartilage. However, because of the periarticular soft tissue involvement the movements of the joints are reduced and may be painful.

Radiography in addition to demonstrating the intrathoracic mass, will reveal the widespread changes of the bone cortex.

Treatment and prevention

Where possible the primary intrathoracic lesion should be treated, usually by excision. If this can be achieved, remission of the bone changes occurs and the skeleton appears normal after a period of a few weeks. However, many of the primary lesions are malignant in character and recurrence is common, with re-establishment of the accompanying bone change, so that euthanasia must be performed. This is also indicated when the primary lesion is inoperable or fails to respond to treatment.

Other bone dystrophies

Hormonal in origin

1 Adrenal

Upset in bone metabolism and renal excretion of minerals produced by hyperactivity of the adrenal cortex leads eventually to bone porosis and sometimes soft tissue calcification. These changes are usually of minor importance compared with electrolyte and water imbalance and upset in glucose metabolism. However they may occasionally become severe enough to be clinically evident. Similarly, long-term treatment with corticosteroid drugs may give rise to skeletal changes.

Aetiology

The exact role of corticosteroids in bone metabolism is not understood but increase in the concentration of hydrocortisone results in reduced formation and increased resorption of bone with decreased absorption and increased urinary excretion of calcium. Thus a progressive reduction in bone tissue is produced. It has been suggested that this is brought about by the effect of corticosteroid on the osteons active in the remodelling of bone such that they increase in number and persist for much longer than normal (Frost 1966). Other authors claim however that the effect is directly on osteoblast precursors.

Pathology

There is thinning of the bone cortex and trabeculae, particularly of the axial skeleton. Weakness of the bone may lead to collapse of a vertebrae but this is extremely rare in animals.

In association with mineral depletion of the skeleton there may be deposition of calcified material in the soft tissues, including the skin, the blood vessels and the kidneys.

Clinical signs and diagnosis

The clinical signs of skeletal abnormalities in this disease are uncommon but may include bone pain, fractures of the long bones or neurological upset due to collapse of one or more vertebrae. Diagnosis of the hormonal abnormality and its treatment are dealt with elsewhere (see Chapter 8). Radiography of the skeleton reveals generalised loss of density but it may be difficult to assess the importance of this finding.

2 Thyroid (see also Chapter 8)

a Hyperthyroidism is associated with increased formation and resorption of bone; the latter predominates so that a degree of osteoporosis ensues. However, clinical evidence of such bone change is rare in animals.

b Calcitonin is a hormone which is secreted by the thyroid and has a specific effect on bone by limiting bone resorption. It has however also been shown to have effect on articular and growth plate cartilage and has been incriminated in the development of osteochondrosis. Hypercalcitonism may be of clinical significance in dogs.

Aetiology

Excessive intakes of calcium may reduce parathyroid activity and stimulate calcitonin production. One result of this may be a tendency towards hypertrophic osteodystrophy. However, calcitonin may also interfere with the normal development of cartilage causing failure of normal mineralisation of the deep layers of articular cartilage, degenerative changes within the cartilage and the formation of fissures leading to separation of fragments in, for example, the humeral head, medial distal humeral condyle, coronoid process of the ulna and medial trochlear ridge of the tibial tarsal bone.

However, other theories have been advanced concerning the aetiology of these changes including direct trauma and interference with blood flow resulting in local ischaemic necrosis. It now seems reasonably certain that osteochondrosis of the femoral head (Legg–Calvé–Perthe's disease) is due to ischaemia of the femoral epiphysis in young dogs, but such vascular change has not been confirmed in osteochondritis dissecans. These joint conditions will be dealt with in the next section of this chapter.

3 Oestrogen

Oestrogen has been shown to produce increased bone formation associated with increased numbers of osteoblasts, and thickening of trabeculae due to reduction of osteoclasis. These findings are reported in mice and rats although interference with endochondral ossification has been seen in dogs given oestradiol (Gustaffson & Beling 1969).

No generalised clinical skeletal defects in dogs have been proven to be due to excess oestrogen but it has been claimed that this hormone is involved in the aetiology of Perthe's disease (Llungren 1967), where it is said to cause ischaemia due to the change in trabecular shape, size and number, and hip dysplasia where its action is claimed to cause increase in laxity of the joint capsule and round ligament. The amounts of oestrogen which were given in the experimental studies were unphysiological and their involvement in clinical manifestations of these abnormalities is open to doubt.

Atrophy

Bone atrophy follows disuse of a limb but usually it gives rise to no specific clinical signs.

Aetiology

Following disuse of a limb due to bone, joint, muscle or nerve damage, there is probably marked reduction in the circulation of blood within the affected limb, due to reduced muscular activity in the area, and also reduced stress applied to the bones. These two factors together contribute to atrophic porosis which is brought about by increased bone resorption rather than reduced formation.

Pathology

There is enlargement of the Haversian canals, thinning of the cortices and reduction in intramedullary cancellous bone.

Clinical signs and diagnosis

Bone atrophy is always secondary to some other lesion and may only be detectable radiographically; the thin, poorly calcified bone is easily detected by comparison with the normal limb (Fig. 6.8).

Bone atrophy becomes clinically important in healing fractures of the radius and ulna in cases of delayed union, particularly in small dogs. Such atrophy may aggravate the relatively poor rate of healing by increasing the bone removal from the fractured ends. For this reason it is important to try to maintain function in the limb during healing.

Treatment and prevention

Splints should be applied in cases in which function can be maintained by their use. In other instances massage and manipulation to maintain blood flow and muscle tone, if possible, will help to reduce the rate of development of atrophy. Administration of sex steroids helps to prevent atrophy but produces undesirable effects elsewhere. Treatment with calcitonin has been found to be beneficial (Pezeshki & Brooker 1977).

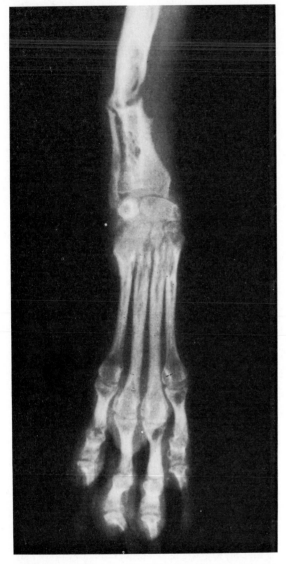

Fig. 6.8 Atrophy: porosis of the carpal and metacarpal bones due to disuse as a result of non-union of a radial fracture.

Craniomandibular osteopathy (temporomandibular periostitis)

This condition occurs primarily in young dogs of small Terrier breeds, notably West Highland White Terriers and Cairn Terriers, although it has occasionally been encountered in larger breeds such as the Doberman Pinscher and Great Dane (Watson *et al* 1975).

Aetiology
The aetiology is unknown.

Pathology
There is marked periosteal reaction which may affect the mandible or the petrous temporal bone or both. Occasionally periosteal new bone plaques are found on the long bones, particularly of the forelimb. The bones are thickened with a reactive, proliferative periosteal covering, under which new bone is formed. There may be some overlying oedema.

Clinical signs and diagnosis
Clinical signs are usually related to the temporomandibular changes. There is localised pain causing disinclination to eat. The thickened mandible can be palpated and is painful on pressure. If the temporal bone is badly involved there may be some luxation of the temporomandibular joint and difficulty in opening the mouth. Occasionally bilateral large swellings of the petrous temporal bones encroach on the pharynx and cause difficulty in swallowing and even difficulty in breathing.

The lesions on the limbs (Fig. 6.9a) are associated with local pain and lameness. No pyrexia is present.

On X-ray the thickened mandibles can be seen with reactive hazy surfaces. Enlargement of the petrous temporal bones is also easily demonstrated and distortion of the temporomandibular joint may be seen (Fig. 6.9b).

Treatment
Response to administration of corticosteroids is good. Reducing doses should be prescribed after a week unless the symptoms reappear. Exacerbations of the condition occur but again respond to treatment. The bone reaction settles down and there may be some remodelling to reduce the thickening of the bone. However, gross temporomandibular distortion, or severe restriction of pharyngeal aperture may lead to residual clinical abnormality.

Recurrences of the condition usually cease once the pup reaches 10–12 months of age, though exacerbations in bitches during early oestral periods have been encountered.

Hypovitaminosis A
This can be produced experimentally in the dog but clinical manifestations of the condition under normal circumstances are unknown. Lack of vitamin A causes proliferation of superficial bone and general retardation of skeletal growth. These changes affect primarily the nervous structures within bony canals, causing pressure necrosis and neural dysfunction, leading to blindness and other disorders.

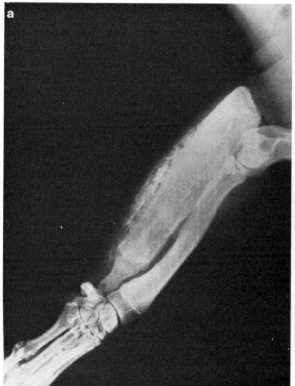 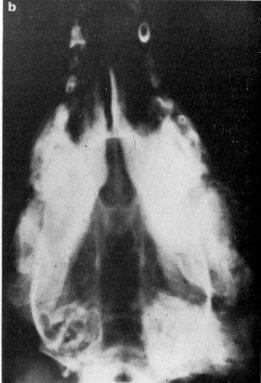

Fig. 6.9 Craniomandibular osteopathy: (a) new bone laid down along the ulna in a West Highland Terrier; (b) bony enlargements on the mandible and petrous temporal bone.

Bone cysts

Developments of large sometimes multinucleated cysts within one or several bones has been described by a number of authors (Carrig *et al* 1975; Jubb & Kennedy 1970; Owen & Walker 1963; Gourlay & Eden 1954).

Aetiology

The cause of the cysts is obscure. The suggestion that parathyroid hyperactivity is associated has not been confirmed.

Pathology

There is a large cavity within the affected bone, filled with gelatinous amorphous fluid or fibrous tissue. Numerous small cysts are often associated with the main cavity which may be multinucleated. No evidence of inflammation or neoplastic reaction is present. Increase in the number of osteoclasts is found around the cyst and there is thinning and porosis of the overlying cortex.

Clinical signs and diagnosis

The only sign may be regional swelling (e.g. in the distal radius or ulna). Occasionally there may be pain though no swelling of the soft tissues is present. Rarely a pathological fracture occurs. Bone cysts, though uncommon, are most likely to occur in larger dogs, particularly Doberman Pinschers.

Radiography reveals the presence of cystic enlargement, usually near the bone ends (Fig. 6.10). The overlying cortex is thinner than normal and displaced outwards but shows no localised areas of necrosis. The cystic cavity may contain intersecting coarse trabeculae which divide the cavity into several compartments. Sometimes more than one cyst can be seen in a particular bone and often more than one bone is affected. Small cysts may occasionally be incidental findings and can usually be ignored.

Treatment

Satisfactory results have been obtained following curettage of the cyst cavity. Transplants of cortical bone (e.g. rib) are indicated in situations where there

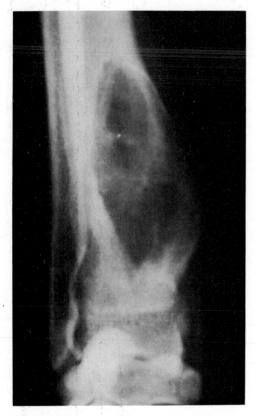

Fig. 6.10 Bone cyst: the destruction of the cortex of the distal radius and division of the cyst into several cavities.

appears to be marked bone weakness. The cyst cavities tend to be filled gradually with cancellous bone and eventually remodelling occurs.

INFLAMMATORY OR INFECTIOUS BONE DISEASE

Osteomyelitis

The infection of bone may involve only the external surface (periostitis) or the medulla but usually severe infection will extend to affect both.

Aetiology
A variety of pathogenic organisms have been implicated in osteomyelitis, notably staphylococci and streptococci of various types although non-pyogenic organisms may also occur. Infection may be haematogenous but much more commonly is introduced via a wound (e.g. a compound fracture or at surgery).

Pathology
The organisms cause an inflammatory reaction which may be very acute with marked local swelling, heat and pain but more commonly is of a chronic nature. There is periosteal inflammation which can occur over the whole length of the bone or be more localised, and gives rise to periosteal new bone deposits. Within the medullary cavity the infection may also spread up and down the length of the bone causing disruption of trabeculae and erosion of cortex, with collection of pus or serous fluid. At the edge of the lesion, if the infection is of a chronic nature, there may be an area of bone sclerosis. Localised areas of cortex may become completely necrotic and may eventually be separated from the surrounding bone, or separated ischaemic fragments may become foci of infection and persist within the affected area. The term sequestrum is applied to such a separate necrotic fragment, which fails to become incorporated in new bone produced in the healing process.

When the infective process is controlled, new bone is laid down and may trap localised foci of infection. Resurgence of infection has been reported, perhaps years later, as a result of liberation of bacteria during remodelling of the bone around such a focus.

Clincal signs and diagnosis
Pain is the most obvious result of such bone infection, particularly when the periosteum is involved. There may be localised heat and swelling.

Most affected animals also develop discharging sinuses as the infection is of a chronic nature in most cases. The sinuses may develop in the skin at a considerable distance from the site of infection, usually more distally but occasionally proximal to the lesion. Such sinuses will persist, although they may close over for variable periods, as long as the infection remains active, and particularly if any sequestra are present.

Radiography reveals bone changes which include periosteal reaction to a variable extent, areas of increased and decreased density in the medullary cavity and possibly an area of sclerosis, due to increased number and thickness of trabeculae, at the edge of the lesion (Fig. 6.11a). Sequestra can be recognised by the fact that they appear relatively dense compared with the surrounding reactive, partly lytic, bone.

Injection of radiopaque material into the sinus may help to indicate the specific area of infection or the position of a sequestrum which may be difficult to detect if small and completely enclosed in a cavity within hyperplastic new bone.

Treatment and prevention
Treatment consists of local and parenteral administra-

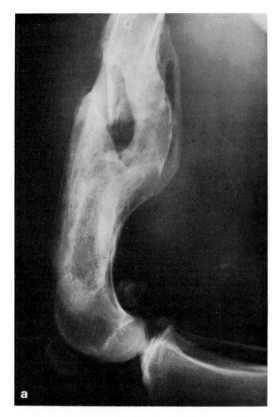

Fig. 6.11 (a) Sequestrum: a healed fracture of a femur, but with a large cavity present in the callus, surrounding two radiodense sequestrated pieces of bone cortex.

tion of antibiotics, preferably following sensitivity tests. A prolonged course of broad-spectrum drugs such as the tetracyclines may be necessary (i.e. lasting 3 weeks or more). Sequestra should be removed surgically; treatment is likely to be ineffective because the drug will not reach the bacteria existing within the necrotic bone. Occasionally sinuses persist in the absence of any sequestra. In such instances, exploration should be carried out to remove any non-absorbable foreign bodies such as suture material. In a minority of such cases no focus of infection can be identified and prognosis in these cases is guarded.

Prevention of osteomyelitis requires prompt treatment of compound fractures or of wounds where bone damage has occurred, and strict aseptic techniques when performing orthopaedic surgery.

Panosteitis (enostosis, eosinophilic panosteitis)
This is a condition which causes bone pain and lameness and which may affect several bones in the same animal, simultaneously or in succession.

Aetiology
The cause of the condition has not yet been elucidated. There appears to be no infective agent responsible although viral organisms cannot be completely ruled out. Similarly no defects of either nutrition, management or genetic predisposition have been confirmed (Bohning *et al* 1970).

Pathology
The disease is associated with localised excessive formation of bone. This is most evident in the medullary cavity which becomes filled to a variable extent with new bone trabeculae and areas of calcification of fibrous tissue. Marked osteoblastic, fibroblastic, and osteoclastic activity is present throughout the affected area, involving periosteum, endosteum and medulla. No inflammatory cells are present nor is there marked infiltration with eosinophilic leucocytes.

Clinical signs and diagnosis
Lameness and localised pain on pressure over one or more long bones of the limbs are the presenting signs. The condition usually occurs in animals between 5 months and 1 year of age and, although it has been said to be self-limiting at around 20 months of age, some cases are encountered up to the age of 5 years. Eighty per cent of affected animals are males and the disease has been described as affecting German Shepherd Dogs more than other breeds.

The lameness may shift from one bone to another, perhaps with a lapse of several weeks between attacks. There appears to be no confirmation of the suggestion that episodes of illness with fever (e.g. tonsillitis) may precede or accompany the disease.

Pain of the long bones is found on firm palpation but usually no muscle atrophy or local hypothermia is present. Radiography of the long bones in the early stages may not provide confirmatory results, particularly if high definition screens are not employed.

The earliest radiographic signs are blurring and increased density of the trabecular pattern within the medulla. Later the medulla assumes a dense, mottled appearance, sometimes localised near the nutrient foramen. Separate affected areas may coalesce to produce a homogeneous density which fills a large portion of the medullary cavity. However, small patches of increased density (less than 1 cm in diameter) may be all that can be detected in some cases. In about 30% of affected animals a periosteal reaction is also seen.

After 4–6 weeks localised bone density gradually diminishes leaving residual coarse trabeculae and roughened inner cortex. By the end of several months even these changes are no longer apparent.

Treatment and prevention
Treatment at present can only be of a palliative nature by means of analgesic drugs commonly used in loco-motor disorders.

NEOPLASIA

Bone can be the site of primary neoplasia or be affected by metastatic spread. Benign tumours of the skeleton are rare though they may respond to surgical treatment (Liu *et al* 1977).

Primary

Single lesions
Primary bone tumours include osteosarcoma, chon-drosarcoma, fibrosarcoma and haemangiosarcoma. Osteosarcomata are by far the most common bone tumours. They can affect dogs of all ages but are more common in middle-aged or older animals, particularly of the large breeds. The occurrence of the tumours in certain predilection sites in the skeleton has been well documented (Wolke & Neilsen 1966) thus in the fore-limb osteosarcomata occur primarily in the proximal humerus and distal radius and ulna, while in the hind-limb the distal femur, proximal tibia and distal tibia are more commonly affected. The reasons for this are not clear but it has been suggested that these are areas of greatest growth during puppyhood or areas of greatest stress.

Multiple
Occasionally osteosarcomata may occur in two sites at the same time but this is extremely rare. Multiple areas of bone destruction due to neoplastic deposits arising within the bone are most likely to be due to multiple myeloma. This disease will be discussed else-where. The skeletal lesions are usually easily identifi-able as local areas of cortical destruction with virtually no new bone formation, leaving a 'punched out' hole in the bone. Such areas of cortical destruction can be found in the long bones, ribs or vertebrae and if the condition is suspected widespread radiographic scan-ning of the skeleton is indicated.

Aetiology
The aetiology of bone tumours, like most other neo-plasms, is still obscure. Previous traumatic damage has often been suggested and the hypothesis of im-mune incompetence has received some support as a result of the response to non-specific stimulation of the immune system by BCG vaccine in the treatment

of osteosarcomata. Viral aetiology is also a possibility in some forms of bone tumour.

Pathology
Primary bone tumours often consist of mixtures of fibrous, cartilaginous and bony tissue, with cell divi-sion occurring in relatively undeveloped precursor cells so that pathological diagnosis is sometimes diffi-cult. If new osteoid tissue is present within the neo-plastic mass, even in small amounts, the diagnosis of osteosarcoma is made. In cases where osteoid is absent, the preponderant abnormal tissue gives the clue to the diagnosis, although in some cases mitotic division in more differentiated cartilage, fibrous tissue or vascular endothelial cells can be identified.

Clinical signs and diagnosis
Primary bone tumours usually cause swelling and lo-calised pain in the area of the new growth. Lameness may be the first indication to the owner that a problem exists, but usually localised pain and swelling will be present as well. The history may be misleading in that traumatic damage is often cited by the owner, but in many instances this may be due to the fact that the

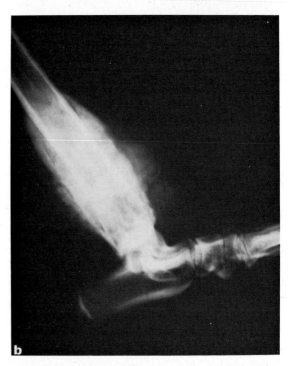

Fig. 6.11 (b) Osteosarcoma: trabecular and cortical de-struction at the distal end tibia, with new periosteal neoplas-tic bone but also well organised, fully formed new periosteal bone (Codman's triangle proximally).

animal shows exaggerated reaction to mild trauma because of the pain already present.

Radiography will usually demonstrate quite clearly that the neoplastic process is affecting the bone. There will be evidence of cortical and trabecular destruction perhaps with periosteal reaction, either neoplastic or simply due to lifting of the periosteum by localised tumour growth (Codman's triangle) (Fig. 6.11b) and new bone formation outwith the skeleton. If a fracture is present, careful scrutiny of the bone end and surrounding tissue is necessary in order to make sure that the fracture is not due to previous pathological change in the bone (Fig. 6.12).

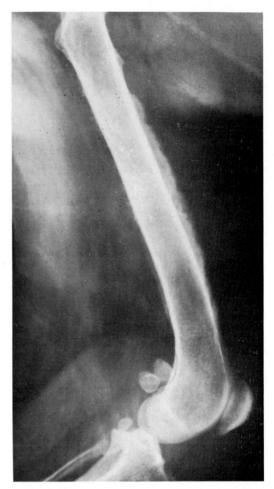

Fig. 6.13 Widespread periosteal reaction affecting only the femur in a dog, with some evidence of trabecular loss distally and areas of thinning and destruction of the distal cortex anteriorly. This tumour was diagnosed histologically as a fibrosarcoma.

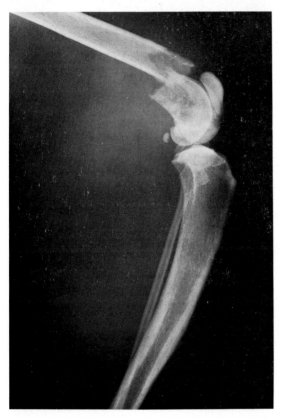

Fig. 6.12 Pathological fracture: on close examination of the radiograph areas of cortical destruction and periosteal reaction can be seen on both fracture ends, in this case of a fibrosarcoma.

Specific diagnosis of the type of tumour on radiography may not be possible. Obvious extraskeletal new bone formation probably indicates that the tumour is an osteosarcoma; if the extraskeletal calcification is very amorphous and of 'snowflake' appearance chon-drosarcoma is a possibility; periosteal reaction extending over the whole or the greater part of the affected bone may suggest fibrosarcoma or haemangiosarcoma (Fig. 6.13). All of these tumours however can produce a predominantly lytic effect with little new bone formation evident on X-ray. Bone tumours seldom cross over a joint and this may be helpful in attempting to reach a diagnosis on the basis of radiographic evidence. In all cases confirmation by histological examination is necessary.

Treatment
Metastatic deposits in lungs and elsewhere are com-

mon with all primary neoplasms of the skeleton. Surgical exploration for biopsy is likely to increase the chance of metastases[1] growth. Occasionally this may be necessary when there is doubt as to whether a given lesion is neoplastic or inflammatory. In most cases the best treatment, in the absence of detectable metastases in the lungs or elsewhere, is amputation of the affected limb. If the owner does not want this performed, euthanasia should be advised, particularly if the animal is showing continual pain.

Amputation followed by treatment with cytotoxic drugs or radiotherapy has so far proved valueless in cases in which metastases are already present. Some response has been achieved by the use of BCG vaccine following amputation but the long-term results are still poor.

Secondary

Metastases from a variety of tumours can cause skeletal changes (e.g. bronchial carcinoma, mammary carcinoma, prostatic carcinoma, haemangio-sarcoma and adenocarcinoma, particularly of structures closely associated with bone such as nasal mucosa). Such metastatic deposits in the skeleton cause local destruction of the bone (Fig. 6.14). There may be some periosteal proliferation present at the edge of the lesion. Deposits may be widespread as in bronchial carcinoma and prostatic carcinoma, or localised as in adenocarcinoma of nasal mucosa. The primary lesion may be evident and causing clinical signs or may be very difficult to identify.

Treatment
Malignant neoplastic deposits in the skeleton carry a very poor prognosis. Metastatic involvement of the skeleton from some other focus is not usually treated, as widespread or inoperable deposits are usual. Amputation of a limb may be possible in an instance such as destruction of a bone end by a metastasis arising within a joint.

INHERITED DEFECTS

Inherited defects are uncommon in small animals. Achondroplasia is occasionally seen (with dwarfism) and some reports of epiphiseal dysplasia have been published (Cotchin & Dyce 1956). Affected puppies are usually destroyed.

In many other abnormalities of the locomotor system genetic factors are suspected but in most cases such a genetic involvement has not been confirmed

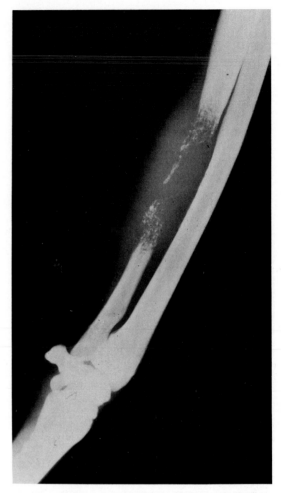

Fig. 6.14 Anaplastic bronchial carcinoma metastases; marked destruction of the bone with little new bone formation.

and specific bone lesions of a heritable nature would appear to be rare in dogs, in comparison to the human where numerous skeletal dysplasias have been shown to be inherited.

MUSCLE DISEASE

The muscles form the largest organ in the body and are commonly affected by disease (myopathies). In many instances a careful pathological examination shows that muscle abnormalities can occur in a large number of diseases although there may be no clinical evidence of dysfunction (e.g. focal fibre necrosis can be found in cases of pyometra). This section will deal

Table 6.2 Primary myopathies

Hereditary or probably hereditary myopathies
Hereditary Myotonia in chows
Myotonia and muscle hypertrophy in black Labradors
X-linked myopathy with myotonia in Irish Terriers
Autosomal recessive myopathy with type II fibre deficiency
    and myotonia in Retrievers.

Inflammatory Myopathies (myositis)
Bacterial myositis
    acute form—pyogenic cocci
    chronic form—pyogenic cocci
    Leptospira Icterohaemorrhagiae
Protozoal Myositis
    Toxoplasma gondii
    idiopathic myositis of the masticatory muscles
    idiopathic polymyositis

Metabolic Myopathies
Mitochondrial myopathy
Glycogen storage diseases

Secondary myopathies
Myopathies in endocrine disease
    Cushing's Disease
Myopathies associated with drugs
    Corticosteroid myopathy
Myopathies associated with malignancy
Myopathies in association with joint disease

primarily with conditions in which muscle disease may be of clinical importance.

A list of diseases is shown in Table 6.2. The most important group of muscle diseases in man are the muscular dystrophies which may be defined as progressive, genetically determined, primary degenerative myopathies. In animals, the term dystrophy has been used to refer to the nutritional myopathies of sheep and cattle. As there is no satisfactory classification of muscle disease in the dog the term 'dystrophy' will be avoided and all the diseases referred to as myopathies. Muscle diseases can be classified as primary or secondary myopathies.

Clinical aspects

Presentation of a case
The animal may be referred because of signs referrable to a myopathy or evidence of muscular abnormality may be detected during an examination for another complaint. Muscle disease tends to cause a fairly limited number of signs.

Weakness. This may be generalised or localised to a single limb or a group of muscles. The weakness may be present continually or only develop on exercise. It is important to realise that in certain myopathies the animal may appear completely normal at rest, signs only developing at exercise.

Stiffness. This may co-exist with weakness or be separate. The stiffness of gait may be continuous or decrease or increase with exercise.

Variation in muscle bulk. Atrophy or hypertrophy may be the reason for referral.

Muscle pain.

History
Besides a 'general history' there are certain special points of interest. How is the condition affected by exercise, rest, heat or cold? Are there other members of the litter affected? Has the dog been receiving any drugs?

Examination
In all cases a general clinical examination should be performed. It is useful to watch the dog walking and, if appropriate, exercising. The muscle bulk should be inspected and palpated and the range of movement checked. Muscle tone and local reflexes (pedal and patellar) should be tested. A partial neurological examination will probably be required. The muscles should be observed for spontaneous movement and in certain diseases percussed for a myotonic dimple. The hair is clipped and the muscle tapped firmly with a pair of artery forceps. In myotonia, a furrow or dimple may form in the muscle and be maintained for up to a minute or more (Fig. 6.15).

Myotonia is defined as 'the continued active contraction of a muscle following cessation of voluntary effort or stimulation' and is basically a failure of the muscle to relax normally. On the EMG myotonia is a high frequency discharge which initially increases and then decreases in both frequency and amplitude. The waxing and waning produces a sound in the loudspeaker similar to a 'dive bomber'. Clinically, it is manifest by stiffness which decreases on exercise ('warming out of it').

A myotonic percussion dimple may be present in some or all muscles. Some animals with myotonia show an abnormal reaction to depolarising muscle relaxants, with a sustained tonic contraction before relaxation (Griffiths & Duncan 1973). Further aspects of myotonia and myotonic diseases have been discussed by Duncan (1980).

Specialised examination
Biochemical, electromyographical and biopsy ex-

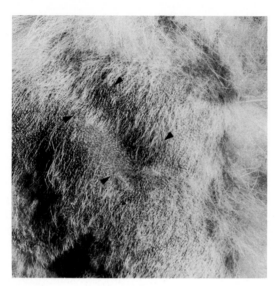

Fig. 6.15 Myotonic dimple (arrows) in the long head of triceps muscle of a Chow with myotonia/muscle hypertrophy syndrome.

aminations are often useful or essential in reaching a diagnosis. It is not intended to discuss them further in this section but the reader may consult the following references or those mentioned with the specific disease (Cardinet 1971; Chrisman *et al* 1972; Griffiths *et al* 1973; Walton 1974).

PRIMARY MYOPATHIES

In primary myopathies, as the name implies, the principal defect exists in the muscle. However, abnormalities of other systems may occur secondarily.

Hereditary or probably hereditary myopathies

At present, all published reports have concerned diseases in which myotonia was present.

Hereditary myotonia in Chows
This disease has been described in Chow Chow dogs in Great Britain (Griffiths & Duncan 1973), New Zealand (Jones *et al* 1977), the Netherlands (Wentink *et al* 1972) and Australia (Farrow & Malik 1981). The signs are present from an early age and have been noted when pups first become ambulatory. Both males and females are affected.

Aetiology
Although still not proven conclusively, it seems highly probable that the disease is inherited, possibly in an autosomal recessive manner. The evidence is the involvement of several dogs from the same litter, and the production of diseased pups by affected animals and their close relations.

Pathology
The main histological abnormality is a marked variation in muscle fibre size with numerous hypertrophic and atrophic fibres. A small proportion of fibres may show evidence of necrosis or regeneration. Internal nuclei are also seen and this feature appears to increase with the duration of the condition.

Clinical signs
There is usually difficulty in rising and marked stiffness of the limbs. The forelegs are abducted and there is a marked inability to flex the forelimbs when moving. This is particularly noticeable when attempting to climb steps or slopes. The hindlimbs may 'bunny-hop'. The degree of stiffness usually decreases with exercise and worsens after resting. The muscles are hypertrophied but tone is not usually increased. A myotonic percussion dimple is readily elicited from most of the muscles. The remainder of the neurological examination is often normal. Patella luxation and stifle arthritis frequently occur as a secondary complication. Serum creatine phosphokinase (CPK) levels may be elevated and hypocholesterolaemia has also been reported (Farrow & Malik 1981).

EMG examination reveals the high frequency discharges typical of myotonia in the majority of striated muscles. Farrow and Malik (1981) have reported more detailed studies of the electrophysiology in these cases. The clinical appearance is so distinctive that the EMG and muscle biopsy are not usually necessary to allow a diagnosis.

Treatment and advice. If left untreated there is usually a slow deterioration over a period of years probably due to the underlying myopathy and secondary complications. Of the various drugs which may stabilise the muscle fibre membrane, procainamide has been reported to produce the best clinical results in reducing muscle stiffness (Farrow & Malik 1981). In view of the suspected inheritance the affected animals, parents and litter mates should not be used for breeding.

Myotonic myopathies in other breeds
Myotonia has been reported in other breeds though not necessarily in association with muscle hypertrophy.

Myotonia and muscle hypertrophy in Black Labradors
A similar muscle hypertrophy/myotonia syndrome to that described in Chow Chows has been seen in Black Labradors. Too few cases have been observed to comment on any hereditary aspects.

X-linked myopathy with myotonia in Irish Terriers
A probable x-linked myopathy in Irish Terriers has been described. The animals, all males, showed dysphagia from 8 weeks of age followed by difficulty in walking, with stiffness and weakness. There was lumbar kyphosis, muscle atrophy and enlargement of the tongue. Muscle necrosis, regeneration, calcification and inflammatory infiltrates were present (Wentink *et al* 1972).

Autosomal recessive myopathy with Type II fibre deficiency and myotonia in Retrievers
A myopathy characterised by a preponderance of Type I fibres and inherited in an autosomal recessive manner has been described. These dogs showed weakness on exercise which was worsened by cold weather and temporarily improved with rest. Priapism was present in males and muscle atrophy was noted (Kramer *et al* 1976, 1981). The clinical signs appeared to stabilise at about 6 months of age and some cases have lived for 6 years with no additional signs.

Inflammatory myopathies (myositis)

Bacterial myositis
This is uncommon and when present is usually masked by other clinical signs of the disease.

Local myositis due to direct spread from a wound. Infection is usually caused by one of the pyogenic cocci and results in a local necrotising myositis and sometimes abscess formation.

The clinical signs are pain and swelling and difficulty in using the affected muscle group.

Treatment is by local wound care and systemic administration of the appropriate antibiotic and the prognosis is usually good.

Chronic myositis often accompanies infected fractures. Sinus tracts form in the muscle and are surrounded by fibrous tissue.

The infecting organism is usually one of the pyogenic cocci.

The predominant clinical signs are referable to the underlying orthopaedic condition. The most serious sequel, as regards the muscle, is the development of a contracture and resultant fixation or limitation of the joint.

Leptospira icterohaemorrhagiae can cause a necrotising myositis with little or no inflammatory reaction (Zenker's degeneration). This can result in painful muscles and weakness although these signs are often unrecognised in the severely ill dog.

Protozoal myositis
The protozoon *Toxoplasma gondii* can cause myositis in both young and old dogs.

Young dogs
The main muscle lesion is a severe necrotising myositis usually with marked mononuclear cell infiltrate. In many cases *T. gondii* cysts are very difficult to find in the muscles. In addition, there is usually myelitis, radiculitis and ganglionitis due to *T. gondii*. As a result, axonal degeneration occurs and there is neurogenic atrophy concurrent with the myositis. Myositis due to *T. gondii* is not uncommon in young dogs and should be strongly suspected in any inflammatory myopathy in this age group even if cysts are not demonstrated in the muscle.

Aetiology. It is difficult to reconcile the severe lesion with the few *T. gondii* cysts and it is possible that some form of immune reaction to toxoplasma or antigen released from damaged muscle is implicated in the aetiology.

Clinical signs. The hindlimbs are usually noted to be affected soon after birth. The puppy is paraplegic or paraparetic, with the limbs in rigid extension. Passive flexion is difficult or impossible. Pain sensation is present but reflexes cannot be evoked due to the rigidity. Some degree of atrophy is often present (Drake & Hime 1967). The above description represents a common and easily recognised clinical picture. Other presentations may include quadriparesis without specific neurological signs and this can in some instances result in the 'swimmer pup' syndrome.

EMG and nerve conduction studies may reveal evidence of denervation following damage to the motor neuron within the cord or ventral roots.

These clinical signs are highly suggestive of *T. gondii* neuromyositis. Further verification may be made by muscle biopsy or serum antibody titres although this is often not necessary.

Treatment. There is no effective treatment for this syndrome and the animal is usually destroyed.

Older dogs

A localised necrotising myopathy is found in some dogs with a CNS infection of *T. gondii*. The clinical signs are often minimal although local pain may be evident. The CNS infection usually dominates the clinical picture and the muscle lesions are chiefly an incidental finding.

Idiopathic myositis of the masticatory muscles

Despite wide clinical recognition, very little is known regarding the aetiology of this disease. Eosinophilic myositis is the form usually described in text books but its frequency appears to be over estimated. Clinically the disease may be acute, subacute or chronic. The chronic form may be a progression from the acute stage or arise without any apparent preceding disease.

As mentioned, the aetiology of the disease is unknown but several suggestions have been made. A virus (perhaps one of the Coxsackie group which are known to cause myositis in man) might be implicated in the acute disease. The same virus has also been implicated in a case of polymyositis in man. Many people have suggested that a hypersensitivity reaction to muscle antigen (or perhaps viral antigen) is involved.

In the acute stages there is severe fibre necrosis and myophagia together with an inflammatory infiltrate, which is commonly mononuclear cells (lymphocytes and plasma cells). Neutrophils may be present in necrotic areas and eosinophils when present usually form a small proportion of the total infiltrate. Regenerative changes are often found even in the acute disease. In the subacute and chronic stages there is an increase in connective tissue, particularly the perimysium. The chronic disease of insidious onset is characterised by an increase in perimysial connective tissue and varying degrees of fibre necrosis and inflammatory infiltrate (Duncan & Griffiths 1980).

The acute disease

The acute disease may cause pain and swelling of the masticatory muscles which in severe cases can cause exophthalmos. There may be consequent pain and reluctance to open the mouth. Systemic signs can include dullness, anorexia, slight pyrexia and mild anaemia. The tonsils and sub-maxillary lymph nodes may be enlarged. Laboratory investigations may show anaemia, leucocytosis (mainly a neutrophilia) and raised plasma globulins. In eosinophilic myositis there is reportedly an eosinophilia although this alone should not be taken as conclusive evidence of eosinophilic myositis.

Subacute and chronic disease

The subacute and chronic disease may follow the acute stage, in which case there can be a history of a preceding period of malaise. In many cases, and in the chronic myositis of insidious onset, there is no such history. The owner usually notices a gradual atrophy of the masticatory muscles which may be either bilateral or unilateral. In a proportion of cases the presenting sign is difficulty in eating. This is caused by inability to open the mouth, which in its severest form may restrict movement to 1 cm or less. Over 50% of affected dogs may have this restriction of jaw opening, although the majority manage to ingest adequate amounts of food.

Diagnosis is based on the clinical signs and preferably a muscle biopsy. The biopsy will confirm the myositis, indicate its severity and duration and may differentiate the idiopathic form from others for which an aetiology can be found, e.g. *T. gondii* myositis. In cases with unilateral muscle atrophy a biopsy will probably distinguish a chronic myopathy from neurogenic atrophy, which on clinical examination is very similar.

Treatment. In cases with jaw restriction the mouth can be forcibly opened by applying traction to the mandible and maxilla. This results in an audible tearing of the excessive fibrous tissue. This procedure must not be performed with excessive enthusiasm as it will then lead to an inability to close the mouth. Opening should only be taken to a limit which will allow the dog to eat. These cases, together with those not requiring this rather severe procedure, should then be given corticosteroid therapy. Betamethazone in doses of 2 mg/day (small dogs) or 4 mg (large dogs) is satisfactory. Maximal doses should be maintained for 2 weeks and decreased over a further 2 weeks. Repeated course(s) may be necessary. It is unlikely that the degree of atrophy will improve greatly but an improvement in the degree of jaw opening can be expected. The corticosteroid therapy will also minimise the formation of fibrous tissue and suppress an autoimmune reaction, assuming that this is involved in the aetiology.

Idiopathic polymyositis

The syndrome of idiopathic polymyositis has been reported more frequently in the USA than the UK, although there is no reason to assume it does not occur here (Averill 1974; Kornegay *et al* 1980).

Aetiology. The aetiology is unknown but, as in masticatory myositis, an immune mechanism has been postulated. The border zone between the two diseases is not necessarily clear cut and both could be different manifestations of the same basic process. It is possible that several aetiologies could produce a similar clinical picture.

Pathology. The changes (which can affect various limb, head, pharyngeal and oesophageal muscles) are similar to those described for masticatory myositis. There is variation of muscle fibre size (often with smaller rather than hypertrophic fibres), necrosis and other degenerative changes, regeneration, internal sarcolemmal nuclei and inflammatory infiltrates. Immunological studies have demonstrated IgG on the sarcolemmal membrane in some cases.

Clinical signs. The signs can be multiple and diverse. The commonest reported signs are muscle pain, weakness (which may be present at rest or exercise-induced), stiffness of gait, and pyrexia. Other signs include muscle atrophy, regurgitation and dysphagia, anorexia and change of bark.

Serum enzymes suggestive of muscle disease (CPK, ALT, AST) may be raised, although this is not constant. EMG may also be abnormal with polyphasic units, spontaneous activity and high frequency discharges. Muscle biopsy may demonstrate the pathological features although, as the severity varies both within and between muscles, it is possible to obtain a misleading appearance.

In reaching a diagnosis the clinical signs, serum enzymes, EMG and biopsy appearance should be considered and the greater the number of abnormalities within these parameters, the more likely is the diagnosis.

Treatment. Corticosteroids (betamethazone or prednisolone) are the suggested drugs. As there is some likelihood of recurrence it may well be necessary to maintain the dog on a low dose of prednisolone. The exact dosage and frequency (e.g. daily or alternate days) will need to be determined in individual dogs.

Metabolic myopathies

Mitochondrial myopathies

Structural and functional abnormalities of mitochondria are common in many muscle diseases and as such are 'non-specific' reactions. However, in mitochondrial myopathies, which appear to be uncommon, the numbers of abnormal mitochondria are excessive and predominate over any other changes. The structural abnormalities are accompanied by changes in mitochondrial function so that there are disturbances in energy production. Normally oxygen consumption is linked to ATP production (oxidative phosphorylation). With abnormal mitochondrial function this relationship is disturbed and leads to uncoupled or loosely-coupled mitochondria. Concurrent abnormalities in glycolysis have also been recorded in some cases.

Aetiology

Defects in mitochondrial function involving the enzyme pyruvate dehydrogenase have been described in Clumber spaniels (Herrtage & Houlton 1979). Single cases in a Collie and Boxer have been seen (Duncan & Griffiths, unpubl. obs.) where the exact enzymal defect was not established.

Clinical signs

The dogs are normal at rest or when moving around a room but when exercised show weakness and collapse. The amount of exercise required varies, but is often only several hundred yards. The dog will take progressively shorter steps and then collapse on all four feet and after a short rest will be able to continue. There is usually no pain or stiffness. Examination at rest reveals no abnormalities. A severe acidosis, causing death in one instance, developed in the Clumber spaniel after exercise.

The main differential diagnosis is myasthenia gravis. In mitochondrial myopathy there is no megaoesophagus or dysphagia and no improvement with a cholinergic or anticholinesterase drug, e.g. neostigmine.

Accurate diagnosis can be made only following muscle biopsy for relevant histochemical and biochemical tests.

Treatment

There is no specific treatment. Experience of the disease is limited but the two cases observed by the author showed complete spontaneous recovery after several months. Provided the animal is not physically stressed it will exist happily.

Glycogen storage diseases (GSD)

At least five forms of GSD affecting muscles have been described in man but to date few have been recognised in dogs.

Aetiology

All forms of GSD are due to enzyme deficiencies ing defects in the glycolytic pathway and a resultant accumulation of stored muscle glycogen. Involvement of different enzymes leads to various clinical syndromes. In dogs, a deficiency of amylo-1, 6-glucos-idase (the glycogen debrancher enzyme) has been described, which would correspond to a type III GSD (Rafiquazzaman *et al* 1976).

Pathology

In the type III GSD excess glycogen was present in various muscles, liver and neurons and glia of the CNS. In the muscles this was located in an interfibrillary position. Biochemical assays of liver demonstrated a severe depletion of the debranching enzyme.

Clinical signs

The four animals reported by Rafiquazzaman *et al* (1976) were young Alsatian bitches which had shown weakness, particularly after exercise, since puppyhood. Hepatomegaly was present, causing abdominal enlargement, and ascites was also present in one case.

Treatment

No successful treatment has been described in these cases.

SECONDARY MYOPATHIES

The myopathy develops secondarily to some other disease, e.g. endocrine disturbance or malignancy. In many instances the myopathy is masked by the original disease.

Myopathies in endocrine disease

Myopathies have been associated with virtually all the endocrine diseases in man. In the dog the only definite association to date is with canine Cushing's disease.

Cushing's disease

Cushing's disease (see also Chapter 8), which results from an excess production of glucocorticosteroids is commonly associated with muscle abnormalities. In many cases the myopathy may be sub-clinical. Various aspects of the canine disease have been described in detail (Duncan *et al* 1977; Greene *et al* 1979; Braund *et al* 1980).

Pathology

Pathological examination may reveal variation in fibre size, focal fibre necrosis and myophagia, regeneration, occasional internal nuclei and fibroplasia. Calcification may also be seen. Sub-sarcolemmal accumulations of mitochondria and glycogen also occur. These abnormalities are focal in nature, only affecting certain areas of some muscles.

Clinical signs

In some milder cases the main signs are weakness and atrophy. The weakness is indicated by the pendulous abdomen and excessive abduction of the elbows and the atrophy is usually most marked in the temporal muscles. Other cases show more marked signs with stiffness of limbs and gait. In the most severe form the limbs, particularly the hindlimbs, become rigid and difficult or impossible to flex, even under general anaesthesia. If the limbs are flexed passively they spring back into extension immediately upon release. The muscles may be hypertrophic rather than atrophic and when percussed a myotonic dimple may be seen.

EMG examination usually demonstrates high frequency discharges, indicating both myotonia and pseudomyotonia (the latter predominating) in multiple muscles. These discharges are usually present even in mild or sub-clinical cases.

Treatment

Treatment is directed at the underlying hyperadrenocorticism (see Chapter 8). Milder cases may well improve or recover but the prognosis in the more severe rigid cases is poor. Greene *et al* (1979) indicate an inverse relationship between response and the duration of clinical signs.

Myopathies associated with drugs

In man a large number of drugs have been reported to be able to cause muscle disease. At present very little is known about drug-induced myopathies in dogs.

Corticosteroid myopathy

A small number of cases have been seen. The corticosteroid was usually administered in a low dosage (0.25–0.5 mg/day) over a long period (a year or more) to suppress various skin reactions.

The clinical signs that have been observed correspond to those described for the severe cases of Cushing's disease with muscle rigidity, myotonia, etc.

Withdrawal of the steroid has not produced remission of signs although the number of cases observed is too small to know if this is always likely to be the case.

Myopathies in association with malignancy

The association between myopathy and malignancy is well known in man. Indeed, an obvious or clinically undetectable malignancy is a common cause of polymyositis or dermatomyositis. In dogs such a relationship has not been proven.

Many cases of canine malignancy show cachexic muscle atrophy usually affecting type II fibres preferentially. Occasionally focal inflammatory infiltrates and fibre necrosis are also present (Griffiths *et al* 1973; Sorjonen *et al* 1982). It is possible that the weakness seen in these dogs is due in some part to myopathic changes.

Myopathies in association with joint disease

Polymyositis may occur in association with inflammatory joint disease. Atrophy is commonly present in muscles and occasionally small focal mononuclear cell infiltrates may also occur. Clinical signs (which may not always be present) consist of weakness, stiffness, muscle pain and atrophy. Treatment of the underlying joint disease is indicated (Krum *et al* 1977).

REFERENCES

Bones

BOHNING R.N., SUTER P.F., HOHN R.B. & MARSHALL J. (1970) Clinical and Radiologic Survey of Canine Panosteitis. *J. Am Vet. Med. Ass.* **156**, 870.

BRODEY R.S. (1971) Hypertrophic osteoarthropathy in the dog: a clinico-pathologic survey of 60 cases. *J. Am. Vet. Med. Ass.* **159**, 1242.

BRODEY R.S., MEDWAY W. & MARSHAK R.R. (1961) Renal osteodystrophy in the dog. *J. Am. Vet. Med. Ass.* **139**, 329.

CARRIG C.B., POOL R.R., McELROY J.M. (1975) Polyostotic cystic bone lesions in a dog. *J. Small Anim. Pract.* **16**, 495.

COTCHIN E. & DYCE K.M. (1956) A case of epiphyseal dysplasia in a dog. *Vet. Rec.* **68**, 427.

FROST H.M. (1966) *Bone dynamics in osteoporosis and osteomalacia.* C.C. Thomas, Springfield, Ill.

FROST H.M. (1968) *Bone formation: a systems analysis.* Orthopedic Research Laboratory, Henry Ford Hospital, Detroit.

GOODSHIP A.E., LANYON L.E. & McFIE H. (1979) Functional adaptation of bone to increased stress. *J. Bone Jt Surg.* **61**, 539.

GOURLAY J. & EDEN C.W. (1954) Bone cyst in a dog. *Vet. Rec.* **66**, 63.

GRONDALEN J. (1976) Metaphyseal osteopathy (hypertrophic osteodystrophy) in growing dogs. A clinical study. *Small Anim. Pract.* **17**, 721.

GUSTAFSSON P.O. & BELING C.G. (1969) Oestradiol-induced changes in Beagle pups. *Endocrinology* **85**, 481.

JUBB K.V. & KENNEDY P.C. (1970) *Pathology of Domestic Animals.* 2nd edn. Academic Press, New York.

LIU S.-K., DORKMAN H.D., HURVITZ A.I. & PATNAIK A.K. (1977) Primary and secondary bone tumours in the dog. *J. Small Anim. Pract.* **18**, 313.

LLUNGREN G. (1967) Legge–Perthes disease in the Dog. *Acta Orthop. Scand. suppl.* 95.

McCANCE R.A. & WIDDOWSON E.M. (1946) *The chemical composition of foods,* 2nd edn. MRC Special Report No. 235. H.M.S.O., London.

OWEN L.N., BOSTOCK D.E. & LAVELLE R.B. (1977) Studies on therapy of osteosarcoma in dogs using BCG vaccine. *J. Am. Vet. Radiol. Soc.* **18**, 27.

OWEN L.N. & WALKER R.G. (1963) Osteitis fibrosa cystica of the radius in an Irish Wolf Hound. *Vet. Rec.* **75**, 40.

PEZESHKI C. & BROOKER A.F. (1977) Immobilisation hypercalcaemia treated with calcitonin. *J. Bone Jt. Surg.* **59A**, 971.

PIERCE K.R., BRIDGES C.H. & BANKS W.C. (1965) Hormone-induced hip dysplasia in dogs. *J. Small Anim. Pract.* **6**, 121.

SUMNER-SMITH G. (1982) *Bone in clinical orthopaedics.* W.B. Saunders & Co, Philadelphia.

TEARE J.A., HINTZ H.F. & KROOK L. (1980) Rapid growth and skeletal disease in dogs, p. 126. *Proc. Cornell Nutr. Conf.*

TEARE J.A., KROOK L., KALLFELZ F.A. & HINTZ H.F. (1979) Ascorbic acid deficiency and hypertrophic osteodystrophy in the dog. A rebuttal. *Cornell Vet.* **69**, 384–401.

TRUETA J. (1963) The role of the vessels in osteogenesis. *J. Bone Jt. Surg.* **45B**, 402.

VAUGHAN J.M. (1981) *The Physiology of bone,* 3rd edn., Oxford University Press, Oxford.

WATSON A.D.J., HUXTABLE C.R.R. & FARROW B.R.H. (1975) Craniomandibular osteopathy in Doberman Pinschers. *J. Small Anim. Pract.* **16**, 11.

WOLKE R.E. & NIELSON S.W. (1966) Site incidence of canine osteosarcoma. *J. Small Anim. Pract.* **7**, 489.

Muscles

AVERILL D.R. Jr. (1974) Polymyositis in the dog. In: *Current Veterinary Therapy,* vol. V. Small Animal Practice, ed. R.W. Kirk, p. 652. W.B. Saunders, Philadelphia.

BRAUND K.G., DILLON A.R., MIKEAL, R.L. & AUGUST J.R. (1980) Subclinical myopathy associated with hyperadrenocorticism in the dog. *Vet. Pathol.* **17**, 134–148.

CARDINET G.H. (1971) Skeletal muscle. In: *Clinical Biochemistry of Domestic Animals,* vol. 2, eds. J.J. Kanero & C.E. Cornelius, 2nd edn, p. 155. Academic Press, London.

CHRISMAN C.L., BURT J., WOOD P.K. & JOHNSON E.W. (1972) Electromyography—small animal clinical neurology. *J. Am. Vet. Med. Ass.* **160**, 311.

DRAKE J.C. & HIME, J.M. (1967) Two syndromes in young dogs caused by *Toxoplasma gondii. J. Small Anim. Pract.* **8**, 621.

DUNCAN I.D., GRIFFITHS I.R. & NASH A.S. (1977) Myotonia in canine Cushing's Disease. *Vet. Rec.* **100**, 30.

DUNCAN I.D. (1980) Myotonia in the dog. In: *Current Veterinary Therapy,* vol. VII. Small Animal Practice, ed. R.W. Kirk, pp. 787–791. W.B. Saunders, Philadelphia.

DUNCAN I.D. & GRIFFITHS I.R. (1980) Inflammatory muscle disease in the dog. In: *Current Veterinary Therapy,* vol. VII. Small Animal Practice, ed. R.W. Kirk, pp. 779–782. W.B. Saunders, Philadelphia.

FARROW B.R.H. & MALIK R. (1981) Hereditary myotonia in the Chow Chow. *J. Small Anim. Pract.* **22**, 451–465.

GREENE C.E., LORENZ M.D., MUNNELL J.R., PRASSE K.W., WHITE N.A. & BOWEN J.M. (1979) Myopathy associated with hyperadrenocorticism in the dog. *JAVMA* **174**, 1310–1315.

GRIFFITHS I.R. & DUNCAN I.E. (1973) Myotonia in the dog: a report of four cases. *Vet. Rec.* **93,** 184.

GRIFFITHS I.R., DUNCAN I.E., McQUEEN A., QUIRK C. & MILLER R. (1973) Neuromuscular disease in dogs—some aspects of investigation and diagnosis. *J. Small Anim. Pract.* **14,** 533.

HERRTAGE M.E. & HOULTON J.E.F. (1979) Collapsing clumber spaniels. *Vet. Rec.* **104,** 334.

JONES B.R., ANDERSON L.J., BARNES G.R.G., JOHNSTONE A.C. & JUBY W.D. (1977) Myotonia in related Chow Chow dogs. *N.Z. Vet. J.* **25,** 217–220.

KORNEGAY J.N., GORGACZ E.J., DAWE D.L., BOWEN J.M., WHITE N.A. & DEBUYSSCHER E.V. (1980) Polymyositis in dogs. *JAVMA* **176,** 431–438.

KRAMER J.W., HEGREBERG G.A., BRUAN G.M., MEYERS K. & OTT R.L. (1976) A muscle disorder of Labrador Retrievers characterised by deficiency of type II muscle fibres. *J. Am. Vet. Ass.* **169,** 817.

KRAMER J.W., HEGREBERG G.A. & HAMILTON M.J. (1981) Inheritance of a neuromuscular disorder of Labrador Retriever dogs. *JAVMA* **179,** 380–381.

KRUM S.H., CARDINET G.H., ANDERSON B.C. & HOLLIDAY T.A. (1977) Polymyositis and polyarthritis associated with systemic lupus erythematosus in a dog. *J. Am. Vet. Med. Ass.* **170,** 61.

RAFIQUZZAMAN M., SVENKERUD R., STRANDE A. & HAUGE J.G. (1976) Glycogenosis in the dog. *Acta vet. Scand.* **17,** 196–209.

SORJONEN D.C., BRAUND K.G. & HOFF E.J. (1982) Paraplegia and subclinical neuromyopathy associated with a primary lung tumor in a dog. *JAVMA* **180,** 1209–1211.

WALTON J.N. (1974) *Disorders of Voluntary Muscle.* Churchill Livingstone, Edinburgh.

WENTINK, G.H., VAN DER LINDE-SIPMAN J.S., KEIJER A.E.F.H., KAMPHUISEN H.A.C., VAN VORSTENBORSCH C.J.A.H.V., HARTMAN W. & HENDRIKS H.J. (1972) Myopathy with a possible recessive X-linked inheritance in a litter of Irish Terriers. *Vet. Path.* **9,** 328.

7
Joint disease

D. BENNETT

ANATOMY AND PHYSIOLOGY

Joints may be classified according to the amount of movement possible (i.e. immovable joints or synarthroses, partially movable joints or amphiarthroses and freely movable joints or diarthroses). The latter are the most important for the present discussion and descriptions of articular anatomy, physiology and pathology will be confined to the diarthrodial type of joint. Diarthrodial joints can be classified according to the type of active movement which they permit:

1 Enarthrosis or ball-and-socket joint which allows flexion, extension, abduction, adduction and rotation (e.g. hip).
2 Condylarthrosis or condyloid joint which allows flexion, extension, abduction and adduction but no active rotation (e.g. carpus).
3 Saddle-shaped or sellar joint which allows flexion, extension, abduction, adduction and a slight rotatory movement.
4 Ginglymus or hinged joint which allows only flexion and extension (e.g. elbow).
5 Trochoid or pivot joint which allows only rotation (e.g. atlas/axis articulation).
6 Arthrosis or plain joint which allows only a slight degree of gliding of one articular surface over another (e.g. between individual carpal and tarsal bones).

Some joints do not conform exactly to one or other of these categories and in some, more than one description may apply (e.g. temporomandibular and stifle joints).

The basic anatomical structure of a diarthrodial joint is shown schematically in Fig. 7.1.

Articular cartilage

This structure covers the articular surfaces of joints and consists of cells (chondrocytes) lying in small cavities or lacunae distributed through an abundant in-

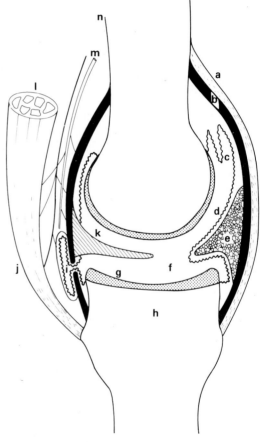

Fig. 7.1 Diagrammatic representation of a diarthrodial joint showing the main anatomical features: (a) ligament; (b) fibrous capsule; (c) synovial fold; (d) synovial membrane; (e) fat pad; (f) articular cavity; (g) articular cartilage; (h) epiphysis; (i) bursa; (j) tendon; (k) meniscus; (l) muscle; (m) blood vessels and nerves; (n) periosteum.

tercellular matrix. It is of the hyaline variety and macroscopically has a shiny, smooth white or pale yellow appearance. Histologically four layers are recognised:

1 Calcified stratum.
2 Radiate stratum.
3 Intermediate stratum.
4 Superficial or tangenitial stratum adjacent to the joint cavity.

Underlying the articular cartilage is a thin layer of compact bone, the subarticular or subchondral bone. The calcified stratum occurs immediately adjacent to the subarticular bone and is characterised by infiltration of the cartilage matrix with calcium. In the calcified and radiate strata the lacunae and chondrocytes are large and spherical and are arranged in radially running rows disposed at right angles to the articular surface. The cells are more oval and arranged in groups in the intermediate stratum and become more and more flattened as they approach the surface of the cartilage with their long axes parallel to the free surface. These cells are generally considered to be constantly removed from the surface during the normal process of 'wear and tear'. In some of the smaller joints, this flattening of the cells towards the surface is not seen and a typical superficial stratum does not exist.

Between the chondrocytes there is an abundance of matrix embedded in which are numerous collagenous, and other, fibres. Despite extensive studies, the exact anatomical arrangement of these fibres is still in dispute. Approximately 70% of the matrix is water, the remainder is proteoglycan, which is mucopolysaccharide material. Many recent investigations into the biochemistry of this matrix have been carried out in both normal and diseased joints and certain well-defined differences are apparent.

Articular cartilage appears to be aneural and therefore insensitive to weight bearing. It is also devoid of blood vessels and lymphatics except in its deepest layer, has no perichondrium and is not covered by synovial membrane. It never ossifies and is only calcified in its deepest layer.

The transitional zone or zone of proliferation refers to the area where the synovial membrane meets with the periphery of the articular cartilage. This region is important since pathological changes, particularly osteophyte development, frequently occur here. The transition from cartilage to synovial membrane and periosteum is gradual. It is suggested that the periphery of the articular cartilage receives nourishment from the blood vessels within the synovial membrane which might explain why this area of cartilage differs in its pathological reaction compared to the more central portions.

Articular cartilage forms a lining layer to the end of a bone at a joint and therefore protects the end of the bone from concussion and provides a smooth surface for the articulation of one bone over another. The articular cartilage also provides a growth zone for the epiphysis in the young animal which contributes to longitudinal growth. Nutrition of the cartilage is thought to arise from the synovial fluid and from the blood vessels which are present in only its deepest layers and at its periphery.

Synovial membrane

The synovial membrane lines the fibrous capsule and intra-articular ligaments and is reflected on to the intracapsular bone. It forms a smooth glistening layer with a few small villi and fringelike folds. Embryonically, the synovial membrane is derived from the mesenchyme of the original skeletal blastema and is therefore a type of connective tissue and does not possess a true epithelial structure. The synovial membrane consists of two layers, the lining or intimal layer adjacent to the joint cavity and the supporting, subintimal or subsynovial layer. With light microscopy the lining layer is seen to be composed of three main cell types within a matrix and the depth of the lining layer varies from one to several cells although occasionally there appear to be interruptions in the integrity of the layer. One type of cell is characterised by having a poorly defined cytoplasm and a large basophilic nucleus, another type has a more defined cytoplasm and a third type is straplike in appearance. The subsynovial layer supports the lining layer and according to its nature the synovial membrane can be classified into three main types: fibrous, areolar and adipose. These different types of synovial membrane can be found within the same joint and it is also common to see overlapping of the different types (e.g. fibro-areolar and areolar-adipose). Various connective tissue elements can be identified within the supporting layer and the predominant components differ with the different types of synovial membrane (e.g. fibroblasts, fibrocytes, adipose cells, collagen fibres and elastic fibres). Mast cells are also seen together with other less specific connective tissue cells. This layer contains several blood and lymphatic vessels.

The synovial membrane with the lining of the capillaries constitutes the blood synovial barrier. Through it must pass that part of the synovial fluid derived from blood as well as any metabolites from the synovial fluid returning to the blood. It is thought that the mucopolysaccharide present in synovial fluid is produced by the synovial cells. The synovial membrane also helps to keep the joint free of detritus by means of the phagocytic cells within it.

Synovial fluid

Normal synovial fluid is a clear or slightly yellow viscous liquid; it is thought to be a dialysate of blood plasma to which mucopolysaccharide is added, The viscocity of synovial fluid is due to its mucopolysaccharide content. It is difficult to aspirate any quantity of synovial fluid from normal joints of the dog. Several hundred nucleated cells per cubic millimetre have been recorded in synovial fluid from normal joints and most if not all of these are mononuclear cells. The mononuclear cells include lymphocytes, monocytes, unclassified phagocytes and synovial cells. A variable number of erythrocytes are also usually found. In addition amorphous particles, probably arising from articular cartilage, cellular debris and unidentified solid material are seen. Synovial fluid as well as forming a fluid medium in the joint for lubrication is probably also concerned with the nutrition of articular structures especially articular cartilage and menisci. Synovial fluid is principally important for soft tissue non-cartilage lubrication which is related to the hyaluronic acid content of the fluid, the molecules of which stick to the surface of the soft tissues such as synovial membrane. Lubrication of articular cartilage is mainly dependent on the extrusion of mucopolysaccharides from the cartilage surface as pressure is applied together with the elastic property of articular cartilage (Marcoux & Lamothe 1977).

Fibrous capsule and ligaments

The fibrous capsule together with the synovial membrane constitutes the articular capsule of the joint. The articular capsule delineates the joint structure and is generally attached to the bones themselves participating in the articulation thus helping to maintain bony relations and restricting and guiding movements. Muscles and tendons also help to limit excursion of joints and prevent damage to articular structures. A proportion of dogs do show an excessive laxity of one or more joints, presumably due to a failure of the capsule, ligaments, etc. to support the joint. Often the dogs manage without any serious inconvenience, although postural abnormalities may be evident and secondary osteoarthritis may be a later complication. Occasionally, defects occur in the fibrous capsule to allow intra-articular tendons to leave the joint or to allow the articular synovial membrane to form a bursa.

Fibrous capsules vary considerably in their degree of development and strength according to the functional demands placed upon them. Thickenings occur within the fibrous capsule and are often referred to as ligaments. However, other ligaments are usually present in most joints distinctly separate from the joint capsule and can be intra-articular or extra-articular. Ligaments help in holding the bones of the joint together, but may also be involved in supporting soft tissue structures within the joint (e.g. menisci) or forming retention bands for tendons. The fibrous capsule and ligaments possess a rich nerve supply and form an important source of pain in many joint diseases. The attachments of ligaments to bone are generally very strong and injury to a joint can frequently result in fracture of the bone adjoining the ligamentous attachment. The fibrous capsule and ligaments are composed of dense fibrous tissue consisting of collagen and reticular fibres, fibroblasts and fibrocytes embedded in an amorphous matrix of mucopolysaccharide and glycoprotein. A few histiocytes, fat cells, pigment cells and an occasional inflammatory cell may also be present.

Intra-articular structures

Intra-articular folds of synovial membrane (i.e. so-called synovial folds), have been regarded as invaginations of synovium by which blood vessels and nerves receive passage to other intra-articular structures and also as remnants of partitions which divided the joint into separate compartments. In certain joints (e.g. the stifle), these folds are particularly prominent. Intra-articular ligaments (e.g. the cruciate ligaments of the stifle and teres ligament of the hip) are surrounded by synovial membrane.

Intra-articular discs and menisci are specialised fibrocartilaginous structures and suggestions for their function have included, facilitation of joint lubrication, shock absorption, increasing the joint stability by improving congruity between the articular surfaces, allowing a combination of different movements at the joint, restriction of excessive movement of a joint, a ball-bearing action, distributing weight across the joint and protection of the joint margins. Many studies have demonstrated degenerative changes within menisci and discs with advancing age. Menisci have been shown to possess a nerve and blood supply restricted to their periphery.

Intra-articular fat pads consist of adipose cells with a considerable amount of elastic tissue and possess a rich blood and nerve supply. It has been suggested that some of these fat pads have developed to fill the dead space which arises during joint movement. Other suggested functions have included cushioning of bony processes, assisting synovial fluid flow across joint

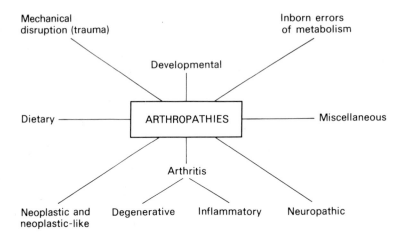

Fig. 7.2 Types of joint pathology seen in the dog.

surfaces and forming storage depots of body fat. The displacement of fat pads between the joint surfaces in certain disease states may be a source of joint pain.

Blood vessels, lymphatics and nerves

Except for articular cartilage and intra-articular discs and menisci, joints have a reasonably good blood supply. Similarly there is a rich lymphatic drainage from the structures well supplied with blood. Coordinated movements of joints depend on the sense of proprioception or awareness; the senses of touch and sight are also of assistance. Joints contain a variety of specialised nerve endings within ligaments and fibrous capsule which provide mechanoreceptor sensation for postural kinaesthetic reception (i.e. providing conscious awareness of joint position and of the amplitude and velocity of joint movement) and which generate reflex influences on the activity of related striated muscle (i.e. arthrokinesis) (Freeman & Wyke 1966, 1967; Wyke 1967, 1972). Different types of nerve receptors have been described in joints and these vary in their exact location within the joint, in their histological and electrophysiological characteristics and in the type of nerve fibre associated with them. With reference to the importance of joint proprioception, it is interesting that persistent postural abnormalities have been observed in human patients suffering articular diseases such as rheumatoid arthritis, possibly due to an interference with the articular nervous system (Dee 1969). Pain receptors are also found within joints, particularly the articular capsule. Joints also receive an autonomic nerve supply principally to the blood vessels where it is important in the control of articular blood flow.

The nerve supply to a joint can be through direct branches from the peripheral nerves or through neighbouring muscle branches (Skoglund 1956).

Occasionally muscle spasm is seen associated with joint pain and is probably reflexly induced by afferent impulses from the joint. In the human patient, it is well known that joint pain may be referred to more remote areas innervated by the same spinal segment or segments.

GENERAL PRINCIPLES OF JOINT PATHOLOGY

An understanding of joint pathology is essential in order to appreciate the problems associated with the clinical diagnosis of joint disease and its treatment. Joints as already discussed are composed of several different tissues and these vary in the way they can react during disease. For example, articular cartilage has no blood supply and therefore cannot be expected to show a true inflammatory reaction. Synovial membrane on the other hand has a rich vascular supply and readily undergoes inflammatory changes. There is also a considerable overlap between different types of joint diseases as far as the pathology is concerned. For example, some cases of osteoarthritis show inflammatory synovial membrane changes just as severe as those seen in rheumatoid arthritis. However, it is generally true that a particular pathological process will predominate in any one type of joint disease and often the pathogenesis of different diseases varies considerably. It is possible for one type of joint disease to accompany another (e.g. osteoarthritis can

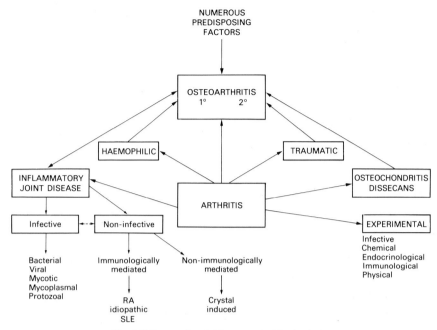

NUMEROUS
PREDISPOSING
FACTORS

OSTEOARTHRITIS
1°   2°

HAEMOPHILIC

TRAUMATIC

INFLAMMATORY
JOINT DISEASE

ARTHRITIS

OSTEOCHONDRITIS
DISSECANS

Infective   Non-infective

EXPERIMENTAL

Bacterial
Viral
Mycotic
Mycoplasmal
Protozoal

Immunologically
mediated

Non-immunologically
mediated

Infective
Chemical
Endocrinological
Immunological
Physical

RA
idiopathic
SLE

Crystal
induced

Fig. 7.3 Types of arthritis recognised in the dog.

develop secondary to other joint diseases such as dysplasia, ischaemic necrosis, osteochondritis dissecans and rheumatoid arthritis, and inflammatory joint disease can develop in a joint already affected with osteoarthritis). These factors can thus make a clear definition of these diseases difficult and often it is necessary to consider several factors together to obtain a definitive diagnosis. The different types of joint diseases are shown in Fig. 7.2. One of the most important is arthritis of which there are again several types (see Fig. 7.3).

The main pathological processes affecting joints can be listed as follows:

Mechanical disruption
This covers the severe traumatic injuries to joints producing luxation (dislocation), subluxation and instability and/or fractures of the articular cartilage or bony components of the joint. Such conditions if left untreated or incorrectly repaired can lead to osteoarthritic change.

Degeneration and infiltrations
Degeneration implies that a tissue loses its proper form and function; it can affect cellular and extracellular components. Cellular degeneration includes necrosis and cloudy swelling. Extracellular degeneration can affect collagen fibres and matrix material. Both cellular and extracellular degeneration can, for exam-

ple, be seen in osteoarthritic articular cartilage. Hyaline degeneration characterised by a loss of cellular and extracellular detail with the presence of acidophilic material is frequently seen in severe inflammation of the synovial membrane.

Infiltration of mucin into extracellular tissues (myxomatous degeneration) can occasionally be seen in inflammation of the articular capsule and accumulation of fibrinoid material in the blood vessel walls of the synovial membrane is very occasionally seen in inflammatory joint disease.

Pathological pigmentations
The main pigment regularly encountered in joints is haemosiderin, derived from haemoglobin, and this most often occurs in inflamed synovial membrane. Jaundice in the dog, irrespective of its origin, can produce yellow discoloration within the joint, particularly of the synovial membrane, and is associated with the deposition of bile pigment.

Circulatory disturbances
Hyperaemia of the synovial membrane is regularly seen in synovitis. This is usually the result of active hyperaemia (i.e. increased blood flowing into the joint rather than a passive hyperaemia due to an obstruction of the blood outflow, although thrombosis of blood vessels is occasionally seen in the inflammatory diseases). Ischaemia can also occur related to joints;

the classic example is Legg–Calvé–Perthe's disease of the femoral head. This disease of unknown aetiology, involves an interruption of the blood supply to the femoral head with a resultant necrosis of bone cells and matrix. Ischaemic necrosis can also arise as a complication of articular fractures where separated fragments can lose their blood supply and become necrotic within the joint.

Blockage of the lymphatic drainage from joints is another important circulatory disturbance. This frequently occurs in the inflammatory conditions particularly rheumatoid arthritis where fibrin is often responsible. Oedema of the articular capsule is often seen during inflammatory disease.

Haemorrhage may be seen within the articular cavity (haemarthrosis) of traumatised joints or within the synovial membrane associated with trauma or inflammatory disease.

Inflammation and repair
The synovial membrane is the best example of a joint tissue which readily shows inflammatory change. The aetiology of the synovitis in some of the inflammatory types of disease such as rheumatoid arthritis is not completely known and it is the persistence of the inflammatory process which becomes important in the pathogenesis of the disease.

Disturbances of growth
These include developmental disorders such as hip dysplasia and congenital dislocation of joints. In many of these cases the exact aetiology may be obscure although hip dysplasia, for example, has a multifactorial aetiology which involves genetic and environmental factors. Neoplasia is also included in this section and various joint neoplasms have been described in dogs, principally of the soft tissues.

Hypertrophy and hyperplasia of the lining layer of the synovial membrane occur in many types of joint disease and hypertrophy of the joint capsule is also frequently seen.

DIAGNOSIS OF JOINT DISEASE

Anamnesis

Details of the case history can be extremely helpful. Certain joint diseases are associated with particular breeds and age of dog, e.g. osteochondrosis. The nature of onset of the disease (sudden or gradual) is relevant and the duration of the problem and whether or not the dog has suffered any known trauma are also important. It is helpful to know if there has been any

progression of the disease, whether it is affected by cold and damp conditions and whether the lameness is intermittent or persistent, shifting from one limb to another and whether it is more apparent after rest or exercise or both. In some cases more than one limb may be permanently affected. The owner should also be questioned regarding the animal's general health; certain forms of polyarthritis in the dog can be associated with disease of other body systems.

On occasions the history may be unhelpful or even misleading. For example, in cases of chronic lameness of several weeks' duration, the owner will often relate the onset of lameness to a traumatic episode which either did not exist or occurred before or after the lameness commenced.

Clinical examination

The animal should be observed whilst standing, walking and if required trotting and galloping. All limbs should be carefully palpated, even though the lameness may be obvious in one particular leg. Joints should be manipulated through their normal ranges of motion and checked for any instability and ligament damage. Any joint enlargement or swellings around and within a joint must be assessed, the presence of joint pain should be noted and if possible related to certain areas of the joint. A single diseased joint can be compared with the same joint on the opposite side. The presence or absence of muscle atrophy is also important. In some dogs, manipulation of a diseased joint is only possible after sedation or even anaesthesia. With certain forms of arthritis and in cases suffering severe trauma, examination of other body systems is relevant.

Radiographical examination

Radiography is the most useful diagnostic aid for joint disease. Several different views are often required—at least a lateral and anteroposterior. General anaesthesia or sedation may be necessary. Weight bearing radiographs of joints are sometimes helpful, particularly for the assessment of alterations in joint space, but are technically difficult to achieve. Manipulated views under anaesthesia ('stress radiographs') are indicated in some cases where the joints are showing clinical instability. Macroradiography is a useful technique for assessing smaller joints, e.g. interphalangeal joints or joints of the smaller breeds where a magnified view allows very slight lesions to be visualised. The technique involves increasing the subject to film distance, e.g. positioning the x-ray film on the floor beneath the dog on the table. Contrast radiography is of limited help.

The radiographs should be examined for any abnormal bony proliferation (exostoses, osteophytes, periosteal reaction), bony destruction seen as discrete erosions, or a more generalised loss of mineralisation or as an irregular joint margin, changes in joint space, increase of soft tissue density, cartilage calcification, soft tissue calcification, calcified joint bodies, presence of fractures and any evidence of joint displacement or deviation. Changes in joint space are difficult to assess in small animals unless weight-bearing radiographs are taken. The joint space in a normal joint is mainly filled with articular cartilage (which is radiolucent), fat, menisci (if present), and synovial fluid. Reduction in joint space may result from loss of articular cartilage and sometimes subchondral bone. Increased joint space may result from an increased amount of synovial fluid, damage to joint capsule and/or ligaments or from a proliferation of synovial membrane within the joint. Advanced cartilage and subchondral bone destruction will also give an appearance of increased joint space in some cases. Causes of increased and decreased joint space can co-exist and the end result will depend on the severity of each. The manner in which the radiograph is taken will also alter the joint space, e.g. weight-bearing, 'stressed' view, manual restraint with traction on the limb of the conscious patient.

Synovial fluid analyses

A synovial fluid sample can be aspirated from most joints with the animal conscious or sedated. Sometimes general anaesthesia is necessary. Strict asepsis should be observed. The laboratory examination of synovial fluid is a useful, but neglected, diagnostic procedure in helping to differentiate various forms of arthritis (see Table 7.3). The following examinations should be made (Bennett 1980):

1 Note its colour and whether it is clear or turbid. Normal synovia is colourless or slightly yellow and is clear.
2 Assess its viscosity. This may be done by the 'string' test, e.g. by allowing a drop to fall from the end of a syringe needle. Normal synovia and synovia from osteoarthritic joints is very viscous and forms a long 'string' before the drop separates. Fluids from joints with an inflammatory arthropathy such as the rheumatoid type generally do not form a long 'string'.
3 Perform the mucin clot test. A drop of synovial fluid is placed into a beaker containing 5% acetic acid.

Normal synovia forms a good compact clot due to the high mucopolysaccharide content. Normally fluids containing a high mucopolysaccharide content also have a high viscosity. Fluids from joints with an inflammatory arthropathy usually give a poor, friable or non-existent clot.
4 Note whether or not the synovial fluid sample clots on standing (fibrinogen clot test). Normal synovia does not clot even though its high viscosity may sometimes suggest this. Only synovia from joints showing a septic or non-septic inflammatory arthropathy will clot on exposure to air.
5 A cytological examination should be performed. A smear of the fluid is made and stained by the Leishman or Papanicolaou methods. Normal synovia has few white cells and most of these are of the mononuclear type (macrophages, lymphocytes). Large numbers of polymorphonuclear cells indicate an inflammatory arthropathy. Osteoarthritic joints generally show slightly increased numbers of mononuclear cells. Large numbers of red cells are more often seen in traumatised joints. Certain other cells may be seen in special circumstances, e.g. cartilage cells, synovial cells, tumour cells, LE-cells, ragocytes. Total red and white cell counts can be done using Thoma diluting pipettes and a haemocytometer; isotonic saline can be used as the diluting fluid and red and white cells counted together.
6 Microbiological examination can be carried out, e.g. bacterial culture in suspected cases of septic arthritis.

Arthroscopy

The endoscopic examination of joints in small animals is a relatively recent introduction to veterinary rheumatology (Kivumbu & Bennett 1981). The technique enables the joint to be examined *in situ* and allows particular assessment of the non-osseous structures of the joint, e.g. articular cartilage, menisci, ligaments, synovium. Anaesthesia is necessary, but the arthroscope can be inserted through a small stab incision in the skin. It is likely to prove a useful additional technique for assessing joint disease and it does allow intra-articular biopsies to be taken. Some examples of the arthroscopic appearance of intra-articular structures are shown in Plate 7.1.

Synovial membrane biopsy

Biopsies can be taken with the arthroscope or by performing an arthrotomy. The histopathological and immunopathological examination of synovial biopsies is helpful in distinguishing certain types of arthritis. The direct immunofluorescent test on frozen sections of synovium is the most useful technique for studying the immunopathology. Such examinations can show the distribution of immunoglobulins (IgG, IgM, IgA), complement, albumin and fibrinogen, within cells, blood vessel walls and free within the tissues. The presence of immune complexes and antiglobulin material can be shown. The biopsy can also be cultured for microbial infections.

Arthrotomy

In some cases an extensive surgical opening of the joint is required in order to identify an intra-articular lesion.

Haematological, biochemical and serological studies

These studies are indicated in certain forms of arthritis, especially those associated with pathology of other body systems, where the arthritis is only one manifestation of a more generalised connective tissue disorder. An assessment of anaemia, the detection of elevated blood globulin and blood enzyme levels and the detection of certain autoantibodies such as rheumatoid factor and antinuclear antibody are all relevant.

Others

Local anaesthetic can be injected into joints or into certain articular structures such as ligaments or joint capsule, as a diagnostic aid to the localisation of the seat of lameness.

TYPES OF ARTHRITIS

The different forms of arthritis seen in small animals are summarised in Fig. 7.3. Confusion has always arisen with the terminology used. Arthritis, which strictly means inflammation of a joint, is used in a broader sense to cover a whole range of well-defined joint disorders. Particular pathological terms are given to the latter and often several terms are applied to the same disorder (e.g. osteoarthritis implying inflammation and osteoarthrosis suggesting degeneration refer to the same clinical disease where both inflammatory and degenerative changes can be identified). These various terms must not be taken in their literal pathological sense (e.g. osteoarthritis does not just mean inflammation within a joint, but includes cartilage degeneration and similarly 'inflammatory joint disease' does not mean that inflammatory processes only exist within the diseased joint). The incidence of different types of arthritis is given in Table 7.1.

Traumatic arthritis ('sprain')

This term is usually restricted to the type of joint reaction produced by a single acute injury to the joint (Ghadially & Roy 1969; Roy *et al* 1966). The lesions produced by such an injury can include a stretched, torn or lacerated joint capsule and/or ligaments, fracture of intra-articular bone, fracture or detachment of articular cartilage and torn and/or displaced menisci. A synovitis is invariably present and there is usually a variable amount of haemorrhagic or serous effusion within the joint cavity. The changes in the synovial membrane include hyperplasia and hypertrophy and infiltration with inflammatory cells, mainly polymorphonuclear leucocytes and lymphocytes. Areas of haemorrhage may be seen within the synovial membrane. Inflammatory infiltrates may also occur

---

Plate 7.1
Some examples of the arthroscopic anatomy of the canine knee.
(a) Arthroscopic appearance of a normal femoropatellar joint. Several elongated villi (sv) are projecting between the patellar (P) and femoral trochlea (FT). Stf-supratrochlea fat. c—joint cavity, a—crescent-shaped area indicating bending of the arthroscope.
(b) Arthroscopic appearance of an osteoarthritic femoropatellar joint. Note roughened area (r) on articular surface of patella (P). The cartilage of the femoral condyle (F) is also roughened (arrow). C—joint cavity, a—bending of arthroscope.
(c) Arthroscopic appearance of the femoropatellar joint

showing mild cartilage erosion. Flakes of articular cartilage (fc) are seen projecting from the patellar (P) into the joint cavity (C). F—femur, sv—synovial villi, a—bending of the arthroscope.
(d) Arthroscopic appearance of the medial femoral condyle (MFC) showing a shallow circular depression (U). RMM—medial meniscus, C—joint cavity, T—tibia, a—bending of arthroscope.
(e) Arthroscopic appearance of the intact anterior cruciate ligament (ANTX). C—joint cavity. a—bending of arthroscope. Arrow indicates blood vessel in synovium covering cruciate.
(f) Arthroscopic appearance of the normal lateral meniscus (LM). LFC—lateral femoral condyle, C—joint cavity, sv—synovial villi.

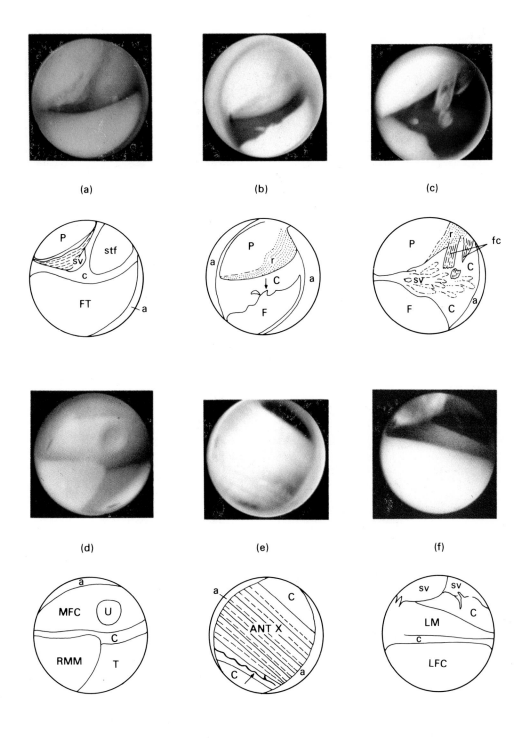

(a)

(b)

(c)

(d)

(e)

(f)

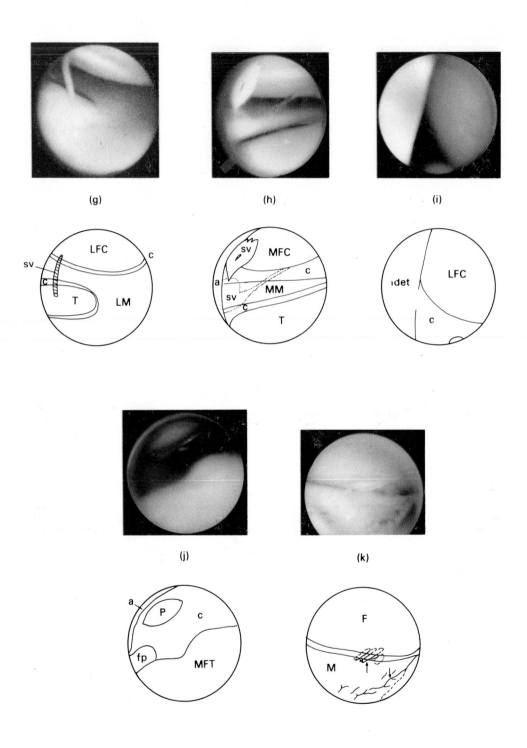

(g)

(h)

(i)

(j)

(k)

Table 7.1 The incidence of arthritis in dogs, based on a referral clinic at the University of Glasgow (Department of Veterinary Surgery). Total number of cases with clinically apparent arthritis—2730 (6 year period).

Type of arthritis	% of cases
Degenerative	
Traumatic	4.2
Osteoarthritis	78.0
Osteochondritis	13.2
Inflammatory	
Infective (bacterial)	1.1
Rheumatoid	0.9
Systemic lupus erythematosus	0.4
Idiopathic	
Type I	1.2
Type II	0.5
Type III	0.3
Type IV	0.2

within the joint capsule and ligaments of traumatised joints and deposits of haemosiderin are often present within the synovial membrane. Radiography may demonstrate joint effusion or show evidence of ligament damage, particularly if a manipulated view is taken. Synovial fluid samples are often haemorrhagic in appearance and the white cells are slightly elevated with variable numbers of synovial and cartilage cells present. The mucin clot test is strongly positive. Treatment will depend on the individual case (e.g. external support of the affected joint, confinement and restricted exercise, surgical exploration of the joint and repair/replacement of damaged ligaments or removal of torn menisci). In some mild cases no treatment other than rest for a few days is required. Some cases of acute traumatic arthritis will develop into osteoarthritis, particularly if joint instability has resulted from the initial trauma. Similarly, repeated trauma to

an individual joint will often produce an osteoarthritis.

Haemophilic arthritis

This is a very rare form of joint disease in the dog (Swanton 1959). The clotting defect in canine haemophilia is similar to that of man and is transmitted as a sex-linked recessive characteristic. Affected animals stand little chance of surviving more than a few months after birth. The dog will show recurring, painful and occasionally swollen joints of the extremities, associated with haemorrhage into the joint cavity and within the joint tissues. Grossly, the synovial membrane appears thickened with visible haemorrhages. Histological examination confirms the presence of haemorrhages and also deposits of haemosiderin. Mild hyperplasia of the lining layer is evident. Articular cartilage damage, intra-articular adhesions and capsular fibrosis with limited joint movement have been recorded. Haemorrhage also occurs within tendon sheaths and fascial structures of the limb, and in many other organs.

Osteoarthritis (osteoarthrosis, degenerative joint disease, hypertrophic arthritis, chronic senescent arthritis)

Osteoarthritis is the commonest form of arthritis which affects the dog, but in spite of this little is known of its exact nature and pathogenesis. There are two main types of osteoarthritis; primary or idiopathic where there is no obvious initiating cause and secondary where the disease follows some other abnormality of the joint. Examples of the latter include osteoarthritis following hip dysplasia, rupture of the anterior cruciate ligament of the stifle joint, patellar luxation,

(g) Arthroscopic appearance of the normal lateral meniscus (LM). Note the sharp inner concave border. LFC—lateral femoral condyle, sv—synovial villi, T—tibia, c—joint cavity.
(h) Arthroscopic appearance of the middle and caudal parts of the medial meniscus (MM). MFC—medial femoral condyle sv—synovial villi, T—tibia, a—bending of the arthroscope, c—joint.
(i) Arthroscopic appearance of the origin of the long digital

extensor tendon (ldet) from the femoral condyle (LFC). c—joint cavity.
(j) Arthroscopic appearance of the femoropatellar joint. P—patella, MFT— medial femoral trochlear ridge, fp—infrapatellar fat c—joint cavity, a—bending of the arthroscope.
(k) Arthroscopic appearance of femorotibial joint. Elongated and thin membranous synovial villi (arrows) are covering the surface of the medial meniscus (M). F—femoral condyle.

collateral ligament ruptures and joint dislocations, osteochondritis dissecans, Legg–Calvé–Perthes' disease, un-united anconeal process, articular fractures and damage to the joint by other types of arthritis. In most of these examples secondary osteoarthritis is associated with an unstable, deformed joint and it is suggested that such joints are susceptible to minor, repeated trauma leading to the development of certain well-defined pathological changes. Other factors are important, for example, excessive exercise or obesity will promote the disease, presumably by increasing the trauma inflicted upon the joint. Primary osteoarthritis would seem to occur in the dog and is possibly more common in certain breeds, e.g. Chow, Dalmatian, Samoyed.

Pathological features

All tissues of the synovial joint affected with osteoarthritis can show pathological changes:

1 Articular cartilage

Biochemical changes. These include hydration and a change in the quantity and quality of proteoglycan (McDevitt 1973; McDevitt & Muir 1976; McDevitt *et al* 1977). The galactosamine-glucosamine molar ratio is increased and there is a higher extractability of proteoglycan aggregate with high molarity calcium chloride solution. Some of these biochemical changes can also be demonstrated by histochemical staining techniques which show a loss of metachromasia.

These biochemical changes have been shown in both natural and experimental osteoarthritis and the latter has included sectioning of the anterior cruciate ligament of the canine stifle joint. Basically, cartilage responds by assuming an immature behaviour, chondrocytes divide and synthesise proteoglycans at a faster rate and synthesise a chondroitin-sulphate-rich immature proteoglycan.

Loss of surface chondrocytes. Cartilage cells are lost from the superficial layers of the articular cartilage.

Flaking and fibrillation. Horizontal flaking of the surface layer occurs, followed by deeper splits extending vertically into the deeper zones and eventually reaching the calcified stratum. Ultimately, cartilage may be sheared off, exposing the underlying subchondral bone. Fibrillation of cartilage involves fragmentation of the collagen network and is associated with proteoglycan depletion and with mechanical softening of the cartilage.

Chondrocyte clumping. This refers to the formation of 'cell nests' of chondrocytes in osteoarthritic articular cartilage. These nests are sometimes associated with deep vertical clefts in fibrillated cartilage and may represent attempted repair of a damaged cartilage.

Other changes. Lacuna resorption, degeneration of cells and matrix and alteration of the collagen fibres may be seen.

2 Bone

Periarticular osteophytes. The presence of marginal proliferation of bone (osteophytes, exostoses, lipping, spurs) is a consistent feature of osteoarthritis (Fig. 7.4). An osteophyte is first recognised as an area of proliferating mesenchymal tissue often in the transitional zone between the synovial membrane and articular cartilage. This tissue undergoes metaplasia to form woven bone, sometimes containing fibrocartilage. Endochondral ossification later becomes a prominent feature of osteophytic growth. A mature osteophyte is one which is covered by fibrocartilage or fibrous periosteum and which consists of cancellous bone with marrow spaces contiguous with the epiphyseal marrow spaces. Osteophytes will develop in other areas of the joint, e.g. at the attachment of the fibrous capsule and ligaments. Osteophyte development is associated with the appearance of numerous blood vessels and can be recognised histologically in the experimental canine (anterior cruciate sectioning) model as early as 3 days after sectioning the cruciate ligament (Gilbertson 1975a, 1975b). This may be compared to a much later appearance of biochemical changes in the articular cartilage (approximately 3 weeks). Thus the initial abnormality of osteoarthritis appears to be a vascular reaction associated with new bone formation and the articular cartilage degenerative changes, normally regarded as the most important pathological feature of osteoarthritis, occur some time later.

Subchondral bone sclerosis. There is a sclerosis of subchondral bone associated with articular cartilage loss in cases of osteoarthritis and the extreme stage of this is eburnation (Bennett *et al* 1942). Sclerosis and eburnation arise from thickening of the subchondral plate, epiphyseal cortex and adjacent trabeculae.

Subchondral bone cysts. These occur not uncommonly in man particularly in the hip joint (Sokoloff 1969). They are not true cysts and arise from the replacement of bone trabeculae and marrow by mixed connective tissue. Subchondral bone cysts are seen in the dog (Riser 1973).

Bone remodelling. Osteophyte production, subchondral sclerosis and cyst formation are all part of the

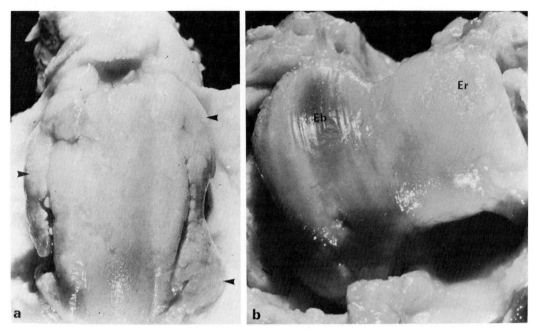

Fig. 7.4 Gross appearance of osteoarthritis. (a) Femoral trochlea, stifle joint: note the advanced osteophyte development (arrows) and the roughened surface of the articular cartilage; the synovial membrane and joint capsule are thickened.

(b) Elbow joint: note the loss of cartilage associated with eburnation of the subchondral bone (Eb) as well as an area of cartilage erosion and roughening (Er).

process of bone remodelling. There is also a general remodelling process of the internal structure of the epiphysis such that it can, with time, take on a completely different shape. This remodelling is brought about by related osteoblastic and osteoclastic activities. Various theories have been suggested to explain the whole of the remodelling process (e.g. altered stress on the joint due to instability or altered mechanics as the pathology of osteoarthritis progresses). Wolff's law has been quoted in this context: it states that the internal architecture of the bone is directly related to the stress distributions to which it is subjected.

It is also interesting that in the experimental cruciate sectioning model in the dog, bone remodelling not only occurs in the unstable joint but also in the contralateral normal stifle joint (McDevitt *et al* 1977; Gilbertson 1975a, 1975b). Subchondral sclerosis has been observed in these joints together with mild histological and biochemical abnormalities of the articular cartilage. This could result from increased loading of the joint due to the loss of use of the other limb with cruciate sectioning. Another explanation suggested has been a reflex increased vascularity to the opposite stifle joint monitoring that of the unstable joint; a similar occurrence has been shown during

fracture healing. The altered vascularity can produce changes in the local tissue conditions (e.g. pH, Po_2, Pco_2).

3 Soft tissue

Synovial membrane. Most reports of the response of the synovial membrane in cases of osteoarthritis describe hypertrophy and hyperplasia of the lining layer and increased thickness of the subsynovial connective tissue. Occasional perivascular accumulations of mononuclear cells are not uncommon (Bennett *et al* 1942). Sometimes a marked inflammatory reaction can occur in the synovial membrane of osteoarthritic joints in both the canine and human patient. This inflammatory reaction is characterised by hypertrophy and hyperplasia of the lining layer and large accumulations of mononuclear cells particularly lymphocytes and plasma cells in the subsynovial layer. There are also increased numbers of blood vessels and lymphatic spaces present. Such changes may represent a response to 'foreign material' such as hydroxyapatite crystals and degenerate cartilage cells, released into the synovial fluid of some osteoarthritic joints.

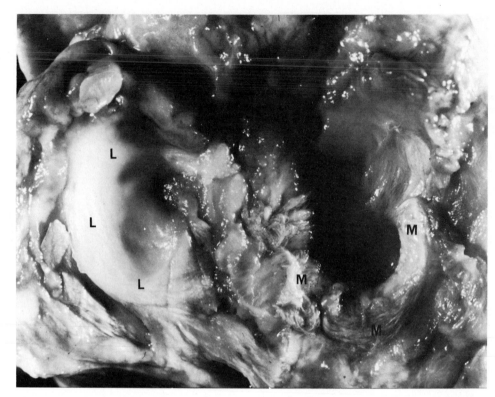

Fig. 7.5 A severely damaged medial meniscus (M), associated with a rupture of the anterior cruciate ligament and secondary osteoarthritis. The meniscus is badly shredded and fibrillated. The lateral meniscus (L) appears relatively normal.

Joint capsule. Fibrous thickening of the joint capsule regularly occurs in osteoarthritis (Marshall & Olsson 1971; Pond 1971).

Menisci. Various changes in the menisci occur such as fibrillation, calcification, splitting, shredding (Fig. 7.5) or tearing and osseous metaplasia (Collins 1949). The significance of the pathological changes in the menisci is, however, obscure, since in several cases of experimental cruciate sectioning in the dog, severe changes in the menisci were not associated with pain or lameness (Gilbertson 1975a, 1975b).

Vascular changes. Hyperaemia of the marrow of the bones of the joint occurs and vascular tufts can be seen penetrating the bone-cartilage interface. Vascular proliferation occurs in association with the osteophyte formation at the transitional zone. Hyperaemia of the synovial membrane and joint capsule is also present and an impaired venous drainage from the bones of osteoarthritic joints is demonstrable by intraosseous phlebography. Changes in blood flow will cause alterations in local tissue conditions which could be important in initiating pathological changes.

Clinical features

Lameness can be an obvious feature of osteoarthritis although many joints affected pathologically with this disease may not show a clinical problem. It is also true that the degree of pathological advancement in osteoarthritis is not always clearly associated with the presence or absence or severity of clinical signs. Generally the lameness is chronic, of insidious onset and may show a progressive deterioration with time. Some cases may show episodes of lameness separated by periods of relative normality and the lameness may be worse after rest or exercise or in cold, damp weather. Lameness in an osteoarthritic joint may be exacerbated by a sudden trauma to the joint. Affected joints are thickened as a result of osteophyte development, bony remodelling and joint capsule fibrosis. Synovial effusion may also be evident although some osteoarthritic joints contain very little synovial fluid. Pain and crepitus are often apparent when the joint is flexed and extended.

When considering secondary osteoarthritis it is important to realise that as well as clinical signs which are attributed to osteoarthritis itself, certain clinical features are also directly related to the predisposing joint problem (e.g. rupture of the anterior cruciate ligament in the stifle joint, hip dysplasia, elbow dysplasia and osteochondritis dissecans). With rupture of the anterior cruciate ligament for instance, an anterior drawer movement will be present.

Radiographic features
One of the most characteristic radiographic features of osteoarthritis is the presence of new bone deposits (Figs. 7.6, 7.7). Depending on the maturity of the osteoarthritic process, these deposits may be visualised as an irregularity or roughening of the bone outline, as obvious masses of bone protruding from the normal bone margins or as irregular densities of bone where the bone deposits are superimposed on the normal osseous architecture. The exact sites of new bone deposition vary according to the different joints and underlying cause and it is interesting that in the experimental cruciate model for example, the very earliest radiographic evidence of osteophytic formation occurs at 2–3 weeks whereas histological evidence of new bone formation occurs as early as 3 days after initiation of the disease process (Gilbertson 1975a, 1975b).

Sclerosis, particularly of the subchondral bone is another feature and is more commonly seen in longstanding cases. Soft tissue changes may also be apparent such as thickening of the joint capsule and synovial effusion. Radiography may also demonstrate obvious ligament damage although this is generally better appreciated by a clinical examination.

Occasionally, free ossified bodies are seen associated with an osteoarthritic joint. Some of these represent ligament avulsion fractures at their bony attachments, others are fractures and separations of osteophytes whereas some are caused by calcification of soft tissues within and surrounding the joint (e.g. menisci, ligaments, joint capsules).

Arthrograms produced by injecting air or positive contrast media into a joint are of limited help in providing further information of any value. A reduction in joint space has consistently been described as a radiographic feature of osteoarthritis (Morgan 1969) although as already explained this is difficult to assess in the canine patient.

Laboratory features
Synovial fluid analysis can be helpful. The fluid is generally viscous and slightly yellow in colour. The white cell count averages 2600/mm³, the majority of which are mononuclear cells (average 85%). Synovial and cartilage cells are sometimes present as also are osteoblasts and osteoclasts. There is no tendency for

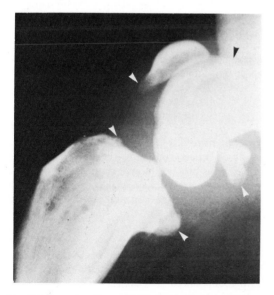

Fig. 7.6 Lateral radiograph of a stifle joint three months after an anterior cruciate rupture. There is extensive osteophyte development (arrows), there is increased density within the joint space, indicating synovial effusion.

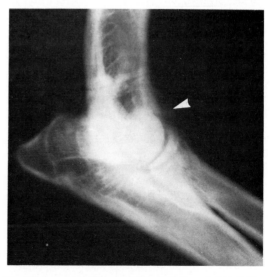

Fig. 7.7 Lateral radiograph of the left elbow joint of a dog with advanced osteoarthritis. Osteophytic development is visible, especially on the anterior aspect of the joint (arrow).

the fluid to clot on standing and the mucin clot test is usually normal.

Treatment

Unfortunately there is no cure for osteoarthritis and treatment is designed (a) to minimise the discomfort suffered by the patient, and (b) to correct the underlying cause if possible in cases of secondary osteoarthritis.

Treatment for the underlying cause of a secondary osteoarthritis depends on the individual case. For example, rupture of the anterior cruciate ligament in the stifle joint may be treated conservatively by strict rest for a couple of months or a prosthetic ligament may be inserted. In cases of Legg–Calvé–Perthes' disease, femoral head excision will prevent progression of the osteoarthritic process.

Once an osteoarthritic joint is showing clinical disease, various approaches to treatment can be considered. Resting the animal or imposing restricted exercise is important. The period of rest will vary between individual cases. The dog is only taken for short walks on the lead and not allowed to have free access to the garden or stairs. In many cases this is very difficult or even impossible to achieve. Sometimes it is easier to apply external support to a limb in the form of bandaging or plastering to support the affected joint and to restrict its movement and use. The feasibility of using this approach depends upon which joint is affected and a potential complication is the development of joint 'stiffness'. Drug treatment can also be used, for which the commonest drugs are acetylsalicylic acid, paracetamol, mefenamic acid, phenylbutazone and melcofenamic acid; most of these drugs have local anti-inflammatory action as well as analgesic property. These drugs are used until clinical improvement occurs; occasionally constant medication is necessary. In the case of the latter, the lowest effective dose should be used and this may involve giving the drug on alternate days or even only once a week. Phenylbutazone is useful, but some dogs show a peculiar sensitivity to it, indicated by frequent vomiting and in these cases the drug should be stopped immediately (Lawson 1971). Acetylsalicylic acid can produce a gastritis although the use of soluble, buffered or enteric-coated preparations can minimise the problem. Melcofenamic acid (Arquel) and the human drug, mefenamic acid (Ponstan) are useful although not licenced for use in the dog. Traditionally, corticosteroids are not recommended for the treatment of osteoarthritis although there is a possibility that if acute 'flare-ups' of the disease are due to a crystal (hydroxyapatite) induced synovitis for example, this inflammatory reaction could be suppressed with advantage by using these drugs. Corticosteroids however have been shown to cause degenerative changes in normal articular cartilage (Behrens *et al* 1975; Mankin *et al* 1972). Recently, the injection of sodium hyaluronate (Healon-vet) into osteoarthritic canine joints has been advocated. Insufficient evaluation exists at the present time although claims for its successful use in the horse have been made.

Certain surgical procedures can be used for the general treatment of osteoarthritis. Joint debridement or cheilectomy is one example where the joint is opened and osteophytes removed particularly if this can be combined with correction of any underlying cause, e.g. replacement of a torn cruciate ligament. Inflamed synovial membrane can also be stripped from the joint. Cheilectomy is only possible for certain joints (i.e. those such as the stifle where the anatomy permits easy surgical access). Another surgical process is arthrodesis. This involves removal of the articular cartilage and application of rigid fixation across the joint (e.g. a stainless steel plate or compression screw), and is most commonly indicated for the radiocarpal and intertarsal joints. Generally, it is sufficient to remove the articular cartilage with a curette. In some cases, arthrodesis of the joint is promoted by the insertion of a bone graft between or across the surfaces to be fused. Excision arthroplasty is another surgical approach to the treatment of osteoarthritic joints of which the commonest example is excision arthroplasty of the hip joint where the diseased femoral head is removed and a fibrous joint allowed to form. Joint replacement is popular in human arthritic patients, but the expense of prosthetic joint replacements and the technical difficulties in the surgery make it unlikely to become a common procedure in veterinary patients.

Osteochondritis (dissecans)

Osteochondritis (dissecans) is one manifestation of the generalised skeletal condition, osteochondrosis which involves a disturbance of endochondral ossification. Osteochondrosis is a disease which affects the growth plate cartilage as well as the articular cartilage of joints (Olsson 1976).

Pathological features

The affected cartilage thickens because normal ossification does not occur and as the cartilage grows without being resorbed it becomes necrotic in its deepest layers, possibly because it 'outgrows' its nutritional supply. Necrosis of the articular cartilage initially appears as areas of focal degeneration. Cracks and fissures occur from the deepest layers to the joint surface and synovial fluid passes along these channels to reach the subchondral bone. Necrotic cartilaginous material also passes along these channels to reach the joint cavity. Mild inflammatory changes occur in the synovial membrane, mainly hyperplasia and hypertrophy of the lining layer with occasional accumulations of mononuclear inflammatory cells in the supporting layer. The term osteochondritis refers to this inflammatory reaction which develops in the joint and the term dissecans relates to the cracks and fissures which develop in the articular cartilage to produce a separate fragment of cartilage forming a flap or loose body within the joint (Fig. 7.8). The latter can receive nutrition from synovial fluid and grow in size. Osteochondritis dissecans is a cause of secondary osteoarthritis in the dog.

Osteochondrosis affects certain well defined areas within specified joints (Arbesser 1974; Bennett *et al*

1981; Grøndalen and Grøndalen 1981; Olsson 1974, 1975a, 1975b; Robins 1970). The lesions which have been attributed to osteochondrosis are shown in Table 7.2, together with other lesions which could possibly be the result of osteochondrosis. Different breeds tend to suffer different forms of osteochondrosis. For example, elbow osteochondrosis is commonly seen in Labradors, Retrievers and Rottweilers and shoulder osteochondrosis in Great Danes and Pyrenean Mountain Dogs.

The aetiology of osteochondritis dissecans is uncertain although the rate of growth is thought to be an important factor. It has been shown experimentally in the pig that the incidence and severity of osteochondritis is directly related to rapid growth (Reiland 1975). Most affected dogs are of the medium-size and large breeds and males show a predisposition (Jones & Vaughan 1970); it is generally true that males grow more rapidly than females. A higher incidence has been

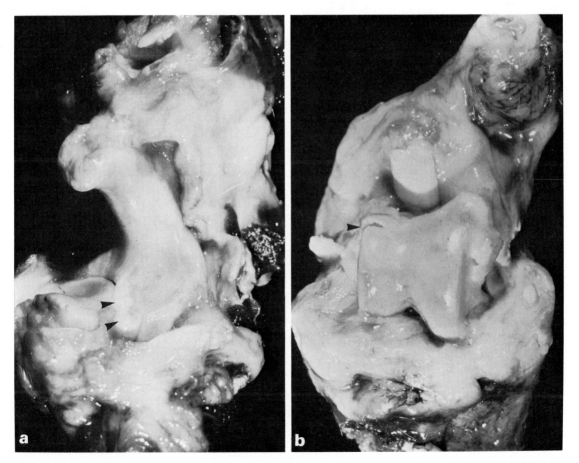

Fig. 7.8 Gross specimens showing osteochondrosis (a) of the coronoid process of the ulna in the elbow (arrows); (b) of the tibial tarsal bone in the hock (arrow).

Table 7.2 Lesions of osteochondrosis seen in the dog

Joint	Area of lesion	Description of lesion	Type of cartilage affected
Shoulder	(a) Caudo-lateral humeral head	Flap of cartilage	Articular
	?(b) Caudo-medial rim of glenoid	Separate body of cartilage and bone	Articular
Elbow*	(a) Medial condyle of humerus	Flap of cartilage	Articular
	(b) Coronoid process of ulna	(i) Fragmentation of the coronoid process (1 or more separate bodies of cartilage and bone)	?Growth plate/articular
		(ii) Fissure of the coronoid process	
	?(c) Anconeus of ulna	Separation of anconeus (separate body of cartilage and bone)	Growth plate
	?(d) Medial epicondyle of humerus	Separation of medial epicondyle (separate body of cartilage and bone)	Growth plate
Stifle	(a) Lateral condyle of femur	Flap of cartilage	Articular
	(b) Medial condyle of femur	Flap of cartilage	Articular
Hock	(a) Medial ridge of tibial tarsal bone	Flap of cartilage	Articular
	?(b) Medial malleolus of tibia	Separate medial malleolus (separate body of cartilage and bone)	?Growth plate/articular
Hip	?(a) Proximal femoral physis	Separation of femoral head (epiphysiolysis)	Growth plate
	?(b) Dorsolateral rim of acetabulum	Abnormal development of acetabulum (Hip dysplasia)	Articular
Spine	? Various intervertebral joints	Instability of intervertebral joints	Growth plate/articular

? Osteochondrosis not definitely proved in these cases.
*(a) and (b) can occur singly or together or with (c)

found in the offspring of certain dogs, although this apparent predispostion may just relate to the growth of the dog. Over-feeding for rapid growth and the genetic capacity for fast growth appear to be important factors in osteochondritis. Trauma to the joint may be another important factor and thus excessive exercise in the young puppy should be discouraged. Related to this could be the pull of the annular ligament on the coronoid process of the ulna which may contribute to the fragmentation of this structure in the elbow. Certain breed postures and stances could predispose a joint to osteochondrosis by causing abnormal loading or trauma.

Clinical features

The disease occurs primarily in the medium-size and large breeds of dog, although osteochondrosis has been reported in the smaller, even toy, breeds. Signs are usually noted between 4 and 8 months of age and males are most often affected. The condition is often bilateral and can even affect different joints in the same animal. Lameness of an insidious onset in one or more limbs occurs and worsens after exercise. Stiffness after rest is another feature. Pain can usually be elicited by palpation, flexion and extension of the affected joint. Sometimes synovial effusion within, and soft tissue thickening around the affected joint is present. Occasionally abnormal posture of the limb is a feature, for example, with lesions of the elbow joint the forelimbs may be held, externally rotated with the elbows close to the chest and in some cases (e.g. of the hock joint), reduced joint movement may be apparent.

Radiographic features

With the shoulder joint, lateral radiographs may reveal a defect in the caudal contour of the subchondral bone of the humeral head (Fig. 7.9) and in the early or mild cases this might only be a flattening of the articular margin. In some cases the defect is located more on the caudolateral aspect of the humeral head rather than caudally and may thus be seen as an area of decreased density in the subchondral bone rather than a defect in the articular margin. In advanced cases sclerosis of the subchondral bone around the defect can be seen. Sometimes calcification of the separated cartilage flap lying over the defect may be visible. If the cartilage flap becomes completely detached it will form a joint 'mouse' which usually becomes lodged in the ventrocaudal pouch of the joint cavity where it will be visible, if calcified. Non-union of the anconeal process is easily recognised on lateral radiographs of the flexed elbow joint. Normally the anconeal process unites with the rest of the ulna by 18–20 weeks of age. Fragmentation of the coronoid process (un-united

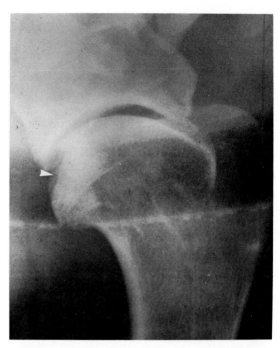

Fig. 7.9 Lateral radiograph of the shoulder joint showing rarefaction of the posterior humeral head (arrow) consistent with osteochondritis dissecans. Superimposition of the air-filled trachea over the shoulder joint aids interpretation.

coronoid process) is usually not visualised by radiography. But this condition can be associated with small osteophytes seen as a roughening of the margin of the anconeal process on a lateral radiograph of the flexed elbow joint (Bennett *et al* 1981) (Fig. 7 10). Generally these changes are not seen until the animal is 7 months of age or more, although clinical signs may have been present since 4–5 months. Fissures of the coronoid process are associated with a milder degree of osteophyte development.

With osteochondritis dissecans of the medial humeral condyle, anteroposterior radiographs of the elbow joint may show a small defect in the subchondral bone of the medial condyle. Sometimes a free calcified body is evident. Osteophyte development on the anconeus is again apparent. Lipping and roughening of the radial head and roughening of the medial aspect of the humerus have also been seen on anteroposterior radiographs of the elbow joint, with the different manifestations of elbow osteochondrosis.

Osteochondritis dissecans of the knee joint is difficult to confirm by radiography. A number of anteroposterior projections of the stifle in different angulations is necessary. The lesion is seen as a defect or

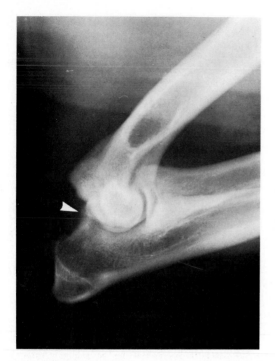

Fig. 7.10 Lateral flexed radiograph of the elbow joint of a dog with osteochondrosis. Note the bony proliferative change on the dorsal aspect of the anconeus (arrow) indicative of secondary osteoarthritic change. This change can only be clearly visualised with a manipulated (flexed) view of the elbow joint.

flattening of the lateral or medial condyle; sometimes flattening of the condyle is seen in the lateral radiograph. The commonest lesion is found on the medial aspect of the lateral condyle. Occasionally a free calcified mass may be seen within the joint. Osteophytes may be visible. A radiolucent defect in the lateral condyle associated with an aberrant cruciate attachment has been mistaken for osteochondrosis (Dueland *et al* 1982).

Anteroposterior views of the hock joint are important in diagnosing osteochondritis dissecans of the tibial tarsal bone. The lesion is seen as a defect of the medial ridge of the tibial tarsal bone and sometimes a calcified or ossified fragment can be seen within the tibiotarsal joint. Soft tissue swelling is often apparent and secondary osteoarthritic changes are common.

Laboratory features
The characteristics of synovial fluid samples are similar to those described for osteoarthritic joints.

Treatment
It is known that some cases of osteochondritis disse-

cans of the shoulder joint will heal spontaneously and this has been explained by the cartilage flap separating and detaching completely to become a free joint 'mouse' which is eventually resorbed from the joint (Olsson 1976). Olsson (1976) suggests this natural cure is more likely if affected animals are encouraged to exercise, rather than rest, with the use of analgesics if necessary; if no improvement occurs within 4–6 weeks surgery should be contemplated. However, the present author favours surgical removal of the loose piece of cartilage as soon as a diagnosis is made. A lateral approach to the shoulder joint is used; the edges of the defect are trimmed and some authorities recommend curettage of the base as well, although this can remove healing scar tissue already present and thus delay the healing period. Cases have been operated on where the cartilage has been cracked and fissured but no separating flap obviously present; in these cases the abnormal cartilage is curetted away. In some cases the cartilage flap has already detached and needs to be flushed out of the joint with a saline wash or grasped with forceps, usually from the ventrocaudal pouch. If a piece of detached cartilage is present in the ventrocaudal joint pouch, and is associated with clinical signs it should be removed. Sometimes pieces of detached cartilage can become lodged in the sheath of the biceps tendon and give rise to pain and lameness and again require to be removed.

Non-union of the anconeal process of the elbow joint is generally treated by surgical removal of the anconeus through a lateral incision between the lateral epicondyle and olecranon. However, some authorities recommend compression screwing of the process back on to the ulna to avoid the instability and eventual osteoarthritis of the elbow joint, which is said to occur following removal of the anconeus. It has also been suggested that surgery should not be done until the animal is 9–12 months of age since if it is done before this, during the rapid growth phase, secondary remodelling and osteoarthritic changes are more likely (Olsson 1976). With osteochondritis dissecans of the medial humeral condyle, surgical removal of the cartilage flap and trimming of the edges of the defect can be performed, using a medial approach to the elbow joint. In some cases no cartilage flap is present and in others it has been converted into a large cartilaginous body adhering to the joint capsule. In some it is difficult to know whether the medial condyle lesion represents osteochondritis or an osteoarthritic ulcer associated with fragmentation of the coronoid; osteochondrosis of the medial condyle and coronoid process do commonly coexist (Bennett *et al* 1981; Olsson 1976). If only a defect is present, the edges are trimmed. Fragmentation of the coronoid process is treated by removal of the fragment or fragments again through a medial approach. The most common finding in these cases is a cartilage-covered ossicle between the coronoid process and head of the radius, although occasionally several small fragments are present; if only a fissure is apparent, this should be curetted. With the medial approach to the elbow it is necessary to section the collateral ligament and occasionally some of the flexor muscle origins in order to achieve sufficient exposure. Robins (1978) describes the approach without sectioning the flexor muscles. Surgery for elbow osteochondrosis should be performed as early as possible, although some cases showing only slight clinical signs can improve with rest and maturity. Surgery of chronic cases showing marked secondary osteoarthritis is of no value. Also surgery is not justified if the joint is free from clinical disease, despite radiographical changes, as may occur with bilateral cases. Surgery of several joints at any one time is not recommended.

Many cases of osteochondritis dissecans in the stifle joint are thought to heal spontaneously without producing obvious clinical signs. Osteoarthritis only seems to occur in a few cases. Surgical removal of the cartilage flap or joint 'mouse' is only indicated in cases showing acute lameness.

Osteochondritis dissecans of the hock joint should again be treated by surgical removal of the detached cartilage or ossicles through a medial approach. It is necessary to section the collateral ligament for sufficient exposure. Involvement of the hock joint carries the worst prognosis and surgery should not be delayed.

In all cases where surgical treatment is used, the dog should be confined for 4–6 weeks postoperatively. In addition, with the hock joint an external support should be provided for 2–3 weeks. Recovery may take up to 3 months. Regular exercise should be given and the amount of exercise should be very gradually increased.

Other considerations

Osteochondrosis has also been associated with the cervical intervertebral joints of Great Danes leading to deformity of the vertebrae ('spondylolisthesis'), and has been reported in the dorsolateral acetabular rim associated with hip dysplasia (Olsson 1976). Separation of the medial epicondyle in the elbow joint of young dogs could possibly be another expression of osteochondrosis. Osteochondrosis of the medial ridge of the tibial tarsal bone is often associated with a radiolucent lesion of the medial malleolus, or an apparent separated ossicle; this has been noted by other workers (Rosenblum *et al* 1978). This ossicle probably represents a separate centre of ossification

since it appears to fuse to the tibia with time. The separation of a small piece of cartilage and bone from the caudo-medial rim of the glenoid in the shoulder joint may be another form of osteochondrosis; the separated body is visible on lateral radiographs.

Osteochondrosis as mentioned can affect growth plate cartilage but in most cases clinical signs do not appear. However, limb deformity can occur in some cases (e.g. lateral deviation of the forefoot where the distal ulna growth plate is affected and its growth reduced, and genu valgum where the distal femoral and proximal tibial growth plates are affected). Slipping of the proximal femoral epiphysis has been associated with osteochondrosis of the growth plate cartilage in pigs and this may also be true in some cases in the dog, especially those associated with no, or minimal, trauma in the larger breeds (Lee 1976).

Bacterial infective (septic) arthritis

Bacterial arthritis is rare in small animals. Diagnosis is based on a positive culture of bacterial organisms from affected joints. Both synovial fluid and synovial membrane should be cultured. Some cases have a positive membrane but negative fluid culture. Thus, culture of the synovial membrane is more reliable than that of the fluid although it is still feasible that some cases of joint infection are missed by false negative cultures, since there are a number of factors which can influence the ability to isolate organisms from infected tissues.

The commonest organisms isolated from dogs' joints are beta-haemolytic *Streptococci* of Lancefield Group G and *Staphylococcus aureus*. Other bacteria have included haemolytic *Escherichia coli*, *Pasteurella* and *Erysipelothrix*. Generally only one joint is affected, although occasionally two joints may be simultaneously infected. Infection of several joints, at the same time would generally indicate bacterial endocarditis (see below).

The route of infection in most cases is uncertain, although it is assumed to be blood borne. The focus of infection is generally obscure although tooth root abscessation, urinary tract and anal sac infections are sometimes present. It is also possible that trauma to the joint, even a minor sprain, may predispose it to infection from the blood. Direct introduction of infection into a joint is possible. Penetrating wounds from bites have caused joint infections. Wounds communicating with joints, particularly the hock joint are frequently seen in association with road traffic accidents but surprisingly persistent infection of these joints is uncommon. Iatrogenic introduction of infection is also a possibility resulting from open joint surgery or from injections/aspirations of joints. The spread of infection into joints from surrounding structures is another possibility (e.g. osteomyelitis can spread to involve a joint) (see Fig. 7.11).

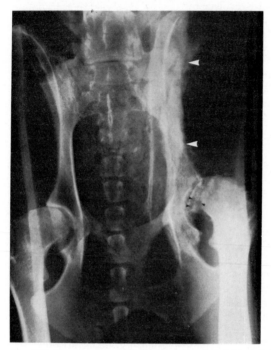

Fig. 7.11 Pelvic radiograph showing an infected hip joint associated with osteomyelitis of the ilium. Rarefied areas within the femoral head are present (black arrows). Bony proliferation is present along the ilial shaft (white arrows). Pelvic fracture lines are also evident.

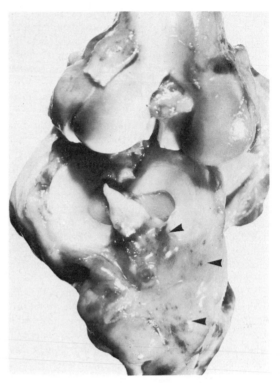

Fig. 7.12 Gross appearance of infected stifle joint. The synovial membrane is thickened and small haemorrhages are visible (arrows).

Pathological features
The principal pathological lesion is a synovitis. Affected joints usually show a thickened and discoloured synovial membrane, sometimes with obvious haemorrhages present (Fig. 7.12). Excess discoloured (usually turbid) synovial fluid is normally present and free fibrin may be present in the joint space. In more advanced cases, articular cartilage becomes covered with granulation tissue (pannus) associated with serious cartilage and bone destruction (Fig. 7.13).

The histopathological characteristics of the synovial membrane vary. In low-grade infections, there is hyperplasia and hypertrophy of the lining cells with a mononuclear cell infiltration (plasma cells, lymphocytes and macrophages) in the supporting layer. The polymorphonuclear cell normally associated with sep-

tic conditions may be present in small numbers or completely absent. Haemosiderin deposits are common. In acute cases the polymorphonuclear cell is normally present in large numbers sometimes forming microabscesses, although mononuclear cells are also seen. Fibrin deposition within and on the outside of the synovial membrane is normally extensive. Cartilage destruction can occur either from proteolytic enzymes released by the inflammatory process or by pannus formation. The latter can lead to subchondral bone destruction. Bony proliferative changes can also occur due to periostitis or secondary osteoarthritic change.

Clinical features
The dogs are generally presented with lameness, either of an acute, sudden onset or of a chronic insidious onset. Dogs of any age can be affected, including very young puppies. Joint infections are mainly seen in the larger breeds of dog (Bennett 1980). The affected joint may be obviously swollen and hot; synovial effusion is often evident. Pain on manipulation may be obvious,

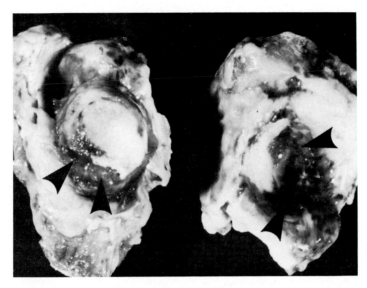

Fig. 7.13 Gross specimen of an infected hip joint. The synovium is obviously inflamed and pannus is seen over large areas of the articular cartilage of both the femoral head and acetabulum (arrows). The pannus is associated with cartilage destruction.

but in many chronic cases pain can be difficult to elicit. Often these dogs are not systemically ill, although younger dogs in particular may show pyrexia, dullness and inappetence.

Radiographic features

It is common for there to be no obvious sign of articular destuction on the radiographs. The joint may appear completely normal or show signs of soft tissue swelling or synovial effusion only. Sometimes there may be decreased mineralisation of the epiphysis of the joint and occasionally subchondral bone erosions may be evident (Fig. 7.11). Bony reaction around the joint may be seen in the form of new bone deposits and periosteal reaction. Occasionally soft tissue calcification is seen. Very advanced cases characterised by varying degrees of epiphyseal destruction with reactive sclerosis of bone and extensive new bone development are only rarely seen in small animals.

Laboratory features

Synovial fluid is generally increased in quantity, cloudy in appearance, less viscous than normal and may clot on exposure to air if much fibrinogen is present. The mucin clot test result is generally poor. The white cell count is increased although in some cases especially the low-grade chronic infections the count may only be in the low thousands. The com-

monest cell type is the polymorphonuclear cell (usually approximately 80% of the total) and some of these may show degenerative changes, particularly nuclear pyknosis. Occasionally bacterial organisms may be seen in the Gram stain of the synovial fluid smear. Cultural examinations of synovial fluid and synovial membrane are important to isolate the organism and determine antibiotic sensitivity. Histological examination of synovial membrane biopsies can help in the diagnosis of infective joint disease. Haematological examinations may or may not show elevation of white blood cells with neutrophilia.

Treatment

Antibiotic therapy is the treatment of choice although the prognosis is always guarded. Long term systemic antibiotics over several weeks are necessary. Aspiration of synovial fluid from affected joints may also help. In cases of single joint involvement and depending upon exactly which joint is affected, open joint surgery can be performed and a drainage/irrigation tube inserted. This allows drainage of fluid as well as infusion of antibiotic solution directly into the joint. Such tubes are often left in place for 1–2 weeks. In conjunction with antibiotic therapy analgesic/anti-inflammatory drugs such as aspirin, meclofenamic acid, and phenylbutazone can be used. Obviously corticosteroids are contraindicated while infection is present. However, they have been used to treat persisting inflammation after the infection has apparently been cleared—this phenomenon being explained by an immune response against persisting bacterial antigens (Bennet 1980). Strict rest of the joint is also advisable and this can be achieved by external support of the limb or confinement of the patient, ideally by hospitalisation.

Other surgical treatment may be required if joint damage is too extensive, e.g. arthrodesis, arthroplasty, amputation.

Bacterial endocarditis and septic arthritis

These dogs, generally adult of the larger breeds, are usually presented with systemic illness (fever, lethargy, anorexia or inappetence), cardiac murmur and lameness. Oral ulceration (probably due to a toxic epidermal necrolysis) is sometimes present—this may cause the dog to salivate and often the saliva is discoloured. Generally several joints are infected, often without bilateral symmetry. The animal may show lameness in one or more limbs and in some cases may have extreme difficulty in standing and walking. Lameness in these animals can also be caused by a septic myositis.

The joint pathology is similar to the description given above for bacterial arthritis; the organisms involved are similar. The pathogenesis of the joint disease involves the spread of organisms and/or septic emboli from the heart lesion to the joints. However, some joints may have a non-infective synovitis caused by a Type III (immune-complex) hypersensitivity reaction where complexes of bacterial antigen and antibody are deposited within blood vessels of the joint

(Bennett 1980) (cf. Type II idiopathic inflammatory arthropathy, see below).

Other pathological lesions are seen, e.g. myositis, retinitis, infarcts in the spleen, brain, kidneys etc., and a vegetative thrombus is generally seen on the endocardium (Fig. 7.14). The explanation for the bacterial colonisation of the endocardium is unclear. The ECG may be abnormal and a leucocytosis is generally present. Bacteria can sometimes be cultured from the blood as well as the joints. Proteinuria and haematuria are frequent findings. Some cases show circulating autoantibodies *viz* rheumatoid factor and antinuclear antibody (Bennett *et al* 1978). These antibodies are normally associated with other types of polyarthritis (see below) and care is needed in interpreting their significance.

The prognosis with these cases is very poor. Very few cases make a recovery and those that do, often relapse. Initial treatment with intravenously administered antibiotics is important; prolonged antibiotic therapy (several weeks) is imperative.

Bacterial discospondylitis

Bacterial infections can localise to the spinal joints, particularly the intervertebral discs. The clinical features include spinal pain, stiffness and lameness and in some cases a neurological deficit (Bennett *et al* 1981). It is again the larger breeds of dog which appear most susceptible. Radiography usually confirms the diagnosis; the lesion is characterised by destruction of bone on either side of the affected disc, giving the intervertebral space an irregular and widened appear-

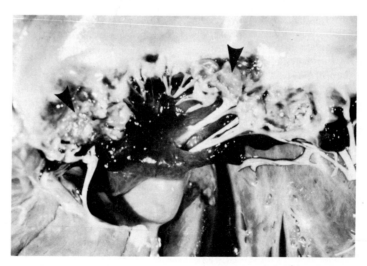

Fig. 7.14 Gross specimen of the heart of a dog with bacterial endocarditis and polyarthritis. The infected thrombus is seen affecting the atrioventricular valve (arrows).

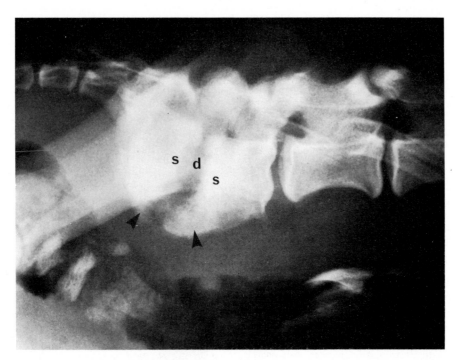

Fig. 7.15 Lateral spinal radiograph showing bacterial infective discospondylitis of L7/S1. The intervertebral disc space is widened and irregular (d). There is sclerosis of the vertebral bone adjacent to the disc space(s) and there is a spondylotic reaction (arrows).

ance (Fig. 7.15). Sclerosis of the vertebral bodies either side of the lytic area is also typical. A spondylotic reaction may be present. *S. aureus* is the commonest organism isolated from these lesions and the infection is presumably blood-borne. There is a suggestion that infections may spread from the urinary tract, so culture of the urine is sometimes relevant. Very occasionally a peripheal limb joint may be affected in addition to the spinal joint. Treatment involves long-term antibiotics together with curettage of the lesion. The latter enables material to be obtained for culture and sensitivity testing. In some cases showing neurological disease such as ataxia, weakness, hyperaesthesia, paresis, paralysis and urinary incontinence, spinal surgery may be advocated, e.g. decompressive laminectomy, spinal immobilisation.

Other infections of joints

Investigations into possible viral and mycoplasmal infections of joints showing inflammatory disease have been carried out by the author, but no evidence yet for the presence of such agents has been obtained. It is obviously not impossible with any microbial infection, but particularly with viruses, to fail to isolate the organism, even though it is present.

Tubercular arthritis can be a feature of tuberculosis in the dog (Hjärre 1939; Olsson 1957). However, this disease is now extremely rare in this species; it is the human type of *Mycobacterium tuberculosis* which is most commonly isolated from the dog.

Mycoplasmal infections of canine joints are reported (Pedersen & Pool 1978) but case reports are lacking. Also, polyarthritis associated with bacterial L-forms has been identified in dogs (Pedersen & Pool 1978). Articular fungal infections are also reported in the dog, e.g. *Coccidioides immitis* (Maddy 1958), *Cryptococcus neoformans* (Kavit 1958), *Blastomyces dermatitidis* (Dr J.F. Prescott, pers. commun.; Maksic 1968) and *Sporotrichum schenckii* (Hutyra *et al* 1938). These however are unlikely to be seen in the UK. Leishmaniasis, a protozoal disease, can also produce joint pathology in dogs (Dr W.C. Pedersen, pers. commun.; Thorson *et al* 1955), and may be seen in imported dogs in the UK.

Rheumatoid arthritis (see also Chapter 10)

This is an inflammatory disease of the joints which until recently was thought to affect only the human population (Boyle & Buchanan 1971). It has now been described in the dog both in the UK (Bennett 1980; Halliwell *et al* 1972) and the USA (Alexander *et al* 1976; Newton *et al* 1976; Pedersen *et al* 1976a).

To help standardise the diagnosis of this disease in man, certain criteria have been compiled, of which seven should be present to justify the diagnosis of classical rheumatoid arthritis and five to diagnose definite rheumatoid arthritis, and as far as criteria 1–5 are concerned, the joint signs must be continuous for at least 6 weeks. The criteria are:

1 Morning stiffness.
2 Pain or tenderness on motion of at least one joint.
3 Swelling of at least one joint.
4 Swelling of one other joint within a 3 month period.
5 Symmetrical joint swelling.
6 Subcutaneous nodules.
7 Radiographic changes suggestive of rheumatoid arthritis (see below).
8 Serological evidence of rheumatoid factor (see below).
9 Abnormal synovial fluid (see below).
10 Characteristic histological changes in the synovial membrane (see below).
11 Characteristic histological changes in subcutaneous nodules.

Until more detailed studies are done, these criteria should be applied when diagnosing rheumatoid arthritis in the dog. Only the classical and definite forms of rheumatoid arthritis are diagnosed in the dog. In addition to satisfying the above criteria as in man, the author also requires two of the criteria, 7, 8, and 10 to be satisfied; these three criteria are the most specific for rheumatoid arthritis. Certain differences between human and canine rheumatoid arthritis have become apparent (e.g. subcutaneous nodules are very rare in the dog, the formation of lymphoid follicles within affected synovium is rare in the dog, and the presence of rheumatoid factor in the blood is less consistent).

The aetiology of rheumatoid arthritis is unknown but is likely to be multifactorial. The synovitis is probably caused by a Type III (immune complex) hypersensitivity reaction involving antigen or antigens unknown, complexing with specific antibody and rheumatoid factor. The involvement of the latter is the reason for describing rheumatoid arthritis as an autoimmune disease. However, genetic factors are possibly also involved, certain tissue types being more susceptible to the disease.

Pathological features

A chronic synovitis, generally affecting several joints simultaneously, characterises this disease. Gross ex-

amination of affected joints shows a thickened and discoloured synovial membrane often with excess, turbid synovial fluid within the joint. Depending on the stage of the disease there may be evidence of cartilage and subchondral bone destruction with deformity and irregularity of the joint surfaces (Fig. 7.16). Lymphocytes and plasma cells are the chief inflammatory cells distributed throughout the supporting layer of the synovium. Macrophages are also seen, but polymorphonuclear cells are rare despite their presence in very large numbers in the synovial fluid. The lining cells generally show hyperplasia and hypertrophy and the synovial surface is thrown into folds and villous projections (Fig. 7.17). Perivascular accumulations of

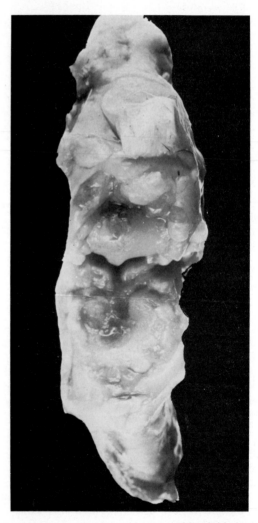

Fig. 7.16 Gross appearance of rheumatoid arthritis (metacarpophalangeal joint). The synovial membrane and joint capsule are thickened and there is loss of articular cartilage.

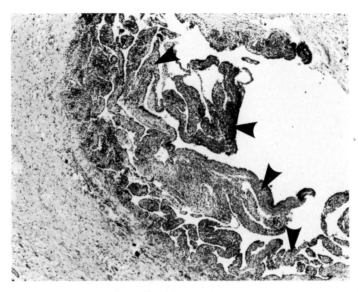

Fig. 7.17 Photomicrograph of the synovial membrane from a dog with rheumatoid arthritis. The lining of the synovium shows villous hypertrophy. The villi (arrows) contain numerous mononuclear inflammatory cells.

plasma cells, haemosiderin deposition, areas of focal necrosis and necrotising arteritis have also been recorded. Fibrin deposits both on the surface and within the synovial membrane are common. Inflammatory fibrovascular proliferations of the synovial membrane (pannus) develop and extend across and beneath the articular cartilage causing destruction of cartilage and subchondral bone (Fig. 7.18). Cartilage destruction can also result from proteolytic enzymes

released during the inflammatory process. In very advanced cases almost total destruction of the joint can occur, with the development of fibrous and bony ankylosis. Involvement of the synovial membranes of tendon sheaths is also possible and in man a generalised vasculitis may complicate the manifestations of rheumatoid arthritis although this has not been reported in the dog.

Electronmicroscopical examination of affected

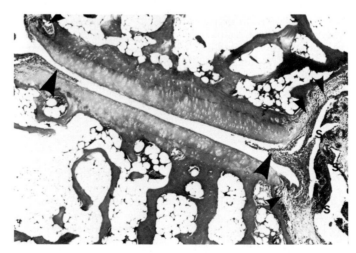

Fig. 7.18 Photomicrograph of a joint from a dog with rheumatoid arthritis. The inflamed synovium, visible at the periphery of the joint(s) is forming a pannus over the articular cartilage (large arrows) and is eroding into and beneath the cartilage, into the subchondral bone at the articular perimeter (small arrows).

canine synovium has revealed tubuloreticular structures, consistent with the appearance of viral particles, in cells within the synovial membrane, although the significance of these findings remains uncertain (Newton *et al* 1974).

Clinical features

The disease is seen more commonly in the small and medium sized breeds of dog (Bennett 1980). Animals are usually adult although the exact age of onset varies; an average of 5–6 years is reported (Bennett 1980). Lameness is the main presenting sign but it varies in severity. There may be a history merely of stiffness, or the patient may be lame in a single limb, or joint involvement may be so severe and widespread that ambulation is impossible. Often the lameness will be of a shifting nature, moving from one limb to another. It is true that many joints may be pathologically, but not clinically, affected and different joints will vary in their involvement with time. A few animals are presented with an acute polyarthritic syndrome accompanied with fever, lethargy and inappetence. Symmetrical joint involvement is typical.

Affected joints are often swollen and painful on manipulation and in advanced cases, gross deformity with abnormal motion and crepitus is apparent. Ligament rupture secondary to the inflammatory process is common and can lead to joint instability and osteoarthritic changes. Any limb joint can be affected although stifle, carpus and metacarpophalangeal are the most common; involvement of the cervical spinal diarthrodial joints has also been recorded. Muscle atrophy may be evident. Other clinical features can be seen, for example, some cases of rheumatoid arthritis in both man and the dog have shown tonsillitis or upper respiratory tract infection. Peripheral lymphadenopathy and renal disease associated with amyloidosis may also be clinically apparent. Pneumonia has been reported and splenomegaly can occur, sometimes associated with leucopenia (Felty's syndrome) (Bennett 1980). Canine rheumatoid arthritis together with 'dry eye' (Sjøgren's syndrome) has also been recorded.

Radiographic features

The classic feature of rheumatoid arthritis is the presence of subchondral bone destruction visualised as an irregularity of the articular surface or as 'punched out' erosions (Figs. 7.19, 7.20, 7.21) (Biery & Newton 1975). Advanced cases may show extensive bone destruction with gross joint deformity. A more generalised loss of mineralisation of the epiphysis can be another feature and soft tissue swelling around or synovial effusion within the joint may be present. Changes in joint space, either an increase or a decrease, may be evident.

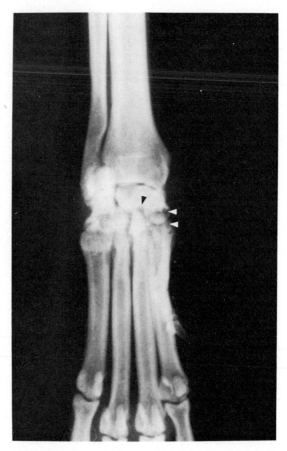

Fig. 7.19 Radiograph of a carpal joint showing rheumatoid arthritis. Subchondral erosions (arrows) are present.

Bony proliferative change may be seen where there has been a periostitis or where secondary osteoarthritis has developed. Calcification of the soft tissues around the joint is also often seen.

In some early cases, radiographic evidence of bone destruction may be absent. Generally such evidence will appear within 6 months.

Laboratory features

Rheumatoid arthritis is commonly but not invariably associated with the presence of circulating autoantibodies against immunoglobulin G, collectively known as rheumatoid factor. Rheumatoid factor however is not specific for this disease since it occurs in other disease states, particularly of a chronic nature where there is antigen–antibody interaction (e.g. bacterial endocarditis and viral infections) (Bennett *et al* 1978). Also, certain dogs in which rheumatoid arthritis can be diagnosed are negative for rheumatoid factor, and

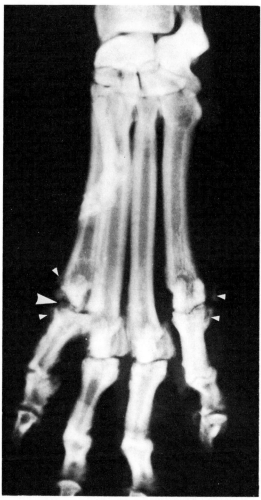

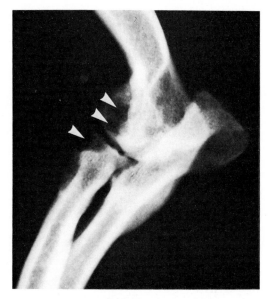

Fig. 7.21 Oblique radiograph of the elbow joint of a Pekingese dog with rheumatoid arthritis. A large erosion is present in the head of the radius (arrow) and there is obvious loss of bone from the distal humerus (arrows).

Fig. 7.20 Anteroposterior radiograph of the metacarpophalangeal joints of a Collie dog with rheumatoid arthritis. In particular, metacarpophalangeal joint of digit 2 shows loss of bone with an irregular joint margin (large arrow). New bone deposits are also visible (small arrows).

some dogs may initially be positive but later become negative, and *vice versa*.

Various tests are used to detect rheumatoid factor in the serum; the author uses a modification of the Rose–Waaler test, where the patient's serum is mixed with sheep red blood cells coated with dog antibodies (Bennett 1980). Rheumatoid factor, which is an antiglobulin, will bind with the globulin on the sheep blood cells and cause their agglutination. The sensitivity of the test varies between laboratories but the author regards a titre of 1/20 as borderline and anything above this as significant. Two separate samples taken within 2 weeks of each other are tested and both should be positive.

It is important to differentiate the polyarthritis of rheumatoid arthritis and systemic lupus erythematosus and thus tests for the latter disease should always be performed (see below). The presence of LE cells or antinuclear antibody in high titre is suggestive of systemic lupus erythematosus although some cases of rheumatoid arthritis can show circulating rheumatoid factor and antinuclear antibody.

Synovial fluid may or may not be present in excessive amounts; it is generally discoloured and usually turbid. Viscosity is decreased and with acetic acid, a flocculent precipitate normally forms. The fluid usually contains fibrin and fibrinogen and may clot on standing if no anticoagulant is added. The white cell count is elevated (average 26 000/mm^3) and the polymorph is the predominant cell (average 85%). Again pyknotic polymorphs may be seen but are usually not as prominent as in cases of septic joint disease. Ragocytes which are neutrophils containing cytoplasmic inclusions, probably altered globulin, are commonly seen in the synovial fluid of human rheumatoid patients and are sometimes seen in dogs.

Other laboratory features have been described (e.g. absolute or relative increases in blood globulin, elevation of serum alkaline phosphatase and sometimes of the liver enzymes alanine transaminase and aspartate

Table 7.3 Aid to the differential diagnosis of arthritis in the dog; NAD, no abnormality detectable; WBC, white blood cell count; PML, polymorphonuclear leucocytes; MN, mononuclear leucocytes.

Type of arthritis	Clinical features	Radiographic features	Synovial fluid analysis	Laboratory features
Traumatic	Single joint. History of injury	NAD. Soft tissue swelling. Synovial effusion. Instability of joint	Often much blood present. Large number of erythrocytes; cartilage and synovial cells	
Haemophilic	Very rare. Immature animal. Easy bruising, haematoma etc. Seldom survive to maturity	NAD. Soft tissue swelling. Synovial effusion. Osteoarthritic changes	Blood may be evident	Blood clotting defect
Osteoarthritis	Can be primary or secondary to some other joint problem. Usually only single joint showing clinical problem. Mature animal	Osteophytes/new bone deposits. Sclerosis. Soft tissue swelling. Synovial effusion	Yellow, clear. Volume normal/ increased. Good mucin clot. Viscosity normal. Negative fibrin clot. WBC 400–7000/mm³. 55–100% MN; cartilage and synovial cells	
Osteochondritis dissecans	Immature animal. Large breed. Usually single joint, can be bilateral, rarely multiple. Mainly shoulder and elbow joints; rarely stifle and hock joints	Defect in articular surface. Calcification of separated cartilage piece. Osteoarthritic change	Similar to osteoarthritis	
Bacterial infections	Single joint or multiple, associated with bacterial endocarditis	NAD. Soft tissue swelling. Synovial effusion. Destruction of subchondral bone in advanced cases. Osteoarthritic changes	Turbid. Volume usually increased. Viscosity low. Poor mucin clot. Positive fibrin clot. WBC 2000–200 000/mm³. 60–90% PMN. Pyknosis of PMN common. May see organisms	Positive culture from synovial fluid and/or membrane
Rheumatoid	Usually multiple joint involvement. Often 'shifting' lameness, stiffness	Subchondral erosions. Loss of epiphyseal mineralisation. Change in joint space. Soft tissue swelling. Synovial effusion. Osteoarthritic changes	Yellow, cloudy. Volume normal/ increased. Viscosity low. Mucin clot poor. Fibrin clot may be positive. WBC 6000–60 000/ mm³. 40–95% PMN. May see PMN inclusions	Serum usually positive for rheumatoid factor

Type of arthritis	Clinical features	Radiographic features	Synovial fluid analysis	Laboratory features
Systemic lupus erythematosus	Multiple joint involvement. May be systemically ill (fever, dull, reduced appetite.) Disease of other body systems (e.g. haemolytic anaemia, glomerulo-nephritis, dermatitis)	NAD. Soft tissue swelling. Synovial effusion. Osteoarthritic changes	Yellow, cloudy. Volume increased. Viscosity normal/low. Mucin clot good/poor. Fibrin clot may be positive. WBC 8000–30 000/mm³. 10–80% PMN. May see PMN inclusions, LE cells	Serum positive for ANA/LE cell phenomenon. Immunoglobulin/C3 deposits in affected tissues
Idiopathic inflammatory	Multiple joint involvement. Usually systemically ill. Some cases also show other disease processes.	Similar to systemic lupus erythematosus	Similar to systemic lupus erythematosus but no LE cells WBC 4000–100 000/mm³. 60–95% PMN.	
Normal joint			Yellow, colourless. Clear and viscous. Small volume (av. 0.25 ml) Good mucin clot. Negative fibrin clot. WBC 400–2400/mm³. 84–100% MN	

transaminase). A mild anaemia is also sometimes identified and some cases show a leucocytosis. Elevation of the erythrocyte sedimentation rate is often recorded. Proteinuria has been found in some patients.

Treatment

Many different therapeutic regimes have been suggested. High doses of analgesic/anti-inflammatory drugs such as aspirin, ituprofen (Alexander *et al* 1976), phenylbutazone, mefenamic acid and meclofenamic acid can be tried. Other authorities recommend immunosuppressive therapy with prednisolone and cytotoxic drugs (e.g. cyclophosphamide and azathioprine) (Pedersen *et al* 1976a). Gold injections (sodium aurothiomalate (Myocrisin)) have also been tried with some success; it is important to use a small test dose before commencing full treatment, to check for any adverse sensitivity to the drug, and to check the animal regularly whilst on treatment for any toxic side-effects. In most cases it is a matter of trial and error with a number of drugs to see if a particular regime is useful in improving the clinical problem in any one patient. Prednisolone often produces marked improvement. Initially, high doses are given (e.g. 2 mg/kg body weight daily in a divided dose) and these are gradually reduced. Eventually, alternate day therapy is used. The author favours a combined therapy with prednisolone and gold. The prognosis is generally poor since the disease will gradually progress although severely affected animals can become relatively free of pain and manage reasonably well. Some authorities are trying to stimulate rather than suppress the immune system by the use of drugs (e.g. levamisole, thymic extract)—stimulation of the suppressor system may help to reduce the inflammation.

Surgical arthrodesis of diseased joints has been attempted with limited success. Synovectomy can afford temporary relief particularly if a single joint is predominantly affected. Replacement of damaged ligaments in joints which have become unstable can sometimes help, as can other surgical procedures such as patellectomy or arthroplasty.

Rest and removal of any stress factors are important adjuncts to treatment.

Systemic lupus erythematosus (see also Chapter 10)

This is a multisystemic disease characterised by the simultaneous or sequential development of auto-immune haemolytic anaemia, immune-mediated thrombocytopenia, leucopenia, glomerulonephritis, dermatitis, polymyositis, pleuritis, CNS disease and symmetrical polyarthritis. It is a disease which has been widely reported in the USA (Lewis 1972, 1974; Lewis *et al* 1965a, b; Pedersen *et al* 1976b). Originally, the commonest sign was haemolytic anaemia, but now symmetrical polyarthritis is regarded as the principal clinical feature. Because the clinical signs are so variable the diagnosis of this disease in the dog can be difficult. It is important to use strict criteria for its recognition.

The author's criteria are as follows:

1 Involvement of more than one body system in the disease syndrome as assessed by clinical examination. Involvement of more than one body system may take time and thus continual reassessment of these cases is imperative.
2 High titres of antinuclear antibody should be present in the blood (see below).
3 The immunopathological features consistent with the clinical involvement should be demonstrable. Thus if haemolytic anaemia, leucopenia or thrombocytopenia are present, antibodies against erythrocytes, leucocytes and thrombocytes, respectively should be demonstrated in the laboratory. Similarly, if the dog has glomerulonephritis, dermatitis or polyarthritis, immunoglobulin and complement deposits should be shown in the glomeruli, skin and synovium respectively.

Criteria 1 and 2 *must* always be satisfied.

All the criteria must be satisfied in order to diagnose *definite* systemic lupus erythematosus. If only 1 and 2 are satisfied, *probable* systemic lupus erythematosus is diagnosed.

The aetiology of systemic lupus erythematosus is obscure, although there is some evidence for an underlying viral infection in the dog (Lewis *et al* 1973, 1974; Lewis & Schwartz 1971; Quimby *et al* 1978) and certain genetic requirements are thought to be important for the expression of the disease (Lewis & Schwartz 1971). The pathogenesis of the disease involves two main components—autoimmunity and immune complex hypersensitivity. Antibodies against red blood cells, platelets and leucocytes are important in producing haemolytic anaemia, thrombocytopenia and leucopenia, and the deposition of immune complexes (possibly nuclear antigen and antinuclear antibody) in the kidneys (glomeruli), joints (synovial blood vessels)

and skin (dermal/epidermal junction) and possibly other organs, explains inflammatory changes in these tissues.

Pathological features

The joint pathology involves a synovitis characterised mainly by infiltrations of lymphocytes, plasma cells and macrophages although polymorphonuclear cells are often seen. The production of pannus with destruction of cartilage and bone is not a common feature. Cartilage degeneration will result from the release of proteolytic enzymes associated with the inflammatory process.

Clinical features

These will vary according to which of the various manifestations of systemic lupus erythematosus are present. Joint involvement is characterised by a symmetrical polyarthritis which causes lameness of varying severity. Affected animals are most often pyrexic, lethargic and anorexic. Joints are swollen, sometimes with obvious synovial effusion and pain on manipulation. Lymphadenopathy is common and muscle atrophy may be present. Polymyositis characterised by painful atrophied muscles has been described in canine systemic lupus erythematosus.

If haemolytic anaemia is present, affected animals may show pale or jaundice mucous membranes and if there is associated thrombocytopenia, petechiae and ecchymoses will be seen in the skin and mucous membranes, sometimes with the presence of haematuria, epistaxis and melaena.

Renal involvement will be associated with clinical signs normally seen with a protein-losing nephropathy. Pleuritis will produce respiratory signs and CNS involvement will result in a variety of neurological abnormalities including personality change and convulsions. Skin lesions are also variable.

Any breed of dog of any age can be affected. It is stated that the disease is more common in females, although reported cases do not always reflect this.

Radiographic features

Joint radiographs may show no obvious abnormalities. Occasionally soft tissue swelling or synovial effusion will be present. Erosive changes within the affected joints are not seen. Other radiographic features may be evident (e.g. splenic enlargement, pleural effusion).

Laboratory features

Systemic lupus erythematosus is characterised by the presence of circulating antinuclear antibody, a group of autoantibodies against nuclear material. However, just as rheumatoid factor is not specific for rheumatoid arthritis, antinuclear antibody is not specific for systemic lupus erythematosus. Antinuclear antibody is released in various chronic disease states including bacterial endocarditis and viral infections (Bennett *et al* 1978). The most significant nuclear autoantibody for systemic lupus erythematosus in man is against native DNA. However, problems exist in the specific identification of this autoantibody in dogs' sera.

One of the most common methods to demonstrate antinuclear antibody is the indirect immunofluorescent test using the patient's serum and rat liver or tissue culture cells as a substrate. A positive result is indicated by fluorescence of the nuclei when viewed under the ultraviolet microscope. In the author's laboratory, a titre 1/16 is borderline and anything above this is significant. Radioimmunoassay techniques exist to identify anti-DNA antibodies in human patients, but these are not satisfactory for the dog.

The LE-cell phenomenon is another test used in the diagnosis of systemic lupus erythematosus (Lewis 1965). This involves the collection and incubation of a blood sample from the patient. If antinuclear antibodies responsible for the LE-cell phenomenon are present, they will react with white blood cells causing their destruction and release of nuclear material, which is then ingested by other white blood cells to form the classic LE-cell. These cells are again not specific for systemic lupus erythematosus, the test is laborious to perform and unlike in the human patient it is insensitive in the dog. It is accepted that some patients with systemic lupus erythematosus can be positive for rheumatoid factor as well as antinuclear antibody although the latter is usually at a very much higher titre than the antiglobulin factor.

Biopsies should be taken from affected tissues (e.g. kidneys, skin and synovial membrane) and subjected to histopathological and direct immunofluorescent examinations (Bennett 1980). The latter will detect immunoglobulin and complement deposits in the tissues consistent with systemic lupus erythematosus. Synovial fluid examination reveals excess, discoloured, sometimes cloudy fluid generally with a poor mucin clot. The fluid may clot on standing if no anticoagulant is added. White cells are increased with a preponderance of polymorphonuclear cells. LE-cells have been reported in synovial fluid smears from affected dogs, as well as polymorphs containing cytoplasmic granules of ingested DNA.

Haematological examinations will show an anaemia with abnormally shaped red cells if autoimmune haemolytic anaemia is present; there may or may not be a reticulocytosis. The Coombs' antiglobulin test performed on a suspension of the patient's red blood cells will be positive in these cases indicating the presence of red cell autoantibodies (Bennett 1980). Occasionally there is a leucopenia and antibodies against white blood cells can be demonstrated using the antiglobulin consumption test (Bennett 1980). Antibodies against platelets are shown with the PF-3 test. Elevation of serum globulin (absolute or relative) may be present. Proteinuria will exist if there is renal involvement and biochemical evidence of renal failure will be present in advanced cases.

Treatment
The prognosis with systemic lupus erythematosus is always guarded and becomes unfavourable if renal involvement develops. Corticosteroid therapy is commonly used and some authorities combine this with cytotoxic drugs (e.g. cyclophosphamide and azathoprine) (Pedersen *et al* 1976b). Again rest and confinement of the dog is important.

Idiopathic arthritis

This type includes a large and somewhat obscure group of dogs. It includes all those cases of inflammatory arthropathy which can not be classified into the other groups, *viz* infective, rheumatoid and systemic lupus erythematosus groups. This group can be divided into 4 sub-categories. As a group, certain breeds seem to be over-represented e.g. Irish Setter, German Shepherd, Shetland Sheepdog and Spaniels.

Type 1: Uncomplicated idiopathic arthritis
This is the most common sub-group, accounting for approximately 51% of the total idiopathic cases. The dogs are presented principally with an arthritic problem, although other body systems may be involved, e.g. skin (dermatitis), kidneys (glomerulonephritis), eyes (uveitis, retinitis). The author has also seen cases of polyarthritis together with polymyositis, which satisfied some of the criteria of dermatomyositis as seen in the human patient (Boyle & Buchanan 1971).

The pathogenesis of the arthritis is possibly immune mediated, i.e. the deposition of circulating immune complexes into the synovial membrane to initiate a Type III hypersensitivity reaction. The underlying aetiology and source of the complexes is obscure. Other explanations are possible, e.g. a primary autoimmune response against the joints or a possible unknown viral attack of the joints.

Type II: Idiopathic arthritis associated with infections remote from the joints
This form accounts for approximately 26% of the idiopathic cases. The common infections are respira-

tory tract infections including tonsillitis (viral and bacterial), urinary tract infections, a variety of bacterial skin infections and certain abscesses such as tooth root infections (Bennett 1980). The dogs usually exhibit a polyarthritis and it is assumed that the infectious process provides an antigenic source for immune complex formation and circulating complexes are deposited within the synovium and sometimes other tissues to initiate inflammation by a Type III hypersensitivity reaction. The clinical features are similar to Type I idiopathic arthritis, but include symptoms associated with the infection. The radiographic and laboratory features are similar to Type I. Treatment is mainly towards controlling the infection; this may involve drug therapy (e.g. antibiotics) or surgical intervention (e.g. removing an abscess or infected tooth). If this is successful, the joint problem will normally resolve. Occasionally corticosteroids may be used to help resolve the arthritis.

It is perhaps of relevance that some cases of rheumatoid arthritis are preceded by, in particular, respiratory infections or tonsillitis in both the dog and human patient. Of some relevance to this group are dogs which show a transient sterile inflammatory polyarthritis following routine vaccination, either with dead or live vaccines. It is rare and seldom serious.

Type III: Idiopathic arthritis associated with gastrointestinal disease
This type accounts for about 13% of the idiopathic cases. Generally a polyarthritis is present, but the number of joints affected is generally smaller than in Types I and Types II and bilateral symmetry may not be apparent. The gastroenteritis is usually characterised by vomiting and diarrhoea although diarrhoea can occur on its own. Sometimes overt blood is present in the diarrhoea. Very occasionally the intestinal disease is an ulcerative colitis. The features are again similar to Type I but symptoms related to the gastrointestinal disease will be present. The aetiology of the gastrointestinal upset is often unknown. It is thought that the diseased gut may show an increased permeability to potential antigens which could stimulate the production of immune complexes which might then be deposited in the joints and sometimes other tissues. Alternatively, the damaged gut may allow the absorption of certain 'toxins', which might have a direct effect in the joints. Treatment of the gastrointestinal disease is important and if this is successful the joint problem will resolve itself. Corticosteroids may help.

In recent years the gut has been incriminated in the pathogenesis of rheumatoid arthritis of man. Abnormal levels of clostridial organisms have been demonstrated in the intestinal tract of such patients. Also, it has been shown experimentally in pigs, that high numbers of clostridia in the gut (caused by feeding a high protein diet) are associated with the development of a rheumatoid-like joint disease.

Type IV: Idiopathic arthritis associated with neoplasia remote from the joints
These dogs which account for about 10% of idiopathic cases have an arthritis (usually multiple), but clinical signs are often not severe. The neoplastic lesion is usually malignant but may not be apparent by clinical assessment; some are only recorded at post-mortem examination. The neoplasms recorded by the author have included squamous cell carcinomata, heart base tumour, leiomyoma, and mammary adenocarcinomata.

Neoplasms can stimulate an immune response by the host and thus circulating immune complexes may again form and be deposited within the joints and other tissues to produce inflammation. If the neoplastic lesion is apparent, and treatment is not possible, euthanasia is often recommended. If the lesion is treatable, the joint problem will generally resolve itself. Corticosteroids may help to relieve the joint inflammation.

The exact importance of infections, gastrointestinal disease and neoplasia in the epidemiology of idiopathic arthritis is not certain and it may be argued that in some cases the association between these is nothing more than coincidence. However, until further studies are completed, the presence of other disease processes should be reported and used to distinguish the different types of idiopathic inflammatory joint disease.

Pathological features
The pathological changes within the joint are similar to those described above for dogs with systemic lupus erythematosus (Fig. 7.22). The synovitis can be variable, e.g. a preponderance of mononuclear cells or polymorphs or a mixture of both (Fig. 7.23); fibrin deposits are not uncommon and a vasculitis is sometimes seen. Some dogs have shown, on gross and histological examination, degrees of articular cartilage and subchondral bone destruction associated with pannus formation, although in most cases this was not suspected on radiographic evaluation and insufficient criteria were satisfied for the diagnosis of rheumatoid arthritis. Occasionally other body systems are involved in the disease process, e.g. a polymyositis, uveitis, retinitis, glomerulonephritis, or dermatitis may also be present. The pathogenesis of these other disease manifestations is likely to be similar to that of the joint disease, i.e. involving an immune complex (Type III) hypersensitivity reaction. Such dogs may

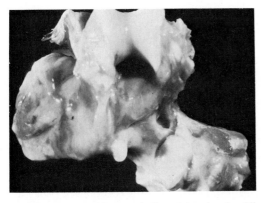

Fig. 7.22 Gross appearance of elbow joint showing idiopathic inflammatory disease. The synovial membrane is thickened and discoloured. The articular cartilage appears normal.

clinically resemble cases of systemic lupus erythematosus, but are negative for antinuclear antibody.

Clinical features

Most of these animals are presented with a bilaterally symmetrical polyarthritis and fever, dullness and loss of appetite. Occasionally an animal is presented with just a chronic lameness and no systemic signs (one third of cases). The degree of lameness can vary markedly and in the least severe cases may be no more than a vague stiffness, whilst more severely affected animals may be unable to stand or walk. Most animals show swollen and painful joints and synovial effusion may be apparent. Tendon sheaths can occasionally be affected. The age of onset can vary from a few months of age to 11 years of age; many are young adults (1–3 years) when first presented. Very occasionally, an idiopathic inflammatory arthropathy may be diagnosed in just a few joints or even in a single individual joint.

Ulceration of the buccal and lingual mucosae is sometimes present, possibly a toxic epidermal necrolysis, often associated with the production of excess, thick, discoloured saliva. Muscle atrophy may be apparent and atrophy of the temporal muscles can often be particularly severe. Other clinical signs may be present if other body systems are involved, e.g. signs associated with polymyositis, glomerulonephritis, dermatitis etc. Symptoms may also be related to the infection in Type II cases, the gastrointestinal disease in Type III and the neoplastic disease in Type IV. A form of idiopathic polyarthritis has been described as an entity in the Greyhound breed in Australia (Huxtable & Davis 1976). The Greyhound has also been

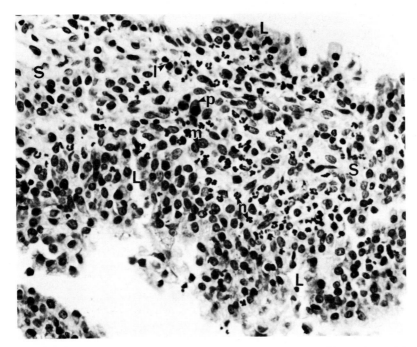

Fig. 7.23 Photomicrograph of the synovial membrane from a dog with idiopathic Type I polyarthritis. There is hyperplasia and hypertrophy of the cells of the lining layer (L) and the supporting layer (S) contains a mixture of inflammatory cells, e.g. plasma cells (p), lymphocytes (l), polymorphonuclear cells (n) and macrophages (m).

associated with a periarticular syndrome in the U.K. (Castell 1969). The author has seen a case of Type I polyarthritis in a Greyhound but recognises no predisposition in this breed. Idiopathic polyarthritis can also be a feature of polyarteritis nodosa (Lewis *et al* 1965b).

Radiographic features

Soft tissue swelling and/or, synovial effusion may be apparent although often there is no abnormality visible (Fig. 7.24); destructive changes are rarely seen.

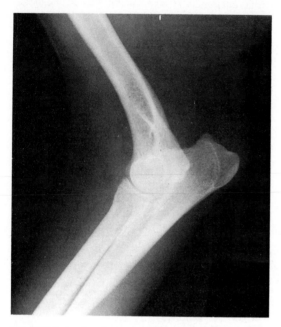

Fig. 7.24 Lateral radiograph of the right elbow joint of a Shetland Sheepdog with idiopathic Type I polyarthritis. No proliferative or destructive changes of bone are visible.

Periostitis is sometimes evident. Occasionally, proliferative bony changes consistent with an osteoarthritis are seen. These may develop with time as a secondary phenomenon if the inflammatory process has damaged the joint in some way (e.g. by producing instability by ligament damage) although cases have been seen where the inflammatory process has been superimposed on a joint already affected with osteoarthritis.

Laboratory features

These dogs are negative for both rheumatoid factor and antinuclear antibody. Some show anaemia, some leucocytosis and others leucopenia. The erythrocyte sedimentation rate may be raised. Serum globulin levels are often absolutely or relatively raised and serum alkaline phosphatase, alanine transaminase and as-

partate transaminase may be increased. Proteinuria may be present.

Synovial fluid examination shows high levels of leucocytes with a predominance of polymorphs. The fluid generally has a poor mucin content and may clot on standing. Synovial membrane biopsy is helpful in confirming the arthritis and identifying immunoglobulin, complement and fibrinogen deposits, within blood vessel walls, inflammatory cells or free within the synovial tissues.

Treatment

The Type I dogs usually respond well to prednisolone. High doses are given for 2 weeks (e.g. 2 mg/kg body weight) and then the dose is gradually reduced over the next 4 weeks. There is generally a marked response within a few days, but it is important to maintain the therapy to help prevent relapses. Relapses are always possible, and therefore the prognosis has to be guarded. Constant corticosteroid medication is sometimes necessary to keep the animal in clinical remission and this is perhaps acceptable if the dose required is only small. Gold therapy can be tried in combination with steroids. Rest and confinement of the animal is important. Certain authorities have also described the use of cytotoxic drugs in combination with prednisolone (Pedersen *et al* 1976b). A very few cases seen by the author have spontaneously recovered within a day or two without any form of treatment other than rest. Analgesic drugs may also be given. Treatment of Type II, III and IV dogs is primarily directed against the infective, alimentary or neoplastic lesion as already referred to above.

NEOPLASIA

Neoplastic disease although very rare can affect joints in one of three ways:

1 Tumours can originate from tissues within the joint.
2 Tumours involving extra-articular structures can erode into the joint cavity.
3 A tumour can metastasise to joint structures although this is rare.

Pathological features

The commonest diagnosed primary neoplasm is the 'synovial sarcoma' (malignant synovioma); other reports of this synovial tumour in dogs have been made (Cotchin 1954; Lieberman 1956). These are highly cellular tumours generally showing large numbers of spindle-shaped cells with a high mitotic rate, with clefts and spaces lined by polygonal cells and multi-nucleated giant cells. Reticular fibres and PAS-positive matrix can often be demonstrated. These tumours can cause extensive bone and cartilage destruction and can metastasise via the blood or lymphatics.

Synoviomas in animals are very rare but have been described arising from tendon sheaths in dogs and cats. Polygonal synovial cells are present in a fibrous stroma with spaces of varying size and shape. Multinucleate giant cells are also present and the mitotic rate is high although these tumours classically show little evidence of local infiltration or metastasis. A synovial chondrosarcoma has also been reported in the dog—an aggressive, infiltrative synovial tumour (Hanlon 1982).

Tumours arising from fatty tissue within the joints have also been seen. These have included both lipoma and liposarcoma. Lipomata tend to form discrete masses of adipose tissue and there is a greater variation in the size and shape of fat cells compared to normal adipose tissue. Even more pleomorphic lipoblasts are seen in liposarcoma together with areas of anaplastic fibrous tissue. Liposarcomata can produce destruction of bone and cartilage and can metastasise via lymphatics.

Tumours which arise outside the joint and which erode the articular space have included a fibrosarcoma arising from extra-articular connective tissue, osteosarcomata arising from the metaphyses and a metaphyseal metastasis of a bronchial carcinoma.

Clinical features

Generally the animal is presented with a chronic persistent lameness. One case of 'synovial sarcoma' of the carpus was initially presented as a lick granuloma problem on the anterior aspect of the affected joint; the dog later became lame. Pain is normally detectable on manipulation of the affected joint and there may be swelling within or around the joint. Joint deformity may be evident in cases of long duration and enlargement of the local lymph nodes may be present.

Radiographic features

Swelling within or around the joint will be seen. Bone destruction may be evident depending on the type and duration of the neoplasm (Fig. 7.25). Bony proliferative change may also be present. Some early cases of destructive joint neoplasia can be confused with inflammatory joint disease. Radiography can also be used to assess the progression of the lesion and to check for any lung metastases.

Laboratory features

Biopsy of the tumour is necessary to obtain a definitive diagnosis and to assess the prognosis.

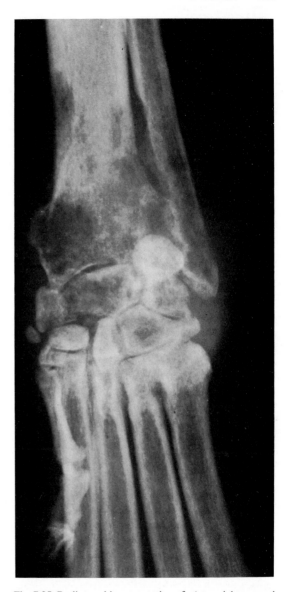

Fig. 7.25 Radiographic presentation of a 'synovial sarcoma' affecting the carpus. Note the widespread bony destruction affecting the distal end radius and ulna and the carpal bones.

Treatment

Local excision of joint tumours can be attempted if this is feasible (e.g. in the case of lipomata). However, if the histological appearance of the tumour is malignant or if there is evidence of local invasion or secondary spread then limb amputation or euthanasia is indicated. Other forms of cancer therapy are possible, but generally not very effective.

MISCELLANEOUS JOINT DISEASE

Various other types of joint disease can be recognised in the dog (see Fig. 7.2), but cannot be dealt with here in detail. Severe trauma to a joint as well as creating traumatic arthritis can produce cartilage or bone damage or such a severe mechanical disruption of the joint with ligament and joint capsule damage that luxation or subluxation of the joint occurs. The abnormal development of a joint in a young animal may result in, for example, hip dysplasia, elbow dysplasia, and congenital patellar, shoulder or elbow luxation. Carpal subluxation has been described as a sex-linked recessive trait in a group of dogs. Abnormalities of growth plates can interfere with normal growth of bone and cause angulation of bones and joints. Ischaemic necrosis of articular structures can occur in association with articular fractures or epiphysiolysis. A well recognised disease of the femoral head, Legg–Calvé–Perthes' disease, basically involves the death of the epiphysis because of a deficient blood supply. The disease occurs in young animals of the toy breeds and can be bilateral. Certain joints have specific abnormalities which can cause articular symptoms, e.g. calcified body on the medial aspect of the elbow joint (Grøndalen & Braut 1976). Pulmonary hypertrophic osteoarthropathy is more a disease of bone but can be associated with pathological changes in the joint capsule. Arthrogryposis has been noted in some new born pups.

A variety of metabolic disorders can cause joint disease. Nutritional secondary hyperparathyroidism for example will result in a loss of bone from the epiphyses of joints and in articular abnormalities. An interesting hereditary disorder of mucopolysaccharide metabolism (a lysosomal storage disease) originally reported in the cat (Jezyk *et al* 1977) has been described in a dog (Schalm 1977; Pedersen *et al* 1983). These animals are lame and show joint pain with enlargement of the metaphyses and epiphyses. Radiography shows proliferation of bone around the joints associated with irregular joint surfaces. Bony proliferative changes can also affect the spine. Other clinical signs may be apparent in mucopolysaccharidosis and circulating neutrophils may be seen to contain numerous metachromatic inclusions. Diagnosis is confirmed by the demonstration of large amounts of mucopolysaccharide in the urine. The bony changes closely resemble hypervitaminosis A as seen in the cat.

A generalised disease of articular cartilage has been reported in a litter of Newfoundland pups (Grøndalen 1981). The condition was described as a generalised fibroid, proliferative degeneration of the joint cartilage. The aetiology was obscure although it was possible that the disease was genetically controlled.

Recently, synovial osteochondromatosis or synovial chondrometaplasia has been described in the dog (Schawalder 1980). Chondroma formation occurs within the synovium and portions of affected synovial villi may detach to form loose bodies. Secondary arthritic changes are common.

Several reports of epiphyseal dysplasia in puppies have been published (Cotchin and Dyce 1956; Hanlon 1962; Lodge 1966; Rasmussen 1971,1972). Affected pups have difficulty in walking with a swaying gait, they fall easily and appear to sag at the joints. Sometimes the limbs are enlarged and dwarfism may result. Radiographically, the epiphyses show numerous punctate areas of increased density.

A rare heritable connective tissue disease known as the Ehlers-Danlos syndrome has been reported in the dog (Gething 1971; Hegreberg *et al* 1969, 1970). It is mainly characterised by fragility and laxity of the skin, but joint laxity and hyperextensibility is also a feature.

Progressive lameness in two Vizsla puppies has been reported associated with periarticular calcinosis of all diathrodial joints (Ellison & Norrdin 1980; Pedersen *et al* 1983). A renal tubular defect, interfering with normal calcium/phosphous transport, has been suggested as the underlying cause.

Inherited dwarfism due to chondrodysplasia has been reported in Alaskan Malamutes and Shetland Sheepdogs and this can be associated with abnormal angulation of joints, particularly the carpi. Achondroplasia, which has been seen in Scottish Terriers and Miniature Poodles, can produce similar problems as can pituitary dwarfism (Scott *et al* 1978; Siegel 1968). Chondrodystrophy is inherent in some breeds of dog such as Bulldogs, Pugs, Pekingese, Basset Hounds and Dachshunds, and in these cases, the conformational abnormalities associated with chondrodystrophy are considered to be normal.

An association between skeletal lesions (including retarded radial, ulnar and tibial growth, ununited and hypoplastic anconeal and coronoid processes, hip dysplasia and delayed epiphyseal development) and eye lesions (retinal dysplasia and detachment and cataracts) has been noted in Labrador Retrievers (Carrig *et al* 1977). The syndrome begins at about 8 weeks of age.

Recently, there has been a suggestion that anterior cruciate ligament rupture in the dog may be accompanied by marked inflammatory changes within the synovium (a plasmacytic lymphocytic synovitis—Pedersen *et al* 1983) and by increased levels of immune complexes in the sera and synovial fluid (Niebauer & Menzel 1982). Such cases of cruciate rupture would seem to have an immunological basis and it is claimed that treatment of the cruciate rupture alone is generally unsuccessful—immunosuppressive drugs, e.g. prednisolone, are required. The author certainly recognises marked inflammatory changes in the synovial membrane of some cases of cruciate rupture but these could be secondary to cartilage debris or hydroxyapatite crystals being released into the joint cavity. Despite the familiarity of this condition, further studies are necessary to fully evaluate the aetiology and pathogenesis of cruciate rupture in the dog.

Joint disease secondary to denervation, e.g. following peripheral nerve injuries is rare in the dog, probably because dogs with such neurological deficits are usually destroyed and not kept long enough for neuropathic arthropathies to develop. The latter include loss of joint support, instability and deformity. The disease probably results from excess trauma to the joint which results from diminished pain and proprioceptive senses.

Disease of the spinal joints is very common in dogs and some references to the spine have already been made. However, it is a specialised field and is better dealt with in a surgical text.

REFERENCES

Joints

ALEXANDER J.W., BEGG S., DUELAND R. & SCHULTZ R. D. (1976) Rheumatoid arthritis in the dog; clinical diagnosis and management. *J. Am. Anim. Hosp. Ass.* **12**, 727.

ARBESSER E. (1974) Osteochondrosis dissecans der Femurkondylen beim Hund. *Weiner Tierärztl Mschr.* **61**, 303.

BEHRENS F., SHEPARD N. & NELSON M. (1975) Alteration of rabbit articular cartilage by intra-articular injections of corticosteroids. *J. Bone Jt. Surg.* **57A**, 70.

BENNETT D. (1980) *The Naturally Occurring Inflammatory Arthropathies of the Dog.* A Clinical, Pathological and Immunological Study, including a Consideration of the Comparative Aspects of these Diseases in Man and the Dog. Vol. I and II. PhD Thesis, Faculty of Veterinary Medicine, University of Glasgow.

BENNETT D., CARMICHAEL S. & GRIFFIFTHS, I. R. (1981) Discospondylitis in the dog. *J. Small Anim. Pract.*, **22**, 539.

BENNETT D., DUFF S. R. I., KENE R. O. & LEE R. (1981) Osteochondritis dissecans and fragmentation of the coronoid process in the elbow joint of the dog. *Vet. Rec.*, **109**, 329.

BENNETT D., GILBERTSON E. M. M. & GRENNAN D. (1978) Bacterial endocarditis with polyarthritis in two dogs associated with circulating autoantibodies. *J. Small Anim. Pract.* **19**, 185.

BENNETT G. A., WAINE H. & BAUER W. (1942) *Changes in the Knee Joint at Various Ages.* N.Y. Commonwealth Fund, New York.

BIERY D. N. & NEWTON C. D. (1975) Radiographic appearance of rheumatoid arthritis in the dog. *J. Am. Anim. Hosp. Ass.* **11**, 607.

BOYLE J. A. & BUCHANAN W. W. (1971) *Clinical Rheumatology.* Blackwell Scientific Publications, Oxford.

CARRIG C. B., MACMILLAN A., BRUNDAGE S., POOL R. R. & MORGAN J. P. (1977) Retinal dysplasia associated with skeletal abnormalities in Labrador Retrievers. *J. Am. Vet. Med. Ass.*, **170**, 49.

CASTELL M. J. H. (1969) Acute periarthritis in a kennel of Greyhounds. *Vet. Rec.* **84**, 652.

COLLINS D. H. (1949) *Pathology of Articular and Spinal Diseases.* Edward Arnold, London.

COTCHIN E. (1954) Further observations of neoplasms in dogs with particular reference to site of origin and malignancy. *Brit. Vet. J.* **110**, 274.

COTCHIN E. & DYCE K. M. (1956) A case of epiphyseal dysplasia in a dog. *Vet. Rec.*, **68**, 427.

COWELL K. R., JEZYK P. F., HASKINS M. E. & PATTERSON D. F. (1976) Mucopolysaccharidosis in a cat. *J. Am. Vet. Med. Ass.* **169**, 334.

DEE R. (1969) Structure and function of hip joint innervation. *Ann. Roy. Coll. Surg. (Eng.)* **45**, 357.

DUELAND R., SISSON D & EVANS H. E. (1982) Aberrant origin of the cranial cruciate ligament mimicking an osteochondral lesion radiographically: A case history report. *Vet. Radiol.*, **23**, 175.

ELLISON G. W. & NORRDIN R. W. (1980) Multicentric periarticular calcinosis in a pup. *J. Am. Vet. Med. Ass.*, **177**, 542.

FREEMAN M. A. R. & WYKE B. (1966) Articular contributions to limb muscle reflexes. *Brit. J. Surg.* **53**, 61.

FREEMAN M. A. R. & WYKE B. (1967) Articular reflexes at the ankle joint: An electromyographic study of normal and abnormal influences of ankle joint mechanoreceptors upon reflex activity in the leg muscles. *Brit. J. Surg.* **54**, 990.

GETHING M. A. (1971) Suspected Ehlers–Danlos Syndrome in the dog. *Vet. Rec.*, **89**, 638.

GHADIALLY F. N. & ROY S. (1969) *Ultrastructure of Synovial Joints in Health and Disease.* Butterworth, London.

GILBERTSON E. M. M. (1975a) *Osteoarthritis: an experimental study in the dog.* PhD Thesis, University of Glasgow.

GILBERTSON E. M. M. (1975b) Development of periarticular osteophytes in experimentally induced osteoarthritis in the dog. *Ann. Rheum. Dis.*, **34**, 12–25.

GRØNDALEN J. (1981) A generalised chondropathy of joint cartilage leading to deformity of the elbow joints in a litter of Newfoundland dogs. *J. Small Anim. Pract.*, **22**, 523.

GRØNDALEN J. & BRAUT T. (1976) Lameness in two young dogs caused by a calcified body in the joint capsule of the elbow. *J. Small Anim. Pract.*, **17**, 681.

GRØNDALEN J. & GRØNDALEN T. (1981) Arthrosis in the elbow joint of young rapidly growing dogs. V A pathoanatomical investigation. *Nord. Vet. Med.*, **33**, 1.

HALLIWELL R. E. W., LAVELLE R. B. & BUTT K. M. (1972) Canine rheumatoid arthritis: a review and a case report. *J. Small Anim. Pract.* **13**, 239.

HANLON G. F. (1962) Normal and abnormal growth in the dog. *J. Am. Vet. Radiol. Soc.*, **3**, 13.

HANLON G. F. (1982) A radiologic approach to bone neoplasms. *Vet. Clinics, N. America*, **12**, No. 2, 329.

HEGREBERG C. A., PADGETT, G. A., GORHAM, J. R. & HENSON J. B. (1969) A connective tissue of dogs and mink resembling the Ehlers–Danlos Syndrome in man. II Mode of Inheritance. *J. Hereditary*, **60**, 249.

HEGREBERG C. A., PADGETT, G. A., OTT R. L. & HENSON, J. B. (1970) A heritable connective tissue disease of dogs and mink resembling Ehlers–Danlos Syndrome of man. I Skin tensile strength properties. *J. Invest. Dermat.*, **54**, 377.

HJÄRRE A. (1939) Ansteckungsquelle für den Menschen über Tuberkulose bei Hunden und Katzen. *Acta tuberc. scand.* **13**, 103.

HUTYRA F., MAREK J. & MANNIGER R. (1938) In *Special Pathology and Therapeutics of the Diseases of Domestic Animals*, 5th edn. Ballière Tindall & Cox, London.

HUXTABLE C. R. & DAVIS P. E. (1976) The pathology of polyarthritis in young Greyhounds. *J. Comp. Path.* **86**, 11.

JEZYK P. F., HASKINS M. E., PATTERSON D. F., MELLMAN W. J. & GREENSTEIN M. (1977) Mucopolysaccharidosis in a cat with arylsulfatase B deficiency. A model of Maroteaux–Lamy syndrome. *Science* **198**, 834.

JONES D. G. C. & VAUGHAN L. C. (1970) The Surgical treatment of osteochondritis dissecans of the humeral head in dogs. *J. Small Anim. Pract.* **11**, 803.

KAVIT A. Y. (1958) Cryptococcic arthritis in a Cocker Spaniel. *J. Am. Vet. Med. Ass.*, **133**, 386.

KIVUMBI C. W. & BENNETT, D. (1981) Arthroscopy of the canine stifle joint. *Vet. Rec.*, **109**, 241.

LAWSON D. D. (1971) Degenerative joint disease. The treatment of canine degenerative joint disease. *J. Small Anim. Pract.* **12**, 101.

LEE R. (1976) Proximal femoral epiphyseal separation in the dog. *J. Small Anim. Pract.* **11**, 669.

LEWIS R. M. (1965) Clinical evaluation of the lupus erythematosus cell phenomenon in dogs. *J. Am. Vet. Med. Ass.* **147**, 939.

LEWIS R. M. (1972) Canine systemic lupus erythematosus. *Am. J. Path.* **69**, 537.

LEWIS R. M. (1974) Spontaneous autoimmune diseases of domestic animals. *Int. Rev. Exp. Path.* **13**, 55.

LEWIS R. M., ANDRÉ-SCHWARTZ J., HARRIS G. S., HIRSCH M. S., BLACK P. H. & SCHWARTZ R. S. (1973) Canine systemic lupus erythematosus; transmission of serologic abnormalities by cell-free filtrates. *J. Clin. Invest.* **52**, 1893.

LEWIS R. M. & SCHWARTZ R. S. (1967) Canine systemic lupus erythematosus: a communicable disease? In *Infection and Immunology in the Rheumatic Diseases*, ed. D. C. Dumande. Blackwell Scientific Publications, Oxford.

LEWIS R. M. & SCHWARTZ R. S. (1971) Canine systemic lupus erythematosus: genetic analysis of an established breeding colony. *J. Exp. Med.* **134**, 417.

LEWIS R. M., SCHWARTZ R. S. & GILMOUR C. E. (1965a) Autoimmune diseases in domestic animals. *Ann. N.Y. Acad. Sci.* **124**, 178.

LEWIS R. M., SCHWARTZ R. S. & HENRY W. B. (1965b) Canine systemic lupus erythematosus. *Blood* **25**, 143.

LEWIS R. M., TANNENBERG W., SMITH C. & SCHWARTZ R. S. (1974) C-type viruses in systemic lupus erythematosus. *Nature* **252**, 78.

LIEBERMAN L. L. (1956) Synovioma of a dog. *J. Am. Vet. Med. Ass.* **128**, 263.

LODGE D. (1966) Two cases of epiphyseal dysplasia. *Vet. Rec.*, **79**, 136.

McDEVITT C. A. (1973) Biochemistry of articular cartilage: nature of proteoglycans and collagen of articular cartilage and their role in ageing and osteoarthritis. *Ann. Rheum. Dis.* **32**, 364.

McDEVITT C. A., GILBERTSON E. M. & MUIR H. (1977) An experimental model of osteoarthritis; early morphological and biochemical changes. *J. Bone Jt. Surg.* **59B**, 24.

McDEVITT C. A. & MUIR H. (1976) Biochemical changes in the cartilage of the knee in experimental and natural osteoarthritis in the dog. *J. Bone Jt. Surg.* **58B**, 94.

MADDY K. T. (1958) Disseminated coccidioidomycosis of the dog. *J. Am. Vet. Med. Ass.*, **132**, 483.

MAKSIC D. (1968). North American blastomycosis. In '*Current Veterinary Therapy. Small Animal Practice*'. p 621. 3rd edn. Edited by R. W. Kirk. W. B. Saunders, Philadelphia.

MANKIN H. J., ZARINS A. & JAFFEE W. L. (1972) The effect of systemic corticosteroids on rabbit articular cartilage. *Arthritis Rheum.* **15**, 593.

MARCOUX M. & LAMOTHE P. (1977) Lubrication of diarthrodial joints: basic concepts. *Can. Vet. J.* **18**, 241.

MARSHALL J. L. & OLSSON S.-E. (1971) Instability of the knee; a long term experimental study in dogs. *J. Bone Jt. Surg.* **53A**, 1561.

MORGAN J. P. (1969) Radiological pathology and diagnosis of degenerative joint disease in the stifle joint of the dog. *J. Small Anim. Pract.* **10**, 541.

NEWTON C. D., ALLEN H. L., HALLIWELL R. E. & SCHUMACHER H. R. (1974) Rheumatoid arthritis. Clinicopathological conference. *J. Am. Vet. Med. Ass.* **165**, 459.

NEWTON C. D., LIPOWITZ A. J., HALLIWELL R. E., ALLEN H. L., BIERY D. N. & SCHUMACHER H. R. (1976) Rheumatoid arthritis in dogs. *J. Am. Vet. Med. Ass.* **168**, 113.

NIEBAUER G. W. & MENZEL E. J. (1982) Immunological changes in canine cruciate ligament rupture. *Res. Vet. Sci.*, **32**, 235.

OLSSON S.-E. (1957) On tuberculosis in the dog. A study with special reference to x-ray diagnosis. *Cornell Vet.* **47**, 193.

OLSSON S.-E. (1974) A new type of elbow dysplasia in the dog. *Sv. Vet.-Tidn.* **26**, 152.

OLSSON S.-E. (1975a) Osteochondritis dissecans in the dog. *Proc. Am. Anim. Hosp. Ass. 42nd Ann. Meeting* **1**, 360.

OLSSON S.-E. (1975b) Lameness in the dog. A review of lesions causing osteoarthritis of the shoulder, elbow, hip, stifle and hock joints. *Proc. Am. Anim. Hosp. Ass. 42nd Ann Meeting*, **1**, 363.

OLSSON S.-E. (1976) Osteochondrosis: a growing problem to dog breeders. *Progress* 1–11.

PEDERSEN N. C. & POOL R. (1978) Canine joint disease. In *Veterinary Clinics of North America*, vol. 8, no. 3, p. 465. W. B. Saunders, Philadelphia.

PEDERSEN N. C., POOL R. C., CASTLES J. J. & WEISNER K. (1976a) Non-infectious canine arthritis: rheumatoid arthritis. *J. Am. Vet. Med. Ass.* **169**, 295.

PEDERSEN N. C., POOL R. R. & MORGAN J. P. (1983) Joint Diseases of Dogs and Cats. Chapter 84. In '*Textbook of Veterinary Internal Medicine. Diseases of the Dog and Cat*'. Vol. II. Edited by S. J. Ettinger. 2nd edn. W. B. Saunders Company, Philadelphia.

PEDERSEN N. C., WEISNER K., CASTLES J. J., LING G. V. & WEISER G. (1976b) Non-infectious canine arthritis: the inflammatory non-erosive arthritides. *J. Am. Vet. Med. Ass.* **169**, 304.

POND M. J. (1971) Normal joint tissues and their reaction to injury. *Vet. Clinics N. Amer.* **1**, no. 3, 523.

QUIMBY F. W., GEBERT R., DATTA S., ANDRÉ-SCHWARTZ J.,

TANNENBERG W. J., LEWIS R. M., WEINSTEIN I. B. & SCHWARTZ R. S. (1978) Characterisation of a retrovirus that cross-reacts serologically with canine and human SLE. *Clin. Immunol. Immunopath.* **9**, 194.

RASMUSSEN P. G. (1971) Multiple epiphyseal dysplasia in a litter of beagle puppies. *J. Small Anim. Pract.*, **12**, 91.

RASMUSSEN P. G. (1972) Multiple epiphyseal dysplasia in beagle puppies. *Acta Radiol. Suppl.*, **319**, 251.

REILAND S. (1975) Osteochondrosis in the pig. *Acta Radiol. Suppl.* 1–118.

RISER W. H. (1973) The dysplastic hip joint: Its radiographic and histologic development. *J. Am. Vet. Radiol. Soc.* **14**, 35.

ROBINS G. M. (1970) A case of osteochondritis dissecans of the stifle joints in a bitch. *J. Small Anim. Pract.* **11**, 813.

ROBINS G. M. (1978) Osteochondritis dissecans in the dog. *Aust. Vet. J.*, **54**, 272.

ROSENBLUM G. P., ROBINS G. M. & CARLISLE C. H. (1978) Osteochondritis dissecans of the tibio-tarsal joint in the dog. *J. Small Anim. Pract.*, **19**, 759.

ROY S., GHADIALLY F. N. & CRANE W. A. J. (1966) Synovial membrane in traumatic effusion. *Ann. Rheum. Dis.* **25**, 259.

SCHALM D. W. (1977) Mucopolysaccharidosis. *Canine Pract.*, **12**, 29.

SCHAWALDER P. (1980) *Synovial osteochondromatosis in the dog.* Schweizer Archiv. für Tierheilkunde **122**, 673.

SCOTT D. W., KIRK R. W., HAMPSHIRE J & ALTSZULER N. (1978) Clinicopathological findings in a German Shepherd with pituitary dwarfism. *J. Am. Anim. Hosp. Ass.*, **14**, 183.

SIEGEL E. T. (1968) Effects of hormones on bone. *Cornell Vet. Suppl.*, **58**, 95.

SKOGLUND S. (1956) Anatomical and physiological studies of knee joint innervation in the cat. *Acta Physiol. Scand.* **36**, suppl. 124, 1.

SOKOLOFF L. (1969) *The Biology of Degenerative Joint Disease.* University of Chicago Press, Chicago.

SWANTON M. C. (1959) Haemophilic arthropathy in dogs. *Lab. Invest.* **8**, 1269.

THORSON R. E., BAILEY N. S., HOERLEIN B. F. & SIEBOLD H. R. (1955) A report of a case of imported visceral leishmaniasis of a dog in the United States. *Am. J. Trop. Med. Hyg.*, **4**, 18.

WYKE B. (1967) The neurology of joints. *Ann. Roy. Coll. Surg. (Eng.)* **41**, 25.

WYKE B. (1972) Articular neurology: a review. *Physiotherapy* **58**, 94.

8

Endocrine System

B. M. BUSH

The system of endocrine glands and their secretions is one of the two major mechanisms (the other is the nervous system) whereby the body regulates and integrates its numerous activities. With the exception of the gonads (dealt with in Chapter 16), those organs that have the production of one or more hormones as a principal function are considered in this chapter. Other organs also produce hormones but are not regarded as being primarily endocrine glands (e.g. liver, stomach, kidney).

Hormones tend to act like catalysts, altering the rate at which reactions proceed, and most act at many different sites in the body. Consequently disorders of the endocrine glands generally affect not just one but a number of body systems, resulting in a variety of clinical signs. Nevertheless not all cases of a particular disorder show every possible clinical sign and at times even a major sign may be absent.

Overactivity of an endocrine gland is almost always associated with an autonomously secreting neoplasm, either of the gland itself or of the pituitary gland which produces a controlling hormone. However, excessive hormone secretion may, on occasion, be a characteristic of a neoplasm elsewhere in the body, either one which involves ectopic tissue of an endocrine gland or a neoplasm of an entirely different tissue which has 'derepressed' and begun hormone production. In the dog, neoplasms of non-endocrine tissue secreting parathormone, insulin, ACTH and erythropoietin (or substances which have identical effects) have been described, though, unlike man, the secretion of cortisol, thyroid stimulating hormone, antidiuretic hormone and growth hormone have not been recorded (Brown 1981). Rarely, cases may be encountered of multiple endocrine neoplasia similar to type 2A in man (thyroid medullary carcinoma, phaeochromocytoma and parathyroid hyperplasia) (Peterson *et al* 1982a).

Accurate methods for directly measuring the levels of some hormones in the dog may not be routinely available, and it may be necessary to employ other diagnostic procedures. The various techniques described here are those which currently appear to be the best for use in canine practice.

Note
Abbreviations are used in the text to represent certain homones and disorders. For ease of reference a list of these abbreviations is given at the end of this chapter.

PITUITARY AND HYPOTHALAMUS

The pituitary gland (or hypophysis) is a small elongated, oval organ connected to the base of the brain by a short stalk (infundibular process). It lies in a depression in the basisphenoid bone of the skull (the hypophyseal fossa) which is the principal part of the sella turcica. The gland is usually described as being divided into an anterior lobe and a posterior lobe, though these names are taken from man, and in the dog the bulk of the anterior lobe lies ventrally. The anterior and posterior lobes in general correspond respectively to the adenohypophysis (derived embryologically from the roof of the mouth) and neurohypophysis (derived from the infundibulum of the brain), with the exception of the pars intermedia which is part of the adenohypophysis included in the posterior lobe. The lobes are partially separated by a cleft (Rathke's cleft) which is all that remains of the cavity of Rathke's pouch when it forms the adenohypophysis.

The neurohypophysis is attached by the pituitary stalk to the overlying hypothalamus and consists of nerve fibres which originate in the hypothalamic nuclei (e.g. supraoptic and paraventricular), plus connective tissue cells known as pituicytes. It is currently believed that the two hormones released from the neurohypophysis are produced in the hypothalamic nuclei and travel along the connecting neurons to the neurohypophysis for storage. These are antidiuretic hormone (ADH), otherwise called vasopressin, which originates principally in the supraoptic nucleus, and oxytocin, which originates mainly in the paraventricular nucleus. Release of each hormone is regulated by nervous stimulation transmitted via the hypothalamus.

The adenohypophysis is composed of chromophobe cells (precursor cells) and chromophil cells. Of the chromophil cells the acidophils produce growth hormone (GH), otherwise named somatotropin, and the luteotrophic hormone (prolactin), and the basophils produce the gonadotrophic hormones: follicle-stimulating hormone (FSH) (which, although the same substance, is known in the male as interstitial cell stimulating hormone, ICSH) and luteinising hormone (LH), plus thyroid-stimulating hormone (TSH) otherwise known as thyrotropin. The chromophobes synthesise adrenocorticotrophic hormone (ACTH) also called corticotropin, and melanocyte-stimulating hormone (MSH).

'Factors' produced in the hypothalamus and conveyed to the adenohypophysis in the hypophyseal portal veins control the secretion of these hormones. In the case of all hormones there is a releasing factor (RF) which stimulates release (e.g. GRF, FSH-RF, LH-RF, TRF, CRF etc.). In the normal animal the production and release of these factors is in each case regulated by a feedback effect of the particular hormone produced by the target organ that is stimulated by the corresponding pituitary hormone (Fig. 8.1). However, no such feedback mechanism operates in the case of prolactin, GH and MSH. Instead, the hypothalamus produces an inhibiting factor (IF) which inhibits release (i.e. PIF, GIF and MIF).

From the above it will be apparent that the hypothalamus is recognised as playing a vital role in the regulation of the output of hormones from both the anterior and posterior lobes.

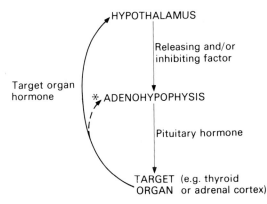

Fig. 8.1 Negative feedback regulating adenohypophyseal hormone release (except in the case of GH, MSH and prolactin). *Most important negative feedback in regulation of thyroid hormone output.

Pituitary disorders

Abnormal rates of secretion, both increased and decreased, of any of the pituitary hormones are possible. Primary tumours of the pituitary gland are not uncommon, especially adenomas. Adenomas of chromophobes and chromophils occur in the approximate ratio 30:1. Chromophil tumours result in increased (autonomous) hormone production whereas chromophobe adenomas may secrete ACTH or compress and invade adjacent tissue, resulting in decreased output of other hormones. Extensive destruction of the pituitary resulting in pituitary cachexia (Simmond's disease) is rare; other signs of panhypopituitarism are the more likely outcome.

In the dog, diseases have been recognised which are attributable to the following:

1 Decreased production of TSH (pituitary hypothyroidism, see thyroid disorders, p. 214).
2 Increased and decreased production of ACTH (see adrenal disorders, p. 226).
3 Decreased production of GH, which gives rise to pituitary dwarfism or, in adults, alopecia and increased GH production resulting in acromegaly.
4 Decreased production of ADH which results in diabetes insipidus.
5 Decreased production of gonadotrophic hormones.

Disorders of the adenohypophysis

Pituitary dwarfism (Fig. 8.2)
Lack of GH during early life will result in reduced production of growth factors (including somatomedins) and stunted growth, although the animal remains normal in its proportions, and throughout life has the dimensions of a puppy. This is in distinction to congenital hypothyroidism (cretinism) where the animal is also dwarfed but has a broad skull, short, thick legs, shortened spine, in severe cases kyphosis (hunchback) and excessive curvature of the frontal and parietal bones. Cretinism is due to a deficiency of the metabolic thyroid hormones and has been recorded chiefly in association with severe iodine deficiency affecting the pregnant bitch and thus intrauterine development. Other disproportionate types of dwarfism are the result of genetic mutations, transmitted as autosomal recessive traits, producing defective growth of the long bones (hypochondroplasia or chondrodysplasia) as in the Alaskan Malamute breed. Other causes of reduced growth include congenital heart disease, familial renal disease and gastrointestinal abnormalities.

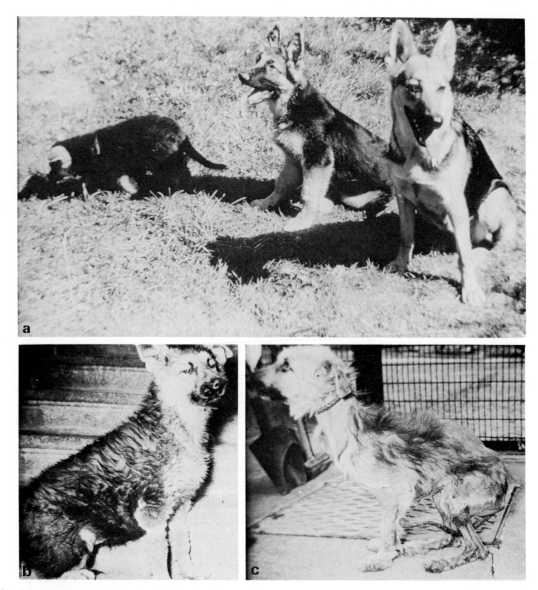

Fig. 8.2 Female German Shepherd pituitary dwarf. (a) At 4 months old (left) compared with her normal littermate (centre) and mother (courtesy of Mr I. Palmer). (b) At 16 months old. Alopecia developed at 6 months of age and the dog started showing aggressive behaviour. RIU at 10 months old confirmed the existence of hypothyroidism and following thyroid hormone therapy a puppy-like haircoat had regrown on all but the thighs and ventral abdomen when this photograph was taken. Oestrus first occurred at $15\frac{1}{2}$ months old and irregularly thereafter. (c) At $3\frac{1}{2}$ years old showing recurrence of the hair loss and severe deterioration in bodily condition.

In addition to their stunted growth, pituitary dwarfs retain their deciduous dentition longer than usual (and may have an undershot mandible), and also retain the shrill puppy bark and the soft puppy haircoat, with the growth of guard hairs restricted to the head and lower limbs or to scattered tufts. Gradually, a bilaterally symmetrical alopecia develops, with hyperpigmentation of the skin which is thrown into exaggerated folds and wrinkles (Scott *et al* 1978). Radiographically these puppies may show failure of the epiphyseal growth plates of the humerus and femur to close for 18 months or more (compared with 9–12 months in normal dogs) and in males failure of the os penis to completely ossify for 12 months or more (compared with 4–5 months in the normal dog).

The range of growth hormone levels in normal dogs determined by specific radioimmunoassay (RIA) is 0.6–4 ng/ml (Eigenmann & Eigenmann 1981). However, the finding of a low level is not conclusive because of overlap with the bottom of the normal range and a clonidine stimulation test is required to clearly distinguish possible GH-deficient individuals. Plasma samples are collected before, and every 15 minutes for an hour after, the intravenous injection of 10μg clonidine/kg body weight (Catapres injection). In normal dogs there is a marked rise in GH levels with a peak above 20 ng/ml after 30 minutes. In contrast, those deficient in GH show little if any response (Eigenmann 1981a).

Even if it is not possible to arrange a GH assay the clonidine stimulation test is still of diagnostic value because also glucose levels rise in normal animals (often by 1.5–2 mmol/l after one hour) but not in pituitary dwarfs. Glucose estimation can also be utilised to distinguish GH deficiency following the intravenous administration of 0.25 iu of neutral soluble insulin (Actrapid MC). In animals lacking in GH glucose levels have fallen 50% after 30 minutes and are still low after 2 hours, whereas in normal individuals the glucose level has been restored almost to normal after 2 hours.

Many pituitary dwarfs also show clinical signs of hypogonadism (atrophic testicles or absence of oestrus) and exhibit reduced activity with tests of thyroid and adrenal function due to decreased TSH and ACTH production. Such animals therefore could be more accurately described as cases of panhypopituitarism.

Pituitary dwarfism most commonly affects German Shepherd Dogs, in which it is inherited as an autosomal recessive condition. Frequently only a single dog in a litter is affected with the others developing normally. Many animals are docile but some are of unreliable temperament, possibly due to associated CNS disturbances.

At *post mortem* examination the majority of cases show gross cystic enlargement of Rathke's cleft causing pressure atrophy of the pituitary; other cases demonstrate pituitary hypoplasia. (Pituitary dwarfism has also been recorded in Weimaraner puppies in association with lack of the thymic cortex, resulting in immunodeficiency and severe wasting (Roth *et al* 1980).

Treatment with bovine or porcine GH (10 iu subcutaneously on alternate days for 1 month or 2 iu on alternate days for longer) has been reported to produce a valuable response, although hypersensitivity reactions may occur. Additional therapy with thyroxine, and possibly corticosteroids, is indicated in cases of proven deficiency of these hormones.

Panhypopituitarism in the adult dog is rare, and in the past has been termed adiposogenital dystrophy. However it is now thought that most such cases were probably primarily cases of hyperadrenocorticism. Affected animals appear obese with marked genital atrophy (e.g. atrophied testicles and flaccid prepuce), polyuria/polydipsia and often a sparse coat. Excess endogenous corticosteroids can suppress GH release, but this is reversible following the successful treatment of hyperadrenocorticism (Peterson & Altszuler 1981).

Recently a growth hormone responsive alopecia has been reported in adult dogs, primarily males of the Pomeranian, Poodle, Chow Chow and Keeshond breeds, which usually develops between 1 and 3 years old. These animals show no other clinical signs apart from typical endocrine alopecia, and demonstrate normal thyroid, adrenal and gonadal function. Laboratory tests show no abnormal features apart from a lowered GH level and, on histological examination of a skin biopsy, a characteristic decrease in elastin fibres. Subcutaneous injections of 5 iu of bovine or porcine GH given on alternate days for 3 weeks results in a re-growth of hair, starting 4–6 weeks after the last injection (Parker & Scott 1980).

Gigantism and acromegaly

Gigantism has been produced experimentally by injecting GH into a growing animal but is rare as a natural disorder in the dog.

Acromegaly is a chronic disorder characterised by the overgrowth of soft tissue, and/or bony structures, resulting from an excessive output of GH in the adult animal after epiphyseal closure. It is thought that some breeds (e.g. Bloodhounds and St Bernards) have been selected for acromegalic characteristics, but as a specific abnormality it has been recorded in middle-aged or elderly bitches, either arising spontaneously during dioestrus or following the use of progestagens (primarily medroxyprogesterone acetate) to control oestrus (Eigenmann & Venker-van Haagen 1981). The clinical signs include (in the order of frequency) snoring, increased amounts of soft tissue (most notably skin folds on the head, neck, or legs and abdominal enlargement), reduced exercise tolerance, enlarged spaces between the teeth and polyuria/polydipsia (Fig. 8.3). On laboratory tests most animals show hyperglycaemia and two-thirds show an elevated SAP level. All have elevated GH levels, usually between 10 and 100 ng/ml, occasionally higher. The snoring (inspiratory stridor) is due to the overgrowth of soft tissues in the orolingual/oropharyngeal region (tongue, larynx, etc.). Hyperglycaemia (responsible in the main for the polyuria/polydipsia) arises because of the metabolic influences of GH on carbohydrate metabolism.

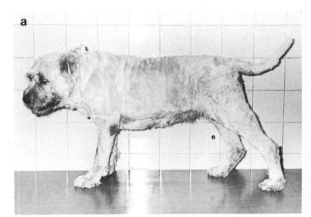

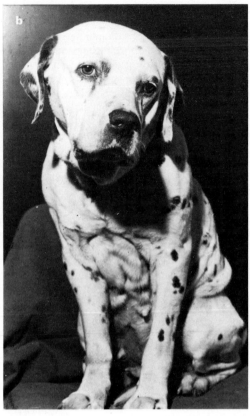

Fig. 8.3   (a) A 6-year-old crossbred Belgian Shepherd bitch showing characteristic features of acromegaly; i.e. thickened trunk and limbs with skin folds around the neck. (Courtesy of Prof. A. Rijnberk and colleagues.)
(b) An 11-year-old Dalmatian bitch with obvious skin folds due to acromegaly. The growth hormone level was extremely high (1476 ng/ml). (Courtesy of Dr. J. E. Eigenmann.)

No abnormalities of the long bones or costochondral junctions is discernible radiographically in the majority of these dogs, in direct contrast to the situation in man and in experimental studies in the dog. It is presumed that this is because in naturally-occurring canine acromegaly exposure to high levels of GH is only intermittent and therefore insufficient to induce marked skeletal change. Ovariohysterectomy, or withdrawing progestagen therapy, is enough to cause regression of the clinical signs.

Disorders of the neurohypophysis

Diabetes insipidus
The antidiuretic effect of ADH (which is arginine vasopressin in the dog) is much greater than its ability to produce a rise in blood pressure. In the normal animal, osmoreceptors in, or connected to, the supraoptic and paraventricular nuclei of the hypothalamus detect changes in the osmolality (tonicity) of the blood plasma and regulate the production of ADH by the nuclei and its release from the neurohypophysis via the supraopticohypophyseal tract. Baroreceptors in the aortic and carotid bodies detect changes in the blood volume and, via the vagus nerve and CNS connections, also influence ADH release. ADH increases the resorption of water from the glomerular filtrate in the distal tubules and collecting tubules of the kidney to reduce water loss from the body.

Diabetes insipidus (DI) is a disease in which there is defective ADH release or action. Two main forms are recognised:

1   Hypothalamic–hypophyseal diabetes insipidus (HHDI) is due to partial or total failure to produce or release ADH. The loss of secretory neurons may be the result of damage to the hypothalamus and/or posterior pituitary by trauma, neoplasia or inflammation, or it may occur for no known cause (idiopathic diabetes insipidus).
2   Nephrogenic diabetes insipidus (NDI), otherwise known as renal diabetes insipidus, is due to a failure of the collecting tubules to respond to ADH. Of the possible causes the best-recognised in the dog is severe renal medullary fibrosis, but it has also been reported in association with other medullary lesions and may rarely be a congenital disorder (Joles & Gruys 1979). NDI is not associated with renal failure and there is no evidence of azotaemia (i.e. high blood urea or creatinine levels).

Diagnosis
The only clinical signs of DI are severe polyuria and compensatory polydipsia. There will be frequent uri-

nation and the history may include inability to retain the large volumes produced (e.g. nocturia), which should be distinguished from true incontinence. Other causes of polyuria and polydipsia (see Table 15.3, p. 420) should be eliminated on the basis of their clinical features and diagnostic tests. In most cases the daily intake and output of water will be much less than in DI. Cases of DI usually show a water intake well in excess of 100 ml/kg body weight per day (i.e. for a 15 kg dog in excess of 1500 ml, or approximately 2.5 pints per day). The output of urine usually exceeds 90 ml/kg body weight per day, and the urine has a specific gravity less than 1.010 (=osmolality less than 335 mosmol/kg); usually much lower.

Some owners may be able to measure water consumption accurately (i.e. amount given minus amount unconsumed) over one or more 24-hour periods; particular difficulties arise where more than one animal has access to the water bowl or when the animal concerned has access to puddles or sinks. Most owners will be unable to collect all the urine which is passed. Hospitalisation to measure water intake and output is therefore preferable, particularly since it will allow further diagnostic tests to be performed and because a change in environment will sometimes result in a markedly reduced intake which suggests psychogenic polydipsia.

Accurate measurement is best made using a metabolism cage, which at its simplest is a cage or kennel with a false floor (of mesh or perforated metal) to allow the urine to be collected uncontaminated by faeces. A sloping underfloor channels the urine into a suitable metal or plastic container. The minimum collection period to obtain meaningful results is 24 hours. Some dogs (usually not DI cases) may be reluctant to consume, and pass, their normal amounts of water when first placed in the cage. If it is suspected that normal behaviour might be inhibited, it is advisable to measure water intake alone for 24 hours before using the metabolism cage so that the intake inside and outside the cage can be compared. The following are other practical points, some of which also apply to the further tests described later:

1 The animal must be hydrated (i.e. not deprived of water) before the test.
2 The bladder must be emptied, preferably by catheter, immediately before and after the test period.
3 The cage should be dried after cleaning and before the dog enters otherwise washing water may also be collected.
4 Bowls or buckets containing drinking water must not leak or allow spillage, since this would produce

results entirely consistent with DI (i.e. apparently increased consumption and apparently increased output of low osmolality). Deep stainless steel buckets bolted to the cage are best for large dogs.
5 Sufficient drinking water should be provided, especially overnight; some should still be present when water containers are refilled.
6 The room temperature should remain constant (18–21°C), especially overnight, since cold may provoke stress and affect the results.
7 Urine should be removed from the collecting vessel at frequent intervals and transferred to a screw-top container. If allowed to stand for 24 hours losses due to evaporation may be significant.

Differential diagnosis
Conditions from which it may be difficult to distinguish the two main types of DI on the basis of this test are hyperadrenocorticism (HAC), liver damage with accompanying polyuria and polydipsia, and psychogenic polydipsia, although only in the last named are similarly large volumes of water consumed and urinated. In liver disease and HAC there is evidence of increased ADH destruction.

Psychogenic (syn. compulsive or primary) polydipsia (PP) is the only condition in which the dog consumes large quantities of water and then needs to eliminate the excess (primary polydipsia and secondary polyuria). In all the other conditions the excessive urine loss precedes the excessive drinking. This compulsive drinking is believed to be an acquired habit in the dog, though in man it may be associated with diseases of the hypothalamic thirst centres which also influence ADH release. The following are clinical pointers to PP:

1 The owner may report that the animal has a neurotic temperament.
2 Drinking may occur as a standard response to certain situations or stimuli (e.g. the entry or departure of the owner or visitors).
3 Water consumption may be normal in hospital, or other newly encountered environments (e.g. kennels at holiday time), and increase again on returning home.

The disorder appears to be more frequent amongst Boxers and German Shepherd Dogs.

Differentiation of the above conditions can almost always be obtained by performing the following two tests with at least a 16-hour interval between them.

Water deprivation test. (This test should not be used, and is indeed unnecessary, in animals suffering from renal failure.) With the dog hydrated, the bladder is emptied and a urine sample collected. The animal is then weighed and placed in the metabolism cage without water. For the duration of the test the dog is unfed. Every hour the animal is removed and reweighed and all the urine formed is collected, which necessitates combining that from both the cage and bladder (free-flow or catheter collection). The specific gravity (or osmolality) of the urine samples is measured. After a loss of 3-6% of the initial body weight the test is stopped. Dogs that are unable to concentrate their urine when deprived of water lose body weight very rapidly.

ADH test (vasopressin test). With the dog hydrated, the bladder is emptied and a urine sample collected. A deep intramuscular injection of vasopressin tannate-in-oil (Pitressin) is given; 5 iu for dogs up to 15 kg body weight, and 10 iu for dogs above 15 kg body weight. Since this product has been discontinued it has been necessary to substitute desmopressin (DDAVP) at a dose rate of 1.3 μg (one-third of a 1 ml vial) for animals up to 15 kg body weight, and 2.7 μg (two-thirds of a 1ml vial) for those above 15 kg body weight. Desmopressin is a structural analogue of natural ADH (arginine vasopressin): the changes in the terminals increase its antidiuretic activity (approximately tenfold) and prolong it compared with natural ADH, and also decrease its pressor effect (to 0.1%). However it is produced in an aqueous solution compared with the oily solution of natural ADH previously used in this test. After injection the dog is placed in a metabolism cage, initially without water, and not fed throughout the duration of the test. Every 60-90 minutes the animal is removed and reweighed and all the urine formed is collected from both the cage and the bladder (free-flow or catheter). In order to keep the animal's weight constant a volume of water should be provided which is equal to the weight loss over the previous period of time. The specific gravity (or osmolality) of the urine samples is measured. The test should be stopped after at least 7 hours.

The important diagnostic features are the maximum specific gravity (or osmolality) attained in both tests, and the time at which the maximum specific gravity (or osmolality) is attained in the ADH test. How the conditions may then be distinguished is shown in Table 8.1. Cases of liver disease and HAC can be confirmed by SAP, SGPT and cortisol estimations (see diagnosis of hyperadrenocorticism, p. 226).

It should be emphasised that the disappearance of polyuria/polydipsia following the administration of desmopressin is not sufficient to confirm the existence

Table 8.1   Differential diagnosis of diabetes insipidus (DI).

	Peak values obtained expressed as SG (osmolality, mosmol/kg)		Time of peak value with ADH test (hours)
	Water deprivation test	ADH test	
Normal dog	1.030 (1000) or more	>1.040 (>1350)*	>5
Hypothalamic-hypophyseal DI	<1.010 (<335)†	>1.021 (>700)	>5
Nephrogenic DI	<1.010 (<335)	<1.010 (<335)	0
Hyperadreno-corticism and/or liver disease	1.010 (335) or more	>1.012 (>400)	<5

(For Normal dog and Hypothalamic-hypophyseal DI, time of peak: usually much later, on average about 12 hours)

*Usually considerably higher values are obtained, but conversion of specific gravity (SG) to osmolality and vice versa loses accuracy above this point. Otherwise values can be converted using the formulae:

osmolality (mosmol/kg) = last two digits of SG $\times$ 33.3

last two digits of SG = osmolality (mosmol/kg) $\times$ 0.03

Older refractometers give SG readings 15-20% higher than those obtained using a urinometer, but more recent models bear a revised scale (marked 'Int' at its base) which provides better correlation. A correction for temperature may also be necessary.

†It has been proposed that a partial deficiency of ADH exists when the urinary concentration increases to more than that of plasma, i.e. SG > 1.010 (>335 mosmol/kg) but is less than that normally expected (SG < 1.027 (<900 mosmol/kg)).

of DI. The same response is seen in dogs suffering from other polyuric disorders (Greene *et al* 1979).

A test is also available which combines the water deprivation and ADH tests, thereby shortening the total procedure. Unfortunately it has the practical disadvantages that it is necessary to estimate the osmolality of each sample soon after collection and that the injection of the ADH and the collection of urine samples may need to be made 12-18 hours or more after starting the test (Mulnix *et al* 1976).

Cases of psychogenic polydipsia (PP) in general show the same response as normal dogs. However in some human cases of PP continual excessive drinking may result in so great a loss of sodium ions from the renal medulla that the collecting tubules cannot respond to ADH (i.e. these individuals behave as NDI cases). Although as yet there is no evidence of such cases in the dog, this type of PP can be distinguished from NDI by the ability to reduce the urine flow as plasma osmolality increases following the intravenous infusion of a hypertonic saline solution (Hickey-Hare test); a response which does not occur in NDI (Lage 1973).

Treatment
There is general agreement that the best control of HHDI in dogs is obtained using vasopressin tannate-in-oil (Pitressin); the intramuscular injection of 5 iu gives control for 1–3 days. Several dogs have been successfully treated in this way for 8–10 years. Unfortunately this product is unavailable to the veterinary profession in the UK, either for diagnosis or treatment. An aqueous synthetic form of natural ADH from the same manufacturers will probably become generally available in late 1983, but it seems unlikely that it will offer any advantages over its analogue desmopressin, which is the drug currently employed in therapy. HHDI cases usually require an intramuscular or subcutaneous injection of up to 1 ml (4 μg) of desmopressin, depending on body size, every day. The observation of increased water consumption determines when a further injection is required; regrettably this often occurs within 18 hours. To decrease the cost and increase the effectiveness, treatment with desmopressin nasal drops have been tried and shown to be very effective in dogs that will accept them. 20 μg (0.2 ml) twice daily is needed in small breeds and correspondingly more in larger animals. The dog's nose is raised vertically and half the dose placed in each nostril using a tuberculin syringe; any transient sneezing seems not to impair the dog's response (Greene *et al* 1979). This product has also been used as eye-drops. Lysine vasopressin nasal spray (Syntopressin) needs to be used more frequently to produce a similar effect. Untreated cases may show a gradual decline in bodily condition and increased susceptibility to other diseases. Cases of hepatic damage may benefit from ADH injection but not as much as HHDI cases.

ADH injection is not effective in NDI cases. For both HHDI and NDI cases an alternative treatment is the oral administration of a thiazide diuretic. The most wisely used is hydrochlorothiazide (1.25–2.5 mg/kg body weight per day). After first decreasing the extracellular fluid volume this drug acts by increasing the re-absorption of sodium and water in the proximal renal tubules and probably also by reducing glomerular filtration. This antipolyuric effect of hydrochlorothiazide is enhanced by a moderate restriction in salt intake, though not a completely salt-free diet. A better response in many HHDI cases is obtained using the oral hypoglycaemic drug chlorpropamide (Diabinese) at a dose of 3 mg/kg body weight once daily, though not in pregnancy because of its teratogenic

effects. Although this drug may enhance deficient ADH formation, it mainly potentiates the renal response to ADH. It may cause vomiting and its long-term use can lead to hypoglycaemia (as with insulin overdosage), so owners should be warned about the appearance of hypoglycaemic signs. Other drugs used orally in man in cases of HHDI are clofibrate (a hypolipaemic drug) at a dose rate of 25 mg/kg body weight per day, and carbamazepine (an antiepileptic drug) at the rate of 8 mg/kg body weight per day, both in divided dosage.

Oral treatment is successful in only a proportion of cases; it is the only treatment available for NDI, but is inferior to ADH injection for cases of HHDI.

Cases of psychogenic polydipsia often respond satisfactorily to a progressively more severe rationing of water to reduce their intake. (Cases of medullary 'washout', if discovered, would require sodium supplementation, at least initially.) Truly psychotic animals when deprived of water may merely exhange polydipsia for another abnormal response (e.g. the chewing of furniture). They may respond to a CNS depressant drug such as chlordiazepoxide (Librium) or behaviour modification methods could be tried (see Chapter 19).

The rare disorder of *inappropriate ADH secretion*, meaning ADH secretion independent of the negative feedback from osmoreceptors and pressure receptors, has been recorded in a dog (Breitschwerdt & Root 1979). It may have been induced by heartworm infection, and resulted in anorexia, weakness and incoordination due to water retention and salt loss.

THYROID GLAND

The canine thyroid gland consists of two separate elongated and encapsulated lobes which lie lateral to the first 5–8 tracheal rings. Only rarely does a connecting isthmus join them anteriorly; most commonly in the brachycephalic breeds. The right lobe is slightly higher, almost touching the larynx. Accessory thyroid tissue occurs in the periaortic fat bodies of approximately 50% of adult dogs and less frequently elsewhere in the midline of the neck, thorax, or even on occasion the abdomen.

Microscopically, the thyroid lobes are composed of numerous near-spherical follicles, each consisting of a single layer of epithelial cells on a basement membrane. The follicles are filled with colloid containing thyroglobulin. The follicular cells are able to 'trap' iodide from the plasma, oxidise it to iodine and link it to tyrosine producing mono- and diiodotyrosine.

These in turn undergo oxidative coupling to form the thyroid hormones thyroxine (T4) and triiodothyronine (T3). T4 and T3 may be either secreted directly into the blood or combined with a protein for storage as thyroglobulin in the colloid. When necessary thyroglobulin can be taken back into the cells and the hormones liberated (by splitting the thyroglobulin molecule with a proteolytic enzyme) and then released into the circulation. Approximately 95% of the circulating hormone of the dog is T4, the rest T3. In the plasma the vast majority is bound to albumin and to specific globulin factions.

The thyroidal uptake of iodide and the production and release of thyroid hormone are increased by thyroid-stimulating hormone (TSH) from the adenohypophysis. TSH release is regulated mainly by the negative feedback effect of thyroid hormones on the adenohypophysis, which decreases the sensitivity of the pituitary to thyrotropin-releasing factor (TRF) (see Fig. 8.1).

Thyroid hormone raises the metabolic rate of the body by increasing transmembrane transport, energy transport and protein synthesis. It causes increased catabolism of carbohydrate, fat and protein and a resultant loss in weight, together with increases in heart rate, blood pressure, body temperature, gut motility and the activity of the central nervous system. It is necessary for the correct growth and development of the young animal, especially the nervous system, and for reproduction.

Arranged between the follicles are larger epithelial cells, designated C (or parafollicular) cells, responsible for production of the hormone calcitonin. They are quite distinct from the cells which synthesise the metabolic hormone, and have a quite different embryological origin. Calcitonin, like parathyroid hormone, is concerned with the regulation of the blood calcium level, but their actions are not identical. It functions as an emergency hormone to prevent hypercalcaemia, which might result from the rapid absorption of calcium after meals.

Calcitonin primarily inhibits bone resorption (which would release calcium and phosphate) and decreases the reabsorption of calcium and phosphate by the kidney, thereby lowering both the calcium and phosphate levels in the blood.

Although calcitonin is being continuously secreted hypercalcaemia provokes a greatly increased output.

Thyroid disorders

The important causes of canine thyroid disorders are summarised in Table 8.2, which also indicates whether

Table 8.2 Canine thyroid disorders: aetiology, presence of goitre and functional status.

Thyroid disorder	Major causes	Presence of goitre	Functional status
Simple goitre	Iodine deficiency	Yes	Euthyroid
Hypothyroidism			
Congenital	Aplasia or hypoplasia	No	
	Iodine deficiency	Yes	
	Dyshormonogenesis	Yes	
Adult primary	Idiopathic atrophy	No	
	End-stage lymphocytic thyroiditis	No	Hypothyroid
	Neoplasia: bilateral, malignant	Yes	
	Iodine deficiency	Yes	
Adult secondary (or pituitary)	Pituitary neoplasia	No	
Thyroiditis	Infection	Possible	Usually euthyroid, rarely hypothyroid
	Lymphocytic (?autoimmune)	Improbable (occasionally very slight enlargement)	Euthyroid, may progress to atrophy and hypothyroid
Neoplasia			
Primary	Unknown	Yes in clinically significant cases (see text)	Mainly euthyroid, sometimes hyperthyroid, rarely hypothyroid
Secondary	Metastasis or local invasion from other organs (rare)	Yes	

there is a change from the normal functional status (i.e. euthyroidism). The most common disorders are hypothyroidism due to atrophy and thyroid neoplasia. Hyperthyroidism in the absence of neoplastic goitre has seldom been reported and never scientifically confirmed.

Goitre

The normal canine thyroid gland is not palpable; a palpable enlargement, whatever its aetiology, is termed 'goitre'. It is most likely to be due to neoplasia which is almost always malignant. Other possible but much less common causes of goitre are an inflammatory reaction (thyroiditis) and iodine deficiency. Bilateral goitre might be expected with severe iodine deficiency although the two lobes need not be equally enlarged. The presence of goitre, considered in isolation, provides no indication of the functional state of the thyroid gland.

The mechanical pressure exerted by a large goitre often results in dysphagia, dyspnoea and dysphonia.

Iodine deficiency

In Table 8.2 iodine deficiency is shown as the cause of simple goitre, and a possible cause of congenital and adult hypothyroidism. In fact some investigators have found great difficulty in producing hypothyroidism, and even goitre, by experimentally depriving adult dogs of iodine. In any case iodine deficiency due to a reduced iodine intake is rare in affluent countries because of the varied diet available; fish and fish products (e.g. cod-liver oil) are naturally rich in iodine, iodised salt is widely used and many commercial pet foods have a very high iodine content. However, dogs fed for a long period solely on meat, or meat and rice diets will not satisfy their iodine requirements, or in the case of a pregnant bitch the iodine requirements of the fetus, and iodine deficiency can develop. An iodine-deficient thyroid gland will endeavour to maintain normal thyroid hormone levels by undergoing hypertrophy and hyperplasia under the influence of TSH thereby increasing the thyroid clearance of plasma inorganic iodine. If by this enlargement the gland is successful in maintaining hormone levels simple goitre will result. If it is not, hypothyroidism, in addition to goitre, may develop.

Treatment

The addition of iodine-containing foods to the diet is usually adequate but one drop of Lugol's iodine (aqueous iodine solution) per 5 kg body weight may be added to the food or water daily. High dosage is contraindicated since this can result in necrosis of the follicular cells.

Hypothyroidism

Hypothyroidism denotes a state of reduced physical and mental activity which results from an inadequate level of circulating thyroid hormone. In over 90% of dogs it is a primary disorder produced by the loss of three-quarters or more of the follicles.

A non-painful lymphocytic autoimmune thyroiditis occurs in dogs and the damage can progress to an end stage form in which the follicles are replaced by fibrous tissue. This may be responsible for almost 50% of cases of primary hypothyroidism (Gosselin *et al* 1981a, 1981b). (The lymphocytic thyroiditis reported in laboratory colonies of Beagles is a less extensive, non-progressive, multifocal and familial disorder which does not give rise to clinical signs of hypothyroidism. Also familial hypothyroidism has been described in Beagles in which the thyroid glands of some animals showed lymphocytic thyroiditis, some atrophy and others neoplastic change (Manning 1979).)

However the overall majority of cases of hypothyroidism show focal or generalised atrophy, with follicles being gradually replaced by adipose tissue. The aetiology of these so-called idiopathic cases is not yet determined, but is not inflammatory.

Less than 10% of cases of hypothyroidism are the result of a reduced output of TSH from the adenohypophysis (secondary, or pituitary, hypothyroidism). This condition often appears to follow destruction of the pituitary by a chromophobe adenoma and as mentioned previously may be part of a generalised lack of pituitary hormones (panhypopituitarism). Thyroid atrophy, lymphocytic thyroiditis and TSH deficiency are not compatible with goitre formation. Hypothyroidism due to other causes (iodine deficiency, dyshormonogenesis, neoplasia or fibrosis following infective thyroiditis) is rare in the UK (Fig. 8.4).

Dogs may be affected from 2 years old onwards but most are presented in middle age (4–8 years old), occasionally older. They usually belong to the larger or medium-sized breeds, particularly Retrievers, Setters, Doberman Pinschers, Airedale Terriers, Beagles, Schnauzers, Boxers, Spaniels and Shetland Sheepdogs (Fig. 8.5). Hypothyroidism appears to be uncommon in miniature or toy breeds.

Diagnosis

Diagnosis is best based on the principal clinical signs of lethargy (i.e. impassive behaviour and inability to exercise due to myopathy), a dry and sparse haircoat with skin thickening, hyperkeratosis and hyperpigmentation, follicular plugging and a bilaterally symmetrical alopecia (usually affecting flank, neck and thighs, Table 8.3), puffy folds on the forehead and neck, increased body weight and an intolerance to cold. Severely affected animals may also show a subnormal body temperature and bradycardia, head tilt, irregularities of the oestrus cycle, decreased libido and fertility, diarrhoea or constipation and occasionally testicular atrophy (with hypospermatism) and umbilical hernia. Electrocardiograms frequently show low voltage and inverted T waves (Nijhuis *et al* 1978). There is also at times an association with pathologic galactorrhoea (spontaneous milk flow) and various

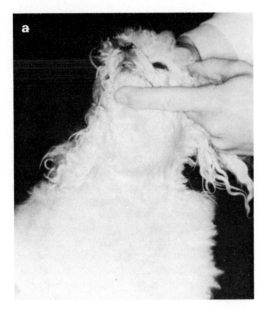

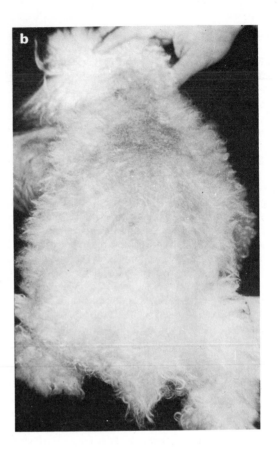

Fig. 8.4 Extensive bilateral thyroid adenocarcinoma in a 7-year-old Toy Poodle bitch which caused such extensive follicle destruction that hypothyroidism resulted. (a) The large bilateral goitre is clearly visible: (b) typical endocrine alopecia over the back.

ocular changes including arcus lipoides (anular infiltration of the peripheral cornea and the perilimbal sclera with lipid) (Chastain & Schmidt 1980; Crispin & Barnett 1978).

Rarely animals may enter a myxoedema coma in which metabolic activity comes to a standstill, often triggered by a very cold environment or a concurrent infectious disease.

Congenital cases of hypothyroidism (cretins) may,

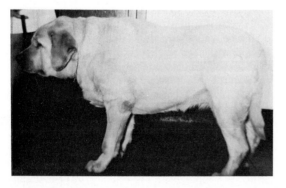

Fig. 8.5 Obese and lethargic 5-year-old male Labrador Retriever suffering from primary hypothyroidism. There are obvious skin folds on the neck and forehead; the latter giving the animal a typical 'worried' expression.

though rarely, occur due to arrested development of the gland or a defect in hormone synthesis (dyshormonogenesis). In addition to many of the above signs they exhibit stunted physical development with a broad skull and short thick legs giving a dwarfed appearance.

The discovery of several signs is a valuable diagnostic indicator but it should be appreciated that one or more of the principal features (skin changes, weight gain) can be absent. The disorder can prove difficult to diagnose and must be distinguished from other conditions, particularly obesity arising from other causes and hyperadrenocorticism. Acromegalic bitches (q.v.) may also be confused because of their increased body size and skin folds.

Supporting evidence from routine laboratory tests would be a mild normocytic, normochromic anaemia (e.g. PCV less than 36%), seen in approximately a quarter of cases, an elevated level of serum creatinine phosphokinase, and particularly a fasting blood cholesterol level above 7.8 mmol/l (300 mg/100 ml), which occurs in about two-thirds of hypothyroid dogs.

However these findings may arise from causes other

Table 8.3 Differential diagnosis of endocrine alopecia.

Endocrine alopecia (i.e. bilaterally symmetrical non-pruritic alopecia of gradual onset) may occur in canine cases of:

Hypothyroidism. Thickened skin

Hyperadrenocorticism. Thin skin

Pituitary dwarfism. Congenital condition with reduced body size

Adult growth hormone deficiency. Hair thinning often not marked. Skin deficient in elastin, and may be reduced in thickness. No other features. Chiefly in males. ⎱ These disorders are described in this chapter

Feminisation (in males). True cases are due to Sertoli cell tumour of the testicle. (Not all cases with a Sertoli cell tumour show alopecia.) Affected dogs can show gynaecomastia, slack prepuce, lack of libido, crouching to urinate and are attractive to other males. Male dogs showing similar signs, but without a Sertoli cell tumour, have been shown not to be true cases of feminisation.

Ovarian imbalance (in bitches)

Type 1. Increased oestrogen production (often associated with cystic ovaries). Unspayed bitches showing enlargement of nipples and vulva, hyperpigmented vulva and often pseudocyesis or anoestrus.

Type 2. Decreased oestrogen production. Spayed bitches with thin pliable skin, infantile vulva and nipples and often showing incontinence.

Notes: (1) Acanthosis nigricans, with lesions arising initially in the axilla (and particularly common in Dachshunds) may also have an endocrine aetiology. (2) Hyperpigmentation is seen in all types of endocrine alopecia except decreased oestrogen production, though less commonly in hyperadrenocorticism. (3) Only hypothyroidism, hyperadrenocorticism and the hyposomatotropic disorders produce histological changes that are sufficiently distinctive to be diagnostic.

Table 8.4 Differential diagnosis of hypercholesterolaemia.

In the dog the fasting total blood cholesterol level is elevated from the normal range, 2.6–7.8 mmol/l (100–300 mg/100 ml), in association with:

Hypothyroidism: in about two-thirds of cases. Values above 13 mmol/l (> 500 mg/100 ml) are primarily due to this disorder. Rarely they may rise to above 52 mmol/l (> 2000 mg/100 ml).

Hyperadrenocorticism: in about half of cases

Diabetes mellitus: in both the early and ketoacidotic stages

Liver disorders: although not in every case (e.g. fatty degeneration, neoplasia)

Nephrosis: there is a reciprocal relationship with the blood albumin level

High fat diet: can produce levels above 10.4 mmol/l (> 400 mg/100 ml)

Notes: (a) Temporary rises in the total blood cholesterol level can follow feeding. (b) Some dogs have an inherited predisposition to increase their blood cholesterol level much more than average when fed on a predominantly meat diet.

than those due to the peripheral action of thyroid hormone (Table 8.4).

None of the *in vitro* tests routinely used to confirm hypothyroidism in man will produce reliable results in the dog without some modification of the test method, except for the measurement of free thyroxine.

Currently the most widely used laboratory tests which will reliably separate normal and hypothyroid dogs are the radioimmunoassays (RIA) of total T4 and T3. These tests were originally designed to provide accurate values over the normal and abnormal ranges likely to be found in man. Modification is necessary because the levels of total T4 and T3 in the normal dog are much lower than those in man (approximately a quarter and a half of human values respectively) and fall even lower in hypothyroidism. Using a validated RIA method total T4 levels less than 19.3 nmol/l (1.5 μg/100 ml) and total T3 levels less than 0.77 nmol/l (50 ng/100 ml)[*] are found in hypothyroid dogs (Belshaw & Rijnberk 1979).

Certain commercial laboratories will perform, with varying degrees of accuracy, RIA of total T4 and T3. One of these[†] currently offers a convenient, and apparently reliable, T4 RIA that is performed on a small quantity of blood absorbed into a special filter paper strip—a feature which greatly simplifies collection and despatch.

Free thyroxine is the unbound and metabolically active fraction, and its measurement is considered to be a more accurate indicator of thyroid function than the measurement of total T4. Although the total amount of T4 in the plasma of man is considerably higher than in the dog, the level of free T4 is of the same order in both species. This makes it possible to measure the level of free T4 in dogs using commercial kits developed for RIA of free T4 in human patients. The first reports of the use of such a kit (Amerlex FT4) are extremely encouraging (Ross & Valori 1982; Eckersall & Williams 1983).

Unreliable *in vitro* tests which have been widely reported are the T3 resin uptake test (RT3 test) and the measurement of serum protein-bound iodine (PBI) levels. In the dog the amount of non-hormonal iodine which is protein bound equals or exceeds the amount of protein bound hormonal iodine and increases with an animal's consumption of iodine, so that the PBI level reflects more a dog's iodine intake rather than its output of hormone.

[*] To convert total T4 values expressed in μg/100 ml to nmol/l (and in the case of free T4, ng/100 ml to pmol/l) multiply by 12.87. To convert total T3 values expressed in ng/100 ml to nmol/l multiply by 0.0154, and to convert those in ng/ml to nmol/l multiply by 1.54.

[†] J.M. Clinical Laboratories, 282, Landis Avenue, Chula Vista, CA 92010, USA

Three other methods can be valuable in diagnosis. The radioiodine uptake (RIU) has generally correlated well with the clinical picture. Whereas euthyroid dogs show a peak uptake of 12–70% of an administered dose of radioiodine after 48, 72, or occasionally 96 hours, hypothyroid dogs usually have a peak uptake of less than 10% occurring before, or at, 24 hours. The diagnostic feature is the lower and earlier peak. The disadvantages of RIU are that it can be performed only at licensed centres and that the uptake will be depressed in normal dogs receiving large amounts of iodine (e.g. as cod-liver oil, cough mixtures containing potassium iodide or simply in commercial diets). If the amount of iodine in the diet is known to be, or could be, excessive, a diet of butcher's meat without supplementation should be fed for the week prior to testing.

Secondly, thyroid scanning (scintigraphy), or the use of a gamma camera, after the administration of radioiodine or pertechnetate, will identify the glands with a poor uptake of the isotope.

Thirdly, thyroid biopsy and subsequent histological examination will very effectively distinguish hypothyroid and normal animals, and also discriminate between primary and secondary causes of hypothyroidism. Excision of the lowest quarter of either lobe is a relatively straightforward procedure, although some clinicians might judge it undesirable to be performed in old animals. The vacuoles (actually an artefact) seen in sections of the normal gland after aqueous fixation are absent in sections from dogs with a deficiency of TSH, and the follicles are distended with colloid.

Primary and secondary hypothyroidism can also be distinguished by repeating the thyroid function test (total or free T4 estimation or RIU) after the injection of TSH. Usually a single dose of 10 iu of TSH (Thytropar) is given intravenously 4 or 8 hours before a T4 estimation, whereas intramuscular injections of 10 iu on each of 3 days before RIU have been employed. In primary hypothyroidism no appreciable change in the result is seen, whereas in secondary hypothyroidism a result equal to, or approaching, that seen in the normal animal is usually apparent. The detection of secondary cases is valuable, especially in older animals, since the pituitary neoplasm which is usually responsible may produce signs of other endocrine disorders and central nervous system disturbances which materially influence the prognosis.

It is not always appreciated that interference with the protein binding of thyroid hormones often causes the plasma levels of total T4 and T3 to be lowered, sometimes markedly so. Dogs with Cushing's syndrome or that have received corticosteroid therapy, and dogs that have received treatment with anti-convulsants (e.g. phenytoin or phenobarbitone), mitotane or phenylbutazone, or that are in the terminal stage of non-thyroidal illnesses, may show low T4 values. Fortunately the plasma T4 response to TSH stimulation allows an unambiguous distinction to be made between these normal (i.e. euthyroid) individuals and cases of primary hypothyroidism. Therefore T4 estimation should be repeated 4–8 hours following an intravenous injection of TSH where there is a history of recent drug therapy or concurrent illness, or indeed whenever borderline 'resting' T4 values are initially obtained. Because of the similar response to TSH stimulation the distinction of such normal dogs from cases of secondary hypothyroidism requires either biopsy or thyroid scanning. Some cases of secondary hypothyroidism will be suffering concurrently from Cushing's syndrome (almost invariably as a result of pituitary neoplasia) and therefore the diagnosis of secondary hypothyroidism is best accompanied by tests of adrenal function (q.v.). (The response to TSH has also been used to distinguish normal dogs from those with primary hypothyroidism when their T4 levels are measured by an enzyme linked immunosorbent assay (Larsson & Lumsden 1980).)

A method of TSH RIA could provide a sensitive and convenient method for diagnosing hypothyroidism and differentiating between primary and secondary cases, but because TSH is species specific it cannot be estimated using the assay for human TSH (Chastain 1978).

In cases where clinical signs and/or laboratory tests produce equivocal results, or where specific diagnostic tests are impossible to arrange, there is justification for a short therapeutic trial with thyroid hormones (see below). If improvement does not result after 4–6 weeks, therapy should be stopped.

Treatment
The best drug for oral replacement therapy is thyroxine (Eltroxin) (0.1 mg/5 kg body weight) given as one dose daily. It is cheaper than liothyronine (which has to be given twice daily) and produces a better clinical response than thyroid extract. Injectable preparations are unnecessary for routine use and also unavailable in the UK. (Animals showing low T4 levels simply because of previous drug treatment do not require thyroid hormone therapy.)

An increase in physical activity and a reduction in blood cholesterol level often occurs 1–2 weeks after beginning treatment, but significant improvements in skin condition and body weight may require several weeks. The start of new hair growth results in the increased shedding of old hairs from the follicles, often accompanied by a transient pruritus that responds to topical corticosteroid creams. Successively descending cholesterol values are a good indicator of successful treatment, though re-estimation of T4 levels provides a specific assessment. Therapy, usually at the same level, will be required for the rest of the dog's life. If a satisfactory response is not forthcoming in a case correctly diagnosed, after 2–3 weeks the daily dose may be raised every week by 0.1 mg thyroxine, but immediately signs of overdosage appear (principally restlessness and polydipsia) the dose should be reduced by 0.1–0.2 mg thyroxine. Some bitches that have been in anoestrus for a year or more may develop severe endometrial hyperplasia in the first oestrus after their return to euthyroidism.

A check-up to establish satisfactory progress should be carried out at least every 6 months.

Thyroid hormone should not be used to correct obesity caused by overfeeding; any weight loss that ensues is more the result of protein breakdown than fat mobilisation, and in addition the normal hormonal feedback mechanism is disturbed (Anderson & Lewis 1980).

Neoplasia

The statement in Table 8.2 that goitre occurs in cases of primary neoplasia refers only to advanced and clinically significant neoplasia. However, over half the primary thyroid tumours are non-goitrous benign neoplasms (adenomas). These occur frequently in older dogs, produce no clinical signs and are only detected, if at all, at *post mortem* examination. The ratio of unilateral neoplastic goitre to bilateral is approximately 6:1.

Goitrous neoplasms are clinically significant because of the mechanical pressure they exert, their almost invariable malignancy (they are chiefly carcinomas) and the fact that they can cause changes in thyroid function. They occur mainly in middle-aged and elderly dogs (Fig. 8.6), especially of the larger breeds and particularly in the Boxer. The sexes appear to be equally affected.

Diagnosis

On palpation most neoplasms feel firm, even hard,

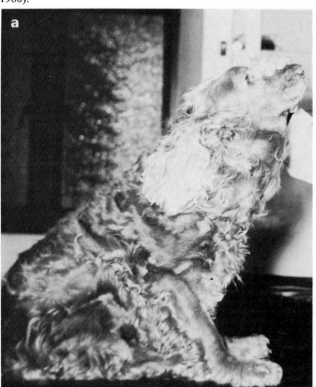
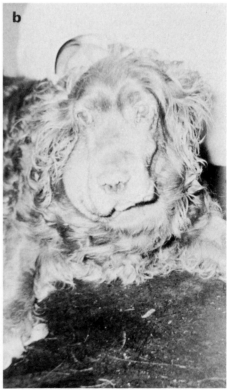

Fig. 8.6 A 12-year-old Cocker Spaniel bitch with a visible bilateral goitre, particularly affecting the right thyroid lobe. The cause was a mixed malignant neoplasm containing elements of spindle-cell sarcoma, haemangiosarcoma and anaplastic carcinoma. The goitre had been first noted only 3 months previously but approximately 25 lung metastases were already present. (a) Lateral view; (b) anterior view, to show the extent of the goitre.

although cystic structures usually have a soft consistency. They are seldom painful. Before they become invasive they can be moved, by palpation, up and down the trachea. An irregular goitre may be due to cyst formation or to extreme malignancy. Metastasis may occur via the lymph drainage to nearby lymph nodes and via the bloodstream, principally to the lungs (present in over 50% of cases). Neoplasia may also affect ectopic thyroid tissue, for example lower down the midline of the neck.

In most cases of thyroid neoplasia no change in functional status is seen. Very rarely bilateral malignant neoplasia, by destroying most of the thyroid follicles, will result in hypothyroidism (Fig 8.4). However, up to 20% of cases may be hyperthyroid due to autonomous hypersecretion of thyroid hormone by the neoplasm. Negative feedback suppresses TSH release and in animals with a unilateral tumour the contralateral lobe atrophies. In these cases the goitre is usually small (up to 5 cm in diameter) and the other principal clinical signs are polydipsia, loss of weight despite polyphagia, intolerance to heat, restlessness, nervousness and panting. Although the femoral pulse is forceful tachycardia is not a consistent feature. Confirmation of neoplasia is possible (by radioiodine scintigraphy, or the failure of the goitre to decrease in size following 2 weeks administration of thyroid hormone), but the probability that the goitre is neoplastic is so great, and the consequences of delay so potentially serious, that immediate removal of the affected lobe(s) is essential.

Treatment
If the tumour is small (3 cm or less) it can probably be easily removed without recurrence. Larger tumours, especially ones which have recently grown rapidly, are more likely to have metastasised. If radiographs confirm lung metastases removal of the thyroid tumour is probably not worthwhile. However if all the neoplastic tissue can be removed, including the cervical lymph nodes if enlarged, a complete cure is possible which gives 2–3 more years of life. Unfortunately in many cases, particularly those due to follicular carcinomas, metastasis has occurred and/or remnants of the original tumour regrow within a few months. Where bilateral neoplasia exists removal of both thyroid lobes requires in addition to subsequent thyroid hormone administration either retaining some intact parathyroid tissue together with its blood supply, which can prove difficult, or undertaking substitution therapy with dihydrotachysterol and calcium lactate. For this reason cases of bilateral neoplasia are often regarded as inoperable, as are cases of very extensive or invasive neoplasia.

The use of radioiodine, to destroy the neoplastic cells of inoperable tumours, metastases and those lobes where only subtotal resection is possible, is limited to licensed centres and to be successful also requires an adequate uptake which does not occur with all tumour types (e.g. solid carcinomas).

Following surgery or radiotherapy, thyroxine administration should be instituted both to maintain normal hormone levels and to decrease the possible stimulatory effects of TSH on tumour growth.

Hypercalcitoninism
Calcitonin-secreting medullary carcinomas, associated with such clinical signs as polyuria/polydipsia and long-standing watery diarrhoea, have been reported in the dog, although this type of neoplasm, involving the C cells of the thyroid gland, appears to be comparatively rare.

A high calcium diet, by stimulating the increased secretion of gastrin, can evoke hypercalcitoninism which leads eventually to hypocalcaemia and the development of skeletal defects (Krook 1977).

PARATHYROID GLANDS

In the dog there are two pairs of parathyroid glands lying in apposition to the thyroid lobes. The larger external glands are oval and about 2–5 mm long. They lie in front of, and slightly lateral to, the upper pole of the thyroid lobe. Each internal gland is smaller and flatter and lies on the medial (tracheal) surface of the thyroid lobe. Accessory glands may at times be present anywhere down the neck to the base of the heart. The parathyroid glands consist of one type of cell, the chief cell, which produces a single hormone (parathyroid hormone or parathormone, PTH). After synthesis the hormone is stored as secretory granules in the chief cells before release. Its function is to maintain the fine regulation of the blood calcium level between 2 and 3 mmol/l (8–12 mg/100 ml) (Fig. 8.7). Blood calcium concentration is also influenced by calcitonin and vitamin D3 (which current opinion regards as a hormone).

There is no nervous or feedback control of PTH production and secretion; these are regulated by the ionised calcium (and to a lesser extent magnesium) concentration in the blood passing through the parathyroid glands. A high calcium level causes reduced PTH release, and conversely a low calcium level increases PTH release.

PTH rapidly exerts an effect on bone and kidney. In bone it increases osteocytic and osteoblastic activity and also, although later, the number of osteoclasts

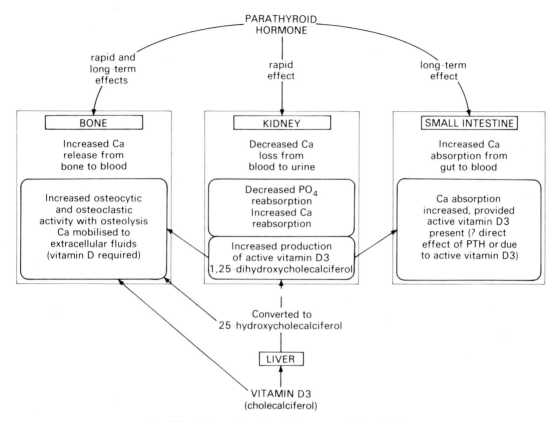

Fig. 8.7 Actions of parathyroid hormone and vitamin D3.

which results in increased bone resorption (osteolysis). Calcium flows from deep in the bone to the bone surfaces and into the extracellular fluids. In the long term the number of osteoblasts may also be increased, but bone resorption always exceeds formation. For PTH to affect bone cells in this way a small amount of vitamin D3, in any stage of its metabolism, must be present.

In the kidney PTH decreases phosphate reabsorption in the proximal tubules and consequently there is increased excretion of phosphate (and sodium, potassium, and bicarbonate) ions. PTH also increases the reabsorption of calcium in the distal tubules so that there is decreased excretion of calcium (and also magnesium, ammonia and hydrogen) ions. In addition PTH promotes the final metabolic stage in the production of active vitamin D3 (1,25-dihydroxycholecalciferol). These effects result in increased blood calcium levels.

Its long-term effect on the small intestine is to increase calcium absorption, provided active vitamin D3 is present. This may be either a direct effect of PTH or

follow from the increased production of active vitamin D3 by the kidney.

Disorders of the parathyroid glands

Hyperparathyroidism
This term embraces four conditions in which there is increased PTH production (Table 8.5). In primary hyperparathyroidism (PHPT) and pseudohyperparathyroidism (PS-HPT) the production of PTH is autonomous and unrelated to pre-existing serum calcium levels, which rise in consequence. In renal secondary and nutritional secondary hyperparathyroidism (RS-HPT and NS-HPT) PTH is produced in response to lowered calcium levels and is often able to restore them to within the normal range. Usually the highest calcium levels and most marked bone changes are seen in cases of PHPT, although this condition is not as commonly encountered as PS-HPT. It is stated (Siegel 1977) that the administration of corticosteroids may lower the calcium level in cases of PS-HPT but

Table 8.5 Differential diagnosis of hypercalcaemia (HCa) and hyperparathyroidism (HPT). Adapted from Osborne & Stevens (1973) and Capen & Martin (1977).
N, values within normal range; ↑, increased; ↓, decreased; * this condition is rarely seen in animals above 1 year old and high SAP values are expected in all growing animals.

		Serum Ca	Serum PO$_4$	SAP	
HCa	Hypervitaminosis D	↑	↑	N	
	Bone metastases from malignant neoplasm	↑	N to ↑	N to ↑	
	Primary HPT	↑	↓ if uraemic	N to ↑	HPT
	Pseudo HPT (ectopic PTH)	↑	↓ N to ↑	N to ↑	
	Renal secondary HPT	N to ↓	↑	N to ↑	
	Nutritional secondary HPT	N to ↓	N to ↑	↑*	

Notes. (1) Normal ranges: serum Ca = 2–3 mmol/l (8–12 mg/100 ml); serum PO$_4$ = 0.8–1.8 mmol/l (2.5–3.5 mg/100 ml); serum alkaline phosphatase (SAP) = < 12KA units/100 ml. (2) Varying degrees of demineralisation occur in HPT, most severe in the primary form. Localised demineralisation occurs with bone metastases, and demineralisation is usually absent (or mild) in hypervitaminosis D.

not in PHPT; the so-called 'steroid suppression test'. Radioimmunoassay of the level of serum PTH has not been routinely employed and values vary according to the method. Using a commercial assay Feldman and Krutzik (1981) found normal dogs to have PTH levels of 65–213 μl Eq/ml, cases with PHPT had slightly higher levels but dogs with RS-HPT, associated with chronic renal failure, generally showed marked elevations with PTH levels between 400 and 2500 μl Eq/ml. (Cases of hypoparathyroidism demonstrated PTH levels below 50 μl Eq/ml.)

The effects of hypercalcaemia are seen in PHPT and PS-HPT, and also in hypervitaminosis D (due to overadministration) and where malignant neoplasms metastasise to bone with increased osteolysis. (Hypercalcaemia can also be a feature of hypoadrenocorticism (Willard *et al* 1982).) High serum calcium levels result in anorexia, vomiting, depression and occasionally constipation (due to intestinal atony). There is generalised muscular weakness, because of decreased neuromuscular excitability. Polyuria and secondary polydipsia, together with dehydration (as a sequel to emesis and polyuria) are commonly seen. Bradycardia, cardiac arrhythmia and ECG abnormalities (often a prolonged PR interval and a shortened QT interval) may also develop. With the excessive passage of calcium through the nephrons the renal deposition of calcium occurs, initially in the medulla and collecting ducts and later in all regions. There is also increased likelihood of calcium uroliths forming (calcium oxalate and calcium phosphate) and of other soft tissue

mineralisation. Marked nephrocalcinosis will show radiographically as increased density and will lead ultimately to chronic renal failure (see Chapter 15).

PHPT (or PS-HPT) resulting in chronic renal failure can be distinguished from chronic renal failure resulting in RS-HPT by the high serum calcium levels in the former, whereas in the latter hypercalcaemia is rare and serum calcium levels are usually normal or slightly lower than normal.

A hypercalcaemic crisis (calcium levels above 3.75–5 mmol/l (15–20 mg/100 ml)), which can prove rapidly fatal, should be treated by the correction of dehydration and the lowering of serum calcium levels. The latter is achieved by peritoneal dialysis (see Chapter 15), and/or the administration of either sodium citrate (100 mg/kg body weight per day orally in divided dosage) or frusemide to produce increased excretion of calcium, and/or the administration of phosphate preparations to promote calcium deposition, provided that blood phosphate levels are not raised (e.g. sodium phosphate 150 mg/kg body weight per day orally in divided dosage).

The effect of PTH on bone is that mineral (chiefly calcium phosphate) is removed and replaced by fibrous connective tissue (fibrous osteodystrophy) throughout the skeleton, but especially in the cancellous bone of the skull. In the mandible and maxilla the bone becomes softened, so-called 'rubber-jaw', and there is loosening and loss of teeth from the alveolar sockets. In older dogs the volume of the bone remains the same but in younger dogs it is often increased producing facial hyperostosis.

Structural weakening of bone results in the occurrence of fractures (often of the compression type in the vertebrae and long bones) after comparatively minor trauma.

Radiographs show subperiosteal resorption of bone and a generalised decrease in bone density, plus in severe cases bone cysts and fractures. These changes are most marked in PHPT.

The aetiology, characteristic features and treatment of the conditions which initiate these changes are described overleaf.

Primary hyperparathyroidism (PHPT)
There is autonomous hypersecretion of PTH from either a parathyroid neoplasm (benign or malignant), or from all four hyperplastic parathyroid glands. Most commonly the lesion is a single adenoma, which can at times arise in ectopic parathyroid tissue near the base of the heart. The condition of PHPT is rare, though more likely in older animals. There is no evidence that in the dog long-standing secondary hyper-

parathyroidism can also result in autonomous PTH secretion ('tertiary hyperparathyroidism').

The parathyroids should be inspected to establish whether there is marked enlargement of 1–3 glands (indicative of neoplasia and requiring total surgical removal of the affected glands) or enlargement of all four glands (suggesting hyperplasia, in which case 3–$3\frac{1}{2}$ glands should be removed). If all the glands appear normal the base of the heart may be explored for evidence of ectopic neoplasia.

In all instances it is vital to retain some parathyroid tissue intact with a competent blood supply. The blood calcium level may fall rapidly after removal of a neoplasm because of decreased bone resorption, accelerated calcium deposition and the previous long-standing suppression of the remaining chief cells. Ideally calcium levels should be monitored and abnormally low levels corrected by the intravenous infusion of calcium gluconate, or preferably calcium borogluconate, and dietary supplementation with calcium salts (e.g. calcium lactate) and vitamin D3.

Pseudohyperparathyroidism (PS-HPT)

This condition results from the excessive production of PTH, or other bone-resorbing substances by a malignant tumour of non-parathyroid tissue. Most cases in the dog have been associated with lymphosarcoma (malignant lymphoma) but there are reports of cases occurring in association with perirectal and perianal adenocarcinomas. All the parathyroid glands are atrophied and the thyroid gland contains prominent areas of C cell hyperplasia. Wherever possible the removal of the offending neoplasm is desirable, followed by monitoring of the blood calcium level and if necessary its correction by calcium and vitamin D administration, as described for PHPT. Corticosteroids may produce a reduction in the serum calcium level, and chemotherapy (e.g. with cyclophosphamide) has also been advocated.

Renal secondary hyperparathyroidism (RS-HPT)

This condition arises in renal failure due to the reduced glomerular filtration rate and continual phosphate release by protein catabolism, both of which contribute to a build-up of serum phosphate. When the serum is saturated with respect to both phosphate and calcium ions a continued increase in one results in a reciprocal decrease in the other (as stated by the mass-law equation). Consequently the serum calcium level falls. In addition renal damage decreases the conversion of vitamin D3 to its active form, and this in turn leads to decreased intestinal absorption of calcium (see Chapter 14). In response to the resultant hypocalcaemia all

four parathyroid glands become hypertrophied, and then hyperplastic, and the output of PTH is increased. By the increase in bone resorption the calcium level is frequently restored to within the normal range, but the phosphate level continues to be elevated.

The treatment required is basically that for chronic renal failure plus supplementation with vitamin D3 and calcium salts, e.g. 10% calcium gluconate, or preferably 10% borogluconate (10–50 ml depending on body weight) by slow intravenous injection, or calcium lactate orally (40 mg/kg body weight per day).

Nutritional secondary hyperparathyroidism (NS-HPT) (juvenile osteoporosis; osteogenesis imperfecta)

The underlying defect in this condition is the lack of dietary calcium, which in practice is almost always aggravated by excess dietary phosphorus. This calcium-phosphorus imbalance is the result of feeding diets rich in meat products. For example the calcium:phosphorus ratio in liver is 1:50, heart 1:40 and horse meat 1:10, whereas the optimum dietary ratio is between 2:1 and 1.2:1. As in RS-HPT an increase in the serum phosphate level produces a reciprocal fall in the serum calcium concentration and PTH production is stimulated, resulting in bone resorption. This PTH release, combined with normal renal function, causes the calcium and phosphate levels to be adjusted to within, or near, the respective normal ranges.

The condition virtually only occurs between 3 and 12 months of age, with most cases being presented when the animals are 6–7 months old (Fig. 8.8).

Lameness is usually the major presenting sign, with pain and weakness especially evident in the hindquarters. Affected animals are unwilling to move, and they take short, hesitant steps. There is splaying of the toes, swelling of the carpus, and the metacarpal and metatarsal bones lie in the horizontal, rather than the vertical, plane.

Clinically this condition may be confused with the now rare disorder of rickets in which both calcium and phosphate levels are low, but is readily distinguished radiographically. One of the main features is that in rickets there is an irregular increase in the thickness of the epiphyseal growth plates whereas in NS-HPT these appear normal (see Chapter 6). The oral administration of aluminium hydroxide gel (or basic aluminium carbonate suspension) to inhibit phosphate absorption, plus dietary supplementation with calcium lactate or calcium borogluconate, have been used as therapy but often it is sufficient to substitute a nutritionally balanced diet (e.g. one which has been commercially prepared) for that containing excessive amounts of meat products. Bone meal, or other calcium supplements with high phosphate levels, should not be used

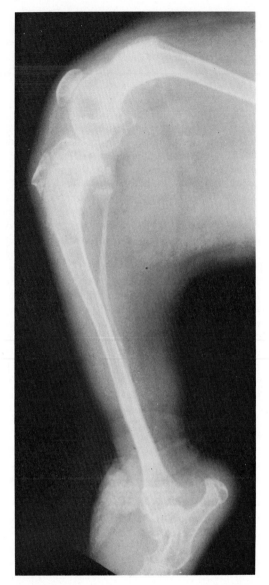

Fig. 8.8 Lateral radiograph of the right hindlimb of a 6-month-old crossbred bitch affected with nutritional secondary hyperparathyroidism. There is evidence of defective demineralisation with thin cortical bone and fractures of the femur and tibia.

and corticosteroids are contraindicated because they further reduce serum calcium levels.

Hypoparathyroidism

This condition is much less common than hyperparathyroidism. It is thought to occur more often in the small terriers, Poodles and Schnauzers, particularly between 2 and 5 years old. Possible aetiologies include agenesis of the parathyroid glands, their removal or damage (including interference to their blood supply) during surgery (particularly of the thyroid lobes), destruction by neoplasia, and parathyroid atrophy in cases of prolonged hypercalcaemia. Other cases, designated idiopathic, may be due to lack of an enzyme required for the synthesis of PTH, or to an auto-immune reaction resulting in lymphocytic parathyroiditis. The latter appears to be the more frequent cause. (Sherding *et al* 1980).

Inadequate PTH production causes an increase in the serum phosphate level, following increased tubular reabsorption of this ion, and a fall in the serum calcium content, due to decreased bone resorption. Polyuria and polydipsia are often evident and cataracts may appear. The low serum calcium level increases neuromuscular excitement and produces the clinical signs of hyperaesthesia, ataxia and weakness (especially when handled) which progress through muscular twitches to generalised tetany and convulsions. Usually the muscle tremors and tetany occur for periods ranging from a few hours to a week at a time. Mild hypocalcaemia can arise in association with a number of disorders (e.g. chronic renal failure, acute pancreatitis, malabsorption and other causes of hypoproteinaemia) but, apart from this condition, hypocalcaemia of sufficient severity to produce tetany appears to arise only in eclampsia (puerperal tetany) and ethylene glycol poisoning (Zenoble & Myers 1977).

The muscle spasms may be controlled in the short term by the intravenous administration of calcium borogluconate. In the long term, the administration of high doses of calcium (up to 5 g/day calcium gluconate) plus vitamin D3 (cholecalciferol) or vitamin D2 (ergocalciferol) (both in 625–2500 μg (25 000–100 000 iu)/day) or dihydrotachysterol (0.2–0.8 mg/day) can be effective. Calcium levels should be monitored every 3–4 months to check that they remain within normal limits.

ADRENAL GLANDS

In the dog each adrenal gland lies in front of and medial to the corresponding kidney; therefore the left gland is the more posterior. The medulla comprises the inner 10–20% of each gland and consists of chromaffin cells which produce the hormones noradrenaline and adrenaline (norepinephrine and epinephrine). Their effects on body organs are identical to those produced by the stimulation of the sympathetic nervous system. Both raise heart rate and systolic blood pressure and cause peripheral vasoconstriction, though noradrenaline is the more potent hypertensive agent. Adrenaline also increases cardiac output, glycogen breakdown in liver and muscle, fatty acid release and skeletal muscle tone, and has the effect of decreasing gut motility. The action of adrenaline and noradrenaline is short lived since they are soon inactivated. Both are regarded as 'emergency hormones' and the adrenal medulla is not essential to life. Functional tumours of the medulla, phaeochromocytomas (producing catecholamines which cause hypertension), appear to be extremely rare in the dog.

In contrast, the presence of the adrenal cortex is vital. This functionally discrete region of the gland surrounds the medulla and consists of three concentric layers: a peripheral zone (zona glomerulosa, comprising 25% of the total); a middle layer (zona fasciculata, 60%) and an inner layer (zona reticularis, 15%).

Table 8.6 Action of corticosteroids.

1 Glucocorticoid effects
On carbohydrate and protein metabolism
Increased glucose formation by gluconeogenesis (i.e. following increased protein breakdown)
Decreased glucose utilisation
Increased glycogen deposition in liver
Protein synthesis increased in liver but decreased elsewhere
  Therefore excess produces: atrophy of skeletal muscles and lymphatic tissue (with lymphopenia), thinning of skin, osteoporosis due to reduced protein matrix in bone and consequential calcium release, hyperglycaemia and negative nitrogen balance

On fat metabolism
Increased fat breakdown
Alteration in sites of fat deposition

On calcium balance
Increased calcium excretion by kidney
Inhibition of vitamin D3 thereby inhibiting calcium absorption

On blood cell production
Increased RBC formation
Increased formation of neutrophils
Decreased production of other WBCs
Possible reduction in levels of circulating antibodies

On inflammation
Prevents or suppresses inflammatory responses provoked by radiation, trauma, infectious agents or immune mechanisms (i.e. inhibits oedema, fibrin deposition, capillary dilatation, WBC migration, capillary and fibroblast proliferation, collagen deposition and cicatrisation)

On cell division
Inhibits or interrupts cell division (e.g. growth and repair)

2 Mineralocorticoid effects
Primarily on electrolytes
Acts on distal tubules of kidney: to increase sodium reabsorption (resulting in hypernatraemia and increased extravascular fluid volume); to increase bicarbonate reabsorption (resulting in alkalosis); and to decrease potassium reabsorption (resulting in hypokalaemia)

The adrenal cortex produces a number of steroid hormones belonging to two groups, the corticosteroids and the adrenal sex hormones (androgens, oestrogens and probably progestagens); the latter are produced only in minute amounts. The corticosteroids are the hormones essential for life. Individual corticosteroids vary in their ability to produce each of the two categories of effects characteristic of the entire group, namely glucocorticoid and mineralocorticoid effects (summarized in Table 8.6).

In the dog the two most important corticosteroids are cortisol (also known as hydrocortisone) which has mainly glucocorticoid effects and aldosterone which has primarily mineralocorticoid effects.

The zona glomerulosa appears to be the only site for the formation of aldosterone. The other two zones both have the capacity to synthesise sex hormones and cortisol, although the zona fasciculata is most concerned with glucocorticoid formation and the zona reticularis with androgen and oestrogen secretion.

Although adrenocorticotrophic hormone (ACTH) from the adenohypophysis has a transient effect on aldosterone production, the secretion of aldosterone is regulated chiefly by the renin–angiotensin system.

ACTH is virtually the exclusive factor controlling the formation of cortisol and androgens, and ACTH production in turn is regulated by corticotropin-releasing factor (CRF) produced by the hypothalamus. The formation of CRF is regulated by the following three factors:

1 Circadian (diurnal) rhythm, controlled by other parts of the central nervous system. This results in minimum cortisol production around midnight and maximum production in the early morning, around 6.00 am.
2 Negative feedback effect of cortisol on the hypothalamus and on the adenohypophysis which directly influences ACTH production.
3 Stress (excitement, fear, pain, injury, hypoglycaemia, pyrexia) which via other parts of the central nervous system increases the output of CRF and therefore ACTH and cortisol.

The first two regulating mechanisms are lost in hyperadrenocorticism (HAC).

Most of the effects of ACTH result from the increased output of adrenal cortex hormones which it stimulates, although increased melanin deposition in the skin (and possibly lipolysis also) is believed to be an independent direct effect. Without any ACTH release, glucocorticoid production is reduced to less than 10% of normal; possibly as little as 1%.

There is virtually no storage of corticosteroids

in the cortex; the rates of release and synthesis are therefore almost identical. In man cortisol is carried in the blood bound to plasma proteins; an alpha-globulin, designated 'transcortin' or corticosteroid-binding globulin, and albumin. All corticosteroids are rapidly removed from the blood by the liver and catabolised.

Disorders of the adrenal cortex

Although occasionally certain adrenocortical neoplasms produce excessive amounts of oestrogens or androgens (which results in feminising or masculinising effects respectively), the major disorders in the dog relate to overproduction or underproduction of glucocorticoids.

Hyperadrenocorticism (HAC; hyperadrenocorticalism; Cushing's syndrome)

Incidence
This disease, which is one of the most common endocrine disorders of the dog, is found in animals from 4 years of age onwards, particularly around 8 years of age. It is most commonly seen in Miniature and Toy Poodles, Boxers, Dachschunds and the small terrier breeds. Slightly more than half of affected animals are bitches. HAC may occur concurrently with hypothyroidism or diabetes mellitus.

Aetiology
Clinical signs arise principally from the excess of cortisol, which may or may not be due to excessive ACTH production. Increased secretion of ACTH occurs in about 85% of cases (pituitary-dependent HAC) causing bilateral adrenocortical hyperplasia. In the majority of these an autonomously secreting neoplasm of the ACTH-secreting cells of the adenohypophysis is probably responsible. Whereas carcinomas are usually large and readily detected at post mortem examination, the much more common adenomas may be microscopic and consequently not easily demonstrable. The other cases where there is overproduction of ACTH ('idiopathic cortical hyperplasia', occurring chiefly in Poodles) are considered to be due to some functional defect in the hypothalamus or adenohypophysis producing insensitivity to the usual negative feedback control. In most of the remaining 15% of dogs with HAC an autonomously secreting tumour (adenoma or carcinoma, and usually unilateral) of the adrenal cortex is responsible for the high blood cortisol level; affected animals are mainly elderly and three times more likely to be female. Due to the negative feedback effect, ACTH secretion is minimal and the cortex of the opposite gland is atrophied. Only one case attributable to both pituitary and adrenal neoplasia has been recorded (Cohen & Kniesşer 1980).

The long-term administration of glucocorticoids in high doses will also produce this disorder (iatrogenic HAC) and because ACTH production is suppressed there is bilateral adrenocortical atrophy. A single intramuscular injection of triamcinolone acetonide (therapeutic dose) will suppress adrenocortical function for 3–4 weeks, methylprednisolone acetate (1.7 times therapeutic dose) gives suppression for 5 weeks, whereas twice the therapeutic dose of prednisolone has no significant effect. However daily intramuscular injections of prednisolone at 4 times the therapeutic dose can result in clinical signs of HAC appearing after a week (Badylak & Van Vleet 1981; Kemppainen *et al* 1981, 1982).

Clinical signs and diagnosis
The major clinical sign, present in virtually every case, is polyuria with secondary polydipsia. This sign is generally attributed to interference with the production, release or action of ADH (probably its effect on the renal collecting tubules), and not to any accompanying damage to the neurohypophysis causing diabetes insipidus.

Many animals (80%) also show polyphagia. (Almost all dogs have at least a good appetite; an indifferent appetite is seldom encountered.) Polydipsia and polyphagia are of course common signs in animals being therapeutically overdosed with glucocorticoids; a situation which may lead to iatrogenic HAC. Their coexistence in the absence of glucocorticoid therapy is indicative of HAC and/or diabetes mellitus.

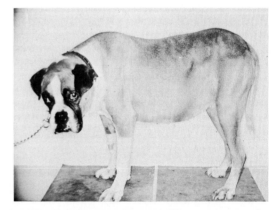

Fig. 8.9 A 4-year-old Boxer bitch with pituitary-mediated hyperadrenocorticism. Weakness of the abdominal muscles resulted in a pendulous abdomen and a pronounced depression between the shoulders and hindquarters. Alopecia and cutaneous hyperpigmentation affected the flanks and back.

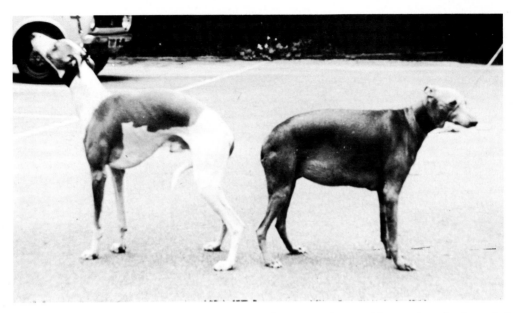

Fig. 8.10 Comparison of a normal 7-year-old male Whippet (left) with an 8½-year-old bitch of the same breed suffering from hyperadrenocorticism, to show the change in bodily contours.

Abdominal enlargement is also common, due to weakness of the abdominal musculature, liver enlargement and increased deposition of fat in the lumbar region. A lateral view shows the abdomen to have descended to, or below, the level of the sternum, and being distended it produces a barrel or 'pot-bellied' appearance (Figs. 8.9 and 8.10).

A high proportion (up to 90%) of dogs show one or more characteristic skin changes (Fig. 8.11). The skin is thin and superficial blood vessels are often clearly visible. There may be wrinkling due to loss of elasticity (as in a dehydrated animal) and follicular plugging with keratin. The latter results in numerous black comedomes over the central abdomen and this, plus increased scaliness, can give the skin the feel of fine sandpaper. Hyperpigmentation may be diffuse or occur in patches (macules) often surrounded by peeling keratin.

Approximately 75% of affected animals show a non-pruritic bilaterally symmetrical alopecia of varying degrees of intensity (see Table 8.3). The majority of hairs enter the telogen phase and there is atrophy of the hair follicles. This results in the easy removal of hairs and occurs first in those areas subjected to great-

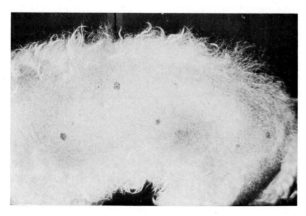

Fig. 8.11 Alopecia of flanks and thighs together with macules (circular pigmented areas) on the skin of an 8-year-old male Miniature Poodle affected with hyperadrenocorticism.

est friction (e.g. flanks, ventral abdomen, posterior thighs, and, if the dog wears a collar, around the neck). The loss may range from only slight thinning of the haircoat to complete hairlessness, except for hairs on the head and lower limbs. Such extensive alopecia may take a year to develop and is most common in the Miniature and Toy Poodles, Scottish Terrier, Skye Terrier, Dandie Dinmont and Cocker Spaniel. The skin may also bruise very easily, because of increased vascular fragility, so that haematomas appear after venepuncture, and wound healing is delayed due to the suppression of inflammatory responses. A number of animals show their dislike of warm surroundings and pant whilst at rest.

The deposition of calcium salts in the cutaneous and subcutaneous tissues ('calcinosis cutis') occurs in about 10% of cases and may be apparent as plaques in the skin, or be seen as erosions of the surface which can bleed and become secondarily infected. They may appear in the ventral midline but in larger breeds (especially the Boxer) the head and neck is often affected (Fig. 8.12). Deposition is thought to follow changes in the structure of collagen and elastin in the skin which attract, and promote the binding of, calcium salts. However hypercalcaemia is not present. The existence of calcinosis cutis, especially with other typical signs, is virtually diagnostic. Calcification can affect other soft tissues (e.g. respiratory tract, alimentary tract, but primarily the kidney pelvis) and if sufficiently prominent may show on radiographs, although this is rare. Osteoporosis is not usually marked in the dog but may be visible radiographically, particularly affecting the lumbar vertebral bodies. Radiography also shows liver enlargement in three-quarters of cases (Huntley *et al* 1982).

Muscular atrophy may be a prominent feature in some dogs, with obvious weakness of the abdominal muscles and wasting of the muscles of the head (Fig. 8.13) and limbs, which leads to trembling and difficulty in walking and climbing stairs. Often the owner reports that the animal can no longer jump, for example on to furniture or into the car. Because such animals prefer to remain recumbent ulceration of the thin skin covering the hocks and elbows is sometimes seen.

Approximately three-quarters of dogs with HAC are depressed and less active than previously. They show increased susceptibility to infection because of impaired inflammatory responses (and a reduction in circulating antibody levels). A number (20–30%) also show testicular atrophy or prolonged anoestrus.

Dogs with pituitary neoplasms may at a later stage show signs attributable to the pressure of the enlarging gland on adjacent areas of the brain, for example

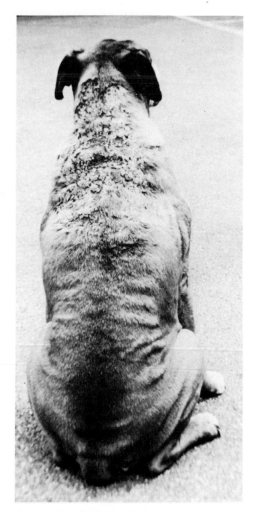

Fig. 8.12 Calcinosis cutis affecting the neck and shoulder region of a 9-year-old female Boxer with hyperadrenocorticism.

apparent blindness, aimless pacing or head pressing against a wall, and difficulty in orientating themselves in familiar surroundings. Rarely signs may appear which are attributable to the invasion or metastasis of an adrenal tumour.

Conditions from which HAC particularly needs to be distinguished are:

1 Hypothyroidism, since many dogs with HAC are depressed and show lowered T4 levels.
2 Acromegaly in bitches, especially in view of the polyphagia, polydipsia, exercise intolerance and increased abdominal size in conjunction with an elevated SAP level and hyper-responsiveness to ACTH stimulation.

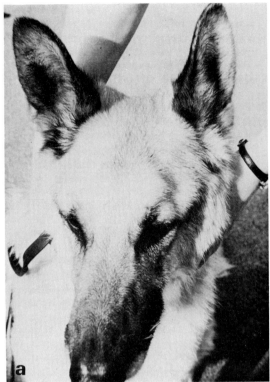

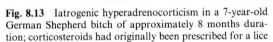

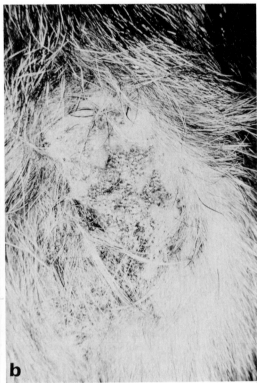

Fig. 8.13 Iatrogenic hyperadrenocorticism in a 7-year-old German Shepherd bitch of approximately 8 months duration; corticosteroids had originally been prescribed for a lice infestation. (a) Marked wasting of the facial muscles, temporals, pterygoids and masseters; (b) erosion of the skin on the flank due to calcinosis cutis.

3 Feminisation in males, because the skin changes appear similar.
4 Other causes of polyuria and polydipsia.
5 Conditions producing ascites.

Diagnostic tests
On routine laboratory scanning tests the most important single diagnostic feature is eosinopenia. The absolute level of eosinophils is usually below 200/mm³ and in the majority of cases no eosinophils are found on the differential WBC count. Lymphopenia (often less than 1500/mm³ and less than 15% on the differential WBC count) usually, but not always, accompanies the eosinopenia. The differential WBC count shows a neutrophilia, due in part to a true increase in absolute numbers and in part to the decreased numbers of eosinophils and lymphocytes. The total number of white blood cells may be elevated but usually not sufficiently to put values outside the normal range (e.g. above 17000/mm³).

Half of the dogs with HAC show an increased level of cholesterol (above 7.8 mmol/l (300 mg/100 ml)), many have an elevated level of alanine aminotransferase (serum glutamic pyruvic transaminase), and all show an elevated level of serum alkaline phosphatase due to the induction of a particular isoenzyme from the liver by the glucocorticoid. Blood glucose levels are usually normal or only slightly raised unless there is accompanying diabetes mellitus. HAC predisposes to the development of diabetes mellitus (DM) and dogs with slight hyperglycaemia should be watched for the later appearance of DM. Such animals show the typical diabetic response to a glucose tolerance test. Poodles are especially likely to suffer from both disorders. In general, the levels of sodium, potassium, calcium and phosphate show no change from normal though almost half of those animals with HAC due to adrenal neoplasia have a blood potassium level of 3.5 mmol/l or less. As would be expected the urinary specific gravity is low.

Specific tests of adrenal function involve measuring either the level of blood cortisol or the urinary output of 17-hydroxycorticosteroids (17-OHCS). However urinary 17-OHCS estimations have proved to be less valuable than those of plasma cortisol.

The radioimmunoassay (RIA) of cortisol is the most

sensitive and accurate method of cortisol measurement. Estimation by fluorimetric determinations are not specific to cortisol and will include other glucocorticoids plus certain other substances which fluoresce. The most important of these is the diuretic spironolactone which should therefore be avoided prior to testing. Estimation by competitive protein binding (CPB) is more specific for cortisol though there is some cross-reactivity with exogenous corticosteroids such as prednisolone, which similarly should be avoided. In general values obtained with fluorimetric techniques are higher than those obtained with CPB or RIA methods.

Unfortunately a 'resting' cortisol level alone is almost never diagnostic because there is a considerable overlap between the range of values commonly found in normal and HAC animals. However if the value is above 330 nmol/l (12 µg/100 ml) it is reasonably certain (and if above 410 nmol/l (15 µg/100 ml) definite) that HAC exists.*

Usually greater discrimination is provided if estimations are repeated after the administration of ACTH (ACTH stimulation test) and/or after dosing with dexamethasone (dexamethasone screening and suppression tests). In addition these tests can enable the cause of the HAC to be determined. Different investigators have used different procedures for these tests; the most common are given below. (Although it might be desirable to assess the result of one test before proceeding to another it is usually more convenient to perform them consecutively and then despatch all the plasma samples to the laboratory at the same time.) Ideally all tests should be started at 9 am with 24 hours between tests. All blood samples should be collected into lithium heparin tubes; usually 5 ml of blood is sufficient but this should be checked with the laboratory beforehand.

1 Distinguishing normal and HAC dogs

ACTH stimulation test. A baseline blood sample is collected and immediately thereafter 0.25 mg tetracosactrin as Synacthen (*not* Synacthen Depot) injected either intravenously or intramuscularly. A second blood sample is collected 2 hours later.

Normal dogs will show an increased cortisol level post-ACTH, but in all cases of pituitary-dependent HAC and many with adrenal neoplasia there is a hyper-response. Values above 550 nmol/l (20 µg/100 ml) are almost always, and values above 970 nmol/l (35 µg/100 ml) always, diagnostic of HAC.†

Unless the dog has been treated with a corticosteroid, which will be estimated by the test method (e.g. cortisol itself), cortisol levels in iatrogenic cases of HAC will be very low (often less than 55 nmol/l (2 µg/100 ml)) initially and barely doubled post-ACTH.

The major problem with this test is that over a third of HAC cases due to adrenal neoplasia show the same order of response to ACTH stimulation as normal dogs. A few cases with adrenal neoplasia show very little increase in cortisol levels and such a finding has diagnostic significance. Repeat tests have also demonstrated that the response of tumours is not necessarily consistent because of spontaneous fluctuations in their secretion of cortisol (Chastain *et al* 1978; Feldman 1981; Peterson *et al* 1982b).

Dexamethasone screening test (as an alternative to the ACTH stimulation test). A baseline blood sample is collected and then 0.01 mg dexamethasone/kg body weight is injected intravenously. Because of the low dose involved this is most conveniently done by adding the contents of a 1 ml vial containing 5 mg dexamethasone/ml (Oradexon injection) to 9 ml isotonic saline, and with a tuberculin syringe injecting 0.02 ml of this dilution /kg body weight. A second blood sample is taken after 8 hours and a cortisol level above 40 nmol/l (1.5 µg/100 ml) is indicative of HAC.

2 Distinguishing pituitary-dependent HAC from adrenal neoplasia HAC

Dexamethasone suppression test. This test is performed initially exactly as is the dexamethasone *screening* test except that 10 times the dose of dexamethasone is employed, i.e. the dog can be injected with 0.2 ml/kg body weight of the diluted dexamethasone solution prepared previously. Blood samples are then collected after 3 and 8 hours. If only one of these demonstrates a cortisol level that is at least 50% lower than the baseline level it indicates pituitary-dependent HAC (in normal dogs *both* samples show this degree of suppression). If the cortisol level in both samples is *more* than 50% of the baseline value it may be due to either an adrenal tumour or incompletely-suppressible pituitary-dependent HAC, usually due to a pituitary neoplasm (Meijer 1980). The ultimate differentiation between these is then usually made by exploratory laparotomy.

A combined dexamethasone suppression and

---

* To convert cortisol values expressed in µg/100 ml to nmol/l multiply by 27.6.
† Where 0.25 mg of tetracosactide (Cortrosyn; Organon Inc., West

Orange, New Jersey, USA—not available in the UK) is injected intramuscularly and a sample taken after 1 hour, values above 825 nmol/l estimated by RIA or above 970 nmol/l estimated fluorimetrically are indicative of HAC.

ACTH stimulation test has also been devised (Eiler & Oliver 1980).

Although the measurement of ACTH levels by RIA in dogs is not yet routinely performed it is capable of distinguishing HAC caused by adrenal neoplasia (low values) from pituitary-dependent HAC (high or high-normal values) (Feldman *et al* 1978; Feldman 1981). Gamma camera imaging is also capable of distinguishing between these possible causes.

Treatment

Obviously in cases due to overadministration of a corticosteroid the drug should be gradually withdrawn. In other cases adrenalectomy, hypophysectomy or chemotherapy may be employed.

Adrenalectomy. This is the treatment of choice for an adrenal tumour (which is usually unilateral). If there is strong evidence, either from adrenal function tests or from the failure of hypophysectomy or chemotherapy to control the condition, that the HAC is due to neoplasia an exploratory laparotomy can be performed. The finding of an obvious enlargement of one gland combined with atrophy of the other appears diagnostic although from their gross appearance alone sometimes there is difficulty in distinguishing between cortical neoplasia and nodular hyperplasia. The bilateral paracostal approach is preferable to ventral midline laparotomy.

A suspected unilateral neoplasm should be completely removed if this is feasible (i.e. if there is no local invasion). If uniform bilateral enlargement is discovered it is suggestive of pituitary-dependent HAC and although adrenalectomy might appear to be the logical course of action, since it would eliminate cortisol production, bilateral adrenalectomy prevents the production of mineralocorticoids as well as glucocorticoids. It has been found more important to replace mineralocorticoids than glucocorticoids, unless hypoglycaemia subsequently develops when they should also be administered. Unfortunately many patients do not survive long after bilateral adrenalectomy, although some surgeons have been more successful than others. During the operation intravenous isotonic saline infusions with added steroids (cortisol sodium succinate 50–100 mg) is essential. Later this is replaced by oral fludrocortisone acetate (Florinef) 0.06 mg/kg body weight twice daily for the remainder of the animal's life. In addition, intramuscular ACTH gel (Acthar) is given for a few days postoperatively. The dosage can be regulated by reference to the plasma levels of sodium and potassium; 50 mg/kg body weight of sodium chloride should be given orally each day. Unilateral adrenalectomy will not be adequate therapy in cases of bilateral hyperplasia, and neither unilateral nor bilateral adrenalectomy will prevent the growth of a pituitary tumour and its subsequent pressure on the brain.

Hypophysectomy. This has been adopted mainly by Dutch veterinarians as an improvement on adrenalectomy in pituitary-mediated cases, although a number of animals (approximately 20%) have died in the critical immediate postoperative stage. Initially substitution therapy is with thyroid hormone, cortisol and ADH, although later the ADH which is still produced by the hypothalamus can be omitted. Approximately 45% of dogs show complete recovery and 20% partial or delayed recovery. Usually polyphagia, and then polyuria, disappear and within the first few months animals become more active and alert and show new hair growth. After this operation many bitches either remain in anoestrus or have abnormal cycles. In about 15% of cases there is no improvement. The procedure demands considerable technical skill. It removes the possibility of further pituitary tumour growth, unless there are tissue remnants, but is unable to influence HAC due to adrenal neoplasia.

Chemotherapy. Undoubtedly this is the treatment of choice for veterinary surgeons in private practice without specialised surgical skill or the facilities for extensive postoperative treatment (Fig. 8.14). Of the drugs so far used in the dog to treat HAC (Lubberink 1977) only mitotane (*op'*DDD; Lysodren) has proved effective.

Mitotane destroys the adrenal cortex; most markedly in the two innermost zones. The oral dose commonly employed is 50 mg/kg body weight given daily for 10 days and then at weekly intervals for a fortnight, then every two weeks for life. Nausea, vomiting, diarrhoea and anorexia may be apparent after approximately 5 days' treatment, and these have been attributed to the sudden change from HAC to low cortisol levels. It is advisable therefore to also administer cortisol orally (Hydrocortone) at the rate of 1.5 mg/kg body weight per day beginning on the third day of treatment and finishing 1 week after the initial 10-day course of mitotane. However some authors believe that these signs are attributable to gastrointestinal irritation caused by the drug and that they can be avoided or minimised by giving each day's treatment in divided dosage. Reported side-effects also include depression, weakness and occasionally neurological signs, which may be wrongly attributed to a pituitary neoplasm.

Successful treatment results in reversal of the clinical signs (in the same order described above in the

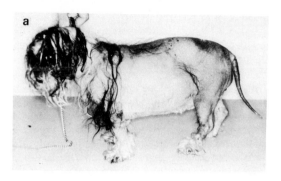

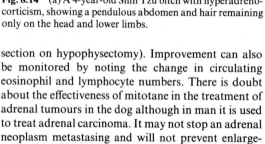

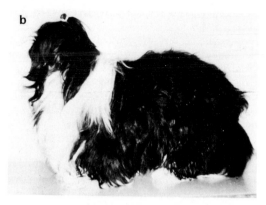

Fig. 8.14   (a) A 4-year-old Shih Tzu bitch with hyperadreno-corticism, showing a pendulous abdomen and hair remaining only on the head and lower limbs.

(b) The same animal 15 months later following continuous mitotane therapy.

section on hypophysectomy). Improvement can also be monitored by noting the change in circulating eosinophil and lymphocyte numbers. There is doubt about the effectiveness of mitotane in the treatment of adrenal tumours in the dog although in man it is used to treat adrenal carcinoma. It may not stop an adrenal neoplasm metastasing and will not prevent enlargement of a pituitary tumour.

In any animal sudden collapse during the initial treatment period is indicative of excessive adrenal suppression and should be corrected immediately by administration of glucocorticoids (preferably by injection), cessation of mitotane therapy and its gradual reintroduction only when polyuria recurs (using a reduced dose of mitotane combined with oral cortisol; 1.5 mg/kg body weight per day).

Treatment for other aspects of the disease (e.g. liver dysfunction, skin erosions due to calcinosis cutis) should be given simultaneously. Where there is concurrent DM an animal will initially have very high insulin requirements which will fall precipitously as soon as mitotane therapy commences. In such instances the initial dose of mitotane should be reduced and supplemented with cortisol to avoid serious hypoglycaemia (Peterson *et al* 1981).

The progress of the animal needs to be reassessed at regular intervals. Depression may occur subsequently due to either under- or overdosing. The presence or absence of polyuria/polydipsia provides the simplest means of differentiation, although reassessment of eosinophil, SAP and cortisol levels provides confirmation. Usually maintaining the same dose of mitotane but increasing or decreasing the interval between doses, as appropriate, is easier for the owner to understand. Where overdosing has occurred further mito-

tane should not be given until polydipsia reappears, and in severe cases prednisolone (0.3 mg/kg body weight/day) should be administered until there is a clinical improvement. Approximately 80% of pituitary-dependent cases make a good recovery, but in only half of these is it maintained for longer than 2 years. In some, central nervous system signs occur later, attributable to the enlargement of a pituitary tumour following reduction of the cortisol levels which removes inhibition of its growth (Schaer 1979). Some animals develop a lack of response to mitotane despite an increasing frequency of administration.

Hypoadrenocorticism (hypoadrenocorticalism; primary cases = Addison's disease)
This is a disease of dogs often undiagnosed in practice which generally affects animals less than 8 years old, especially those around 4 years old. Three-quarters of affected animals are bitches but there is no known breed incidence. The features of Addison's disease are non-specific and easily confused with those of renal or gastrointestinal diseases.

Aetiology
The majority of cases are primary (i.e. with adreno-cortical damage and a reduced output of both mineralocorticoids and glucocorticoids). Of these 90% show bilateral cortical atrophy, believed to be due to an autoimmune mechanism. Such cases are described as idiopathic. Less common causes are destruction of the cortices by neoplastic metastases, amyloidosis, chronic inflammation and fibrosis (including fibrosis following extensive haemorrhage) and thrombosis of the adrenal vessels. The disease may also follow treatment of HAC with mitotane or adrenalectomy.

Destructive lesions of the pituitary or hypothalamus

can result in reduced ACTH secretion and secondary hypoadrenocorticism, with the reduced secretion of glucocorticoids alone. The sudden cessation of long-term corticosteroid administration which has suppressed ACTH production, or the exposure of animals on long-term corticosteroid therapy to acute stress (e.g. infection or trauma), can have the same effects and in cases of overdosage will be accompanied by signs of iatrogenic HAC (Scott 1980).

Clinical signs and diagnosis

Clinical signs may be sudden in onset (shock and renal failure) or develop progressively. In the latter instance hormone levels may only be clearly inadequate at times of stress (trauma, other illness, surgery) resulting in the characteristic 'waxing and waning' of signs.

The lack of glucocorticoids results in anorexia in three-quarters of cases, vomiting in two-thirds, and depression in approximately one-half (Willard *et al* 1982). It can also be responsible for muscular weakness with trembling, diarrhoea and abdominal pain. Aldosterone deficiency causes increased excretion of sodium (accompanied by chloride, bicarbonate and water) and increased retention of potassium. Often, though not in every case, the serum sodium level is below 135 mmol/l and that of potassium above 5.5 mmol/l, leading to a sodium: potassium ratio of less than 27:1 which is diagnostically valuable. The increased potassium level initiates typical ECG changes (peaked T waves, flattened P waves and increased QT intervals) and, if severe, bradycardia (less than 70 beats/minute). Increased fluid loss provokes dehydration and weight loss, a reduction in blood pressure, cardiac output and heart size (discernible on radiographs), and decreased renal perfusion leading to prerenal acute renal failure (see Chapter 15). In some animals the increased fluid loss produces obvious polyuria and polydipsia and the femoral pulse may be weak. Ultimately there is peripheral circulatory collapse known as an 'Addisonian crisis'. Chronic cases most commonly show anorexia, vomiting, depression and muscular weakness of fluctuating severity.

Diagnostic tests

As well as the changes in sodium and potassium levels an increased number of eosinophils occurs in some, though not all, affected animals (more than 1250/mm³, corrected for dehydration) and absolute lymphocytosis may also occur (more than 4800/mm³, corrected for dehydration). Hypercalcaemia may be present.

Three-quarters of cases show azotaemia (increased blood levels of urea and creatinine). However the most valuable diagnostic test which can be performed is the ACTH stimulation test previously described. The initial ('resting') cortisol level is usually well below 135 nmol/l (5 µg/100 ml), although it may be higher measured fluorimetrically, and, most significantly, the cortisol level 1 hour after Synacthen injection shows no or very little increase (certainly not as much as three-fold) and generally does not rise above 190 nmol/l (7 µg/100 ml). Indeed with the stress of the test the cortisol level often falls.

ACTH assay by RIA will discriminate between primary cases (very high levels) and secondary cases (very low levels).

Treatment

Acute cases: Addisonian crisis. Emergency treatment of a collapsed animal is essential. If the history is consistent with this disorder blood samples should first be collected (for haematology, sodium, potassium, urea, glucose and cortisol estimation and ideally through an intravenous catheter), one 0.25 mg vial Synacthen should be injected intramuscularly and immediately thereafter sufficient 0.9% saline solution infused intravenously to correct the dehydration. The required amount of fluid is 10 ml/kg body weight for each 1% deficiency. It is preferable to leave an indwelling catheter in the bladder during this procedure to check that the animal is not anuric. If urine is not produced frusemide should be administered (see acute renal failure, Chapter 15). After 1 hour a second blood sample for cortisol estimation is collected (ACTH stimulation sample). Then corticosteroids can be administered; a soluble glucocorticoid by slow intravenous injection (cortisol sodium succinate (Solu–Cortef) at 7 mg/kg body weight repeated in 4 hours if necessary) and a long-acting (3–4 week) mineralocorticoid given intramuscularly (deoxycortone pivalate (Percorten M) 6 mg/kg body weight).

Further intravenous saline may be necessary to replace fluid losses during the following days.

This regimen allows samples to be collected unaffected by treatment, and the therapy will not prove harmful if the crisis is later shown not to be Addisonian. If there is evidence which suggests, or confirms, hyperkalaemia (e.g. bradycardia, ECG findings, blood level) or acidosis (e.g. uraemia established with a rapid blood urea test, such as Urastrat) treatment should be given with, respectively, intravenous dextrose and intravenous bicarbonate solutions (see acute renal failure, Chapter 15).

Chronic cases (maintenance therapy following crisis, or in absence of crisis). Oral mineralocorticoid treatment with fludrocortisone acetate is given, initially at the rate of 0.1–0.5 mg/day depending on size. This dose can be gradually raised if routine sodium and potassium estimations show that levels have not yet returned to within their respective normal ranges. The minimum dose required to maintain normal electrolyte levels is given daily thereafter and will probably require little adjustment throughout the rest of the animal's life. Additional salt (1–5 g/day as tablets or in the diet) should be provided, and additional glucocorticoids are required if anorexia and lethargy persist (e.g. prednisolone 0.3 mg/kg body weight per day normally, but doubled or trebled at times of stress).

Only if vomiting occurs is it *necessary* to use injectable preparations but an alternative treatment is the long-acting deoxycortone pivilate previously mentioned.

Every 3–6 months the stabilisation should be checked by redetermining the sodium and potassium values and then if necessary adjusting the dosage of the steroids.

PANCREAS

In the dog the pancreas is an irregularly lobulated V-shaped gland lying in the upper part of the abdominal cavity. The two lobes which form the arms of the V are united behind the pylorus of the stomach and diverge as they pass backwards, the slender right lobe alongside the duodenum and the shorter, thicker left lobe along the medial surface of the stomach. Ectopic pancreatic tissue may occur elsewhere in the abdomen, chiefly in the gall bladder and mesentery.

The acinar cells which form the bulk of the lobules secrete pancreatic juice, the digestive exocrine secretion of the gland, which is carried to the first part of the duodenum by the dorsal and ventral pancreatic ducts.

Scattered throughout the pancreas are small groups of cells, the islets of Langerhans, responsible for endocrine production. They consist chiefly of alpha cells, secreting glucagon, and beta cells, secreting insulin, though occasionally other types (delta cells, F cells) of uncertain function are discovered.

The production of proinsulin and its conversion to insulin occurs within the beta cells. Insulin release is stimulated chiefly by glucose, but also by amino acids, fatty acids, other sugars and ketone bodies. Although a rise in blood sugar will provoke insulin release, glucose in the alimentary tract causes an even greater release of insulin due to the additional stimulation of the pancreas by hormones from the alimentary mucosa; secretin and gastrointestinal glucagon. Certain hormones (glucagon, glucocorticoids, ACTH, oestro-

gens, progesterone and growth hormone), by stimulating gluconeogenesis and other actions, provoke increased insulin secretion, which if prolonged can lead to beta cell exhaustion and diabetes mellitus. Insulin secretion is inhibited by adrenaline and noradrenaline.

The three primary target organs for insulin are liver, adipose tissue and skeletal muscle. Insulin enhances the movement of glucose into these cells and stimulates the anabolism of carbohydrate, fat and protein. There is increased synthesis of glycogen in liver and muscle, increased protein synthesis in muscle, increased fat production in adipose cells and increased nucleic acid formation, whilst gluconeogenesis, lipolysis and proteolysis are diminished.

Conversely pancreatic glucagon increases glycogenolysis, gluconeogenesis and lipolysis, increasing the blood glucose level. Its secretion is triggered primarily by a lowered blood sugar level.

Both hormones are degraded principally by the liver and kidneys.

Disorders of pancreatic endocrine function

Diabetes mellitus (hypoinsulinism)

Aetiology
Diabetes mellitus (DM) is a complex disorder of carbohydrate, fat and protein metabolism which results from an inability to produce or utilise adequate amounts of insulin. Some breeds have a genetic predisposition towards DM; the Miniature Poodle, Scottish Terrier, Samoyed, King Charles Spaniel, Rottweiler, and in particular the Dachshund. Many cases are associated either with destruction of the beta cells, especially as the result of chronic relapsing pancreatitis (or occasionally neoplasia or trauma), or with an idiopathic reduction in the number of beta cells and the disappearance of many of the islets. Rarely DM is due to aplasia of the islets. Functional phaeochromocytomas, by secreting catecholamines, inhibit insulin secretion. The drugs phenytoin and hydrochlorothiazide also have an insulin-inhibitory effect, though one which is reversible. DM arising from these causes is characterised by a low plasma insulin level.

However DM can arise in association with a high insulin level, resulting from either the synthesis of insulin which is biologically inactive (secondary hormone resistance) or diminished responsiveness of the target tissues (primary hormone resistance). The latter condition may be due to the presence of anti-insulin antibodies or (better recognised in the dog) the presence of excess glucocorticoids or growth hormone which induce peripheral resistance to the effects of insulin.

Spontaneous DM in the dog can be classified into three types by measuring the plasma insulin level and its response to glucose administration (Kaneko *et al* 1978). It seems likely that DM first develops as covert or 'chemical' diabetes (Type III) in which the 'resting' insulin concentration is normal or high, rises in response to a standard dose of glucose, but fails to return to its initial level as rapidly as normal. This stage of DM is the only one likely to respond to treatment solely with diet and/or hypoglycaemic drugs.

Subsequently this early stage progresses to one of two types of overt diabetes. Type I, the equivalent of human juvenile DM, is the most severe, showing a virtual absense of plasma insulin and no rise in response to a glucose load. Most dogs presented for treatment are of this type (though in contrast to man most are middle-aged or elderly) and will require insulin injections to control the condition. Type II (similar to human maturity-onset DM) shows a normal or high insulin level which fails to rise in response to glucose administration. The fact that such cases *also* respond to insulin therapy suggests that the underlying problem is failure to produce an effective insulin, or insulin inactivation by antibodies, or peripheral resistance to the effects of insulin.

The overall incidence of DM varies between 0.1 and 0.6% of the total dog population. Incidence rises with age and it is seen most frequently in dogs 8 years old and over, though occasional cases are seen in animals under 1 year old. DM was discovered to be an inherited disorder in a line of Keeshonds with onset occurring between 2 and 6 months old (Kramer *et al* 1980).

DM is 3 times as common in bitches as in males and its onset often follows oestrus. This is because the increased synthesis of progesterone in dioestrus stimulates an increased output of growth hormone (GH). GH in turn creates DM by inducing insulin resistance in the target tissues, restricting glucose transport and by directly stimulating the beta cells to increase their output of insulin, ultimately causing beta cell exhaustion (Eigenmann 1981b). Long term, low dose, therapy with a progestagen (e.g. methylprogesterone acetate) has a similar diabetogenic effect, again through stimulating the overproduction of GH. High levels of glucocorticoids, either naturally produced (i.e. in hyperadrenocorticism) or administered (particularly long term) can also initiate or aggravate DM by inducing peripheral insulin resistance. Consequently high plasma insulin levels are a feature of DM caused by GH or glucocorticoids.

Clinical signs
Polyuria and polydipsia are prime clinical signs. The renal threshold for glucose in the dog lies between 9.7–12.2 mmol/l (175 and 220 mg/100 ml) and usually when the blood glucose level exceeds 10 mmol/l (180 mg/100 ml) glucose is incompletely reabsorbed from the renal tubules resulting in glycosuria and, because of osmotic diuresis, increased urine production and frequency of micturition. Additional water is consumed to compensate for this loss. Failure to retain the increased amount of urine over long periods, particularly overnight, is frequently the factor which provokes the owner to seek advice. Polyphagia is often present, though not invariably, until the ketotic stage is reached. Other common clinical signs are cataract (usually bilateral) in about 25% of cases, an enlarged liver (established by palpation and radiography) in up to 50%, and muscle wasting which produces weight loss. A number of dogs show impairment of pancreatic exocrine function, which is also characterised by polyphagia and weight loss. Capillary microangiopathy resulting in retinopathy, glomerulosclerosis and occlusive vascular disease can also be demonstrated in long-standing cases in the dog. Most dogs with DM have some degree of peripheral neuropathy (Steiss *et al* 1981).

In the terminal (ketoacidotic) stage fat breakdown is increased, and because fatty acids are produced faster than they can be oxidised acetoacetic acid is formed and then converted to acetone or beta-hydroxy-butyric acid. These three substances constitute the ketone bodies which are excreted in the urine, and in addition acetone is exhaled. The acids produce metabolic acidosis and acetoacetic acid and acetone are also directly toxic to the central nervous system. In this stage the clinical signs are inappetence, increased rate and depth of breathing, vomiting, dehydration and listnessness progressing to ketoacidotic (diabetic ketotic) coma and ultimately death. Animals which are markedly acidotic, depressed and dehydrated when presented are most likely to die and therefore have a very poor prognosis. There may be abdominal pain due to pancreatitis which Ling *et al* (1977) found to be the most common complication of ketoacidosis in dogs that were vomiting more than two or three times per 48 hours. Severe dehydration may lead to the onset of acute renal failure.

The severity of DM is related more to the tendency to develop ketosis than to the initial blood sugar level or to insulin requirements.

Diagnosis
Diagnosis is based chiefly on the clinical signs plus the findings of glycosuria and hyperglycaemia.

Glucose is usually absent from canine urine and its presence is mainly associated with DM; in 75% of newly diagnosed cases the glucose level is above 2%. (Other causes of hyperglycaemia and glycosuria are listed in Table 8.7.) Ketone bodies are often present in DM and tests should be made for them. The urinary specific gravity may be raised though often not sufficiently to put it above the normal range (1.015–1.045) since 4% glucose will add only 0.015 to the specific gravity.

A fasting blood glucose level above 7.2 mmol/l (130 mg/100 ml) (normal range 3.3–5.6 mmol/l (60–100 mg/100 ml)) is most commonly due to DM, although the possibility that it is due to hyperadrenocorticism, or the effects of severe stress, should be eliminated. Blood cholesterol, SAP and ALT (SGPT) levels also rise, though these findings are not specific. Radioimmunoassay of insulin has not been widely employed in the dog and has only recently become routinely available.

A glucose tolerance test is valuable in doubtful cases, chiefly where the blood glucose level is between 6.7–9.7 mmol/l (120–175 mg/100 ml), and where there is glycosuria without apparent hyperglycaemia, or where glucose is not consistently present in the urine

Table 8.7 Differential diagnosis of hyperglycaemia and glycosuria.

Hyperglycaemia (results in glycosuria when the renal threshold is exceeded)
Diabetes mellitus—always present, in all 3 types
Acute pancreatitis (rapid onset follows glucagon release)
Hyperadrenocorticism—rarely
Acromegaly in bitches (in dioestrus or on progestagen therapy)
Following the parenteral administration of sugars or other carbohydrates (e.g. i.v. dextrose) or of adrenaline
Convulsions due to a hypocalcaemia or primary CNS disorders
Severe stress
Chronic liver disease—rarely
Hyperthyroidism—rarely
Serious insulin overdosage may result in a transient hyperglycaemia (Somogyi effect)
Following pancreatic surgery to remove an insulinoma
Occasionally after a high carbohydrate meal
(Following the use of certain drugs; e.g. streptozotocin)

Glycosuria without hyperglycaemia
Primary renal glycosuria
Fanconi syndrome
Chronic renal failure—very rarely
Poisoning with lead or anticholinesterases (e.g. organophosphates)
(Following the use of certain drugs; e.g. phlorizin)

There is normally a minute amount of glucose in urine (much less than can be detected with conventional methods) which forms the basis of the hypoglycosuria screening test for significant bacteriuria.

(or even because there is a familial history of DM). However this test is not necessary as a routine, and indeed may precipitate ketoacidosis in animals with marked diabetes.

The oral glucose tolerance test (OGTT) is relatively simple to perform and usually provides a clear distinction between normal and diabetic dogs. After 12 hours fasting the dog is dosed with glucose (2.2g/kg body weight orally) dissolved in as little warm water as possible. If the dog will not consume it voluntarily (e.g. following administration with a disposable syringe) a stomach tube is employed, if necessary under tranquillisation. Just before glucose administration and 30 minutes, 1, 2 and 3 hours afterwards, blood is collected (in fluoride-oxalate tubes) for glucose estimation. In normal dogs the peak value (usually below 8.9 mmol/l (160 mg/100 ml)) is reached after 30–60 minutes, and the level falls to near the fasting level in 2 hours. In diabetics the level at 1 hour is usually above 8.3 mmol/l (150 mg/100 ml) and does not fall rapidly. Any effects of malabsorption or delayed stomach emptying can be overcome by the slow intravenous injection (lasting 30 seconds) of a smaller dose of glucose (0.5 g/kg body weight), as a 50% sterile solution (intravenous glucose tolerance test; IVGTT). An immediate rise in the blood glucose level will occur (above 16.6 mmol/l (300 mg/100 ml) at 15 minutes), which in the normal dog will return to the fasting level in approximately 1 hour but in the diabetic dog may not do so for 2 or 3 hours. Diagnosis of DM can also be based on the time required for the plasma glucose concentration to fall by one-half following glucose administration. (An IVGTT should not be performed in an anaesthetised dog because the reduced blood flow through the pancreas decreases insulin release.)

The measurement of glycosylated haemoglobin to aid the diagnosis and monitoring of canine DM in the future appears promising (Wood & Smith 1980; Mahaffey & Cornelius 1982).

Treatment

In mild (Type III) diabetes mellitus the reduction of carbohydrate intake (and, if obese, of fat intake also) is often sufficient to control hyperglycaemia and glycosuria. Moderate cases may need, in addition, an oral hypoglycaemic drug to stimulate insulin secretion. The most commonly employed are sulphonylureas; in the dog tolbutamide is markedly hepatotoxic and it is preferable to use chlorpropamide.

Unfortunately, most diagnosed cases in the dog are severe Type I (over half already show ketonuria) and the above therapy alone will not control the disease. Successful treatment requires the routine (i.e. daily) subcutaneous injection of insulin after urine testing.

Following initial stabilisation this will need to be carried out by the owner, which must be made clear at the outset. If the owner is unwilling to perform this task, or the animal's temperament makes success unlikely, the most humane course of action is euthanasia.

In the author's opinion stabilisation (i.e. assessing and regulating the animal's insulin requirements) is best performed with the dog hospitalised. A depot insulin with 24 hour action is preferable for both stabilisation and maintenance (e.g. Zinc Suspension Lente insulin of beef origin; a mixture of insulin zinc suspensions). Isophane insulin, otherwise known as Neutral Protamine Hagedorn (NPH), has an action which lasts slightly under 24 hours, and Protamine Zinc Insulin (PZI) lasts for slightly longer than 24 hours and daily doses can have a slight cumulative effect; however both show considerable variation in the time of peak activity in dogs (Church 1981). Other insulin zinc suspensions are unsuitable; Semilente (amorphous insulin zinc suspension) acts for approximately 16 hours and Ultralente (crystalline insulin zinc suspension) acts for around 36 hours.

Soluble insulin (Insulin Injection) with a rapid, short-acting effect, should be reserved for the emergency treatment of ketoacidotic coma (see p. 238).

In March 1983 the changeover to human patients to U100 insulin (100 units/ml) began in the UK, to reduce the chances of dosage error involved in using a variety of insulin strengths (20, 40 and 80 units/ml) with a standard syringe graduated in terms of 20 units/ml insulin. Such a change has already been completed in Canada, Australia and New Zealand and is almost complete in the USA. Consequently all *new* canine diabetics should from the outset be treated with U100 insulin and existing cases should be changed over as soon as is practicable.

Glass (re-usable) and plastic (disposable) syringes are available for measuring U100 insulin doses; both are available in two sizes—$\frac{1}{2}$ ml (with a graduation every 1 unit) and 1 ml (with a graduation every 2 units). Disposable insulin syringes, with needles attached, are preferable to glass-barrelled syringes which require sterilisation before use, with the risks of infection and insulin inactivation by heat or spirit. In a temperate climate insulin will keep for months at room temperature and will sting less if not chilled (Watkins 1982). However in tropical countries, or if there are large stocks, it should be refrigerated, though never frozen. The bottle should be well shaken before withdrawing a dose.

Urine samples should be collected first thing in the morning (after overnight fasting). When commencing insulin treatment it is valuable to know the exact glucose concentration and because commercial tests do not distinguish between any of the levels which are over 2% it is preferable to use Benedict's quantitative test for this first estimation. Routine testing thereafter, especially that performed by the owner should employ the convenient Keto-Diastix strips. The 'glucose band' is specific for glucose, gives a percentage reading and is unaffected by ascorbic acid, which may be present in large amounts in canine urine, and the 'ketone band' allows a check on ketones to be maintained.

As a simple guide the number of units in the first subcutaneous injection should be twice the percentage glucose concentration (i.e. if the glucose concentration is 4%, 8 units should be given), or alternatively $\frac{1}{2}$ unit/kg body weight.

Subsequent daily injections are regulated according to that morning's urinary glucose level and the following rules:

1 Urinary glucose = 1% or more: give previous day's dose plus two units. (If values above 2% are detectable animals should receive the previous day's dose plus 4 units.)
2 Urinary glucose = 0.1–0.5%: give previous day's dose.
3 Urinary glucose = 0%: give previous day's dose minus 2 units (to avoid overdosage).
4 If hypoglycaemic signs or coma occurred on previous day: give previous day's dose minus 4 or more units. (To convert mmol/l to % multiply by 0.018.)

Stabilisation on a more or less constant dose may take 3–4 weeks; the case may then be allowed home to follow the same regimen. The owner should be given a demonstration of correct syringe filling, subcutaneous injection technique and urine testing, and should be provided with a prescription for the insulin preparation. The importance of ketones should be emphasised and the owner advised to return the dog for further treatment if they apppear in the urine.

A single daily injection of insulin should be given in the midmorning (10.30–11.00 am) whilst at the same time feeding about a quarter of the daily food intake. This may also encourage the animal to accept the injection more readily. This timing will allow any untoward effects of the insulin occurring later to be observed during the daytime. It is best to inject after the food has been consumed so that if the animal refuses to eat no injection has been given. The remaining food should be given as the main meal of the day about 8–9 hours later when the insulin will exert its maximum effect.

Dietary control and the regulation of exercise are important. The diet should be low in fat and consist of approximately 80% meat and 20% carbohydrate (e.g. biscuit meal or rice) fed at the rate of 28 g/kg normal body weight per day (i.e. allowance should be made for wasting or obesity). Regular weighing should be encouraged and titbits must not be given. Water should be available *ad lib.* and its reduced consumption indicates successful therapy. The same moderate amount of exercise should be given each day since any appreciable variation can affect insulin requirements.

In bitches where the onset of DM follows progestagen therapy or oestrus, prompt diagnosis and treatment (by respectively progestagen withdrawal and ovariohysterectomy), before beta cell exhaustion occurs, can result in restoration to normality.

Complications

Insulin resistance. Where animals require high levels of insulin (3 or more units/kg body weight per day) checks should be made to ensure that the insulin is being correctly stored and administered and is not out-of-date or inactivated. If no fault can be found the possibility of concurrent hyperadrenocorticism (q.v.) should be investigated. In proven cases mitotane therapy causes a dramatic fall in insulin requirements. Also in acromegaly GH causes diminished responsiveness to insulin.

Hypoglycaemic coma. This results from insulin overdosage and is preceded by signs of drowsiness, weakness and ataxia. One or two tablespoons of honey, or concentrated glucose solution (which should be kept in the refrigerator for emergency use), given orally results in a rapid return to normality. However a careful watch should be maintained because when this sugar is metabolised the signs can reappear, necessitating further treatment. Owners should be made aware of these signs and of the corrective measures to take. If they are untreated the animal will collapse and have convulsions which require prompt subcutaneous or preferably intravenous, glucose administration (e.g. 10–12 ml/kg body weight of either 5% dextrose injection or 5% dextrose and 0.9% sodium chloride injection).

In some instances serious overdosage with insulin will lead to a temporary hyperglycaemia and glycosuria, accompanied by polyuria and polydipsia (Somogyi effect). This is because the initial extreme fall in blood glucose triggers physiological mechanisms to raise it, but in the absence of any compensatory insulin secretion this leads to hyperglycaemia (Feldman & Nelson 1982). The extreme fluctuation in blood glucose levels can be reduced by decreasing the daily insulin dose.

Ketoacidosis. An animal may be presented with this condition or it may develop in a dog which is receiving inadequate treatment. The clinical signs have already been described.

From the packed cell volume and clinical signs the fluid deficit should be assessed (see acute renal failure, Chapter 15). This must lie between 5 and 15% and is most likely to be of the order of 10%. To this figure should be added any additional volume of fluid subsequently lost by vomiting. Each 1% deficit will require 10 ml/kg body weight of intravenous fluid to correct it. The administration of fluid (drip rate) should be adjusted to achieve correction within the first hour if possible, up to a maximum of 75 ml/kg body weight per hour (i.e. which is sufficient to correct a 7.5% deficit). A greater deficiency should be corrected over 2 hours (e.g. a 10% deficiency can be corrected by 50 ml/kg body weight per hour for 2 hours). After this, normal water loss should be balanced by providing intravenous fluid at the following rates:

1 For animals up to 9 kg body weight: 2.5 ml/kg body weight per hour.
2 For animals between 9 and 20 kg body weight: 2 ml/kg body weight per hour.
3 For animals over 20 kg body weight: 1.7 ml/kg body weight per hour.

Additional fluid should be given to replace that lost by vomiting.

The first 500 ml of the intravenous replacement fluid should be 0.9% sodium chloride injection, and thereafter 0.45% sodium chloride injection (half normal saline).

The use of an indwelling urinary catheter allows a check to be kept on urine production, and if urine is regularly drained from the bladder the glucose content of the urine can be monitored. Severe dehydration may result in prerenal acute renal failure, which if prolonged could lead to acute tubular necrosis. If oliguria is present fluid administration should cease (see Chapter 15).

If ketones are present in 'large' amount soluble insulin should be administered (2 units/kg body weight for animals up to 20 kg body weight and above that weight 1 unit/kg body weight), half intravenously and half intramuscularly. This dose should be repeated every 3–4 hours until the level of ketones falls from 'large' to 'moderate' or 'small'. Then the dose can be halved, giving it all by the intramuscular route. This should be repeated every 3–4 hours until ketones completely disappear from the urine. At this stage a depot insulin should be substituted, with the initial dose depending on the glucose concentration in the urine as mentioned previously.

Opinions vary as to whether bicarbonate is advisable to correct the acidosis. Most authors prefer to provide lactate (e.g. in lactated Ringer's solution) although it may give rise to paradoxical acidosis of cerebrospinal fluid. If bicarbonate is used 2.5 ml/kg body weight of 4.2% sodium bicarbonate injection should be given after the first 4 hours and repeated every 12 hours for 2 days.

As the acidosis is corrected, and potassium accompanies glucose into the cells as insulin is given, the potassium level in the serum will fall. To correct this after the first 4 hours of fluid therapy (and following the administration of bicarbonate injection if employed) the fluid then administered should be 0.20% potassium chloride and 0.9% sodium chloride injection. If blood glucose levels can be monitored with a simple test (e.g. Dextrostix or Reflotest-Glucose) then when the blood glucose levels falls below 13.9 mmol/l (250 mg/100ml), 5% dextrose solution can be administered alongside the potassium chloride/sodium chloride solution; the rate of administration of each solution is the same, with a total rate not exceeding the figures given above. ECG monitoring may be valuable to indicate the presence of hypokalaemia (i.e. depressed T waves and a prolonged QT interval).

Pancreatitis. A doubling of normal serum amylase or lipase activity in a vomiting ketoacidotic diabetic dog is indicative of pancreatitis. Oral fluids should be limited and atropine sulphate administered subcutaneously at the rate of 0.05 mg/kg body weight four times daily to decrease the pancreatic exocrine secretion in addition to the therapy for ketoacidosis.

Hyperosmolar (hyperglycaemic non-ketotic) coma. Weakness, polyuria/polydipsia, severe dehydration, anorexia and glycosuria progressing to coma in a non-ketotic animal is indicative of a rare hyperosmolar diabetic condition.

Blood glucose levels are markedly elevated (e.g. 50 mmol/l (900 mg/100 ml) or more), levels of sodium and blood urea are also increased and the serum osmolality is in excess of 320 mosmol/kg, often above 375 mosmol/kg. Treatment requires the slow administration of sufficient 0.45% sodium chloride injection to correct the dehydration. An initial injection of soluble insulin (1 unit/kg body weight half intravenously and half intramuscularly) should be given but not be repeated unless essential because this condition is more responsive to insulin than ketoacidotic DM.

Glomerulosclerosis. Dogs with long-standing (2 years plus) DM which has been poorly regulated may develop glomerulosclerosis, with proteinuria and mild polyuria, which can lead to chronic renal failure.

Fatty degeneration of the liver. This is frequently a feature of canine DM and should receive concurrent therapy (see Chapter 14). If the condition is of long standing, cirrhosis may develop.

Urinary tract infection (UTI). Although emphysematous cystitis is more likely to affect the bladder of diabetic animals there appears to be no greater incidence of UTI in diabetic dogs than in the canine population as a whole. This impression may be simply due to the fact that both diabetes mellitus and UTI are more common in older animals.

Further progress of diabetes mellitus
The owner should record each day: time of urine collection, urinary glucose level (and presence, if any, of ketones), number of units of insulin injected, times of injection and feeding, quantity of food, and any other features (e.g. dietary changes, amount of exercise or illness). These records should be inspected when the dog is presented for regular check-ups every 3–4 months. Any anomalous results should be investigated and any errors in procedure corrected. Examination is best performed in the late afternoon, several hours after the last insulin dose.

Periods of stress (with the release of glucocorticoids) result in considerable fluctuation in insulin dosage. The high levels of progesterone produced after oestrus (in dioestrus) and during pregnancy also cause fluctuation in insulin requirements. In addition in pregnancy an insulinase is produced by the placenta, and fetal GH output is stimulated, resulting in fetuses larger than normal, which could provoke dystocia. Consequently ovariohysterectomy of intact bitches is advisable. During surgery one-half of the calculated dose of insulin for that day is given and the animal maintained on intravenous 5% dextrose injection during the procedure.

On average, treatment increases the lifespan of diabetic dogs by about 2 years.

Hyperinsulinism
Dogs, above 4 years of age, may develop an autonomous insulin-secreting neoplasm of the beta cells of the pancreas, which occasionally can be present in ectopic pancreatic tissue. The term 'insulinoma' may be used to describe such a neoplasm, although this has been held to designate an adenoma, whereas 70% or more are carcinomas. There is a slightly higher incidence in Boxers, German Shepherd Dogs, Irish Setters,

Collies, Poodles, German Short-Haired Pointers and terriers, but no sex predisposition.

Clinical signs
The clinical signs are those of hypoglycaemia, i.e. restlessness, weakness, disorientation and ataxia proceeding to a variety of neurological signs including uncontrolled barking, incontinence, twitching and convulsions. Hypoglycaemic attacks become more frequent and severe, ultimately ending in a coma. These attacks are particularly likely to occur after fasting, exercise or excitement, and also after eating, which stimulates insulin release. However owners often report a more rapid recovery if animals are fed early in an attack.

Diagnosis
During a hypoglycaemic episode the blood sugar level is almost always below 2.8 mmol/l (50 mg/100 ml) and usually below 2.2 mmol/l (40 mg/100 ml). The initial diagnosis is based on the finding of a low fasting blood glucose level. Fasting for longer than 8 hours is usually unnecessary (and potentially dangerous), although it may be necessary in *some* suspected cases to starve for 24 (even 48) hours before such low levels become apparent. However, the condition needs to be distinguished from other causes of hypoglycaemia which are summarised in Table 8.8.

The glucagon tolerance test may cause profound hypoglycaemia and is not recommended for routine use. (It involves taking blood samples before and at 5, 15, 30, 45 and 60 minutes after an intravenous injection of glucagon (Glucagon injection) (0.03 mg/kg body weight) to a fasting animal. In dogs with insulinomas the blood glucose level remains below 8.3 mmol/l (150 mg/100 ml) and returns to the hypoglycaemic range within an hour.)

Immunoreactive insulin levels are generally elevated but can be in the normal range if the excessive secretion is predominantly proinsulin.

The most accurate diagnostic index of hyperinsulinism is a value of > 30 μU/mg glucose obtained from the expression

$$\frac{\text{serum insulin (in } \mu\text{U/ml)} \times 100}{\text{plasma glucose (in mg/100 ml (}or\text{ mmol/l} \times 18))} - 30$$

(Caywood *et al* 1979; Kruth *et al* 1982).

Treatment
In a severe hypoglycaemic attack 50% dextrose injection should be administered through a catheter inserted into the jugular vein until improvement occurs.

Table 8.8 Differential diagnosis of hypoglycaemia.

Hyperinsulinism
Insulin-secreting tumour of pancreatic beta cells
Overdosage of insulin (or similarly overdosage of other hypoglycaemic drugs)

Neoplasia of other organs
Production of insulin or an insulin-like substance
Rapid utilisation of blood glucose

Severe liver damage (destruction of liver enzymes)
(e.g. toxic hepatitis, cirrhosis, neoplasia or vascular anomalies)

Hypoadrenocorticism
Reduced glucocorticoid secretion by adrenal glands
Inadequate ACTH secretion by adenohypophysis

Inadequate uptake of glucose
Malabsorption of glucose
Starvation to point of emaciation
Anorexia, associated with toxaemia or other debilitating disease

Von Gierke syndrome in puppies (Type I glycogen storage disease)

Functional hypoglycaemia of hunting dogs (possible Type III glycogen storage disease)

Transient juvenile hypoglycaemia

Neonatal hypoglycaemia

Severe sepsis

Ketotic hypoglycaemia during pregnancy

Hypoglycaemia can also be induced by ethanol administration

There is a risk of thrombophlebitis from administering this concentration of dextrose into smaller blood vessels. The simultaneous intramuscular injection of prednisolone (4 mg/kg body weight) is advisable plus aqueous glucocorticoids intravenously in high doses (e.g. 50–500 mg cortisol), and diazepam (Valium) (1 mg/kg body weight intravenously) for sedation.

An exploratory laparotomy should be performed as soon as possible to minimise the risk of metastatic spread. The tumours are usually very small, can be difficult to find, and may be in ectopic pancreatic tissue. Metastases of malignant neoplasms, particularly to the spleen, liver and local lymph nodes, may occur and these secondary tumours may become functional up to 18 months later. If the tumour cannot be identified and removed either resection of the entire right lobe (which bears 60% of all pancreatic tumours) or, preferably, complete pancreatectomy is advisable. Clearly permanent substitutional therapy with insulin and pancreatic enzymes is then required. The mean life expectancy after surgery is a little over a year. To minimise the possibility of further hypoglycaemic attacks occurring in animals awaiting surgery they should be well, and frequently fed, and diazoxide

(Eudemine) administered orally (up to 7 mg/kg body weight 3 times per day). Also, by blocking insulin release diazoxide can give temporary control where metastasis has occurred or surgical removal of the primary tumour is not feasible (Parker *et al* 1982). Corticosteroids do not provide effective control, and whilst the cytotoxic drug streptozotocin is purported to selectively destroy beta cells it has a fairly narrow safety margin and can easily cause renal toxicosis.

The control of convulsions of hypoglycaemic origin is most likely to be successful using phenytoin (Epanutin) 10 mg/kg body weight per day (in divided dosage).

During surgery equal volumes of 10% dextrose injection and 10% dextran 40 in 0.9% sodium chloride injection should be infused (and for up to 2 hours afterwards) to reduce the risk of pancreatitis and hypoglycaemic shock following the release of large amounts of insulin from the tumour. The injection of 0.2 mg/kg body weight atropine sulphate per hour also helps prevent postoperative pancreatitis.

Because of the rapid spread of metastases which become functional, the possible occurrence of permanent hypoxic brain damage if surgery is delayed, and the increased hazards of surgery, the prognosis for cases of hyperinsulinism is poor.

ABBREVIATIONS USED IN TEXT

ACTH: adrenocorticotrophic hormone
ADH: antidiuretic hormone
ALT: alanine aminotransferase (= SGPT)
CPB: competitive protein binding
CRF: corticotropin releasing factor
DI: diabetes insipidus
DM: diabetes mellitus
FSH: follicle stimulating hormone
FSH-RF: follicle stimulating hormone releasing factor
GH: growth hormone
GIF: growth hormone inhibiting factor
GRF: growth hormone releasing factor
HAC: hyperadrenocorticism
HHDI: hypothalamic-hypophyseal diabetes insipidus
ICSH: interstitial cell stimulating hormone
IVGTT: intravenous glucose tolerance test
LH: luteinising hormone
LH-RF: luteinising hormone releasing factor
MSH: melanocyte stimulating hormone
MIF: melanocyte stimulating hormone inhibiting factor
NDI: nephrogenic diabetes insipidus
NPH: Neutral Protamine Hagedorn
NS-HPT: nutritional secondary hyperparathyroidism

OGTT: oral glucose tolerance test
17-OHCS: 17-hydroxycorticosteroids
op′DDD: ortho-para-prime DDD (mitotane)
PBI: protein bound iodine
PHPT: primary hypoparathyroidism
PIF: prolactin inhibiting factor
PP: psychogenic polydipsia
PS-HPT: pseudohyperparathyroidism
PTH: parathyroid hormone
PZI: Protamine Zinc Insulin
RIA: radioimmunoassay
RIU: radioiodine uptake
RS-HPT: renal secondary hyperparathyroidism
RT3 test: T3 resin uptake test
SAP: serum alkaline phosphatase
SGPT: serum glutamic pyruvic transaminase
T3: triiodothyronine
T4: thyroxine
TRF: thyrotropin releasing factor
TSH: thyroid stimulating hormone

Note

All the intravenous fluids mentioned in this chapter are obtainable from Travenol Laboratories Ltd, Thetford, Norfolk, with the exception of 10% calcium borogluconate solution. This may be prepared by dilution of the standard commercial 20% solution.

REFERENCES

ANDERSON G. L. & LEWIS L. D. (1980) Obesity. In *Current Veterinary Therapy VII, Small animal practice*, p. 1034, ed. R. W. Kirk. W. B. Saunders, Philadelphia.

BADYLAK S. F. & VAN VLEET J. F. (1981) Sequential morphologic and clinicopathologic alterations in dogs with experimentally induced glucocorticoid hepatopathy. *Am. J. Vet. Res.* **42**, 1310.

BELSHAW B. E. & RIJNBERK A. (1979) Radioimmunoassay of plasma T4 and T3 in the diagnosis of primary hypothyroidism in dogs. *J. Am. Anim. Hosp. Assoc.* **15**, 17.

BREITSCHWERDT E. B. & ROOT C. R. (1979) Inappropriate secretion of antidiuretic hormone in a dog. *J. Am Vet. Med. Assoc.* **175**, 181.

BROWN N. O. (1981) Paraneoplastic syndromes of humans, dogs and cats. *J. Am. Anim. Hosp. Assoc.* **17**, 911.

CAPEN C. C. & MARTIN S. L. (1977) Calcium metabolism and disorders of parathyroid glands. *Vet. Clinics N. Am.* **7**, 513.

CAYWOOD D. D., WILSON J. W., HARDY R. M. & SCHULL R. M. (1979) Pancreatic islet cell adenocarcinoma: clinical and diagnostic features of six cases. *J. Am. Vet. Med. Assoc.* **174**, 714.

CHASTAIN C. B. (1978) Human thyroid stimulating hormone radioimmunoassay in the dog. *J. Am. Anim. Hosp. Assoc.* **14**, 368.

CHASTAIN C. B., MITTEN R. W. & KLUGE J. P. (1978) An ACTH-hyper-responsive adrenal carcinoma in a dog. *J. Am. Vet. Med. Assoc.* **172,** 586.

CHASTAIN C. B. & SCHMIDT B. (1980) Gallatorrhoea associated with hypothyroidism in intact bitches. *J. Am. Anim. Hosp. Assoc.* **16,** 851.

CHURCH D. B. (1981) The blood glucose response to three prolonged duration insulins in canine diabetes mellitus. *J. Small Anim. Pract.* **22,** 301.

COHEN S. J. & KNIESSER M. (1980) Hyperadrenocorticism in a dog with adrenal and pituitary neoplasia. *J. Am. Anim. Hosp. Assoc.* **16,** 259.

CRISPIN S. M. & BARNETT K. C. (1978) Arcus lipoides corneae secondary to hypothyroidism in the Alsatian. *J. Small Anim. Pract.* **19,** 127.

ECKERSALL P. D. & WILLIAMS M. E. (1983) Thyroid function tests in dogs using radioimmunoassay kits. *J. Small Anim. Pract.* **24,** 525.

EILER H. & OLIVER J. (1980) Combined dexamethasone suppression and cosyntropin (synthetic ACTH) stimulation test in the dog: a new approach to testing of adrenal gland function. *Am. J. Vet. Res.* **41,** 1243.

EIGENMANN J. E. (1981a) Diagnosis and treatment of dwarfism in a German Shepherd Dog. *J. Am. Anim. Hosp. Assoc.* **17,** 798.

EIGENMANN J. E. (1981b) Diabetes mellitus in elderly female dogs: recent findings on pathogenesis and clinical implications. *J. Am. Anim. Hosp. Assoc.* **17,** 805.

EIGENMANN J. E. & EIGENMANN R. Y. (1981) Radioimmunoassay of canine growth hormone. *Acta Endocrinologica* **98,** 514.

EIGENMANN J. E. & VENKER-VAN HAAGEN A. J. (1981) Progestagen-induced and spontaneous canine acromegaly due to reversible growth hormone overproduction: clinical picture and pathogenesis. *J. Am. Anim. Hosp. Assoc.* **17,** 813.

FELDMAN E. C. (1981) Effect of functional adrenocortical tumours on plasma cortisol and corticotropin concentrations in dogs. *J. Am. Vet. Med. Assoc.* **178,** 823.

FELDMAN E. C. & KRUTZIK S. (1981) Case reports of parathyroid levels in spontaneous canine parathyroid disorders. *J. Am. Anim. Hosp. Assoc.* **17,** 393.

FELDMAN E. C. & NELSON R. W. (1982) Insulin-induced hyperglycemia in diabetic dogs. *J. Am. Vet. Med. Assoc.* **180,** 1432.

FELDMAN E. C., TYRRELL J. B. & BOHANNON N. V. (1978) The synthetic ACTH stimulation test and measurement of endogenous plasma ACTH levels: useful diagnostic indicators for adrenal disease in dogs. *J. Am. Anim. Hosp. Assoc.* **14,** 524.

GOSSELIN S. J., CAPEN C. C. & MARTIN S. L. (1981a) Histologic and ultrastructural evaluation of thyroid lesions associated with hypothyroidism in dogs. *Vet. Pathol.* **18,** 299.

GOSSELIN S. J., CAPEN C. C., MARTIN S. L. & KRAKOWKA S. (1981b) Induced lymphocytic thyroiditis in dogs: effect of intrathyroidal injection of thyroid autoantibodies. *Am. J. Vet. Res.* **42,** 1565.

GREENE C. E., WONG P. L. & FINCO D. R. (1979) Diagnosis and treatment of diabetes insipidus in two dogs using two synthetic analogs of antidiuretic hormone. *J. Am. Anim. Hosp. Assoc.* **15,** 371.

HUNTLEY K., FRAZER J., GIBBS C. & GASKELL C. J. (1982)

The radiological features of canine Cushing's syndrome: a review of forty-eight cases. *J. Small Anim. Pract.* **23,** 369.

JOLES J. A. & GRUYS E. (1979) Nephrogenic diabetes insipidus in a dog with renal medullary lesions. *J. Am. Vet. Med. Assoc.* **174,** 830.

KANEKO J. J., MATTHEEUWS D., ROTTIERS R. P. & VERMEULEN A. (1978) Glucose tolerance and insulin response in diabetes mellitus of dogs. *J. Small Anim. Pract.* **19,** 85.

KEMPPAINEN R. J., LORENZ M. D. & THOMPSON F. N. (1981) Adrenocortical suppression in the dog after a single dose of methylprednisolone acetate. *Am. J. Vet. Res.* **42,** 822.

KEMPPAINEN R. J., LORENZ M. D. & THOMPSON F. N. (1982) Adrenocortical suppression in the dog given a single intramuscular dose of prednisolone or triamcinolone acetonide. *Am. J. Vet. Res.* **43,** 204.

KRAMER J. W., NOTTINGHAM S., ROBINETTE J., LENZ G., SYLVESTER S. & DESSOUKY M. I. (1980) Inherited early onset insulin requiring diabetes mellitus of Keeshond dogs. *Diabetes* **29,** 558.

KROOK L. (1977) Nutritional hypercalcitonism. In *Current Veterinary Therapy VI: Small animal practice*, p. 1048, ed. R. W. Kirk. W. B. Saunders, Philadelphia.

KRUTH S. A., FELDMAN E. C. & KENNEDY P. C. (1982) Insulin-secreting islet cell tumours: establishing a diagnosis and the clinical course for 25 dogs. *J. Am. Vet. Med. Assoc.* **181,** 54.

LAGE A. L. (1973) Nephrogenic diabetes insipidus in a dog. *J. Am. Vet. Med. Assoc.* **163,** 251.

LARSSON M. & LUMSDEN J. H. (1980) Evaluation of an enzyme linked immunosorbent assay (ELISA) for determination of plasma thyroxine in dogs. *Zbl. Vet. Med.* A **27,** 9.

LING G. V., LOWENSTINE L. J., PULLEY L. T. & KANEKO J. J. (1977) Diabetes mellitus in dogs: a review of initial evaluation, immediate and long-term management, and outcome. *J. Am. Vet. Med. Assoc.* **170,** 521.

MAHAFFEY E. A. & CORNELIUS L. M. (1982) Glycosylated hemoglobin in diabetic and non-diabetic dogs. *J. Am. Vet. Med. Assoc.* **180,** 635.

MANNING P. J. (1979) Thyroid gland and arterial lesions of beagles with familial hypothyroidism and hyperlipoproteinemia. *Am. J. Vet. Res.* **40,** 820.

MEIJER J. C. (1980) Canine hyperadrenocorticism. In *Current Veterinary Therapy VII, Small animal practice*, p. 975. ed. R. W. Kirk. W. B. Saunders, Philadelphia.

MULNIX J. A., RIJNBERK A. & HENDRIKS H. J. (1976) Evaluation of a modified water-deprivation test for diagnosis of polyuric disorders in dogs. *J. Am. Vet. Med. Assoc.* **169,** 1327.

NIJHUIS A. H., STOKHOF A. A., HUISMAN G. H. & RIJNBERK A. (1978) ECG changes in dogs with hypothyroidism. *Tijdschr. Diergeneesk.* **103,** 736.

OSBORNE C. A. & STEVENS J. B. (1973) Pseudohyperparathyroidism in the dog. *J. Am. Vet. Med. Assoc.* **162,** 125.

PARKER W. M. & SCOTT D. W. (1980) Growth hormone responsive alopecia in the mature dog: a discussion of 13 cases. *J. Am. Anim. Hosp. Assoc.* **16,** 824.

PARKER A. J., O'BRIEN D. & MUSSELMAN E. E. (1982) Diazoxide treatment of metastatic insulinoma in a dog. *J. Am. Anim. Hosp. Assoc.* **18,** 315.

PETERSON M. E. & ALTSZULER N. (1981) Suppression of growth hormone secretion in spontaneous canine hyperadrenocorticism and its reversal after treatment. *Am. J. Vet. Res.* **42,** 1881.

PETERSON M. E., NESBITT G. H. & SCHAER M. (1981) Diagnosis and management of concurrent diabetes mellitus and hyperadrenocorticism in thirty dogs. *J. Am. Vet. Med. Assoc.* **178**, 66.

PETERSON M. E., RANDOLPH J. F., ZAKI F. A. & HEATH H. (1982a) Multiple endocrine neoplasia in a dog. *J. Am. Vet. Med. Assoc.* **180**, 1476.

PETERSON M. E., GILBERTSON S. R. & DRUCKER M. D. (1982b) Plasma cortisol response to exogenous ACTH in 22 dogs with hyperadrenocorticism caused by adrenocortical neoplasia. *J. Am. Vet. Med. Assoc.* **180**, 542.

ROSS R. J. M. & VALORI R. M. (1982) Measurement of thyroid hormones in Labradors. *Vet. Rec.* **111**, 329.

ROTH J. A., LOMAX L. G., ALTSZULER N., HAMPSHIRE J., KAEBERLE M. L., SHELTON M., DRAPER D. D. & LEDET A. E. (1980) Thymic abnormalities and growth hormone deficiency in dogs. *Am. J. Vet. Res.* **41**, 1256.

SCHAER M. (1979) Treatment of canine Cushing's syndrome with op'-DDD. *Canine Pract.* **6**, (6) 38.

SCOTT D. W. (1980) Systemic glucocorticoid therapy. In *Current Veterinary Therapy VII, Small animal practice*, p. 988, ed. R. W. Kirk. W. B. Saunders, Philadelphia.

SCOTT D. W., KIRK R. W., HAMPSHIRE J. & ALTSZULER N. (1978) Clinicopathological findings in a German Shepherd with pituitary dwarfism. *J. Am. Anim. Hosp. Assoc.* **14**, 183.

SHERDING R. G., MEUTEN D. J., CHEW D. J., KNAACK K. E. & HAUPT K. J. (1980) Primary hypoparathyroidism in the dog. *J. Am. Vet. Med. Assoc.* **176**, 439.

STEISS J. E., ORSHER A. N. & BOWEN J. M. (1981) Electrodiagnostic analysis of peripheral neuropathy in dogs with diabetes mellitus. *Am. J. Vet. Res.* **42**, 2061.

WATKINS P. J. (1982) ABC of diabetes. *Br. Med. J.* **285**, 866.

WILLARD M. D., SCHALL W. D., McCAW D. E. & NACHREINER R. F. (1982) Canine hypoadrenocorticism: report of 37 cases and review of 39 previously reported cases. *J. Am. Vet. Med. Assoc.* **180**, 59.

WOOD P. A. & SMITH J. E. (1980) Glycosylated hemoglobin and canine diabetes mellitus. *J. Am. Vet. Med. Assoc.* **176**, 1267.

ZENOBLE R. D. & MYERS R. K. (1977) Severe hypocalcemia resulting from ethylene glycol poisoning in the dog. *J. Am. Anim. Hosp. Assoc.* **13**, 439.

FURTHER READING

General

ETTINGER S. J. (ed.) (1983) *Textbook of Veterinary Internal Medicine, Diseases of the Dog and Cat*, 2nd edn. Vol II, Section XI, The Endocrine System, p. 1522. W. B. Saunders, Philadelphia.

FELDMAN E. C. (ed.) (1977) Symposium on Endocrinology. *Vet. Clinics N. Am.* **7**, 431.

McDONALD L. E. (1980) *Veterinary Endocrinology and Reproduction*, 3rd edn. Lea & Febiger, Philadelphia.

MARTIN S. L. & CAPEN C. C. (1979) The Endocrine System. In *Canine Medicine* Vol II, 4th edn., p. 1087, ed. E. J. Catcott. American Veterinary Publications Inc., Santa Barbara.

MULNIX J. A. (consult. ed.) (1980) Endocrine and metabolic disorders. In *Current Veterinary Therapy VII; Small Animal practice*, p. 974. ed. R. W. Kirk. W. B. Saunders, Philadelphia.

SIEGEL E. T. (1977) *Endocrine Disorders of the Dog.* Lea & Febiger, Philadelphia.

Diabetes insipidus

RICHARDS M. A. (1974) The diabetes insipidus syndrome in dogs. In *Current Veterinary Therapy V; Small animal practice*, p. 805, ed. R. W. Kirk. W. B. Saunders, Philadelphia.

Thyroid disorders

GOSSELIN S. J., CAPEN C. C., MARTIN S. L. & KRAKOWKA S. (1982) Autoimmune lymphocytic thyroiditis in dogs. In *Advances in veterinary immunology 1982*, p. 185. eds. F. Kristensen & D. F. Anczak. Elsevier, Amsterdam.

ROSYCHUK R. A. W. (1982) Thyroid hormones and antithyroid drugs. *Vet. Clinics N. Am.* **12**, 111.

RIJNBERK A. (1971) *Iodine metabolism and thyroid disease in the dog.* PhD thesis, University of Utrecht.

Parathyroid disorders

BENNETT D. (1976) Nutrition and bone disease in the dog and cat. *Vet. Rec.* **98**, 313.

Adrenal cortex disorders

KELLY D. F. (1973) Functional disorders of the adrenal gland in dogs. In *Veterinary Annual*, 13th edn., p. 174, eds. C. S. G. Grunsell & F. W. G. Hill. John Wright, Bristol.

LUBBERINK A. A. M. E. (1977) *Diagnosis and treatment of canine Cushing's syndrome*. PhD thesis, University of Utrecht.

SCOTT, D. W. (1979) Hyperadrenocorticism. *Vet Clinics N. Am.* **9**, 3.

WILCKE J. E. W. & DAVIS L. E. (1982) Review of glucocorticoid pharmacology. *Vet. Clinics N. Am.* **12**, 3.

Diabetes mellitus

LAUDER I. (1973) Canine diabetes mellitus. In *The Veterinary Annual*, 13th edn., p. 152, eds. C. S. G. Grunsell & F. W. G. Hill. John Wright, Bristol.

9

Skin and Associated Structures

B. G. BAGNALL

INTRODUCTION

It has been estimated that, on average, the British small animal practitioner will treat nearly 30 dogs each week for skin disease. The abundance of cases can be satisfying for the enthusiastic clinician who has developed a special interest in the skin, but it is not uncommon to find that the inevitable accumulation of chronic patients becomes a wearisome burden. Progress in some countries has led to a number of practising veterinary specialists in dermatology who welcome difficult cases referred for a second opinion. Until this type of service becomes widely available there remains one major source of help and guidance: the indispensable textbook, *Small Animal Dermatology* (Muller, Kirk & Scott 1983).

Skin biology

A working knowledge of skin function can be of real benefit in understanding why disease conditions lead to lesions of widely varying superficial morphology and which treatments are likely to provide symptomatic relief.

Compared to human skin that of the dog is rather fragile. Devoid of protective hair its total thickness may be less than 1mm and the vital epidermis covering it may be scarcely one-tenth as thick. The basal epidermal cells adhere to the relatively acellular collagenous connective tissue of the underlying dermis but, without the number of rete ridges seen in man, the adhesion is not as good and it takes little rubbing to dislodge the epidermis and cause ulceration. The canine epidermis is comprised of a layer of only four or five interlocking 'prickle' cells which divide off the basal layer and are pushed upwards to be shed 10–14 days later as dead keratin flakes from the stratum corneum. The process of keratinisation of epidermal cells is still not fully understood. Under normal conditions, it provides a waterproof barrier but if defective can lead to the abnormal scaling of parakeratosis,

invasion of microorganisms and the formation of cracks and fissures.

The epidermis has considerable powers of healing and at the first sign of damage can rapidly increase its cellular 'turnover time' to as little as 2–3 days. Repeatedly assaulted on the surface, it will protect itself by hyperkeratosis of the stratum corneum (e.g. the normal elbow callus seen on most larger dogs). Extensive damage to the epidermis can heal without scarring, but if the dermis is severely injured fibrous repair will result in a visible scar because hair follicles do not regenerate once they have been destroyed.

Hair growth
Hair growth is a complex cycle regulated by hormones and many other factors not yet evaluated. A period of active growth of the follicle is followed by regression of the hair bulb and then a resting phase when the hair shaft remains in place until development of a new hair. Most hair follicles in the dog are part of what is called a compound follicle. A central large primary 'guard' hair grows out from the major follicle with several surrounding smaller secondary follicles providing the woolly hairs of the undercoat. Detailed knowledge of hair replacement in dogs is lacking; some breeds like the Poodle grow hair continuously and need clipping, while short-haired breeds such as the Dalmatian grow frequent replacement hairs and shed the old ones all over the house.

Each hair follicle, regardless of size, possesses a sebaceous gland which secretes waxy sebum into the follicle which gives the hair a glossy sheen and the epidermis some added surface protection and moisture. In certain laboratory animals it has been shown that male sex hormones stimulate sebum secretion, but it is difficult to demonstrate this effect clearly in the dog and more complex regulatory mechanisms are suspected. Each primary hair follicle has an associated apocrine sweat gland which secretes sweat of the type found in the human armpit and is responsible for a characteristic odour. Eccrine sweat glands which produce most human sweating are rare in the dog, occurring only on the footpad and nose. Body cooling in dogs is achieved primarily by the respiratory tract in the form of panting.

Diagnostic aids for skin cases

Time is the most pressing requirement because examination of the entire skin of a dog is a lengthy process. The animal should be placed on a table and every area searched for skin lesions or parasites. A simple regular routine of examination is a good idea to ensure that no part is missed, including ventral thorax, abdomen, legs, feet, ears, lips and perineum.

Electric clippers. Fast, sharp and efficient electric clippers are a great asset. Unless the dog is to be exhibited at shows, do not be afraid to clip off hair which is concealing skin lesions. This will allow detailed examination of skin changes as well as easy application of topical treatments.

Good lighting. This is essential for seeing small parasites and observing subtle lesions. Of great benefit is an illuminating lamp with a central magnifying lens. Equipment of this type can be mounted on the wall and suspended over the dog when needed.

Skin scraping. This is the basic laboratory aid which is frequently omitted because it is time consuming. This is regrettable as it can confirm a diagnosis of Sarcoptes, Demodex, Cheyletiella or ringworm, all of which are not uncommon and require specific treatment. Potassium hydroxide (KOH) 5% is a versatile medium for mounting the scraping; when gently heated for a minute or two over a flame or after standing for an hour or more it 'clears' keratin debris and hair, which allows detection of both parasites and dermatophyte fungal spores. If consulting sessions are busy, it is good practice to take a skin scraping when the dog is on the table but to leave the microscopic examination until time is available to spend at least 5 minutes scanning the slide. Alternatively, nursing staff can be trained to carry out the microscope work. A quality microscope is essential for successful skin scrapings.

The following is a suitable routine for taking a skin scraping:

1   Clip the hair off the chosen area of skin.
2   Apply 1–2 drops of 5% KOH direct to the skin surface.
3   Scrape gently with a clean blunted scalpel blade until sufficient material is collected (Fig. 9.1).

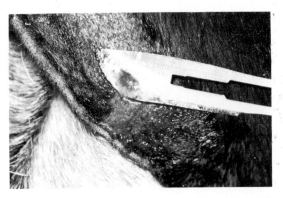

Fig. 9.1. Skin scraping. The most valuable aid to diagnosis in canine dermatology. An essential step for investigating all cases of scaling, hair loss or pustules.

4   Stop scraping at the first sign of blood.
5   Transfer the accumulated debris to a clean glass slide.
6   Add extra drops of KOH and mix thoroughly.
7   Cover with a clean coverslip.
8   Swab the scraped area of skin with damp cotton wool.
9   Heat slide over flame or leave to stand for an hour.
10   Examine slide with reduced microscope iris diaphragm for maximum visual contrast.

Bacteriology. This is frequently needed to investigate deep skin infections and if incubation facilities are available simple testing for antibiotic sensitivity may be useful. In recurrent cases, however, it is preferable to send swabs to a laboratory which offers more sophisticated identification of organisms. Samples should always be taken from freshly extruded purulent material; swabbing of ulcerated open skin lesions will be very misleading due to overgrowth of many nonspecific contaminants.

Fungal culture. On Sabouraud's medium at room temperature fungal culture is extremely easy, but the correct identification of fungal colonies requires expertise. If hair samples are to be sent to a diagnostic laboratory they should not be placed in sealed containers or wrapped in plastic as the retained moisture will result in rapid growth of saprophytes. Samples are best wrapped in paper or placed in a small paper envelope where they will remain dry.

Biopsy. This remains the definitive laboratory aid to dermatological diagnosis. It is unfortunate that so few histologists are familiar with skin pathology and their interpretation of dermatoses may not help. Nonetheless, the taking of skin biopsies should be encouraged and contact with enthusiastic histologists established. Biopsy is often reserved for tumours which are fairly well defined by histology.

Skin biopsy can be carried out in the consulting room using an intravenous sedative and subcutaneous local anaesthetic for all but the most unmanageable dogs. A small ellipse of the skin lesion is excised with a small blade, taking care not to damage the sample of skin with forceps. Closure of the wound with a single suture is usually all that is necessary.

DISEASE CONDITIONS OF CANINE SKIN

Compared to other body organs, the skin possesses the ability to exhibit a wide variety of clinical signs and symptoms. The changes in themselves are not diagnostic because some diseases cause superficially similar lesions. Demodectic mange is a great mimic and is, for example, able to produce lesions identical to ringworm, pyoderma, hormonal alopecia or seborrhoea.

The aim in examining the skin patient is to determine the aetiology so that specific treatment can be given. In many skin cases a precise cause cannot be found and treatment may be symptomatic or empirical (i.e. a scientific basis for the therapy cannot be explained). Novel and imaginative treatments sometimes result in unexpected improvement which may help elucidate new disease syndromes.

The remainder of this chapter is devoted to the discussion of canine skin diseases. However, instead of the usual classification by aetiology (available in full detail in Muller, Kirk & Scott 1983), the predominating clinical sign will be used as the starting point. There will not be an exhaustive list of all canine dermatoses; only the more commonly occurring ones are included, leaving rarer conditions to further reading.

HAIR LOSS

Loss of hair is a frequent clinical sign. The term alopecia in medical terminology implies specific failure of hair growth. Hair loss often causes no distress to the dog, but considerable anxiety to its owner because the lesions are so plainly visible and disfiguring. The question of possible contagion will need to be answered as quickly as possible.

Hormonal alopecia complex

This large group of diseases presents a critical diagnostic challenge for clinical practice.

The classical sign of hormonal alopecia is bilateral symmetry of the hair loss. Early changes such as thinning of the haircoat and abnormal pigmentation or scaling of the epidermis may precede eventual bald patches by some months. Commonly affected areas of the body are the flanks, chest, thighs and also the neck, where rubbing of the collar may exaggerate the failure of hair to grow normally.

Hormonal alopecia is more common in the dog than any other domestic animal and the wide variety of causes is testimony to the complex endocrine mechanisms which regulate hair growth in the various breeds. As a general rule, the appearance of the skin lesions alone does not allow a precise diagnosis to be made and careful attention must be paid to the history, full clinical examination of the patient and laboratory tests. Patchy hair loss which is not typical of hormonal alopecia should always have a skin scraping taken to exclude the possibility of mange or ringworm. Patchy lesions which show greasy scaling and inflammation are more likely to give a diagnosis of seborrhoeic dermatitis, based on negative results to specific tests.

The underlying endocrine disturbances which are well-recognised causes of hormonal alopecia can be listed as follows:

Thyroid-related alopecia
Confirmation of true hypothyroidism is not easy in the dog (see Chapter 8). Patients with alopecia which are proven subsequently to have normal thyroid function may nonetheless benefit from thyroxine administration, giving rise to a diagnosis of thyroid-responsive alopecia.

Adrenal-related alopecia
Cushing's disease is the term popularly used to describe hyperadrenocorticism caused by a number of factors, including neoplasia or hypertrophy of the adrenal cortex and/or pituitary gland (see Chapter 8). Iatrogenic Cushing's syndrome resulting from prolonged therapeutic dosage of corticosteroids is well recognised, but not as common as one might fear when considering the large quantities of these drugs dispensed to control chronic itching dermatoses in the dog. Hypoadrenocorticism (Addison's disease) was formerly a rare condition which sometimes had associated hair loss and abnormal skin pigmentation (see Chapter 8) but is now a not uncommon result of treating patients with Cushing's disease with the adrenocorticolytic compound o,p'DDD (Lysodren).

Oestrogen-related alopecia

Hyperoestrogenism is classically seen in male dogs with a testicular Sertoli cell tumour. Less well understood is a condition in bitches traditionally described as 'ovarian imbalance'. Cystic ovaries and 'functional' ovarian tumours may be the cause. Bitches of certain breeds, particularly Boxers and Bulldogs, may show recurrent alopecia of the thorax and flank regions which is possibly dependent on the oestrous cycle and spontaneously regresses (Fig. 9.2). These cases nonetheless often respond to thyroxine therapy.

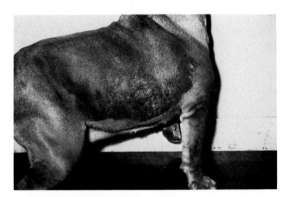

Fig. 9.2 Hormonal alopecia ('ovarian imbalance'). A Bulldog with bilateral recurrent thyroid-responsive alopecia.

Miscellaneous endocrine alopecia

Despite attempts at differential diagnosis, including circulating hormone estimations, there remains a group of ill-defined 'hormonal' alopecias which defy accurate classification. Poodles are notorious in this regard and are probably a special case with their woolly continuous-growth type of hair. Empirical treatment with a wide variety of hormones such as testosterone and anabolic steroids sometimes dramatically restores hair growth. This may be an example of breaking an 'imbalance' rather than true endocrine insufficiency. Experiments with laboratory animals have shown that external factors such as photoperiod and temperature may influence hair growth and replacement using complex hormonal mechanisms to induce seasonal moulting. Clear evidence now exists to show that thyroxine increases the rate of hair growth but reduces the duration of the active growing period, whereas oestrogens decrease both the rate and duration of hair growth. Corticosteroids appear to prolong the period of follicular resting. Interrelationship of the moulting cycle with the reproductive cycle illustrates that it may take many years before the precise endocrine mechanisms of non-spècific hormonal alopecias are explained. Re-growth

of hair in mature male dogs treated with experimental bovine or porcine growth hormone has led to description of growth hormone—responsive alopecia in Poodles, Pomeranians and Chows. The role of this hormone in hair growth will need further evaluation.

Differential diagnosis

Differential diagnosis of hormonal alopecia often relies on the accumulation of circumstantial evidence, because definitive endocrine assays are beyond the scope of the clinical laboratory. Skin biopsy gives similar results in many cases, with keratin debris filling the hair follicles. The most characteristic histopathological change is calcinosis in the case of hyperadrenocorticism.

The following associations help to make a diagnosis:

Hypothyroidism. Lethargy, fatigue, obesity, infertility and intolerance of cold. Dry, sparse haircoat with skin thickening and hyperkeratosis. Middle-aged dogs of larger breeds. Fasting blood cholesterol in excess of 350 mg/ml (see Chapter 8 for specific endocrinological diagnosis).

Hyperadrenocorticism. Polydipsia and polyuria with urine specific gravity of less than 1.012. Lethargy, muscle atrophy and weakness, unusual barrel-like body fat disposition, abdominal enlargement and excessive appetite. Paper-thin dry skin with areas of calcinosis and patchy pigmentation. Prominent superficial blood vessels with skin atrophy and striae over abdomen. Eosinopenia, hyperglycaem, and cholesterolaemia with increased serum alkaline phosphatase (see Chapter 8 for specific endocrinological diagnosis).

Hyperoestrogenism. Gynaecomastia and enlargement of scrotal or abdominally retained testicle in male dogs with Sertoli cell tumour. Mammary and vulval enlargement with abnormal oestrus in bitches. Specific assay of plasma sex hormones is a task for specialist research laboratories; their advice for collection of blood samples is usually necessary.

Treatment

Treatment of hormonal alopecia will depend on whether a specific diagnosis has been possible (see Chapter 8 for hypothyroidism and hyperadrenocorticism).

Dogs with Sertoli cell tumours should be bilaterally castrated and treated with testosterone by implant, injection or tablet until hair growth returns. Bitches with hyperoestrogenism or 'ovarian imbalance' should have bilateral ovariectomy or total hysterectomy performed. Follow-up treatment with oral thyroxine may hasten the return of hair growth.

Non-specific hormonal alopecia should be treated according to clinical judgement. Trial thyroxine therapy (0.4–0.8 mg/day for average-sized dogs) should be continued for at least 4–8 weeks to allow time for hair growth to begin again. Ideally, the dosage should be gradually implemented over a period of 2 weeks and 'tailed-off' over a period of 4 weeks when discontinued. Nonetheless, there appears to be much less danger of metabolic disturbances arising from thyroxine therapy in the dog than in man. Desiccated thyroid tablets are an outdated form of treatment with an unreliable shelf life and should not be used. Undiagnosed cases of hormonal alopecia which deteriorate or fail to respond to treatment should be referred to a specialist centre where endocrinological expertise is available.

Excessive hair shedding

Some dogs appear to shed abnormally large amounts of hair without suffering from detectable alopecia or even thinning of the haircoat. Owners of these animals may seek veterinary advice because the shed hair has become a nuisance around the house, collecting on furniture, carpets and clothing. Conscientious owners will attempt daily brushing of the dog on a heroic scale without noticeable reduction in the hairy pollution.

Most cases are normal variations of breed-dependent moulting which usually has seasonal peaks but may continue throughout the year. Dogs with light-coloured hair such as Dalmatians and Golden Retrievers are often the subject of complaint for the sole reason that their shed hairs are so visible.

When the shedding definitely exceeds normal limits for a particular breed of dog, the animal should be given a full clinical examination to rule out obvious disease or endocrine disturbance. Specific treatment to reduce shedding is not possible, although improvement is occasionally reported following non-specific hormonal therapy, particularly the administration of thyroxine. Supportive therapy in the form of multivitamins and fatty acid supplements may help and certainly do no harm. Centrally heated houses are sometimes blamed for causing excessive hair shedding. Although scientific proof is lacking for this theory, it may provide a useful excuse for restricting the offending dog to colder areas such as the garage, workshop or barn.

Demodectic mange

The follicular mite *Demodex canis* is a normal inhabitant of canine hair follicles, but in smaller numbers which cause no damage. For reasons which are still largely unexplained, this parasite can become pathogenic and multiply rapidly to produce massive populations of mites which destroy hair shafts, provoke skin scaling and seborrhoea, and mildly inflame the skin. The clinical result is patches of hair loss which may become generalised.

Factors which favour the development of demodectic mange include heredity, with short-haired breeds (e.g. Dachshunds) appearing more susceptible and certain bitches producing litters of puppies which have a high incidence of the disease. It has been shown experimentally that immunosuppressed pups are likely to develop demodectic mange, which suggests that failure of an immune mechanism is responsible for the naturally occurring disease.

Demodectic mange can be localised to only one or two patches of mild hair loss and sometimes restricted to only the head or legs. It may slowly spread or suddenly erupt as the generalised form of the disease with widespread disfiguring loss of hair. Two main types of skin damage are recognised:

1   Squamous lesions of scaling and waxy seborrhoea with either partial or complete loss of hair (Fig. 9.3).

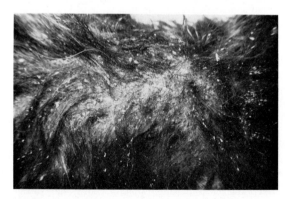

Fig. 9.3   Demodectic mange. Diffuse hair loss and marked skin scaling were features of demodicosis on this Yorkshire Terrier, although some pustules were also present.

2   Pustular lesions which result from rupture of mite-filled hair follicles into the dermis with subsequent foreign-body granulomatous inflammation and frequent secondary bacterial infection. Severe cases of generalised pustular demodectic mange will show marked ill health and may die or require euthanasia.

Demodectic mange is a common disease of young dogs and is often not diagnosed because it can appear in a wide variety of forms and thus mimic almost any other skin condition.

Diagnosis

Diagnosis of demodectic mange will present few problems provided careful skin scrapings are taken from *all* lesions which show any suspicious hair loss, surface scaling or pustule formation. It can be extremely embarrassing to refer a chronic skin case for second opinion without having examined a skin scraping. Failure to detect demodicosis by neglecting to take a scraping will lead to wasted expense on ineffective treatments, resentment by the worried owner and even accusations of malpractice.

The following points will help to make a diagnosis:

Age. Most dogs (but not all) will be under 1 year.

Itching. Pruritus is not a feature of the disease although pustular lesions may be irritable.

Fluorescence. Routine examination by Wood's light should be made to exclude *M. canis* ringworm.

Contagion. In-contact dogs will not become affected and lesions will not develop on the owners.

Positive skin scraping. The mites are relatively easy to detect and are the sole proof of diagnosis.

Duration of lesions. Chronic demodectic mange may persist for years, ringworm usually regresses within weeks.

All breeds. The 'susceptibility' of short-haired breeds may merely reflect the visibility of demodectic lesions on them. Long-haired breeds are not immune and risk misdiagnosis.

Treatment

Treatment of demodectic mange is a needlessly controversial subject. Published therapeutic suggestions range from the non-insecticide nutritional support approach to the subtoxic administration of topical and systemic organophosphorus insecticides. The fact that many dogs suffering from demodectic mange will eventually recover spontaneously, even without treatment, has probably led to the conflicting claims about therapeutic efficacy. Rotenone, an insecticidal compound, is generally recognised to be the treatment of choice for demodicosis. In the author's experience the following method of treatment is recommended:

1   Clip hair surrounding all lesions; in generalised mange this may mean a total body clip.
2   Wash the entire dog using a selenium sulphide shampoo and allow to remain 20–30 minutes on the skin before rinsing off. Local washing will suffice if minor lesions are present on a large dog. It is omitted for solitary or periocular lesions.
3   When the dog is dry, apply a spirit solution of rotenone (0.75%) to localised lesions *once every four days* using a small brush. For generalised mange paint *one-quarter of the body every day* so that all lesions will receive the solution once every 4 days.
4   Repeat the selenium shampoo every fourth day followed by rotenone application.

Do not exceed the dosage by applying the rotenone solution to more than one-quarter of the body at one time, otherwise toxicity may occur in the form of ataxia, hyperaesthesia and convulsions. Deeply ulcerated areas of skin should not be painted with solution which will cause stinging and allow toxic absorption; apply a soothing antibiotic cream instead.

5   Dogs suffering from the pustular form of the disease should receive appropriate long-term systemic antibiotic treatment.
6   Continue the shampoo and rotenone treatment for at least four weeks. Chronic generalised cases may require up to 3 months' treatment or more. Because the treatment is tedious and messy, it should be adequately explained to owners who may not be able to carry it out themselves.
7   Simultaneous treatment with corticosteroids to reduce erythema is contraindicated, however tempting.
8   Avoid topical greasy ointments which prevent rotenone penetration of parasitised hair follicles. Mange preparations which contain mixtures of other insecticides may be efficacious in mild localised cases.
9   The prognosis is very good for all but the most severe chronic pustular cases. Permanent scarring may result from destruction of hair follicles where pustules were prominent.
10   Administration of hormones or oral insecticides does not produce added benefit.
11   An agricultural miticide, amitraz, is now available in veterinary formulation for the treatment of demodectic mange. It may be a useful alternative when rotenone is not obtainable.

Ringworm

Certain fungi have evolved an affinity for growing on

keratin and are called dermatophytes in recognition of the damage they can cause to keratinised skin components such as hair, nails and epidermis. Many are thought to originate from soil saprophytes whose functions may have included breakdown of naturally shed hair, feathers and skin scales. Some species of dermatophytes are now wholly adapted to a parasitic life on skin and their reservoirs are not in the soil but on carrier animals or man.

In the dog, three species of dermatophyte are commonly capable of causing skin lesions which are sometimes circular with a raised inflammatory rim; hence the popular but misleading term, 'ringworm'.

Microsporum canis is a zoophilic fungus best adapted to the skin of the cat where it may persist for years in a carrier state producing little or no skin damage. Lesions are also seen in man and the dog where the infection is self-limiting by provoking an inflammatory response and susequent immunity. *M. canis* is responsible for more than 50% of canine ringworm.

Trichophyton mentagrophytes is also zoophilic but best adapted to rodent skin. Infection is mostly derived from carrier reservoirs in rats and mice. Together with its hedgehog-adapted variant *T. erinacei*, this fungus is the second most frequent cause of canine ringworm.

Microsporum gypseum is a geophilic fungus (i.e. a soil saprophyte), but in some countries, particularly those of warm climate, it occasionally causes ringworm in dogs. The lesions are usually inflammatory and the infection is self-limiting. Multiple spontaneous lesions suggest that dogs are infected direct from the soil; it is rare for dog-to-dog transmission to occur.

Pathogenesis
The pathogenesis of dermatophytosis is the result of fungal hyphae invading hair shafts, follicles and the stratum corneum of the epidermis. The keratin is actually digested by the fungus causing hair to fall out and skin scaling to occur. The hyphae do not invade living cells, but their toxic products may induce quite a severe local inflammatory reaction. Young dogs are more frequently infected because older animals develop immunity.

Lesions
The lesions of ringworm are·variable according to the breed of dog, age and the species of fungus infecting them. Hair loss is usual although it may not result in obvious patches but only areas of thinning or abnormal hair. Skin scaling is sometimes severe. Classical ringworm-shaped lesions are in fact the exception; numerous surveys have shown that 'typical' lesions confirm less than 10% of cases as positive for ringworm. Areas of the body most commonly affected are the head, feet and legs.

Diagnosis
The diagnosis of ringworm rests entirely on identification of the infection by Wood's light fluorescence, skin scraping and/or culture of the dermatophyte fungus. *All* cases of hair loss should be routinely examined by Wood's light in a dark room. Most infections with *M. canis* will show greenish fluorescence of affected hairs. Allow time for the lamp to warm up and examine areas of hair loss carefully as small fluorescing stumps of hair are easily overlooked. Infections of *T. mentagrophytes* or *M. gypseum* do not exhibit fluorescence. If scrapings are taken in KOH and allowed adequate time or heat to 'clear', accumulations of fungal arthrospores can be detected around infected hair shafts to provide a positive diagnosis. Mycological culture of suspect hair samples is highly desirable for all cases of possible ringworm but regrettably this simple laboratory technique is all too often neglected in practice. Plates of Sabouraud's medium should incorporate an inhibitor such as cycloheximide to suppress growth of saprophytic fungi. Bacterial contamination can be controlled by first swabbing the skin with 70% alcohol before taking hair samples. Normal hairs are unlikely to be infected; the chances of isolating a ringworm fungus will be increased if samples are taken of broken or abnormal hairs from the advancing edges of lesions. After incubation of culture plates at room temperature for at least 1–2 weeks, identification of dermatophyte colonies can be attempted. This requires some knowledge of mycology, but the task is not too difficult and good descriptions are available in textbooks. *M. canis* colonies are characteristically woolly with a yellowish undersurface; *T. mentagrophytes* colonies have a powdery granular surface with brownish undersurface; *M. gypseum* colonies are buff coloured with chamois-leather texture. Dark or black fungal colonies are usually contaminants.

A new technical problem has arisen from the widespread use of a so-called 'dermatophyte test medium' (Fungassay). It is basically Sabouraud's agar with added phenol red indicator which is supposed to reveal its colour when dermatophyte fungi form colonies and release alkaline metabolites. Its use by diagnostic laboratories has led to the erroneous assumption that all red-releasing colonies are dermatophytes and as a result reports of over 50% positive samples for ringworm are now common. Considering that the incidence of ringworm in the dog is very low, the false overdiagnosis of ringworm from using the colour indicating medium presents serious implications for both the veterinary clinician and the dog owner who believe the laboratory result. The problem can only be resolved by a return to the use of conventional media combined with an adequate knowledge of colony identification. Incorrect laboratory diagnosis of ringworm is leading to unjustified complaints of ineffective griseofulvin therapy.

Treatment

The treatment of ringworm in the dog is much easier than in the cat, where endemic *M. canis* infections in catteries call for heroic measures. Griseofulvin is the drug of choice in the dog and it should be remembered that because it is incorporated into keratin at least 4–6 weeks therapy will be required for full efficacy. The daily dosage should be 15 mg/kg body weight given once with some high fat food to aid absorption from the gut.

Topical treatment of ringworm lesions is not very effective but is additionally desirable to reduce the risk of transmission of the infection to human skin, especially that of children. Hair should be clipped away and a non-irritating fungicidal cream such as tolnaftate applied once or twice daily. Generalised ringworm in the dog is an indication for total hair clip and twice weekly bathing with a water soluble povidone-iodine solution (Pevidine). A decision to commence specific ringworm therapy should never be taken unless the diagnosis is confirmed by Wood's light, skin scraping or fungal culture. It is paradoxical that a number of non-fungal skin diseases, particularly seborrhoeic dermatitis, produce lesions which are more 'ringworm-like' in appearance than ringworm itself.

PIGMENTARY DISORDERS

The basal layer of the epidermis contains a number of dendritic cells called melanocytes which produce masses of tiny melanin pigment granules. The colour of the skin is determined by the quantity of melanin and the rate at which it is taken up by the epidermal prickle cells as they move towards the surface and are keratinised. Actively growing hair bulbs also contain melanocytes which produce a variety of melanin granules incorporated into the hair shafts to provide the spectacular variety of coat colours.

Pigment production is under complex genetic and hormonal control and is a relatively trouble-free part of skin biology in the dog. Abnormalities of hair pigmentation are extremely rare except for the inevitable greying which age ultimately brings to us all. On the other hand, hair staining is an almost unavoidable cosmetic complaint in breeds such as Poodles and Maltese Terriers. White hair beneath the eyes, tail, perineum and axillae can take up a pink-brown stain following secretion of tears, sweat and mucus. In some animals the degree of staining, particularly beneath the eyes, can be disfiguring and can lead to justifiable use of dilute hydrogen peroxide or sodium hypochlorite as bleaching agents. Abnormalities of skin pigmentation are not all that uncommon, but unless accompanied by hair loss usually remain hidden beneath the coat. An example of normal skin failing to pigment adequately is nasal depigmentation. Otherwise, too much or too little pigmentation is seen mostly in association with abnormal skin changes such as acanthosis, hyperkeratosis or hormonal alopecia.

Acanthosis nigricans

This condition occurs predominantly in Dachshunds but can also be seen in Poodles, Terriers and other breeds. A typical case will show marked thickening of the epidermis (acanthosis) in both axillae with accompanying hair loss and excessively dark pigmentation. Dogs as young as 6 months of age can develop bilateral lesions not only in the axillae but also across the ventral chest which may resemble demodectic mange or ringworm. Older dogs may suffer from a more chronic form of the disease which can slowly lead to thick greasy folds of blackened skin under the neck, axillae, chest, flanks, hocks and medial limb surfaces. In these cases, seborrhoea and an unpleasant skin odour may be additional problems.

Aetiology

The aetiology of acanthosis nigricans is unknown. Response to a variety of hormones and steroids suggests a complex pathogenesis.

Diagnosis

Diagnosis of acanthosis nigricans relies on the presence of typical changes in both axillae. Similar lesions may also be seen in dogs suffering from hormonal alopecia but more widespread hair loss will usually be evident.

Treatment

Treatment is of necessity somewhat empirical. Although the thyroid glands may be functioning normally, administration of thyroxine will often benefit the younger patient with early lesions. Older dogs with advanced skin changes should also receive systemic corticosteroids, with long-term therapy needed in many cases. Topical application of corticosteroid creams will aid resolution. Shampoos will help chronic seborrhoeic lesions but complete cure of advanced cases should not be expected; the aim is to make them comfortable.

Nasal depigmentation

Black-nosed dogs may lose their attractive appearance when the prominent shiny nasal pad loses its black pigment.

Trauma

Trauma is a nasal occupational hazard because the snout is regularly used as a digging, burrowing and pushing tool. Despite its thickness the dorsal surface of the snout is easily damaged and bacterial infection can follow. Nasal pigment may be temporarily 'washed out' by rapid turnover of epidermal cells during the inflammatory process. Deeper damage to the nasal surface will often produce scarring with a local area of permanent depigmentation. Chronic ulceration of the nose is not uncommon in German Shepherds and Collies with subsequent risk of chronic sunburn ('Collie nose'), particularly in hot climates. Differential diagnosis from nasal pyoderma due to chronic bacterial infection is not always easy. Failure to heal in chronic cases of nasal ulceration may herald the onset of precancerous changes. A variety of newly-described autoimmune diseases may present with nasal ulceration in the dog (see Chapter 10).

Generalised nasal depigmentation

This is a cosmetic curiosity which can worry owners of show dogs. A previously jet-black nose fades to light brown in the absence of any clinical skin lesions. Sometimes the pigment returns several months later and recurrent nasal depigmentation is seen. Without an adequate aetiological explanation, no treatment can be recommended for this condition. A hormonal mechanism is possible.

Other pigmentary disorders

Hyperpigmentation often accompanies chronic skin inflammation or irritation, irrespective of the cause. Many persistent skin lesions will eventually darken, especially during the final phases of resolution or defensive thickening. This type of abnormal pigmentation will normally fade if the skin condition heals. Hyperpigmentation, often of a patchy variety, is to be expected with any of the hormonal alopecias and will usually disappear if endocrine treatment is successful.

Hypopigmentation is a natural consequence of many inflammatory skin conditions. The basal melanocytes simply cannot produce sufficient melanin to pigment the rapidly reproducing epidermis and it is 'washed out'. When the epidermis resumes a normal turnover time pigmentation of previously coloured skin will return. Vitiligo is the term for disfiguring patches of skin which cease pigmenting and are embarrassingly visible on black human skin. An autoimmune mechanism is suspected. The term is occasionally used to describe patches of animal skin which are otherwise normal but fail to produce normal pigment. In dogs, such patches are most commonly the sign of scarring after previous trauma.

PRURITUS

This latin-derived noun used to describe itching is often misspelt to end -*itis*, nonetheless it is a widely used clinical term in veterinary practice. In human medicine however, the word prurigo is used to describe any skin eruption which is accompanied by persistent severe itching.

The itching dog is probably the most important problem facing the veterinary dermatologist. Owners will not tolerate an animal which continually scratches, rubs and bites itself. It is distressing to observe and, in addition, disturbing at night if the dog sleeps inside the house. The inevitable result of canine pruritus is self-inflicted trauma to the fragile skin. The damaged epidermis can heal quickly if it is left alone and is not subject to secondary infection but the repair process is irritable and so the itch-scratch cycle unfortunately gathers momentum. All too often this results in unsightly skin lesions and a self-perpetuating disease although the initial cause of the original itching (e.g. fleas) may have departed. Certain breeds of dog, particularly those which have a highly strung temperament or unusually sensitive skin, can develop a habit of itching and scratching which leads to chronic problems.

Pathophysiology
The pathophysiology of canine pruritus has received little study and it remains to be determined if the skin of the dog is in fact intrinsically more prone to itch sensations. Receptors and nerve endings transmit impulses to the brain from the skin but it is also possible that a central medullary 'itch centre' may exist, as exemplified by animal infections such as scrapie and Aujesky's disease. Biochemical mediators such as histamine undoubtedly play a major role in the generation of pruritus but a specific antipruritic drug remains to be found. Scratching temporarily relieves itching by

producing overriding pain sensations, but the skin damage usually results in release of further prurito-genic mediators and hence the itch-scratch cycle begins. The 'itch threshold' of the central nervous system should not be overlooked. General 'neuronal excitement' can raise this threshold, suggesting that physical activity and mental diversion can help alleviate pruritus. On the other hand boredom and inactivity are well-recognised factors which favour the development of itch-scratch problems in the dog.

Causes

The causes of canine pruritus are many and varied. Skin damage or inflammation of any kind is likely to produce itching. Allergic conditions in which hypersensitivity reactions occur in the skin are notorious for the severity of pruritus they induce. Simple dryness or superficial scaling of the skin is frequently pruritic.

Finally, ectoparasitic infestations will usually produce pruritus merely by crawling about the skin surface. Certain clinical syndromes are notable by the fact that pruritus itself is the major manifestation in the absence of other significant changes such as dermatitis, pustules or scaling. These predominantly pruritic conditions will now be discussed in detail.

Scabies (sarcoptic mange)

The parasitic mite *Sarcoptes scabiei* var. *canis* burrows into the superficial layer of the epidermis and it is here that the female lays her eggs. For reasons which are still not fully understood, the infestation results in intolerable pruritus of distressing intensity. Because the itching does not develop until a few weeks after the mites have become established, it is thought by some that the itching may be due to the development of hypersensitivity to their secretions and excretions.

Scabies is readily transmissible between dogs although close body contact is necessary. The general incidence of the disease shows cyclical peaks of infection with periods of many years when little scabies is reported. In areas where dogs receive routine insecticidal flea-control baths scabies may become quite rare. Foxes act as the natural reservoir for the disease in some countries. Human scabies caused by *Sarcoptes scabiei* is not transmissible to dogs but the canine variety is capable of surviving on the skin of individual dog owners for several days, sufficient to cause irritable papules whilst close contact with an infected dog is maintained.

Although canine scabies is not common in most cities it occurs more often than many veterinarians believe. Outbreaks are sometimes seen in kennel establishments and puppies purchased from pet shops may subsequently show clinical signs. All dogs which are brought to a veterinary clinic suffering from intense pruritus should be closely examined for the possibility of scabies.

The following points may help to establish a diagnosis:

1 Unlike demodectic mange, scabies is seen in dogs of all ages and breeds.
2 A recent stay in boarding kennels should arouse suspicions of scabies.
3 The owners should always be asked if they have noticed any irritable papules on their own skin. The presence of small red lesions on the arms or trunk will necessitate a careful search for either Sarcoptes or Cheyletiella mites on the suspect dog.
4 The hallmark of canine scabies is persistent and intense pruritus which may exhaust the dog from irresistible scratching. Although any area of the body can be infested with mites the ears, elbows and hocks are most noticeably affected. Scratching by the hindleg becomes an almost involuntary reaction and if the ear is rubbed with fingers a so-called 'scratch reflex' is almost diagnostic of scabies.
5 The ears, head and elbows may be severely mutilated from continual hindlimb scratching, thus obliterating any of the tiny lesions caused by the Sarcoptes mites themselves. Close examination of the skin of non-traumatised areas will usually reveal the papules typical of canine scabies (Fig. 9.4). Reddened 'tunnels' in the skin which are diagnostic of human scabies do not occur on the much thinner skin of the dog.
6 Affected skin may also be hot, inflamed and partially hairless as a result of scratching and biting.
7 Every effort should be made to confirm a diagnosis of scabies by identifying Sarcoptes mites in a skin scraping. Chances of doing this are improved if 2–3 scrapings are taken from non-traumatised sites, preferably those which show typical papules. Sarcoptes mites are comparatively large so time can be saved by using a very low-powered microscope objective (e.g. × 4) for examination of the preparation.
8 If scabies is suspected but mites cannot be found despite several skin scrapings it is sensible to begin trial acaricidal treatment for a few weeks to assess the response.

Treatment

Treatment of scabies is not simple because the life-cycle of the mite is about 3 weeks and reinfection from contaminated bedding can occur. Sarcoptes mites are relatively easy to kill with a variety of chemical compounds. Successful therapy will largely depend on its

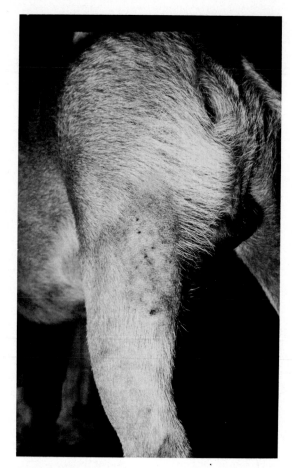

Fig. 9.4 Scabies. The hair has been clipped away from the hindlimb to reveal *Sarcoptes* papules.

duration; at least 4 weeks are needed to bring the infestation under control. The following treatment routine can be recommended:

1   Thoroughly wash the entire dog with a BHC-containing shampoo (Quellada) and leave it on the skin for 30 minutes before rinsing off, if possible.
2   Apply a final rinse containing another suitable insecticide, such as bromocyclen (Alugan) or lime-sulphur (available from garden centres, dilute to approximately 0.7%).
3   When the dog is dry, apply topical benzyl benzoate lotion to the worst affected areas of skin.
4   Repeat the above treatment each week for at least 4 weeks or longer until the pruritus has abated. Destroy or wash infested bedding and spray kennels with an insecticide.
5   Initial administration of corticosteroid tablets for

4–5 days will dramatically relieve the pruritus and allow traumatised skin to heal. Undiagnosed cases of scabies which receive long-term corticosteroid therapy to suppress pruritus (without the benefit of acaricides) may develop bizarre forms of generalised Sarcoptes infestation ('scabies incognito') aggravated by immuno-suppression.
6   Canine scabies papules on human skin will benefit from application of crotamiton lotion (Eurax).
7   Injectable ivermectin provides good control of scabies in sheep, cattle and pigs. Although further evaluation is needed, this compound promises to be the first injectable treatment for canine scabies.

Flea infestation

The truism 'common things commonly occur' is highly relevant to fleas on dogs. Some veterinarians firmly believe that fleas cause 90% of canine pruritus and even go so far as to prescribe trial insecticidal treatment before wasting further clinic time investigating the itchy patient. Certainly mild itching and scratching centring on the backline area will invariably turn out to be due to infestation with fleas. These parasites are now becoming resistant to older insecticides and flea infestations in household dogs and cats present a growing problem.

Fleas cause pruritus from simple mechanical irritation by crawling on the skin, but their bites can also irritate. A percentage of dogs will eventually develop fleabite hypersensitivity with the result that only one or two fleas can provoke severe bouts of itching and dermatitis. This allergy to flea saliva can provoke intense immunological skin reactions including immediate-type antibody-mediated hypersensitivity (wheal and flare), delayed-type cell-mediated hypersensitivity (induration), or a combination of both.

Clinically, flea allergy dermatitis ('summer eczema') is invariably characterised by marked pruritus with an exudative dermatitis along the backline and base of the tail. Aggravated by self-inflicted biting and rubbing, these areas of skin soon show hair loss. Chronic cases which suffer from recurrent seasonal flea allergy may exhibit permanent backline scarring, thickening and pigmentation which can become bizarre ('elephant hide'). Owners of such dogs sometimes doubt that simple fleas can cause such a disfiguring skin condition.

Diagnosis
The diagnosis of flea infestation is not difficult if the following points are considered:

1 Fleas ingest much more blood than is necessary for their survival and pass frequent faeces comprised of almost pure dried blood ('flea dirts'). Detection of flea faeces is usually possible with the naked eye, particularly along the backline and tail-base favoured zones. Nonetheless, a useful diagnostic aid is the wet paper flea test (Fig. 9.5). A sheet of white paper is wet

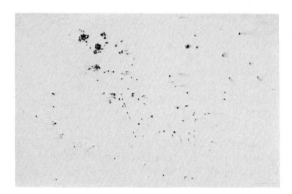

Fig. 9.5 Wet paper flea dirt test. Bloodstained streaks identify flea faeces.

and placed under or near the dog. The haircoat is brushed with the fingers and any dislodged debris collected on the paper. Flea faeces quickly give rise to bloodstained streaks on the paper which are more readily visible than the tiny black 'dirts' themselves.

2 It is normally unnecessary to hunt for live fleas on the animal. If certain owners need further convincing a brief application of a 'knockdown' flea spray will usually result in dead fleas becoming detectable on the dog or the examination table. This procedure is not routinely advisable because of possible long-term toxicity risks to the veterinarian.

3 Most fleas found on dogs are the common cat flea *Ctenocephalides felis felis*. The dog flea *C. canis* is less frequent. Hedgehog and rabbit fleas are sometimes found on dogs which have contact with these animals or their territories.

Treatment and prevention
The treatment and prevention of uncomplicated flea infestations can be tedious if the owners do not participate enthusiastically in the eradication programme. In many instances cats provide the reservoir of parasites and must also be treated.

1 The choice of insecticides and the methods of application will depend on a variety of factors including the size and temperament of the dog, facilities available at home (e.g. bath), ability of the owner, and

cost. Residual insecticide rinses following a bath are most effective but are least practical, especially in winter. Aerosol sprays are convenient and effective if properly used. Many proprietary flea powders sold at pet shops are ineffective or of very short persistence. Availability of new synthetic pyrethroid insecticides such as resmethrin promise to revolutionise flea control with their low toxicity, lack of odour and high efficacy.

2 Flea collars and medallions are a useful aid to parasite control but are rarely sufficient alone.

3 Most of the flea life-cycle is spent off the host and treatment of the dog's environment is essential if control is to be achieved. Weekly vacuum-cleaning of infested household rooms is advisable, followed by application of a persistent insecticide aerosol. Kennels and bedding must also be washed and treated.

4 Explanation of the life-cycle of fleas to the owner will be necessary to ensure their full cooperation. A printed leaflet will save time. Local authorities or professional pest exterminators should be contacted for control of fleas in severely infested houses.

5 Dogs suffering from suspected flea-bite hypersensitivity require exceptionally rigorous flea control as even a single parasite can trigger severe skin lesions. Initial corticosteroid therapy is indicated to relieve acute dermatitis. Some clinicians favour simultaneous administration of an antihistamine for added benefit. A topical steroid cream will hasten resolution of intensely inflamed backline lesions. Hyposensitisation therapy by injection of whole-flea antigenic extracts has been tried in several countries, but results are usually disappointing and short lived.

Other parasite infestations

Many arthropod parasites are capable of inducing pruritus in the dog.

Lice
Lice are occasionally a problem, particularly in populations of puppies such as in breeding kennels or pet shops. Infestations usually cause marked pruritus around the head and neck. Severely parasitised animals may need clipping of matted hair to allow adequate treatment. Anaemia may be present in very young pups.

Cheyletiella
These mites also cause pruritus in the dog. Scaling of the skin is the prominent clinical sign however and the condition is described later in this chapter (see p. 206).

Trombicula

Trombicula harvest mites can be a problem in some areas.

Ticks

Ticks, particularly the larval forms, may cause noticeable itching in some dogs.

Miscellaneous

Miscellaneous free-living arthropods are found in large numbers in straw, hay, grass and even carpets. Their role as causes of pruritus in the dog is ill defined and worthy of further investigation: the straw itch mite *Pyemotes tritici* commonly infests straw, hay and grain and can cause skin eruptions in both man and animals. Non-specific insecticidal treatment may be helpful in suspect cases.

Non-specific pruritus (prurigo)

When all commonly recognised causes of primary pruritus have been eliminated there remains a group of dogs whose persistent itching defies a specific diagnosis. Effective therapy is not difficult to find: the corticosteroids usually provide rapid relief of symptoms. Worry over the consequences of long-term steroid administration combined with a natural desire to find a cause may lead the veterinarian to attempt a plausible diagnosis in the absence of convincing scientific proof. The art of clinical judgement when assessing chronic canine pruritus is frequently stretched to the limits. The major areas of controversy are discussed below.

Allergy

More than 20 years ago, before immunology became such a special science, allergic reactions were just being defined. Many previously mysterious skin eruptions were shown to be caused by hypersensitivity to a variety of antigens which were more popularly termed 'allergens'. The precise immunological mechanisms are now better understood, and further reading on this complex subject is essential for full understanding. Several basic concepts remain clear however.

Allergy requires a period of sensitisation to induce the appropriate immunological state. A common misconception is that an allergic reaction occurs on first exposure to an antigen, whereas in fact it is usual for an allergy to develop gradually following prolonged and repeated contact with the antigen. Some substances are potent sensitisers and will induce hypersensitivity fairly soon in most individuals. Other substances are weak sensitisers and hypersensitivity only develops in susceptible individuals after months or even years of regular contact.

Sensitisation can induce two common types of hypersensitivity state. The first is mediated by specific circulating antibody (IgE) which has the unique ability to attach itself to skin mast cells. Further contact with the specific antigen results in immediate hypersensitivity which occurs within minutes and typically produces in the skin a wheal and flare reaction that subsides an hour or two later. The second type of state is mediated by sensitised cells, usually lymphocytes, which are part of the body's cellular immunity system. Further contact with the specific antigen requires migration of cells from the blood and lymphatic systems to produce, about 48 hours later, a delayed hypersensitivity reaction which starts an inflammatory skin reaction with accompanying induration and frequently exudation or vesiculation. Both types of hypersensitivity induce release of numerous biochemical mediators, with histamine predominating in immediate-type reactions. Pruritus is a clinical feature of both states.

In the dog it is often impossible to recognise which type of hypersensitivity is occurring in a suspected clinical allergic skin condition. Not only does hair obscure visibility, but self-inflicted damage also confuses the picture. A well-recognised allergic syndrome is generalised skin urticaria which may follow an insect sting or ingestion of a particular substance, plant or food to which the dog has been sensitised. Immediate-type hypersensitivity is the underlying mechanism.

Diagnosis

Diagnosis of allergy is regularly attempted in man by means of intradermal prick or injection tests for determining the presence of specific circulating IgE antibody. A positive result is indicated by a wheal and flare reaction in the skin. Interpretation of the overall results is difficult as many people have specific antibodies to a variety of antigens without any symptoms whatsoever. Intradermal tests in dogs are frequently unreliable because antigen supplies are usually not standardised and responses by different breeds vary widely. The true incidence of allergic-based pruritus in the dog is thus unknown, but deserves further scientific investigation.

Treatment

The treatment of allergy aims, if possible, to avoid the antigen(s) responsible for the clinical syndrome. Antihistamines are of some use in preventing immediate-type reactions, but once hypersensitivity has occurred it is only the corticosteroids which are regularly useful in dogs. Acute urticaria and facial swelling will require intravenous injection of a soluble steroid and perhaps adrenaline as well if respiratory distress or shock is present. Chronic allergic conditions such as flea hypersensitivity or contact allergic dermatitis can be suppressed by administration of corticosteroids although more specific drugs may eventually be developed. Hyposensitisation therapy by injection of repeated large doses of antigens was at one time very popular in human medicine. The theory was that 'blocking' antibodies were produced which reduced the hypersensitivity reaction. In general, the benefits are small and of short duration, but treatment of this nature is still frequently prescribed on the basis that although it may do little good, it generally does no harm. Enthusiastic reports of successful hyposensitisation therapy in dogs continue to appear in the literature, but the evidence is generally anecdotal. Recently it has been suggested that crude extracts of household vacuum-cleaner dust give 'good results' in cases of suspected non-specific allergic pruritus. Such recommendations belong more to folk-medicine than science and as such are similar to herbalism, homeopathy or acupuncture, all of which have their advocates in veterinary medicine.

There is a risk that allergy and dermatology will become separate veterinary specialities, as in human medicine, unless more scientific and experimental data are offered to substantiate the claims for hyposensitisation therapy, restrictive diets and withdrawal of suspected household contact sensitisers and so on.

The differences between contact irritants and contact sensitisers in the dog are poorly understood. Atopy is becoming a popular diagnosis but, contrary to popular belief, it cannot be scientifically based solely on a positive intradermal test. Its incidence outside the USA, in countries where ragweed hypersensitivity does not occur, remains a matter of conjecture. Atopic individuals possess an innate ability to produce abnormally large amounts of IgE antibody to a wide variety of inhaled or in-contact antigens. The presence of these circulating antibodies does not imply that any disease ensues; indeed the majority of human atopics are symptomless. Because laboratory assay of antigen-specific IgE in serum is time consuming and expensive, the only practical method of assessing atopy in man is to perform skin prick testing to a battery of common antigens such as the house dust mite, grass pollen, animal epithelial extracts and fungal derivatives. One or more positive tests arbitrarily defines an atopic individual and on this basis about 30% of the population are thus considered atopic, although essentially normal.

The diseases associated statistically with atopy in man are hay fever, asthma and infantile eczema but the precise role of IgE antibodies is far from clear. Atopy in the dog is a clinical diagnosis which should be restricted until further research clarifies this somewhat academic subject.

Diet

Dog food manufacturers have some data on the role of nutrition in canine pruritus but little has been published. Essential fatty acid deficiency was described several decades ago and is discussed later as a possible cause of skin scaling and sometimes pruritus. Vitamin deficiencies are based on similar assumptions but may well occur in dogs not fed modern commercial 'complete' dog food. The administration of balanced vitamin and fatty acid supplements to dogs suffering from non-specific pruritus is thus a harmless and perhaps beneficial practice. There is clearly a pressing need for further research into the whole subject of nutrition and its influence on canine skin. Occasional reports of so-called zinc-responsive dermatosis in dogs indicate that this mineral plays a role in skin health.

Food allergy as a cause of pruritus in the dog is frequently overdiagnosed on circumstantial evidence. In the absence of alimentary allergic symptoms or urticaria it probably does not occur.

Environment

Many breeds of dog were bred to thrive in subarctic climates and it is not surprising that during the summer in warm climates they suffer from a variety of skin disorders. Centrally heated houses are often thought to disrupt the normal skin biology of many thick-coated dogs, with non-specific pruritus being a frequent complaint. It is difficult to estimate the role played by temperature and humidity but experience shows that as a general rule such pruritus will be reduced by colder conditions. Excessive dryness which develops in centrally heated homes can also increase the degree of pruritus suffered by dogs with an abnormally dry and scaly skin. Confinement to a colder area of the house may benefit the dog and satisfy the owner.

The texture of surfaces on which a dog lies will also influence the development of pruritus. Abrasive materials such as concrete are notorious causes of skin irritation in kennelled dogs where outbreaks of scabies-like pruritus with hair loss, callus formation, ulceration and superficial infection are not uncommon. Unusual skin problems in dogs which frequently lie on concrete should be suspect and a trial period of removal from the concreted surfaces should be considered. Newly laid concrete can be particularly irritant to canine skin. Treatment of troublesome concrete is possible and advice should be sought from an expert in cement surfacing.

Straw, hay, grass, wood shavings and sawdust are all potential irritants to some dogs with sensitive skins. The irritation may be due to associated mites or chemicals or merely to the prickly nature of these materials. Mats made of seagrass or synthetic fibre can also possess abrasive surfaces. Some carpets are occasionally irritating to dogs but there is little justification for the household disruption and anxiety brought on by trial removal. Allergy to carpets is very rare although frequently proffered as a diagnosis for chronic pruritus. Itchy skin disease has natural periods of regression which render circumstantial evidence meaningless and can lead to unjust incrimination of harmless fabrics.

Neurosis

Although difficult to diagnose with certainty, some cases of non-specific pruritus are of central nervous origin.

Neurotic dogs may possess a very low itch threshold and also perhaps derive satisfaction from scratching and self mutilation. This complaint is frequently seen in Poodles in which chewing of the dorsal surfaces of the feet may be a characteristic feature. Dogs of this temperament are also candidates for the eventual development of lick granulomas.

Systemic disease

It is well recognised in man that pruritus may accompany a variety of internal illnesses including jaundice, neoplasia, diabetes and uraemia. Such associations are rarely reported in dogs but should nonetheless be considered in the investigation of pruritus. Generalised neoplasia such as mastocytosis or lymphoma will usually be detected by the presence of some skin plaques or ulcerative lesions. A skin biopsy is necessary to provide a histological opinion. Internal parasites such as intestinal or heart worms can provoke pruritus by the migration of larvae through skin blood vessels.

Treatment

The treatment of non-specific pruritus should be flexible to allow variation by the owner according to the severity of itching at the time.

The following points may be considered:

1 Corticosteroids are potent suppressors of pruritus in the dog. Administration for 1–2 weeks is harmless and will often break the itch-scratch cycle to allow healing. Oral treatment is preferable to depot-type injections as it ensures full control of daily dosage. Long-term corticosteroid therapy should only be considered when all diagnostic procedures have been ex-

hausted. Alternate-day dosage can often control pruritus without inducing serious side-effects. Intelligent owners can be given a liberal supply of corticosteroid tablets if they are able to use them sparingly according to the need of the dog. High doses for 2–3 days may induce regression of symptoms for more than a week and are preferable to needless routine daily dosage.

2 Antihistamines are disappointing drugs for the control of pruritus in dogs. Any beneficial effect is more likely to be due to concurrent sedation and specific tranquillisers may do a better job. Nonetheless, many veterinarians favour a combination of corticosteroid and antihistamine therapy for the control of pruritus.

3 Regular bathing and shampooing will often benefit dogs with non-specific pruritus. A tar-based shampoo is preferable. Rinsing with a water-miscible 'bath oil' sometimes aids the inherent itchiness of dry skins.

4 Dietary supplementation with fatty acids plus vitamins will sometimes bring unexpected benefit to dogs suffering from non-specific pruritus. The soothing effect may be due to increased skin oiliness which often follows their administration. A change of diet can also be considered, particularly if the previous one is suspected to be deficient in any way.

5 Exercise, games and fellow canine companions will help to distract the pruritic dog's attention from his skin. A holiday can benefit the dog as well as its owner.

SKIN SCALING

A small amount of skin scaling ('scurf') is normal in the dog. Just as dandruff affects some people, excessive skin scaliness becomes noticeable in some dogs, particularly those with contrasting black hair. Mild scaling alone is rarely a problem unless cosmetically unacceptable to the ówner. More frequently skin scaling is accompanied by pruritus and/or hair loss and a veterinary consultation may be sought.

Ichthyosis (dry skin)

Strictly speaking, the term ichthyosis is used in man to describe scaling of the skin which is genetically determined and present throughout life. Various types are recognised (e.g. dominant, recessive and sex-linked). The most common variety expresses itself simply as 'dry' skin with fine surface scaling. Such skin tends to be irritable and more prone to damage and infection.

In the dog the situation has scarcely been studied, and it is not possible to classify ichthyosis with any precision. Nonetheless some dogs do appear to possess a dry scaly skin from birth with occasional severely affected animals.

Dogs which develop skin scaling later in life may be suffering from no more than the equivalent of human dandruff. The role of surface bacteria and yeasts in this condition is still not understood but certain lipophilic yeasts are frequently implicated.

Diagnosis

The diagnosis of canine ichthyosis is uncertain and more often is arrived at by elimination of more well-defined causes of scaling such as *Cheyletiella* mites, seborrhoeic dermatitis complex and squamous demodectic mange.

Treatment

Ideally, treatment is aimed at restoring normal epidermal keratinisation and removing accumulated defective scales. True ichthyosis can, of course, never be cured so relief of symptoms is all that can be hoped for.

1 Regular baths will often be sufficient to remove unsightly scaling. Shampoos which contain tar derivatives will also slow down the rate of scaling. Selenium-based shampoos will help to remove the scaly layer, but if used regularly may increase skin dryness; they are better suited to seborrhoeic skin.
2 Scaling skin which is particularly dry will often benefit from a post-bath final rinse with a water-miscible bath oil sold for human use.
3 Dry ventral skin may benefit from topical application of simple lanolin-based creams. Newer urea-based hydrating creams developed for man may be worth trying in problem cases.
4 Administration of essential fatty acid supplemets is justified if skin scaling due to a deficient low-fat diet is suspected.

Hyperkeratosis

When the stratum corneum of the epidermis becomes abnormally thickened it is usually obvious as hardened hyperkeratotic skin. As mentioned previously, hyperkeratosis may be a natural defence against trauma as typified by the formation of calluses over bony prominences. Hyperkeratosis may also develop as a secondary change in a variety of canine dermatoses including hormonal alopecia, acanthosis nigricans and chronic dermatitis.

Primary hyperkeratosis is an unusual entity but is well recognised in the nasodigital form ('hard pad'). Although an association with the canine distemper virus was proven some years ago, the majority of cases of nasodigital hyperkeratosis nowadays have no clinical history with distemper. The nose alone may be affected with extraordinary thickening and fissuring or the footpads may be the only affected sites. The rigidity and cracking of the hard keratin can impede walking.

'Corns' in the footpads are a not uncommon cause of lameness. The aetiology is obscure but lesions produced by the canine papilloma virus are strikingly similar and outbreaks of digital warts and corns have been described in racing Greyhounds.

Treatment

The treatment of hyperkeratosis depends on the cause. If secondary to other skin conditions the hyperkeratotic skin can slowly return to normal once the primary cause is removed.

1 Corticosteroids, particularly if applied topically, will generally reduce the degree of hyperkeratosis.
2 Topical antibiotics will also be necessary if fissuring is present.
3 Long strands and crusts of keratin can be trimmed carefully from the footpads with scissors after softening the pads in warm water.
4 Nasodigital hyperkeratosis often becomes a permanent condition so therapy should be directed towards keeping the dog mobile and comfortable.
5 Unsightly calluses are often the result of sleeping on hard abrasive surfaces and, if they are to be avoided, provision of soft bedding for large bony dogs is essential.

Seborrhoea (seborrhoeic dermatitis)

Excess sebum secretion by the skin's sebaceous glands is termed seborrhoea. In man, the nose and facial area is prone to oily adolescent seborrhoea, which is a condition with no real parallel in the dog. When skin scaling is marked by a waxy yellowish surface deposit the term dry seborrhoea is used; this type of abnormality is very common in dogs. Whether sebum secretion is elevated is, in fact, doubtful but accurate measurements have not been reported. The syndrome in dogs is most likely to be a combination of abnormal keratinisation (parakeratosis) with resultant scaling as well as sebum deposition. Canine seborrhoea is characterised by greasy scaling and a distinct 'mousy' rancid odour. It is often secondary to other skin diseases, notably demodicosis and hormonal alopecia.

Primary seborrhoea is more or less normal on the dorsal 'tail gland' area of some male dogs. Seborrhoea as a skin problem is detected by finding the typical greasy deposits on the skin surface of the backline, legs, perineum, neck and external ear. Cocker Spaniels, West Highland White Terriers, and wire-haired breeds are particularly susceptible. In the majority of cases the condition becomes complicated by other skin changes, especially scaling, hair loss, dermatitis and mild pruritus. The term seborrhoeic dermatitis then applies (Fig. 9.6). Patchy lesions may develop which lead to confusion with ringworm or demodectic mange. Many dogs have a 'seborrhoeic' tendency and may develop a wide variety of skin lesions over the years; the term seborrhoea complex covers the basic problem.

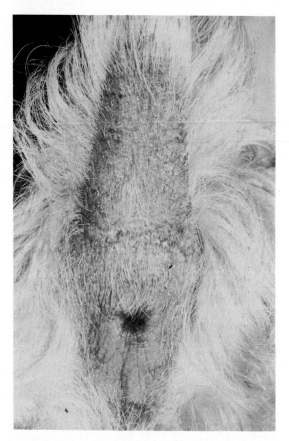

Fig. 9.6 Seborrhoeic dermatitis. Yellow waxy scales, inflammation and loss of hair are typical of seborrhoeic lesions as seen here under the tail of a West Highland White Terrier.

Aetiology
The aetiology of primary canine seborrhoea is unknown despite a frequent incidence in clinical practice. Research into the disease is urgently required to inves-

tigate common theories such as hormonal abnormality, dietary deficiency, genetic predilection or superficial infection.

Diagnosis
The diagnosis of seborrhoea is one of clinical judgement, no specific test or pathognomonic lesion can assist. Because secondary seborrhoea is also common, every effort should be made to exclude all other diagnostic possibilities. A skin scraping is warranted from *every* case. There is obviously considerable uncertainty about the whole question of the canine seborrhoea complex: most chronic skin cases referred to specialist centres are seborrhoeic patients.

Treatment
In the absence of a primary cause, treatment is basically symptomatic. Affected dogs are likely to suffer recurring episodes of seborrhoea and a permanent cure should not be anticipated.

1 Antiseborrhoeic shampoos with selenium or tar bases are of most benefit. The shampoo should be left on the skin for 30 minutes before rinsing off.
2 Systemic corticosteroid therapy will provide dramatic relief where seborrhoeic dermatitis predominates. Long-term administration may be unavoidable.
3 Multivitamin and fatty acid supplements to the diet may greatly benefit some cases.
4 Systemic antibiotics will be needed where superficial exudation or infection has occurred. Severe cases of seborrhoeic dermatitis can be quickly controlled by the simultaneous administration of generous doses of oral antibiotic and corticosteroid for 1–2 weeks.
5 Topical application of a potent combined corticosteroid/antibiotic preparation will greatly assist local lesions and may be all that is necessary in mild cases or for maintenance therapy. Non-greasy lotions or creams are preferable.
6 Hormonal therapy with thyroxine or sex hormones is questionable but may be tried as a last resort in chronic cases. Castration or ovariectomy should not be expected to be of benefit unless an endocrine disturbance is strongly suspected.
7 Seborrhoea is often first manifest by external otitis (Fig. 9.7). As a result, all otitis cases should receive a full skin examination.

Cheyletiella mite infestation

This worldwide ectoparasite has only attracted attention in recent years when it was recognised that it

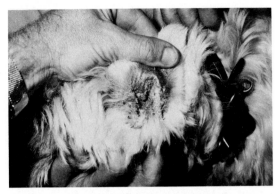

Fig. 9.7 Seborrhoea complex. Dogs with a seborrhoeic skin predisposition are frequent candidates for external otitis.

exists as a variety of host-adapted species and not just as the rabbit fur mite *Cheyletiella parasitivorax*. The species primarily adapted to dogs is *C. yasguri*. The mite lives on the surface of the skin where it feeds on tissue fluid and lays eggs which adhere to the hair similar to louse nits. The entire life-cycle of about 5 weeks is spent on the host.

Curiously, this parasite causes little damage to the dog's skin even when present in massive numbers. The main result of an infestation is marked skin scaling which, together with the just-visible mites and their eggs, gives rise to the popular term 'walking dandruff'.

Diagnosis
The diagnosis is simple because the mites are large (0.4 mm) and usually numerous, particularly along the backline. With good lighting and a magnifying lens it is not difficult to observe the parasites moving about on the skin. Rapid confirmation of the diagnosis is possible merely by pressing a piece of adhesive transparent tape several times on the skin then sticking it to a glass slide for examination under the microscope.

Cheyletiella mites are distinctive with large hooks on their mouthparts. Skin scrapings will allow more detailed microscopic examination and the numerous eggs of the parasite will be seen. Young puppies are most commonly affected although older dogs will carry a small population of mites. Outbreaks of cheyletiellosis may be seen in kennel establishments. The Boxer breed is peculiarly susceptible to this parasite. Apart from causing dandruff, Cheyletiella will produce varying degrees of pruritus and subsequent self-inflicted trauma.

Almost more important than the effects of the mites on the dog is the public health risk. Like Sarcoptes, transfer of Cheyletiella mites to human skin frequently results in highly irritating papules. It is therefore wise to question the owners about possible lesions on their own arms and trunk where mites are transferred whilst fondling an infested puppy.

The rabbit fur mite *C. parasitivorax* is ubiquitous and pet rabbits may carry massive infestations. This parasite is capable of transient habitation on both canine and human skin occasionally causing prurigo in all members of a household and exactly mimicking an outbreak of scabies. The cat-adapted species *C. blakei* may cause similar problems, thus all pet animals in the household may need to be examined.

Treatment
The treatment of Cheyletiella infestations is relatively straightforward as the parasite is susceptible to most insecticides. Because the life-cycle is rather long, weekly treatments should be continued for 4–6 weeks. Bedding and kennels should also be kept clean and treated with insecticides. Regular insecticidal baths or sprays should be maintained where the problem has arisen in dog colony establishments. Affected human skin usually requires no treatment as the papules regress quickly once the infested animal has been located and treated.

DERMATITIS AND ECZEMA

Canine dermatology is burdened with a terminology largely derived from our medical colleagues as many skin lesions in dogs which morphologically resembled human lesions were given the same name. The terms dermatitis and eczema are the most notorious examples. A diagnosis of eczema in a dog may cause anxiety to an owner who knows that the condition in man is likely to be a lifelong series of unsightly lesions with uncertain aetiology. Language is defined ultimately by common usage so dermatitis and eczema in dogs are here to stay along with other anachronisms like ringworm and mange.

Dermatitis describes inflammation of the skin, whatever the cause. Eczema in the dog describes inflammatory lesions which are superficial and characterised by weeping, oozing and crusting. Both words are non-specific and somewhat vague but serve a useful descriptive purpose in the absence of histological definitions like those in man.

Both conditions are inflammatory by nature and will usually cause discomfort and irritation to the dog. It is not possible here to discuss all the causes; virtually any external agent is capable of damaging the skin either by primary irritation or secondary induction of hypersensitivity.

Investigation of an inflammatory skin condition

requires time and clinical judgement to elucidate a full and relevant history. Laboratory tests should be utilised to help arrive at a correct diagnosis. Care should be taken to recognise demodicosis, scabies, fleas and self-inflicted trauma from the itch-scratch syndrome.

Contact irritant dermatitis

The ventral areas of skin in the dog are generally lacking the thick layer of hair which so effectively protects other parts of the body against physical contact with external agents. In many breeds of dog the abdominal skin is often completely hairless and thus exceptionally vulnerable to damage. Every time the dog lies or sits down this area comes into contact with a wide variety of underlying surfaces such as grass, concrete, tarmacadam, vinyl, floorboards or carpets. These materials may, in themselves, be abrasive or irritant but may also be coated with chemical substances such as weedkillers, insecticides, disinfectants, detergents or polishes. Bearing in mind that the canine epidermis is more fragile than that of man, it is not unexpected to find that contact dermatitis is a well-recognised clinical condition. Far more difficult to determine, however, is whether the offending agent is a primary irritant capable of harming most dogs or an allergen which can induce hypersensitivity only in certain susceptible dogs after repeated exposure. From the clinician's point of view the difference may be purely academic as the treatment for both contact irritant and contact allergic dermatitis is the same (reduce the inflammatory response and avoid further contact with the cause). The problem is comparable to housewife's hand dermatitis.

Lesions
The lesions of contact irritant dermatitis are variable but include acute erythema, scaling, crusting, reddened papules and moist oozing which may be secondarily infected. Self-inflicted trauma from licking and biting the affected areas is a usual complicating factor. The abdomen, thighs, sternum and axillae are invariably involved; the feet, lips and perineum less so.

Diagnosis
The diagnosis of contact irritant dermatitis is not easy to make with any confidence. Sophisticated and standardised patch tests available for human diagnostic use are not suitable for dogs. Circumstantial evidence or provocative exposure testing is unreliable and thus the clinical history becomes very important.

1   Seasonal recurrence of contact dermatitis suggests implication of grasses, probably the most common cause in dogs with access to gardens and fields.
2   Sudden acute erythema suggests a potent irritant such as floor disinfectant.
3   Regression of lesions during a stay in boarding kennels or a holiday is a useful guide.
4   Contact dermatitis is far less common in dogs than endogenous skin disease such as seborrhoeic dermatitis which frequently involves ventral skin surfaces. Patchy lesions found elsewhere on the body suggest a diagnosis other than contact dermatitis.
5   German Shepherds, Retrievers and other dogs with tucked-up moist abdominal skin frequently develop irritation of this area during the summer. The role of heat and sweating is uncertain but these factors may provoke self-inflicted damage from chewing and licking in the absence of any contact irritant.

Treatment
The treatment of contact irritant dermatitis is aimed at suppression of inflammation, to stop pruritus and to encourage healing.

1   Generous dosages of corticosteroids, preferably given twice daily by mouth for 7–10 days, are invaluable. Because secondary bacterial infection commonly accompanies contact dermatitis, improved clinical results can be achieved by simultaneous administration of a broad-spectrum antibiotic such as a tetracycline.
2   Small areas of severely affected skin can be treated with a topical steroid/antibiotic cream or lotion. The best results will be seen by using a potent fluorinated steroid (Synalar) as weaker preparations may be ineffective when much is licked off the skin by the dog. Owners who apply these topical steroids should be advised to wash their hands afterwards.
3   Maintenance or repeat dosage of drugs may be indicated for chronic cases or where the skin is severely affected, thickened and pigmented.

Secondly, every effort should be made to identify the contact irritant and eliminate it from the dog's environment. This usually means trial-and-error judgement and is often unrewarding. Avoiding grass should be the first step in evaluating uncertain cases. Carpets are rarely the cause of contact irritant dermatitis and needless removal of suspected furnishings should be discouraged.
4   Allergic contact dermatitis is difficult to confirm as a diagnosis. In man, the problem has been overcome by an internationally standardised system of patch testing. Samples of suspected contact-sensitising substances are applied under an occlusive dressing and 48

hours later the patches of skin are examined for signs of delayed-type hypersensitivity (inflammation, thickening and vesiculation). Patch testing of dogs is generally impractical and false-positive reactions from overriding primary irritant effect are an added disadvantage. The true incidence of allergic contact dermatitis in dogs is thus unknown, but it is almost certainly much less common than irritant dermatitis.

Intertrigo (skin-fold dermatitis)

Excessive moisture at the skin surface prevents normal keratinisation and weakens the natural barrier against superficial damage and infection. When combined with a certain degree of friction, a moist dermatitis termed intertrigo is frequently found where skin-folds are deep or tight. In dogs these folds are usually ge-

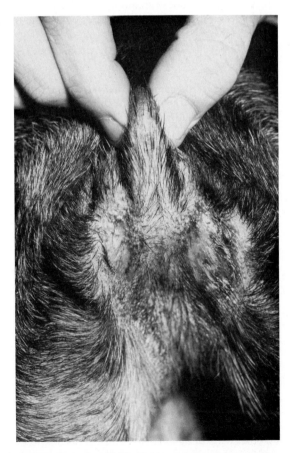

Fig. 9.8 Intertrigo. Folds of skin where moisture and friction occur are liable to develop an inflammatory condition termed intertrigo. An affected vulval fold is demonstrated here by lifting up the vulva.

netically determined such as the facial skin of brachycephalic dogs, the screw-tail of the Bulldog or the pendulous lips of Spaniels. Obesity can also result in the formation of skin folds and spayed bitches may exhibit a fold of skin around the atrophied vulva (Fig. 9.8). Initially the skin shows some erythema and irritation but the problem may go unnoticed because the affected skin is hidden in the fold. Oozing and secondary superficial infection usually result in more severe inflammation with eventual malodour and ulceration. Interdigital and perianal skin may become similarly affected due to chronic friction, moisture and bacterial contamination.

Treatment

The treatment of intertrigo is aimed at controlling moisture, friction and infection.

1 The affected area should be gently cleansed and dried followed by twice daily application of a potent steroid/multiantibiotic/antifungal lotion or cream (Panalog).

2 Once the lesions have substantially regressed a daily maintenance application should be continued for a few weeks to allow complete healing.

3 Troublesome skin folds should routinely be kept clean and lubricated with a smear of ointment. Only as a last resort in recurrent cases should surgical excision of the offending fold of skin be attempted.

4 Chronically infected 'lip folds' in Spaniels may benefit from cauterisation with silver nitrate. Otherwise surgical excision is preferred as a permanent solution to this condition.

5 Interdigital dermatitis is complicated by frequent licking and the regular wear and tear of walking. Clipping of long digital hair will aid ventilation and allow easier cleansing. In wet weather the feet should be washed with water to remove mud or foreign material and dried with a towel. Application of astringent antiseptic paints is sometimes more effective than treatment with creams or ointments.

6 Intertriginous skin which has become severely purulent may require specific systemic and topical antibiotic therapy.

Acute moist dermatitis ('wet eczema')

This condition is an example of the serious consequences which can ensue when the microclimate of the skin surface is disturbed in favour of bacterial overgrowth. Clinically, wet eczema presents itself as an acute painful inflammatory skin lesion which spreads rapidly. Within 24 hours it can become a large area of red, swollen, wet, purulent skin with no hair in the centre and sticky crusted matted hair around the periphery (Fig. 9.9). The condition is prevalent in breeds of dogs which have a dense woolly underfur, especially German Shepherds and Retrievers, and occurs mainly in the summer months.

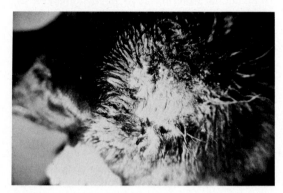

Fig. 9.9 'Wet eczema'. This large lesion on the head developed over 2 days and shows central hair loss, a purulent surface, peripheral crusting and matting of hair.

Pathogenesis
The pathogenesis has not been studied in detail but the following sequence of events appears likely:

1 Some initiating trauma to the skin damages the fragile epidermis causing local inflammation and a small zone of surface exudation. The initial minor trauma is usually self-inflicted biting, chewing or scratching at an area of irritation (e.g. fleas, otitis or impacted anal sacs). However, identical lesions can follow trauma by electric clipper blades ('clipper rash'), fencing wire or cat scratches.
2 The microclimate at the skin surface is excessively warm and moist and acts as an incubator to produce rapid proliferation of surface bacteria. These organisms include a variety of species which provoke sloughing of the superficial layers of the epidermis and hair, further exudation, the formation of surface pus and, invariably, acute pain when the tense inflamed skin is touched.
3 Some dogs are particularly susceptible to development of wet eczema and may suffer from multiple and recurrent lesions.

Treatment
Treatment is aimed at cleaning up the debris and allowing fresh air to dry the surface.

1 The matted hair surrounding the lesion should be clipped away with scissors for at least an inch around the lesion. If electric clippers are used the blades must be thoroughly cleaned and disinfected afterwards. Dogs with very painful lesions may require sedation.
2 The surface of the lesion is gently cleansed with an antiseptic detergent to remove all exudate and crusts, then allowed to dry.
3 Whilst most lesions once cleaned up and dried will heal rapidly without further treatment, it may be advisable to apply a mild steroid/antibiotic cream.
4 Highly strung dogs which persist in licking or chewing the lesions should be sedated for 1–2 days or restrained with an Elizabethan collar.
5 The underlying causes of skin irritation, if they are detected, should be treated at the same time as the main lesion. Owners of recurrent cases can be advised to treat lesions as soon as they begin.
6 Hair follicles are not usually damaged, despite the apparent severity of the lesions and regrowth of hair will be seen within a few weeks. Some long-standing lesions, however, may cause follicular damage and heal with some permanent scarring.

Vesicular ventral dermatitis (nummular eczema)

Some dogs, especially West Highland White Terriers, develop coin-shaped ('nummular') eczematous lesions which are noticeable on the less hairy ventral skin but may occur all over the body. Quite commonly the condition is chronic with fresh lesions breaking out as others are healing.

Lesions
These appear to begin as a small skin vesicle or tiny weeping pustule. They enlarge over a few days to resemble classical patches of ringworm with a reddened peeling margin and central scaling. Irritation may be absent or moderate. In about a week the lesions heal centrally leaving a characteristic pigmented mark. Numerous lesions may be present at one time (Fig. 9.10).

Aetiology
The aetiology is obscure. One popular belief is that these lesions are bacterial infections ('staphylococcal rings'). Some relationship to seborrhoeic dermatitis is likely, however, because not only are the lesions rather waxy but there is frequently evidence of seborrhoea on other parts of the body (e.g. ears, perineum, feet.)

Treatment
This is somewhat empirical. Systemic antibiotics alone often fail to give a response and best results are seen

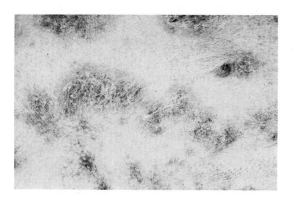

Fig. 9.10 Nummular eczema. Characteristic coin-shaped lesions on ventral skin show crusting and peripheral inflammation with central resolution followed by pigmentation.

when systemic corticosteroids are administered simultaneously. If only a few lesions are present on the abdomen, topical treatment with a steroid/antibiotic cream will cause rapid regression. More severely affected dogs may require 1–2 weeks on systemic steroid and antibiotic followed by reduced dosage for another few weeks to allow complete resolution. Weekly tar-based or selenium-based shampoos can aid in the control of this condition. Remission may continue for several months but recurrent bouts of lesions are usual.

PYODERMA

When pus forms *within* the skin the term pyoderma is both descriptive and appropriate. It implies a condition in which bacterial infection and necrosis are playing primary roles in skin damage. Exudative dermatoses which exhibit a wet purulent *surface* are often erroneously called pyoderma but in most cases any bacterial involvement is secondary to another primary cause (e.g. intertrigo). There have been few studies on the normal bacterial flora of canine skin, although the external auditory meatus has been the subject of many surveys. A major potential source of pathogenic bacteria is the mouth of the dog, particularly in view of the frequent incidence of grossly infected periodontal disease. Normal intact skin is extremely resistant to invasion by pathogenic bacteria.

Impetigo

Superficial infection of the epidermis with staphylococci and streptococci can lead to intraepidermal pus-

tules, vesicles and scab formation. Epidemics are common in school children but such transmissibility is rare in dogs except perhaps within some litters of puppies.

Small, whitish, superficial pustules are regularly seen on the abdominal skin of young dogs, sometimes accompanied by surrounding inflammation and irritation. Less frequently more widespread lesions may be seen on the body, particularly around the mouth or feet.

Diagnosis
The diagnosis of impetigo in dogs is generally by clinical observation to ensure that the pustules and vesicles are superficial. Typically these exude pus and serum which dries to form yellowish crusts. Debilitated puppies are more prone to impetigo than older animals. Bacteriological culture may be confusing because of surface contamination but if an intact pustule can be sampled, a meaningful culture can be obtained.

Treatment
Treatment of impetigo is generally encouraging. Small lesions will respond to topical antibiotic treatment alone as drug penetration of the superficial infection is not difficult. Simultaneous administration of systemic antibiotic is advisable for more widespread lesions. If there is accumulation of crusts and debris, irrigation of the affected areas should precede the topical application.

Furunculosis (deep pyoderma)

Bacterial infection of the hair follicles, dermis and subcutaneous fat is of serious consequence. Hairy canine skin can be likened to that of the human scalp or beard where deep infections are frequently intractable. The key factor determining the severity is the involvement of large hair follicles which subsequently abscessate and release necrotic material deep into the dermis. Hair shafts are thus dispersed into dermal tissues where they set up a further complication: a foreign-body reaction to keratin itself. Damaged hair follicles do not easily repair and pockets of bacterial infection can remain to perpetuate a chronic pyoderma with scarring as an inevitable result.

Folliculitis
Folliculitis is inflammation around a hair follicle and occasionally in the dog it may be detectable as reddish papules or pustules with a central hair or follicular opening. It is thought that folliculitis is a precursor to

more severe pyoderma because formation of a follicular pustule invariably involves further spread of infection to other follicles.

Acne

This is a term borrowed from man where lesions characteristically occur on the face. Male hormone secretion in adolescents gives rise to blockage of the pilosebaceous orifices with formation of comedones ('blackheads'), pustules and deep granulomas. Some dogs, especially brachycephalic breeds such as Bulldogs and Boxers, develop lesions on the face which clinically resemble human acne. Whether a hormonal mechanism is involved is doubtful as it can affect dogs of all ages.

Furunculosis

Furunculosis describes the formation of deep follicular abscesses which often coalesce to create large dermal and subcutaneous pus-filled cavities and sinuses. Clusters of deep pustules which exude pus and blood are typical of canine lesions (the equivalent of human 'boils' and 'carbuncles' are rare). Furunculosis is most common in short-haired breeds of dog, particularly those with stout hair such as the Bulldog, Boxer, Dobermann and Great Dane. Lesions can occur anywhere on the body but are more frequent on areas where pressure and trauma may aggravate the infection (i.e. lateral chest and limbs and particularly over bony prominences). The latter may develop callus pyoderma where distorted follicles form deep purulent foci (Fig. 9.11). Pain is not a prominent sign in most cases of pyoderma.

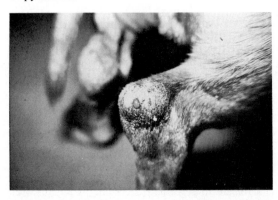

Fig. 9.11 Callus pyoderma. The development of a callus over a bony prominence may result in deep infection of blocked hair follicles. Discharge of pus to the surface is visible here over the hock.

Chronic deep pyoderma

In the dog chronic deep pyoderma is a distressing condition which can involve large areas of the body. Hair loss becomes evident and foul-smelling lesions exude purulent material which forms dried crusts on the skin surface. Freshly cleansed lesions will often reveal considerable local necrosis with honeycomb-like interconnecting furuncles. It is generally accepted that bacteria, especially staphylococci, are the primary cause of such pyoderma although it is known that experimental reproduction of the disease by inoculation of pathogenic bacteria is usually unsuccessful. The conclusion to be drawn is that dogs suffering from chronic pyoderma are somehow unable to mount an adequate immunological defence perhaps due to illness, malnutrition or immune system dysfunction.

Interdigital pyoderma

This is a disabling form of the disease which can cause sufficient pain to inhibit walking, especially in heavy dogs. Interdigital dermatitis may initiate pyoderma and, once established, deep furuncles can develop over the entire foot. Another precursor to pyoderma is the interdigital granuloma ('cyst') (Fig. 9.12). This lesion occurs precisely between the toes and commonly enlarges with fluid before rupturing and releasing bloodstained or purulent material. The origin of these so-called 'cysts' is thought to be a foreign-body reaction to deeply penetrating coarse hair shafts which puncture the delicate skin of the interdigital web (a similar condition occurs in hairdressers).

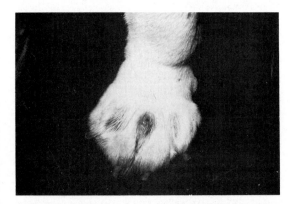

Fig. 9.12 Interdigital granuloma. Coarse short hair can penetrate the interdigital web and produce a foreign-body granuloma. These lesions often enlarge ('cysts') before rupturing and releasing bloodstained or purulent material. Recurrent lesions are best excised.

Nasal pyoderma

This is another form of furunculosis which is most common in German Shepherd dogs. The vulnerable and fragile dorsal skin is doubly aggravated by licking and rubbing.

Anal furunculosis
This is almost exclusively seen in German Shepherd dogs. A moist condition due to low tail carriage over the anus is probably an initiating factor. Once established, the lesions can become large and deep with resulting pain on defaecation.

Treatment
The treatment of pyoderma aims at drainage of the deep pus combined with long-term administration of an antibiotic to which the offending bacteria are sensitive.

1   Cleansing and irrigation of all pyoderma lesions is essential. Unless this is enthusiastically carried out each day, dried exudate will quickly block drainage of purulent material. Once the raw lesions have been cleaned, it is unnecessary and possibly deleterious to continue using antiseptics in the irrigating water. Two teaspoonsful of common salt per litre of warm water will provide a better solution for treating affected areas. Dogs suffering from severe generalised pyoderma will require hospitalisation and daily full-soak baths. Sedation or Elizabethan collars may be needed to prevent added self mutilation.
2   Debridement of devitalised skin is desirable to encourage drainage and healing. Curettage of particularly deep lesions may be necessary.
3   Topical application of an antibiotic cream or lotion is only practical where small areas of skin are involved. Large areas can be treated inexpensively with an antiseptic preparation (e.g. chlorhexidine obstetric cream).
4   Systemic antibiotics should be selected on the basis of both bacterial sensitivity and cost. High doses should be administered for at least 2 weeks followed by further long-term dosage for up to 3 months or more. If a good response is seen to antibiotic therapy it is important to continue the treatment long enough to eliminate deep foci of infection.
5   Swabs for bacteriological sensitivity testing should be taken from freshly extruded deep pustules (not from open contaminated lesions). A simple Gram stain of a smear will provide a valuable clue to the specific cause of the infection.
6   The prognosis for some cases of generalised pyoderma is poor. Euthanasia may be preferable to very expensive treatment of dogs which fail to respond.
   Re-examination for Demodex should be obligatory in all non-responding cases of pyoderma.
7   Autogenous bacterial vaccines or toxoids are still popular for treating canine pyoderma despite the absence of any worthwhile evidence of efficacy. This type of treatment for humans was abandoned many years ago. Nonetheless, a course of such injections is thought by some to be worthwhile and unlikely to cause much harm. It should not be generally recommended.
8   Anal furunculosis is a special surgical problem which appears to respond best to cryosurgery. Several sessions of freezing may be necessary to obtain complete resolution.
9   Chronic intractable generalised pyoderma may respond to combined systemic corticosteroid and antibiotic therapy.
10   Pyoderma characterised by acute and severe skin necrosis should arouse suspicions of an infection with bacteria such as Clostridia, Pseudomonas or other unusual organisms.

Pustular demodectic mange

For reasons which are not clear, some dogs with demodicosis develop the pustular form of the disease. Mite-filled follicles rupture into the dermis where a severe foreign-body type inflammatory process is started. Secondary infection with a variety of bacteria is not uncommon.
   Pustular demodectic mange should be considered in the differential diagnosis of *all* cases of pyoderma (with the exception of anal furunculosis). Mites are not difficult to detect in skin scrapings even of purulent material.

Treatment
The treatment of pustular demodectic mange has been considered earlier in this chapter (see p. 249). Severe cases will need similar antibiotic and irrigation therapy to deep pyoderma patients, combined with acaricidal treatment for the mites. The prognosis is often better than might be expected.

ULCERATION

Chronic skin ulceration is not a common clinical condition in the dog. Repair of the epidermis is facilitated in hairy skin by the epidermal lining of the hair follicles growing upwards to replace denuded areas.

Lick granuloma

Some dogs, notably Yellow Labradors and Great Danes, have a tendency to develop chronic ulcerated plaques as a result of continual self-inflicted damage from licking and chewing. Lick granulomas occur on those areas of the body which can be licked with ease and comfort (i.e. the dorsal foreleg and lateral hindleg regions). The initiating cause of lick granulomas is obscure. Many undoubtedly follow traumatic damage to the skin but some appear to arise spontaneously from licking alone. Boredom, neurosis and sexual frustration have been suggested as additional factors leading to excessive licking of the skin.

The lesions of lick granuloma are characterised by painless thickening of the affected skin; a moist, red, hairless, granulomatous plaque develops together with an indolent epithelial edge. The size of the granuloma varies from early lesions of 1 cm diameter to chronic massive areas over the entire lateral thigh.

Treatment
The treatment of lick granuloma is a complex task aimed at defeating the desire and ability of the dog to continue the damage by licking. The lesions themselves are thought to be intensely itchy.

1   Small early lesions may respond to topical application of steroid under an occlusive dressing for a week. Dogs which remove bandages will require an Elizabethan collar.
2   Larger lesions are best treated by cryotherapy. Several sessions of freezing may be needed. No dressings or collars are applied although the response at first appears unsightly. The freezing probably destroys irritable nerve endings as well as excessive granulation tissue.
3   Regular exercise and play will help prevent lesions recurring by providing mental diversion and physical fatigue. It is worth remembering that guide dogs for the blind almost never suffer from lick granulomas.

Mucocutaneous ulceration

Chronic ulceration of the mucocutaneous junctions is occasionally seen in the dog. Painless raw lesions occur around the lips, nose, eyes, anus, vulva, and prepuce. Treatment with antibiotics usually fails to arrest the condition and large areas of the face may end up ulcerated.

The cause is obscure. Chronic cases which have been extensively investigated have yielded no clues as to aetiology although involvement of the immune system seems likely. Canine pemphigus, an autoimmune disease with similarities to the human condition, has been described with mucocutaneous ulceration occurring among other skin changes (see Chapter 10). Further

research will be required before this newly described entity is fully evaluated. Over-diagnosis is to be expected as a result of the frequent reports of canine pemphigus-like syndromes now being published by the immunology-oriented academic community.

Treatment
The treatment of mucocutaneous ulceration remains empirical. Simultaneous administration of oral corticosteroid and tetracycline has given the best results. A similar topical application is given to the affected skin. Healing is slow and therapy may need to be continued for some weeks.

SKIN TUMOURS

Lumps on the skin are very common on dogs, particularly in older animals. Several neoplasms are recognisable by their clinical appearance and will be discussed below.

Epidermoid cyst ('sebaceous cyst')

These round cysts can arise anywhere on the body but mostly they occur along the backline. Sometimes a number of them appear spontaneously. They are slightly soft when squeezed and, if ruptured, will reveal caseous contents. Unless particularly large these cysts remain unnoticed until ruptured by abscessation or self mutilation. Epidermoid cysts are derived from hair follicles (not sebaceous glands) and possess a keratinising epidermal lining which generates the contents. This, the entire cyst, although benign, should be excised otherwise it may recur.

Sebaceous adenoma

Older dogs frequently exhibit several of these small benign tumours. They are superficial, firm, pale, multilobular and usually hairless. If accessible to the dog's mouth they may be damaged and ulcerated. Some animals develop large numbers of these sebaceous gland tumours. Excision is advisable if they become unsightly or ulcerate.

Mastocytoma

Mast cell tumours are very common, especially in the Boxer breed. Beginning as firm nodules they slowly enlarge and may become denuded of hair and ulcerate.

They can occur anywhere on the body but are particularly seen around the perineum and genitalia. Older dogs are generally affected.

These tumours should be widely excised as more than 30% of them may be potentially malignant. A useful diagnostic aid is the impression smear; rapid staining with Giemsa or toluidine blue will reveal numerous mast cells.

Corticosteroid and radiation therapy is indicated for recurrent or metastatic tumours.

Histiocytoma ('button tumour')

This benign tumour grows rapidly over a few weeks and is often recognisable as a partly ulcerated nodule with a well-demarcated epithelial edge. It occurs predominantly in young dogs under two years of age, usually on the face or legs as a solitary tumour.

Although histiocytomas will often regress spontaneously they are best excised for cosmetic reasons. The histological diagnosis requires some expertise.

Papilloma

Viral papillomatosis is occasionally seen affecting the oral cavity of young dogs. Isolated skin papillomas are common in older dogs and often occur as small skin 'tags', particularly on the head. If these benign tumours bleed or ulcerate they should be excised.

Basal cell tumour

A slow-growing mass on the face or limbs may be a basal cell tumour, particularly in Spaniels. They can become quite large and ulcerate. Some form keratinised centres and are termed trichoepitheliomas. Others may heavily pigment and be confused with melanomas. Basal cell tumours are usually benign and local recurrence after excision is rare.

Cutaneous lymphoma

Some dogs with a systemic lymphoma may develop cutaneous involvement. This diagnosis should be considered when erythema, alopecia and scaling lesions fail to respond to conventional therapy in the older dog. Multiple skin biopsies may be required to confirm the diagnosis by histology.

Other tumours

A histological diagnosis is desirable.

A pigmented tumour suggests a diagnosis of melanoma. Those which occur in the mouth are frequently malignant but those on the skin are generally benign.

An ulcerated tumour on the feet, nose or lips may be a squamous cell carcinoma. This tumour is often locally invasive but metastases are less common.

Anal tumours are usually perianal adenomas. They occur mostly in male dogs and administration of oestrogens causes temporary regression. Although generally benign they often recur after excision unless simultaneous castration is carried out. Radiotherapy is advisable for difficult cases.

A multilobular, firm, closely attached tumour on an old dog may indicate neurofibroma. Wide excision is advisable as local recurrence is common.

A firm, fleshy tumour which is anchored to the dermis and bleeds or ulcerates suggests fibrosarcoma. Despite wide excision this type of tumour frequently recurs and metastasises.

FURTHER READING

MULLER G. H., KIRK R. W. & SCOTT D. W. (1983) *Small Animal Dermatology*. 3rd edn. W. B. Saunders, Philadelphia.

10
Diseases Associated with Autoimmunity

L. L. WERNER AND
R. E. W. HALLIWELL

At a critical time in an animal's development (about the 42nd day of gestation in the case of the dog) an inventory is taken of all antigenic material present, and this is designated 'self'. Any antigens introduced later on in life are then recognised as foreign and an immune response is mounted against them. The mounting of a response against 'self' tissue is a concept which should be completely foreign to an effective immune system. This system has been finely orchestrated and programmed to distinguish between self and non-self, and the destruction of autologous tissue represents the ultimate failure.

Although autoimmune diseases can probably result from any of the established mechanisms of immunological damage (Gell & Coombs 1968), disease resulting from Type I (immunoglobulin E mediated) reactions are very uncommon. The Type II, or cytotoxic reaction, mediated by autoantibody and complement is most commonly implicated, causing, for example, primary autoimmune haemolytic anaemia and immune-mediated thrombocytopenia. In the case of Type III (immune complex) reactions, the tissue damaged is often not antigenically involved in the antigen-autoantibody interaction. For example, complexes of DNA and anti-DNA in systemic lupus erythematosus can cause both renal and skin disease by what has been termed an innocent bystander reaction. Complement is activated at the site of deposition, and inflammatory cells are drawn to the site. In an analogous manner, both erythrocytes and platelets can be damaged by circulating immune complexes which become non-specifically attached. Reticuloendothelial cells will then operate to destroy the innocent bystander cell. Type IV (cell-mediated) reactions may also be involved, with a good example being autoimmune thyroiditis. The destructive mechanism involves the release of lymphokines upon contact of immunocompetent lymphocytes with the appropriate antigen. These substances attract macrophages and other inflammatory cells to the site in a cascade reaction, and the activities of the involved tissue are rapidly compromised.

The function of the immune system is, in its simplest terms, the protection of the individual against foreign antigenic material. Thought must be given to the reasons why such a sophisticated system can go astray and result in a highly damaging immune response directed against self tissue. A number of possibilities exist.

1 Diseases of the lymphoid system whose role in part is to distinguish between 'self' and 'not self' are sometimes responsible. There is a high incidence of autoantibodies and of autoimmune diseases seen in association with neoplastic conditions affecting this system.

2 The emergence of new antigens during the animal's development also has the propensity to lead to autoimmunity (e.g. myelin, lens protein and spermatozoa). So long as such antigens are sequestered from the body as a whole, no problems arise, but when the barriers are broken down, autoimmunity may result. For example, in the encephalomyelitis associated with canine distemper, anti-myelin antibodies may develop which are pathogenic *in vitro* and may well contribute to the pathogenesis of the disease *in vivo*.

Similarly, some hidden antigenic determinants may become exposed by various means leading to an autoimmune response. An example is rheumatoid factor which is an antibody directed against determinants on immunoglobulin molecules which become exposed as a result of steric changes following combination with antigen.

3 Drugs can lead to immune-mediated disease by a number of mechanisms. Firstly, they may act as haptens and become attached to proteins such as those forming cell walls. This can produce a new antigen, and the resulting immune response which is directed both against drug and against cell wall can readily damage the latter; penicillin-induced autoimmune anaemia is caused by such a mechanism. Secondly, they may become complete antigens by binding to plasma proteins. The resulting immune response leads to the development of circulating antigen–antibody complexes which can become secondarily attached to red

cells or blood platelets which are hence damaged via an 'innocent bystander reaction'. Finally, drugs can also incite a true autoimmunity via shared antigenicity. An example in man is the antihypertensive drug α-methyldopa which apparently has antigenic similarity to Rh determinants on RBCs of man.

4 Antigenic modification can occur by action of enzymes, attachment of viruses or by physical means such as heat or ultraviolet light. The resulting immune response may be reactive not only with the altered antigens, but also may have reactivity against the original undamaged tissue. The presence of a virus in association with a cell may furthermore be pathogenic via an innocent bystander reaction, as the antibody response to the virus can damage the cell with which it is associated. Possible examples of both types of mechanisms occur in systemic lupus erythematosus in which there is some evidence of viral infection.

5 The role of suppppressor T cells may be very important. The antibody response is controlled by a number of humoral and cellular mechanisms. Central to the regulation is the role of thymus derived (T) lymphocytes that are responsible for both initiating and controlling antibody production. There is evidence that autoantibody production is present to a limited extent in all individuals, but is kept controlled by powerful inhibitory forces from suppressor T cells. The emergence of damaging levels of autoantibody in autoimmune diseases is often associated with markedly impaired suppressor T cell function.

6 The incidence and severity of disease in some of the laboratory animal models of autoimmunity can be affected by hormones. In the SLE-like condition seen in the F_1 cross between the New Zealand black and the New Zealand white mouse, both androgens and antioestrogens are inhibitory. It is thus noteworthy that both autoimmune haemolytic anaemia and immune-mediated thrombocytopenia in dogs are far more common in females. In the case of SLE, however, no sex predisposition is evident, which is in marked distinction to the situation in man where the disease is seen predominantly in young adult females.

The relevance of the foregoing concepts to clinical autoimmune disease is essentially speculative, although all are probably incriminated to some extent in a number of disease processes. In some instances two or more mechanisms may be implicated. In yet others, the reaction against 'self' occurs in the presence of an immune system that can be regarded as in impeccable working order by all accepted parameters.

It is important to point out that the demonstration of autoantibodies against 'self' tissue does not necessarily imply that they are responsible for the disease.

They may be the result rather than the cause. Four criteria should be considered when assessing their relevance to the pathogenesis.

1 Autoantibody or autoreactive immunocompetent cells should be demonstrated in all cases of the disease.
2 If antibody is deposited in a tissue there is a greater likelihood of its being pathogenic if complement is also deposited.
3 If antibody is found fixed to tissue or cells, upon elution that antibody should be shown to be reactive against the same cells or tissue.
4 The pathogenicity of the antibody or the immunocompetent cells should be demonstrable by a cytopathogenic effect upon transfer to the same tissue of a homologous or heterologous species.

It will become apparent that these criteria have been applied to a greater or lesser extent to the diseases described in this chapter. In some instances the disease is truly autoimmune, but in others their description as such is based on highly tenuous grounds.

The diagnosis of autoimmune diseases often involves the use of antisera to canine immunoglobulins or other serum proteins such as C3 (the third component of complement). These antisera are conjugated to fluorescein isothiocyanate when used for fluorescent antibody studies. An alternative that is increasing in popularity is the use of enzyme labelling. It is of the utmost importance that these antisera are properly prepared and species specific. The use of antihuman sera for diagnosis of canine immune-mediated disease is quite invalid.

AUTOIMMUNE HAEMOLYTIC ANAEMIA

Red blood cell (RBC) membrane antigen-antibody systems have long been a subject of intense investigation because of their importance in blood transfusion and maternal–fetal incompatibility. It is not surprising, therefore, that autoimmune haemolytic anaemia (AIHA) is one of the earliest and best documented examples of autoimmune disease in man and animals (Coombs *et al* 1945; Lewis *et al* 1963). AIHA represents yet another example of antibody-mediated destruction of RBCs, unique in that failure of self tolerance, and not isoantibody or isoimmunization to RBC antigens, accounts for the haemolytic event and subsequent anaemia. AIHA includes a heterogeneous group of immunohaematological disorders in which a number of different autoantibody types and physicochemical properties have been demonstrated. It is the most common autoimmune disorder seen in the dog, and likewise, the incidence in the canine species far exceeds that reported in other domestic animals (Halliwell 1978; Switzer & Jain 1981).

Aetiology and pathogenesis

AIHA is mediated by autoantibodies, with or without complement activation, which produce cytolytic damage to RBC membranes via the type II immunological injury of Gell and Coombs (1968). IgG alone, or in combination with the third component of complement (C_3), is the most commonly demonstrated immune reactant in canine AIHA (Slappendel 1979). IgM is less frequently involved, and IgA autoantibodies are exceedingly rare. Destruction of RBCs occurs in two ways. First, and most prevalent, is phagocytosis by macrophages of the reticuloendothelial system (RES), referred to as extravascular haemolysis. In this instance, macrophage receptors for the Fc portion of IgG or for C_3b affix RBCs opsonised by either, resulting in phagocytosis or RBC membrane damage via release of lysosomal enzymes. Secondly, both IgG and IgM autoantibodies, when present on RBC membranes in sufficient quantity, can bind and activate complement, causing intravascular haemolysis, and more fulminant haemolytic disease.

Distinction has been made between true or primary AIHA, and secondary AIHA. Primary AIHA is the result of a breakdown in the immunoregulatory mechanisms which maintain the normal state of self-tolerance. Secondary AIHA, on the other hand, is associated with an immunological response to exogenous insults, such as infectious, parasitic or chemical (drug-induced). Drug-induced AIHA can result from chemical alteration of RBC membrane antigens which elicits antibody formation against the 'new' hapten (as in the case of penicillin and cephalosporins). Alternatively, drugs can act as haptens upon combination with serum proteins and elicit an antibody response resulting in circulating immune complexes that nonspecifically bind to cell membranes. This type of immune-mediated RBC damage is referred to as an innocent bystander reaction and can occur with other exogenous antigens such as viral or bacterial. Drugs which have been shown to cause this latter type of secondary AIHA in man include quinidine, dipyrone, phenylbutazone, and chlorpromazine. Other types of secondary AIHA include infectious agents which share antigenic determinants with RBC membrane proteins, in which a so-called 'cross-reacting' antibody response occurs. Organisms such as Haemobartonella and Babesia which parasitise RBCs can cause an antibody-mediated haemolysis. Finally, toxic or infectious insults can damage external RBC membranes,

exposing previously sequestered or 'hidden' membrane antigens which elicit an antibody response.

Regardless of whether the immune-mediated haemolysis is primary or secondary, the RBC destruction is manifested in one or more of five possible ways. These five classifications of AIHA are defined by the physicochemical properties of the involved antibodies and by the extent of complement activation involved (Dacie & Worledge 1975).

Class I. These autoantibodies are referred to as in-saline acting autoagglutinins. They can be either of class IgG or IgM, and result in direct or intravascular haemagglutination at body temperature (37–39°C). Agglutination can be observed immediately upon withdrawing blood into a syringe or glass vial, or when a drop of anticoagulated blood is placed on a glass slide (Fig. 10.1). Diluting the blood sample with an

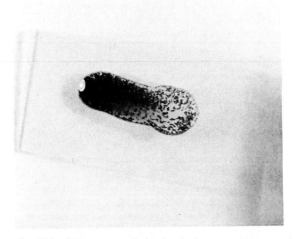

Fig. 10.1 Direct autoagglutination is demonstrated on a glass slide. Courtesy of John W. Harvey, University of Florida, College of Veterinary Medicine, Gainesville, FL.

equal volume of physiological saline is necessary to distinguish true agglutination from rouleaux formation. The latter is particularly common in blood samples drawn from cats and horses, and is frequently associated with elevations in serum proteins leading to hyperviscosity, or resulting from elevations in inflammatory proteins. Ultimately, microscopic examination is indicated to differentiate rouleaux from agglutination, and to detect microscopic agglutination. The finding of in-saline acting autoagglutination is virtually diagnostic for AIHA, and precludes the necessity of running a direct Coombs' test to confirm the diagnosis.

Class II. Intravascular haemolysins refers to those antibodies, IgG or IgM, which initiate the classical complement pathway, resulting in activation of sequences C_5-C_9, to cause intravascular haemolysis. Such patients show icterus, haemoglobinaemia and haemoglobinuria.

Class III. Incomplete antibody is the term used to designate the majority of cases of AIHA in which neither autoagglutination nor intravascular haemolysis occur. The antibody, either IgM or IgG, occurs in insufficient quantity or avidity to cause agglutination or haemolysis, and is therefore detected only by the performance of a direct Coomb's antiglobulin test. The haemolytic anaemia seen in Class III AIHA is usually of more insidious onset, and is less fulminant than that seen in Class I or Class II.

Class IV. Cold agglutinin disease is frequently less fulminant than the Class I in-saline acting or 'warm agglutinin' type of AIHA. Affected individuals usually display a mild to moderate anaemia and may show distal extremity ischaemic lesions involving the ears, feet, and tail (Fig. 10.2). The temperature dependency of the autoantibody (often IgM) reaction in this instance is less than core body temperature and occurs over a wide range of temperatures. Bouts of cold environmental temperature are sometimes, but not always, associated. Agglutination of blood at less than body temperature, and dispersion upon rewarming to 37°C are virtually diagnostic for cold agglutinin disease.

Class V. Cold acting, non-agglutinating antibodies result in a paroxysmal type of haemoglobinuria which is temperature related and associated with only a mild to moderate anaemia. Thus, Class V AIHA is usually a mild clinical syndrome, and performance of the direct and indirect Coombs' antiglobulin test at 4°C is necessary in order to confirm the diagnosis.

Clinical signs

The chief presenting clinical signs of AIHA are referable to the progressive anaemia. Thus weakness, lethargy, and occasionally syncope are reported. In the more acute or fulminant cases, seen in Class I and Class II AIHA, fever, icterus and emesis are sometimes associated. Hepatomegaly, splenomegaly and lymphadenopathy can accompany any case of AIHA. Haemoglobinaemia and haemoglobinuria are less common and accompany Class II or Class V AIHA. Cold agglutinin disease (Class IV AIHA) usually has a more moderate clinical course, but life-threatening exacerbations of haemolytic anaemia do occur. The distal extremity lesions are due to ischaemic necrosis from temperature-dependent agglutination of RBCs at these sites. The most common clinical presentation is Class III AIHA. The clinical course tends to be more insidious in onset, but nonetheless, profound anaemia can be associated.

AIHA can be the sole disease process, or can be accompanied by or secondary to other systemic disorders, including those that are immune mediated, such as thrombocytopenia and systemic lupus erythematosus (SLE). Other abnormalities which have been associated with some cases of canine AIHA include bacterial infections (pyometra, pyuria), polyarthritis, proteinuria, nephropathy, hepatopathy, systemic rickettsial and parasitic disorders and neoplasia (Slappendel 1979; Werner 1980; Switzer & Jain 1981).

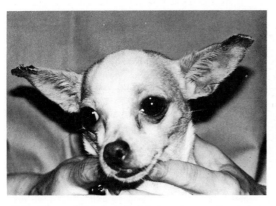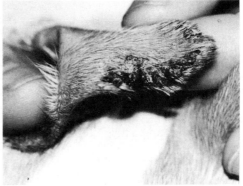

Fig. 10.2 Bilaterally symmetrical ischaemic, crusting lesions on pinnae of a two-year-old female Chihuahua with cold agglutinin disease. Frontal and close-up views.

There is no accepted breed predilection for AIHA, and the disease affects a broad range of ages from less than one year to geriatric. Most of the sizeable case surveys on canine AIHA agree that there is a female predisposition. Interestingly, Switzer and Jain (1981) have reported a male predominance for AIHA cases occurring at less than a year of age, while in the middle age onset group (4–7 years), there was a 2:1 female predominance over males.

Diagnosis

Coombs' Test
The observation of cold or warm agglutination of the patients' RBCs is virtually diagnostic for AIHA, providing rouleaux formation is ruled out by saline dilution (1:1) and microscopic examination. Performance of the direct Coombs' antiglobulin test (Coombs *et al* 1945) is necessary to confirm the presence of antibody or C_3 on the RBCs of patients with Class II, III, and V AIHA. The blood sample is collected in heparin or EDTA. The RBCs are separated, washed three times in phosphate buffered saline (PBS), and resuspended to a 2% cell volume in PBS. The Coombs' reagent is an antiserum made in a heterologous species (e.g. rabbit) against IgG, IgM and C_3 of the species under test. Polyvalent antisera can be used, or ideally, monospecific antisera which detect each immune reactant separately. Doubling dilutions of the Coombs' antisera are made in PBS, an equal volume of the patient's RBC suspension is added, and the samples are incubated for one hour in a 37°C water bath. For detection of cold reacting autoantibodies, care must be taken to perform every step of the entire procedure under cold conditions, generally 4°C. Following incubation, the samples are checked for agglutination both macroscopically and microscopically.

Although the Coombs' test is a reliable test in most cases, there are instances of both false negative and false positive reactions which should be noted. False negative Coombs' results can occur for a variety of reasons, not the least of which include improperly prepared or non-species-specific antisera. Secondly, it is possible that the concentration of autoantibody present on the RBCs is below the level of sensitivity of the Coombs' reagent, or alternatively, that there is Coombs' reagent antibody excess relative to amount of autoantibody present on the RBCs. The latter instance is referred to as a prozone effect and can be avoided by utilising serial dilutions of the Coombs' antisera. The ideal Coombs' reagent(s) should include antisera to detect IgM and C_3, in addition to IgG. Detection of C_3 on RBC membranes is particularly important in cases where the autoantibody concentra-

tion is below the level of sensitivity of the Coombs' reagent, or in cases of cold-reactive antibody which may elute from the RBC membrane if temperature dependency conditions are not met. Switzer and Jain (1981) reported a rather high incidence (33.7% of 77 cases) of canine AIHA in which the Coombs' test was negative. The diagnosis was made using other clinicopathologic criteria supportive of AIHA, exclusion of other causes of haemolytic anaemia, and ultimately by a favourable response to corticosteroid therapy.

False positive Coombs' results can occur due to failure to absorb the Coombs' antisera with a pool of normal canine RBCs, antisera activity against transferrin, activity against non-specific serum proteins adsorbed onto RBC membranes, and recent incompatible blood transfusion. Experience with the 4°C Coombs' test in the authors' laboratory indicates a 50% incidence of positive reactions in over two hundred non-anaemic dogs. Thus, a positive direct Coombs' test at 4°C must be interpreted in light of other evidence suggestive of cold haemolytic disease (Wintrobe *et al* 1974).

Clinicopathological findings
Haemogram findings consistent with a diagnosis of AIHA generally include spherocytosis and evidence of a regenerative anaemia such as polychromasia, macrocytosis, and an elevated reticulocyte index. In most cases, there is a concomittent neutrophilic leucocytosis, often profound and frequently accompanied by a regenerative left shift. This so-called leucomoid response can also be seen in severe bacterial infections and myeloproliferative disorders, both of which must be ruled out as underlying diseases causing a secondary AIHA. Contributing causes of the leucomoid response in uncomplicated AIHA probably include bone marrow regeneration at a pleuripotential stem cell level and chemotactic factors associated with the heightened immune response. Platelet counts are indicated due to the possibility of concurrent immune-mediated thrombocytopenia. Thrombocytosis is sometimes seen in evidence of the overall regenerative bone marrow response.

Non-regenerative anaemias are occasionally seen in AIHA. Contributing factors include peracute onset of the haemolytic crisis in which insufficient time has elapsed for enhanced erythrogenesis, recent blood transfusion (Schalm 1975), and autoantibody directed against RBC precursors in the bone marrow. Indirect evidence for the latter has been encountered in canine AIHA where a regenerative erythroid response was seen following induction of aggressive immunosuppressive therapy (Stockham *et al* 1980). This type of AIHA with delayed erythroid regeneration is similar to pure red cell aplasia (PRA), a human autoimmune disorder (Marmont *et al* 1975).

Bone marrow aspiration or biopsy in most cases of AIHA shows a hyperplastic or regenerative response with a normal to decreased M:E ratio, and evidence of erythrophagocytosis. Erythroid hypoplasia or maturation arrest can be seen in cases of AIHA with a non-regenerative anaemia (Stockholm *et al* 1980).

Haemoglobinaemia and hyperbilirubinaemia usually accompany only those cases of AIHA with significant intravascular haemolysis. In such cases haemoglobinuria and bilirubinuria are also present. In cases showing only extravascular haemolysis, haemoglobin and/or bilirubin may be detected in the urine due to their rapid renal clearance, but are generally not present in serum. Hepatic or non-organ specific enzymes may be elevated as a result of intercurrent disease, hypoxaemia, or ischaemia due to intravascular haemagglutination. Serum haptoglobin determinations can be helpful in differentiating between haemolytic and non-haemolytic causes of anaemia in cases where more routine diagnostic tests yield equivocal results. Serum haptoglobin values are reduced during haemolytic episodes. In the absence of a positive Coombs' test, other causes of haemolytic anaemia must be considered as well when serum haptoglobin levels are low.

Differential diagnosis

Cases of suspected or confirmed AIHA should be thoroughly evaluated to identify the presence of other associated diseases requiring specific therapy. When other autoimmune diseases are suspected, tests for antinuclear antibody, LE cells or antiplatelet antibody are indicated. Unless there are strong supportive findings for AIHA, including marked spherocytosis, auto-agglutination or a positive Coombs' test, other non-immunologic causes of regenerative anaemia should be considered in the differential diagnosis. These would include chronic blood loss, bleeding disorders, parasites, and bleeding tumours such as haemangiosarcoma or gastrointestinal neoplasia. Haemangiosarcoma is of particular interest, since often the haematological findings are that of profoundly regenerative anaemia (active reticulocytosis). In addition, false positive Coombs' tests have been associated with haemangiosarcoma of the spleen and liver (Halliwell 1978).

Treatment and prognosis

The aims in treatment of AIHA are to manage the acute anaemic crisis, inhibit the sequestering and phagocytosis of RBCs in the RES, treat specifically any underlying disease, and lower the production of anti-RBC antibody in lymphoid tissue. Corticosteroids (prednisone and prednisolone), at an initial dose of 1–2 mg/kg every 12 hours, are used to suppress erythrophagocytosis and lymphoid tissue. Blood transfusion should be avoided except in life-threatening anaemia, since it may precipitate or accelerate haemolytic crisis, enhance antibody production or suppress the normal response of bone marrow to anaemia. Good supportive care, the elimination of stress factors and oxygen supplementation, if necessary, will often sustain patients during a haemolytic crisis until steroid therapy takes effect. When blood transfusion is deemed necessary to save the patient during anaemic crisis, cross-matched blood should be given, along with immunosuppressant therapy. Antibiotic therapy should be instituted in patients with bacterial infections. Corticosteroid therapy in the presence of infection is not recommended unless the anaemia is life-threatening.

If significant stabilisation or gain in PCV is not achieved during the first 48–72 hours of steroid therapy, more potent immunosuppressant agents should be utilised. These include the cytotoxic drugs such as cyclophosphamide or azathioprine (Table 10.5). The authors prefer to begin cytotoxic therapy from the outset in patients showing severe autoagglutination or intravascular haemolysis. The cytotoxic drugs are potent inhibitors of antibody formation by lymphocytes. When a patient is stabilised on immunosuppressant therapy, the PCV should rise steadily towards normal over a period of 1–4 weeks. It is not uncommon during the first week of therapy to find an increase in the number of spherocytes due to suppression of erythrophagocytosis by corticosteroids. Drug doses should be tapered over a period of 1 to 3 months once clinical remission has occurred. Alternate day steroid therapy at 25–50% of the starting dose should be maintained while periodic haemograms are performed to evaluate for progress or signs of exacerbation, and for evidence of myelosuppression when cytotoxic drugs are used.

Splenectomy should be considered in those cases which respond inadequately to steroid therapy, tolerate immunosuppressant therapy poorly, or tend to exacerbate frequently in spite of proper medical management. Removal of the spleen eliminates both a concentrated source of antibody-producing lymphocytes as well as a major portion of the RES.

Classes I and II AIHA yield the poorest prognosis and have the highest percentage of deaths. In all cases, attempts should be made to treat specifically any underlying disease or infection, and to eliminate any drug therapy which may be responsible for a drug-induced AIHA. Although some cases of AIHA tend to recur intermittently, it is worthwhile to taper and withdraw animals in remission from all therapy for a period of 2–3 months and recheck periodical haemograms and Coombs' tests for evidence of exacerbation. Cold-acting forms of AIHA should be managed in the same way as the more common types and, in addition, these animals should be protected against exposure to cold temperatures.

IMMUNE-MEDIATED THROMBO-CYTOPENIA

Immune-mediated thrombocytopenia (IMT) is one of the most common causes of reduced platelet production and life span in the dog. Previously termed idiopathic thrombocytopenic purpura (ITP), IMT has been designated a more appropriate term for cases of thrombocytopenia for which no underlying non-immune aetiology can be found, and which are either corticosteroid-responsive or associated with the finding of antiplatelet antibodies. The ability of antiplatelet antibody, sometimes in conjunction with complement, to cause platelet destruction was first demonstrated as an unidentified human serum factor by Harrington in 1951. Identification of this serum thrombocytopenia factor as antibody was made by Shulman *et al* in 1965. With the advent of the platelet factor 3 assay (Karpatkin & Siskind 1969) and its modification for canine use (Wilkins *et al* 1973), numerous cases of canine IMT have been documented.

Aetiology and pathogenesis
Immune-mediated thrombocytopenia can occur as the result of several types of immunological interactions involving platelets. As in AIHA, there can be autoantibody against platelet membrane antigens, drug- or microorganism-induced antigenic modification of the membrane, crossreacting antibody, and 'innocent bystander' types of immunological injury. Both primary (true) and secondary types of IMT are recognised. Approximately 25% of canine IMT cases in one study were designated as primary (Jain & Switzer 1981). IMT associated with or secondary to underlying disease has been attributed to viral infections, drug interactions, rickettsial parasite infections, neoplasia and other autoimmune disorders such as AIHA and systemic lupus erythematosus (Jain & Switzer 1981). Drug-induced IMT has been suspected in several canine cases exposed to therapeutic agents such as digoxin, phenylbutazone, chlorpromazine, and sulpha drugs (Wilkins *et al* 1973; Schalm 1975).

IgG antibody is responsible for the majority of human and canine cases of IMT (Dixon & Rosse 1975;

Dodds & Wilkins 1977). Although complement fixation and activation leading to direct platelet lysis has been demonstrated in some cases, sequestration, membrane damage and phagocytosis of platelets in the RES are the primary causes of reduced circulating platelets in IMT. The spleen is the major organ responsible for these three main contributing factors in reduced platelet survival, as well as for the production of anti-platelet antibody. That antiplatelet antibody by itself causes morphological and functional alterations in canine platelets has been demonstrated by Shebani (1982).

Platelet production can also be reduced in IMT, owing to autoantibodies which crossreact with megakaryocyte membrane antigens in the bone marrow. Thus, cases of IMT with low megakaryocyte activity can also be found. Localisation of IgG antibody to megakaryocytes in dogs with IMT has been reported (Jain & Switzer 1981).

There is a 2:1 female predilection in canine IMT (Wilkins *et al* 1973; Jain & Switzer 1981), and the average age is about five years. The poodle breed appears over-represented among other breeds in the incidence of IMT (Dodds & Wilkins 1977), however no statistical adjustments have been made which take breed popularity into account.

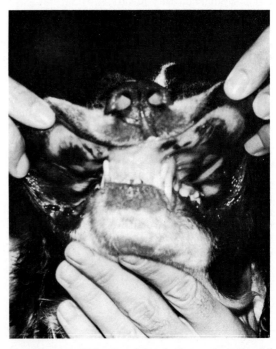

Fig. 10.3 Petechial and ecchymotic haemorrhages in oral mucous membranes of a four-year-old male Britany Spaniel with immune mediated thrombocytopenia.

Clinical signs

Petechial and ecchymotic haemorrhages (Fig. 10.3) are the hallmarks of thrombocytopenia. Though IMT may be acute, chronic, or cyclic in its course, clinical signs of haemorrhage often do not occur spontaneously until the platelet count falls below $50\,000/mm^3$ (Jain & Switzer 1981). Petechial and ecchymotic haemorrhages can be localised or disseminated. Favoured distribution sites include the mucous membranes, pressure points or areas of excessive trauma. Some patients will present with excessive bleeding following trauma. Retinal haemorrhages, epistaxis, prolonged bleeding during oestrus, haematuria or haemorrhagic diarrhoea can be present, sometimes without associated cutaneous petechiae or ecchymoses. Other clinical signs such as neurological dysfunction and cardiac dysrhythmias can accompany fulminant IMT, presumably the result of haemorrhage into these tissues. Other clinical findings include lethargy and weakness, particularly if blood loss is profound. Fever, hepatosplenomegaly and lymphadenopathy can also occur.

Clinicopathological findings

Haemogram findings compatible with IMT include a decreased platelet count, normal to increased neutrophil count, and normal to decreased PCV. The platelets seen on blood smears are often abnormally large and excessive clumping is sometimes observed. When anaemia is present, it can be either regenerative or non-regenerative, depending on the chronicity of either blood loss due to haemorrhage, concommitant autoantibody-mediated erythrolysis, or both. There are no particular biochemical abnormalities associated with IMT, but routine biochemical screening tests are indicated to evaluate possible involvement of other body systems due to haemorrhage, anaemic hypoxia or intercurrent disease.

In most cases, bone marrow aspirates show normal to increased megakaryocytes in response to the thrombocytopenia, and a normal to decreased M:E ratio if there is active erythrogenesis. Less commonly, reduced megakaryocytes are evident, suggesting their involvement in the immunological injury. IgG antibody has been demonstrated by direct immunofluorescence of megakaryocytes from dogs with IMT (Jain & Switzer 1981). Because the haemostatic defect involves only the platelets, clotting times are expected to be normal in uncomplicated cases, while bleeding time is prolonged.

Immunologic tests

A diagnosis of IMT is confirmed when antiplatelet antibody is demonstrated by the platelet factor 3 (PF_3) test (Wilkins *et al* 1973). This test system utilises platelets from a normal dog (platelet-rich plasma or PRP) which are incubated with both normal dog globulin fraction (control) and the patient's globulin fraction in the presence of canine contact product (activated clotting factors XI and XII). If antiplatelet antibody is present in the globulin fraction of the test serum, the antibody injures the platelet membrane and releases the procoagulant substance termed platelet factor 3. The clotting time of the PRP (initiated by the addition of 0.025 M $CaCl$) is shortened by at least 10 seconds as compared with the normal control. Up to 60-70% of thrombocytopenic dogs show a positive PF_3 test (Wilkins & Dodds 1974; Joshi & Jain 1976). False negative PF_3 tests have been reported after 2-3 days of corticosteroid therapy (Wilkins *et al* 1973), however Jain and Switzer (1981) have reported positive PF_3 tests in dogs on corticosteroid therapy for up to two weeks. In instances where the PF_3 test fails to demonstrate antiplatelet antibody, a good response to corticosteroid therapy and elimination of other causes of thrombocytopenia are the basis for a presumptive diagnosis of IMT.

Direct immunofluorescence (DIF) using fluorescein-conjugated anticanine IgG on ethanol fixed bone marrow smears is a sensitive method for detection of antiplatelet antibodies on megakaryocytes (Joshi & Jain 1976). The incidence of a positive DIF test on bone marrow preparations from canine cases of IMT is not known. Since IMT is often coexistent with other autoimmune diseases, a Coombs' positive anaemia is sometimes encountered. IMT may be associated with systemic lupus erythematosus. In this instance, a positive antinuclear antibody (ANA) test, or LE-cell preparation is expected.

Differential diagnosis

The finding of thrombocytopenia should bring to mind all of the possible aetiologies of decreased platelets. In general, thrombocytopenia may result from decreased platelet production in the bone marrow, increased utilisation or consumption of platelets, and decreased life-span of platelets. Thrombocytopenia may result from myeloproliferative disease, bone marrow hypoplasia, lymphoproliferative disorders, septicaemia, viral infection, consumptive coagulopathy, incompatible blood transfusion, malignancies, and certain drugs or toxins. Two rickettsial organisms, *Erlichia canis* and a platelet-specific rickettsia, as yet unnamed (Harvey 1978), cause thrombocytopenia. It is important to rule out any underlying disease which may be responsible for increased platelet destruction or utilisation regardless of whether or not the thrombocytopenia is immunologically mediated.

Treatment and prognosis

Therapy of IMT is aimed at controlling haemorrhage when necessary, suppressing the reticuloendothelial destruction of platelets, suppressing the formation of the autoantibody, and specific treatment for underlying disease. Specific antimicrobial therapy for any existing bacterial infection is paramount in animals who are candidates for corticosteroid or other immunosuppressant therapy. Corticosteroids should be discouraged when possible if bacterial infection exists.

Most cases of IMT will not require intensive crisis management or transfusion. The degree of active haemorrhage must be assessed with each patient regardless of the actual platelet count. Platelet counts as low as 2000/mm³ are compatible with clinical compensation, providing stress factors and the activity of the patient are limited. Likewise, severe haemorrhagic compromise can complicate the clinical course in patients with less severe thrombocytopenia.

Prednisone or prednisolone therapy is initiated at a dose of 2–4 mg/kg in two divided doses per day. Platelet counts should start to rise within 48–72 hours as the RE system is suppressed. With prolonged therapy, the amount of antiplatelet antibody is reduced. Therapy is maintained at the starting dose until remission is achieved. This should be based on both clinical and haematological evaluation since clinical signs may disappear long before the platelet count rises to within normal range. Upon remission, therapy should be tapered and continued on an alternate-day basis. If drug-induced IMT or viral infection are suspected aetiologies, therapy need not be prolonged after remission. Withdrawal from the offending drug will usually result in good response to therapy. Recurrence of IMT which is drug- or virus-related is not expected except in unique circumstances.

When anaemia and thrombocytopenia present as true medical emergencies, fresh whole blood or platelet-rich plasma transfusions may be necessary. Haemostatic measures and supportive care measures are based upon thorough patient evaluation and monitoring. Multisystemic involvement, either secondary to haemorrhage (particularly CNS and cardiac) or due to intercurrent disease, should be recognised and treated as specifically as possible.

In some instances, corticosteroid therapy is ineffective in increasing platelet counts significantly. More potent immunosuppressive therapy may be required to adequately inhibit antiplatelet antibody production. Drugs such as cyclophosphamide and azathioprine have been used to restore platelet counts in dogs who do not respond satisfactorily to steroids. The vinca alkaloids (Table 10.5), vincristine and vinblastine are known to have a thrombogenic effect on bone marrow in man and the dog (Hwang *et al* 1969; Klener *et al* 1974).

Vincristine has been successfully used in canine IMT cases which were poorly responsive to glucocorticoid therapy (Greene *et al* 1982). The proposed thrombogenic effect is mediated by the action of the vinka alkaloid in altering peripheral platelet morphology and function, thereby inducing a reactive megakaryocyte hyperplasia (Jackson & Edwards 1977).

Splenectomy is advocated by some in the management of recurrent IMT. This is often of considerable benefit, since the spleen is a major site of platelet destruction, and is also a rich source of antibody-producing lymphocytes. Patients must have adequate clotting function before a surgical procedure is attempted. Ovariohysterectomy is recommended during remission phases in females who tend to exacerbate the thrombocytopenia and haemorrhage during oestrus.

The overall prognosis for IMT is favourable in properly managed patients who do not have serious underlying disease or organ failure.

SYSTEMIC LUPUS ERYTHEMATOSUS

The name systemic lupus erythematosus (SLE) derives from the wolfish appearance imparted to human patients suffering from the erythematous rash that may accompany the disease. The condition however is not confined to the skin and a plethora of autoantibodies are present which often lead to multisystem disease.

Aetiology and pathogenesis

Autoantibodies associated with SLE include antibodies directed against red blood cells, platelets, polymorphs, lymphocytes, thyroid antigens, coagulation factors and various nuclear components. Of great interest is the fact that lymphocytotoxic antibodies are directed largely, if not exclusively against suppressor T cells and the loss of activity of these cells may well be responsible for the development of significant levels of other autoantibodies. In the pathogenesis of the disease, damage to, for example RBCs and platelets, via a direct complement-mediated cytotoxicity (type II reaction) is of obvious importance. An additional major feature of the pathogenesis is the presence of immune complexes of DNA and anti-DNA which lead to the associated arteritis, glomerulonephritis and also skin lesions, via a type III reaction.

There is increasing evidence from studies in both man and dog that a viral agent is implicated in the disease. C-type viral particles have been recently demonstrated in man in immune complexes in both kidney and skin and there is a high incidence of both ANA and lymphocytotoxic antibodies in workers in rheumatology laboratories concerned with analysing samples from patients with SLE. However, there is no apparent increase in the incidence of clinical SLE in these individuals.

Experimental studies in dogs have yielded somewhat parallel findings. The work of Lewis and Schwartz (1971) and Lewis *et al* (1973) has established that the serological abnormalities associated with canine SLE, namely positive ANA and positive LE-cell preparation, can be transmitted by cell-free filtrates to other dogs and also to mice. Some of the mice developed lymphosarcoma, and cell-free extracts of this could again induce the same serological abnormalities when passaged back into dogs. This can be taken as evidence that the serological abnormalities at least may be associated with a virus, but no disease has resulted in these animals. Also, high titres of ANA are sometimes found in completely normal people and dogs. Breeding experiments on dogs affected with clinical SLE also have been undertaken, and after 10 years and 5 inbred generations, some animals have developed SLE and other autoimmune diseases (Schwartz *et al* 1978). This data collectively suggests that the aetiology of SLE involves a virus in a genetically susceptible individual. The virus on its own can produce serological changes, but no overt disease.

Pathology

The pathological findings in SLE are often somewhat unremarkable. The most characteristic and specific changes are a thickening of the glomerular basement membrane of the kidney and hyaline thrombi and haematoxylin bodies in the arterioles and a periarteriolar fibrosis in the spleen. There may also be a generalised arteritis with thickening, necrosis and fibrinoid deposits in the medium-sized arterioles and a periarteriolar inflammatory infiltrate. This vasculitis may be diffuse or localised. Dermal changes are characterised by necrosis of collagen and a proliferation of elastic tissue. There may be either a thickening or a thinning of the epidermis and a characteristic periadnexal and/or lichenoid infiltration with mononuclear cells.

Histology of the synovial membrane of affected joints reveals proliferation of the lining cells, an inflammatory infiltrate rich in polymorphs and a necrotising vasculitis.

Clinical signs

The first report of SLE in the dog was that of Lewis *et al* (1965). This described a haematological form of the disease, but later work by many investigators has confirmed that this disease, as in man, is multisystemic and can present with a wide range of clinical signs either alone or in combination and which can develop in random sequence. The disease often has an insidious onset and presents a considerable diagnostic challenge.

The clinical signs associated with the disease in dogs can be divided into major signs, which are of the greatest diagnostic significance, and minor signs that are either less frequently encountered or are less specific for the disease.

Major signs

Musculoskeletal. Involvement of this system commonly takes the form of a polyarthritis which is usually symmetrical and may be sudden or gradual in onset. The disease is not as rapidly progressive as rheumatoid arthritis, and is usually, but not always, non-deforming. Nonetheless it may be quite severe. A diagnosis of myositis is difficult in the dog, but cases may be encountered in which the stiffness and difficulty in ambulation is hard to relate exclusively to joint disease and myositis may be suspected.

Skin disease. The skin changes associated with canine SLE are many and varied and often bizarre (Fig. 10.4). They are commonly symmetrical with a predilection for the head and ears (Fig. 10.4). Sometimes they may be more extensive and involve the feet and the mucocutaneous junctions. They are not usually ulcerative in distinction to pemphigus, but are more often erythematous and/or atrophic, with crusting being common.

Anaemia. This is a haemolytic anaemia and is truly autoimmune in nature. It is usually of the incomplete antibody type, and has a gradual onset, but autoagglutination with an acute onset is sometimes seen.

Glomerulonephritis. This is manifested initially by proteinuria which may lead to hypoalbuminaemia and subsequent oedema. Renal failure may ensue.

Thrombocytopenia. In some instances the presenting sign is either petechial or ecchymotic haemorrhages or an even more massive haemorrhage which can be life threatening. This can ensue when the thrombocyte count falls much below 45 000/mm³.

Leucopenia. Changes in leucocyte count are not uncommon in SLE and may be in either direction. Leucocytosis is commonly seen in so many diseases that it

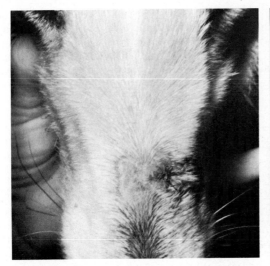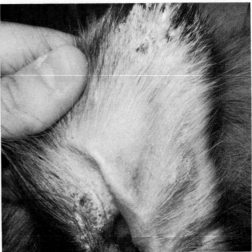

Fig. 10.4 Cutaneous manifestations of SLE. There are crusting lesions on the ear and nose. (Reproduced with permission from *The Compendium on Continuing Education for* *the Practising Veterinarian*, Veterinary Learning Systems Co., Inc., Princeton, N.J.)

is of little diagnostic help. Leucopenia, however, is much rarer in clinical medicine but is not uncommon in SLE. A WBC count below 7000/mm³ which cannot be ascribed to any other aetiology is strong supportive evidence.

Minor signs

Fever. This may be intermittent or continual and is usually corticosteroid responsive but it responds less well to antipyretics such as aspirin.

Central nervous signs. These may be manifested as symptoms of encephalitis, meningitis or myelitis.

Pleuritis. This is not uncommonly seen in man, but it is difficult to diagnose in the dog as it is clinically mild and minor chest pain only may result. Radiographs, chest taps and cytology are needed to support the diagnosis.

Oral ulcers. Again, although this is a common sign in man, oral or pharyngeal ulcers have only recently been documented in canine SLE.

The incidence of clinical signs in 116 cases of canine disease diagnosed as SLE in the literature has recently been documented by Scott *et al* (1983) and is recorded in Table 10.1.

Diagnosis

In order to qualify as a major sign supporting a diag-

Table 10.1 Clinicopathological signs in 116 cases of canine SLE abstracted from the literature (After Scott *et al* 1983).

Sign	Number	Percentage
(a) *Major signs*		
Polyarthritis	89/116	76.7
Proteinuria	56/116	48.2
Anaemia	30/86	34.9
Skin lesions	38/116	32.8
Leucopenia	11/39	28.2
Thrombocytopenia	10/86	11.6
(b) *Minor signs*		
Fever	89/116	76.7
Respiratory signs (particularly pleuritis)	6/116	5.2
Oral ulcers	5/116	4.3
Neurologic disease	5/116	4.3

nosis of canine SLE, certain characteristics must be fulfilled in each instance. The polyarthritis is not usually erosive and deforming although cases are sometimes encountered which are. Biopsies of the joint synovial membrane reveal an infiltrate which is less exclusively mononuclear than that of rheumatoid arthritis. However, joint fluid analysis is very similar in the two diseases and rheumatoid factor may be present. Radiographic changes may be absent, but if present are less severe than those seen in rheumatoid arthritis.

When there is skin involvement direct immunofluorescence on affected and sometimes adjacent normal skin should reveal deposits of IgG and/or complement at the dermoepidermal junction. Histopathology of the skin lesions should reveal the changes documented earlier.

An important feature of the anaemia is that it must be Coombs' positive if it is truly part of SLE, and likewise the thrombocytopenia should be PF3 positive.

When there is renal involvement, biopsies processed for immunofluorescence should reveal a deposition of IgG and complement along the basement membrane in a 'lumpy-bumpy' immune complex pattern and histopathology should show a classical immune complex glomerulonephritis.

The relative incidence of the varying clinicopathologic signs of canine SLE is documented in Table 10.1.

A diagnosis of definite active SLE is not tenable without evidence of autoantibody activity directed against nuclear antigens. Amongst these are double-stranded (native) DNA, soluble and insoluble nucleoproteins, saline extractable nuclear antigens (notably the Sm antigen and ribonucleoprotein) and synthetic polyribonucleotides. Although studies in canine SLE have confirmed the existence of autoantibody activity against specific nucleoproteins, for practical purposes the demonstration of broad antinuclear antibody activity is sufficient. Originally this was assessed by the LE cell phenomenon. Briefly heparinised blood is taken, vortexed in order to fragment some cells and permit free nuclear material into the cell suspension, and incubated for varying times at 37°C. If antinuclear antibody is present, it will opsonise the nuclear material causing it to be engulfed by a polymorph. A

buffy coat preparation is then made and stained appropriately. The classic LE cell is a polymorph which has ingested nuclear material (see Fig. 10.5a). It is now believed that this test is not as sensitive as the ANA by immunofluorescence.

Antinuclear antibodies have reactivity which crosses the species barrier and thus the source of nuclei is immaterial. Fresh frozen or acetone preserved sections of mouse liver are often employed and tissue culture preparations of mammalian cell lines are a convenient alternative. To perform the test, dilutions of the patient's serum and a positive and negative control are placed on the nuclear source, incubated, washed, and overlaid with a fluorescein conjugated anticanine IgG. After further washing, the preparation is viewed with an ultra violet microscope (Fig. 10.5b). Fluorescent patterns noted include ring, homogeneous and diffuse speckled, all of which may be seen in SLE. Nucleolar fluorescence is less specific for the disease in man, but has been encountered in canine SLE.

Low titred ANA activity is found in many normal sera, and the level that constitutes a significant titre varies with the substrate. At the University of Florida a titre of 1/20 or greater is considered significant when employing mouse liver, but the titre should be 1/100 or greater in the case of mammalian cell lines. It must also be remembered that high titres of ANA are sometimes found in normal animals (and people), and so a positive ANA in no way constitutes a diagnosis of SLE. Another substrate in use in man is the protozoan *Crithidia lucidae* with its kinetoplast of double-stranded DNA. However, for reasons that are not

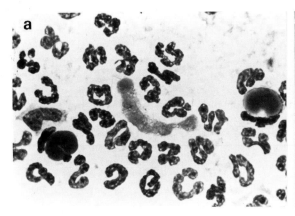

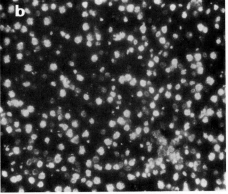

Fig. 10.5(a) A positive LE cell test. Pictured are two neutrophils which have phagocytised a large homogeneous inclusion body consisting of opsonised nuclear material. (Reproduced with permission from *The Compendium on Continuing Education for the Practising Veterinarian*, Veterinary Learning Systems Co., Inc., Princeton, N.J.; Original

photo courtesy of Dr John Harvey, University of Florida, College of Veterinary Medicine, Gainesville, FL.)
(b) Positive ANA (indirect immunofluorescence) test using mouse liver section and fluorescein conjugated sheep anticanine IgG.

readily apparent, this has proved to be very insensitive in canine studies.

The ANA titre may or may not fluctuate with the intensity of the disease and will be low or absent if the patient is in spontaneous remission. Successful therapy, however, does not necessarily cause a marked reduction in titre.

Other methods of diagnosing antinuclear antibody in man include radioimmunoassay and agglutination of latex particles coated with DNA. These methods are not in general applicable to the dog due to the presence of an anionic protein which binds DNA and which is not antibody in nature. False positives with these techniques may result.

The authors propose the following diagnostic scheme, for canine SLE.

I. *Definite SLE*. This diagnosis is justified in cases presenting with two major signs and supportive serologic evidence, or with one major and two minor signs together with positive serology.

II. *Probable SLE*. This diagnosis is justified if one major sign is present with positive serology, or when two major signs are present but without evidence of positive ANA.

Treatment and prognosis
Once the diagnosis of definite SLE has been reached it is likely that lifelong therapy will be required. However, some cases do go into remission and once the condition has been stabilised it should be safe to discontinue therapy so long as careful patient monitoring is practised. On the other hand, if a high titre ANA still persists, it is probably unwise to attempt to withdraw the patient from therapy.

Therapy of canine SLE involves the use of corticosteroids and immunosuppressive agents. SLE is not necessarily a fatal disease with good management, although a reduced life expectancy is usual resulting either from the disease process itself or from side-effects of therapy. Bacterial infections are common, in both treated and non-treated SLE.

Public health aspects
As noted earlier, the finding of a high incidence of serological abnormalities in workers in rheumatology laboratories raises the possibility of viral involvement in the disease. Assuming one of these individuals was genetically susceptible, the possibility for disease theoretically exists, although such an occurrence has yet to be documented.

The somewhat anecdotal report of familial SLE which implied that the disease might be transmissible

from man to dog (Beaucher *et al* 1977) was quickly refuted by three controlled studies (e.g. Kristensen *et al* 1979).

Discoid lupus erythematosus
This benign relative of SLE is associated only with cutaneous disease (Griffin *et al* 1979). Not only is there no internal organ involvement but ANA tests are negative.

This disease is clinically similar to pemphigus erythematosus, and resembles descriptions of Collie nose. Lesions are exacerbated by sunlight, and consist of pigment loss, erythema, alopecia and crusting. Histopathology is similar to the cutaneous lesions of SLE, and deposits of immunoglobulin are seen in involved skin. The aetiology is unclear, but it probably involves deposition of immune complexes. There is no autoimmune reactivity against skin tissue. Sunscreens and topical corticosteroids are often effective in therapy, although systemic corticosteroids are necessary in some cases.

RHEUMATOID ARTHRITIS

Rheumatoid arthritis (RA) is a chronic systemic inflammatory disease which preferentially involves articular structures. Joint involvement is frequently multiple or symmetrical beginning with acute synovitis and progressing to an erosive, highly destructive and disabling arthritis. The disease has been described in man as early as the seventeenth century, and was first reported in the dog by Liu *et al* (1969).

The discovery of rheumatoid factor (RF) in human sera (Waaler 1940) launched an era of intense investigation of the immunologic events participating in the pathogenesis of RA. Though considered an autoimmune disease, exhaustive research efforts have as yet failed to discern precisely the inciting aetiology of RA. The recognition of spontaneously occurring rheumatoid-like arthritis in dogs has provided a unique model for additional investigative efforts over the past ten years (Newton *et al* 1976, 1979; Pedersen *et al* 1976; Schumacher *et al* 1980).

Aetiology and pathogenesis
The proposed autoimmune nature of rheumatoid arthritis stems chiefly from the high correlation in man (80-90%) with the presence of elevated titres of rheumatoid factor in patient's sera. RF is immunoglobulin (usually IgM and/or IgG) with specificity for antigenic determinants of autologous IgG, i.e. RF is an autoantibody. The fact that both human and canine RF crossreact well with heterologous IgG is the basis for

not only the accidental discovery of its existence, but also the routine laboratory methods for its detection (see RF test under diagnosis). One of the central questions regarding the aetiology of RA has always been the role of RF in the pathogenesis of the polyarthritis, i.e. what instigates the formation of autoantibody against native IgG, and does RF initiate the inflammatory process, perpetuate it, or merely result as a by-product? Two basic lines of investigation have attempted to address these questions for nearly four decades. The first involves the search for an insidious infectious agent which incites a local immune response that sterically alters native IgG rendering it non-self, thereby initiating the production of RF both locally within the synovium and ultimately systemically. Although an attractive concept, research has produced conflicting and ambiguous evidence for the existence of an infectious agent in the pathogenesis of RA (Olhager 1975; Schumacher *et al* 1980). Because certain spontaneous human and animal forms of infectious arthritis can produce a self-perpetuating reactive arthritis similar to RA, the search for a similar aetiology in human and canine RA continues (Wager 1975; Ennis *et al* 1972; Hjerpe & Knight 1972). The second and major line of investigation involves the role of immunologic events in the initiation and perpetuation of RA (Table 10.2). Once again, a wealth of data, sometimes with conflicting results, has been accumulated. A fairly consistent map of certain immunological events has been outlined and has withstood the test of time and continued investigation.

Table 10.2 Immunological events in RA.

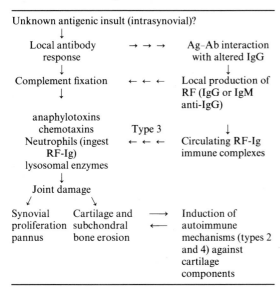

Participating in the events which ultimately lead to synovitis and joint destruction are circulating immune complexes consisting of RF-IgG or self-aggregates of RF, the local production of RF by immune synovial cells, consumption of complement within the synovium, phagocytosis of immune complexes and release of damaging lysosomal enzymes. Less certain aetiologic participants include autoantibodies against articular cartilage, T lymphocyte interactions, and the role of prostaglandins.

Epidemiological and genetic studies have implicated a probable polygenic heritability factor in the incidence of human RA. No such factor has been associated in canine RA.

It is presently unknown whether the pathoaetiology of canine and human rheumatoid arthritis is identical or dissimilar. However, there appear to be sufficient similarities in clinical, histopathological and immunological criteria to justify the application of 'rheumatoid arthritis' to the canine model.

Pathology

Synovial changes in the early stages of canine rheumatoid arthritis include proliferation of the synovial lining cells (hyperplasia) with overlying fibrin deposition, villous hypertrophy, and diffuse inflammatory infiltrates of the underlying connective tissue consisting predominantly of lymphocytes and plasma cells. The degree of neutrophil invasion varies, but may be a more prominent finding in canine RA than in human RA (Schumacher *et al* 1980). With more advanced disease, erosions of articular cartilage and subchondral bone, beginning at the margins of synovial attachment, progress with the extension of a pannus-type granulation tissue over the articular surface and dissecting under cartilage into subchondral bone.

Clincal signs

The clinical signs of rheumatoid arthritis include shifting leg lameness, weakness, muscle atrophy, multiple joint tenderness with soft tissue swelling, and later on, excessive joint laxity with angular deformity and degenerative changes (Fig. 10.6). Because RA is a systemic disorder, fever, lymphadenopathy and splenomegaly can also be encountered. Cardiopulmonary involvement, seen in some cases of human RA, has not been reported in the dog. Rheumatoid nodules, which are a distinguishing feature of human RA, are not seen in the canine disease.

Canine RA appears to be a more rapidly progressive disease, unlike human RA which is often more insidious and slowly progressive. Favoured joint distributions in the dog are the carpal and tarsal joints,

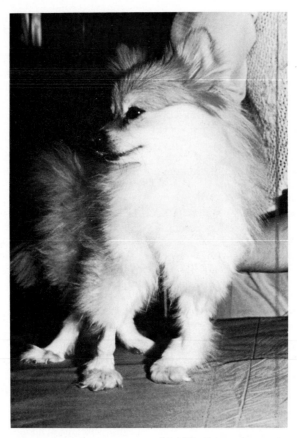

Fig. 10.6 A Pomeranian with rheumatoid arthritis. Pictured are bilateral carpal swelling and angular deformities of the left carpus and right tarsus. (Reproduced with permission from *The Compendium on Continuing Education for the Practising Veterinarian*, Veterinary Learning Systems Co., Inc., Princeton, N.J.)

elbow and stifle joints, with the interphalangeal joints affected less often than in man.

Diagnosis

Rheumatoid arthritis is associated with a variety of immunological events (both humoral and cell mediated) which are not specific for this particular immunologic disorder. Therefore , there is no single test which reliably determines a diagnosis of RA. Rather, the diagnosis is achieved by fulfillment of a number of criteria which may not be satisfied in every individual case at a certain point in time. These criteria include clinical evidence, radiographical evidence, serological evidence (RF), and ideally, histopathological evidence. Equally important is the exclusion of other causes of polyarthritis such as infectious, SLE and idiopathic immune-mediated polyarthritis.

The criteria established by the American Rheumatism Association for the diagnosis of human RA have been applied successfully in most reported cases of canine RA (Table 10.3). A diagnosis of classical RA is

Table 10.3 ARA criteria for diagnosis of rheumatoid arthritis (After Ropes *et al* 1958).

1	Morning stiffness
2	Pain on motion of at least one joint
3	Soft-tissue swelling
4	Swelling of at least one other joint within a 3-month period
5	Symmetrical joint swelling
6	Subcutaneous nodules
7	Radiographic findings suggestive of RA
8	Serological evidence of RF
9	Poor mucin precipitate from synovial fluid (when added to glacial acetic acid)
10	Characteristic histological changes in synovial membrane
11	Characteristic histological changes in nodules

justified when seven or more of the eleven criteria are met. Definite RA is justified when five criteria are met, providing any of criteria 1–5 are of at least six weeks duration.

The early radiographic changes in canine RA are often limited to periarticular soft tissue swelling, and juxta-articular osteopenia characterised by an enhanced trabecular bone pattern. Thus, the early stages of the disease can be radiographically indistinguishable from other forms of polyarthritis. With disease progression, subchondral and periarticular rarefaction or cystic lesions become apparent, the joint capsule becomes thickened, and there is diminution of the joint spaces signifying destruction of articular cartilage (Fig. 10.7). Secondary hypertrophic degenerative

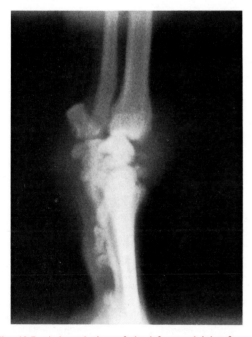

Fig. 10.7 A lateral view of the left carpal joint from a seven-year-old male Sheltie. Pictured are soft tissue swelling, erosion and collapse of cartilage, rarefaction of subchondral bone, and proliferative osteophyte formation.

changes with sclerosis and osteophyte formation accompany the progression of joint instability and ligamentous rupture. Bone atrophy appears with time and disuse.

Synovial fluid analysis is useful in establishing whether a particular arthropathy is inflammatory, septic or sterile, or non-inflammatory. Synovial fluid changes are by no means a specific indicator for RA. Generally synovial fluid in RA has less viscosity than

normal (poor mucin clot quality), and has increased numbers of predominantly neutrophils, as well as macrophages and occasionally lymphoid and plasma cells (rarely). Routine stains and light microscopy seldom reveal the presence of phagocytised immune complexes in macrophages or neutrophils (ragocytes) in canine RA.

Haematological and biochemical testing seldom contribute to the diagnosis of RA except as indicators of general health or concomittant problems. Reported haematological changes include a low-grade normochromic, normocytic anaemia, elevated RBC sedimentation rate, neutrophilic leucocytosis and elevations in acute phase reactants such as fibrinogen.

The presence of rheumatoid factor is not specific for RA in either man or dogs, since detectable serum levels occur in some normal individuals as well as in other systemic and arthritic disorders (Wager 1975; Halliwell 1978). The presence of high serum titres of RF *in conjunction with* satisfaction of the above mentioned ARA criteria are necessary for the diagnosis of RA. Titres of rheumatoid factor in canine RA tend to be much lower than in man as a general rule. Reports of positive RF tests in canine RA range over 25–70% . (Pedersen *et al* 1983; Halliwell 1978). Experience at the University of Florida Veterinary Medical Teaching Hospital over the past five years parallels the lower figure of approximately 25% incidence of positive RF tests in canine RA. There are several explanations, borne out by recent laboratory experiments (Halliwell *et al*, unpubl. obs.), for lower serum RF titres and a higher incidence of seronegative RA in the dog. First, canine RF is frequently IgG antibody, and unlike IgM, is a much poorer agglutinating antibody (see RF test below). Second, rheumatoid factors can exist as immune complexes by either self-association or by complexing with native IgG, thereby decreasing the availability of free RF for detection by routine agglutination tests. Third, more sensitive tests than simple agglutination systems, may be necessary to detect canine RF, such as prior pepsin digestion or acid dissociation of immune complexes, immunodiffusion or radioimmunoassay.

Rheumatoid factor test

The most popular method of detection of canine RF remains the rabbit Rose–Waaler test. In this system sheep red blood cells (SRBC) are sensitized with a subagglutinating titre of rabbit anti-sheep RBC (IgG). Serial two-fold dilutions of the test sera are incubated with the IgG-coated SRBC, incubated at 37°C for one hour and examined for agglutination. Titres of 1:16 or greater in the dog are considered significant (Halliwell 1978), while a 1:8 titre is equivocal. Latex particle agglutination is another popular screening test for human RF, however experience with this test is more limited in canine RA, and it is considered a less specific test in the dog.

Differential diagnosis

Rheumatoid arthritis must be differentiated from other causes of inflammatory joint disease including infectious, systemic lupus, idiopathic, and secondary to underlying systemic disease processes such as viral, parasitic and neoplastic (Pedersen *et al* 1976, 1976a). When RF tests are negative or equivocal, and radiographic change is minimal, synovial biopsy is the more definitive diagnostic test. Serological tests for ANA and LE cells should be routinely performed in all cases of chronic polyarthritis, for a diagnosis of SLE excludes the diagnosis of RA.

Treatment and prognosis

The aims in the treatment of RA are to reduce inflammation and pain, promote ambulation, and to delay the progression of destructive lesions. There is no cure for RA and progression of the disease with time is the rule rather than the exception, in spite of treatment. Instances of spontaneous remission are rare, and in such cases the diagnosis is in question.

There are a multitude of treatment modalities, some accepted and some experimental, in man. They range from salicylates and other non-steroidal anti-inflammatory drugs, to gold salts, corticosteroids, immunosuppressive cytotoxic drugs, immune stimulating compounds, sulphhydryl compounds, venoms, lymphopheresis, antilymphocyte serum and others. Of these, only salicylates, penicillamine and gold salt therapy have withstood the test of time.

There are widely differing opinions on the efficacy of aspirin in canine RA. It is the first line drug in early, non-aggressive RA in man. Although salicylates have a place in the treatment of canine RA, rapid progression of this disease in the dog does not justify their use as sole therapy (Pedersen *et al* 1983). Salicylates do not impede the production of RF or the progression of cellular and pannus-type infiltration of synovium, cartilage and bone. The recommended dose of aspirin in canine RA is 25–35 mg/kg every eight hours (Yeary & Brant 1975).

The use of corticosteroids remains very controversial in the treatment of erosive joint disease. There is no question that they achieve significant clinical improvement, especially early in the course of the disease; however their efficacy over the long-term is not sustained and their contribution to articular breakdown has always been of great concern to rheumatologists. For this reason, the use of corticosteroids

in canine RA should be cautious and reserved for cases in which rapid progression of the disease is manifest, or where acute active inflammation renders the animal non-ambulatory and generally ill in spite of other nonsteroidal therapy. The recommended starting dose of short-acting corticosteroid (prednisone or prednisolone) is 2–4 mg/kg orally in divided doses every twelve hours (Pedersen *et al* 1983). Upon significant clinical response, every effort should be made to gradually taper the dose to an alternate day schedule of 25–50% of the starting dose. As in the case of aspirin, corticosteroids used alone are not considered very satisfactory over the long term. In man, the use of corticosteroids in conjunction with aspirin is not recommended due to a drug interaction which significantly reduces the level of salicylate achieved in the synovium (Gifford 1973).

Cytotoxic immunosuppressive drugs in combination with initial corticosteroid therapy have been the most satisfactory treatment for canine RA according to Pedersen *et al* (1976, 1983). The rationale of using immunosuppressive drugs to inhibit lymphocyte (both B and T cells) interactions in the progression of RA appears justified, and once again the early response is often profound. Clinical remission is usually more long-lived than with aspirin or steroids used alone. However toxic side effects and disease exacerbation upon tapering doses or discontinuation are frequently the case in canine RA. Cyclophosphamide and azathioprine are the two recommended cytotoxic drugs in immune-mediated polyarthritis. Starting doses for each drug are 50 mg/m² daily. For cyclophosphamide a cycle of four days of treatment, and three days of 'rest' each week is recommended. Following good clinical response, the drugs should be tapered (this, as with other drugs, remains empirical or individual according to each case) and discontinued following sustained remission. Treatment duration is variable, but should not exceed four months, and interval check-ups to monitor for clinical response *and* toxicity are mandatory (see further details in section on drug therapy).

Although experience with gold salt therapy in canine RA is limited, initial observations by Newton *et al* (1979) would indicate their potential benefit in canine patients. The disadvantage for severely afflicted dogs is their more latent onset of efficacy (weeks to months). However, a possible advantage might be a more prolonged remission time. The recommended dose of gold sodium thiomalate (Myocrysin) is 1 mg/kg intramuscularly once a week. Upon remission, the injections can be reduced to biweekly. If remission is sustained, withdrawal from therapy should be attempted. Dogs on gold salt therapy should be monitored for haematological abnormalities and renal toxicity. Although anaphylaxis has not been experienced in gold salt therapy in dogs, a test dose under close observation is recommended.

Surgical arthrodesis, frequently of multiple joints, is sometimes performed to restore function as much as possible. Surgical candidates should be in a state of clinical remission prior to arthrodesis. Synovectomy rarely has application in canine RA, due to the multiple joint involvement.

Patient management for RA is a long-term commitment both for the dog owner and the attending veterinarian. Maintenace of the ambulatory state depends upon judiciously applied physical therapy in addition to specific therapy. Short periods of leash exercise, passive joint manipulations, and swimming or hydrotherapy may prove beneficial in preserving as much joint mobility and function as possible. Unfortunately, the prognosis for canine RA is guarded in regard to long-term quality of life. Euthanasia is the most common cause of death in canine RA.

BULLOUS AUTOIMMUNE SKIN DISEASES

A number of these diseases, which were previously thought not to occur in domestic animals, have been recognised in the dog in recent years, and have been the subject of a recent extensive review (Scott & Lewis 1981). The very thin canine epidermis renders the bullous phase very short and so affected animals usually present showing ulcerative lesions with resultant crusting and scarring. This has delayed their recognition clinically as bullous diseases and it is only improved histological and immunological techniques that have confirmed their existence in the dog. The pathogenesis derives from autoimmune reactions against skin antigens. The specificity of the autoantibodies in the various diseases differs, and this leads to a variety of clinicopathological findings. The four major aids to diagnosis in these diseases are:

1 Histopathology
2 Cytology of blister fluid
3 Direct immunofluorescence for the demonstration of deposits of antibody and complement
4 Indirect immunofluorescence in a search for evidence of circulating autoantibodies

It is important that all biopsies for both immunofluorescence and routine histopathology are taken from the edge of fresh lesions or by excision of complete bullae if these are evident. The classical pathology for each disease is often very transitory, and many sections through many biopsies may be required before the diagnostic changes are encountered.

Biopsies fresh frozen in isopentane cooled in solid CO_2 provide the best starting point for direct immunofluorescence as formalin fixation destroys the antigenicity of the immunoglobulins deposited, and biopsies so preserved are unsuitable. There is some suggestion that formalin-fixed tissues may be acceptable for performing enzyme-linked antibody studies, but definitive evidence is awaited. If freezing is impractical, biopsies may be preserved for transport to the laboratory via the mail in a medium developed by Michel *et al* (1971). Indirect immunofluorescence on serum using fresh frozen canine buccal mucosa or oesophagus as the substrate may also be employed, but positive results are rarely obtained. This is in marked distinction to the situation in man where high titres, which tend to parallel the disease activity, are the rule.

A recent retrospective study undertaken at the University of Florida compared the value of histopathology and of direct immunofluorescence in achieving a definitive diagnosis (Werner *et al* 1983). It was reached by means of histopathological findings in some 69% of cases and by immunofluorescence in 53%. Thus both techniques should be employed in order to optimise the clinician's chances. As lifelong therapy with potentially lethal drugs is employed, the importance of achieving the correct diagnosis is clear.

Pemphigus vulgaris

This was the first of the bullous diseases to be described in the dog (Stannard *et al* 1975; Hurvitz & Feldman 1975). Clinically it is the most severe. Indeed, the disease in man was invariably fatal prior to the advent of corticosteroids.

Clinical signs
The onset may be either acute or chronic and is characterised classically by the development of bullae involving the mucocutaneous junctions and the oral mucosa. Nail beds may be affected, leading to shedding of the nails, and the disease may generalise and involve any area of the body. The bullous phase is very short, however, and most animals will be presented with circumscribed areas of superficial ulceration, exudation and crust formation. Secondary bacterial infection is common and affected animals may become febrile and systemically ill.

Diagnosis

Histopathology. The major pathological change of all the pemphigus group is acantholysis, which can be defined as loss of cohesion between epidermal cells leading to their rounding off as individual darkly staining cells. In the case of pemphigus vulgaris a cleft appears within the epidermis which is suprabasilar, leaving the basal cell layer intact. It must again be emphasised that this histopathology, which is absolutely diagnostic for pemphigus vulgaris is rarely encountered in a single routine biopsy, and diligent and patient searching on the part of clinician and pathologist alike is necessary.

Immunofluorescence. Intercellular deposits of immunoglobulin and complement may be found within the epidermis (Fig. 10.8). Circulating autoantibodies may sometimes be demonstrable using fresh frozen dog oral mucosa or oesophagus as the substrate. Titres in the dog are not high, however, and it is not unusual for cases positive by all other parameters to lack evidence of positive indirect immunofluorescence.

It is not necessary that all of these diagnostic criteria be fulfilled. The histopathological signs outlined above are absolutely diagnostic for pemphigus vulgaris, and positive direct or indirect immunofluorescence alone indicates that the disease is in the pemphigus family. This may be sufficiently close for all practical purposes. It is important, however, not to rely solely on clinical impressions, for the condition may be readily confused with mucocutaneous candidiasis. Immunosuppressive therapy, which is required for pemphigus, could have fatal results in candidiasis as the latter is usually associated with an immunodeficient state.

Pemphigus foliaceous

This more recently described variant (Halliwell & Goldschmidt 1977) is being recognised with increasing frequency, and is the commonest of the pemphigus group.

Clinical signs

In contrast to pemphigus vulgaris, the distribution shows no apparent predilection for the mucocutaneous junctions, and mucosal involvement is exceedingly rare. The onset is usually gradual. The bulla is very shallow, being subcorneal in position, and as it readily becomes infiltrated with neutrophils, it resembles a pustule that is often no larger than that associated with a staphylococcal infection. The head, nose and ears are often involved, and the condition may generalise (Fig. 10.9). Pruritus is variable, but may be quite intense. The patient usually suffers no systemic involvement.

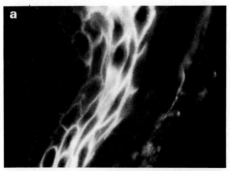

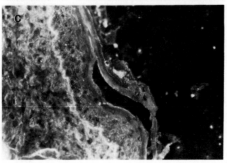

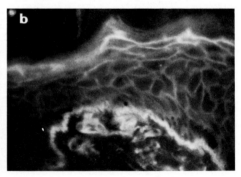

Fig. 10.8 (a)   Positive direct immunofluorescence in sections of skin from a dog with pemphigus foliaceous showing intercellular deposits of IgG.

(b)   Positive direct immunofluorescence in a skin biopsy section from a dog with pemphigus erythematosus. IgG deposits are located both intercellularly within the epidermis and along the dermoepidermal junction. (Reproduced with permission from *The Compendium on Continuing Education for the Practising Veterinarian*, Veterinary Learning Systems Co, Inc., Princeton, N.J.)

(c)   Immunoglobulin deposition at the dermoepidermal junction on direct immunofluorescence from a dog with bullous pemphigoid.

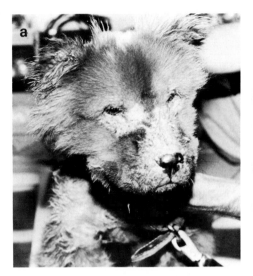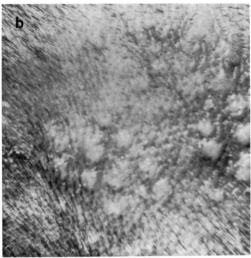

Fig. 10.9 Clinical signs of pemphigus foliaceous. (a) The face of an affected Chow. (b) Bullous lesions on the flank of a mongrel.

Diagnosis

Histopathology. A subcorneal bulla should be visualised if an intact lesion is biopsied. The blister is rich in acantholytic cells and neutrophils (Fig. 10.10). The former cells are absent or rare in subcorneal pustular dematosis (Halliwell *et al* 1977), which is a pustular disease of unknown aetiology, and also in staphylococcal pyoderma. Bacterial organisms are usually visualised in the latter disease, and may occur also as secondary invaders in pemphigus foliaceous and subcorneal pustular dematosis.

Immunofluorescence. Direct immunofluorescence may show deposits of epidermal intercellular immunoglobulin in a pattern indistinguishable from pemphigus vulgaris. Some cases are encountered in which the antibody is deposited in the more superficial layers of the epidermis which would account for the more superficial cleft in pemphigus foliaceous. Indirect immunofluorescence rarely may be positive.

Other diagnostic criteria
An unequivocal diagnosis of pemphigus foliaceous is often very difficult to achieve, and clinical, histopathological and immunological findings all should be considered. Sometimes a retrospective diagnosis is made after trial therapy. The differential diagnostic criteria are summarised in Table 10.4.

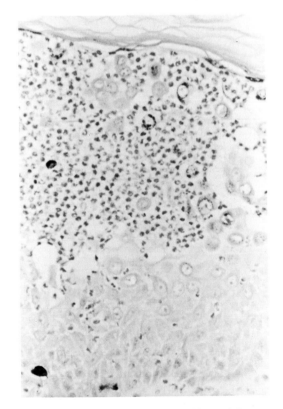

Fig. 10.10 Histopathology of pemphigus foliaceous. Numerous acantholytic cells are seen within a subcorneal bulla.

Table 10.4 Diagnostic criteria in autoimmune skin diseases.

Disease	Histopathological changes	Direct immunofluorescence	Indirect immunofluorescence	Other findings	Occurrence in dogs
Systemic lupus erythematosus	**1** Hydropic degeneration of the basal cells **2** Thinning or hyperkeratosis of the epidermis **3** Periadenexal and periarterial mononuclear infiltrate	Deposits of IgG at dermoepidermal junction of involved and normal skin	Negative	ANA usually positive greater than 1:100; LE preparation usually positive	Yes
Pemphigus vulgaris	Acantholysis prominent with a suprabasilar cleft	Epidermal intercellular deposits of IgG and C3 always demonstrable	Circulating autoantibodies against intercellular substance cement sometimes demonstrable	—	Yes
Pemphigus foliaceous	Acantholysis with subcorneal bulla formation	Intercellular epidermal deposits of IgG and C3 always demonstrable	Circulating autoantibodies against intercellular cement substance sometimes demonstrable	—	Yes
Bullous pemphigoid	Subepidermal bullae with predominantly mononuclear infiltrate	Linear or globular deposits of IgG at dermoepidermal junction	Circulating autoantibodies against 'basement zone substance' sometimes demonstrable	—	Yes
Discoid lupus	Hyperkeratosis; hydropic degeneration of basal cells; atrophy of stratum malpighii; patchy periadenexal lymphoid infiltrate; dermal oedema and vasodilation	Deposits of IgG at dermoepidermal junction of involved skin only	None	None; ANA and LE preparations are negative	Possibly

Pemphigus vegetans

This rare variant of pemphigus vulgaris has been the subject of two reports in the dog (Schultz & Goldschmidt 1980; Scott 1977). A severe disease, it is characterised by ulcerative and proliferative lesions affecting the oral mucosa, mucocutaneous junction and tending to readily generalise.

Histopathology reveals intraepidermal, suprabasilar abscesses which contain acantholytic cells and become invaded with neutrophils and eosinophils. Direct and indirect immunofluorescence may be positive.

Pemphigus erythematosus

This is a variant of pemphigus foliaceous which has some features of SLE.

Clinically, the condition resembles old descriptions of Collie nose, with crusting and alopecia, which is usually symmetrical. It involves the nose and ears, and may spread to involve much of the head.

The histopathology is indistinguishable from that associated with pemphigus foliaceous, but direct immunofluorescence may reveal immunoglobulin deposits concomitantly at the dermoepidermal junction and intercellularly within the epidermis (Fig. 10.8b). ANA is often evident in moderate titres.

Bullous pemphigoid

This disease, whose name literally means 'pemphigus-like', is the latest of the bullous diseases to be described in detail in the dog (Kunkle *et al* 1978).

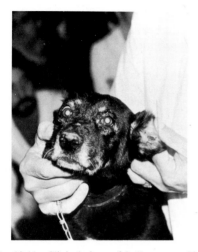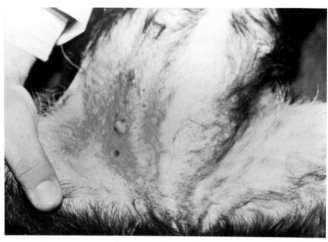

Fig. 10.11 Clinical signs of bullous pemphigoid. (Reprinted with permission from *Journal of The American Veterinary Medical Association*.)

Clinical signs

1 The acute and severe form. The onset is usually sudden and the eruption involves the oral mucosa, the mucocutaneous junctions and sometimes the ears (Fig. 10.11). Clinically it is very similar to pemphigus vulgaris except that intact bullae are more likely to be encountered as they are subepidermal in origin and involve other parts of the body surface.

2 The chronic and benign form has been recorded as lacking any predilection sites. There are mild bullous and then ulcerative lesions which tend to heal spontaneously only to break out again in close proximity. There is crusting and exudation.

Diagnosis

Histopathology. In contrast to the pemphigus group, acantholysis is not a feature of this disease and the bulla is subepidermal in origin (Fig. 10.12).

Direct immunofluorescence. Immunoglobulin and complement deposits are readily demonstrable at the dermoepidermal junction, but again in distinction to pemphigus there is no staining of the epidermis (Fig. 10.8c). Circulating autoantibodies reactive against antigenic material in the basement membrane zone are sometimes present and may be demonstrated by indirect immunofluorescence.

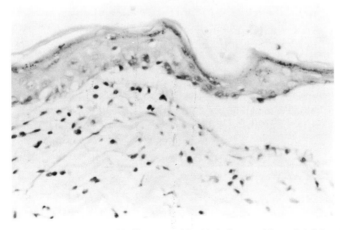

Fig. 10.12 Histopathology of bullous pemphigoid. A dermoepidermal cleft is evident.

Therapy of bullous autoimmune skin diseases

No two cases of autoimmune skin disease are the same, and definitive statements should not be made. The therapy can be conveniently considered in two parts, namely induction of remission and maintenance.

Corticosteroids are the therapeutic cornerstone, and should be given in doses of 2–4 mg/kg of prednisone or prednisolone in two daily divided doses. The newer and more expensive corticosteroids seem to offer little advantage. Some clinicians advocate simultaneous therapy with cyclophosphamide at 1.5–2.0 mg/kg for the first two weeks. Concomitant antibiotic therapy may be indicated, particularly if the animal is febrile or if large areas of ulceration are present, as is sometimes seen in pemphigus vulgaris and bullous pemphigoid.

Injectable gold therapy with sodium aurothioglucose (Solganol) has been advocated and may be used with corticosteroids to assist in induction of remission and for maintenance. Weekly test doses of 5 mg and 10 mg are given, and then weekly injections of 1 mg/kg. The therapy is tapered to monthly injections once remission is achieved. Response has been variable in the authors' hands. Some patients respond quite well, but in others the drug is apparently ineffective.

Maintenance with corticosteroids alone is clearly impractical at the initial dosages, for cushingoid side-effects will rapidly ensue. Some patients can be tapered to alternate day therapy at a dose of around 1–2.5 mg/kg and can be maintained relatively free of side-effects. However, combination therapy of corticosteroids and azathioprine has proved quite useful. In the early stages the two drugs may be given on the same day, and once remission is achieved, azathioprine can be given at a dose of around 1–1.5 mg/kg every other day alternating with prednisone or prednisolone.

The prognosis for the bullous autoimmune skin diseases is not good, and lifelong therapy is usually required. Occasional cases are encountered which apparently go into spontaneous remission enabling withdrawal from therapy. Thus, if the condition has been stabilised it is wise to gradually reduce the levels of drugs in order (1) to establish the minimum effective maintenance dose, and (2) to verify that continued therapy is in fact needed.

OTHER AUTOIMMUNE DISEASES

Autoimmune aspects of neurologic diseases

Myasthenia gravis
This is a neostigmine responsive muscular weakness in which circulating autoantibodies against muscle tissue, which incidentally crossreact with thymus, develop. The pathogenicity of these antibodies was long in doubt, but their relevance to the disease has recently been demonstrated unequivocally by the induction of a myasthenic type of syndrome in mice following injection of serum from patients with the disease.

More recent studies have shown that the majority of cases in man are characterised by development of autoantibodies against the acetylcholine receptor and that the resultant ultrastructural damage to the receptor tissue is related to the severity of the disease process. Presence of antireceptor antibodies has also been shown in canine myasthenia gravis (Lennon *et al* 1978).

Clinically, the condition in the dog is similar to that in man, and is characterised by weakness and considerably reduced exercise tolerance (Fraser *et al* 1970). Dilatation of the oesophagus may be an additional complication.

Diagnosis is readily achieved by observing the response to injection of neostigmine and atropine. Intramuscular doses of 1–2 mg/20 kg of neostigmine methylsulphate given with atropine may be used, and a response should be noted within 30 minutes.

Neostigmine may be given orally in higher doses for long-term control, but the recent unequivocal demonstration of the autoimmune pathogenesis suggests that immunosuppression should play a part in any therapeutic regimen.

Autoantibodies associated with distemper
Myelin protein is ordinarily sequestered from the reticuloendothelial system and so is not recognised as 'self'. When the blood–brain barrier is compromised as a result of inflammation, development of antimyelin antibodies may result. This has been shown to be the case in the encephalomyelitis associated with distemper, and the antibodies have been shown to be pathogenic *in vitro*. It is thus likely that they contribute to the pathogenesis of the disease.

Autoimmune thyroiditis

Histological evidence of lymphocytic infiltrates in the thyroid glands of Beagles has long been documented as incidental finding, but no endocrine disturbance was believed to result (Maudesley-Thomas 1969). More recently, however, evidence has emerged that autoimmune thyroiditis analogous to Hashimoto's disease of man is a major cause of hypothyroidism in dogs. In a recently published study, 48% of dogs with confirmed hypothyroidism (as judged by abnormal response in thyroxine levels following stimulation with thyroid stimulating hormone) had significant levels of antibodies to thyroglobulin (Gosselin *et al* 1982).

Canine Sjögren's syndrome

This disease in man is characterised by keratoconjunctivitis sicca (KCS) and reduction or absence of saliva. It is often associated with other autoimmune diseases, and the pathogenesis at least in part involves autoantibodies against lacrimal and salivary gland tissue.

The condition has been tentatively documented in the dog (Quimby *et al* 1979). The two dogs described had severe KCS, and dental caries. Immunological findings included positive ANA and the presence of autoantibodies against the epithelial cells of the nictitating membrane, but not against salivary or lacrimal tissue. The true role of autoimmunity in the rather common condition of KCS awaits the results of further studies.

Polyarteritis

One definitive report has appeared in the literature concerning polyarteritis of immune or possibly autoimmune aetiology (Harcourt 1978).

The age of onset in this Beagle colony was 3–15 months, and affected animals were depressed, febrile and reluctant to move. Gait and posture was altered, and the animals appeared markedly uncomfortable. Their condition was temporarily responsive to corticosteroid therapy. Histopathological examination revealed that meningeal and cardiac arteries were most often involved.

Autoimmune aspects of ocular disease

The role of autoimmune phenomena in recurrent uveitis as being partly or solely responsible for the pathogenesis has long been controversial and most studies are inconclusive.

Of particular interest is the possible canine model for the Vogt-Koyanaghi-Harada syndrome of man which is characterised by recurrent uveitis and depigmentation of the skin. A very similar syndrome has been seen particularly in Siberian Huskies and Akitas. It has been hypothesised that the condition results from autoimmune reactions against melanocytes and immunosuppression is clearly important in the therapy.

CONSIDERATIONS IN THE TREATMENT OF AUTOIMMUNE DISEASES

Progress in specific therapy of immune-mediated diseases has long been hindered by lack of complete understanding of the aetiopathological mechanisms involved, and by lack of significant data to establish relative efficacy of certain types or combinations of therapy via controlled clinical trials in veterinary medicine. Traditionally, we have been limited to using anti-inflammatory and immunosuppressive drugs which are not specifically aimed at the abnormal link in the immunological chain of events leading to autoimmune disease, and which furthermore have potentially undesirable immune modulating effects.

Because many instances of secondary immune-mediated disease occur, whenever possible underlying infection or disease should be eliminated by specific therapy against the offending agent, whether it is bacterial, parasitic or any other organism. This might include surgical treatment in the case of closed cavity or deep infection. Specific treatment of a known infection may preclude the necessity of less specific therapy with anti-inflammatory or immunosuppressive drugs. It is important to recognise drug-induced autoimmune disease since removal of the offending drug is often the only treatment necessary.

Anti-inflammatory drugs such as salicylates, phenylbutazone, ibuprofen and indomethacin provide varying degrees of analgesia, antipyretic effect, and anti-inflammatory potency in the treatment of the immune-mediated rheumatic diseases such as polyarthritis and polymyositis. However, it is important to remember that these drugs do not alter the underlying immunological abnormalities, but merely suppress some of the pain and inflammation which account for many of the clinical signs. Platelet dysfunction and gastrointestinal side-effects (emesis, haemorrhage, ulceration) are the major toxicities of these drugs.

In the absence of infection, corticosteroids are the first drug of choice in the treatment of many autoimmune diseases. Corticosteroids remain the most potent anti-inflammatory drugs available and are used primarily for this effect, and for suppression of the RE phagocytic system. The immunosuppressant effects of corticosteroids are considerably less potent than the effects of antimetabolites or alkylating agents, but are none the less significant.

The recommended initial dose of corticosteroid is 2–4 mg/kg in two divided doses daily. Shorter-acting preparations, prednisone and prednisolone, given per os are preferable. Initial doses should be tapered as the condition of the patient allows, and given once daily on an alternate-day basis to minimise the possibility of harmful side-effects. Continuous treatment with corticosteroids is not recommended.

Cytotoxic immunosuppressant drugs such as cyclophosphamide and azathioprine have been widely used in veterinary cases of autoimmune disease for nearly a decade. Immunosuppressant drugs are not a panacea for the treatment of these diseases, because they nonspecifically suppress many phases of the immunological response, and may in fact enhance certain undesirable lymphocyte interactions. Many patients with autoimmune disease are already compromised by inadequate function of their normal immune responsiveness. This puts them at high risk of acquiring infection. This risk is compounded by the addition of immunosuppressant agents to the treatment regime. For this reason caution is essential when using these agents.

Combination therapy with corticosteroids at a lowered dose, cyclophosphamide, and/or azathioprine are recommended when remission is not attained by corticosteroid therapy alone, or when steroid intolerance arises. This combination has been useful in treating refractory cases of AIHA, IMT, SLE, pemphigus and rheumatoid arthritis in the dog.

Cyclophosphamide is an alkylating agent which suppresses both humoral and cell-mediated immunity by interfering with replication through crosslinking with DNA. The end result may be cell death, or interference with blast transformation in response to antigenic stimulus. Azathioprine is a purine derivative which has both anti-inflammatory and immunosuppressive activity. It acts as an antimetabolite by causing the incorporation of abnormal purine bases into DNA, RNA, and coenzymes, thus interfering with both cellular and humoral immune response.

The vinca alkaloids, vincristine, and vinblastine arrest cell division by inhibiting microtubule formation in the mitotic spindle. They have less potent immunosuppressive effects than the alkylating agents or antimetabolites and have application only in cases of refractory IMT, where they are known to stimulate megakaryocytosis in the bone marrow.

Patients on immunosuppressant therapy must be monitored at frequent intervals while on full dose therapy. Weekly examination and haemograms are recommended to ensure that possible toxic side-effects are recognised as early as possible. In that event these drugs are tapered or withdrawn, depending on the severity of the encountered drug toxicity. The known and speculated side-effects of these drugs in the dog and in man are listed below:

1   Myelotoxicity
2   Increased susceptibility to infection
3   GI disturbances
4   Haemorrhagic cystitis, bladder fibrosis (cyclophosphamide)
5   Alopecia (cyclophosphamide)
6   Ovarian failure, aspermatogenesis (cyclophosphamide)
7   Neuromuscular weakness (vinca alkaloids)
8   Effects on genetic apparatus?
9   Predisposition to neoplasia by inhibiting immune surveillance?

Hepatorenal disease increases the possibility of toxic side-effects. Because these drugs affect cells most severely in increasing order of their turnover rates, the lymphoid cells are particularly sensitive to their actions, as are certain tumour cells. Because bone marrow cells are also rapidly dividing cells, myelotoxicity is an important side-effect of these agents. Patients who experience a drop in WBC to less than $4000/mm^3$, or a platelet reduction to $<100\,000/mm^3$ while on combination immunosuppressant therapy should be immediately withdrawn from therapy until these counts return to normal. Prolonged therapy is not recommended.

Table 10.5   Recommended canine doses for immunosuppressant drugs.

Cyclophosphamide	2 mg/kg (50 mg/m²) per os	Once daily four consecutive days each week
Azathioprine	2 mg/kg (50 mg/m²) per os	Once daily
Vincristine	0.015 mg/kg (0.5 mg/m²) IV	Once a week
Vinblastine	0.03 mg/kg (1.0/m²) IV	Once a week

Note: Doses should be empirically lowered when hepatic or renal failure is present

In general, disease remissions can be achieved during a period of 2–4 weeks on full doses and doses should be tapered and discontinued as soon as stabilisation warrants.

Although the era of pharmacological immunomodulation is now well established, much remains to be discovered regarding the effective, safe manipulation of immune responses. Parallel efforts at ellucidating the more subtle pathoaetiological events leading to autoimmune disorders must continue as well if significant therapeutic advances are to be made. Newer areas of immunopharmacology research include the identification, characterisation and purification of lymphocyte-derived substances (lymphokines) which have enhancing or suppressing activity at a more confined or discreet level of immune response. The goals of improved therapy for immunological disorders are to increase and prolong therapeutic efficacy and to reduce undesirable side-effects. The reader is referred to articles by Koller (1982), Gainer (1982), and Hooks *et al* (1982) for further details on the subject of immunomodulation therapy.

REFERENCES

Beaucher W. M., Garman R. H. & Condemi J. J. (1977) Familial lupus erythematosus antibodies to DNA in household dogs. *New Eng. J. Med.* **296**, 982.

Brown D. L., Dacie J. V. & Worledge S. M. (1983) Auto-allergic blood diseases. In *Clinical Aspects of Immunology*, 4th edn., eds. P. J. Lachmann & D. K. Peters. Blackwell Scientific Publications, Oxford.

Coombs R. R. A., Mourant A. E. & Race R. R. (1945) A new test for the detection of weak and 'incomplete' Rh agglutinins. *Br. J. Exp. Pathol.* **26**, 255.

Dacie J. V. & Worledge S. M. (1975) Autoallergic blood diseases. In *Clinical Aspects of Immunology*, 3rd edn, eds. P. G. H. Gell, R. R. A. Coombs & P. J. Lachmann. Blackwell Scientific Publications, Oxford.

Dixon R. H. & Rosse W. F. (1975) Platelet antibody in autoimmune thrombocytopenia. *Br. J. Haematol.* **31**, 129–34.

Dodds W. J. & Wilkins R. J. (1977) Animal model of human disease: canine and equine immune-mediated thrombocytopenia and idiopathic thrombocytopenia purpura. *Am. J. Pathol.* **86**, 489–91.

Ennis R. S., Dalgard D. *et al* (1972) Mycoplasma hyorhinis swine arthritis. II. Morphological features. *Arthritis Rheum.* **14**, 202.

Fraser D. C., Palmer A. C., Senior J. E. B., Parres J. D. & Yealland M. F. T. (1970) Myasthenia gravis in the dog. *J. Neurol. Neurosurg. Psychiat.* **33**, 431.

Gainer J. H. (1982) Suppressor factors and their potential for immunotherapy, and chemical influences on interferons. *J. Am. Vet. Med. Assoc.* **181**, 1107–10.

Gell P. G. H. & Coombs R. R. A. (1968) In *Clinical Aspects of Immunology*, 2nd edn., eds. P. G. H. Gell & R. R. A. Coombs. Blackwell Scientific Publications, Oxford.

Gifford R. H. (1973) Corticosteroid therapy for rheumatoid arthritis. *Med. Clin. N. Am.* **57**, 1179–90.

Gosselin S. J., Capen C. C., Martin S. L. *et al* (1982) Autoimmune lymphocytic thyroiditis in dogs. *Vet. Immunol. Immunopathol.* **3**, 185–201.

Greene C. E., Scoggin J. *et al* (1982) Vincristine in the treatment of thrombocytopenia in five dogs. *J. Am. Vet. Med. Assoc.* **180**, 140–3.

Griffin C. E., Stannard A. A., Ihrke P. J. *et al* (1979) Canine discoid lupus erythematosus. *Vet. Immunol. Immunopathol.* **1**, 79–87.

Halliwell R. E. W., Schwartzman R. M., Ihrke P. J., Goldschmidt M. H. & Wood M. G. (1977) Dapsone for treatment of pruritic dermatitis. (Dermatitis herpetiformis and subcorneal pustular dermatosis) in dogs. *J. Am. Vet. Med. Assoc.* **170**, 697.

Halliwell R. E. W. & Goldschmidt M. H. (1977) Pemphigus foliaceous in the canine: a case report and discussion. *J. Am. Anim. Hosp. Assoc.* **13**, 431.

Halliwell R. E. W. (1978) Autoimmune disease in the dog. *Adv. Vet. Sci. Comp. Med.* **22**, 221–63.

Halliwell R. E. W., Werner L. L. *et al* (1983) Unpublished data.

Harcourt R. A. (1978) Polyarteritis in a colony of Beagles. *Vet. Rec.* **102**, 519–22.

Harrington W. J., Minnick V. *et al* (1951) Demonstration of thrombocytopenic factor in the blood of patients with thrombocytopenic purpura. *J. Lab. Clin. Med.* **38**, 1–9.

Harvey J. W., Simpson C. F. & Gaskin J. (1978) Cyclic thrombocytopenia induced by a Rickettsia-like agent in dogs. *J. Infect. Dis.* **137**, 182–8.

Hjerpe C. A. & Knight H. D. (1972) Polyarthritis and synovitis associated with mycoplasma bovomastitides in feedlot cattle. *J. Am. Vet. Med. Assoc.* **60**, 1414.

Hooks J. J., Hooks B. D. & Levinson A. I. (1982) Interferons and immune reactivity. *J. Am. Vet. Med. Assoc.* **181**, 1111–14.

Hurvitz A. I. & Feldman E. (1975) A disease in dogs resembling human pemphigus vulgaris: case reports. *J. Am. Vet. Med. Assoc.* **166**, 585.

Hwang V. F., Hamilton H. E. & Sheets R. F. (1969) Vinblastine-induced thrombocytosis. *Lancet* **ii**, 1075–6.

Jackson C. W. & Edwards C. C. (1977) Evidence that stimulation of megakaryocytopoiesis by low dose vincristine results from an effect on platelets. *Br. J. Haematol.* **36**, 97–105.

Jain N. C. & Switzer J. W. (1981) Autoimmune thrombocytopenia in dogs and cats. *Vet. Clinics North. Am. (Small Anim. Pract.)* **2**, 421–34.

Joshi B. C. & Jain N. C. (1976) Detection of antiplatelet antibody in serum and on megakaryocytes of dogs with autoimmune thrombocytopenia. *Am. J. Vet. Res.* **37**, 681–5.

Karpatkin S. & Siskind G. W. (1969) *In vitro* detection of platelet antibody in patients with idiopathic thrombocytopenic purpura and systemic lupus erythematosus. *Blood* **33**, 795.

Klener P., Donnes L., Hyncica V. *et al* (1974) Possible mechanism of vinblastine-induced thrombocytosis. *Scand. J. Haematol.* **12**, 179–84.

Koller L. D. (1982) Chemical-induced immunomodulation. *J. Am. Vet. Med. Assoc.* **181**, 1102–6.

Kristensen S., Flagstad A., Jansen S., Bendixen G., Manthorpe R., Oxholin P. & Wiik A. (1979) Absence of evidence suggesting that systemic lupus erythematosus is a zoonosis of dogs. *Vet. Rec.* **105**, 423.

Kunkle G., Goldschmidt M. H. & Halliwell R. E. W. (1978) Bullous pemphigoid in a dog: a case report with immunofluorescent findings. *J. Am. Anim. Hosp. Assoc.* **14**, 52.

Lennon V. A., Palmer A. C., Pflugfelder C. & Indrieri R. J. (1978) Myasthenia gravis in dogs: acetylcholine receptor deficiency with and without antireceptor autoantibodies. In *Genetic Control of Autoimmune Disease*, eds. N. R. Rose, P. E. Bigazzi & N. L. Warner. Elsevier, Amsterdam.

Lewis R. M., Henry W. B., Thornton G. W. *et al* (1963) A syndrome of autoimmune hemolytic anemia and thrombocytopenia in the dog. *J. Am. Vet. Med. Assoc.* **1**, 140.

LEWIS R. M., SCHWARTZ R. S. & HENRY W. B. (1965) Canine systemic lupus erythematosus. *Blood* **25**, 143.

LEWIS R. M. & SCHWARTZ R. S. (1971) Canine systemic lupus erythematosus. Genetic analysis of an established breeding colony. *J. Exp. Med.* **132**, 417.

LEWIS R. M., ANDRE-SCHWARTZ J., HARRIS G. S., HIRSCH M. S., BLACK R. H. & SCHWARTZ R. S. (1973) Canine systemic lupus erythematosus. Transmission of serologic abnormalities by cell-free filtrates. *J. Clin. Invest.* **52**, 1893.

LIU S., SUTER P. F., FISCHER C. A. & DORFMAN H. D. (1969) Rheumatoid arthritis in a dog. *J. Am. Vet. Med. Assoc.* **154**, 495–502.

MANNING T. O., SCOTT D. W., KRUTH S. A. *et al* (1980) Three cases of pemphigus foliaceous and observations on chrysotherapy. *J. Am. Anim. Hosp. Assoc.* **76**, 189–202.

MARMONT C., PESCHLE M. & SANGUINTI M. (1975) Pure red cell aplasia (PRCA): response of three patients to cyclophosphamide and/or antilymphocyte globulin (ALG) and demonstration of two types of serum IgG inhibitors to erythropoiesis. *Blood* **45**, 247–61.

MAWDESLEY-THOMAS L. E. (1969) Lymphocytic thyroiditis in the dog. *J. Small Anim. Pract.* **9**, 539.

MICHEL B., MILNER Y. & DAVID R. (1971) Preservation of tissue fixed immunoglobulin in skin biopsies of patients with lupus erythematosus and bullous diseases. Preliminary report. *J. Invest. Derm.* **59**, 449.

NEWTON C. C., LIPOWITZ A. J., HALLIWELL R. E. W. *et al* (1976) Rheumatoid arthritis in dogs. *J. Am. Vet. Med. Assoc.* **168**, 113–21.

NEWTON C. C., SCHUMACHER H. R. & HALLIWELL R. E. W. (1979) Gold salt therapy for rheumatoid arthritis in dogs. *J. Am. Vet. Med. Assoc.* **174**, 1308–9.

OLHAGER B. (1975) On the aetiopathogenesis of rheumatoid arthritis. *An. Clin. Res.* **7**, 119–28.

PEDERSEN N. C., POOL R. C., CASTLES J. J. *et al* (1976) Noninfectious canine arthritis: rheumatoid arthritis. *J. Am. Vet. Med. Assoc.* **169**, 295.

PEDERSEN N. C., WEISNER K., CASTLES J. J. *et al* (1976a) Non-infectious canine arthritis: the inflammatory, non-erosive arthritides. *J. Am. Vet. Med. Assoc.* **169**, 304.

PEDERSEN N. C., POOL R. R. & MORGAN J. P. (1983) Joint diseases of dogs and cats. In *Textbook of Veterinary Internal Medicine Diseases of the Dog and Cat*, ed. S. J. Ettinger, pp. 2187–235. W. B. Saunders, Philadelphia PA.

QUIMBY F. W., SCHWARTZ R. S., POSKITT T. *et al* (1979) A disorder of dogs resembling Sjögrens syndrome. *Clin. Immunol. Immunopathol.* **12**, 471–6.

ROPES M. W., BENNETT G. A., COBB S. *et al* (1958) Revision of diagnostic criteria for rheumatoid arthritis. *Bull. Rheum. Dis.* **9**, 175–6.

SCHALM O. W., JAIN N. C. & CARROLL E. J. (1975) *Veterinary Hematology*, 3rd edn., pp. 336–55. Lea and Febiger, Philadelphia.

SCHALM O. W. (1975) Autoimmune hemolytic anemia in the dog. *Canine Pract.* **2**, 37–45.

SCHULTZ K. T. & GOLDSCHMIDT M. H. (1980) Pemphigus vegetans in a dog: A case report. *J. Am. Anim. Hosp. Assoc.* **16**, 579–82.

SCHUMACHER H. R., NEWTON C. & HALLIWELL R. E. W. (1980) Synovial pathologic changes in spontaneous canine rheumatoid-like arthritis. *Arthritis Rheum.* **23**, 412–23.

SCHWARTZ R. W., QUIMBY F. & ANDRE-SCHWARTZ J. (1978) Canine systemic lupus erythematosus: Phenotypic expression of autoimmunity in a closed colony. In: *Genetic Con-*

SCHWARTZ R. W., QUIMBY F. & ANDRE-SCHWARTZ J. (1978) Canine systemic lupus erythematosus: Phenotypic expression of autoimmunity in a closed colony. In: *Genetic Control of Autoimmune Disease*. Eds. N. R. Rose *et al*, p. 287. Elsevier North Holland, Amsterdam.

SCOTT D. W. (1977) Pemphigus vegetans in a dog. *Cornell Vet.* **67**, 431–6.

SCOTT D. W., MILLER W. H. LEWIS R. M. *et al* (1980) Pemphigus erythematosus in the dog and cat. *J. Am. Anim. Hosp. Assoc.* **16**, 815–23.

SCOTT D. W., WALTON D. K., MANING T. O., SMITH C. A. & LEWIS R. M. (1983) Canine lupus erythematosus. I. Systemic lupus erythematosus. *J. Am. Anim. Hosp. Assoc.* **19**, 461–79.

SHEBANI O. I. (1982) Autoimmune thrombocytopenia in the dog: interaction of heterologous and isologous platelet antibody with canine platelets. *Dissertation Abstracts International* **42**, 3202–B.

SHULMAN N. R., MARDER V. J. & WEINRACK R. S. (1965) Similarities between known antiplatelet antibodies and the factors responsible for thrombocytopenia in idiopathic purpura: Physiologic, serologic, and isotopic studies. *Ann. N.Y. Acad. Sci.* **124**, 499–542.

SLAPPENDEL R. J. (1979) The diagnostic significance of the direct antiglobulin test (DAT) in anemic dogs. *Vet. Immunol Immunopathol.* **1**, 49–52.

STANNARD A. A., GRIBBLE D. H. & BAKER B. B. (1975) A mucocutaneous disease in the dog resembling pemphigus vulgaris in man. *J. Am. Vet. Med. Assoc.* **166**, 575.

STOCKHAM S. L., FORD R. B. & WEISS D. J. (1980) Canine autoimmune hemolytic disease with a delayed erythroid regeneration. *J. Am. Anim. Hosp. Assoc.* **16**, 927–31.

SWITZER J. W. & JAIN N. C. (1981) Autoimmune hemolytic anemia in dogs and cats. *Vet. Clinics North Am.* (*Small Anim. Pract.*) **11**, 405–20.

WAALER E. (1940) On the occurrence of a factor in human serum activating the specific agglutination of sheep blood corpuscles. *Acta. Pathol Microbiol. Scand.* **17**, 172.

WAGER O. (1975) Immunological diagnosis of rheumatoid arthritis and systemic lupus erythematosus. *Ann. Clin. Res.* **7**, 168–82.

WERNER L. L. (1980) Coombs' positive anemias in the dog and cat. *The Compend. Cont. Ed. Pract. Vet.* **2**, 96–101.

WERNER L. L., BROWN K. A. & HALLIWELL R. E. W. (1983) Diagnosis of autoimmune skin diseases in the dog: Correlations of immunologic, histopathologic and clinical findings. *Vet. Immunol. and Immunopathol.* (In press.)

WERNER L. L., HALLIWELL R. E. W., JACKSON R. F. & NEEDHAM T. (1983) The incidence of positive Coombs' antiglobulin reactions in heartworm infected and non-infected dogs. Proceedings of the 1983 Heartworm Society Symposium, Orlando, Fl. Feb. 11–13. (In press.)

WILKINS R. J., HURVITZ A. J. & DODDS-LAFFIN W. J. (1973) Immunologically mediated thrombocytopenia in the dog. *J. Am. Vet. Med. Assoc.* **163**, 277.

WILKINS R. J. & DODDS W. J. (1974) Idiopathic (immunologic) thrombocytopenia purpura. In *Current Vet. Therapy V*. Ed. R. W. Kirk, pp. 365–7. W. B. Saunders, Philadelphia.

WINTROBE M. W., LEE G. R., BOGGS D. R. *et al* (1974) *Clinical hematology*, 7th edn. Lea and Febiger, Philadelphia.

YEARY R. A. & BRANT R. J. (1975) Aspirin dosages for the dog. *J. Am. Vet. Med. Assoc.* **167**, 63–4.

11
Clinical Haematology

D. J. MEYER AND J. W. HARVEY

The haemogram is a routine adjunct to the clinical evaluation of the dog. Interpretation of the blood picture requires an understanding of the production, kinetics and functions of the various cell types. The haematological information gained can be used to confirm a diagnosis or, more commonly, direct further investigation.

Disorders involving the erythrocyte and leucocyte cell types are classified and discussed. Platelet disorders and coagulation factor deficiencies which result in bleeding disorders are also covered.

The discussions are intended to maximise the information gained from the haemogram and further develop the differential diagnosis of haematological disorders. The reader is referred to the reading list for more detailed references.

PRODUCTION AND FUNCTIONS OF BLOOD CELLS

The bone marrow is the site of production of all blood cell types, although lymphocytes are also produced in peripheral lymphoid organs. Continued production of blood cells is dependent on the presence of haematopoietic stem cells that are capable of self-replication as well as differentiation. The most primitive stem cell type has the capacity to form all blood cell types (Fig. 11.1). There is good evidence for the existence of one stem cell with the potential to form lymphocytes and another with the capacity to form the other blood cell lines. Committed or unipotential stem cells also exist with the ability to form only one cell line (Fig. 11.1). Little is known about factors regulating stem cells.

Erythropoietin, granulopoietin(s) and thrombopoietin(s) are specific inducers of terminal maturation for erythrocytic, granulocytic and megakaryocytic cell lines. In disease states such as anaemia, thrombocytopenia and inflammation, the marrow is selectively stimulated to increase the production of the blood cell type(s) needed to alleviate the condition. The adequacy of the response can determine whether a dog lives or dies.

Erythrocytes

Over a period of approximately 4 days, nucleated erythroid precursors in the bone marrow progress through a series of divisions and maturation processes which result in the production of approximately 16 anucleated immature erythrocytes (reticulocytes) from each initial rubriblast. Reticulocytes normally remain in the marrow for one or two days before release into the blood. Final maturation (approximately one day) occurs in the blood and spleen. Maturation events occurring during the reticulocyte stage include the completion of haemoglobin synthesis, loss of ribosomes and mitochondria and development of the biconcave shape typical of mature erythrocytes.

Tissue hypoxia is the fundamental stimulus for erythropoiesis, which is mediated by the hormone erythropoietin. Erythropoietin is formed from the interaction of proteins produced in the kidney and liver. Erythropoietin stimulation increases erythrocyte production by increasing the number of cells entering the erythroid maturation series and shortening the time needed for production and release of reticulocytes from the marrow. Other hormones, including androgens, growth hormone, thyroid hormones and corticosteroids, appear to potentiate the effects of erythropoietin, although they have no intrinsic activity.

Canine erythrocytes normally have a life span in the circulation of approximately 110–120 days. They function in the transport of oxygen and carbon dioxide and in the buffering of hydrogen ions. Aged or damaged erythrocytes are removed primarily by macrophages in the spleen, liver and bone marrow.

Granulocytes and monocytes

There appears to be a separate stem cell compartment capable of giving rise to both granulocytes and mono-

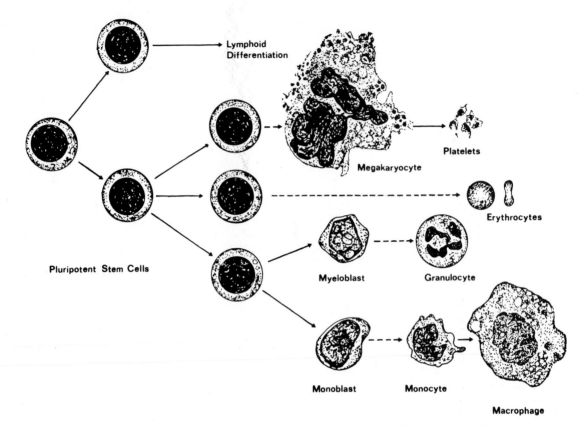

Fig. 11.1 Schema of blood cell production from pluripotential and committed stem cells (from Harvey J. W. (1981) *Vet.* *Clin. North Am.* **11,** 349–81, reprinted with permission).

cytes (Fig. 11.1). Factors which induce production of granulocytes and monocytes have been called colony-stimulating factors or colony-stimulating activities. These substances are needed for both the proliferation and maturation of cells committed to the granulocyte and monocyte cell lines. Thus far, monocytes, macrophages, activated lymphocytes, and endothelial cells have been shown to produce or release these factors. Depending on the types of mediators released, the production of one or more of the granulocyte types and/or monocytes will be increased in response to foreign substances (e.g. bacteria and allergens).

Bone marrow granulocytic cells are produced from myeloblasts. Maturation results in clumping of the nuclear chromatin and indentation of the nucleus (metamyelocyte); at this stage the cells are no longer capable of division. Further nuclear maturation progresses through the band-shape to form the mature segmented nucleus. The development time from myeloblast to mature granulocyte is approximately 5 days. Mature granulocytes may remain in the marrow for

an additional day or two under normal conditions, but can be released immediately upon demand.

Granulocytes circulate in the blood (half-life of about 6 hours) before entering the tissues. The total blood neutrophil pool includes the circulating and the marginating neutrophil pools. Approximately one-half of the neutrophils in the blood vasculature system are adherent to the vascular endothelium (marginating neutrophil pool), while, in normal dogs at any given time the other half is in circulation (circulating neutrophil pool). The absolute number of neutrophils measured when blood samples are taken can be altered dramatically by shifts to or from the marginating pool.

The primary function of neutrophils is the phagocytosis and destruction of microbes, especially bacteria. For optimal phagocytosis, microbial agents must first be coated with antibodies and complement. Substances released from bacteria and inflamed tissue, antigen–antibody complexes, and certain components of complement can stimulate neutrophil migration.

Once the organism is engulfed, it is destroyed by an oxidative metabolic pathway and non-specific enzymes from the cytoplasmic granules. This mechanism is protectively useful; however, the pathological release of the powerful cytoplasmic enzymes may cause unwanted tissue damage.

The function of eosinophils is not well understood. Eosinophils are attracted to sites of mast cell degranulation and appear to neutralise substances released during immediate-type hypersensitivity reactions. Eosinophils also appear to participate in the destruction of parasites which migrate through the tissues.

Basophils are rich in histamine and heparin. Their physiological function is unknown.

Monocytes are produced rapidly in the marrow, undergo limited maturation and are released into the blood within a day or so. Monocytes spend a number of hours in the blood, then enter the tissues and mature into macrophages (e.g. pulmonary macrophages and Kupffer cells).

Macrophages are phagocytes that are particularly important in the protection against viruses, fungal infections and certain facultative intracellular bacteria such as mycobacteria. Besides their protective phagocytic functions, macrophages phagocytise aged cells, devitalised tissues and endotoxins, process antigens for interaction with lymphocytes, store iron and synthesise a number of substances (e.g. colony-stimulating activity and certain complement components).

Lymphocytes

Lymphocytes are broadly classified as being involved either in antibody production (B-lymphocytes) or cell-mediated immunity (T-lymphocytes). The bone marrow contains stem cells which give rise to uncommitted lymphocytes. The adult mammalian bone marrow appears to further orient some of the lymphocytes into the B-cells. Following antigen stimulation in lymphoid organs, B-lymphocytes differentiate into plasma cells with the capacity to produce large amounts of antibody.

The thymus produces substances which direct the T-lymphocyte commitment on the lymphocyte stem cells from the marrow. Various populations of T-lymphocytes with diverse, complex functions exist within the body. In addition to being cytotoxic for certain parasites, virus-infected cells and neoplastic cells, populations of T-lymphocytes regulate B-lymphocyte function, and are involved in granulocyte and monocyte production. A substantial portion of blood lymphocytes are long-lived recirculating T- and B-memory cells.

Platelets

Platelets are produced from the cytoplasm of megakaryocytes in the bone marrow. Megakaryocyte maturation and platelet production requires 3–5 days and involves nuclear duplication without cell division. It is estimated that several thousand platelets are produced from the cytoplasmic fragmentation of each megakaryocyte. Platelet production is controlled by the number or the mass of platelets in the circulation. Increased platelet production occurs in response to thrombocytopenia, as the result of both increased size and numbers of megakaryocytes.

Circulating platelets normally survive for 10–12 days and are an integral part of haemostasis. Platelet function involves the formation of a platelet plug at the site of vessel damage and providing platelet factor 3, a membrane-bound phospholipid which accelerates blood coagulation.

HAEMATOLOGICAL METHODS

Equipment

The minimum equipment required for haematological measurements include a high-quality microscope with flat-field objectives, a microhaematocrit centrifuge with a reader, a refractometer with a direct reading scale for the plasma protein concentration, and a method for counting leucocytes. A variety of electronic cell counters are available in price ranges the private practitioner can afford. Leucocytes and platelets can be counted manually using a commercial reservoir (Unopettes) and a haemocytometer chamber; however, erythrocyte counts should be done with an electronic cell counter. The haemoglobin concentration can be accurately determined with a spectrophotometer using the cyanmethaemoglobin method.

Blood sample collection and handling

Blood should be collected from animals fasted overnight to avoid postprandial lipaemia. *In vitro* haemolysis often occurs in lipaemic samples and lipaemia produces artifactually high plasma protein and haemoglobin values.

Blood films should be quickly prepared to avoid changes in cell morphology caused by the anticoagulant. The collection of blood samples directly into 2 ml vacuum tubes using vacuum tube holders circumvents two common problems. First, platelets easily aggregate *in vitro*. These platelet aggregates may be left behind in a syringe, resulting in an artifactually low platelet count. Second, the chance of submitting a clotted blood sample to the laboratory is minimised.

Platelet counts and reticulocyte counts should be done as soon as possible after sample collection. Time is not as critical for leucocyte and erythrocyte counts, the PCV or the plasma protein determinations. These measurements can be delayed a couple of hours until there are other samples.

Blood samples for most coagulation tests are collected with citrate as the anticoagulant. Samples should be kept cool and the coagulation tests should be done as quickly as possible after the sample is collected. It is essential that (a) the correct ratio of blood to citrate is used, and (b) blood from a normal dog is collected at the same time and in the same manner for use as a control. Special tubes are required for the activated clotting time (ACT) (Vacutainer) and fibrin degradation products tests.

Microhaematocrit tube interpretation

The centrifuged microhaematocrit provides the packed cell volume (PCV), the easiest, most reproducible indicator of red cell mass. There is additional information provided by the microhaematocrit tube. The height of the buffy coat roughly correlates with the total leucocyte count. A severe leucopenia or marked leucocytosis may be suspected from its appearance. The buffy coat may appear reddish due to the presence of a marked reticulocytosis which occurs secondary to a regenerative anaemia.

The plasma in the microhaematocrit tube is normally clear and colourless. Hyperlipaemia is indicated if the plasma appears white and cloudy. A layer of lipid may also be seen at the top of the plasma column. The presence of lipaemia is frequently the result of a recent meal (postprandial lipaemia). Idiopathic or primary hyperlipaemia is uncommon but has been described in the Miniature Schnauzer. Secondary hyperlipaemia can be associated with hypothyroidism, diabetes mellitus, acute pancreatitis and hyperadrenocorticism.

An increase in the plasma bilirubin concentration imparts a yellow colour to the plasma. A yellow plasma with a normal PCV suggests liver disease. Hyperbilirubinaemia associated with a marked decrease in the PCV suggests an increased destruction of erythrocytes.

The presence of haemoglobin is indicated if the plasma appears red in colour. The haemoglobinaemia can result from the lysis of erythrocytes during the collection of the blood sample or from a true intravascular haemolytic disease. The presence of haemoglobinuria supports intravascular haemolysis.

After the PCV is measured and the appearance of the plasma and buffy coat are noted, the microhaematocrit capillary tube is broken just above the buffy coat and the plasma is placed in a refractometer for plasma protein determination. Plasma protein values are low in the newborn (approximately 4.5–5.5 g/dl) and increase to the adult range by 3–4 months of age. The presence of lipaemia or haemolysis will result in a falsely increased plasma protein concentration.

Normal haematological values for adult dogs are given in Table 11.1. The PCV in puppies is in the adult

Table 11.1 Mean and ranges of normal haematological findings in adult dogs*.

Parameter	Units	Mean	Range
Haemoglobin	g/dl	15	12–18
Erythrocytes	$\times 10^{12}$/litre	6.8	5.5–8.5
PCV	litre/litre	0.45	0.37–0.55
MCV	fl	70	60–77
MCHC	g/dl	34	32–37
MCH	pg	22.8	19.5–24.5
Total leucocytes	$\times 10^9$/litre	11.5	6.0–17.0
Band cells	$\times 10^9$/litre	0.07	0–0.3
Neutrophils	$\times 10^9$/litre	7.0	3.0–11.5
Lymphocytes	$\times 10^9$/litre	2.8	1.0–4.8
Monocytes	$\times 10^9$/litre	0.7	0.1–1.3
Eosinophils	$\times 10^9$/litre	0.5	0.1–0.8
Basophils	$\times 10^9$/litre	rare	
Platelets	$\times 10^9$/litre	400	200–600
Plasma proteins	g/dl	7.0	6.0–8.0
Serum iron	μg/dl	149	84–233
TIBC	μg/dl	391	284–572

* Derived, with slight modification, from Schalm *et al* (1975) and from Harvey *et al* (1982). PCV, packed cell volume; MCV, mean cell volume; MCHC, mean cell haemoglobin concentration; MCH, mean cell haemoglobin; TIBC, total iron-binding capacity in serum.

range at birth, but decreases (PCV of 25–35%) by 3–4 weeks of age. There is a gradual increase to the adult range by the time sexual maturity is reached.

The capacity of the dog spleen to expand and contract can result in substantial changes in the PCV. Excitement or exercise immediately before sampling can increase the PCV by 20% or more. Conversely, sedation or anaesthesia (especially with barbiturates) can cause splenic enlargement and the PCV may drop below the normal range. Packed cell volumes are occasionally measured above 55% in individuals from certain breeds of dogs (i.e. Poodle, German Shepherd, Boxer, Beagle, Dachshund and Chihuahua). These values are believed to result from splenic contraction in animals with a high normal erythrocyte mass. The normal range for the PCV in Greyhounds (49–65%) is higher than that of other breeds.

Maximum information can be gained by interpretation of the PCV and plasma protein concentrations simultaneously. Various combinations of low, normal or high PCV values may occur with low, normal or high plasma protein concentrations. The various combinations and examples of how they can be interpreted are given in Table 11.2

Table 11.2 Concomitant interpretation of packed cell volume (PCV) and plasma protein (PP) concentration.

Normal PCV with:
  (a) Low PP—gastrointestinal protein loss, proteinuria, severe liver disease
  (b) Normal PP—normal
  (c) High PP—dehydration-masked anaemia, increased globulin synthesis

High PCV with:
  (a) Low PP—protein loss with splenic contraction
  (b) Normal PP—splenic contraction, primary or secondary erythrocytosis, dehydration-masked hypoproteinaemia
  (c) High PP—dehydration

Low PCV with:
  (a) Low PP—substantial ongoing or recent blood loss, overhydration
  (b) Normal PP—increased RBC destruction, decreased RBC production, chronic blood loss
  (c) High PP—anaemia of chronic disease, lymphoproliferative diseases

---

Blood cell counting, haemoglobin determinations and erythrocyte indices

Of the three indicators of erythrocyte mass (PCV, haemoglobin concentration and erythrocyte count), the PCV is the most practical test. Consequently, it is probably not worth the effort to do automated erythrocyte counts or measure haemoglobin concentrations unless erythrocyte indices are calculated and used to classify anaemias. In addition, electronic cell counting systems adjusted to count human erythrocytes may not be satisfactory for counting and sizing dog erythrocytes, owing to the smaller size of canine erythrocytes. This is particularly true for dogs with microcytic erythrocytes. It is important, therefore, that cell counters be adjusted to optimally count canine erythrocytes.

Erythrocyte indices

Erythrocyte indices (Table 11.1) are commonly provided by commercial veterinary laboratories. The most useful of the indices is the mean cell volume (MCV). The MCV can be determined electronically by cell counters or can be calculated by dividing the PCV by the total erythrocyte count and multiplying by ten. A low MCV indicates the presence of small erythrocytes. Microcytic erythrocytes can occur in normal Japanese Akita dogs and in dogs with chronic iron deficiency anaemia or portosystemic vascular anomalies. Macrocytic erythrocytes (MCV > 77 fl) are most frequently associated with regenerative anaemias and represent the immature erythrocytes (reticulocytes). Macrocytic erythrocytes also occur in Alaskan Malamutes with hereditary stomatocytosis, dogs receiving long-term treatment with diphenylhydantoin which is a folate antagonist, and in some normal Toy and Miniature Poodles.

The mean cell haemoglobin concentration (MCHC), calculated by dividing the blood haemoglobin concentration by the PCV and multiplying by 100, can provide useful information. Low MCHC values (< 32%) can occur in association with macrocytosis in regenerative anaemias with markedly increased reticulocyte counts. A low MCHC is frequently associated with the microcytosis in chronic iron deficiency anaemia. High MCHC values (> 37%) are always artifactual in that the haemoglobin concentration within erythrocytes cannot actually increase. Increased values are recorded when free haemoglobin is present in the plasma as a result of intravascular haemolysis or poor sample collection. Increased values can be obtained in association with marked hyperlipidaemia or the presence of Heinz bodies within erythrocytes. Haemolysates prepared for haemoglobin determination in these conditions can be sufficiently turbid to inhibit light transmission in the spectrophotometer, thereby giving an erroneously high haemoglobin value.

The mean cell haemoglobin (MCH) is frequently recorded on haematology forms but provides little information in the dog.

Examination of stained blood films

Blood films are generally examined following methanol fixation and staining with Romanowsky-type stains such as Giemsa, Wright or Leishman. These stains allow for examination of erythrocyte and leucocyte morphology. A second stain is needed to stain for Heinz bodies and reticulocytes. The recommended stain consists of 0.5% new methylene blue in 0.85% NaCl, to which 1 ml of full-strength formaldehyde has been added per 100 ml. Dry, unfixed blood films are stained by placing a drop of stain between a coverslip and glass slide. Platelets are accentuated by this stain, making it very useful in estimating the adequacy of platelets (Plate 11.1a). Although this stain is not optimal for differential leucocyte counts, the number and type of leucocytes present can be appreciated.

Blood films should first be scanned using a low power objective to get an overall impression of cellularity, to examine for the presence of platelet aggregates, and to look for microfilaria and abnormal cells. After finding a uniform, well-stained area, the blood film is examined using high power objectives.

Platelets

The presence and adequacy of platelets, including clumping, should be evaluated first. Canine platelets are quite uniform in size. Large platelets are generally indicative of young platelets and increased numbers suggest increased platelet production. Megaplatelets and hypogranular platelets may also be seen in myeloproliferative disorders.

Erythrocyte morphology

The biconcave shape of normal canine erythrocytes results in the appearance of prominent central pallor on stained-blood films. In contrast to horses and cats, rouleaux formation by erythrocytes is minimal in normal dogs, but becomes prominent in immune-mediated haemolytic disorders, inflammatory conditions and hyperglobulinaemia.

Reticulocytes are called polychromatophiles on routinely stained canine blood films (Plate 11.1b). The large, bluish-red erythrocyte comprises 1% or less of the red blood cells in normal dogs. Since there is a direct correlation between the degree of polychromasia and reticulocytosis in the dog, the magnitude of the polychromasia provides useful information in the differential diagnosis of anaemia.

Small numbers of nucleated erythrocytes are often seen on the blood film in association with regenerative anaemias; however their presence is a less useful indicator of a regenerative response than the degree of reticulocytosis. Nucleated erythrocytes are occasionally seen in lead poisoning in which there is minimal or no anaemia, in conditions where bone marrow is damaged (such as endotoxic shock), and in myeloproliferative disease in which there is minimal reticulocy-

tosis. Low numbers are seen for unexplained reasons in some dogs with liver disease, haemangiosarcomas and in some normal Miniature Schnauzers.

Anisocytosis is the term used to describe variation in erythrocyte size on stained blood films. The most common cause of increased anisocytosis is the presence of large immature cells in regenerative anaemias (Plate 11.1b). Moderate anisocytosis may also be present in iron deficient or folate deficient conditions and in myeloproliferative disease.

Poikilocytosis is a term used to describe the presence of abnormally-shaped erythrocytes. More specific terminology is frequently used for certain abnormal shapes. Crenation is used to describe the presence of erythrocyte with regularly shaped and spaced membrane projections. Crenation is usually an artifact which results from excess EDTA or improper smear preparation, and may also be seen in uraemia, immediately after transfusion of stored blood or in pyruvate kinase deficiency. Cells with irregularly spaced projections of varying shapes and lengths are called acanthocytes or spur cells (Plate 11.1c). They are seen most consistently in dogs with haemangiosarcoma.

Spherical erythrocytes (spherocytes) result from erythrocyte swelling and/or loss of cell surface. Spherocytes occur most frequently in association with immune-mediated haemolytic anaemia in the dog (Plate 11.1b).

Shizocytes are fragmented erythrocytes which can be seen in dogs with microangiopathic haemolytic anaemia associated with disseminated intravascular coagulation (Fig. 11.2). Leptocytes are thin, flat

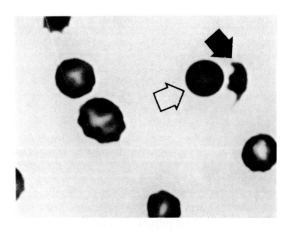

Fig. 11.2 A shizocyte (closed arrow) and spherocyte (open arrow) in blood from a dog with disseminated intravascular coagulation, Wright-Geimsa stain, × 1500 (from Harvey J. W. (1980) *J. Am. Vet. Med. Assoc.* **176**, 970–4, reprinted with permission).

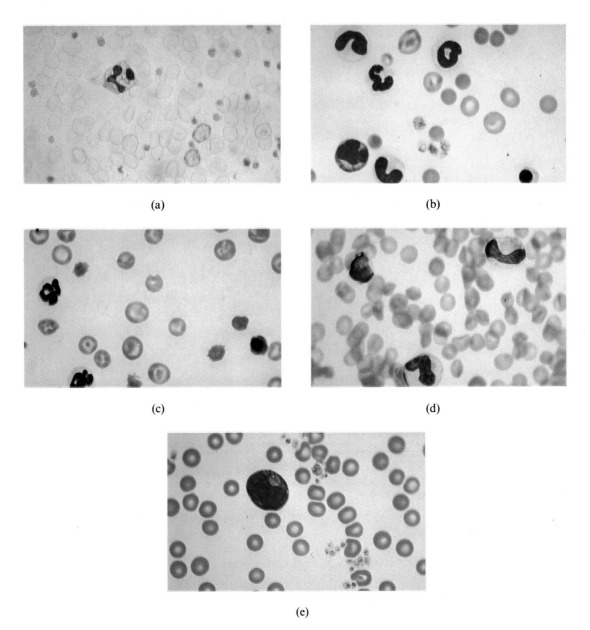

(a)

(b)

(c)

(d)

(e)

Plate 11.1 (a) Numerous blue staining platelets, two reticulocytes and an eosinophil in a new methylene blue-stained wet preparation. Eosinophilic granules and erythrocytes are unstained.
(b) Small spherocytes, large polychromatophilic erythrocytes and a nucleated erythrocyte in blood from a dog with autoimmune haemolytic anaemia. A mature neutrophil, three band neutrophils and a monocyte are also present. Wright–Giemsa stain.

(c) Three acanthocytes, several large polychromatophilic erythrocytes and a nucleated erythrocyte in blood from a dog with haemangiosarcoma. Two neutrophils and an erythrocyte containing a Howell–Jolly body are also present. Wright–Giemsa stain.
(d) Two-band neutrophils with toxic cytoplasm and a lymphocyte in blood from a dog with a bacterial abscess. Wright–Giemsa stain.
(e) Atypical lymphocyte in blood from a dog with parvovirus infection. Wright–Giemsa stain.

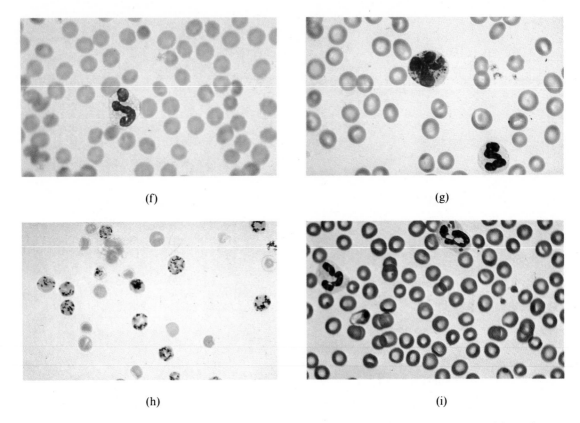

(f)   (g)

(h)   (i)

(f) Eosinophil in blood from a Greyhound dog. Wright–Giemsa stain.
(g) Canine basophil and neutrophil. Wright–Giemsa stain.

(h) Reticulocytes in blood from a dog with autoimmune haemolytic anaemia. Reticulocyte stain.
(i) Red-staining distemper inclusions in two erythrocytes and a neutrophil. Diff–Quick stain.

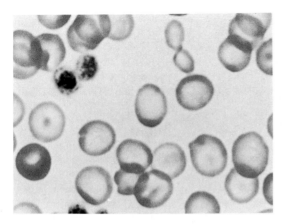

Fig. 11.3 Hypochromic leptocytes in blood from a dog with chronic iron deficiency anaemia. Wright–Geimsa stain, × 1500.

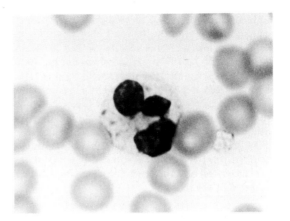

Fig. 11.4 Neutrophil with toxic cytoplasm containing several Döhle bodies, Wright–Geimsa stain, × 1500.

hypochromatic erythrocytes most commonly associated with iron deficiency (Fig. 11.3).

Leucocyte morphology

Canine neutrophils are easily recognised by the segmentation of their nucleus and the colourless to pale-pink staining of their cytoplasm and granules. Low numbers of neutrophils without nuclear segmentation (bands) occur in normal dogs. Increased numbers of bands are referred to as a left shift (Plate 11.1b). In some disorders, especially septicaemia and endotoxaemia, toxic changes are observed in the cytoplasm of neutrophils and neutrophilic precursors. Manifestations of toxicity include diffuse basophilia, foamy vacuolation of the cytoplasm (Plate 11.1d), and prominent Döhle bodies (Fig. 11.4). Occasionally neutrophils are observed with increased numbers of nuclear lobes (four or more). These hypersegmented neutrophils occur during prolonged stress, following glucocorticoid therapy, in hyperadrenocorticism or during late stages of chronic inflammatory disease.

Lymphocytes generally have round nuclei with scant blue cytoplasm, although medium-sized lymphocytes may have more abundant cytoplasm and be confused with monocytes. Atypical lymphocytes (transformed lymphocytes, reactive lymphocytes, immunocytes) may be observed in association with infections or autoimmune diseases where antigenic stimulation is occurring. These cells have intense cytoplasmic basophilia and occasionally a pale Golgi zone. The nucleus may be round, but is frequently pleomorphic (Plate 11.1e).

Monocytes are generally larger than other leucocyte types. The cytoplasm of monocytes is basophilic, abundant and often contains vacuoles. Fine dust-like reddish azurophilic granules may be observed in the cytoplasm. The nucleus can be almost any shape, but is not as segmented and has less nuclear condensation than neutrophils (Plate 11.1b).

Eosinophils are easily identified in most dog breeds due to their segmented nuclei and variably-sized red-to-orange granules. Eosinophils in Greyhounds are less easily recognised because the granules stain poorly, giving them the appearance of vacuolated neutrophils (Plate 11.1f).

Basophils in dogs contain sparse numbers of purple granules within a light-blue cytoplasm (Plate 11.1g). Basophils may degranulate and give the cytoplasm a purplish colour.

Differential leucocyte counts

A differential leucocyte count is performed by identifying 200 consecutive leucocytes. The percentage of each type is multiplied by the total leucocyte count to get the absolute number per microlitre of blood. The absolute number of each leucocyte type is important when evaluating the leucogram. Relative values (percentages) can be misleading if the total leucocyte count is abnormal. Let us consider two dogs, one with 7% lymphocytes and a total leucocyte count of 40×10^9/litre, and the other with 70% lymphocytes and a total leucocyte count of 4×10^9/litre. The first case would be said to have a 'relative' lymphopenia and the second case would be said to have a relative lymphocytosis.

Both cases, in fact, have the same normal absolute lymphocyte count (2.8×10^9/litre). Greyhounds normally have lower total leucocyte ($4-11 \times 10^9$/litre), neutrophil ($2-7 \times 10^9$/litre) and lymphocyte ($0.8-3.5 \times 10^9$/litre) counts than other species (Table 11.1).

If nucleated red blood cells (nRBC) are noted on the peripheral blood film, the total leucocyte count will need to be corrected downward, since they are included in the total leucocyte count. The number of nRBC seen during the differential leucocyte count are recorded per 100 leucocytes counted (e.g. 20 nRBC/ 100 leucocytes) and the total leucocyte count is then corrected by the formula:

Corrected total leucocyte count =
$$\frac{100 \times \text{uncorrected leucocyte count}}{100 + \text{nRBC}}$$

where nRBC is the number detected per 100 leucocytes. The corrected total leucocyte count is used to determine the absolute leucocyte number for each type.

Reticulocyte counts

Reticulocyte numbers may be estimated using Schalm's new methylene blue-stained wet preparations (Plate 11.1a), but generally reticulocyte counts are made on films prepared after blood and one of several vital stains are incubated together. One satisfactory technique involves the incubation of equal parts of blood and stain (0.5 g new methylene blue and 1.6 g potassium oxalate in 100 ml distilled water) together for 15 minutes at room temperature. This procedure causes ribosomes to aggregate together for visualisation (Plate 11.1h). The percentage of cells containing blue staining material is determined after examining 500 cells.

Serum iron determinations

Iron is very efficiently conserved and recycled in the dog. Iron is carried from its site of absorption in the small intestine and from storage sites in the body to the developing erythroid cells by a transport protein called transferrin. Serum iron is measured by direct means, while transferrin is usually measured indirectly as the total iron-binding capacity (TIBC) in serum (Table 11.1). In dogs, transferrin iron-binding sites are 25 to 50% saturated with iron.

Serum iron studies are useful at times in the differential diagnosis of anaemia. Substantial decreases in serum iron concentrations, but normal TIBC, have been reported in iron deficiency in dogs. Serum iron values may be low-normal to moderately decreased in the anaemia of inflammatory disease, but the TIBC is generally also decreased. High serum iron values are generally measured in haemolytic anaemia.

INFECTIVE AGENTS AND INCLUSIONS OF BLOOD CELLS

Howell–Jolly bodies

Howell-Jolly bodies are small spherical blue-staining inclusions of erythrocytes (Fig. 11.5). These DNA-containing nuclear remnants are visible with all routine blood stains. Increased numbers occur in dogs with regenerative anaemias, splenectomised dogs, dogs given glucocorticoids and in Poodles with macrocytic erythrocytes.

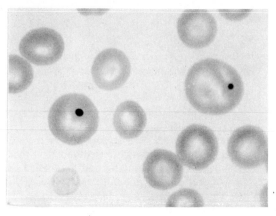

Fig. 11.5 Two large erythrocytes, each containing a Howell–Jolly body. Wright–Geimsa stain, × 1500.

Heinz bodies

Heinz bodies, which consist of denatured haemoglobin, are usually spherical, vary in size, and occur within erythrocytes. They do not stain with routine Romanowsky-type blood stains, but may be recognised at times as light staining areas within, or nipple-like projections from erythrocytes. They are easily visualised as blue-staining inclusions after staining with new methylene blue (Fig. 11.6) or the reticulocyte stains. Low numbers of Heinz bodies may be seen in splenectomised dogs, but their occurrence in intact dogs indicates a prior exposure to oxidants.

Basophilic stippling

Basophilic stippling is seen on Romanowsky-stained blood films as multiple, small, dark-blue to black in-

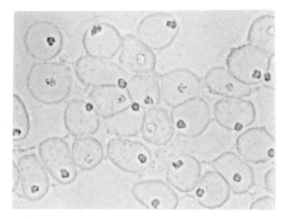

Fig. 11.6 Erythrocyte 'ghosts' each containing a Heinz body. New methylene blue wet preparation × 1500.

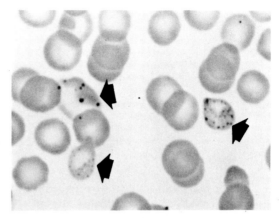

Fig. 11.7 Basophilic stippling in erythrocytes (arrows) in blood from a dog with lead poisoning. Wright–Geimsa stain, × 1500.

clusions in normochromic erythrocytes (Fig. 11.7). It represents the aggregation of reticulocyte ribosomes. Basophilic stippling is classically observed in lead poisoning. Blood films made without an anticoagulant and stained without prior methanol fixation accentuate their presence. Blood smears should be quickly made from blood collected without an anticoagulant in suspected cases of lead toxicity. The amount of stippling is reduced proportionally to the concentration of, and the length of time of exposure to EDTA.

Siderotic inclusions

Blue-black aggregates of iron-containing granules (Pappenheimer bodies) can be seen in Romanowsky-stained blood films (Fig. 11.8). Siderotic inclusions can be differentiated from basophilic stippling by the Prussian blue stain for iron. The significance of siderotic inclusions has not been adequately studied in dogs.

Distemper inclusion bodies

Inclusions associated with canine distemper may be seen in both erythrocytes and leucocytes (Plate 11.1i). The aggregates of viral nucleocapsids vary in size and shape. Distemper inclusion bodies stain bluish-white, blue, or red depending on the staining techniques. A multi-purpose quick stain (Diff-Quick; Harleco, Gibbstown, New Jersey, USA) is available which gives consistently good results.

Döhle bodies

Döhle bodies are light-blue angular inclusions in the cytoplasm of neutrophils (see Fig. 11.4). They are considered to be a sign of defective cytoplasmic maturation and are most frequently observed in association with severe bacterial infections.

Infective agents

Three species of *Babesia* infect erythrocytes of dogs. *B. canis* (Fig. 11.9) and *B. vogeli* are large pyriform protozoa which often appear in pairs or multiples of two. *B. gibsoni* is a much smaller ring-shaped organism.

Haemobartonella canis is a small rickettsial epicel-

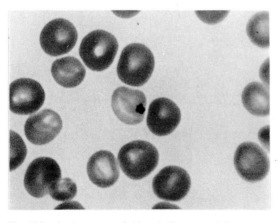

Fig. 11.8 An aggregate of siderotic (iron-containing) granules in a canine erythrocyte. Wright–Geimsa stain, × 1500.

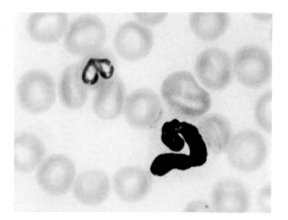

Fig. 11.9 Two *Babesia canis* organisms in an erythrocyte. Wright–Geimsa stain, × 1500 (from Harvey J. W. (1980) *J. Am. Vet. Med. Assoc.* **176**, 970–4, reprinted with permission).

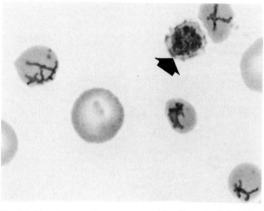

Fig. 11.10 Four erythrocytes parasitised by epicellular *Haemobartonella canis* organisms. A large platelet (arrow) is also present. Wright–Geimsa stain, × 1500.

lular parasite of erythrocytes. These blue-staining organisms may appear as small individual coccoids, rings or rods, but more commonly form chains of organisms extending across the erythrocyte surface (Fig. 11.10).

Ehrlichia canis organisms are blue-staining rickettsial organisms which occur in multiples within membrane-lined vacuoles (morulae) of mononuclear leucocytes (Fig. 11.11). They are often difficult to find in the blood of dogs with ehrlichiosis. A rickettsial organism has been recently discovered within dog platelets (Fig. 11.12). This new agent causes a cyclic thrombocytopenia and has been classified as *Ehrlichia platys*.

Lastly, one must be aware of the common pseudo-parasites such as stain precipitation and platelets which overlay erythrocytes; their appearance is similar to the less commonly encountered infective agents.

ANAEMIA

Anaemia is defined as the presence of an abnormally low erythrocyte count or haemoglobin concentration. Anaemia always occurs secondarily to another disorder. The clinical signs associated with anaemia are dependent on the degree of anaemia and the rapidity of its development. Pale mucous membranes, weak-

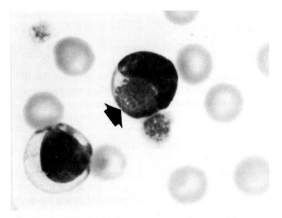

Fig. 11.11 A large *Ehrlichia canis* morula (arrow) is present in the cytoplasm of a mononuclear leucocyte from a blood buffy coat smear. Wright–Geimsa stain, × 1500.

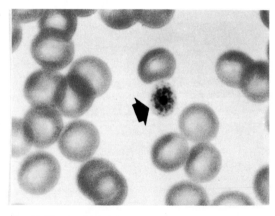

Fig. 11.12 An *Ehrlichia platys* morula in the cytoplasm of a large platelet (arrow). Wright–Geimsa stain, × 1500.

ness and an increase in the heart and the respiratory rates may be noted in anaemic dogs. Acute haemolytic episodes may cause fever, haemoglobinuria, and icterus; pale mucous membranes may not be initially noted due to the haemoglobinaemia caused by the haemolytic event.

Classification of anaemia

A classification of anaemia is helpful because it allows the laboratory findings to be used as a guide to the diagnosis of the underlying disorder. Anaemias can be classified according to erythrocyte morphology, bone marrow response and the pathophysiological mechanism responsible for the reduced erythrocyte number. Each classification has its advantages and disadvantages and often a combination is used to define the anaemia.

Regenerative and non-regenerative anaemia

Anaemia is first characterised by whether or not there is a bone marrow response. A regenerative response suggests blood loss or increased erythrocyte destruction. Two to three days are required for the increased erythroid activity in the bone marrow to be reflected in the blood. A non-regenerative blood picture suggests defective or reduced erythrocyte activity in the bone marrow (Table 11.3).

Table 11.3 Causes of reduced (hypoproliferative) or defective (hyperproliferative) erythrocyte production.

Reduced erythropoiesis	Defective erythropoiesis
Chronic renal insufficiency (Lack of functional erythropoietin)	Iron deficiency Lead toxicity
Endocrine Hypothyroidism Hypoadrenocorticism Hyperoestrogenism Sertoli cell tumour Exogenous administration	Folic acid deficiency Diphenylhydantoin
Chronic inflammation	
Infections Ehrlichiosis—chronic infection	
Haematopoietic neoplasia	

Blood loss

Acute blood loss will initially appear as a non-regenerative anaemia due to the time required for the increased erythroid production to be observed in the blood. However acute blood loss is usually associated with a readily identifiable site of haemorrhage while the site of chronic blood loss can be difficult to identify. Parasitism and gastrointestinal disorders, e.g. bleeding ulcers and neoplasms, are the more common causes of chronic blood loss.

The regenerative response in blood loss anaemia may be associated with a decreased plasma protein concentration. Following a single episode of blood loss, the haematocrit and plasma protein decrease together and return to normal within 1–2 weeks. The persistence of a regenerative response and a low plasma protein indicates continued blood loss. Ultimately chronic external blood loss results in the depletion of iron. After weeks to months of iron deficiency the regenerative response changes to a poorly regenerative blood picture. This transition occurs more rapidly in the young because of minimal iron stores. Thus a mild parasitic infection, e.g. fleas or hookworms, can readily cause an iron deficiency anaemia in the young dog.

Increased erythrocyte destruction

Increased erythrocyte destruction is a common cause of a regenerative anaemia in the adult dog. Erythrocyte destruction usually occurs by phagocytosis in the mononuclear phagocyte system (extravascular haemolysis). In some disorders, however, the erythrocyte destruction occurs primarily within the blood vascular system (intravascular haemolysis). Intravascular haemolysis characteristically has an acute onset resulting in haemoglobinaemia and haemoglobinuria. Disorders in which intravascular erythrocyte destruction may be prominent include some cases of autoimmune haemolytic anaemia, Heinz body anaemia, acute babesiosis, the venae cavae syndrome of dirofilariasis and disseminated intravascular coagulopathy.

Hyperbilirubinaemia will occur if the haemolytic episode is severe enough to overwhelm the liver's ability to remove the unconjugated bilirubin from the blood. The bilirubinuria associated with the haemolytic anaemia is due to an increase in the unbound bilirubin component in the plasma which subsequently appears in the urine.

The regenerative response to haemolytic anaemia is usually more intense than the response stimulated by blood loss, because the iron from the haemolysed erythrocytes is efficiently recycled for erythropoiesis. The increased bone marrow activity may cause an increased granulopoiesis. A regenerative left shift, similar to the one seen with an infectious disease, can develop. This response is most consistently seen in autoimmune haemolytic anaemia.

A regenerative response is indicated by a prominent

reticulocytosis (or polychromasia), increased aniso-cytosis, and the presence of a few nucleated red blood cells. Several factors should be kept in mind when assessing the magnitude of the regenerative response to anaemia. Reticulocytes or polychromatophilic cells are the primary indicators of a regenerative response. Several days are required for a regenerative response to be observed in the blood and the peak response occurs in about one week. The more severe the anaemia, the greater will be the regenerative response; a haemolytic anaemia usually results in a greater regenerative response than a blood loss anaemia of equal severity. Finally, the reticulocyte count should be corrected for the degree of anaemia by dividing the patient's PCV by 45 (normal canine PCV) and multiplying by the reticulocyte count. The corrected reticulocyte count helps to standardise the interpretation of the regenerative response.

Immune-mediated haemolytic anaemia
Immune-mediated haemolytic anaemia is common in the dog and may be primary, i.e. no identifiable aetiology, or may occur in association with diseases such as systemic lupus erythematosis; viral, rickettsial, protozoal, and bacterial infections; and neoplasia, especially lymphoproliferative disorders. The erythrocyte destruction is the result of antibodies directed against antigens associated with the erythrocyte membrane. These antibodies can function as haemolysins which result in intravascular haemolysis or cause agglutination and/or phagocytosis of the erythrocytes.

There are certain laboratory findings which support a diagnosis of immune-mediated erythrocyte destruction. Erythrocyte agglutination may be seen in a freshly drawn drop of EDTA-blood placed on a glass slide. The autoagglutination associated with immune-mediated anaemia may appear similar to rouleau formation. Rouleau formation, but not autoagglutination, is often dispersed by washing the erythrocytes in physiological saline or by diluting a drop of blood with a drop of saline on a glass slide. A Coombs' antiglobulin test is a more sophisticated procedure for the detection of antibodies on the erythrocyte membrane. A negative Coombs' test does not negate a clinical diagnosis of immune-mediated anaemia due to limitations of the test procedure. Specific testing for canine immunoglobulins at 4 and 37°C will indicate the presence of complement, IgG, or IgM. The reader is referred to Chapter 10 for more details.

Babesiosis
Babesiosis is an infectious cause of haemolytic anaemia (Fig. 11.9). The spectrum of the disease varies from a fulminant disorder with marked depression and clinicopathological findings consistent with disseminated intravascular coagulopathy, to a mild clinically inapparent anaemia. Concurrent infection with *Ehrlichia canis* can occur. Drugs recommended for the treatment of babesiosis include diminazene aceturate and imidocarb dipropionate.

Heinz body haemolytic anaemia
The presence of Heinz bodies in erythrocytes results in a haemolytic anaemia. The formation of Heinz bodies is the result of oxidant damage to haemoglobin. The Heinz bodies are readily observed with the new methylene blue (Fig. 11.6) or reticulocyte stains. Reported causes of Heinz body haemolytic anaemia include the consumption of onions and the administration of large doses of methylene blue. Palliative treatment with transfusions is usually adequate until the inciting cause is metabolically eliminated.

Haemobartonellosis
Haemobartonella canis is an epierythrocyte infection which causes an accelerated extravascular removal of the erythrocyte (Fig. 11.10). The disease is uncommon in the dog and is usually associated with splenectomy. Stain precipitate may be confused with the organisms on the blood films.

Erythrocyte pyruvate kinase deficiency
Pyruvate kinase deficiency is a recessive hereditary disorder in the Basenji and Beagle. The resultant haemolysis is usually insidious with myelofibrosis, replacement of the bone marrow with fibrous connective tissue, and/or liver failure due to haemochromatosis as the terminal events. Carriers of the disorder can be identified by measuring the pyruvate kinase level in the erythrocyte.

Microangiopathic haemolytic anaemia
Microangiopathic haemolytic anaemia results from the pathological deposition of fibrin in small blood vessels, predominantly arterioles. The fibrin strands 'slice' pieces off the erythrocytes as the blood flows through the affected vessels. The shizocytes (Fig. 11.2), characteristic of the disorder, are often observed in association with haemangiosarcoma and the venae cavae syndrome of dirofilariasis. The abnormal fibrin deposition is probably related to a more general disorder of the haemostatic mechanisms, disseminated intravascular coagulopathy, which always occurs secondary to another disease process.

Vena cavae syndrome of dirofilariasis
The venae cavae syndrome occurs in certain dogs

which have a large number of heartworms in the right atrium and venae cavae. The disorder is acute with clinical signs of marked weakness, respiratory distress and pale mucous membranes. Anaemia, fragmented erythrocytes, haemoglobinaemia, and/or haemoglobinuria are common findings. The occurrence of prolonged coagulation tests and thrombocytopenia suggests that disseminated intravascular coagulopathy may be involved in the pathogenesis of the disorder.

Haemangiosarcoma
Haemangiosarcoma is a common neoplasm in the dog which frequently causes characteristic haematological findings. A regenerative mild anaemia is associated with acanthocytes (Plate 11.1c) and in some cases fragmented erythrocytes. Nucleated red blood cells are present, dramatically out of proportion to the anaemia.

Reduced and defective production of red blood cells
Reduced erythropoiesis and defective erythopoiesis are insidious disorders which result in non-regenerative anaemia. The anaemia can be further classified by the examination of the bone marrow. The bone marrow appears hypoproliferative if there is reduced erythropoiesis. Abundant erythroid precursors are observed in the bone marrow associated with defective erythropoiesis.

Renal failure and endocrine causes
A differential diagnosis of renal and endocrine causes of reduced erythropoiesis can usually be made from a combination of the history, physical examination and appropriate laboratory tests. The blood picture which results from the exogenous administration of oestrogen (e.g. for mismating or from increased endogenous production by a Sertolli cell tumour) is noteworthy. Oestrogens, especially oestradiol cypionate, have an adverse effect on all bone marrow cell lines. Thrombocytopenia followed by neutropenia usually develops within two to four weeks. A progressive non-regenerative anaemia develops slowly unless complicated by haemorrhage. Once the aplastic anaemia develops it is usually not reversible. Spontaneous recovery occasionally occurs after weeks of supporting the patient with transfusions and monitoring the patient for infections. Bone marrow recovery following the surgical removal of a Sertoli cell tumour is, likewise, accompanied by a guarded prognosis.

Anaemia of inflammatory disease
The mild anaemia associated with chronic inflammation or neoplasia is attributed to an ineffective mobilisation of iron stores for erythropoiesis. The serum iron concentration is low-normal to mildly decreased and abundant iron stores are seen in the bone marrow. This is in contrast to the poorly regenerative anaemia associated with chronic blood loss in which the serum iron concentration is markedly decreased, no iron stores are observed in the bone marrow, and a low MCV usually develops.

Ehrlichiosis
A mild to moderate anaemia associated with leucopenia and/or thrombocytopenia is associated with ehrlichiosis. Ehrlichiosis is a common cause of these haematological abnormalities in dogs exposed to ticks. The acute infection with *Ehrlichia canis* is usually associated with a fever and mild clinical signs which last about two weeks. Thrombocytopenia develops rapidly which may result in bleeding episodes. Examination of the bone marrow shows normal to increased cell numbers with increased megakaryocytes. The chronic form of ehrlichiosis takes several months to develop and is haematologically characterized by thrombocytopenia, neutropenia, non-regenerative anaemia and an elevated serum globulin concentration. The pancytopenia is associated with a hypocellular bone marrow, often with an apparent increase in plasma cells. Serological confirmation is required for the diagnosis and the haematological abnormalities slowly (weeks to months) improve with tetracycline therapy.

Iron deficiency anaemia
Iron deficiency anaemia is generally caused by bloodsucking internal and/or external parasites. Iron deficiency can result from chronic haematuria or gastrointestinal haemorrhage. The MCV is normal in early iron deficiency but eventually decreases below normal. The MCHC may be decreased in association with the low MCV. Serum iron concentrations are 8–60 mg/dl in iron-deficient dogs with microcytic anaemias (Harvey *et al.* 1982). Although the reticulocyte response is inadequate in severe cases, corrected reticulocyte counts are usually above normal. Therapy consists of treating the source of blood loss and administering oral iron supplements.

Lead toxicity
Lead toxicity often causes a characteristic blood picture. An apparent dichotomy in this non-regenerative anaemia is the presence of inappropriate numbers of nucleated erythrocytes and minimal polychromasia associated with a mild anaemia. The classic finding of basophilic stippling (Fig. 11.7) supports the diagnosis. Dogs, especially young, with neurological and/or gastrointestinal signs and these haematological abnor-

malities should have the blood lead concentration measured.

Folic acid deficiency
Impaired folic acid metabolism is a poorly documented cause of defective erythropoiesis in the dog. A deficiency of the vitamin impairs nuclear maturation but not the cytoplasmic maturation of the erythrocyte. This disturbance in the bone marow results in large erythrocytes in the blood associated with a non-regenerative anaemia. Diphenylhydantoin is an antagonist of folic acid which can cause the disorder in dogs on long-term therapy.

POLYCYTHAEMIA (ERYTHROCYTOSIS)

Polycythaemia refers to an increased number of circulating erythrocytes. Polycythaemia may be relative or absolute. Relative polycythaemia is commonly associated with dehydration in which both the PCV and plasma protein appear increased due to the loss of plasma volume. Splenic contraction in an excited dog at the time of blood sampling may result in a moderate increase in the PCV. This transient increase in the PCV is associated with a normal plasma protein concentration.

Absolute polycythaemia refers to an increase in the red cell mass with a normal plasma volume. The plasma protein concentration usually remains normal. Hypoxia, secondary to the right-to-left shunting in congenital heart disorders and circulatory insufficiencies, is a common cause of an absolute increase in the PCV. Renal carcinomas in dogs have also been associated with an absolute increase in the erythrocyte mass. The tumours are suspected of producing an erythropoietin-like hormone; the PCV returns to normal following their surgical removal.

Polycythaemia vera is an uncommon neoplastic disorder involving the erythroid tissue of the bone marrow. The proliferative disorder results in a progressive increase in the erythrocyte cell numbers.

METHAEMOGLOBINAEMIA

Methaemoglobinaemia is formed when the iron in haemoglobin is oxidised from the ferrous to the ferric state. Methaemoglobin is unable to bind oxygen resulting in hypoxaemia. The formation of methaemoglobin in the dog may be drug-induced or may be caused by a congenital enzyme defect in the erythrocyte. Drug-induced methaemoglobinaemia is com-

monly associated with the application of benzocaine-containing topical preparations to ulcerative skin lesions. The dogs exhibit cyanotic mucous membranes and variable clinical signs including weakness and respiratory distress. A venous blood sample appears dark with a brownish tinge. Gentle shaking of the venous blood sample after exposing the tube to air does not result in the anticipated reddening of the sample, but instead accentuates the brown colour. Similarly, a drop of blood from the patient can be placed on a white filter paper next to a drop of venous blood from a normal dog. The blood spot from the patient will remain chocolate-brown in colour while the control blood reddens. The diagnosis is confirmed by measuring the methaemoglobin concentration (normal $<2\%$). Treatment usually consists of removing the drug remaining on the skin and resting the dog in a cage for a day or two. Animals with severe respiratory distress may be transfused with packed erythrocytes or treated with low-dose methylene blue intravenously ($1–2\,mg/kg$). Methylene blue can enhance Heinz body formation, therefore the PCV should be followed daily as a monitor for the development of a haemolytic anaemia. Congenital methaemoglobinaemia is usually a serendipitous finding and requires no specific treatment other than avoiding exertion.

BLEEDING DISORDERS

Haemostatic mechanisms involve the interaction of blood vessels, platelets and coagulation factors. A deficiency or defect in one or more of these components is manifested as a bleeding disorder. The clinical sign characteristically associated with a platelet disorder is petechial and ecchymotic haemorrhages of the skin and mucous membranes. Melaena and haematuria can also be the result of a platelet disorder. Disorders of the coagulation factors more commonly result in haemorrhage into a body cavity (haemothorax), a joint (haemarthrosis) or the eye (hyphaemia).

Screening tests

The initial laboratory tests used to evaluate the bleeding disorders include the platelet count, the prothrombin time (PT), the activated partial thromboplastin time (PTT) and the activated coagulation time (ACT). Coagulation Factors X, V, II and I comprise the common pathway in the coagulation sequence. The PT evaluates Factor VII (extrinsic pathway) plus the common pathway factors. The PTT and the ACT evaluate Factors XII, XI, IX, VIII (intrinsic pathway) plus the common pathway factors. These coagulation tests are independent of the platelet numbers.

Special tests are required to diagnose certain bleeding disorders and are discussed with the particular disorder. Recommendations for sample collection and handling have been previously discussed and should be carefully followed (p. 300).

Platelet disorders

Platelet disorders involve either abnormal platelet numbers (Table 11.4) or abnormal platelet function.

Table 11.4. Causes of thrombocytopenia.

Increased destruction
  Immune-mediated
    Primary (autoimmune)
    Secondary
      Autoimmune haemolytic anaemia
      Systemic lupus erythematosis
      Lymphoproliferative disorders
      Drug-induced
  Infectious
    Ehrlichia canis (acute stage)
    Ehrlichia platys
Decreased production
  Drug-induced
    Oestrogen
    Phenylbutazone
    Cancer chemotherapeutic agents
  Infectious
    Ehrlichia canis (chronic stage)
  Cyclic haematopoiesis in grey collies
Increased utilisation
  Disseminated intravascular coagulopathy
  Pulmonary thromboembolism
  Septicaemia

Decreased platelet numbers, thrombocytopenia, can result from an increased destruction, a decreased production, or an increase in their utilisation. Abnormal platelet function can be a hereditary disorder or an acquired disorder.

Increased destruction

The destruction of platelets in which no underlying disorder can be identified is termed idiopathic thrombocytopenia. A specific antiplatelet antibody is detectable in the majority of these patients, justifying a diagnosis of autoimmune thrombocytopenia. The platelet factor 3 test* indirectly reflects the presence of this antibody. Autoimmune thrombocytopenia is usually

* Performed by Dr Jean Dodds, Division of Laboratories and Research, New York State Department of Health, Albany, New York.

responsive to glucocorticoid therapy. Lack of platelet response is an indication for a bone marrow aspirate to evaluate the megakaryocyte population.

Rickettsial infections frequently cause a thrombocytopenia. The pancytopenia which develops in ehrlichiosis is consistently highlighted by a mild-to-severe thrombocytopenia. The decreased platelet numbers in ehrlichiosis are probably the combined result of direct platelet injury, immunological mechanisms and a decreased platelet production depending on the time course of the infection. A platelet-specific rickettsial organism classified as *Ehrlichia platys* (Fig. 11.12) has been described by Harvey *et al* (1978). Infection of normal dogs with the rickettsial agent under controlled conditions causes a cyclic thrombocytopenia which resolves spontaneously. The clinical importance of this infectious agent is currently being studied.

Decreased production

Oestrogens, phenylbutazone and cancer chemotherapeutic drugs can cause myelotoxicity. The toxic effect of oestrogens on canine bone marrow is reflected initially by thrombocytopenia. A fatal aplastic anaemia is a common sequelae in those dogs which develop oestrogen-induced myelotoxicosis. The myelotoxicity of phenylbutazone appears to be an idiosyncratic reaction characterised by a severe agranulocytosis in the acute form and neutropenia and thrombocytopenia in the chronic form. Lastly, drugs used in the treatment of cancer often cause a myelotoxic-induced thrombocytopenia.

Increased utilisation

Increased platelet utilisation resulting in thrombocytopenia is associated with disseminated intravascular coagulopathy, septicaemia and pulmonary thromboembolism.

It is important to remember that thrombocytopenia can be an indication of neoplastic disease. Over 50% of dogs with advanced neoplasia of the lymphoid tissue have thrombocytopenia, the cause of which may be one or more of the mechanisms discussed.

Abnormal platelet function

Hereditary

Von Willebrand's disease is a hereditary defect of platelet adhesion commonly seen in Doberman Pinschers. The disorder has also been reported in inbred lines including the German Shepherd, Golden Retriever, Miniature Schnauzer, Scottish Terrier and Pembroke Welsh Corgi. The platelet adhesion defect is related to an abnormal Factor VIII molecule. In addition to the coagulant activity of Factor VIII which is assessed by the PTT and ACT, a portion of the Factor VIII molecule (the von Willebrand factor) is required for normal platelet adhesion. The von Willebrand factor is assessed by the measurement of Factor VIII-related antigen. In an affected dog, the coagulant activity of Factor VIII and the Factor VIII-related antigen concentration are both decreased. Because the disorder is variably expressed genetically, clinical signs vary from ease of bruising to severe haemorrhage. Surgical procedures or disease may initiate severe bleeding in a dog which appears clinically normal. The PTT and ACT may be normal in mild cases. The bleeding time can be used to assess platelet function in this disorder, but lack of standardisation of technique makes it unreliable.

A hereditary defect in platelet aggregation has been reported in Otter Hounds and Basset Hounds. Special tests are required to confirm this defect.

Acquired

Certain drugs adversely affect platelet function. Commonly used ones include aspirin, phenylbutazone and penicillin.

Several disease syndromes can cause abnormal platelet function. These include uraemia, hepatic cirrhosis, myeloproliferative disorders and multiple myeloma.

Coagulation disorders

Hereditary coagulation factor deficiencies

Intrinsic pathway
Hereditary deficiency of coagulation factors involving the intrinsic pathway includes Factors VIII, IX, and XI. One of these factor deficiencies is suspected when the PTT and ACT is prolonged and the PT is normal. An assay for the specific factor is required to confirm the diagnosis. Factor VIII deficiency (classic haemophilia A) is common in many purebred and mixed breeds. In contrast to von Willebrand's disease, only the Factor VIII coagulant activity is deficient. Factor IX deficiency (haemophilia B) is reported in the Beagle, Cairn Terrier, St. Bernard, Alaskan Malamute, Cocker Spaniel, French Bulldog, and Coonhound. Factor XI deficiency has been reported in the Springer Spaniel.

Extrinsic pathway
Factor VII constitutes the extrinsic pathway. A prolonged PT with the other screening tests remaining normal suggests a Factor VII deficiency. A specific

assay confirms the diagnosis. Factor VII deficiency is reported in the Beagle and Malamute.

Common pathway
Factor X is the only reported coagulation deficiency involving the common pathway in the dog; occurring in the Cocker Spaniel breed. The deficiency is suspected when the PTT, ACT and PT are prolonged.

Acquired coagulation factor deficiencies

Common pathway
A number of disorders cause multiple coagulation factor deficiencies resulting in a prolonged PTT, and PT with normal platelet numbers. These disorders include vitamin K antagonism (e.g. warfarin toxicity) and vitamin K deficiency (e.g. associated with the malabsorption syndrome and severe liver disease). In warfarin toxicity, vitamin K1 therapy results in normal coagulation tests within 4–12 hours. Some anticoagulant rat poisons have longer half-lives than warfarin. Following parenteral vitamin K1 therapy,* oral vitamin K should be given for 1–2 weeks and the coagulation tests monitored following its discontinuation.

Disseminated intravascular coagulopathy is a common acquired cause for a prolonged PTT, ACT and PT. In addition the platelet numbers are usually decreased, abnormal erythrocyte shapes (shizocytes) may be observed on the blood smear (Fig. 11.2) and an increased concentration by fibrin degradation products may be demonstrated by a test kit (Thrombo-Wellcotest). The accelerated, uncontrolled consumption of the coagulation factors and platelets always occurs secondarily to another pathological process. Some of these disorders include septicaemia, venae cavae syndrome of dirofilariasis, heat stroke, severe liver disease, disseminated neoplasia, acute babesiosis and pulmonary embolism (often subsequent to the treatment for heartworms). Treatment of the coagulopathy necessitates management of the inciting disorder.

TRANSFUSION AND CROSS-MATCHING (See also Chapter 12)

The objective of the blood transfusion is to maintain the circulating haemoglobin concentration at a level which provides adequate tissue oxygenation. A PCV of 15% or less is an arbitrary guideline for which a

---

* Intravenous vitamin K may cause an anaphylactic reaction. The drug should be administered slowly over 5 to 8 minutes.

transfusion may be beneficial. This depends on the rate of development of anaemia and the presence of disorders involving the cardiovascular and pulmonary systems. Autoimmune haemolytic disease poses a special concern. A decision to transfuse a dog with immune-mediated anaemia should be made after careful deliberation. The anti-erythrocyte antibodies may rapidly (hours) haemolyse the transfused cells. Intravenous glucocorticoids should precede the transfusion if it must be given.

Dogs have multiple blood types but only one is strongly antigenic. Fortunately there is a low incidence of naturally-occurring autoantibodies to this blood type. Cross-matching is suggested whenever possible but is especially advisable prior to transfusing a dog which has previously received blood.

The transfusion can be given at a rate of 5–10 ml per kilogram body weight per hour. The transfusion should be terminated if urticaria develops soon after the transfusion is initiated.

Sedimented erythrocytes may be given when volume expansion of the recipient is not desirable. Storing the blood container upside down results in a concentration of erythrocytes at the transfusion outlet. The transfusion is stopped when mostly plasma remains in the container.

Stored blood is not a source of platelets. Fresh blood, collected in plastic, must be used when platelets are required. Fresh blood is also required for the replacement of deficient coagulation factors.

LEUCOCYTES

The term leucocytes refers to all the nucleated blood cells including neutrophils, eosinophils, basophils, monocytes, lymphocytes and their precursors. Leucocytes are routinely examined by performing total and differential counts along with evaluation of leucocyte morphology. Leucocytosis refers to an increase and leucopenia refers to a decrease in the total leucocyte count from the normal range. Nucleated erythrocytes are not considered part of the total leucocyte count and if present should be subtracted from the total count. It is important to identify which of the leucocytes are responsible for the leucocytosis or leucopenia. The term leucocyte response refers to the changes in leucocyte numbers and morphology.

Neutrophils

The neutrophil comprises the majority of leucocytes in the dog. The function of the neutrophil is to phagocytise particulate material and destroy bacteria. Neutrophils are continuously produced in the bone mar-

row, spend several hours in the peripheral blood, marginate (stick) along blood vessel walls and then migrate into the tissues. Normally the bone marrow releases mature, segmented neutrophils into the blood. As the demand intensifies in response to infections the bone marrow reserve of mature neutrophils becomes depleted and immature neutrophilic precursors are released (left-shift). A left-shift may include the presence of bands, metamyelocytes and myelocytes in order of increasing immaturity. An increase in immaturity is associated with a corresponding decrease in functional ability.

Neutrophilia

An absolute neutrophilia refers to an increase in the number of circulating neutrophils. A regenerative left-shift indicates an increased number of immature neutrophils associated with a neutrophilia. A degenerative left-shift indicates a marked increase in the number of immature neutrophils associated with a neutropenia or normal neutrophil count; the number of immature neutrophils may exceed the number of segmented neutrophils. The magnitude and change of these events provides a clinical indicator which reflects the course of an inflammatory process.

Physiological neutrophilia refers to an increase in circulating mature neutrophils as a result of demargination. Physiological exertion, e.g. struggling during sampling, causes the release of adrenaline (epinephrine) which results in temporary (hours) demargination. There is no left-shift and the lymphocyte count remains normal or is slightly elevated. The condition is less common in the dog than it is in the cat.

Stress-induced neutrophilia is very common in the dog and is associated with non-inflammatory disorders, e.g. trauma. The administration of exogenous glucocorticoids causes a similar blood picture. A monocytosis, lymphopenia and an eosinopenia are frequently associated with the stress-induced neutrophilia. Endogenous and exogenous glucocorticoids cause demargination of neutrophils, impede the migration of neutrophils into the tissues and increase the rate of release of these cells from the bone marrow.

The neutrophilia of inflammation haematologically represents a local or generalised tissue demand for neutrophils. Evaluation of the leucocyte blood picture allows for the detection of an inflammatory process and provides a monitor of its course. The magnitude of the neutrophilia crudely parallels the extent of the inflammatory process. In addition to infectious agents, non-infectious disorders, such as immune-mediated diseases, may simulate the neutrophilia of inflammation.

The number and maturity of neutrophils observed

in the blood during the inflammatory process represents a balance between the demand for the cells and the rate of release from the bone marrow. A neutrophilic leucocytosis with a left-shift (regenerative response) indicates that the production and the release exceed demand. The magnitude of the left-shift is a reflection of the intensity of the inflammatory process. A normal-to-decreased number of segmented neutrophils associated with a marked left-shift (degenerative response) suggests that the demand exceeds the production and release capacity of the bone marrow—an unhappy situation! If the inflammatory process subsides, the neutrophil count will stabilise and fewer immature neutrophils and some hypersegmented neutrophils will comprise the neutrophilia. Fig. 11.13 summarises the discussion.

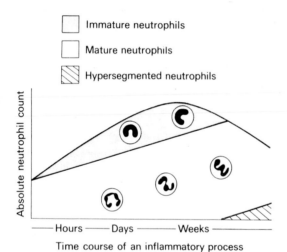

Time course of an inflammatory process

Fig. 11.13 Circulating neutrophil response to a chronic suppurative inflammatory process when the bone marrow reserve can meet the demand.

Neutropenia

Neutropenia refers to a decrease in the absolute number of neutrophils and is usually attendant to a serious disorder. In addition to suggesting a serious disorder, the low neutrophil count predisposes the animal to infection by opportunistic organisms. A persistent neutropenia (days) implies a guarded prognosis. Neutropenia may be caused by an excessive utilisation or a decreased production by the bone marrow.

A massive tissue demand for neutrophils quickly depletes the reserves in the blood and the bone marrow resulting in a neutropenia from excessive utilisation. If the inflammatory process can be controlled, e.g. surgical repair of a perforated intestine, the degenerative left-shift will improve to a regenerative left-shift. Continued neutrophil production following the control of the inflammatory process often results in a marked neutrophilia (termed leucomoid response) for a few days; a favourable response. A bone marrow examination during neutropenia from excessive utilisation indicates intense granulopoiesis.

Neutropenia associated with a decreased bone marrow production is most commonly caused by an infectious agent (e.g. ehrlichiosis, parvovirus), or myelotoxicity (e.g. oestrogens, cancer chemotherapeutic agents). Less commonly, neoplasms invading the bone marrow and idiopathic aplastic anaemias may cause the neutropenia. Often other cell types in the blood are also noted to be decreased in numbers. A bone marrow examination reveals decreased granulocytic cell numbers and often indicates a decreased production of other cell types.

Lymphocytes

An absolute lymphopenia is usually a consequence of some type of stress. The decrease in lymphocyte numbers roughly parallels a progressive inflammatory disorder. A rising lymphocyte count is generally associated with clinical improvement. Lymphopenia may occur secondarily to a rupture of the thoracic duct or an extravasation of lymph associated with intestinal lymphangiectasia, in which case the plasma protein is also decreased. Glucocorticoids, endogenous or exogenous, will result in a temporary decrease in lymphocyte numbers.

An absolute lymphocytosis is uncommon in the dog. An increase in lymphocyte numbers may be associated with immune-mediated disorders, following vaccination and with lymphocytic leukaemia. An occasional atypical lymphocyte is commonly observed in association with antigenic stimulation such as viral infections, vaccinations and immune-mediated disorders.

Monocytes

A monocytosis is frequently associated with increased levels of glucocorticoids and chronic inflammatory disorders characterised by suppuration and necrosis. Monocytosis is also a common finding in deep mycotic infections.

Eosinophils

Eosinophilia is associated with the presence of certain parasites, mast cell tumours, allergic disorders involving the skin and lungs, and eosinophilic infiltration of the gastrointestinal tract.

Eosinopenia is difficult to define since a normal dog may not have eosinophils observed in a blood sample.

The absence of eosinophils is frequently a component of the 'stress pattern' (neutrophilia, lymphopenia, monocytosis) previously described and attributed to the effects of glucocorticoids. In a sick dog, if a stress leucocyte pattern is absent, the unexpected presence of eosinophils is suggestive of adrenal insufficiency (Addison's disease).

Basophils

Basophilia is uncommonly observed, except in dogs with dirofilariasis and hypothyroidism.

Primary leucocyte disorders

Primary non-neoplastic disorders involving the leucocyte are uncommon in the dog. The Pelger–Huet anomaly is a hereditary disorder in which the nucleus of the granulocyte fails to become segmented. The immature-appearing cells suggest a marked left shift. The abnormality does not appear to predispose the dog to infections.

Cyclic haematopoiesis is a hereditary disorder in the grey-coloured Collie breed. In addition to several anatomical abnormalities there is a primary stem cell defect. Cyclic decrease of the neutrophil and the platelet numbers are prominent haematological findings.

HAEMATOPOIETIC NEOPLASIA

Lymphoproliferative disorders

Neoplasms that begin in the marrow and involve lymphocytes and plasma cells have been classified as lymphoproliferative disorders. Lymphocytic neoplasia may involve either poorly-differentiated lymphocytes (acute lymphocytic or lymphoblastic leukaemia) or normal-appearing mature lymphocytes (chronic lymphocytic or well-differentiated lymphocytic leukaemia). The bone marrow is, by definition, involved in lymphocytic leukaemia but the total blood leucocyte count may not be increased. In the case of acute lymphocytic leukaemia, even the absolute lymphocyte count may not be increased. A bone marrow biopsy is often required to make a definitive diagnosis.

A leukaemic blood phase, with variable marrow infiltration, occurs at times in association with lymphoid tumours (lymphomas or lymphosarcomas) developing in lymph nodes, spleen, or thymus. Neoplastic cells in lymphocytic leukaemias can infiltrate peripheral lymphoid organs making it difficult to determine whether a specific animal has lymphocytic leukaemia or a lymphoma with a leukaemic blood picture.

Multiple myeloma (plasma cell myeloma) is a disorder in which there is a proliferation of plasma cells and their precursors. A diagnosis of multiple myeloma is considered in dogs with increased plasma proteins, especially if a serum protein electrophoresis has demonstrated a monoclonal band ('spike') in the β or γ region. Definitive diagnosis is usually dependent on examination of a bone marrow biopsy. Low numbers of neoplastic plasma cells may occasionally be seen on blood films.

Myeloproliferative disorders

The term 'myeloproliferative disorders' is used to describe a group of neoplastic disorders involving non-lymphoid precursor cell line in the bone marrow. Myeloproliferative disorders are characterised by abnormal proliferation of one or more of granulocytic, monocytic, erythrocytic or megakaryocytic cell lines in the marrow, with subsequent abnormalities usually observed in the blood. Abnormal findings in the blood include cytopenias (neutropenia, thrombocytopenia, anaemia) and/or leukaemia. If a particular cell line(s) dominates the picture, more specific terminology is used, e.g. granulocytic leukaemia, monocytic leukaemia, megakaryocytic myelosis. Myeloproliferative disorders are less common in the dog than in the cat (Harvey 1981).

Inflammatory-induced leukaemoid responses must be differentiated from leukaemia. A leukaemoid response is characterised by a dramatic neutrophilia with an orderly left-shift secondary to an inflammatory response such as pyometra. A bone marrow biopsy is often needed before a diagnosis can be made with confidence.

ACKNOWLEDGEMENT

The authors acknowledge Pam Miller for her invaluable assistance in the preparation of the manuscript and the technicians in clinical pathology who absorbed more of the clinical burden during our increased absence as a result of this project.

REFERENCES

ADEYANJU B. L. & ALIU Y. O. (1982) Chemotherapy of canine ehrlichiosis and babesiosis with imidocarb dipropionate. *J. Am. Anim. Hosp. Assoc.* **18,** 827.
GREENE C. E. (1975) Disseminated intravascular coagulo-

pathy in the dog: a review. *J. Am. Anim. Hosp. Assoc.* **11,** 674.

This reference reviews the disseminated intravascular coagulopathy syndrome.

HARVEY J. W. (1980) Canine hemolytic anemias. *J. Am. Vet. Med. Assoc.* **176,** 970.

HARVEY J. W. (1981) Myeloproliferative disorders in dogs and cats. *Vet. Clin. N. Am.* **11,** 349.

This reference reviews haematopoietic neoplasia in the dog.

HARVEY J. W., FRENCH T. W. & MEYER D. J. (1982) Chronic iron deficiency anemia in dogs. *J. Am. Anim. Hosp. Assoc.* **18,** 946.

This reference reviews the clinicopathologic parameters and response to therapy for iron deficiency anaemia.

HARVEY J. W., SIMPSON C. F. & GASKIN J. M. (1978) Cyclic thrombocytopenia induced by a Rickettsia-like agent in dogs. *J. Infect. Dis.* **137,** 182.

MEYER D. J. (1983) The technique of bone marrow biopsy. In *Current Techniques in Small Animal Surgery*, M. J. Bojrab (Ed.), pp. 1068–1073. Lea and Febiger, Philadelphia.

This reference describes various techniques for obtaining a bone marrow biopsy.

MOORE D. J. (1979) Therapeutic implications of *Babesia canis* infection in dogs. *J. S. Afr. Vet. Med. Assoc.* **50,** 346.

These references (Adeyanju & Moore) review the use of several drugs for the treatment of babesiosis and ehrlichiosis.

SCHALM O. W., JAIN N. C. & CARROLL E. J. (1975) *Veterinary Hematology*, 3rd edn. Lea and Febiger, Philadelphia.

This reference provides a complete, detailed discussion of haematological techniques and disorders in the dog.

12

Disorders of Fluid and Electrolyte Balance

A. E. WATERMAN

Disturbances of fluid and electrolyte balance are inevitable consequences of many disease processes and correction of these imbalances is often empirical in practice. Normally both the volume and composition of body fluids are maintained within narrow limits but pathological impairment of regulating mechanisms by disease processes may result in depletion of body water, electrolyte imbalances and acid–base disturbances. The aim of fluid therapy is to correct these disorders.

GENERAL PRINCIPLES

Normal Water Balance

Water constitutes approximately two-thirds of body weight, the exact proportion varying with the fat content of the body. Fat dogs have a lower body water content (approx. 50%) whereas immature animals have a much higher water content (approx. 70-80%). Two-thirds of the water is intracellular (ICF) (44% of body weight), the rest is extracellular (ECF). Extracellular water is subdivided into plasma water (25% of ECF or approx. 5% of body weight), and interstitial fluid (75% of ECF or approx. 16% of body weight).

The distribution of water within the body is governed by a balance of the opposing forces of hydrostatic and osmotic pressure. The electrolyte composition of the ECF and ICF are quite different. Sodium and chloride are the principal extracellular ions whereas potassium and phosphate predominate intracellularly. Interstitial fluid resembles plasma except for the absence of significant amounts of protein.

Water and electrolytes are gained and lost from the body through four routes, namely the gastrointestinal tract, kidneys, skin and lungs. In health the gastrointestinal tract is the sole route for gaining water and electrolytes. A small quantity of water, approx. 10% of total water intake, is also produced by oxidation of food. Although more water is produced per gram from fat than from protein or carbohydrate, more water is produced *per calorie* by carbohydrates, hence carbohydrates reduce the need to drink, and by sparing the oxidation of protein and fat, reduce the urinary solute load and therefore urinary water losses.

On average, dogs ingest (free water + water in food) 55.9 ml water/kg body weight (English & Filippich 1980), with total water intake being estimated to be 72.9 ml/kg body weight (free water + combined water + metabolic water).

Water intake and output are finely balanced and regulated by centres in the hypothalamus which control the sensation of thirst and the urge to drink. Dogs will regulate the amount of free water drunk according to the moisture content of their food so that their total intake remains constant. This is in contrast to cats which do not increase their water intake if fed on dry food (Anderson 1982). There is also some element of voluntary control, but excessive drinking is extremely rare and normally dogs drink when they reach a certain degree of dehydration.

Water is lost via the faeces, urine, expired air and in secretions. Faecal losses are normally minimal unless there is diarrhoea. There is a continuous obligatory water loss through the kidneys which continues even in severe dehydration. The ability of the kidneys to conserve water depends on their concentrating ability which varies from species to species. Antidiuretic hormone, which is released from the pituitary when osmoreceptors in the lateral hypothalamus are stimulated promotes renal conservation of water, while electrolyte regulation is under the influence of aldosterone which acts on the distal tubules to retain Na^+ and excrete K^+, further enhancing water conservation.

The respiratory system accounts for a significant amount of water loss in dogs, because evaporative cooling from the airways and mouth by panting is an important way of losing heat in this species. Losses through the skin, on the other hand, are minimal because dogs have poorly developed sudoriferous glands.

Water lost through the skin and via the respiratory tract is often termed the 'inevitable water loss' because it is dependent on external factors such as temperature and humidity and cannot be deliberately reduced by homeostatic mechanisms. Its magnitude obviously increases with temperature and increased activity.

It is generally estimated that half the daily water intake is required to meet 'inevitable water losses' while the rest is lost via the urine. Exact daily requirements depend on the ambient temperature, relative humidity, as well as on the animal's renal concentrating ability.

Tables are available for calculation of normal maintenance requirements based on the animal's body weight (Finco 1972), but generally the average adult dog requires a volume of approximately 40–60 ml/kg body weight (mean 50 ml/kg body weight). Maintenance requirements will obviously be higher in smaller dogs with a relatively large surface area, immature animals, lactating or pyrexic animals or if the ambient temperature is high.

Similar estimates of electrolyte requirements suggest that to this fluid should be added 1 mmol/kg per 24 hours Na^+ ions and 2 mmols/kg per 24 hours K^+ ions.

Disorders of water and electrolyte metabolism

Disorders are often classified as follows:

1 Primary water depletion
2 Mixed water and electrolyte depletion
3 Acid–base disturbances

In practice, disorders are nearly always combinations of two or more of these three categories, although one may predominate.

Primary water depletion
This occurs when intake is insufficient and inevitable losses continue. Intake may be curtailed by conditions of drought or neglect or when disease prevents the animal drinking or swallowing, e.g. tetanus, oesophageal obstruction, fractured mandible. Primary water depletion due to excessive *renal losses* is less common but does occur, e.g. osmotic diuresis with glycosuria in diabetes mellitus and failure of ADH activity leading to production of dilute urine in diabetes insipidus.

Primary water loss will first affect the ECF which becomes hypertonic. Water is drawn into the ECF from the ICF, thus the loss is evenly distributed throughout the body. Tissue catabolism liberates even more intracellular water so that the ICF contracts even further. Initially electrolytes are excreted to maintain ECF tonicity, but later, if losses continue, the need to maintain ECF volume results in oliguria with a urine of a high specific gravity, and haemoconcentration.

Thirst is usually marked and the mucous membranes are dry, but there is no significant hypotension or tachycardia unless the deficit is massive. Death occurs when approximately 40% of body water has been lost and is due primarily to medullary failure.

Since the ECF is usually hypertonic replacement fluids should aim to provide water in excess of electrolytes and the most appropriate fluid to use is N/5 saline (0.18%) with 4.3% dextrose.

Mixed water and electrolyte depletion
This develops when body secretions are lost in vomitus or diarrhoea, or as exudates from discharging wounds, and burns, or when extensive pleural or peritoneal effusions develop.

Water plus electrolytes (mainly sodium and chloride but also potassium and bicarbonate) are lost, but if the animal continues to drink, the plasma sodium concentration will tend to fall so that the ECF becomes hypotonic. This provokes a diuresis and also causes water to move into the ICF in an attempt to maintain ECF osmolality. This results in an early decrease in ECF (and therefore plasma volume), so that signs of circulatory failure develop fairly early. After the initial diuresis the hypovolaemia affects renal function so that oliguria occurs. The cellular overhydration resembles water intoxication and affects cerebral, intestinal and renal function. Thirst is not a marked feature of this disorder as plasma sodium and chloride levels are either normal or low. These animals are dull and weak, their mucous membranes are moist but their saliva is often viscous. Treatment should be aimed at replacing electrolyte losses, so isotonic or even hypertonic electrolyte solutions are used.

Potassium metabolism
Potassium (K^+) is the major intracellular cation and is held within the cell in proportion to proteins, carbohydrates and water. Losses of these cellular constituents cause a concomitant loss of K^+ ions from the cell into the ECF. This K^+ is excreted very quickly by the kidney as long as renal function is normal, but if renal function is impaired plasma K^+ levels will rise. Hyperkalaemia (levels in excess of 7 mmol/l) will

therefore develop in animals which become anuric or oliguric from any cause. The main clinical signs are those of impaired cardiac function characterised by depressed myocardial excitability and conduction velocity which lead to arrhythmias, bradycardia and eventually, when levels reach 8–9 mmol/l, ventricular fibrillation or asystole, possibly without warning.

Hypokalaemia (plasma levels less than 2.5 mmol/l) develops when intake is curtailed or losses via secretions are increased while urinary excretion continues. It therefore tends to develop with prolonged anorexia and with severe vomiting and diarrhoea. Hydrogen ions and potassium ions exchange across the cell membrane during buffering processes, hence in an alkalosis, plasma K^+ levels will fall (whilst an acidosis may provoke a hyperkalaemia). Symptoms of hypokalaemia include glucose intolerance, skeletal muscle weakness (which can affect the muscles of respiration giving rise to dyspnoea), intestinal atony, inability to concentrate urine and alterations in cardiac conduction. The ECG findings are less reliable than those accompanying hyperkalaemia but atrial or ventricular tachycardia and eventually ventricular fibrillation can occur.

Acid–base disturbances

The regulation of the concentration of free hydrogen ions in the body is essential for the maintenance of cellular function. Hydrogen ions are generally produced by oxidation of food and tissues and are immediately buffered by the buffering systems of the body so that the actual concentration of free hydrogen ions is very low (40 nmol/l). Conventionally hydrogen ion concentration (H^+) is measured as the pH, which is the negative log_{10} of the $[H^+]$, and blood pH is normally maintained within relatively narrow limits (7.35–7.45). Deviations below 6.8 or above 7.8 are generally incompatible with life. There are many buffering systems within the extracellular and intracellular compartments but the most important in terms of its ability to make rapid adjustments is the bicarbonate-carbonic acid system.

The ratio of undissociated acid to its dissociated salt in any system is governed by the Law of Mass Action, thus:

$$\frac{[H^+] \times [Base^-]}{[Acid]} = \text{Constant}$$

For the bicarbonate system this can be rewritten as:

$$[H^+] = \frac{[H_2CO_3]}{[HCO_3^-]} \times \text{constant (Ka)}$$

Converting this to the pH system gives:

$$pH = pKa + \log \frac{[HCO_3^-]}{[H_2CO_3]}$$

which is known as the Henderson–Hasselbach equation, which may also be written

$$pH = pKa + \log \frac{[HCO_3^-]}{aP_{CO_2}} \quad \frac{\text{(Metabolic)}}{\text{(Respiratory)}}$$

where 'a' is the solubility coefficient for carbon dioxide and P_{CO_2} is the carbon dioxide tension (partial pressure).

The importance of this equation is that it illustrates that the pH is directly proportional to the bicarbonate concentration and inversely proportional to the P_{CO_2} and it is the ratio of $[HCO_3^-]$ to CO_2 which determines pH (normally the ratio is 20:1). Thus a gain or loss of hydrogen or bicarbonate ions (metabolic disturbances) first causes an alteration in the ratio of bicarbonate to carbonic acid, which then provokes an alteration in pulmonary ventilation so that carbon dioxide is retained or eliminated until the *ratio* and therefore the blood pH is returned to near normal. Renal adjustment of base excretion or retention then follows more slowly. A metabolic acidosis occurs when there is increased production or retention of acid metabolites or excessive loss of bicarbonate base. In shock, for example, reduced tissue perfusion leads to the accumulation of acid metabolites, whilst in diarrhoea, large quantities of bicarbonate are lost. A metabolic alkalosis is less common but develops if H^+ ions are lost, as in severe vomiting, and if excessive bicarbonate is administered during treatment of an acidosis.

Respiratory disturbances affect the P_{CO_2} tension of blood primarily and alterations in the ratio provoke a secondary renal adjustment of bicarbonate concentrations. A respiratory acidosis occurs if pulmonary ventilation is impaired for any reason, while an alkalosis will result from hyperventilation.

Diagnosis of disorders

History and clinical signs

An accurate history can give valuable information on the *type and size* of deficit present. Mixed depletion states occur in vomiting, diarrhoea or intestinal obstruction whereas comatose animals tend to develop a primary water loss. It is important to ask about all the factors which may have contributed to the disorder.

Hence, it is important to determine the presence or absence of signs such as diarrhoea or vomiting, polyuria, anorexia, panting, pyrexia. Using this information the size of the accumulated deficit may be estimated. Alternatively a rough estimate of the degree of dehydration may be made by physical examination. Examination of the texture and elasticity of the skin and the appearance of the mucous membranes has been suggested by Finco (1972) and Cornelius (1980). However, a loss of water equivalent to less than 5% of body weight is undetectable clinically and, at the other extreme, when losses are greater than 15% the animal is usually moribund. The first sign of dehydration is a loss of skin elasticity and pliability (7% deficit). This becomes more severe with a 10% deficit and is accompanied by a sinking of the eye into the orbit and a slowed capillary refill time. A 12–15% deficit results in hypovolaemia and the onset of circulatory collapse. There are pitfalls associated with this method of assessing disorders:

1 Cachetic animals' skin loses elasticity as a result of fat and protein loss even when not dehydrated
2 Fat animals' skin tends to retain elasticity even when dehydrated (Cornelius 1980).

Changes in body weight can be a useful guide to the extent of the loss, if the normal body weight is known.

Dryness of the oral mucous membranes can indicate dehydration but panting will also cause dryness even though hydration may be normal (Cornelius 1980). Capillary refill time is another rough indication of the adequacy of perfusion. A refill time of over 2 seconds indicates hypotension, hypovolaemia or peripheral vasoconstriction. This, together with cool extremities and a rapid weak pulse indicates oligaemic shock, which if due to dehydration, suggests a very large body fluid deficit.

Laboratory tests

Haematological estimations
Packed cell volume (PCV), haemoglobin concentration (Hb) and total plasma protein (TPP) measurements are all of value in assessing the severity of the dehydration. All these parameters rise as a result of dehydration, but single estimations are open to misinterpretation. Pre-existing disease can cause changes which will influence the value of any of these tests, for instance a pre-existing anaemia will cause the PCV and Hb levels to appear normal if the animal subsequently becomes dehydrated. Similarly, TPP will be apparently normal in a dehydrated dog which is also hypoproteinaemic. However, assessment of both PCV

and TPP is likely to be valuable in substantiating the clinical appraisal of the degree of dehydration present and it is less likely that both parameters will be similarly affected by a disorder unassociated with the dehydration. The 'normal' range for these parameters varies from laboratory to laboratory but a general guide is given in Table 12.1.

Table 12.1 Normal blood values in the dog.

Constituent	Mean	Range
PCV (%)	45.0	37.0–50.0
Haemoglobin (g/dl)	13.0	9.0–16.0
Total serum protein (g/l)	59.0	53.0–69.0
Plasma urea (mmol/l)	5.3	2.5–6.7
Sodium (mmol/l)	145.0	127.0–153.0
Potassium (mmol/l)	4.0	3.7–5.8
Chloride (mmol/l)	110.0	100.0–120.0

Serial estimates of these parameters are invaluable in monitoring response to treatment.

The PCV may be used to calculate fluid requirements. Approximately 10 ml/kg should be infused for each 1% rise in the PCV over 45%. (In anaemic dogs 5–10% should be added to the measured PCV figure.) Blood urea concentration also rises in dehydration, but renal disease and excessive tissue catabolism will also cause this parameter to increase and must be excluded first.

Plasma electrolytes
Determination of plasma electrolytes is of limited value as they do not necessarily reflect the total body content of these ions. Low plasma levels will always indicate a large deficit but normal concentrations do not rule this out. Plasma sodium [Na^+] concentrations will provide information on the relative deficit of water and electrolytes in the ECF and, by inference, on the state of intracellular hydration. A raised [Na^+] (hypernatraemia) indicates a severe net water deficit.

Since most of the potassium in the body is intracellular, estimations of plasma levels will not reflect the total body store of this cation. Plasma K^+ levels can remain normal even when intracellular K^+ is depleted, although a hypokalaemia indicates a severe total body deficit of this cation. Hyperkalaemia usually indicates a failure of potassium excretion which may be associated with low or normal cellular K^+ concentrations. It is nevertheless as important to know the concentration of potassium in the plasma as the total body content because of the influence that this ion has on the resting cell membrane potential and therefore function of skeletal and, more importantly, cardiac muscle.

Acid–base estimations

The accurate assessment of acid base balance depends on the measurement of arterial blood pH, bicarbonate ion concentration $[HCO_3^-]$ and arterial CO_2 tension ($Pa\,CO_2$). Normal values for the dog are given in Table 12.2.

Table 12.2 Normal acid–base values in the dog (arterial blood).

Parameter	Mean	Range
pH	7.35	7.31–7.45
PCO_2 (mmHg) (kPa)	36.0	29.0–40.0
	(4.79)	(3.86– 5.32)
Standard bicarbonate (HCO_3^-) (mmol/l)	25.0	22.0–28.0

In clinical cases, it may not be possible to obtain an arterial sample and a jugular venous sample may be almost as informative (Speirs 1980). In the absence of a blood gas and pH analyser a simple titration method of measuring plasma bicarbonate is available using the Harleco apparatus which will provide information on any metabolic disturbances which may have occurred.

Metabolic disorders are reflected in $[HCO_3^-]$ whereas respiratory imbalances alter $Pa\,CO_2$ levels. Therefore in a simple metabolic acidosis, pH and $[HCO_2^-]$ will be low but $Pa\,CO_2$ will be normal. In a primary respiratory acidosis pH and $Pa\,CO_2$ are affected while $[HCO_3^-]$, although initially unaltered, later tends to rise. Conversely a metabolic alkalosis is reflected in an increased $[HCO_3^-]$ with a raised pH and a normal or raised $Pa\,CO_2$.

Urinalysis

If there is no urinary tract infection and the kidneys are healthy, the pH of the urine can serve as a rough indicator of the animal's acid–base status (Finco 1972) especially at the extreme ends of the scale (<5.0, >7.5). However, this estimate should always be interpreted with extreme care, as acid–base status is not invariably reflected in urinary pH.

The specific gravity of the urine will also give some indication of hydration status providing the kidneys are normal and there are no abnormal constituents in the urine to raise S.G. spuriously (e.g. glucose or protein).

Osmotic pressure

Measurement of the osmolality of blood can indicate whether the animal is suffering from hypotonic or hypertonic dehydration. The normal range for heparinised blood is 280–310 mosmol (Green 1978) but hypovolaemia is also possible in the presence of normal osmolality.

Clinical measurement

The observation, measurement and recording of physiological variables is an essential part of the treatment of the critically ill animal. The application of appropriate monitoring techniques enables the clinician to judge the condition of the patient and promptly detect any changes which might necessitate alterations in therapy.

Central venous pressure (CVP). The CVP gives a guide to the efficiency of the cardiac pump, and to the volume of blood returning to the heart. A high CVP therefore indicates either cardiac pump failure or circulatory overload, while a low CVP can indicate hypovolaemia. As CVP is determined by both blood volume and the state of the vascular bed, if venous constriction occurs, hypovolaemia may not be accompanied by a fall in CVP. It is a poor guide to cardiac output as so many other factors such as peripheral resistance, heart rate and contractility are also involved.

Nevertheless, in conditions of circulatory insufficiency the measurement of CVP, and the observation of the effect of transfusion upon this parameter is a valuable method of assessing the state of the circulation. It is essential that the catheter tip is in the anterior vena cava, at the level of the right atrium. The catheter is then connected via a three-way stop-cock to a saline manometer and saline drip which is used to prime the system (see Fig. 12.1). If the catheter is correctly placed, the saline level in the manometer will fluctuate with each respiration. Measurements are made from a reference point level with the right atrium (midsternal when the dog is laterally recumbent). Normal absolute values in the dog vary widely from 0 to 6 or 7 cm of water and, as with most tests, serial measurements are of far greater value than a single estimation in detecting a trend which may be significant. A falling or low CVP implies a lack of blood returning to the heart and therefore a relative or absolute hypovolaemia; a rising CVP that remains consistently above 15 cm H_2O indicates severe fluid overload or heart failure. In fluid overload, however, the CVP will tend to fall once the infusion is stopped. An impression of CVP can be obtained by observing peripheral veins such as the jugular vein or tarsal vein provided there is no obstruction between them and the heart; in the unconscious animal, the tongue veins may also be used.

In relation to the prevention of pulmonary oedema by monitoring CVP, it must be remembered that the

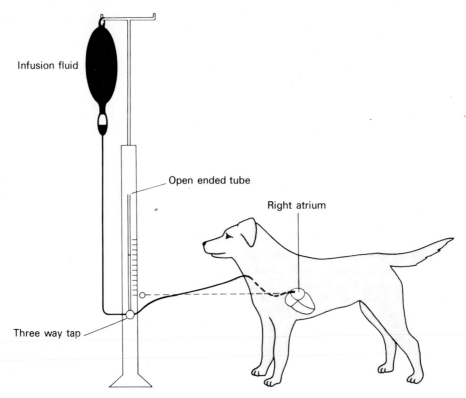

Infusion fluid

Open ended tube

Right atrium

Three way tap

Fig. 12.1   The measurement of central venous pressure.

condition can develop as a result of excessive crystalloid infusions in the absence of heart failure and therefore without any change in CVP.

Urine output. The rate of urine production is proportional to the glomerular filtration rate (GFR) and therefore to renal perfusion. Thus, the rate of urine production may be used as a very sensitive measure of the adequacy of tissue perfusion. GFR falls drastically when arterial pressure falls below 60 mmHg so that indirectly urine production is also a measure of arterial blood pressure.

Urine output is best measured by inserting an indwelling urinary catheter. In male dogs the catheter may be secured by a piece of tape attached to the catheter and sutured to the prepuce, while in bitches a Foley catheter is ideal. After placement of the catheter, the bladder is emptied and monitoring begins. Measurement may be continuous by connecting the catheter via tubing to a reservoir bag or bottle, or in more active animals the bladder may be emptied hourly with the catheter tip being occluded with a plastic plug at other times. Urine is normally produced at a rate of 1–1.5 ml/kg per hr, and a flow of less than

0.5 ml/kg per hr may be considered to constitute oliguria. Fluid therapy should improve urine flow fairly rapidly and if there is no response after two hours, the use of a test dose of a diuretic may be considered. A negative response indicates the presence of acute renal failure.

Treatment

General principles

Treatment may be divided into three phases:

Restoration of circulating blood volume

This is the first consideration in all cases of fluid depletion. In animals in oligaemic shock an infusion must be set up at once, preferably using a colloid solution. The volume which should be infused depends on the state of the animal but a rough estimation may be made by calculating the total water deficit from the history and from this obtaining the plasma volume loss. For example: a 10 year old bitch weighing 20 kg, off food and water for five days and vomiting about four times a day for the last three days; oliguria has been present for the last few days.

Deficit

1 5 days inevitable water loss at 20 ml/kg per 24 hr

$$20 \times 20 \times 5 \qquad = 2000 \text{ ml}$$

2 Urinary loss (allow for 1 day's normal loss at 20 ml/kg per hr)

$$20 \times 20 \times 1 \qquad = 400 \text{ ml}$$

3 Water lost in vomit (approx. 4 ml/kg per vomit)

$$4 \times 20 \times 4 \times 3 \qquad = 960 \text{ ml}$$

Total water loss	$= 3360$ ml
ECF deficit (1/3)	$= 1120$ ml
Plasma deficit ($\frac{1}{4}$ of ECF)	$= 280$ ml
(or $\frac{1}{12}$ of total loss)	

Thus this dog would need approximately 250 ml of plasma or plasma volume expander in order to improve its circulation.

If such a rough estimate cannot be calculated but the state of the dog indicates the presence of circulatory collapse, then a colloid solution should be infused at a rate of 5–10 ml/kg for 15–20 minutes; this should improve the animal's condition and allow time for a more careful assessment.

Maintenance of normal daily requirements

Normal total daily water requirements to meet urinary and inevitable losses are approximately 40 ml/kg body weight. Requirements may be increased in critically ill patients and up to twice this amount should be supplied. These requirements must be met daily until the animal is able and willing to drink voluntarily again.

Replacement of existing deficits and continuing abnormal losses

The calculation of the existing deficit will give a rough guide as to the amount of fluid to be replaced (approximately 3 litres in the example given). The method used here is that described by Hall (1967); other ways have been devised based on an estimation of percentage dehydration from the loss of skin elasticity and other clinical signs (Gross & McCrady 1977) but such methods are probably less accurate. However, all methods of calculating fluid requirements are approximate and the only way to decide if sufficient fluid has been given is to monitor the response to treatment.

Ideally, existing deficits should be made up within the first 24 hours of treatment. Thereafter, the volume of fluid given should cover daily requirements plus any abnormal losses. Abnormal losses include diarrhoea, vomit, polyuria and these should be replaced on a volume-for-volume basis. When possible losses should be measured and a 'fluid balance' chart kept, which records input and output. However, it is not always possible to measure diarrhoeic losses and it is worth

bearing in mind that losses of the order of 200 ml/kg per day can be anticipated with this condition.

Volume and rate of infusion

The calculation of the volume of the infusion has already been discussed. The rate of the infusion will depend on the severity of the dehydration and there is no hard and fast rule. In severe hypovolaemic shock in a large dog replacement needs to be as fast as possible and several veins may be cannulated simultaneously. In small dogs with a relatively small deficit the drip rate must be slower. In hypovolaemic shock, the initial infusion rate must be very fast—up to 4 ml/kg per min for the first 20–30 minutes until the animal's circulation starts to improve. Unless hypovolaemic shock is present, however, a gradual restoration of fluid and electrolyte deficits is obviously preferable. Even with severe dehydration, if the total deficit is scheduled for replacement over 24 hours, the rate of administration need not exceed 10 ml/kg per hr and for more moderately dehydrated animals and for administering normal maintenance requirements, a rate of 5 ml/kg per hr is ideal. However, it is often not practicable to give fluids over 24 hours and then a faster infusion rate of about 15 ml/kg per hr is often employed. In fact, it has been shown that in mildly dehydrated dogs (8–14% dehydration) without cardiovascular disease, it is possible to infuse crystalloid infusions at a rate of 90 ml/kg per hr with a substantial margin of safety (Cornelius *et al* 1978).

The flow rate in ml/kg bodyweight per hr may be converted to drops/min by the following formula:

$$\text{Drops/min} = \frac{\text{drops/ml delivered by infusion set}}{60} \times \text{ml/kg bodyweight}$$

Most giving sets deliver 15 drops/ml but this should be checked. Thus a flow rate of 10 ml/kg dog will require a drip rate of

$$\tfrac{15}{60} \times 10 \times 12 = 30 \text{ drops/min}$$

Route of administration

The route chosen depends on the nature and severity of the illness, the condition of the patient, and the time and the equipment available.

Oral route

This should be used whenever feasible as the bowel mucosa acts as a barrier for selective absorption of water and electrolytes. Force feeding of large volumes of fluid is time consuming and difficult and daily stomach tubing by the oral or nasal route, although possible, is often distressing for the animal. Therefore, if therapy is likely to last for several days or more, as in the case of animals with injuries to the head or neck or those recovering from oral, nasal, laryngeal or oesophageal surgery, the insertion of a pharyngostomy tube is undoubtedly indicated. This allows both fluid and food to be administered with ease. Properly inserted pharyngostomy tubes will remain in place for 4–6 weeks. They are well tolerated and cause few complications provided they are inserted correctly. The technique for placement of pharyngostomy tubes was described by Böhning *et al* (1970) and has also been detailed by Lane (1977).

Fluids given via the oral route need not be sterile but must be hypotonic. However, if the animal is vomiting or suffering from gastrointestinal obstruction the oral route cannot be used.

Subcutaneous route

Fluids may be given rapidly and easily and it may be the only practicable route in tiny puppies and dogs which are difficult to restrain for intravenous infusion. Absorption is slower than by the intravenous route, but provided the volume given is not large and the animal is not severely ill this is not a serious disadvantage. The use of hyaluronidase has been advocated (Hall 1967) to aid absorption from this site but it is not essential. Only isotonic solutions should be infused subcutaneously. Hypotonic saline or glucose solutions are contraindicated as they may produce diffusion of electrolytes into the subcutaneous tissue and precipitate circulatory collapse. Hypertonic solutions should also be avoided.

The presence of oedema, severe oligaemia or hypothermia (which retards absorption considerably) are all contraindications to the use of this route.

Intraperitoneal route

Large volumes may be given rapidly but there is a danger of puncturing viscera or causing peritonitis. Absorption is delayed in hypovolaemic states. Isotonic solutions only should be infused (unless for peritoneal dialysis). Electrolytes and water are absorbed well and blood may also be given by this route.

Intravenous route

This is the parenteral route of choice as it is the most effective. It is the only practicable means of rapidly restoring the circulation in animals with severe dehydration. Isotonic or hypertonic solutions may be used by this route.

The site of intravenous infusion. The cephalic vein is the most accessible and most commonly used, but it should not be used for the infusion of hypertonic fluids because of the danger of thrombophlebitis. The medial and lateral saphenous veins are more difficult to cannulate and needles or cannulae in these veins are more difficult to secure in place. These veins are generally used only if the cephalic veins have been rendered useless. The jugular vein is the most suitable for long-term fluid administration and for the infusion of hypertonic solutions. It also permits the measurement of CVP and is often the only vein large enough in young or miniature dogs.

Type of catheter to use. *Needles* are difficult to secure firmly except in the cephalic vein. Their rigidity and sharp bevel edge cause damage to the vein wall and the vein may be torn if there is much movement. Needles tend to become dislodged easily and are only suitable for short-term fluid infusion such as during anaesthesia. *Butterfly needles* are easier to insert but are still rigid and tend to become dislodged with long-term use. *Intravenous catheters* are preferred for long-term fluid administration. There are three main types: over the needle units (ONC); through the needle units (TNC); and 'cut down' intravenous cannulae.

Over the needle units (ONC) e.g. Jelco i.v. catheter (Johnson & Johnson); Abbocath-T (Abbot Lab.); Angiocath (Deseret, Warner-Lambert Ltd). These are designed for percutaneous introduction but with thick skinned dogs it is better to make a small skin incision first to avoid damaging the tip of the catheter. These cannulae are all made of flurorethylene propylene (teflon) which is associated with a much lower incidence of thrombophlebitis than the older PVC cannulae. ONC units are made in a wide variety of sizes from 24 gauge to 10 gauge and are either short (i.e. up to about 3–4 inches) and suitable for use in the cephalic or saphenous veins, or long (>8 inches) and suited for insertion into the jugular vein.

Through the needle units (TNC) e.g. 'Intracath' (Deseret, Warner-Lambert Ltd). These consist of a needle, catheter, needle guard and plastic sleeve. The catheter is longer (8″–24″) and is designed for insertion into the jugular vein for long-term fluid therapy, delivery of irritant fluids or for CVP measurement. Since the needle remains attached, despite being withdrawn from the skin, there is a risk of the sharp bevel shearing off the catheter causing a catheter embolus, unless the needle is properly secured. Also, since the needle is bigger than the catheter, there is more likely to be perivenous leakage of blood and fluids with this type of catheter.

'Cut-down' *cannulae* are inserted by cut down and are used only in the jugular vein when venous collapse necessitates such a procedure.

Practical considerations for intravenous catheterisation
1   Follow strict aseptic technique when inserting any i.v. catheter: prepare the site and your own hands.
2   Infiltrate local anaesthetic if a large bore cannula is being inserted.
3   Secure catheter firmly to the skin, covering skin puncture site with a *sterile* dressing. Bandage limb or neck so that only catheter tip is exposed: this reduces the likelihood of contamination and damage to the catheter.
4   Change the dressing daily, and the catheter and giving set every 48–72 hours.
5   Change the giving set after giving blood, plasma or lipid emulsion.
6   Ensure patency of the catheter by flushing with heparinised saline (1:100) once daily after completion of infusion.
7   If the catheter becomes clogged, aspirate but do not irrigate. Irrigation may cause local damage and expel a clot into the general circulation.
8   If there is evidence of infection or phlebitis, remove the catheter and use a new catheter and another vein.
9   Avoid giving viscous or irritant fluids via a small bore catheter in a small vein and use instead the jugular vein (N.B. remember antibiotics are irritant).
10   Warm fluids to 37°C before administration. Cold fluids not only cause venospasm which will reduce their effective flow rate, but also impose a 'thermal debt' on the animal, which can be extremely detrimental to an already sick animal.

Giving sets. Three basic types should be available: one suitable for crystalloid infusions; one incorporating a filter suitable for blood administration; and a burette type for giving small volumes of fluid accurately to very small dogs. Ideally, a micropore filter should also be available for infusing old stored blood or scavenged autologous blood.

Type of infusion to use
The type of fluid used depends on the deficit present. Deficiencies should be replaced 'in kind'. Thus blood is indicated in haemorrhage, plasma in hypoproteinaemia and crystalloid solutions in other cases. Table 12.3 summarises the composition of the various crystalloid solutions which are available and indicates their uses.

In animals suffering from profuse, prolonged vomiting, severe, protracted diarrhoea or prolonged starvation, potassium reserves are often severely d   29

although for reasons already discussed, plasma values may be normal. If plasma concentrations of potassium fall, however, clinical signs of hypokalaemia may become evident and specific replacement of potassium will be necessary. Mild hypokalaemia may be treated by offering foods high in potassium (e.g. citrus juices, meat) or by using oral preparations such as potassium gluconate. More severe deficits (<3.0 mmol/l) in the anorexic or vomiting animal usually require parenteral therapy. When administering potassium-containing fluids it is the rate of administration which is critical; the maximum infusion rate should not exceed 0.5 mmol/kg body weight per hour. Since fluids are often given at about 10–15 ml/kg per hour, this means that the K^+ concentration of the fluid should not be more than 35 mmol/l in order to avoid exceeding this rate of K^+ administration. For reasons already discussed, the quantity of K^+ required to restore the body deficit of the ion cannot be determined; it is therefore essential to monitor the plasma concentration of K^+ repeatedly during therapy and to monitor the heart throughout the infusion in order to avoid producing hyperkalaemia. As a guide, it is generally recommended that a dose of 3–5 mmol K^+/kg per 24 hours should not be exceeded (Shaer 1982).

Hyperkalaemia is more immediately life threatening as it can cause sudden cardiac arrest. The most common causes of hyperkalaemia are acute renal failure, urethral obstruction of over 24 hours duration, excessive administration of potassium-containing fluids and severe metabolic acidosis. (In this latter condition cellular K^+ enters the ECF in exchange for H^+ ions.) Certain conditions exaggerate the effects of a mild (6.0 mmol/l) to moderate (<8.0 mmol/l) hyperkalaemia and produce life-threatening arrhythmias. These include a rapid increase in plasma K^+ concentration, a co-existing hypocalcaemia and the presence of an acidosis.

The treatment of hyperkalaemia must be aimed at correcting any cardiac irregularities (as indicated by the ECG) and at the same time treating the underlying cause. In the absence of cardiac abnormalities, and plasma levels <8.0 mmol/l, mere correction of the dehydration and acidosis and restoration of renal function is all that is required. However, in severe cases (>8.0 mmol/l) or where arrhythmias are present (ECG shows progressively peaking of T wave, shortening and widening of P wave, prolongation of P-R interval, complete loss of P wave, and widening of QRS complex giving a 'biphasic' ECG with superimposed heart blocks, idioventricular complexes and escape beats and rhythms) more specific therapy will be required. This treatment aims to reverse the membrane abnormalities, restore the transcellular

Table 12.3 Composition of intravenous fluids (mmol/l).

Solution	Tonicity	Calories/l	Na$^+$	K$^+$	Ca^{2+}	Mg^{2+}	Cl$^-$	Lactate	HCO$_3^-$	Comments	Indications
5% Dextrose	Isotonic	200	—	—	—	—	—	—	—	Causes glycosuria. May produce haemolysis. Dilutes plasma Na$^+$ ∴ may produce oliguria	Used to replace 1° water loss
Normal (0.9%) saline	Isotonic	0	154	—	—	—	154	—	—	Large volumes give excess of Cl$^-$	Useful in vomiting—large Cl$^-$ loss. Use to replace half total water loss. Use to replace continuing loss of secretions especially prepyloric losses
N/5 Saline (0.18%) with 4.3% Dextrose	Isotonic	170	31.0	—	—	—	31.0	—	—	Large volume produces water overload and Na$^+$ deficit. Causes glycosuria	Use to cover normal daily requirements
Ringer's	Isotonic	0	147	4	2.5	—	156	—	—	Provides K$^+$ and Ca^{2+}	Better than saline for vomiting and any dehydration associated with an alkalosis
Lactated Ringer's (Hartmann's)	Isotonic	9	131	5	2.0	—	111	29	—	Approximates closely to composition of ECF lactate metabolised to bicarbonate	Fluid of choice for restoring ECF volume. Use for postpyloric losses and whenever in doubt
Sodium bicarbonate 5%	—	600	—	—	—	—	—	—	600	Provides 0.6 mmol/ml	Use to correct metabolic acidosis.
2.5%	—	300	—	—	—	—	—	—	300	Provides 0.3 mmol/ml	Add to infusion
Potassium chloride (vials)	—	—	—	2.0 mmol/ml	—	—	2.0 mmol/ml	—	—	Avoid if there is oliguria. use with care i.v. only if absolutely necessary. Give slowly in a large volume of fluid	Hypokalaemia (<2.5 mmol/l). Do not exceed ½ mmol/kg/hour i.v.

gradient by moving potassium back into the cells and removing excess potassium from the body. Membrane excitability can be restored by administering calcium as the gluconate salt at the rate of about 0.5–1.0 ml of 10% solution/kg i.v. slowly over about 10 minutes at the same time as monitoring the ECG. However, the effect of calcium is transient as the ion is soon excreted and it should be used only to reverse a life threatening arrhythmia.

Movement of K$^+$ back into the cells may be encouraged by giving glucose in combination with soluble insulin. A dose of glucose of 0.75–1.5g/kg as a 10–20% solution together with ½ iu of insulin/g glucose will cause a fall in potassium levels within about half an hour. Administration of sodium bicarbonate, by correcting the acidosis which usually accompanies hyperkalaemia will also promote the return of K$^+$ into the cells, as well as enhancing renal excretion of the ion. A dose of about 1–2 mmol/kg given slowly i.v. will usually produce a considerable improvement in the animal's condition. Excess potassium can also be removed by means of rectal or oral administration of cation exchange resins, or if the animal's condition is very critical by peritoneal dialysis.

All these measures are used to improve cardiac function temporarily while other specific forms of treatment are used to correct the animal's underlying disorder; they are seldom used repeatedly.

Correction of acid–base imbalances is essential if the changes are severe. Treatment is directed at restoring the bicarbonate deficit by the administration of solutions containing bicarbonate or its precursors (acetate, gluconate, lactate, citrate). Bicarbonate has an immediate effect but cannot be added to polyionic solutions as it cannot be autoclaved during manufacture. Therefore, sodium lactate is used in polyionic solutions as an alternative source of bicarbonate. Lactate and other precursors have to be metabolised to bicarbonate first, hence there is some delay before they are effective. Lactate is metabolised solely in the liver whereas acetate ions are also metabolised by other tissues; Ringer's acetate–gluconate is therefore probably preferable to Ringer's lactate in treating animals in shock which may have impaired liver function.

The amount of bicarbonate required to correct the acidosis is determined by the following formula:

$$\frac{\text{Body wt(kg)}}{3} \times \text{Base deficit} = \text{mmol bicarbonate required}$$

Base deficit is the 'normal' minus the actual plasma bicarbonate level in mmol/l with the normal level taken to be 25 mmol/l. By using this formula one is aiming to correct only the extracellular deficit of bicarbonate. It allows for a more cautious approach to restoration of imbalances and is less likely to result in over-correction of a deficit than other formulae.

If the plasma bicarbonate level is not known, correction must be empirical. As a rough guide, in a mild acidosis there is likely to be a base deficit of 5 mmol/l; in a severe acidosis it can be as much as 15 mmol/l. It is wise to be cautious in the empirical administration of bicarbonate, however, for although an acidosis may be suspected from the history it need not necessarily be present. It is always safer to err on the side of under-correction if in doubt. Excessive bicarbonate administration raises the blood pH (metabolic alkalosis) which results in respiratory depression and a shift in the haemoglobin dissociation curve, thus reducing the ability of haemoglobin to transfer oxygen to the tissues. Overzealous correction of an acidosis will also shift potassium into the intracellular space and cause a hypokalaemia, as well as decreasing the concentration of ionised calcium in the blood which may precipitate hypocalcaemic tetany. Also, too rapid an increase in arterial blood pH will be accompanied by a paradoxical fall in cerebrospinal fluid (CSF) pH as CSF bicarbonate levels lag behind plasma levels, but CO_2 levels do not. This CSF acidosis causes a deterioration in cerebral function, respiratory disturbances and even tetany and convulsions.

A primary metabolic alkalosis, which may develop with severe vomiting, is treated by correcting the underlying cause, and restoring volume depletion by the administration of 0.9% saline. Specific acidifying agents are not required.

Monitoring response to treatment

The only criterion to use in judging the efficacy of treatment is the animal's response. Laboratory tests and clinical measurements should be continually repeated to assess whether or not the patient's condition is improving.

SPECIFIC DISORDERS

Gastrointestinal disease

Vomiting

The stomach secretes a large volume of fluid rich in hydrogen and chloride ions as well as sodium and potassium ions. The hydrogen ion concentration increases when the parietal cells are stimulated and falls when the animal is fasted, and sodium ion concentration varies inversely with the hydrogen ion concentration in gastric secretions (Twedt & Grauer 1982). Mild or infrequent vomiting does not cause serious fluid or electrolyte imbalances but profuse or prolonged vomiting, especially that associated with a pyloric or high intestinal obstruction, will cause a considerable loss of acid gastric secretions. Thus a metabolic alkalosis together with a hypochloraemia tends to develop. Hypokalaemia also develops, partly because of losses in vomitus but also because the kidney, in an attempt to conserve hydrogen ions, excretes potassium instead in the distal tubule, in exchange for sodium. The hypochloraemia also means that, paradoxically, in the case of a metabolic alkalosis, an acid urine is produced. This is because in the kidney any sodium which is reabsorbed has to be accompanied by an anion; normally Cl^- is reabsorbed, but if the concentration of this ion is low then bicarbonate ions are reabsorbed instead in order to maintain electrical neutrality. Hence the metabolic alkalosis is perpetuated, and an acid urine is produced.

Treatment of vomiting is directed at the primary cause but it is also essential to withhold oral intake of food or water, in order to diminish gastric secretions and minimise further loss. Parenteral fluid therapy must also be instituted. The fluid of choice should contain adequate chloride and potassium ions. The ideal is therefore Ringer's solution, although with an illness of short duration 'normal' saline will probably suffice, because with volume replacement and enough chloride, the kidney will usually be able to restore any electrolyte imbalances itself. With severe, longstanding vomiting (3+ days) the hypokalaemia may be severe enough to indicate the need for supplementation of the fluids with 20–30 mmol/l of KCl, but this should only be carried out if the plasma $[K^+]$ has been measured.

Milder vomiting associated with gastroduodenal reflux and loss of alkaline duodenal fluid will tend either to produce no metabolic imbalance or a mild metabolic acidosis and should be treated by the administration of lactated Ringer's solution.

Diarrhoea

Diarrhoea results in a net loss of fluids and electrolytes from the intestinal tract. Animals quickly become dehydrated as not only normal secretions but abnormal exudates from the intestinal mucosa are lost. The intestinal fluid lost is rich in sodium, potassium, chloride and especially bicarbonate ions, so that a metabolic acidosis soon develops. Normally the large intestine absorbs potassium but in diarrhoea it can secrete this cation (Phillips 1972) and losses can be significant.

In mild diarrhoea oral replacement therapy with a proprietary mixture of electrolytes, glucose and glycine (e.g. Ionaid) may suffice but in severe cases the disturbance to normal absorptive mechanisms will be such that oral therapy will merely exacerbate the diarrhoea and then the parenteral route should be employed. In order to restore the existing deficit and meet continuing losses, a balanced electrolyte solution such as lactated Ringer's solution should be used, while the normal daily requirements may be met by giving N/5 (0.18%) saline with 4.3% dextrose solution.

In severe cases, additional bicarbonate may be required to correct the acidosis, and water soluble vitamins (B complex and C) should also be provided parenterally, as their absorption will be impaired. There is often a marked body deficit of K^+ ions, although there may not be a hypokalaemia because of the acidosis, but it is wisest to delay potassium supplementation until the correction of any hypovolaemia, the reversal of the acidosis and the restoration of adequate urinary output have been achieved.

Acute haemorrhagic gastroenteritis and parvovirus enteritis

Both syndromes are characterised by the sudden onset of a severe diarrhoea, marked dehydration and hypovolaemia, which can rapidly be fatal. Indeed, large volumes of protein-rich or even haemorrhagic fluid can be effectively lost from the circulation into the intestinal lumen so rapidly that severe hypovolaemic shock develops before clinical signs of diarrhoea become apparent. Haemoconcentration is severe in these cases and intravenous fluid therapy is essential. Disruption of the intestinal mucosa leads to considerable protein and even whole blood loss. Loss of epithelial integrity also leads to bacterial and endotoxin uptake and septic or endotoxin shock often becomes superimposed on a primary hypovolaemic shock. Intravenous fluid therapy should be instituted immediately, using either a balanced electrolyte solution such as lactated Ringer's or if protein and/or blood loss is marked, a colloid solution or even whole blood. Vigorous replacement therapy is continued until the circulation improves and the PCV, which may be as high as 60–80% initially, falls to around 45–50%, when the infusion rate may be slowed.

Hypoglycaemia often accompanies severe diarrhoea where there is secondary endotoxin shock and if it develops, an infusion of 5% dextrose solution should be given as well as the lactated Ringer's during the initial phase of therapy (Twedt & Grauer 1982). Once the hypovolaemia and existing deficit has been corrected, daily fluid therapy is then required to meet daily requirements and continuing abnormal losses, and up to 200 ml/kg/day may be required until the animal starts to improve. This is ideally given by the intravenous route but if the dehydration is mild (PCV 50–55%) and the animal's condition not severe, fluids may be given subcutaneously, up to 90 ml/kg per day, in four or five divided doses.

Severely dehydrated dogs (PCV >60%) are also almost certainly severely acidotic and additional sodium bicarbonate i.v. (1–3 mmol/kg body weight) should be given slowly (Burrows 1977).

Gastric torsion and dilatation complex

Various approaches to the treatment of this syndrome have been advocated, but all are agreed on the vital importance of combating the life-threatening circulatory collapse which develops so rapidly. At the same time as instituting measures to decompress the stomach, a large bore intravenous catheter should be inserted and rapid fluid therapy started. Ideally, a colloid solution such as dextran 70 or a gelatin solution should be infused initially but the type of fluid matters less than the rate of infusion, which should be fast (80–100 ml/kg in first 1–2 hours) and lactated Ringer's may be used from the outset if no colloid solution is available. Once the circulation starts to improve, the infusion should be changed to lactated Ringer's and the infusion rate slowed. Experimentally-induced gastric dilatation and torsion in the dog causes a severe metabolic acidosis (Wingfield *et al* 1975) but recent measurements in clinical cases (Wingfield *et al* 1982) have shown that this is not always so in the naturally occurring disease, although those which died tended to have a lower blood pH. It appears that in the clinical disease, the tendency to metabolic acidosis caused by the hypovolaemia and reduced tissue perfusion is offset by the metabolic alkalosis induced by loss of H^+ ions into the lumen of the dilated stomach.

Additional bicarbonate therapy may not therefore be required although the absence of monitoring facilities, supplementation at a rate of 2–3 mmol/kg, will help correct an acidosis if it is present, without causing harm if the pH is normal.

A transient hyperkalaemia frequently results from rapid decompression (Wingfield *et al* 1975) and this can result in cardiac arrhythmias and even sudden death. The heart should therefore be monitored during this period and if necessary appropriate measures taken to counteract the effect of the hyperkalaemia. After decompression and/or surgery, fluid therapy should continue until the animal is able to drink voluntarily again, which may be several days later. In this period, potassium deficits may develop and provided that urinary output is normal (1.0 ml/kg per hour) additional K^+ may be administered (20–30 mmol/l fluid).

Bowel obstruction
When the lumen of the gut is occluded, massive amounts of fluid and electrolytes are lost from the ECF. Gastric and intestinal secretions are lost in vomitus, and fluid accumulates in the intestine proximal to the obstruction. (Functional obstruction or ileus will produce a similar sequestration of fluids in the lumen of the bowel.) The fluid consists of normal secretions together with an effusion from the mucosa of the obstructed bowel. Shields (1965) has shown that the intestinal mucosa immediately proximal to an obstruction first loses its ability to absorb water and electrolytes and then within 12 hours begins to secrete fluids. The intestinal lumen proximal to the obstruction becomes distended and this in turn provokes vomiting, which further exacerbates the dehydration. Intestinal obstruction therefore leads very rapidly to hypovolaemia and circulatory collapse. A metabolic acidosis also tends to develop unless the obstruction is in the proximal duodenum when a metabolic alkalosis is more likely because of profuse vomiting.

Before surgery, fluid therapy is aimed merely at supporting the circulation; restoration of the total deficit may be deferred until the obstruction has been relieved. Oral therapy is obviously contraindicated in these cases. The most effective way of restoring the blood volume is by the intravenous administration of a colloid solution. Once the circulation improves anaesthesia can be induced and the operation may proceed. During and after surgery the dehydration may be corrected by the continued intravenous infusion of a balanced electrolyte solution (lactated Ringer's). Parenteral therapy should be continued for 24–48 hours post-operatively, especially if an enterotomy or enterectomy has been performed, and certainly until oral fluids are retained and peristalsis returns.

As these cases are generally recent in origin, additional potassium therapy is not indicated. Unless blood pH measurements indicate otherwise, additional bicarbonate is not required, the lactate provided by the lactated Ringer's solution being sufficient.

Pancreatitis
The exact sequence of pathological events which result in pancreatitis is still not clear but the result is damage to the gland and the massive release of proteolytic and lipolytic enzymes and vasoactive kinins from the pancreatic tissue. Large amounts of fluid are lost from the circulation into the pancreas, peritoneal cavity, intestinal lymphatics and omentum (Hill 1978). Hypovolaemic shock develops rapidly and will prove fatal in severe cases unless treated. Vomiting and sequestration of fluid as a consequence of the ileus which can develop secondary to the peritonitis further exacerbate the circulatory collapse (Twedt & Grauer 1982).

The fluid lost is similar in composition to extracellular fluid and should be replaced by a balanced polyionic solution (lactated Ringer's). If hypovolaemic shock is present a colloid solution or plasma should be infused initially. Acid–base disturbances are variable but if hypovolaemic shock is present an acidosis is very likely and additional bicarbonate will be required. Hypocalcaemia may occur in pancreatitis although clinical signs are rare because the concurrent acidosis increases the proportion of the ionised active form of the ion and loss of plasma protein decreases the protein bound fraction. Rapid over-enthusiastic correction of the acidosis should therefore be avoided as it may precipitate hypocalcaemic tetany. If this does occur a slow i.v. infusion of 10% calcium gluconate 0.5–1 ml/kg bodyweight should correct the condition. Other therapeutic measures may also be indicated. These include the use of clofibrate to inhibit the release of the vasoactive kinins which contribute so markedly to the development of hypovolaemic and endotoxin shock, the administration of analgesics and antiemetics and the possible use of peritoneal lavage to minimise the damaging effect of the released pancreatic enzymes.

Urogenital system

Acute renal failure (ARF)

Acute renal tubular necrosis will follow a period of renal ischaemia resulting from prolonged hypotension or hypovolaemia. Most oliguric animals will start producing urine once they are rehydrated but if oliguria persists after a few hours of fluid therapy then it must be assumed that ARF has supervened. Uraemia develops quickly and any urine which is produced has a low specific gravity (<1.012). The prognosis in these cases is generally good provided that water overload does not occur. Water intake must be restricted to that required to replace extra renal losses (i.e. 20 ml/kg/day) plus a volume equal to the amount of urine produced, and should be given by the oral route if possible.

Metabolic acidosis and hyperkalaemia are likely to develop in these cases and should be treated appropriately.

Diuretic therapy should be tried using mannitol or preferably frusemide. If there is no response however, a regime of fluid, electrolyte and protein restriction should be instituted and peritoneal dialysis may be carried out to control the uraemia, hyperkalaemia and acidosis. Although a potentially useful technique, it is not without hazard and should be embarked on only after careful assessment of the case. Detailed accounts have been published elsewhere (Jackson 1964; Osborne & Low 1972; Gourley & Parker 1977) and it is not proposed to discuss the technique further here.

Recovery from ARF is marked by the onset of a diuresis which can last several days. During this period it is essential to maintain an adequate fluid intake.

Chronic renal failure

Chronic renal failure is common but rarely diagnosed because of the large functional reserve of the kidneys. Such animals are unable to produce concentrated urine so that if water intake is curtailed for any reason (e.g. before surgery), dehydration develops quickly and may cause oligaemia, reduced renal perfusion and renal failure. Such animals should therefore never be allowed to become dehydrated. They should be allowed water pre-operatively and renal perfusion should be maintained by the intravenous infusion of a crystalloid solution such as N/5 saline with 4.3% dextrose or 5% dextrose during and after surgery. Episodes of hypotension and oligaemia during surgery should be anticipated and urine output must be monitored throughout. A fluid intake of 80–160 ml/kg per day is often required and must be maintained until the animal drinks voluntarily.

If oliguria and uraemia develop, treatment should be along the lines noted earlier. However, the prognosis in such animals is not good and it is doubtful if they should be treated for long. If uraemia and vomiting persist for more than 4 days, then euthanasia is the most humane course.

Ruptured urinary bladder and urethral obstruction

Both these conditions require prompt surgical correction and give rise to a broadly similar picture of fluid and electrolyte derangements characterised by dehydration, metabolic acidosis and hyperkalaemia. The clinician is posed the question of whether to operate immediately or correct the derangements first. Experience suggests that anaesthesia and surgery should not be carried out until the life-threatening hyperkalaemia and metabolic acidosis have been corrected. Correction of the acidosis by administration of bicarbonate will also help to correct the hyperkalaemia and rehydration will lower plasma $[K^+]$ by mere dilution. In severe cases peritoneal dialysis will not only help to rectify these metabolic and electrolyte derangements but will also reduce blood urea levels. Arrhythmias are common with both hyperkalaemia and metabolic acidosis and can lead to a fall in cardiac output and a compromised cerebral circulation. Anaesthesia can only increase the likelihood of sudden cardiac arrest or cerebral hypoxia in such cases. There is nothing to be lost and much to be gained by correcting these imbalances first before embarking on corrective surgery.

Pyometritis

Bitches suffering from this disorder are frequently severely dehydrated. There is a loss of secretions into the uterus which may or may not be apparent, and these secretions are rich in electrolytes and protein and may also contain blood. Vomiting and polyuria are also frequent features of the illness and result in further fluid loss. Polyuria is thought to be associated with immune complex membrane-proliferative glomerulonephritis (Obel *et al* 1964). The antigen is thought to be either bacterial or derived from damaged uterine tissue. Happily, these changes are structurally and functionally reversible following ovariohysterectomy, although repair may take several days.

Ideally the dehydration ought to be corrected before surgery but the operation should not be delayed unduly, as until it is carried out, excessive losses will continue. If surgery is to be performed before rehydration is complete, the deficit in the circulating blood volume at least must be restored first by the intravenous administration of a colloid solution; total replacement may then continue during and after surgery by the administration of a balanced electrolyte solution. Until the polyuria subsides urinary losses should be replaced on a volume-for-volume basis, and urine output ought therefore to be measured.

Diabetes mellitus

The aetiology and pathophysiology of this condition are discussed elsewhere in this book. Severe water and electrolyte depletion, ketosis and acidosis often accompany this condition and until these derangements are corrected carbohydrate metabolism cannot be restored to normal. Fluid therapy must therefore be combined with insulin treatment. Initial treatment should consist of lactated Ringer's or 0.9% saline administered intravenously at a dose rate of up to 20–30 ml/kg for the first hour if the depletion is severe. Once blood glucose levels fall to below 13–14 mmol/l the infusion may be changed to 5% dextrose or N/5 saline with 4.3% dextrose. Although there is usually a severe acidosis, sodium bicarbonate should be administered with care. As insulin treatment proceeds, ketones are metabolised and the pH of the blood rises. The base deficit should therefore be calculated and approximately 25% of the calculated bicarbonate only should be given during the first 6 hours of therapy. Blood levels should then be checked before further bicarbonate is administered to avoid the danger of overcompensation and the development of metabolic alkalosis. After 3–4 hours' treatment serum potassium levels tend to fall as the potassium moves intracellularly with the glucose and insulin. If levels fall below 2.5 mmol/l (or 3.5 mmol/l if rehydration is incomplete) then replacement is indicated. Approximately 20–30 mmol should be added to one litre of infusion fluid so that the potassium is administered slowly.

Congestive heart failure

Congestive heart failure (CHF) results in an increase in total body water and sodium expanding the ECF volume. Venous pressure rises and plasma protein concentration falls so that there is a tendency to transudation of fluid into interstitial tissue and body cavities. Although the plasma sodium concentration is usually normal the total body content of this ion is increased because of renal sodium retention. Dogs in CHF do not therefore excrete a saline load and when fluid therapy is indicated a low (0.45% NaCl) or even sodium-free solution (5% dextrose) should be used. Diuretics are important in the management of CHF but one consequence of using a loop diuretic such as frusemide is that excessive K^+ loss will in time lead to hypokalaemia. This may be avoided by administering a potassium supplement (1–1.5 mmol/kg per day) or by using K^+ sparing diuretics such as spironolactone or triamterene. Should such animals require surgery great care must be taken not to overload the circulation or to provoke antidiuresis, and fluid replacement should be matched exactly to intraoperative losses post-operatively. Close monitoring of urinary output is essential as oliguria will indicate water retention and the likelihood of pulmonary oedema.

Young puppies

Neonates are more susceptible to dehydration for several reasons. They have a high surface area to body weight ratio and a high basal metabolic rate, both of which increase inevitable water losses. Puppies have poorly developed renal function at birth. Their kidneys have short loops of Henle and relatively avascular connective tissue, so that the countercurrent mechanism is underdeveloped. Thus, they are unable to produce a concentrated urine in response to water deprivation, nor can they excrete a water load since their GFR is fixed at a relatively low level. Neonatal kidneys are also unable to excrete a strongly acid urine making neonatal animals particularly vulnerable to acidosis and uraemia (Dalton 1969). As a general rule isotonic solutions are best avoided in neonates. Hypotonic saline ($\frac{1}{4}$ to $\frac{1}{2}$ strength) with added glucose (5–10%) should be used. Daily requirements are 100–150 ml/kg bodyweight given in small divided doses, preferably by the oral route. If intravenous administration is indicated a combination of 5% dextrose in half strength lactated Ringer's solution is probably the most appropriate to use.

Acid-base adjustments must be made with great care as the immature kidney cannot easily deal with excess bicarbonate. Remember also that renal immaturity makes urine output a less reliable guide to the adequacy of therapy. Fortunately renal efficiency improves considerably by the time of weaning and the management of fluid disorders becomes easier.

Neonatal animals have around 85 ml of blood per kg bodyweight. Thus a 2 kg pup will have a circulating blood volume of only 170 ml. It can tolerate a loss of only a very small percentage of this (5–10%) before replacement becomes necessary. For this reason pups subjected to surgery should always have an intravenous line in place before losses commence. Losses of less than 10% may be replaced by a crystalloid solution but greater deficits should be met with a colloid infusion. A special burette-type of giving set will allow the relatively small volumes of fluid to be given accurately and slowly.

Pups are born with small glycogen reserves. Failure to feed results in rapid depletion of these reserves and the onset of hypoglycaemia within two days. It is essential therefore to include 5–10% glucose in the fluid intake of sick pups.

Parenteral nutrition

Serious injury initiates a series of cardiovascular and metabolic changes within the body. The cardiovascular changes are dealt with later, but the metabolic changes, although slower in onset, are nonetheless important. Changes in circulating levels of various hormones such as cortisol, ACTH, glucagon and catecholamines, result in an increased state of catabolism. Body protein is broken down to provide calories, while glucose utilisation is impaired. The rapid loss of protein and excretion of nitrogen leads to marked muscle wasting and it is essential to provide these animals with an alternative source of calories if this loss of body tissue is to be minimised.

Critically ill animals are also frequently unwilling or unable to eat and unless fed forcibly will rely on their body reserves of fat and protein.

Enteral or parenteral feeding is therefore very important in sick or injured animals. The oral route is the easiest and also the safest to use. Palatable liquidised food should be offered several times a day. If it is refused, the animal should be fed via a stomach tube or preferably through a pharyngostomy tube. If gastrointestinal disease precludes enteral feeding the intravenous route must be used. Parenteral diets must contain a source of calories (fats, carbohydrates) plus a source of protein (amino acids) as well as essential vitamins. Sufficient calories must be provided to avoid wasteful utilisation of amino acids for gluconeogenesis. Calorific requirements increase exponentially with body weight (see Finco 1972) but on average 60–80 cal/kg per day will suffice. Larger dogs will require less, puppies and pyrexic animals will need more. Daily nitrogen requirements are approximately 12.5 mg protein/calorie per day or 2 mg nitrogen/calorie per day (Finco 1972).

Source of calories

Carbohydrates such as glucose and fructose provide only 4 calories per gram. Thus one litre of 5% dextrose provides 200 calories. A 20 kg dog would therefore need at least 6 litres per day to meet its calorific requirements. Glucose is therefore used as a 20–25% solution, but such solutions are irritant and cause thrombophlebitis if infused into a small, peripheral vein. In addition unless it is given very slowly throughout the day the renal threshold for glucose will be exceeded, causing an osmotic diuresis.

Ethanol provides 7 cal/gram and has a nitrogen sparing effect, but its rate of administration is limited by its pharmacological actions. Its utilisation is optimised by combination with fructose or sorbitol and amino acids (as in Aminoplex 5) which accelerate its clearance from the bloodstream. Fat emulsions made isotonic with glycerol or sorbitol are excellent sources of calories. Cottonseed oil emulsions have proved unsatisfactory (patients developed liver damage and even died) and are no longer marketed. Soya bean oil emulsions, on the other hand, are in widespread use in man and animals. Intralipid is such an emulsion which contains either 10 or 20% soya bean oil with 1.2% egg yolk phospholipids, 2.25% glycerine and water. It provides either 1.1 or 2.2 cal/ml and has the advantage of being non-irritant to peripheral veins. Fat emulsions should not be used in animals suffering from hepatic dysfunction as they are unable to utilise the chylomicrons. Unfortunately the high cost and short shelf life of fat emulsions often preclude their use.

Amino acids

Amino acid mixtures are either hydrolysates of casein or fibrin or pure solutions of synthetic L-amino acids. Enough nitrogen for an average sized dog will be provided by 400–500 ml of a 5% solution, but additional calories will be required. Some amino acid preparations also contain sorbitol or ethanol or fructose as a source of calories as well as electrolytes and so are suitable for complete parenteral nutrition (e.g. Aminofusin L600, Aminoplex 5, Vamin fructose, Synthamin 7S).

Other additives

In addition to energy and nitrogen, provision must be made for electrolytes, phosphorus, trace elements and vitamins. B vitamins are essential for metabolism and vitamin C assists wound healing. These vitamins should therefore be added to any regime of parenteral feeding. Remember that B vitamins degrade on exposure to light and solutions to which they have been added should be protected from light; the vitamins should preferably be given i.v. as a bolus.

Shock

'Shock' is a term used to describe a syndrome characterised by tachycardia, pale mucous membranes, cold periphery, delayed capillary refill, oliguria, collapsed superficial veins and an altered level of consciousness. The mechanism underlying these signs is a fall in

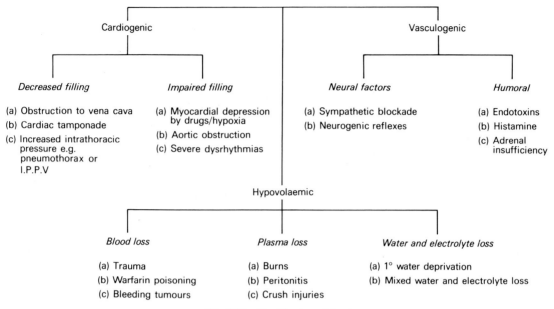

Fig. 12.2 Classification of shock.

cardiac output and therefore blood flow such that tissue perfusion becomes inadequate. Thus, insufficient oxygen is delivered to the tissues to meet requirements for normal cell metabolism and cellular dysfunction and ultimately death will result.

There are many causes of this acute decline in tissue perfusion which for convenience are often classified into one of three categories:

1 Cardiogenic—pump failure ⎫ Inadequate
2 Hypovolaemic ⎱ Peripheral ⎬ cardiac
3 Vasculogenic ⎰ circulatory ⎭ output.
             failure

The important causes of these three types of shock are summarised in Fig. 12.2 and it is not proposed to discuss them in detail here.

Cardiogenic shock is rare in dogs but can occur as a result of anaesthetic overdose. In vasculogenic shock the blood volume is normal but the capacitance of the circulation is increased so that there is relative hypovolaemia. This occurs when there is loss of sympathetic tone (e.g. epidural blockade) or release of vasodilator substances (histamine, vasoactive kinins released by endotoxins, etc.).

Hypovolaemic shock is the most commonly encountered form of shock in dogs. Normal blood volume is 70–80 ml/kg, although the figure tends to be higher in neonatal animals and lower in females. A 10% blood loss may be tolerated but the sudden loss of 15–25% will precipitate shock. A 40% deficit will produce severe circulatory failure from which only 50% of animals will recover if untreated. Loss of more than half the circulating blood volume is almost always fatal.

Pathophysiology of shock

It is not intended to give a detailed account here of the events which underlie the development of shock. However, in order to understand the rationale of therapy a brief consideration of the changes which occur in the circulation must be included. The failure of cardiac output activates the sympathetic nervous system to cause widespread vasoconstriction and also initiates the release of hormones which promote water and salt retention by the kidneys. In mild cases, these mechanisms are sufficient to restore circulating blood volume and cardiac output to an adequate level. However, if the original insult is severe, these are the very mechanisms which serve only to perpetuate and worsen the condition. At the microcirculatory level, the vasoconstriction which increases the net inward flow of fluid from the ECF to the vascular compartment also results in a reduction in tissue perfusion which, if it persists for any period of time, leads to cellular hypoxia, cell damage and death. Hypoxic cells switch to anaerobic metabolism and acid metabolites accumulate. Eventually cell damage leads to loss of capillary endothelial integrity and extravasation of fluid occurs, thus exacerbating the original condition.

The other consequence of this stagnation of tissue blood flow is that microthrombi tend to form which can block capillaries and cause local areas of cell death and tissue necrosis or initiate widespread clotting and the consumption of clotting factors (disseminated intravascular coagulation or D I C). These microaggregates may also be transported to the lung where they have been implicated in the development of a progressive syndrome of hypoxia, oedema and progressive pulmonary insufficiency known as 'shock lung' (Ledingham & Routh 1979).

In dogs particularly, prolonged vasoconstriction and ischaemia lead to intestinal mucosa damage and breakdown of the 'gut' barrier so that endotoxin shock is often superimposed on the primary process. Myocardial depression too is an accepted feature of established shock. Several mechanisms are involved, the most important of which are ischaemia due to hypoxia and hypotension, the effects of a peptide produced by hypoxic pancreatic acinar cells known as myocardial depressant factor and the depressant effect of the metabolic acidosis. A fall in GFR and therefore urine production is an inevitable consequence of shock and prolonged renal ischaemia will lead to acute renal failure; its onset is not, however, predictable.

Treatment of shock

1   Adequate volume replacement is the single most important measure in treating shock. Initially the type of fluid matters less than the speed of administration. Ideally the solution used should mimic that which has been lost (e.g. colloid solution for blood loss) but in an emergency set up an infusion with whatever is available. Up to 3 ml/kg per min may be infused for the first 10 minutes or so, slowing to a rate of 1 to 1½ ml/kg per min for the next 30 minutes. As the animal's condition improves, the infusion rate may be further slowed. In order to achieve these high flow rates, it is essential to use a large gauge needle or catheter placed in the jugular vein or to set up several infusion lines.

There is considerable evidence that a mild degree of haemodilution is beneficial in shock. Blood loss need not require transfusion with whole blood initially, although if losses are severe it will become necessary. E C F volume contracts in shock whatever its cause so ideally even whole blood loss should be replaced by a combination of a crystalloid and colloid infusion. Monitoring is vital in shock; assessment should be made on clinical signs such as pulse rate and volume, capillary refill time, urinary output and the temperature of the periphery in relation to body core temperature. In shock, reduced tissue perfusion leads to a widening of this gradient: a narrowing of the gradient

will indicate that tissue perfusion is improving. Laboratory estimations, for reasons already discussed, are of limited value in assessment in the early stages of shock. Haematocrit estimations following initiation of fluid therapy can be of value, however, in deciding whether to change to whole blood transfusion.

2   Since blood viscosity increases in shock, the infusion of a low molecular weight dextran may be indicated, although usually fluid replacement by virtue of causing a degree of haemodilution is all that is required.

3   Sodium bicarbonate will be required to correct the metabolic acidosis. If the base deficit cannot be measured, 2–5 mmol/kg may be administered fairly safely.

4   Oxygen may be beneficial, but the advantages must be weighed against what the animal will tolerate. If restraint is required, this often provokes struggling, which is obviously counter-productive.

5   There is *no* place in the treatment of shock for vasopressors such as adrenaline. Indeed, their use may be positively harmful as they further reduce tissue perfusion.

6   If tissue perfusion does not improve despite adequate fluid replacement therapy, *vasodilator agents* such as phentolamine, thymoxamine and acepromazine may be helpful. However, their use in hypovolaemic animals must be avoided as the generalised vasodilation they induce can cause a disastrous fall in venous return.

7   *Corticosteroids* in massive doses are reported to be beneficial in endotoxin and septic shock (Wright 1972). Their value in hypovolaemic shock is more equivocal. In large doses they improve tissue perfusion in the same way as vasodilator drugs; they also enhance myocardial contraction and stabilise cell membranes. If they are to be effective, they must be given in adequate dosages which means 30 mg/kg of methylprednisolone succinate every 4–6 hours or 50 mg/kg of hydrocortisone succinate initially followed by dexamethasone (5–10 mg/kg) 4-hourly. The cost of such treatment is therefore considerable and in view of their side-effects and the controversy surrounding their value in shock, their use must be hard to justify (Hall 1980).

8   If myocardial function deteriorates, the use of inotropic agents such as dopamine or dobutamine can be beneficial. Dopamine has the added advantage of improving mesenteric and renal blood flow.

9   Some workers recommend the use of *heparin* in patients who are not bleeding, to prevent the development of D I C. It would seem more sensible to reserve the use of this drug for established cases of D I C and thus avoid the serious danger of iatrogenic haemorrhage.

10 Broad spectrum *antibiotic* therapy is essential when sepsis is evident or suspected, and in view of the susceptibility of dogs in shock to intestinal mucosal damage antibiotic cover is probably indicated whatever the primary cause. Treatment should be immediate and intravenous using continuous, high doses of bacteriocidal drugs.

11 Body heat should be conserved. If the animal is hypothermic further heat loss should be avoided by covering the animal, but do not rewarm rapidly as this will provoke peripheral vasodilation. It is better to warm slowly (1° C/hr), provide a high ambient temperature (27-29° C) and warm all intravenous fluids to 37° C before administration.

Blood transfusion

Blood transfusion may be indicated in acute haemorrhage, severe anaemia or when specific constituents of blood are lacking, e.g. platelets, clotting factors. There is no justification for giving small volumes of blood especially to young animals and those likely to require further transfusions, and whenever possible plasma or a plasma substitute solution should be used instead. Severe blood loss, however, reduces the red cell mass so that the oxygen-carrying capacity of the blood is impaired and a whole blood transfusion becomes essential. If severe intra-operative blood loss is anticipated, prior collection of autologus or homologous blood can be carried out. In an emergency there may be no time to crossmatch homologous blood and in general the first transfusion a dog receives is safe since naturally occurring isoantibody titres are low. There are at least seven different isoantibody systems in dog blood (Swisher & Young 1961) but the only important factor known to cause transfusion reactions is the A factor. Approximately 63% of dogs are A + ve and 37% are A − ve. Thus A − ve dogs are 'universal donors' and A + ve dogs are 'universal recipients'. A − ve dogs will form antibodies to A + ve blood and will develop a transfusion reaction to a subsequent infusion.

Crossmatching detects incompatibility if the recipient has been previously sensitised and is essential if repeated transfusions are given. Sensitised dogs destroy transfused red cells very quickly (7-10 days) and the pups of bitches so sensitised may develop haemolytic disease if they are A + ve and are allowed to suck colostrum.

There are several techniques described for crossmatching of blood. Exact methodology varies from laboratory to laboratory but basically blood is collected from both donor and recipient and allowed to clot. A red cell suspension (5%) of each is prepared following washing with saline and

1 Donor cells (2 drops) are mixed with recipient serum (2 drops) (major match)
2 Recipient cells (2 drops) are mixed with donor serum (2 drops) (minor match)
3 Donor cells (2 drops) are mixed with 2 drops of saline (control)

Following incubation at 37-38° C for up to one hour the tubes are gently centrifuged and examined for evidence of haemolysis. The cells are then resuspended and examined for evidence of agglutination on a *warm* slide. All reagents *must* be kept at 38° C.

Collection of blood
Blood may be obtained from:

Live donors—bled as required
Advantages
1 Blood is fresh, therefore it has a longer post-transfusion life and the platelets and white cells are functional.
2 Known health status of donors.
3 A dog with a good temperament may be chosen.
Disadvantages
1 Dog must be large and therefore costly to feed.
2 Delay in collection may be critical in emergency.

Live donors—regular collection and storage
Advantage
1 Blood is always at hand.
Disadvantages
1 Blood may become out of date before it is used.
2 No value for clotting factors and platelets.

Collection from euthanasia cases and storage
Advantages
1 Large volumes may be collected and stored.
2 Always at hand.
Disadvantages
1 Health status of animal uncertain.
2 Legal owner may object.
3 Blood may contain drugs.
4 Blood may become outdated before use.

The choice between these three methods depends on the volume of blood required over a given period. If small amounts only are needed a live donor, bled as required, is best. For requirements greater than 500 ml every 6 weeks, a donor may be bled every 3 weeks and the blood stored. More frequent use demands the need for several donors or for exsanguination of euthanasia cases.

The technique of blood collection is important and proper aseptic precautions should always be observed. Either the jugular vein or femoral artery (euthanasia cases) should be cannulated with a large bore needle so that the blood flows freely. Local anaesthetic should be infiltrated at the site of venepuncture in conscious donors. Proprietary blood collecting kits are undoubtedly the easiest and most convenient ways of collecting blood. These plastic packs contain sufficient anticoagulant for 500 ml blood and have plastic tubing and needle attached. The anticoagulant chosen depends on whether the blood is to be stored. Heparin (20–30 mg/500 ml) or EDTA (400 mg in 30 ml water) will suffice if the blood is to be used immediately. Acid citrate dextrose (ACD) or citrate phosphate dextrose (CPD) must be used if the blood is to be stored. CPD is superior to ACD if the blood is to be stored more than 3 weeks, as post-transfusion red cell viability is maintained for longer (Eisenbrandt & Smith 1973). Although Owen and Holmes (1972) noted no significant deterioration in canine red cell viability after up to 6 weeks storage in ACD at 4° C, in general a three week limit should be observed for keeping ACD blood and a four week limit for CPD stored blood. If, however, 4–6 week old blood is all that is available it can be used, but it should be given cautiously and preferably via a micropore filter in order to prevent the microaggregates which form in stored blood entering the circulation and causing pulmonary capillary damage. 'Shock lung' and even DIC are thought to be possible sequelae to this lung damage.

Blood storage should always be stored at 4° C, as storage at a higher temperature dramatically reduces post-transfusion red cell viability (Shields 1972).

Storage of blood results in several biochemical changes which reduce the quality of the blood. These 'storage lesions' include a fall in pH, Po_2, glucose and bicarbonate levels and a rise in Pco_2 and lactate. Intracellular and extracellular potassium and sodium tend to equilibrate so that plasma K^+ concentration rises slightly, but this increase is insignificant compared to that which occurs in stored human blood (Owen & Holmes 1972). There is an increased tendency to haemolysis as the erythocytes swell and white cells, platelets and clotting factors do not survive more than 24 hours.

Microaggregates of platelets, leucocytes, fibrin strands and red cell fragments begin to develop within a few hours of storage, increasing dramatically in numbers after the first week of storage, and by the end of the third week there can be over 10×10^7 microaggregates, ranging in sizes of 10–40 μm in each unit of blood. Although the clinical significance of the pulmonary effects of these particles is unresolved, recent studies (Loong 1980) have indicated that they can cause pulmonary microvascular occlusion and pulmonary oedema and that these changes are prevented by filtering the blood through a 20 μm diameter filter before administration.

Administration of blood

Sterile, disposable equipment is readily available for giving blood. All incorporate a nylon net filter of 170–200 μm and some include a device for infusion under manual pressure.

Blood should be warmed to 37° C before administration; cold blood is more viscous, tends to cause vasoconstriction, lower body temperature and may cause cardiac arrhythmias. Direct warming of the bag should be avoided, rather warm the blood as it passes through the giving set by immersing the tubing in a warm water bath. Excessive warming (>45° C) will cause haemolysis.

Hazards of transfusion

Incompatibility. This may occur in a dog subjected to a second transfusion of incompatible blood. Signs vary in severity from immediate hypotension, vomiting, convulsions, salivation, tachycardia, haemolysis and haemoglobinuria followed by massive bleeding as clotting factors are consumed, to milder reactions where transfusion is followed by slight jaundice and anaemia. In the most severe form, death will occur within three days or so as a result of acute renal failure as agglutinated red cells block capillaries and haemoglobin is precipitated in the renal tubules.

Pyrogenic reactions and infections. Pyrogens in the equipment or bacterial contamination of the blood may cause a pyrexia. Viral or parasitic agents may also be unwittingly transfused.

Biochemical effects. Rapid transfusion of large volumes of stored blood may cause a metabolic acidosis and citrate intoxication. Citrate intoxication occurs if the transfusion is so rapid that the liver is unable to cope and will cause a potentially dangerous hypocalcaemia. If this is likely, calcium gluconate should be injected intravenously (10 ml of 10% per litre of blood given).

Circulatory overload. If the blood volume is increased too rapidly the heart may be unable to cope. Pulmonary congestion will develop and the CVP will rise.

This is more likely in older dogs with a history of cardiac disease or in chronically anaemic animals where the myocardium is already compromised. Previously healthy animals can usually tolerate a moderate degree of overtransfusion. In susceptible animals blood should be transfused slowly and if circulatory overload develops measures to promote vasodilation such as warming the animal may help, as will the administration of suitable inotropic agents.

Autologous blood transfusion

Reinfusion of the animal's own blood may be considered as an alternative to homologous transfusion in certain situations. In premeditated surgery where large blood losses are anticipated, blood may be collected 1–2 weeks pre-operatively or peri-operatively, after induction of anaesthesia, when it is replaced by an equal volume of a synthetic colloid solution (i.e. normovolaemic haemodilution). This blood is reinfused when losses begin during surgery.

Shed blood can be scavenged and re-cycled. This can be difficult to carry out during surgery but if there has been haemorrhage into a body cavity, the blood may be aspirated and reinfused via a micropore filter. The blood must be collected into sterile containers and should not be used if it is contaminated with intestinal contents, fat, bile or pus. Blood which has been in contact with pleural or peritoneal surfaces for over 24 hours should not be reinfused because it will contain too many microaggregates and will be too haemolysed (Crowe 1980). There are obvious hazards associated with autologous blood transfusion of shed blood but when large volumes have been lost and haemorrhage is continuing, it may be the only way that the requirement for blood can be met.

Use of blood products and plasma substitutes

Plasma. Plasma from stored blood may be decanted aseptically into sterile containers and stored for several months in a refrigerator or two years if frozen. Plasma is indicated if there is hypoproteinaemia or hypovolaemia not caused by acute blood loss. It is as efficient as whole blood in these circumstances and carries a much lower risk of antigenic sensitisation.

Packed red cells

Red cells may be removed from fresh blood and resuspended in a small volume of saline (up to 70% suspension). Such a preparation is indicated in cases of anaemia with haemodilution where whole blood would overload the circulation.

Blood and plasma substitutes

Various artificial colloids have been used as plasma volume expanders. All contain molecules of varying sizes which are large enough to remain within the circulation and exert an oncotic pressure comparable to that of plasma proteins.

Dextrans. These are polysaccharides produced by bacterial fermentation of agar-sugar compounds. Partial hydrolysis yields molecules of appropriate molecular weight. There are 3 main sizes of dextrans: (a) high molecular weight dextrans (M.W. 110000–150000) which are not used therapeutically these days because they increase blood viscosity, and tend to cause rouleaux formation and intravascular coagulation; (b) medium molecular weight dextrans (dextran 70, M.W. 70000); and (c) low molecular weight dextrans (dextran 40, M.W. 40000).

The dextrans have been in use for over 30 years and considerable experience has been gained in their use. The commonly used preparations, 10% dextran 40 and 6% dextran 70 are hypertonic and will therefore tend to draw fluid into the vascular compartment from the ECF thus causing ECF depletion unless a crystalloid solution is also infused.

The time which a dextran molecule remains in the circulation depends on its size, smaller molecules being excreted more rapidly than larger ones. Thus dextran 70 has a half-life of about 6 hours while dextran 40 lasts only 1½–2 hours. This rapid renal excretion of dextran 40 leads to high concentrations of the molecules in the renal tubules and it has been implicated as a cause of acute renal failure in humans (Isbister & Fisher 1980). The magnitude of the plasma volume expansion depends primarily on the amount of dextran present—each gram will bind 20–25 ml of water compared to 12 ml/gram of albumin (Ricketts 1973). Dextrans therefore are remarkably efficient at restoring circulating blood volume, though this is often at the expense of the rest of the ECF, especially with dextran 40 (vide supra).

Dextran 70 solutions are used widely primarily to treat hypovolaemia, whereas dextran 40 solutions, by virtue of their greater ability to decrease blood viscosity and reduce platelet aggregation, tend to be used more to improve peripheral blood flow and reduce the likelihood of thrombus formation. As both dextran 70 and dextran 40 have this anticoagulant effect, the volume administered should be limited to 15–20 ml/kg per 24 hour.

Gelatin

Gelatins were the first preparations to be used clinically. Problems relating to sterilisation, antigenicity and gel formation prevented their widespread use until the development of modified gelatin solutions. There are three types of preparations available, urea-linked gelatin, modified fluid gelatin and an oxypoly-gelatin. 'Haemaccel' (urea crosslinked gelatin) is the most widely used solution in the UK. It is a 3.5% solution which is isotonic with plasma so that interstitial dehydration is not a problem. It does not interfere with blood clotting either so that, unlike dextran solutions, there is no danger of producing bleeding or of interfering with crossmatching. Because the average size of the molecules in Haemaccel is only 35 000, their intravascular half-life is relatively short (2–3 hours in normovolaemic patients). However, in hypovolaemic states renal clearance will obviously be delayed, prolonging the effective half-life of the colloid considerably. This shorter half-life compared to dextran 70 is of little importance as repeat infusions can be given, with no total dose limit, until homoeostasis is achieved. Its longer shelf life, ease of storage and greater spectrum of usefulness compared to dextran solutions has led to Haemaccel becoming the most widely used plasma volume expander in veterinary practice in recent years.

Anaphylactoid reactions to gelatin solutions do occasionally occur and are due to histamine release.

Starch

Hydroxyethyl starch is available as a 6% solution. It has a half-life of 6 hours and appears to be similar to dextran 70 in its action. It is not widely available and results of clinical trials are equivocal. Reactions to its infusion have occurred and are thought to be mediated by activation of complement and release of kinins.

Perfluoro chemical blood substitutes

Fluorocarbon emulsions dissolve and carry oxygen, but exert insufficient oncotic pressure to maintain blood volume. The addition of a *poloxamer* solution overcomes this problem. Such preparations have been used experimentally in animals and in controlled clinical trials in humans and show great promise.

REFERENCES

ANDERSON R.S. (1982) Water balance in the dog and cat. *J. Small Anim. Pract.* **23**, 588.

BÖHNING R.H., DeHOFF W.D., McELHINNEY A. & HOFSTRA P.C. (1970). Pharyngostomy for maintenance of the anorectic animal. *J. Am. Vet. Med. Assoc.* **156**, 611.

BURROWS C.F. (1977) Canine haemorrhagic gastroenteritis. *J. Am. Anim. Hosp. Assoc.* **13**, 451.

CORNELIUS L.M., FINCO D.R. & CULVER D.H. (1978). Physiologic effects of rapid infusion of Ringer's Lactate solution into dogs. *Am. J. Vet. Res.* **39**, 1185.

CORNELIUS L.M. (1980) Fluid therapy in small animal practice. *J. Am. Vet. Med. Assoc.* **176**, 110.

CROWE D.T. (1980). Autotransfusion in the trauma patient. *Vet. Clinics North Am. [Small Anim. Pract.]* **10**, (3), 581.

DALTON, R.G. (1969). Renal function in neonates. *M & B Vet. Review* **XXI**, 2.

EISENBRANDT D.L. & SMITH J.E. (1973). Evaluation of preservative and containers for storage of canine blood. *J. Am. Vet. Med. Assoc.* **163**, 988.

ENGLISH P. B. & FILIPPICH L.J. (1980). Measurement of daily water intake in the dog. *J. Small Anim. Pract.* **21**, 189.

FINCO D.R. (1972). Fluid therapy-detecting deviations from normal. *J. Am. Anim. Hosp. Assoc.* **8**, 155.

GREEN R.A. (1978). Perspectives of clinical osmometry. *Vet. Clinics North Am.* **8** (2), 298.

GOURLEY J.M. & PARKER H.R. (1977). Peritoneal dialysis. In *Current Veterinary Therapy VI*, pp 1144–1149. ed. R.W. Kirk. W.B. Saunders, Philadelphia.

GROSS D.R. & McCRADY J.D. (1977). General concepts of fluid therapy. In *Veterinary Pharmacology and Therapeutics*, 4th Edn, p. 556. Eds. L. Meyer Jones, N.H. Booth & L.E. McDonald. Iowa State University Press, Iowa.

HALL L.W. (1967). *Fluid balance in canine surgery—An Introduction*. Baillière Tindall, London.

HALL L.W. (1980). Chapter 40 'Shock'. In *Scientific Foundations of Veterinary Medicine*, p. 322. Eds. Phillipson A.T., Hall L.W. & Pritchard W.R. Heinemann Med. Books Ltd., London.

HILL F.W.G. (1978). Acute pancreatic necrosis. In *The Veterinary Annual*, 18th Issue, Eds. C.S.G. Grunsell & F.W.G. Hill. John Wright, Bristol.

ISBISTER J.P. & FISHER M. McD. (1980). Adverse effects of plasma volume expanders. *Anaesthesia and Intensive Care* **VIII** (2), 145.

JACKSON R.F. (1964). The use of peritoneal dialysis in the treatment of uraemia in dogs. *Vet. Rec.* **76**, 1481.

LANE J.G. (1977). Pharyngostomy intubation of the dog and cat. In *Veterinary Annual*, 17th Edn, p. 164. Eds. C.S.G. Grunsell & F.W.G. Hill. Wright-Scientechnica, Bristol.

LEDINGHAM I. McA. & ROUTH G.S. (1979). The pathophysiology of shock. *Br J. Hosp. Med.* **21**, 472.

LOONG E.D. (1980). Microfiltration of stored blood. *Anaesth. Intensive Care* **VIII** (2), 158.

OBEL A, NICAUDER L. & ASHEIM A. (1964). A reversible mixed membrane proliferative glomerulonephritis. *Acta Vet. Scand.* **5**, 146.

OSBORNE C.A. & LOW D.G. (1972). The application of principles of fluid and electrolyte therapy to patients with renal disease. *J. Am. Anim. Hosp. Assoc.* **8**, 181.

OWEN R. ap. R. & HOLMES P.H. (1972). An assessment of the viability of canine blood stored under normal veterinary hospital conditions. *Vet Rec.* **90**, 231.

PHILLIPS S.F. (1972) Diarrhoea. A current view of the pathophysiology. *Gastroenterology* **63**, 495.

RICKETTS C.R. (1973). Blood substitutes. *Br J. Anaesth.* **45**, 958.

SHAER M. (1982). A practical review of simple acid–base disorders. *Vet. Clinics North Am. [Small Anim. Pract.]* **12**(3), 439.

SHIELDS C.E. (1972). Application of isotopic methods for measuring post-transfusion survival of stored blood in dogs. *Lab. Anim. Sci.* **22**, 196.

SHIELDS R. (1965). The absorption and secretion of fluid and electrolytes by the obstructed bowel *Br. J. Surg.* **52,** 774.

SPEIRS V.C. (1980). Arterovenous and arterocentralvenous relationships for pH, *P*co$_2$ and actual bicarbonate in equine blood samples. *Am. J. Vet. Res.* **41,** 199.

SWISHER S.N. & YOUNG L.E. (1961). The blood grouping systems of dogs. *Physiol. Rev.* **41,** 495.

TWEDT, D.C. & GRAUER G.F. (1982). Fluid therapy for gastrointestinal, pancreatic and hepatic disorders. *Vet. Clinics North Am. [Small Anim. Pract.]* **12**(2), 463.

WINGFIELD W.E., CORNELIUS L.M. & DE YOUNG D.W. (1975). Experimental acute gastric dilation and torsion in the dog. 1. Changes in biochemical and acid base parameters. *J. Small Anim. Pract.* **16,** 41.

WINGFIELD W.E., TWEDT D.C., MOORE R.W., LEIB M.S. & WRIGHT M. (1982). Acid–base and electrolyte values in dogs with gastric dilatation-volvulus. *J. Am. Vet. Med. Assoc.* **180** (9), 1070.

WRIGHT C.J. (1972) Septic shock in abdominal disorders. In *Conference on Shock*, p. 169, Eds. I. McA. Ledingham & T.A. McAllister. Henry Kimpton, London.

ACKNOWLEDGEMENTS AND SUGGESTED FURTHER READING

The literature on fluid therapy is voluminous and the author wishes to acknowledge the many texts and papers which have been consulted in the preparation of this chapter. Readers are recommended to refer to the following publications for a more detailed appraisal of the subject:

HALL L.W. (1967) *Fluid Balance in Canine Surgery—An Introduction.* Balliere, Tindall & Cassell, London.

Journal of the American Animal Hospital Association **8** (1972)—The whole issue is devoted to fluid balance.

Journal of the American Veterinary Medical Association **175** (1979). Several papers in this issue devoted to 'shock'.

Veterinary Clinics of North America **2** (1972). 'Shock'.

Veterinary Clinics of North America (*Small Animal Practice*) **10** (1980). 'Trauma'

Veterinary Clinics of North America (*Small Animal Practice*) **12** (1982). 'Fluid and Electrolyte Balance'.

13
Specific Infections

H. J. C. CORNWELL

Infectious diseases of the dog are usually grouped into categories based on the nature of the aetiological agent. Thus it is normal to classify infection as bacterial, viral, parasitic, etc.

Not every agent, however, always limits itself to a single clinical entity: thus canine adenovirus can be associated with a systemic infection (hepatitis) or respiratory disease, rarely both at the same time. Canine parvovirus produces myocarditis in susceptible puppies infected during the first 2–3 weeks of life, but enteritis in weaned pups and young adult dogs. On the other hand, a clinical syndrome such as contagious respiratory disease may be associated with a number of different viruses and bacteria, each a primary pathogen in its own right. Furthermore, more infectious agents have been isolated from dogs than can be linked with recognised distinct clinical entities and some agents have yet to be allocated to a definite syndrome. Until that time they are often classified as secondary invaders or opportunistic pathogens, and they are only promoted to the category of primary pathogens when Koch's postulates have been fulfilled.

There are certain periods in the dog's life when it is particularly susceptible to a whole range of infectious processes:

1 The immediate postnatal period (neonatal disease).
2 Following waning of protective maternal antibody (systemic disease).
3 When concentrated with other dogs in kennels, breeding and boarding establishments (respiratory disease).

In the dog population as a whole, most of the important generalised infections occur in the young dog. This is hardly surprising as by the time the animal reaches adulthood, it has acquired protective immunity, either by contact with infection or by vaccination. It is only the occasional dog which slips through this protective net of immunity to acquire infection in later life. Bearing in mind the above considerations, the important infectious diseases in the dog will be discussed not on the usual aetiological basis but taking account of the major disease patterns which the dog is likely to encounter during its life. This chapter deals mainly with the important generalised infections. With the exception of respiratory disease, local infectious diseases involving mainly a single system or organ are dealt with elsewhere in the relevant chapter.

NEONATAL INFECTIONS

Aetiology

Puppies are particularly at risk during the first 3–4 weeks of life. The causes of infant puppy mortality are legion. They include congenital defects, trauma, haemolytic disease, hypothermia, poor kennel management and *Toxocara canis* infestation. Certain other infectious agents have also been implicated but their relative importance is unknown: all the evidence to date suggests that they probably account for only a relatively small percentage of deaths.

Bacterial infections

The search for causal bacteria has received the greatest attention and beta-haemolytic streptococci have been the most commonly isolated organisms. Other bacteria that have been isolated from cases of puppy death are *Escherichia coli*, haemolytic staphylococci, *Pasteurella septica*, *Bordetella bronchiseptica*, Haemophilus spp., Proteus spp., Pseudomonas spp. and *Brucella canis*. It is clear that most reports on the isolation of bacteria from cases of puppy mortality give little if any information on either the gross pathological or histological changes, and there is little direct experimental evidence that most of these organisms cited are indeed capable of inducing neonatal disease in puppies. Much of the earlier work on bacterial aetiology must be questioned on the grounds that at the time virology was in its infancy and the presence of virus infection could not be excluded. Nevertheless it would be dangerous to underestimate the importance of bacteria and there is some experimental evidence that at least beta-haemolytic streptococci and *E. coli* can be considered primary pathogens for the neonatal puppy.

Canine brucellosis

Brucella canis can also be considered a cause of infant puppy mortality and, although primarily associated with abortion in bitches and epididymitis and infertility in adult male dogs, the bacterium has been isolated from the blood and organs of weakly or dead puppies born to infected dams. Canine brucellosis appears to be fairly widespread in the USA and there is a report of its occurrence in the UK. Transmission in the adult is by ingestion of infective discharges or by venereal spread. Puppies are most probably infected *in utero* following a bacteraemia and localisation of the organism in the placenta. As the infected dam may shed the bacteria in vaginal discharges and in the urine, such animals are a potential hazard for other in-contact neonates and adult dogs, and possibly also for man. Evidence of infection in the bitch can be demonstrated by culture of blood, placenta, urine or vaginal discharges and by the demonstration of a rise in circulating agglutinins. There is no specific treatment; antibiotics have been used with mixed success.

Viral infections

Many cases of neonatal mortality have proved to be bacteriologically sterile and this has led to the suggestion that other agents might be involved. It is now known that canine distemper virus (CDV) can cross the placenta, with varying consequences. At the one extreme, abortion may occur though the virus may not be demonstrable in the aborted fetuses. At the other, the bitch may remain healthy and apparently normal puppies may be born, only to develop typical distemper when anything up to 6 weeks of age. From studies carried out in the USA, some workers believe that transplacental infection by CDV may be more common among random-source pregnant bitches than is generally recognised. Canine parvovirus (CPV) can also cross the placenta of non-immune pregnant bitches but the full consequences are not yet understood. Infection of susceptible neonatal puppies results in myocarditis but this is unlikely to be revealed clinically until animals reach 3–6 weeks of age and may not be seen until much later.

Two other viruses have been studied closely in relation to their role in canine infant mortality. These are canine adenovirus type 1 (CAV-1) and canine herpesvirus (CHV). The incidence of viral infection of the neonate whether it be associated with CDV, CPV, CAV-1 or CHV is, however, unknown, but it is reasonable to assume that virus infections account for at least a small proportion of deaths among puppies during the first 2 weeks of life.

Canine adenovirus infection

There are a number of reports on the isolation of CAV-1 from cases of neonatal mortality and there is ample experimental evidence that the virus can cause a systemic infection similar to that in older puppies. Although there is some evidence too that the virus can cross the placenta the probable route of infection is by ingestion, possibly of virus shed in the urine of a recovered bitch. Carrier bitches, therefore, may act as a continual source of infection for newborn puppies. Dual infection of CAV-1 and beta-haemolytic streptococci has also been recorded.

Canine herpesvirus infection

This virus has been implicated in mild local infections of the respiratory and genital tracts. In the neonate, however, CHV is associated with a severe generalised, usually fatal infection within the first 3 weeks of life. Generalised infection in older dogs has never been recorded.

Morphologically, the virus is a typical herpesvirus and grows well in dog kidney tissue culture. Its growth characteristics *in vitro* would appear to be relevant to the disease process in the host animal since it replicates at 37°C, but not at 39°C, which is approximately the temperature of the adult. The newborn puppy may be particularly susceptible because it cannot control its body temperature. On the other hand, the ability of the virus to replicate in the adult animal in the respiratory tract but not in internal organs may be a reflection of the lower temperature in that region. Puppies may be infected *in utero* or in passage through the vaginal canal. In other instances, newborn puppies may acquire infection by contact with other infected puppies, probably by inhalation of virus. CHV has been isolated from recurrent lesions on the external genitalia of bitches; although the existence of latent infection is one of the hallmarks of herpesvirus infections in other species, it has been recorded that bitches which lose a litter from CHV infection may produce normal litters subsequently.

Clinical signs

There is no well-recognised clinical pattern for any of the infectious agents associated with neonatal mortality and diagnosis rests usually on laboratory findings. Puppies may be born dead or weakly to survive for a few hours or days. Other puppies appear quite bright and normal at birth but gradually become dull, are reluctant to suck, cry persistently, and die between 7 days and 14 days after birth. These are often termed 'fading puppies' but it is by no means certain that they are always suffering from an infection.

Diagnosis

At necropsy, a distinctive *post mortem* picture is found only in CHV infection. Here, focal renal cortical haemorrhages together with splenomegaly, pulmonary oedema, generalised lymphadenitis and effusions into the body cavities are lesions considered characteristic of the disease. In other neonatal infections, necropsy findings are often inconclusive. In CAV-1 infection generalised congestion, pulmonary oedema and intestinal haemorrhages have been recorded in some cases while in others no gross changes are evident.

Histological and immunofluorescence examinations readily distinguish CHV from CAV infections. In the former, focal areas of necrosis and haemorrhage are found in the kidneys, liver, spleen, lungs, adrenal glands, intestine and brain. The most severe lesions are found in the kidneys where as many as two-thirds of the cortical tubules may be destroyed. Intranuclear inclusion bodies are rarely found, but immunofluorescence studies reveal abundant virus antigen in the necrotising lesions. In CAV infections, on the other hand, necrotising lesions are confined to the liver although there may be haemorrhages elsewhere. In contrast to CHV infection, however, intranuclear inclusion bodies are often plentiful, particularly in the hepatic parenchymal cells. Thus, a section or smear of liver stained with Giemsa's method for inclusions may produce a rapid diagnosis.

Histological examination of bacterial infections is usually inconclusive and diagnosis rests with bacterial culture methods. Consideration should also be given to examining swabs taken from the vagina of the dam.

Both CHV and CAV-1 grow well in dog kidney tissue cultures and produce distinctive cytopathic effects; attempts at virus isolation from the liver in both these virus infections are often successful.

Treatment and prevention

There is no specific treatment for any of the neonatal infections. As a proportion of cases are of bacterial origin it is always wise as a first step to give an antibiotic cover. Antibiotic treatment of the bitch 2–3 days prior to parturition and for a few days afterwards has also been suggested, particularly where beta-haemolytic streptococci are concerned. In the case of CAV and CHV infections the administration of hyperimmune globulin to the puppies immediately at birth may help to allay the effects of the virus, but it should be remembered that in both infections some puppies may be born already affected and in these cases hyperimmune serum will probably be of no help. Whether or not administration of serum to the dam prior to parturition is effective is not known. It has been suggested that as CHV does not grow well at 39°C, keeping puppies in a high ambient temperature may be useful in preventing the disease. Some workers, however, have found this has no effect. There are currently no commercially prepared vaccines available against CHV or against any of the potential bacterial pathogens. Bitches vaccinated against CAV should confer immunity to the puppies via the colostrum. It is generally not considered advisable to immunise a pregnant bitch as the effect of the vaccine on the fetus is unknown. If the antibody level in the bitch is low and vaccination is considered necessary it may be safer to use a dead vaccine.

In neonatal infections, consideration should always be given to thorough disinfection of infected pens, and bitches which have produced infected litters should be sequestered in view of the fact that some may be carriers of CAV-1 and CHV.

SYSTEMIC DISEASES IN THE YOUNG DOG

Canine parvovirus infection

Aetiology

As its name implies, canine parvovirus (CPV) is an extremely small virus, only 22 nm in diameter. Its DNA genome is likewise very small and lacks the gene that codes for the DNA polymerase enzyme required for its replication. In consequence, CPV can only replicate in cells in which cellular DNA polymerase is present, i.e. those in the S (synthesis of DNA) phase of the mitotic cycle, a phase which lasts for a few hours only. Virus replication therefore occurs most readily in tissues containing large numbers of actively dividing cells; virtually no replication occurs in tissues with a low mitotic index. This explains the apparent tropism of the virus for embryonic and lymphoid tissues, for the myocardium of the young puppy and for the intestinal epithelium which, in the weaned dog with its varied nutrients and fluctuating bacterial flora, has a high turnover of cells.

CPV is very closely related antigenically to feline panleucopenia virus and seems to have arisen as a result of mutation of the feline virus. In the laboratory, it can be grown in rapidly growing cell cultures derived from a variety of species, but feline cells seem to be more sensitive than dog cells. Growth is not accompanied by the production of a gross cytopathogenic effect but intranuclear inclusions may be seen in certain types of cell by Giemsa staining. Replication is normally detected by immunofluorescence and by the production of a haemagglutinin for pig red blood cells. This haemagglutinin can also be detected in the faeces of dogs with CPV enteritis. CPV is an extremely resistant virus, being able to survive outside the body for over a year.

Pathogenesis and pathology

In 1978, the entire canine population was susceptible to CPV. Consequently infection occurred in all ages of dogs from neonate pups to aged animals and both myocardial and enteric forms of the disease were seen. In breeding kennels at this time, the myocardial form of CPV was commonly found, as susceptible pups from non-immune bitches met infection in the perinatal period. As the pattern of disease has become enzootic rather than epizootic, CPV myocarditis has become less common since most kennelled bitches are now immune. These immune bitches provide protection for their pups *in utero* and via colostrum in the first few weeks of life when infection will result in myocarditis, although as colostral immunity wanes, the pups will be susceptible to the development of CPV enteritis. Myocarditis is now seen predominantly in the pups of individual, non-immune, pet bitches which, for some reason, e.g. caesarian section, are brought into an infected environment at whelping. CPV enteritis is now the major form of the disease, occurring in both kennelled and individual animals. In kennels with a regular throughput or turnover of dogs, CPV enteritis tends to become enzootic. In such kennels, the resident adult dogs are immune and active infection and disease is seen in pups as their maternal antibody wanes (usually between 6 and 14 weeks) and in newly-introduced, non-immune dogs.

Infection with CPV occurs by ingestion and in many cases probably takes place by direct contact between dogs. However, since CPV is extremely resistant, and is excreted into the environment in large amounts in the faeces of infected dogs, indirect transmission, by contact between a susceptible dog and faecally-contaminated objects, e.g. kennels, wellington boots, lab. coats, waste ground, can easily occur. Some cases of myocarditis may result from *in utero* infection.

In general, animals with enteritis do not have myocarditis and *vice versa*. The main reasons for the occurrence of two distinct forms of the disease are:

1 The virus can only replicate in dividing cells and

2 As an animal develops, the cells in different tissues multiply at different rates.

Consequently, the susceptibility of different tissues to CPV infection depends upon the age at which infection occurs. Early in life, either prenatally or during the first few weeks, the myocardium is still expanding rapidly, but intestinal epithelial cell turnover appears to be relatively low. Infection during this period results in myocarditis. By weaning, multiplication of heart cells has stopped but intestinal epithelial cell turnover has increased. Thus infection in weaned and older animals results in enteritis. In both groups, i.e. neonate pups and weaned pups and adults, the lymphatic system and bone marrow also provide cell populations with a high turnover. Infection therefore also results, in the initial phase at least, in lymphocytolysis (seen as thymic atrophy in young animals) and leucopenia.

In weaned pups and older dogs, experimental infection by the oral route produces enteritis. In most cases, ingestion of virus results in invasion of the body via the oropharyngeal lymphoid ring and an initial period of viraemia (3–5 days PI). This is followed by localisation and multiplication of virus in the lymphoid organs with generalised lymphocytolysis and leucopenia (3–6 days PI). The intestinal Peyer's patches are amongst the lymphoid sites attacked and spread of virus from these to the overlying intestinal epithelium results in the development of enteric lesions (5–10 days PI). The epithelial cells attacked are the rapidly dividing cells at the base of the intestinal crypts. Consequently, there is distortion of normal epithelial production with, in severe cases, crypt aplasia and virtually total mucosal collapse. In recovering animals, there is reactive hyperplasia of both lymphoid tissues and intestinal epithelia.

The severity of the intestinal lesions depends in large part on the mitotic rate of the epithelial cells at the time of infection. In gnotobiotic dogs, with a limited and stable intestinal flora, the mitotic rate is low and, although initial viraemia and leucopenia are easily induced, clinically significant enteritis is rare. In more conventional animals, with a more varied and fluctuating flora, the mitotic index is higher and, correspondingly, clinical disease is much more common.

Oral infection of colostrum-deprived neonatal pups results in the same initial phase of viraemia and lymphopenia, but virus also localises in the myocardium where, at this time, mitotic activity is prominent. CPV appears to persist in the heart muscle and by $3–3\frac{1}{2}$ weeks of age a non-suppurative myocarditis is present. Depending on the severity and extent of this, affected pups may die very rapidly in acute heart failure, usually between 3 and 6 weeks of age, or may gradually develop more subacute heart failure at anything up to 1 year or more.

At postmortem examination of fatal cases of enteritis, the carcase is usually thin and dehydrated. There is usually intestinal congestion which may be mild or severe, although in young pups the intestines may appear rather blanched. Typically, the intestines feel thickened or inelastic and the serosal surface has a roughened, granular appearance. The mucosa may appear ragged with a catarrhal or even diphtheritic exudate and the contents may be fluid, containing floccules of mucosal debris, blood tinged or even frankly dysenteric. The ileum is often the most severely affected portion although duodenal lesions are usually prominent in animals which have suffered protracted vomiting. The lymph nodes may be swollen and oedematous or congested and in young dogs there is frequently thymic atrophy.

Histological examination reveals a severe degenerative enteritis with necrosis and sloughing of intestinal crypt epithelial cells, areas of crypt aplasia with dilatation of remaining crypts and shortening or even total loss of villi. Inclusion bodies are difficult to find. There is frequently extensive superficial necrosis with secondary bacterial invasion. In Peyer's patches, lymph nodes, spleen and thymus there is severe lymphocytolysis, often with the formation of pale-staining, histiocytic nodules in the germinal follicle areas of the lymphoid tissues.

Postmortem examination of pups with myocarditis which have died suddenly or in acute heart failure may reveal little macroscopically other than severe pulmonary oedema. Microscopy reveals a severe and diagnostic myocarditis. The earliest lesion (3–4 weeks) is focal degeneration of the myocardial fibres with interstitial oedema and sarcolemmal reaction, but this is rapidly followed (4–6 weeks) by an intense interstitial mononuclear cellular infiltration. Intranuclear, basophilic inclusion bodies are commonly present in cardiac myocytes in the early stages and electron microscopy reveals parvovirus particles in these nuclei.

In older animals with subacute heart failure (8 weeks onwards), pulmonary oedema likewise occurs, but there is also hydropericardium and ascites with hepatic enlargement and congestion. The heart itself is enlarged and dilated with pale streaks or more definite patches of fibrosis. Histological examination shows these lesions to be of long-standing duration with extensive myocardial scarring but little cellular infiltration, thus proving that the initial infection took place weeks or even months previously. The lymphoid tissues in such cases show reactive hyperplasia rather than lymphocytolysis, again indicating that initial infection took place some time before the development of myocarditis.

Clinical signs

1 *Enteritis syndrome*

All ages of dog can be affected by CPV enteritis but it is commonest in pups. The morbidity and mortality vary according to the age of the animal, the severity of challenge, the presence of intercurrent disease problems etc. In 12-week-old pups mortality averages 10%, but in otherwise healthy adults the *overall* mortality (as opposed to the mortality in presented cases) is probably only about 1%.

There is a wide range in the severity of clinical signs from the asymptomatic case (common in otherwise healthy adults) to the peracute dysenteric animal which collapses and dies within 24 hours. However, most commonly there is sudden onset vomiting with marked depression and anorexia. Vomiting is often severe and protracted and many practitioners have initially suspected the presence of an intestinal foreign body, until diarrhoea has developed. Diarrhoea is usually seen within 24–48 hours of the onset of vomiting. The faeces are usually profuse and fluid, often with flecks or streaks of blood. However, they can vary from being simply soft or pasty to grossly haemorrhagic. Dehydration and weight loss are usually marked. The rectal temperature is variable.

Without the institution of fluid therapy, death may occur in 48–72 hours. In many animals recovery is surprisingly rapid but in a proportion of cases prolonged therapy is required and some dogs are left with soft faeces or intermittent diarrhoea for some time.

2 *Myocarditis syndrome*

CPV myocarditis has so far been recognised only in dogs between 3 weeks and 1 year of age and is nearly always a litter problem. Approximately 70% of pups from affected litters die by 8 weeks of age and the remaining 30% may subsequently die at up to a year of age. Within a litter, the individual pups are likely to exhibit a number of different manifestations of the disease.

Sudden death. This is often the first and is certainly the most dramatic manifestation. It usually occurs in young pups about 4 weeks of age following a period of stress or excitement, such as feeding or play. Apparently healthy pups collapse and die within minutes. Pale mucosae, cold extremities and terminal convulsions have been noted.

Acute heart failure with respiratory distress. This again occurs in relatively young pups of 4–6 weeks of age. They are collapsed, cold and dyspnoeic with tachycardia, a weak pulse and pallor or cyanosis of the mucosae. They usually die within 24 hours.

Subacute heart failure. This usually occurs in older pups (8 weeks or more) and there may be a history of earlier sudden deaths in littermates. The pups are tachypnoeic or dyspnoeic (especially on exercise); they may become cyanotic or show pallor with cold extremities. The abdomen is swollen as a result of hepatomegaly (chronic venous congestion) and ascites. The ascitic fluid is frequently haemorrhagic. There is tachycardia and sometimes arrhythmias with a weak pulse. Electrocardiography shows low, slurred or notched QRS complexes, sometimes with extra systoles and occasionally with abnormally shaped P waves.

Radiologically, the heart appears enlarged but this is due to dilatation rather than hypertrophy. Radiology also shows evidence of pulmonary oedema.

Superficially normal. Some pups from affected litters appear clinically normal at rest. Electrocardiographic examination may or may not reveal abnormal QRS complexes with slurring and notching, arrhythmias and/or extra systoles. Some of these pups may become exercise intolerant, may collapse on exercise or may subsequently develop subacute heart failure with radiographic cardiomegaly. Other pups will show no clinical evidence of disease. Unfortunately, it is at present impossible to predict which will survive and which will not. Furthermore, whether these dogs are more likely to develop degenerative heart disease in middle and old age is also unknown.

Diagnosis

The differential diagnosis of CPV enteritis on purely clinical grounds is difficult. Some early cases may resemble intestinal obstruction by foreign bodies and it is virtually impossible to differentiate between CPV infection and such diverse causes of vomiting and diarrhoea as dietary upsets and infection with other agents, e.g. coronavirus, Salmonella or Campylobacter. Mixed viral/viral or viral/bacterial infections are not uncommon. Virological examination is therefore required for a definitive diagnosis.

In dogs with enteritis, virus can be isolated from fresh faecal samples. It can also be visualised by electron microscopy using negative staining techniques. The simplest test, however, is to examine a faecal sample for the presence of viral haemagglutinin, using a suspension of pig red blood cells. The peak period of virus excretion is early in infection and in dogs which have been ill for 2–3 days, virus excretion may have dropped to below detectable levels. However, in CPV enteritis there is a very rapid and high antibody response corresponding to the drop in virus excretion so that in animals which have been ill for a few days serology (haemagglutination-inhibition test) will indicate the presence of active infection. 5 ml samples of both faeces and clotted blood (for serum) will usually give a definite answer for any individual dog. In fatal cases, histological examination of the intestines and lymphoid tissues will provide confirmation of diagnosis.

A history of sudden deaths in a group of previously healthy puppies 3 weeks of age or older is highly suggestive of CPV myocarditis. An electrocardiograph can be used to screen suspected puppies but a quality machine is required. In the case of young dogs with subacute heart failure or mild cardiac abnormalities, the history of their littermates and of the kennels in which they were bred is of major importance in establishing a diagnosis. *Postmortem* examination with histopathology of the heart muscle is diagnostic. The lung and liver will show changes indicative of heart failure, i.e. pulmonary oedema and passive venous congestion.

Treatment and prevention

Prompt fluid replacement therapy is essential in CPV enteritis and Hartmann's solution (Ringer/lactate) is the fluid of choice since there is severe electrolyte imbalance as well as fluid loss. In severely dysenteric animals in circulatory collapse, whole blood or plasma volume expanders may be used in preference, at least initially. Supportive antibiotic or antibacterial chemotherapy is advisable since these animals are immunosuppressed and frequently have secondary or concomitant bacterial invasion of the bowel wall.

In mild cases only standard symptomatic antiemetic/antidiarrhoeal therapy may be required. The use of lactobacilli preparations as an aid to the restoration of normal intestinal flora is currently fashionable.

The only logical treatment for cases of myocarditis is enforced rest and diuresis, possibly with oxygen therapy, and antiarrhythmic drugs. Dogs in acute heart failure seldom respond, but quite marked improvements may be obtained in dogs with subacute heart failure. Unfortunately, these animals invariably relapse when enforced rest is ended and exercise and stress recur, so that treatment of myocarditis is not recommended.

When CPV first became a major problem it was suggested that, because of its close antigenic relationship with feline panleucopenia virus (FPV), the vaccines developed against feline panleucopaenia should be used in dogs. Experimental studies showed that a single dose of modified live panleucopenia vaccine provided substantial protection against CPV and the first live vaccine specifically licensed for use in dogs in the UK was a modified live FPV vaccine (Felocell). Although excreted by the recipient dog, FPV, paradoxically, has only limited powers of replication in the dog so the immune response tends to be dose-dependent, as with an inactivated vaccine. Indeed, it has been recommended that two doses of vaccine be given simultaneously to ensure the presence of sufficient antigenic mass. Another vaccine licensed for use in the UK consists of inactivated, adjuvanted CPV which produces a similar immune response to that given by the live FPV vaccine. Provided there is no maternal antibody to interfere with vaccination, antibody appears in the serum of most recipients 7–10 days after one dose of either vaccine. With the haemagglutination-inhibition test, titres range from 4 to 512 with a mean range of 64–128. Antibodies disappear within 6–12 months, the exact time depending on the initial titre. Dogs with a titre of greater than 64 are fully resistant to challenge, i.e. they remain clinically and pathologically normal, do not excrete virulent virus and show no change in their serum titre. Vaccinated dogs with titres of less than 64 remain clinically normal but excrete virus and develop a rising titre. The response to booster doses of vaccine is likewise dependent upon the existing antibody titre. A live attenuated CPV vaccine has been developed in the United States and has been shown to produce more rapid protection and much higher and longer lasting antibody titres than were attainable with previous vaccines. It is probable that this vaccine will soon become available in Britain.

Whatever vaccine is employed, certain principles should be borne in mind. Dogs may be vaccinated at any age but in pups pre-existing maternal antibody blocks the response to vaccination. Consequently, in pups vaccinated before 12–14 weeks of age, vaccination must be repeated after this age in order to ensure that a satisfactory immune response occurs. In individual pups, vaccination (with inactivated CPV or live FPV) at 8, 12 and 16 weeks will usually prove adequate. Where possible, immunisation, especially with regard to boosters, should be timed to meet expected exposure to challenge, e.g. a stay in boarding kennels. Live vaccines should not be used in pregnant bitches.

In enzootically infected premises, it is almost impossible to eliminate the disease problem in weaned pups solely by vaccination. The blocking effect of maternal antibody combined with the heavy burden of infection on such premises make it impossible to get all the pups to respond to vaccination before they come in contact with natural challenge. In such prem-

ises, thorough disinfection, combined with batching of pups to reduce the burden of infection and prevent a constant turnover of infection, is also necessary to control the problem effectively. In disinfecting, it should be remembered that CPV is resistant to many commonly used compounds. Only formalin and hypochlorites (bleach) have high activity against CPV and both are rapidly inactivated by organic material. Formalin fumigation of previously cleaned, isolated and sealable kennel units is probably the most effective but is not often feasible. Thorough scrubbing down of kennels in a bleach solution (Chloros 1:30–1:40) is probably more practical in most instances. Runs should also be disinfected.

Distemper

Aetiology

In unvaccinated populations in large urban centres, the incidence of distemper remains high and its spectre still haunts the small animal veterinarian. The disease usually occurs in dogs less than 1 year of age with a peak between 3 and 6 months of age, although neonatal puppies and middle-aged dogs are occasionally affected.

CDV is now classified as a morbillivirus, this name denoting its relationship to measles (and rinderpest) virus. The virus particle, which shows great variation in size (110–550 nm), consists of two main components, the filamentous nucleocapsid core containing the genome of the virus and a lipid outer envelope which is derived from the host cell membrane. The envelope has a fringe of radial projections which allow attachment of the virus to a target cell. Neutralising antibody produced against the envelope prevents attachment to new cells and is therefore important in immunity. Nucleocapsid is often produced in the cytoplasm of infected cells in large amounts and forms the eosinophilic inclusion bodies which are useful in the histological diagnosis of the disease. Free nucleocapsid is not infective and antibody directed against it alone is non-protective; perhaps only about 5% of viral nucleocapsid produced by the cell is enveloped at the cell surface to produce infectious virus.

Replication of CDV in the highly susceptible lymphoid cells is only now being studied in depth but it is clear that in epithelial cells the viral growth cycle is a relatively slow and insidious process, the latent period · being around 18 hours and budding continuing for at least a further 50 hours, the amount of virus present at any one time being small. It is therefore not surprising that *in vivo*, virus may be present in small amounts in epithelial tracts for periods of several weeks.

Distemper virus is a very delicate structure and is readily inactivated by heat and light; the lipid coat is sensitive to bile salts and, as it is also inactivated by acid pH, the virus is unable to survive passage through the stomach and small intestine. Hence it is unlikely that ingestion is an important route of infection.

Pathogenesis and pathology
CDV can replicate in a variety of cell types but lymphoid cells and macrophages seem to be particularly susceptible. Indeed, the outcome of infection is dependent upon what happens during the early interaction of virus with lymphoid tissue. Epithelial cells, especially those of the respiratory and alimentary tracts and nervous tissue are also susceptible and consequently the clinical picture depends largely on the degree of viral activity in these sites. However, there is now firm experimental evidence that some strains of virus have a greater ability than others to produce a demyelinating encephalitis.

Most dogs are probably infected by inhalation of virus and the earliest sites of viral activity are the palatine tonsils and the bronchial lymph nodes. From there, virus reaches the blood stream in about 2 days, probably carried there by macrophages passing along the lymphatic vessels; following transportation by circulating mononuclear cells virus is found multiplying in the bone marrow, spleen and other lymphoid tissues within a week of infection. Multiplication of virus in these areas is responsible for the lymphocytolysis and leucopenia which are common features of the disease. Subsequently, carried there by migrating mononuclear cells, virus begins to appear in epithelial structures throughout the body and, after a period of multiplication there, usually a few weeks, clinical signs referable to epithelial damage begin to appear.

Virus can be found in the brain as early as 8–10 days after first exposure to infection but usually some weeks elapse before clinical nervous signs begin to appear. The degree of epithelial and nervous involvement varies from animal to animal. In some cases it is minimal, whereas in others severe respiratory disease, gastroenteritis, conjunctivitis, hyperkeratosis and encephalitis ensue. Some dogs show a particular involvement of one system, such as the respiratory tract, but little evidence of activity elsewhere. Thus, the eventual clinical picture often shows a wide variation in pattern from animal to animal. This variation is probably related to the target sites where the virus is the most active, the stage of the disease when the animal is examined and the inherent susceptibility of the individual dog. Whether or not the development of immunity is delayed or rapid also affects the final clinical picture. Thus, if a full immune response occurs quickly

the virus may be eliminated before it has a chance to penetrate the brain.

As the disease progresses and the dog develops some degree of immunity, virus is first eliminated from the lymphoid tissues and bloodstream but can still persist in the epithelial cells of the respiratory and alimentary tracts, and in the brain where circulating antibody cannot penetrate. Eventually virus may be cleared from all tissues but may persist for longer periods in the central nervous system. This virus persistence may account for the development of nervous signs in a dog long after (sometimes many months after) it has recovered from the systemic effects of the virus.

Clinical signs
The clinical picture is variable and is dependent on a number of factors, some of which have already been discussed. A further important consideration which may influence the final pattern of events is the activity of organisms such as *Bordetella bronchiseptica* which is responsible for the development of exudative pneumonia which so often accompanies severe distemper. Not all animals therefore show the classical generalised disease which often culminates in nervous signs. In general, the clinical signs of distemper can be divided into three broad groups:

1   Mild infection
Such dogs show minimal signs which (solely on clinical examination) cannot be conclusively attributed to distemper. The clinical picture is usually of a previously normal bright puppy becoming listless and inappetent. There may be a mild pyrexia but other catarrhal signs of distemper are absent. Such puppies recover without developing generalised signs of infection.

2   Generalised infection
The wide spectrum of clinical features which characterise generalised distemper is due to the ability of the virus to multiply in a variety of cell types in a wide range of organs. Although an initial febrile reaction (usually not exceeding 40°C) develops about 1 week after initial exposure, clinical signs associated with the presence of virus in epithelial cells of the respiratory and alimentary tracts are usually delayed for several weeks. The first signs are often a serous nasal and conjunctival discharge, intermittent coughing and vomiting. In the early stages the dog may remain bright but usually as the respiratory and alimentary involvement increases it becomes listless and its appetite is depressed. Diarrhoea occurs frequently and the faeces may contain small flecks of blood. At this stage there is often a second febrile response and there-

after the rectal temperature may show periodic fluctuations.

In progressive cases of the disease, all the cardinal signs of distemper may be well developed by 4 weeks after first exposure to the virus. The nasal and conjunctival discharges eventually become purulent and greenish-yellow flecks of pus may cake the nostrils and line the eyelids; the conjunctiva are often hyperaemic.

The presence of virus in the skin is reflected by hyperkeratosis of the footpads ('hard pad'). This common lesion varies in severity from minor involvement, which can only be detected on histological examination, to cases where there is a marked build-up of keratin on the pads which become thickened with a decidedly firm edge. Irregular fissures may develop in the thickened keratin and, if deep, may be painful and cause the dog to become lame. When the pads are thickened, the dog may make a distinct clicking noise when walking on hard surfaces. Wet pavements and wet kennel floors soften the keratin so that the abnormality may be partially masked. Later in the disease, hyperkeratinised pad-tissue exfoliates, with the central and extreme periphery the last areas to do so. Although the footpads are particularly affected, the nose is also frequently involved although not usually to the same degree. In some cases of distemper, particularly in kennel populations, respiratory disease is the main presenting feature. Indeed, distemper and contagious respiratory disease due to other agents may coexist in the same population and it may be difficult to separate clearly the two diseases on clinical examination. Respiratory signs associated with distemper vary from an intermittent soft dry cough which may be accompanied by a serous or seropurulent discharge to severe bouts of coughing which may be precipitated by excitement or exercise. Coughing may persist over a period of weeks. Some dogs develop an exudative pneumonia usually associated with *Bordetella bronchiseptica* and these animals show an increased respiratory rate, an increased rectal temperature and sometimes extreme depression. The prognosis in these cases is poor.

3   Nervous disease

One of the hallmarks of distemper is the development of nervous signs which usually appear from the fourth week onwards in more than 50% of the generalised cases. The type and severity of nervous signs vary from animal to animal and depend to some extent on the region of the brain and spinal cord involved.

It is not always realised that distemper is responsible for some, if not most, of the sporadic cases of encephalitis in mature and old dogs ('old dog encephalitis'). Nervous manifestations in distemper may be delayed for months or years after a clinical episode earlier in the animal's life. Indeed severe neurological disturbances can develop quite suddenly in dogs which have had no history of systemic distemper. In these cases, virus is confined to nervous tissue of the brain and spinal cord and the animal often has measurable levels of circulating antibody.

Diagnosis

There are a number of laboratory tests which can be used in the live animal to confirm a clinical diagnosis. These tests are of course not always available to the practitioner but in an outbreak of disease in which distemper is suspected to be involved it is helpful to know what steps can be taken without recourse to a necropsy.

In the early stages of the disease (i.e. 2–3 weeks after infection) air-dried smears of buffy coat, conjunctival and tonsillar scrapings can be used for immunofluorescence tests for distemper virus antigen or for the histological demonstration of inclusion bodies. Immunofluorescence is much more sensitive than histological examination for inclusions. As the disease progresses the success of these tests diminishes. Attempts can be made to isolate virus from the buffy coat by inoculation of dog kidney tissue culture cells. This procedure is lengthy, requiring an overall observation period of at least one month before discarding the cultures as negative. Attempted isolation of virus from nasal and tonsillar swabs meets with very limited success. Since they are much more susceptible to CDV than kidney cells, cultures of canine alveolar macrophages are now used for virus isolation whenever possible, but unfortunately they are not always readily available.

In theory, diagnosis can be confirmed retrospectively in the mild case by demonstrating a rise in serum-neutralising antibody in paired serum samples. In practice, the acute phase sample may not have been taken sufficiently early to permit the demonstration of a significant rise. In more severe cases, the virus will have produced a partial immunosuppression, so the antibody titre of the second sample will be little higher than that of the first. The results of neutralisation tests are therefore seldom of diagnostic value.

Haematological investigations in the generalised disease often reveal a lymphopenia and neutropenia, a reflection of viral activity in the bone marrow but hardly a diagnostic finding. Biochemical investigations are likewise unhelpful.

At necropsy, macroscopic changes are variable and often inconclusive, even in dogs showing severe clinical signs. Atrophy of the thymus, considered by some to be pathognomonic of distemper, is not a consistent finding, particularly in the mild case. Although the lungs are often normal in appearance, a variety of changes do occur from diffuse pulmonary oedema to plum-coloured areas of secondary bacterial bronchopneumonia or raised yellowish-grey lesions of alveolar epithelial hyperplasia affecting primarily the cranial and middle lobes.

The histological diagnosis of distemper often rests with the demonstration of eosinophilic intracytoplasmic inclusion bodies, particularly in lymphoid and epithelial tissues. Of the latter sites, the respiratory mucosa and the mucosa of the urinary bladder are particularly fruitful areas for inclusions at the height of the disease. A common microscopic finding is lymphocytolysis, particularly in the thymus, tonsils, spleen and retropharyngeal lymph nodes; germinal centres are sparse.

As the disease progresses, plasma cells infiltrate the medullary cords of lymph nodes, there is increasing lymphoid hyperplasia and the appearance of germinal centres. In some tonsils, however, lymphoid activity remains dormant and macrophages and giant cells appear in large numbers. Apart from the presence of inclusion bodies and lymphoid changes the histological diagnosis is based on catarrhal and purulent changes throughout the respiratory tract with bronchiolitis and epithelial metaplasia in the lungs. Histological examination of the brain of puppies suffering from generalised distemper shows demyelination and malacia particularly in the pons, medulla, midbrain and cerebellar folia. Glial cells proliferate and, as in other tissues, intracytoplasmic inclusion bodies can be demonstrated in glial cells and in neurons. These changes may be found whether or not the dog is showing nervous signs. Some animals develop extensive areas of malacia in various parts of the brain with a predominance of intranuclear as well as intracytoplasmic inclusion bodies.

Immunofluorescence tests for distemper virus antigen in lymphoid tissues, lungs and brain provide a sensitive yet rapid means of diagnosing the disease. It is always advisable to examine a range of tissues as the amount of virus may vary and in some cases virus may be absent from some tissues yet abundant in others.

Where possible, small portions of tissue sent to the laboratory for histological or immunofluorescence examination (in 10% formalin for the former and fresh tissue for the latter) should include lung, thymus, spleen, retropharyngeal lymph node, urinary bladder, kidney, tonsil, stomach, ileum and brain (particularly cerebellum, pons and medulla oblongata).

In general, the results of attempted virus isolation by inoculation of cell cultures with tissue homogenates from infected dogs have proved disappointing. More success has been achieved by direct cultivation of kidney or cerebellum from infected animals. Undoubtedly the most rapid yet sensitive method of virus isolation is by direct cultivation of macrophages which have been flushed from the lungs of infected dogs. This sometimes permits a diagnosis to be made within 24 hours but, since viable cells are required, the lungs must be received within a few hours of death.

Treatment and prevention

In common with all virus infections there is no specific cure and treatment is symptomatic. Broad-spectrum antibiotics probably help to control secondary infections but have no effect on the virus itself. Nervous signs may be temporarily abated with sedatives and anticonvulsant drugs. The administration of specific hyperimmune sera is of little or no value once clinical signs develop. Indeed, there is some experimental evidence that this may increase the severity of damage to the central nervous system. The importance of good nursing should not be underestimated. Distemper can be an unpleasant disease not only for the affected animal but also for the owner who may have to cope with a coughing, vomiting and diarrhoeic pet which, in addition, may have periodic convulsions. In particular, affected dogs should be kept in quiet surroundings and ocular and nasal discharges gently cleaned with moist cotton wool or swabs.

As distemper is a disease of the young animal it is vital that vaccination procedures are carried out as soon as possible in the dog's life. Here the influence of maternal antibody controls the time when the animal may be safely vaccinated without fear of neutralisation. If a bitch has antibody to distemper her puppies will acquire a small amount of antibody *in utero* (approximately 3% of that of the dam). After taking colostrum, however, the level of antibody in the puppy reaches approximately 80% of that of the dam. This passively acquired immunity is lost exponentially, the titre halving every 9 days. Thus, the higher the antibody titre of the bitch the longer it takes for antibody levels in the puppy to fall and the longer they are resistant to vaccination. It is generally accepted that by 12 weeks of age virtually 100% of puppies have lost their maternal antibody. Vaccination is therefore most effective at this time but there may be some puppies whose maternal antibody has waned earlier and will be at risk.

Until neutralising antibody appears in the blood (around the eighth day after vaccination) no guarantee can be given as to the immune status of the dog. There is evidence, however, that the vaccinated puppy may develop resistance long before detectable antibodies appear in the blood, in some cases as early as 24 hours after vaccination. In areas where distemper is uncommon, the best course may be to delay vaccination until 12 weeks, but where infection is endemic the safest procedure is to vaccinate at 8 weeks and then again at 12 weeks.

All distemper vaccines currently in use in the UK consist of freeze-dried live attenuated virus grown in tissue cultures of whole chick embryo (Onderstepoort strain), in monkey kidney cultures (Snyder Hill strain) or dog kidney cultures (Rockborn strain). They are available alone or combined with adenovirus and leptospiral antigens. A measles vaccine (heterotypic vaccine) is also available for use in the dog. Measles virus which is antigenically related to distemper virus is non-pathogenic for the dog and the virus used in the vaccine is attenuated with respect to man. The measles vaccine was introduced to overcome the problem of maternal antibody. Since distemper serum has little or no neutralising activity against measles virus, the latter agent can be used to vaccinate puppies which have maternal antibody to distemper. Measles virus sensitises the immune system to CDV so that when the latter agent is introduced an accelerated humoral immune response occurs. A cell-mediated immune reaction to CDV is also set up but other immunological processes invoked are not understood. Some doubts have been expressed as to the efficacy of this vaccine but it should be remembered that it was designed to be used as a prior step to immunisation with CDV at 12–13 weeks of age; without this subsequent inoculation, the immunity produced by measles vaccine is likely to be of very limited duration.

A single dose of distemper vaccine at 12 weeks probably confers immunity which lasts for years, although the actual duration may vary from animal to animal. Repeated vaccination at yearly or 2-yearly intervals, although often recommended, is probably unnecessary although it covers the eventuality of a dog not responding to earlier vaccinations or the event of immunity waning early in a small proportion of dogs.

The efficacy of passive administration of distemper serum to confer immediate immunity when a susceptible dog has been exposed to distemper is doubtful and may possibly even be harmful. Early protection may be obtained by immediate vaccination anyway.

Canine adenovirus infections

Aetiology
Two antigenically closely-related, but nevertheless distinct, adenoviruses are associated with infections in the dog: type 1 and type 2.

Canine adenovirus type 1 (CAV-1)
This virus is responsible for the generalised disease known as infectious canine hepatitis or Rubarth's disease and is also one of the viruses implicated in contagious respiratory disease. It is also associated with nephritis, neonatal and ocular disease and possibly with chronic liver damage.

Canine adenovirus type 2 (CAV-2)
This virus is implicated in some cases of contagious respiratory disease but not with systemic infection.

The relative prevalence of the two strains of adenoviruses is unknown. Both agents have a typical adenovirus structure and differ only in the length of the fibre antigen. Characteristically, they produce large basophilic intranuclear inclusion bodies in infected cells, a finding which is useful in the histological diagnosis of the disease. The canine adenoviruses are much more stable than distemper virus. They can be distinguished by haemagglutination-inhibition tests although partial cross-neutralisation occurs. Under moist conditions, but out of direct sunlight, the virus may be expected to remain infective for up to 10 days. This is important when considering transmission of CAV-1, which is often excreted in the urine.

Systemic CAV-1 infection (infectious canine hepatitis)
All strains of CAV-1 are very closely related antigenically so that for all practical purposes the virus can be regarded as existing in only one antigenic type. However, very minor antigenic differences can be demonstrated among strains of CAV-1 when the kinetics of neutralisation are compared.

Serological studies have indicated that infection with CAV-1 is widespread in the unvaccinated dog population in the UK. The proportion of dogs which become obviously ill with systemic CAV infection is, however, very small; within this small proportion, mortality is high. Like distemper, systemic adenovirus infection is a disease principally of the young dog and most cases occur in animals of less than 1 year of age. CAV-1 is also involved in some cases of neonatal and respiratory disease.

Pathogenesis and pathology
Virus can be excreted in the saliva, faeces and urine and therefore these are all possible sources of infection. The importance of urine as a vehicle for transmission of virus should not be minimised as virus can be excreted in the urine for more than 6 months after a dog has recovered from infection. Ingestion is the most likely route of infection. Inhalation of virus is important in the respiratory form of the disease but whether or not it is an important factor in the spread

of the systemic form of disease is unknown. From experimental studies, it has been shown that susceptible puppies will not develop the systemic form of the disease if kept in separate pens from infected dogs, provided adequate measures are taken to prevent mechanical transmission of infected faeces and urine. Thus actual dog-to-dog contact or contact with infected material must occur before transmission can take place. Respiratory and systemic forms of CAV-1 infection rarely, if at all, occur in the same animal and it is likely that the development of respiratory signs or systemic infection may depend on the route of infection.

Initial viral multiplication appears in the tonsils and subsequently the retropharyngeal and cervical lymph nodes. There is also some evidence to support the view that virus may bypass the pharynx to reach the intestine where initial multiplication of virus occurs in the Peyer's patches and subsequently in the mesenteric lymph node. Viral multiplication in lymphoid tissue reaches a peak 2–3 days after infection. At this time there may be a low grade tonsillitis and regional lymphadenitis. Virus then appears in the bloodstream and viraemia reaches a peak about 5–7 days after infection. In the blood, the virus is associated with circulating mononuclear cells. Viraemia heralds the appearance of the clinical phase of the disease, and at this time there is a leucopenia probably associated with the presence of virus in the bone marrow. In mild cases, the animal may recover at this stage, with few if any clinical signs and elimination of virus from lymphoid tissues and blood. In severe cases, virus is transported by the mononuclear cells to invade three main target areas: the liver, vascular endothelium and lymphoid tissue. It is the prolific multiplication of virus in these areas that gives rise to most of the clinical features of the disease. The main organ for virus attack is the liver where focal areas of hepatocellular destruction sometimes coalesce into widespread areas of necrosis. The liver becomes enlarged and mottled in appearance due to the necrotising lesions. Characteristically, numerous intranuclear inclusion bodies are found in the hepatic and Kupffer cells. In approximately 35% of severe cases, jaundice develops as a result of both damage to liver cells and obstruction to biliary channels. Widespread invasion of vascular endothelial cells throughout the body results in leakage of fluid, fibrin and red cells into the perivascular spaces. Serous or serofibrinous effusions are found in the pericardial sac and in the thoracic and abdominal cavities. Strands of fibrin are often found adhering to the surface of the liver and between its lobes. In some cases there may be marked haemorrhage into the abdominal cavity, and small ecchymotic haemorrhages are often found

in the thymus, lungs, brain, epicardium and endocardium. Further evidence of vascular damage can often be seen in the thymus and wall of the gall bladder which are often markedly oedematous. Generalised lymph node involvement is seen in most cases; the lymph nodes are enlarged, oedematous and often show pinpoint haemorrhages. A striking feature on histological examination of the medullary sinuses is erythrophagocytosis. At this stage of the disease (i.e. between the sixth and eighth day), severely affected animals succumb. In less severe cases which are destined to recover (probably the majority of animals) virus has disappeared from the liver, vascular endothelium and lymphoid tissue by 10 days after infection.

At the time antibody begins to appear in the blood, a number of immunologically linked lesions are superimposed on the existing systemic infection. During the initial period of antibody production (i.e. from about 6 days after infection), circulating immune complexes are formed. These are deposited in the mesangial region of the renal glomeruli to produce an immune complex glomerulonephritis. IgG, complement and viral antigen can all be detected by immunofluorescence in the glomeruli and, at the same time, there is some degree of mesangial proliferation. This lesion, which is associated with an elevation in blood urea levels and a proteinuria, is transient in nature and as far as is known does not lead to any permanent glomerular damage, although deposition of IgG may persist for some weeks.

In addition to an immunologically mediated glomerular lesion and often occurring at the same time, the kidneys of recovering dogs may show a focal interstitial nephritis associated with persistence of infectious virus in the renal tubules. Approximately 70% of recovering dogs show this lesion, which reaches a peak between 10 and 15 days after infection. It has been recognised for many years that dogs recovering from systemic CAV infection may excrete virus in the urine for many months despite the presence of circulating antibody. Although there is no conclusive evidence that virus may be associated with progressive renal disease, the shedding of infectious virus by recovered dogs proves a constant threat to unvaccinated animals. Unlike the glomerular lesion which is a type 3 hypersensitivity reaction, the interstitial lesion bears many of the hallmarks of a cell-mediated type 4 hypersensitivity reaction in which epithelial cells containing virus antigen are surrounded by large populations of macrophages, lymphocytes and plasma cells; the latter cells are known to produce antiviral antibody.

A further hurdle for the recovering dog to surmount before complete recovery is ensured is the development of corneal oedema ('blue eye'). This is quite a common sequel to systemic CAV infection, and occurs in approximately 20% of recovering animals within 2–3 weeks of infection and reflects a local immunological reaction in the anterior segment of the eye. The corneal opacity may be unilateral or bilateral, but fortunately it is usually transient and disappears within a few days. Occasionally, the lesion may become more protracted with severe ocular reactions and permanent impairment of vision. The lesion occurs in all breeds although it has been suggested that the Afghan Hound is particularly susceptible. Oedema of the cornea appears to follow the interaction of virus antigen in the corneal endothelium and antibody which has leaked into the aqueous humour. Immune complexes are formed which together with complement factors attract macrophages and neutrophils into the anterior chamber. Damage to the corneal endothelium allows fluid to accumulate in the corneal stroma with consequent opacity of the cornea.

Finally, some experimental work has suggested the possibility that infection of partially immune dogs may be followed by progressive liver disease. There is, however, no evidence as yet that natural cases of chronic liver disease are directly or indirectly associated with CAV-1 infection.

Clinical signs

Mild forms of the disease are difficult to diagnose solely on clinical examination. In these cases a slight malaise, partial anorexia and transient elevation in rectal temperature may be the only features. These mild cases invariably recover and sometimes the disease may be diagnosed retrospectively by the appearance of unilateral or bilateral corneal opacity.

In severe cases, the clinical picture is much more conspicuous with usually the sudden onset of extreme depression, total anorexia and thirst. Some animals die suddenly without any previous clinical signs. Intermittent emesis invariably occurs and, in terminal cases, the vomitus may contain blood. Extreme pallor of the mucosae is also a feature and examination of the oral cavity may show tiny gingival haemorrhages. In the later stages of the disease, the dog is sometimes jaundiced. Early in the course of the disease an elevated temperature which reaches more than 40°C is a common finding; terminally, the temperature drops to below normal and at this time the pulse is fast and weak. Examination of the abdomen is very important. Palpation of the anterior abdomen usually elicits pain and, because of the abdominal discomfort, the animal is often restless. Abdominal pain is associated with enlargement of the liver which may extend well beyond the last rib. In some cases there may be massive abdominal effusions which may be detected by percus-

sion. Other signs which occur less frequently are hyperaemia of the tonsils, diarrhoea sometimes flecked with blood and nervous signs in the form of hyperexcitability, posterior incoordination and convulsions. Nervous signs are, however, uncommon and appear to be related to the occurrence of perivascular haemorrhage in the brain. The prognosis in these severe cases is extremely poor.

Diagnosis

A young dog which shows sudden collapse, pallor of the mucosae, high rectal temperature and abdominal pain suggests systemic adenovirus infection. Only cases of severe early CPV infection, warfarin (and other) poisoning and major abdominal catastrophies such as intussusception and acute alimentary obstruction may be confused with the severe form of the disease. Cases which show jaundice may be confused with *Leptospira icterohaemorrhagiae* infection while those showing pyrexia, vomiting and convulsions may be suspected of suffering from canine distemper infection. A pyrexic animal showing abdominal pain and a palpably enlarged liver may also be confused with salmonellosis or the rare case of generalised toxoplasmosis. In the less severe case, the development of corneal opacity may help in retrospect to identify a previously undiagnosed mild infection.

In a suspected case of systemic adenovirus infection a number of steps can be taken to confirm the diagnosis in the live animal. On haematological examination, one of the features of the disease is a marked reduction in the number of circulating leucocytes. This leucopenia usually accompanies the febrile response and the viraemic phase of the disease; total white cell count may fall to less than 3000 mm³. There is both a neutropenia and lymphopenia. This reduction in the number of white cells is usually followed by a lymphocytosis during the recovery period of the disease. In addition to leucopenia an elevation in erythrocyte sedimentation rate and an increased clotting time may also be expected. Examination of buffy coat smears by immunofluorescence for the presence of virus antigen in circulating mononuclear cells is a rapid but not very reliable test. Similar tests can also be applied to smears of tonsillar scrapings, but this is usually even less reliable. Serum biochemical analysis often shows elevation in enzymes such as glutamic oxaloacetic transaminase (aspartate transaminase) and glutamic pyruvic transaminase (alanine transaminase); the latter is due to necrosis of hepatic tissue. There is often an elevation in circulating bilirubin and an associated bilirubinuria. Biochemical analysis of urine often shows a moderate proteinuria due, in the main, to lytic damage to the glomeruli by the virus and, during the early recovery period of the disease, to the deposition in the glomeruli of circulating immune complexes. This leakage of protein rapidly disappears with the waning of the glomerular lesions. In a similar fashion, bilirubin reflecting liver damage can also be detected in urine samples. The levels of albumin and bilirubin in the urine, however, vary from animal to animal. Haematological and biochemical tests although helpful are time consuming, expensive and are often inconclusive. Their value is therefore limited and a clear-cut laboratory diagnosis can only be achieved by other methods such as virus isolation from blood or urine samples or even from a liver biopsy.

Diagnosis can be confirmed retrospectively in the recovered animal by demonstrating a rise in circulating antibody; paired serum samples taken at an interval of at least 2 weeks are used. The serum neutralisation test is unquestionably the most sensitive test but meaningful results have also been achieved with the haemagglutination-inhibition, complement fixation, gel diffusion and indirect immunofluorescence tests.

In severe cases, a clinical diagnosis is usually confirmed at necropsy where a characteristic picture of hepatitis, lymphadenitis and perivascular haemorrhage is often found. An enlarged mottled liver with strands of fibrin between the lobes and oedema of the wall of the gall bladder is usually thought enough to confirm a clinical diagnosis. The most characteristic feature on histological examination is the presence of intranuclear inclusions which are particularly prevalent in the liver parenchymal cells. A rapid diagnosis can be achieved at necropsy by examining smears of liver for the presence of these inclusions using Giemsa's stain or, better still, immunofluorescence. Inclusions and virus antigen are also found throughout the vascular endothelium but particularly in that of the renal glomeruli. As the virus grows well in dog kidney tissue culture with the characteristic cytopathic effect appearing in a few days, virus isolation from the liver is often successful. As virus persists in the kidneys for long periods after infection, isolation from kidney homogenates or, if possible, by direct cultivation of a kidney removed from an animal as soon as possible after death, often meets with success.

Treatment and prevention

There is no useful treatment directed specifically against the virus. Large doses of hyperimmune serum have been used, mainly without success, as by the time the animal is clinically ill the virus has already invaded its target cells where antibody cannot penetrate. Administration of antiserum to unvaccinated puppies exposed to an infected dog will give protection for a short time which depends on the titre of antibody, but it may interfere with subsequent vaccination. Treatment is thus usually directed against individual clinical signs. Intravenous administration of glucose saline, and where possible whole blood, may help to control the haemorrhage and fluid loss. The progress of the disease is so rapid that secondary bacterial invasion is not usually a problem and antibiotics, consequently, are not usually indicated. In general terms, the use of corticosteroids in virus infections is not considered beneficial nor indeed safe. Treatment of the occasional protracted ocular lesion is dealt with in Chapter 4.

The two types of CAV are closely related antigenically so that a solid immunity to one gives an almost equally solid immunity to the other. CAV-1 vaccine is either formol-inactivated or attenuated by prolonged passage in dog kidney and pig kidney tissue culture. Several manufacturers now produce adjuvanted inactivated CAV-1 vaccines and claim that they can be given in a single dose though, even after two doses, the antibody titres tend to be lower than those produced by live vaccines and do not last for so long. Nevertheless, it has been shown experimentally that inactivated CAV-1 provides a solid immunity against hepatitis even when challenge is delayed until as late as 12 months after the antibody titre has fallen to a non-detectable level. On the other hand, inactivated virus does not produce such a good immunity to respiratory adenovirus infections. The live vaccine provides a solid immunity within about eight days, not only to hepatitis but also to the respiratory form of CAV infection. In some dogs at least, high antibody titres may persist for life, even in the absence of re-exposure.

The advantage of using dead vaccine is that it is free from side-effects. The use of the live attenuated virus vaccine has been associated with two unwanted, although not necessarily serious, side-effects. There is now good evidence that the use of the live vaccine may result in some cases in a mild nephropathy characterised by focal infiltrates into the renal interstitium of lymphocytes and plasma cells. There is no evidence that this lesion progresses to produce renal failure or indeed that it is a common occurrence. However, virus may be excreted in the urine of these dogs and while there is yet no evidence of reversion to virulence, the shedding of virus, albeit attenuated, into the environment is not acceptable to some veterinarians. Of more clinical importance and the subject of great controversy, is the association of the use of live attenuated vaccine and corneal oedema ('blue eye'). There is no doubt that this association exists but it is still not clear how many dogs develop this lesion following vaccination. The lesion, which may be unilateral or bilateral, usually appears within a month after vaccination and usually disappears in a few days (see also Chapter 4). The mechanism by which the lesion is produced is similar to that observed in natural cases of systemic adenovirus infection by virulent virus. This has led to the suggestion that all cases of corneal oedema following vaccination are due to the dog's exposure to virulent virus at about the same time. All the evidence, however, clearly points to a relationship between vaccinal strains and corneal oedema.

In order to preserve the benefits inherent in the use of a live CAV vaccine and at the same time overcome the undesirable side-effects which follow its use, two quite independent developments have recently taken place. By passage in a canine cell-line, a stable variant of CAV-1 that does not produce a viraemia and hence cannot reach the eye or kidney has been selected and forms the basis of the vaccine now marketed by one pharmaceutical company. Other manufacturers now use live CAV-2 virus which provides an excellent immunity to hepatitis and to respiratory infection and which has no tropism for the eye or kidney.

As with distemper vaccine, the influence of maternal antibody must be considered and it is usual to administer both vaccines at the same time (i.e. at 12 weeks of age). Most evidence indicates that the live attenuated vaccine does not interfere with establishment of immunity to distemper virus where both are administered in a dual vaccine. Unlike the distemper vaccine, CAV vaccines do not induce early protection, and at least 8 days, preferably 10, should be allowed for the development of immunity.

The role of canine adenoviruses in neonatal and respiratory diseases will be dealt with elsewhere.

Leptospirosis

Aetiology

Leptospirosis has a worldwide distribution and is an important zoonosis. Although many pathogenic serotypes have now been recognised in man and animals only two are considered to be of importance in the dog:

1   Serotype *canicola* which is mainly associated with acute interstitial nephritis.
2   Serotype *icterohaemorrhagiae* which principally affects the liver and is associated with jaundice and haemorrhage.

It is true to say, however, that there may be no clear-cut distinction between these diseases as serotype *canicola* can be associated with jaundice and serotype *icterohaemorrhagiae* with kidney disease.

Before the introduction of antibiotics and vaccination procedures, the incidence of infection by these serotypes was high but it is now probably much lower. The two serotypes are indistinguishable from each other morphologically. Special methods such as dark-ground microscopy or silver impregnation techniques are needed to visualise them as they are extremely slender organisms. Special culture methods are also necessary to grow the organisms. Leptospirae can penetrate the mucosa of the alimentary tract, conjunctivae and nasopharynx. Transplacental and venereal transmission has been recorded in leptospiral infections in other species with different serotypes. Whether or not this occurs in the dog is uncertain. The organisms are also able to pass through the skin, especially if the latter is traumatised. Infected urine appears to be an important vehicle of transmission and infected dogs can shed the organisms in the urine for long periods. The acid nature of canine urine, however, rapidly destroys leptospirae and their prolonged survival in voided urine is consequently dependent on dilution with water. Leptospirae are readily inactivated by direct sunlight, desiccation, and disinfection and appear to require adequate moisture, neutral pH and a temperature of 25°C or below for survival outside the host. It must be remembered, too, that both serotypes can infect man and therefore their presence in the dog population is of importance to public health.

1   *Leptospira canicola* infection: acute interstitial nephritis

Although the incidence of this disease is now fortunately low, it still occurs sporadically in young dogs in urban areas. It is likely, however, that most infected dogs suffer from a mild or subclinical infection rather than the severe acute infection which sometimes leads to renal failure. It is largely a disease of the town dog.

Pathogenesis and pathology

Ingestion or inhalation of infected material, particularly urine, is probably the most likely route of infection. There follows a period of leptospiraemia which usually lasts for about a week before the organisms penetrate the proximal epithelial tubules of the renal cortex. These respond by becoming swollen and necrotic. It is the presence of large numbers of leptospirae in the tubules which stimulates the massive cellular infiltration into the renal interstitium. The infiltrates consist of large numbers of macrophages, lymphocytes and plasma cells. These cellular infiltrates are manifest at necropsy as white foci in the renal cortex; in severe cases these foci coalesce to produce much more extensive white deposits in the deep cortex. At this stage, the kidneys are often markedly swollen. Immunofluorescence tests demonstrate leptospiral antigen in the kidneys as whole leptospirae in the renal tubules, as granular deposits of antigen in the cytoplasm of macrophages and as large extracellular clumps in the interstitium. The latter which also contain IgG appear to represent necrosed leptospirae-containing tubules flooded with antileptospiral antibody. Acid eluates of homogenised renal cortex show the presence of antileptospiral antibody when examined by the agglutination-lysis test. The cellular infiltrate appears to fulfil two important functions: the production by plasma cells of antibody directed against *L. canicola*; and phagocytosis by macrophages of cell debris and presumably leptospiral antigen–antibody complexes. At this time, affected animals shed leptospirae into the urine where they can be detected by dark-ground microscopy. Leptospiruria may persist in some cases for many weeks. There is still some controversy as to whether or not acute leptospiral nephritis is succeeded, in those dogs which recover, by progressive renal fibrosis and the end-stage kidney, usually referred to as chronic interstitial nephritis. Although direct experimental evidence is lacking some natural acute cases have been followed through to the chronic stage and it is now generally accepted that at least some cases of chronic interstitial nephritis are associated with a prior leptospiral infection. Chronic renal nephropathy will be considered in Chapter 15.

Clinical signs

Mild cases may show only a vague illness of a few days and subsequent recovery. Severe cases are pyrexic in the early stages and develop extreme depression and thirst. Vomiting and oliguria are often noted and there may be abdominal pain associated with swelling of the kidneys. Examination of the mouth of uraemic cases often shows lingual and/or oral ulcers and there is usually halitosis. Occasionally a dog may show jaundice but this is more usually associated with infection by serotype *icterohaemorrhagiae*.

Diagnosis

Mild cases are difficult to diagnose purely on clinical examination. A young unvaccinated dog which suddenly becomes depressed, vomits and shows uraemic stomatitis or glossitis, strongly suggests *L. canicola* infection. These cases have to be differentiated from the severe case of systemic adenovirus infection, particularly as abdominal pain may be found in both cases, although in the latter there are no uraemic oral lesions.

Severe intoxication should also be considered in the differential diagnosis.

In life, a number of steps can be taken to confirm the clinical diagnosis. In the leptospiraemic phase of the disease, the organism may be demonstrated directly in blood smears by means of dark-ground microscopy, silver staining techniques or immunofluorescence. The value of these tests, however, is limited. Suitable laboratory culture media such as Schuffner's medium may be inoculated with blood or urine, but prolonged culture is often necessary before successful isolation of leptospirae is obtained. Possibly the simplest yet most sensitive aid to diagnosis is the demonstration of raised antibody levels when paired serum samples are examined by the agglutination-lysis test. Likewise, the demonstration of leptospirae in urine sediments by dark-ground microscopy, silver techniques or immunofluorescence is a useful diagnostic method. Where the renal lesions are well established, impairment of renal function can be demonstrated by marked elevation in blood urea, retention of phosphate and creatinine and oliguria. Moderate degrees of proteinuria are often present and examination of the urine sediment often shows red cells, leucocytes and granular casts. In cases of less severe renal involvement there may be only a mild proteinuria with very little alteration in serum biochemistry, although large numbers of organisms can still often be demonstrated in the urine.

At necropsy, post mortem findings may be inconclusive in mild cases. The presence of a few white foci or more extensive lesions in the deep cortex of the kidney is highly suggestive of *L. canicola* infection and this can usually be confirmed on histological examination, particularly if silver staining techniques or immunofluorescence tests are employed. In cases of severe acute interstitial nephritis there are often extensive extrarenal lesions indicative of uraemia in the form of lingual and oral ulceration, atrial necrosis and haemorrhagic gastritis.

Treatment and prevention

Antibiotics, especially penicillin, streptomycin and the tetracyclines, are all effective in clearing *L. canicola* from the circulation and from the kidneys. In the vomiting dog, intravenous administration of glucose saline is useful supportive therapy and when uraemia is marked, peritoneal dialysis should be considered.

Killed vaccines incorporating serotypes *canicola* and *icterohaemorrhagiae* are now widely used and, since their introduction, the incidence of severe acute interstitial nephritis appears to have been markedly reduced. Leptospiral bacterins, however, produce a relatively short-lived immunity and annual revaccination is normally recommended. There is some experimental evidence too, that although immunised dogs develop circulating antibody and are protected against clinical illness, some may excrete leptospirae in the urine after challenge. The vaccine is usually administered separately or incorporated with distemper and adenovirus antigens. The first dose is usually given at 12 weeks, and the second dose 2–3 weeks later. Titres which result from vaccination seldom exceed 1:1000 and soon fall to below 1:100. In the unvaccinated dog a titre of 1:100 and above is generally accepted as indicating possible infection and, for this reason, some countries will not accept for import from the United Kingdom dogs with such titres.

2 *Leptospira icterohaemorrhagiae* infection

This is a very serious leptospiral infection of the dog and is similar to the disease known as Weil's disease in man. Its overall incidence in the dog population, however, is small.

Pathogenesis and pathology
The route of infection and initial course of the disease is similar to serotype *canicola* infection. Thus, there is an initial leptospiraemia which lasts for approximately 1 week. Thereafter the courses of the two diseases diverge: serotype *canicola* produces a nephropathy and serotype *icterohaemorrhagiae* induces acute hepatitis and perivascular haemorrhage. The prime lesion in serotype *icterohaemorrhagiae* infection is varying degrees of hepatocellular degeneration and necrosis and, although similar degenerative changes may also occur in the kidneys, there is usually only a sparse cellular infiltrate. Perivascular haemorrhages are often found, particularly in the lungs and gastrointestinal tract.

Clinical signs
There is often a sudden onset of fever, jaundice and extreme depression. Infected dogs may also show vomiting, thirst and bloodstained diarrhoea. There may be petechial haemorrhages in the mucous membranes of the conjunctivae and oral cavity; the conjunctivae are often also severely congested. Death can occur in as little as 2–3 hours after the onset of clinical illness or the condition of the affected dog can deteriorate rapidly over a few days.

Diagnosis
The sudden onset of jaundice and fever in a young dog is suggestive of serotype *icterohaemorrhagiae* infection, although it must be remembered that occasionally serotype *canicola* can cause similar signs. In the differential diagnosis, systemic CAV-1 infection is the main consideration and it may not be possible to distinguish between the two diseases on clinical examination alone.

At necropsy, the most constant findings are icterus and perivascular haemorrhages, particularly in the lungs. Laboratory tests are identical to those used in the diagnosis of serotype *canicola* infection.

Treatment and prevention
Antibiotic therapy, if given early enough, may prevent invasion of the liver and kidneys and prevent the subsequent development of the disease. The course of the disease is usually so rapid, however, that by the time clinical signs develop prognosis is considered grave. Whole blood transfusions may help to contain the haemorrhage. Vaccination is protective against the clinical disease and has already been discussed.

CONTAGIOUS RESPIRATORY DISEASE

Aetiology
It is now well recognised that dogs kept in pet shops, research establishments, boarding and breeding kennels, indeed any situation where they are concentrated in groups, are likely to develop a respiratory infection characterised by a mild but sometimes intractable cough. This is particularly true of the open type establishments where there is a constant movement of animals into and out of a central pool. In this situation, newcomers introduce new infectious agents into the central pool or, in turn, may acquire infection from the pool and transfer it to other establishments or to household contacts. In this way, the microbial flora responsible for the condition may be constantly changing. It is also as well to remember that respiratory disease in general consists of two sometimes overlapping clinical syndromes. Firstly, it is one of the main features of distemper and in some instances CDV is involved alone, while in others it is present in concert with other respiratory infectious agents; in some of these cases the other clinical manifestations of distemper may be overlooked. It has been recorded that in one large kennel of random-source dogs where CDV, CAV-2 and canine parainfluenza virus (CPIV) were present, the incidence of respiratory disease was much higher in dogs without antibody to CDV than in those with antibody to CDV; prevention of distemper seemed to be the key to the control of severe, prolonged and often fatal respiratory disease. Secondly, there is a group of well-defined agents which affect the

respiratory tract and which individually or together and in the absence of distemper can cause outbreaks of respiratory disease. It is the second clinical condition which is known as contagious respiratory disease, tracheobronchitis or 'kennel cough'. Unlike distemper, all the agents involved in contagious respiratory disease confine their activities largely to the respiratory tract and there is no general systemic involvement.

Early interest in the disease centred around the role of bacteria, and a long list of bacterial organisms has been isolated from the respiratory tract of affected dogs. The organisms most commonly found are *Bordetella bronchiseptica*, beta-haemolytic streptococci, staphylococci, Klebsiella spp., Proteus spp. Pseudomonas spp., Neisseria spp. and Pasteurella spp.

All of these agents can also be recovered from the nasopharynx of clinically normal dogs; many, if not all, probably act as secondary invaders. Only *Bordetella bronchiseptica* has been shown to be a primary pathogen for the respiratory tract although it may also act as a secondary invader in respiratory virus infections and in distemper. Mycoplasms have also received much attention and although a number of different strains have been isolated from animals with respiratory disease it is still uncertain whether or not they act as primary pathogens.

More recent interest has focussed on viruses and a number of different agents have now been implicated: these are CAV-1 and CAV-2, CHV, CPIV and reovirus. Details of individual agents which are important in canine respiratory disease are given below, but it should be remembered that clinically, respiratory disease is often multifactorial and a 'pure' infection with only one agent may be the exception rather than the rule. The relative incidence of all these respiratory agents is unknown.

Bordetella bronchiseptica infection

The fortunes of this organism have waxed and waned over the years insofar as its importance as a primary pathogen is concerned. Early workers considered the organism to be the cause of distemper as it could often be isolated from the respiratory tract of such cases. However, the demonstration that distemper infection was due to a virus was followed by the relegation of *Bordetella bronchiseptica* to the role of a secondary invader. It occupied this position until quite recently when it was clearly proved to be a primary pathogen of the respiratory tract and to be one of the agents involved in 'kennel cough'. There are now a number of experimental studies which have conclusively

shown that inhalation of the organism results in a rapid colonisation of the respiratory mucosa, particularly that of the trachea and bronchi, where masses of the organism attach to the ciliated mucous surface. Although the organism does not appear to penetrate the mucosal barrier its presence stimulates an acute inflammatory reaction as early as 4 days after infection. The resulting tracheobronchitis is characterised by a mucous or mucopurulent exudate in the tracheobronchial tree and patchy areas of pneumonia. These lesions, which are associated with varying degrees of coughing and nasal discharge resolve within 2–3 weeks, but the organism can persist in the respiratory tract for months. The disease is highly contagious and spreads rapidly to in-contact animals. Recovered dogs are immune to subsequent challenge but the duration of this immunity is not known. Since virtually all cases survive unless complicated by other infections, detailed epidemiological and pathological studies of 'pure' bordetellosis in the field have not yet appeared in the literature. However, the lesions found in the experimental studies are similar to those previously described in some natural cases of contagious respiratory disease and to those found in dogs with kennel cough which have died of other diseases. There is experimental evidence that the duration of the disease is considerably extended when concurrent CPIV infection is present.

Canine adenovirus

Two distinct canine adenoviruses CAV-1 and CAV-2 are associated with naturally occurring respiratory disease in the dog and, under experimental conditions where dogs are infected by aerosol, both induce a mild respiratory infection, characterised by coughing and tachypnoea. The experimental infection is indistinguishable from that seen in mild cases of natural respiratory disease.

CAV-1 is usually associated with an acute systemic infection and whether or not susceptible dogs develop this or the more limited respiratory infection appears to be related to the route of infection. CAV-2 on the other hand has so far only been associated with respiratory infections. The relative importance of the two adenoviruses in canine respiratory disease is unknown. Both viruses induce similar lesions in the respiratory tract with necrotising bronchiolitis and focal necrosis of the turbinates and tonsillar epithelium. These lesions resolve quickly and recovered dogs are immune to subsequent challenge. The duration of immunity is unknown. In both infections intranuclear inclusion bodies can be detected in the respiratory mucosa.

Canine herpesvirus

This virus is best known for the serious generalised disease it induces in young puppies. In the older animal it is associated with mild respiratory infection with a serous nasal discharge and sometimes coughing. Pathological changes in the respiratory tract are usually milder than those found in adenovirus or *Bordetella bronchiseptica* infections, but focal epithelial necrosis at all levels from the turbinate mucosa to the tracheobronchial tree have been described. The number of intranuclear inclusion bodies in epithelial cells varies from animal to animal but they are usually sparse.

Canine parainfluenza virus

This is considered to be an important cause of contagious respiratory disease in the United States where it is associated clinically with a nasal discharge and coughing, and pathologically with catarrhal rhinitis and bronchiolitis. Its presence has been established in outbreaks of respiratory disease in the United Kingdom but usually in association with other respiratory agents. In general, it appears that 'pure' infections with the virus are mild or subclinical.

Canine reovirus

Although there is serological evidence that reovirus infection is prevalent in the dog population there is no evidence that the virus plays any significant role in clinical outbreaks of contagious respiratory disease. The virus has been isolated from the respiratory tract of normal dogs and dogs with respiratory disease, but under experimental conditions produces only an extremely mild or subclinical infection.

Clinical signs

It is impossible to distinguish between the respiratory agents mentioned above on clinical grounds alone. An intermittent soft dry cough is often the only sign of infection although coughing bouts are precipitated by excitement, exercise or by pinching the trachea. In severe cases, bouts of paroxysmal coughing may occur. Usually the animal remains bright and maintains its appetite. Coughing develops in a susceptible animal between 5 and 10 days after contact with infected dogs and although it may last for only a few days it occasionally persists for months. Some cases may also show a serous or seropurulent nasal discharge. Recovery is usually uneventful but occasion-ally severe bronchopneumonia develops with attendant pyrexia and depression, gradual deterioration in health, and death.

Diagnosis

As clinical signs of contagious respiratory disease are common to a number of respiratory pathogens, identification of the causal agent rests with laboratory findings. In life, nasal and pharyngeal swabs may be sent to the laboratory for bacteriological and virological examination. Paired serum samples may be examined by the tube agglutination test for antibody to *Bordetella bronchiseptica*. Elevation in serum antibody to the different respiratory viruses may also be detected. At necropsy, the presence of bronchopneumonia or a mucopurulent exudate in the trachea and bronchi may indicate the presence of *Bordetella bronchiseptica*. There are no specific macroscopic findings in the case of the respiratory viruses. An important feature of the histological diagnosis of adenovirus respiratory disease is the presence of basophilic intranuclear inclusions in respiratory epithelial cells. Likewise in CHV infection, eosinophilic inclusion bodies may be encountered particularly in the turbinate and tracheal epithelium. In the absence of inclusion bodies, the histological diagnosis of the different forms of respiratory infection may be difficult. For all the respiratory viruses, examination of the respiratory tract by immunofluorescence is usually more sensitive than a search for inclusion bodies. *Bordetella bronchiseptica* infection is usually characterised by tracheobronchitis and the appearance of masses of organisms on the luminal aspect of the ciliated respiratory epithelium. Finally, bacteriological and virological examination of the respiratory tract should be carried out.

The main problem in the differential diagnosis is the exclusion of distemper virus. In any one kennel population with successive outbreaks, each instance may be associated with a different respiratory agent or mixture of agents. The occasional case of *Filaroides osleri* infection may also have to be considered, but the use of bronchoscopy and faecal larval examination should exclude that condition.

Treatment and prevention

As a general rule, the use of antibiotics parenterally or by aerosol should be considered even where the primary agent is a virus, in order to prevent any secondary bacterial activity. There is of course no specific treatment against viral agents themselves.

Clinical signs are usually treated symptomatically; codeine compounds are often used to allay coughing. Most cases are not severe enough to warrant further action.

There is at present no commercially available vaccine that incorporates all the known respiratory pathogens. In *Bordetella bronchiseptica* and CPIV infections, and possibly in others, the main defences lie in the local secretory antibody response and in local cell-mediated immunity; serum antibody titres have little correlation with resistance. In these instances, administration of vaccine by the intranasal route is far more effective than by the subcutaneous route. On the other hand, subcutaneous inoculation of live CAV vaccines, especially CAV-2, provides complete or almost complete protection against CAV respiratory disease. In general terms, it is wise to ensure that all dogs are vaccinated against distemper and adenovirus.

The vaccine licensed for the protection of dogs against *Bordetella bronchiseptica* consists of the live avirulent strain S55 and is inoculated intranasally. Multiplication of the organism results in the formation of local secretory IgA antibody in the respiratory tract and it is this antibody which confers immunity to subsequent infection with virulent strains of the organism. Humoral antibody is also formed but there is no correlation between the serum titre and resistance to infection. Vaccination gives complete or almost complete protection against the clinical disease, lowers the number of organisms present and reduces the period during which they are shed. About 20% of dogs may be protected in as little as 48 hours, 85% by 5 days and at least 95% by 14 days after vaccination. Preliminary studies have shown that immunity lasts for at least 10–12 months, though the manufacturer of the vaccine is rather more cautious in its claim.

Experimentally, CPIV produces a fairly mild disease but it has been shown to increase the severity and duration of *Bordetella bronchiseptica* infection so vaccination may be useful in the overall control of kennel cough. The vaccine consists of a live attenuated strain of CPI virus, grown in a canine kidney cell-line, and is inoculated by the subcutaneous or intramuscular routes, preferably by the latter route since higher antibody titres are produced. Two doses of vaccine are recommended because the antibody titres decrease rather rapidly after a single dose. The vaccine reduces the period of shedding of virulent virus following challenge but does not eliminate it completely.

CANINE INFECTIOUS DIARRHOEA

Aetiology

Outbreaks of infectious enteritis or gastroenteritis, like outbreaks of kennel cough, occur regularly in groups of kennelled dogs. In general, there is only a low mortality and because of this and because of the difficulties involved in isolating and identifying significant microorganisms from the mass of normal gut flora, infectious canine enteritis has, in the past, been a neglected area of veterinary research. Investigations of infectious enteritis outbreaks are now providing more definite information about the aetiology and pathogenesis of this condition and it is likely that much more information will become available over the next few years. Details of individual agents which are associated with infectious diarrhoea are listed below but it should be remembered that, like respiratory disease, diarrhoea is often multifactorial and a 'pure' infection with only one agent may be the exception rather than the rule. The relative incidence of all these intestinal agents is unknown.

Canine parvovirus

CPV has been implicated in many outbreaks of infectious diarrhoea over the past few years. The virus attacks the actively multiplying cells in the intestinal crypts causing a severe, degenerative enteritis with necrosis of intestinal crypt cells and villous atrophy.

Canine coronavirus

Canine coronavirus has also been shown to cause diarrhoea in dogs. The pathogenesis of this infection is similar to that of transmissible gastroenteritis (TGE) of pigs and coronavirus infection of calves. The virus attacks the mature epithelial cells of the intestinal villi causing villous atrophy, hypercellularity of the lamina propria and depression of epithelial enzyme function; the ileum is the most severely affected region. The incidence of coronavirus infection is unknown but, in one survey, over 50% of dogs had serological titres to TGE virus which cross-reacts strongly with canine coronavirus.

Other viruses

CDV infection often results in enteritis which is usually catarrhal in nature. Other evidence of distemper is usually present. Rotavirus and adenovirus particles have been identified in the faeces of dogs with diarrhoea, but as yet their significance is unknown. In other species, rotaviruses predominantly affect young animals; in the dog, they have been isolated from fatal cases of enteritis in neonatal pups.

Campylobacter jejuni infection

Campylobacter jejuni has seldom been isolated from individual household dogs without enteric disease but has been found in the faeces of about 10% of dogs with enteritis. However, when the organism is present in kennels, it can be isolated from virtually all dogs whether they have diarrhoea or not. In experimentally infected adult dogs, uncomplicated infection resulted in a mild transient diarrhoea within seven days of infection. On histopathological examination, the enteritis was non-specific in appearance, with congestion and inflammatory cell infiltration of the lamina propria, particularly in the ileum, and superficial colonisation by the organism. The enteritis was accompanied by a mesenteric lymphadenitis and both were similar to those found in naturally occurring cases. Natural infections in pups appear to be rather more severe but even so are seldom fatal. In untreated cases, the organism seems to persist in the alimentary tract for about 5–7 weeks and in some cases for longer. Suitable chemotherapy with neomycin, erythromycin or tylosin is effective in eliminating the organism from the alimentary tract.

Campylobacter jejuni can cause enteritis in man and is therefore of zoonotic importance. It seems likely that although the dog can act as a source of infection for man, many cases of dual pet and human infection represent exposure to a common source rather than straightforward dog to human transmission. The source is seldom clear. In kennels, contamination of water and food bowls by birds, many of which excrete the organism in their faeces, is one possibility, while another is the feeding of contaminated meat or offal. Surveys have shown that 60% or more chicken carcases may be contaminated with the organism, and it can also be found in the water of marshlands and ponds from which individual pet dogs may drink.

Other bacteria

Certain pathogenic serotypes of *Escherichia coli* have been found in association with diarrhoea in the dog, usually in younger animals. However, there is little published evidence to show that this bacterium is important in adult canine enteritis. As in other animals, Salmonella spp. are an occasional cause of enteritis in dogs (see later). Clostridia spp. have been isolated from the gut of dogs with severe, necrotising or haemorrhagic enteritis. It is uncertain whether they are primary pathogens or secondary invaders. Spirochaetes, Proteus spp. and Pseudomonas spp. have all been isolated from diarrhoeic dogs but are of unknown significance.

The relative importance of the above agents or of others should become clearer over the next few years. It is probable that, as in kennel cough, more than one agent may be involved in any particular outbreak. It should be remembered that protozoa and helminth infestations can also give rise to an apparently infectious enteritis, especially in young dogs.

Clinical signs

Many cases are apparently self-limiting: the animal does not appear ill and the diarrhoea resolves spontaneously. In more severe cases, especially if diarrhoea is very profuse, there are more obvious clinical signs, with dullness, inappetence, vomiting and the development of dehydration and electrolyte imbalance. In some cases, there may be dysentery and rapid collapse. The rectal temperature may be raised, especially with acute bacterial infections, but is often within normal range or, in profusely diarrhoeic and collapsed animals, subnormal. Abdominal palpation reveals fluid- and/or gas-filled intestinal loops. There is usually excessive bowel motility and loud borborygmi.

Diagnosis

It is relatively simple to make a diagnosis of infectious enteritis on the basis of history and clinical signs. However, infectious enteritis should be differentiated from dietary upset which is the commonest cause of transient diarrhoea in the dog.

On clinical grounds it is virtually impossible to decide which of the numerous aetiological agents are involved. It is seldom worthwhile undertaking exhaustive bacteriological or virological investigations in individual animals, but these may be worthwhile in severe kennel outbreaks or if there is a possiblity of zoonosis. Special media or conditions are required for the detection of Salmonella spp., Campylobacter and Clostridium spp. and many enteric viruses do not grow well in tissue culture and are best detected by direct visualisation using an electron microscope. Full investigations can thus be expensive and time consuming. In fatal cases, specific pathological changes may be detectable (e.g. parvovirus and coronavirus enteritis).

Treatment and prevention

In mild cases, little specific treatment is required. Simple reduction in food intake for 24–48 hours may be sufficient, but adsorbents such as kaolin or bismuth, or drugs inhibiting bowel motility (e.g. atropine, codeine phosphate) can be given. In more severe cases, more active therapy is required and antibiotic cover should be given. Neomycin acts mainly within the gut lumen but broad spectrum, systemically active compounds should be used if septicaemia is suspected. If specific organisms are isolated, sensitivity tests should be carried out. Fluid therapy is essential in animals which are dehydrated and in electrolyte imbalance. Lactated Ringer's solution (Hartmann's solution) is suitable and is best given warmed, by the intravenous route. In collapsed, shocked animals, plasma expanders can also be used.

Control and prevention are best achieved by, where possible, vaccination and by the methods of hygiene, batching and disinfection already described under canine parvovirus infection.

SPECIAL INFECTIONS

Tuberculosis

Aetiology

Cases of tuberculosis in the dog are now fortunately rare but the disease remains a potentially important public health consideration. Infection of the dog occurs with *Mycobacterium tuberculosis* (human) and *Mycobacterium bovis*. Infections with other types are extremely uncommon.

Pathogenesis and pathology

Pulmonary tuberculosis is the usual form of the disease. Inhalation of the organism, usually after contact with an infected dog or owner, is followed by localisation in the lungs and in the regional lymph nodes (primary complex); in many cases only the lymph nodes are involved. Ingestion of the bovine type, usually in milk, can result in the alimentary form of the disease, with lesions mainly in the mesenteric lymph node. Subsequent dissemination of the primary lesion in the thorax or abdomen can produce multiple foci in many organs and tissues, particularly the serous membranes, liver and kidneys.

Enlargement of the tracheobronchial nodes is the commonest thoracic lesion. Affected nodes are firm and fibrous and may have central areas of necrosis and cavitation; caseation is not a feature of canine tuberculosis. Pulmonary lesions, when present, take the form of small nodules or more confluent areas of bronchopneumonia; in severe pulmonary lesions cavitation may occur. In some cases pleural effusions accompany the pulmonary lesions. The pleural fluid in these cases may be milky or straw-coloured and the serosal surface may show widespread granulation tissue. Abdominal lesions take the form of mesenteric

lymphadenitis, with or without accompanying peritonitis and ascites.

Clinical signs

These are extremely variable and depend on the site of the primary lesion. Thus, thoracic tuberculosis is associated with respiratory signs such as tachypnoea and coughing. There is usually a fluctuating pyrexia but the first presenting sign is often simply progressive weight loss and general loss of condition. In the abdominal form, the mesenteric lymph node may be palpable and the abdomen may be tender on palpation.

Diagnosis

In life, a diagnosis may be obtained by microscopic examination of pleural or peritoneal effusions (obtained by paracentesis) for the presence of acid-fast bacilli (Ziehl–Neelsen method). Radiographic examination may show a thoracic or abdominal mass which is often mistaken for a malignant tumour. As the growth of tubercle bacilli *in vitro* is slow, this is seldom helpful in the initial diagnosis but is essential when ascertaining the type of bacillus involved. Skin reactions to BCG have been used for the diagnosis of tuberculosis in the live dog. In infected animals, the intradermal inoculation of between 0.1 and 0.2 ml of BCG results within 72 hours in local erythema, induration and necrosis, all of which are indications of the presence of cell-mediated immunity to tubercle bacillus.

Final diagnosis is usually based on necropsy and histological findings where the chronic granulomatous lesions in the lymph nodes and other organs are highly suggestive of the disease. Acid-fast bacilli can be found in varying numbers in these lesions. A search for multinucleated giant cells may also be rewarding.

Differential diagnosis must take into account malignant neoplasia and the rare cases of chronic mycosis, both of which diseases may involve primarily the thoracic or abdominal lymph nodes. Two other diseases which are sometimes associated with tuberculosis and indeed are considered sequelae to it are hypertrophic pulmonary osteoarthropathy and renal amyloidosis.

Treatment

Isoniazid and streptomycin have been used with some success in the treatment of canine tuberculosis. Because of the danger of transmission to man, however, treatment of canine tuberculosis must be considered inadvisable, indeed hazardous, and the owner should be advised of the risk to himself or other household contacts.

Salmonellosis

Aetiology
There are many reports on the isolation of different serotypes of salmonellae from the faeces of clinically normal dogs, or dogs suffering from enteritis. Young dogs in particular are more likely to be affected. Over 40 different serotypes have been recovered from dogs, and of these *Salmonella typhimurium* appears to be the organism most often associated with clinical disease. Many infected dogs remain symptomless carriers and may shed the organism in the faeces intermittently for long periods; these dogs are a potential danger to contact animals and of course to man. Infection is usually via contaminated food.

Pathogenesis and pathology
Little is known of the pathogenesis of salmonellosis in dogs and why, in some cases, the organism confines its activity to the intestine, while in others septicaemia occurs. The presence of organisms in the intestinal wall results in varying degrees of enteritis with or without petechial haemorrhages. In septicaemic cases, pulmonary oedema with exudation of fibrin into the alveolar spaces has been found. Focal necrotising hepatitis and meningitis have also been recorded.

Clinical signs
These vary from the asymptomatic carrier to the severe septicaemic case with anorexia, pyrexia, vomiting, diarrhoea, rapid prostration and death. Abdominal pain associated with intestinal or liver lesions may also be present. Nervous signs and jaundice have also been observed. Mild cases may show only slight diarrhoea.

Diagnosis
Clinical and histological examinations are often inconclusive, particularly in the mild case. The severe case with fever, abdominal pain and rapid prostration has to be differentiated from systemic adenovirus and *parvovirus* infections.

Final diagnosis rests with the isolation of Salmonella organisms from the faeces, blood or internal organs such as the liver and gall bladder. Repeated attempts may have to be made before successful isolation of the organism is possible. Once a successful culture is achieved, the organism should be retained for subsequent typing.

Treatment and prevention
Salmonella infections respond well to sulphonamides and chloramphenicol, but although clinical signs subside the animal may continue to excrete the organism in the faeces. Thus it is important to culture the faeces for some time after therapy has been discontinued to ensure complete clearance of the organism from the alimentary tract.

Rabies

Rabies is a virus disease of the central nervous system. The signs in dogs are diverse, but for the sake of convenience they may be divided into two categories: 'furious' and 'dumb'. Furious rabies has always been comparatively easy to diagnose, and there are numerous graphic and accurate descriptions that date back beyond the third century BC. The dumb form, which is characterised by paralysis, is not spectacular and is difficult to diagnose despite being more common than the furious form. In those parts of the world where the disease in dogs has been brought under control, cases of rabies are rarely seen and consequently there are few experienced observers. There is, therefore, the danger that recognition of the disease may be delayed should it appear in countries where it is not enzootic.

Epidemiology
Rabies is present in all continents except Australasia and Antarctica. There are, however, several countries including the United Kingdom, Eire, Portugal, Finland, Norway, Sweden, Iceland and Japan which at present are free.

Because of its highly specialised mode of transmission, rabies virus can survive only when suitable hosts are numerous and in sufficiently close contact for the virus to be readily transmitted. Until the turn of the century, dogs were the most important vectors and indeed still constitute the greatest danger to man. However, rabies has long been enzootic in a number of species of wildlife in many parts of the world, notably racoons and skunks in the USA, vampire bats in Central America, the mongoose in South Africa and the red fox in Europe. Although cases in foxes were frequently reported from areas of Europe over the centuries, it was following the major disturbance caused by the Second World War that the fox population increased considerably and enabled a wave of rabies to spread from Eastern to Western Europe. Flocks of backyard poultry have virtually disappeared from some countries such as England, consequently foxes are now tolerated and even encouraged in periurban areas, and they have become numerous enough to constitute a major potential reservoir for rabies.

Aetiology

Rabies virus is a member of the group of bullet-shaped viruses, now known as rhabdoviruses. While the old concept that all rabies viruses are identical is no longer tenable, the great majority of those that affect man and dogs are so closely related that vaccines prepared from a single type of virus are suitable for protection against them all. Minor differences demonstrable by serum neutralisation tests (but not by complement-fixation or fluorescent antibody tests) can be shown between classical rabies virus and the viruses of the West African disease of dogs 'Olou fato', the vampire bat strain of South America, a strain isolated from a bat in South Africa, and possibly most strains adapted to existence in wild animals. The Lagos bat virus, the Mokola virus obtained from shrews in Nigeria, and two strains isolated recently from insects, have differences sufficient to warrant their separate classification as 'rabies-related viruses'.

Pathogenesis

Following inoculation of virus by a bite, it enters the axon sheath of an afferent nerve within 5 hours and, by 10 hours, is no longer at the bite site or in the nodes. It travels up to the spinal ganglion where it multiplies for a few days, after which it enters the dorsal horn of the cord and soon reaches the ependymal cells. From the segment of the cord first involved, the virus ascends to the brain by cell-to-cell infection. Once the brain is involved, infection spreads centrifugally down the cranial nerves to reach the salivary glands and other organs. The fox is so susceptible that it may die before virus has left the brain and infected the salivary glands. In less severe infections, the virus reaches the salivary glands where it multiplies further. It is also recorded as multiplying to a lesser extent in the lungs and kidneys. Virus is usually excreted in the saliva for only a few days before death occurs. The dog requires a high dose of virus before it becomes infected, but fox saliva can be so rich that the massive dose given to a dog it bites may be so overwhelming that the dog dies before its saliva has become infective. Fortunately virus excretion in the saliva occurs in only 50% of rabid dogs.

Pathology

The lesions of rabies are surprisingly mild compared with the severity of the signs. Rabies is characterised by perivascular accumulations mainly of lymphoid cells in the spinal cord, the brain stem (particularly the pons and medulla) and the basal ganglia. In addition, neuronal degeneration is seen associated with infiltration of microglia. Negri bodies, so highly characteristic of rabies, are frequently found in the cytoplasm of neurons in those areas of the brain (notably the hippocampus and cerebellar Purkinje cells) where little inflammatory reaction is visible. Although cytoplasmic bodies had been seen by earlier workers it was the meticulous work published by Negri in 1903 which established their significance.

Clinical signs

Dogs have been classed as being of intermediate susceptibility to rabies, with adult dogs more resistant than pups. The incubation period is variable and depends on several factors: the most important of which are the site of infection, severity of the bite, and the dose of virus inoculated. The amount of virus inoculated is greater if entry occurs at a point where there is little hair to absorb the saliva which carries it, and the virus reaches the brain more rapidly if the wound is near the head.

The incubation period is rarely less than 10 days or more than 4 months but may be as short as 5 days and incubation periods as long as 10 months have been reported. Some exposed dogs never develop rabies; some delayed and sometimes atypical cases may occur, influenced possibly by the animals' immune response. Fortunately, such cases are rare. Severe stress has been shown to be a precipitating factor in these cases.

Most cases of rabies commence with a change of temperament. During this prodromal phase there is usually an elevation of temperature. Dogs that are normally friendly tend to seek solitude and may hide away in such places as under beds or in cupboards; others which are normally placid may become excessively affectionate and make persistent attempts to lick the hands and faces of their owners. In a few cases the site where the virus gained entry may itch intensely. As the saliva of dogs may contain large amounts of virus up to 3 days before the onset of clinical signs, the hazard of contact with these cases is obvious and dogs in known infected areas or those which have recently been released from quarantine and which show sudden changes in temperament should be handled with caution and treated with suspicion.

In about 25% of rabid dogs the disease gradually develops into a phase of marked hyperexcitation, but the percentage may possibly vary with different strains of virus, as in the case of Olou fato. Dogs which show the furious forms of rabies become highly restless and irritable and snap at any restraint and even at imaginary objects. They may show depraved appetite and chew and swallow stones, wood, carpet or straw. If confined they may bite at chains or iron bars so fiercely as to break their teeth and gums, and may howl in a peculiar way. Spells of hyperexcitability may be short and infrequent but may last about 5 hours and recur after periods of quiescence when the dog may be friendly. If free to wander, rabid dogs may travel long distances, 25 miles or more, after which they may attempt to return home. Because of their dishevelled state the owner may think they have been involved in a motor car accident or a fight. Generalised signs of paresis gradually become apparent as weakness of legs and tail, difficulty in swallowing, and drooping jaw and eyelids. Great care should be taken in handling such animals and they should be securely confined pending examination by a Ministry Veterinary Officer. Although affected dogs develop difficulty in swallowing, they do not go into spasms at the sight of water. Therefore the term 'hydrophobia' does not apply to the dog as it does to man. Dogs affected with the furious form of rabies may die during a convulsive seizure but in most, the paralysis becomes accentuated and the animal usually dies in a state of coma.

In most cases of rabies in dogs only the dumb form of the disease is seen and this may be difficult to diagnose with prodromal and furious phases either absent or of short duration. Rather, a progressive paralysis of all muscles develops. The jaw and eyelids droop and the eyes tend to squint. Conjunctival congestion is usually marked and saliva may drool from the sagging jaws. There is difficulty in swallowing, and because food and saliva collect in the pharynx the animal may appear to be choking. The signs may be mistaken for those caused by foreign bodies in the throat. Therefore great caution should be used when examining such a dog because scratches on the examiner's hands could become infected with the virus.

The course of the disease is seldom more than 15 days from the start of the clinical syndrome, and death usually follows within 5 days of signs becoming apparent. However, it should be remembered that cases of the West African Olou fato type may linger on for 25 days.

Where possible any dog in which rabies is suspected should not be killed but should be confined immediately and the suspicion reported to the responsible authority, because diagnosis in the laboratory is more satisfactory in advanced cases. If a suspected animal cannot be captured with safety and has to be shot, care must be taken, if possible, not to damage the brain which is required for establishing a diagnosis. Furthermore, any in-contact dogs or cats should be held in isolation pending receipt of the results of diagnostic tests.

Diagnosis

Specific diagnosis of rabies is seldom possible in live animals. Sometimes fluorescent antibody can be used to detect virus antigen in corneal impression smears and high levels of serum antibody would be indicative of recovery from infection; but such cases are extremely rare.

Veterinary surgeons should consider the possibility of rabies whenever a dog is presented showing nervous signs including unexplained paresis. If there is a chance that the dog has rabies, the animal should not be killed but should be securely confined and the matter reported in accordance with the regulations of the country concerned.

Rabid dogs seldom live more than 5 days after the onset of nervous signs, but where there is any suspicion of rabies the animal should be held for a further 10 days before release. In the past it was necessary to let rabid dogs die so that a diagnosis based on the demonstration of Negri bodies could be made. However, nowadays dogs may be killed once characteristic symptoms are present and the diagnosis established by the fluorescent antibody technique.

Furious rabies is usually clinically obvious but as most cases show little or no signs of fury the possibility that a dog is infected with rabies should be considered whenever an animal is presented with a history of sudden change of temperament accompanied by progressive paralysis. There is usually a moderate rise in temperature in the early stages followed by a fall to subnormal. This and the marked congestion of the conjunctivae should help to exclude the possiblitity of a foreign body in the throat.

Many cases show signs of gastritis, and rabies should be considered when the stomach is found at necropsy to contain such items as wood, stones or leaves in dogs with a history of nervous signs and paralysis.

The fact that a dog has been vaccinated against rabies does not preclude the possibility that it is rabid; and it should be remembered that very occasionally the incubation period can be more than the 6 months that imported dogs are held in quarantine.

If the animal dies or is killed, the head should be removed by an authorised person and transported intact to a diagnostic laboratory. It should be packed in a sealed container, held at low temperature but not frozen. At the laboratory the brain is removed under conditions designed to protect the operator, and tests are carried out to determine the diagnosis.

The most reliable test for rabies is the intracerebral inoculation of brain suspensions into newly weaned white mice; but this test usually takes 10–12 days for a positive result and should be allowed to go 21 days before a negative diagnosis can be accepted. Impression smears of the hippocampus may be stained, usually with Sellers' stain, and examined for Negri bodies which are found in most cases provided the dog was left to die of the disease or was killed *in extremis.*

Nowadays laboratory diagnosis of rabies is based on the demonstration of the viral antigen in brain smears by the fluorescent antibody test or the immunoperoxidase technique. These methods are quick and accurate. Because they are less accurate, histological methods of diagnosis are falling into disuse in well-equipped diagnostic laboratories.

Vaccines

Modern vaccines, properly used, are capable of inducing a high degree of protection against rabies. Once rabies has become established in an area or in a country, a programme of canine vaccination is a most useful adjunct to other control measures (e.g. the control of movement of dogs, the elimination of strays and the destruction of wildlife). To have any significant effect in the control of canine rabies at least 70% of the dog population must be vaccinated.

Vaccines containing live attenuated virus are cheaper to prepare than those with inactivated virus, and have been used with very satisfactory results in the USA, Africa and Malaysia. A single dose of live Flury LEP vaccine prepared in eggs was shown to protect adult dogs for at least 3 years. Unfortunately, heat lability causes problems in hot climates, and the vaccine virus is pathogenic for some young puppies; furthermore the high tissue content of the vaccine may be harmful.

In Western Europe and Japan there has been a reluctance to disseminate live rabies virus, and reliance has usually been placed on inactivated virus vaccines. Most have been prepared from fixed virus grown in nervous tissue of adult animals. The use of other strains of virus and propagation in the brains of suckling animals, or more recently in cell cultures, has led to the development of safe potent vaccines of both live and inactivated types. However, it should be remembered that indiscriminate use of either live or inactivated vaccines in countries free from infection might mask the disease should it enter, and so delay its recognition.

In an attempt to standardise procedures used in different countries, a WHO Committee has recommended that dogs should be vaccinated primarily at 3-4 months of age (once in the case of live virus vaccines but twice at a month's interval with inactivated types). A booster dose must be given at 1 year of age and thereafter every 2-3 years depending on the virus strain used in the vaccines. Live virus vaccines must be injected intramuscularly in the hindleg but the subcutaneous route is acceptable for inactivated vaccines. Should it be necessary to protect younger puppies, inactivated vaccines must be used and the pups subjected to the procedure outlined above once they are 3 months old. In all cases at least a month should be allowed for the development of immunity. During this time, animals in infected areas must be kept confined.

Now that safe human vaccines are available, people exposed to increased risk of infection by nature of their work should be protected by prophylactic vaccination. At the present time, the most satisfactory for this purpose is believed to be an inactivated virus vaccine prepared from human diploid cell cultures.

ACKNOWLEDGEMENTS

This text is a revised version of the one prepared by Professor N.G. Wright for the first edition of this book. The writer is grateful to Dr D.A. Haig for his help in providing the section on rabies and to Drs I.A.P. McCandlish and H. Thompson and Professor E.W. Fisher for assistance with canine parvovirus infection, contagious respiratory disease and infectious diarrhoea.

FURTHER READING

Neonatal diseases

CORNWELL H.J.C. & WRIGHT N.G. (1969) Neonatal canine herpesvirus infection: a review of present knowledge. *Vet. Rec.* **84**, 2.

WRIGHT N.G. & CORNWELL H.J.C. (1969) Role of bacteria and viruses in neonatal canine mortality. *Vet. Bull.* **39**, 815.

Canine parvovirus infection

APPEL M.J.G., SCOTT F.W. & CARMICHAEL L.E. (1979) Isolation and immunisation studies of a parvo-like virus from dogs with haemorrhagic gastroenteritis. *Vet. Rec.* **105**, 156.

McCANDLISH I.A.P., THOMPSON H., CORNWELL H.J.C., LAIRD H. & WRIGHT N.G. (1979) Isolation of a parvovirus from dogs in Britain. *Vet. Rec.* **105**, 167.

McCANDLISH I.A.P., THOMPSON H., FISHER E.W., CORNWELL H.J.C., MACARTNEY L. & WALTON I.A. (1981) Canine parvovirus. *In Practice* **3**, 5.

Distemper

APPEL M.J.G. & GILLESPIE J.H. (1972) Canine distemper virus. In *Virology Monographs*, **11**, p. 1. Springer-Verlag, New York.

CORNWELL H.J.C., CAMPBELL R.S.F., VANTSIS J.T. & PENNY W. (1965) Studies in experimental canine distemper. I. Clinicopathological findings. *J. Comp. Path.* **75**, 3.

CORNWELL H.J.C., VANTSIS J.T., CAMPBELL R.S.F. & PENNY W. (1965) Studies in experimental distemper. II. Virology, inclusion body studies and haematology. *J. Comp. Pathol.* **75**, 19.

KRAKOWKA S., HIGGINS R.J. & KOESTNER A. (1980) Canine distemper virus: Review of structural and functional modulations in lymphoid tissues. *Am. J. Vet. Res.* **41**, 284.

LAUDER I.M., MARTIN W.B., GORDON E.D., LAWSON D.D., CAMPBELL R.S.F. & WATRACH A.M. (1954) A survey of canine distemper. *Vet Rec.* **66**, 607, 623.

WRIGHT N.G., CORNWELL H.J..C., THOMPSON H. & LAUDER I.M. (1974) Canine distemper: current concepts in laboratory and clinical diagnosis. *Vet. Rec.* **94**, 86.

Adenovirus infections

CORNWELL H.J.C., KOPTOPOULOS G., THOMPSON H. & McCANDLISH I.A.P. (1982) Immunity to canine adenovirus respiratory disease: a comparison of attenuated CAV-1 and CAV-2 vaccines. *Vet. Rec.* **110**, 27.

HAMILTON J.M., CORNWELL H.J.C., McCUSKER H.B., CAMPBELL R.S.F. & HENDERSON J.J.W.P. (1966) Studies on the pathogenesis of canine virus hepatitis. *Br. Vet. J.* **122**, 225.

SWANGO L.J., WOODING W.L. & BINN L.N. (1970) A comparison of the pathogenesis and antigenicity of infectious canine hepatitis virus and the A26/61 virus strain (Toronto). *J. Am. Vet. Med. Assoc.* **156**, 1687.

WRIGHT N.G. (1976) Canine adenovirus; its role in renal and ocular disease: A review. *J. Small Anim. Pract.* **17**, 25.

WRIGHT N.G., CORNWELL H.J.C., THOMPSON H., ARMITAGE A. & MORRISON W.I. (1972) Canine adenovirus respiratory disease: Isolation of infectious canine hepatitis virus from natural cases and the experimental production of the disease. *Vet. Rec.* **90**, 411.

Leptospirosis

McINTYRE W.I.M. & MONTGOMERY G. L. (1952) Renal lesions in *Leptospira canicola* infection in dogs. *J. Path.* **64**, 145.

MICHNA S.W. (1970) Leptospirosis. *Vet. Rec.* **86**, 484.

MORRISON W.I. & WRIGHT N.G. (1976) Canine leptospirosis: An immunopathological study of interstitial nephritis due to *Leptospira canicola. J. Path.* **120**, 83.

Contagious respiratory disease

APPEL M.J.G., PICKERILL P.H., MENEGUS M., PERCY D.H., PARSONSON I. M. & SHEFFY B.E. (1970) *Current status of Canine Respiratory Disease.* Gaines Veterinary Symposium, Kansas.

BEY R.F., SHADE F.J., GOODNOW R.A. & JOHNSON R.C. (1981) Intranasal vaccination of dogs with live avirulent *Bordetella bronchiseptica:* Correlation of secretory IgA with protection against experimentally induced infectious tracheobronchitis. *Am. J. Vet. Res.* **42**, 1130.

THOMPSON H., WRIGHT N.G. & CORNWELL H.J.C. (1975) Contagious respiratory disease in dogs. *Vet. Bull.* **45**, 479.

THOMPSON H., McCANDLISH I.A.P. & WRIGHT N.G. (1976) Experimental respiratory disease in dogs due to *Bordetella bronchiseptica. Res. Vet. Sci.* **20**, 16.

WRIGHT N.G., THOMPSON H., CORNWELL H.J.C. & TAYLOR D.J. (1974) Canine respiratory virus infections. *J. Small Anim. Pract.* **15**, 27.

Infectious diarrhoea

CARMICHAEL L.E. & BINN L.N. (1981) New enteric viruses in the dog. *Adv. Vet. Sci. Comp. Med.* **25**, 1.

HOLT P.E. (1980) Incidence of *Campylobacter, Salmonella* and *Shigella* infections in dogs in an industrial town. *Vet. Rec.* **107**, 254.

MACARTNEY L., McCANDLISH, I.A.P., AL-MASHAT R.R. & TAYLOR D.J. (1982) Natural and experimental enteric infections with Campylobacter jejuni in dogs. In *Campylobacter, Epidemiology, Pathogenesis and Biochemistry.* Proceedings of an International Workshop on Campylobacter Infections, University of Reading, March 1981, p. 172. MTP Press Limited, Lancaster.

Tuberculosis

JARRETT W.F.H. & LAUDER I.M. (1957) A summary of the main points in tuberculosis in the dog and cat. *Vet. Rec.* **69**, 932.

SNIDER W.R. (1971) Tuberculosis in canine and feline populations. *Am. Rev. Resp. Dis.* **104**, 877.

Salmonellosis

GALTON M.M., SCATTERDAY J.E. & HARDY A.V. (1952) Salmonellosis in dogs. I. Bacteriological, epidemiological and clinical observations. *J. Infect. Dis.* **91**, 1.

THOMPSON H. & WRIGHT N.G. (1969) Canine salmonellosis. *J. Small Anim. Pract.* **10**, 579.

Rabies

BAER G.M. (1975) *The Natural History of Rabies.* Vols. I and II. Academic Press, New York.

FLEMING G. (1872) *Rabies and Hydrophobia.* Chapman & Hall, London.

KAPLAN C. (ed.) (1977) *Rabies, the Facts.* Oxford University Press, Oxford.

MINOR R. (1977) Rabies in the dog. *Vet. Rec.* **101**, 516.

SIKES R.K. (1970) In *Infectious Diseases of Wild Mammals,* eds. J.W. Davis, L.H. Karstad & D.O. Trainer. Iowa State University Press, Ames, Iowa.

TAYLOR D., BEDFORD P.G.C., CRICK J. & BROWN F. (1976) Rabies: epizootic aspects; diagnosis; vaccines; notes for guidance; official policy. *Vet. Rec.* **99**, 157.

TURNER G.S. (1977) An assessment of the current position of rabies vaccination in man. In *Recent Advances in Clinical Virology,* ed. A.P. Waterson. Churchill Livingstone, Edinburgh.

WEST G.P. (1972) *Rabies in Animals and Man.* David & Charles, Newton Abbot.

WHO (1973) *Expert Committee on Rabies, 6th Report.* WHO Technical Report Series No. 523. World Health Organisation, Geneva.

14

Alimentary Tract and Associated Glands

D. B. MURDOCH

This chapter will cover diseases affecting the alimentary canal from the oesophagus distally. In addition, hepatic and exocrine pancreatic problems will be discussed.

Diseases of the alimentary canal produce a limited range of clinical signs, the commonest being vomiting and diarrhoea. Rather than discuss each disease as an isolated entity, an attempt has been made to establish lists of differential diagnoses under the broad headings 'vomiting' and 'diarrhoea' and the conditions considered within this framework.

Exocrine pancreatic and hepatic problems will be dealt with in separate sections.

VOMITING

There are three patterns of vomiting, although there may be an overlap between one type and another.

1   True vomiting. Active vomiting which involves movement of the abdominal, thoracic and diaphragmatic muscles, resulting in forceful ejection of vomitus from the mouth, is by far the commonest form.
2   Regurgitation. The act of regurgitation is more passive than true vomiting with little movement of the thoracic and abdominal muscles. The animal lowers its head and a 'cast' of food, frequently tubular in shape, falls from the mouth. This type of vomiting is associated with oesophageal lesions.
3   Pharyngeal retching. Following normal prehension of food, the animal has obvious difficulty in swallowing and indeed may become distressed. There is immediate retching of partially masticated boluses of food plus saliva, usually followed by a bout of coughing due to ingesta passing down the trachea.

Aetiology of vomiting

This is summarised in Fig. 14.1.

Visceral. Many conditions cause direct stimulation of the vomiting centre in the brain. These diseases may be divided into two groups:

1   Those which produce irritation or inflammation of the mucosa of the alimentary tract.
2   Those which produce pathological changes in visceral organs.

Vestibular stimulation. Motion affects the semicircular canals with subsequent stimulation of the vomiting centre. The most common example of this is travel sickness.

Central. Located in the brain is an area, the chemoreceptor trigger zone, which can stimulate the vomiting centre to produce emesis. The stimulants of this zone can be divided into two categories:

1   Drugs which may produce vomiting as a side effect (e.g. digitalis, aspirin, phenylbutazone).
2   The toxins or toxic substances produced during the course of a large number of conditions (e.g. uraemia).

Emotional.   The higher centres of the brain can stimulate the vomiting centre. This is rare in domestic animals but may occur in both cats and dogs due to fear, changes in surroundings or routine.

Diseases associated with vomiting

These conditions will be grouped under two broad headings: persistent vomiting and transient vomiting. The term 'persistent vomiting' is applied to any condition which has produced vomiting for many weeks. 'Transient vomiting' indicates a short duration with the outcome either recovery or death. With such an arbitrary classification, there are obviously many conditions which are difficult to classify.

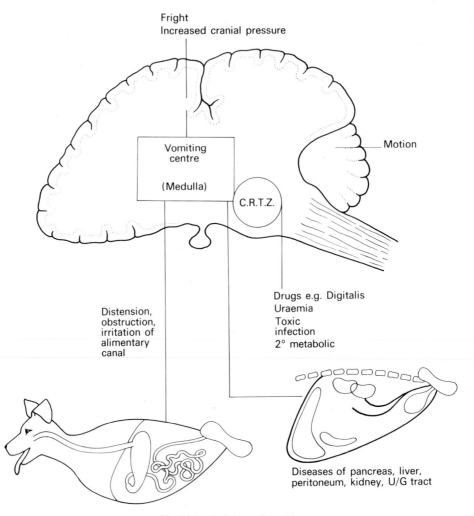

Fig. 14.1   Aetiology of vomiting.

Persistent vomiting

Persistent vomiting first noticed at weaning
1   Megaoesophagus
2   Pyloric stenosis/pylorospasm
3   Incomplete obstruction with a foreign body (see p. 373)
4   Vascular rings
5   Cricopharyngeal achalasia

Megaoesophagus. Considerable confusion has arisen regarding the terminology applied to this condition. For many years it was assumed that the condition resulted from a failure of the distal oesophagus to relax. It has now been demonstrated that the dog does

not have a true sphincter between the oesophagus and the stomach. Further, Rogers *et al* (1979) showed that the pressure in the caudal oesophageal segment was similar in normal dogs and in those with a congenital or acquired megaoesophagus, i.e. affected dogs do *not* have achalasia of the lower oesophageal segment. Thus the terms 'achalasia', 'chalasia' and 'oesophageal paralysis' have been abandoned in favour of the general term 'Megaoesophagus'. These cases may be divided into two distinct categories.

1   Idiopathic congenital megaoesophagus. This is a disease of the young dog characterised by megaoesophagus, failure of progressive peristalsis and asynchronous function of the lower oesophageal segment

(both the latter changes can only be detected using contrast studies and fluoroscopy).

The condition has been described in many breeds including the Newfoundland, Red Setter, Miniature Schnauzer, Doberman and Retriever. In 1980, Cox suggested that the mode of inheritance was either an autosomal dominant or an autosomal recessive with incomplete penetration. The hereditary nature of the problem is potentially very serious as all the dogs in an affected litter may not exhibit clinical signs, i.e. if fluoroscopic examination of litters with idiopathic congenital megaoesophagus is performed at a few weeks of age, all the pups may exhibit the abnormalities described above. In most dogs, however, the condition has resolved by 4–6 months of age, leaving a very small percentage showing clinical signs. This means that clinically normal adults will carry the gene for idiopathic congenital megaoesophagus.

2 Acquired megaoesophagus. This form of the disease affects the mature dog without a history of prior oesophageal neuromuscular dysfunction. As above, these dogs show a lack of progressive peristalsis with asynchronous function of the lower oesophageal segment, but do not develop clinical signs till several years of age.

The affected animals exhibit regurgitation frequently accompanied by reconsumption of the vomitus. A cough is frequently noted as inhalation pneumonia results from the abnormal swallowing and regurgitation.

Confirmation of the diagnosis is by radiography. Following administration of a mixture of meat and barium sulphate, early cases will show the neuromuscular defects described above. When the condition becomes more advanced, the entire thoracic and frequently the cervical oesophagus becomes dilated (Fig. 14.2). The inhalation pneumonia is usually most obvious in the apical lobes.

Treatment. There is universal agreement that the congenital form of the disease should be treated by gravity feeding, i.e. the dog is fed from an elevated bowl so that its head is higher than the stomach, thus, gravity aids the passage of ingesta down the oesophagus. It is beneficial to feed these dogs frequently on small quantities of soft, moist food (Fig. 14.3).

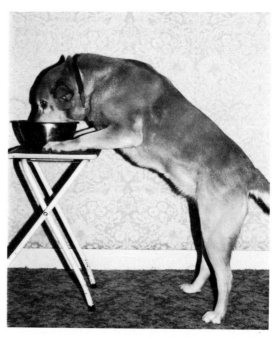

Fig. 14.3 Eight-year-old Labrador eating from an elevated bowl to assist the passage of ingesta into the stomach.

With the acquired form of the disease, the controversy regarding medical versus surgical treatment has been debated for many years. Protagonists of the modified Hellers operation concede that the surgical procedure does not restore synchronous oesophageal function, but the dogs improve clinically as the oesophagus can empty more easily.

Pyloric stenosis/pylorospasm. Pyloric stenosis is seen as a congenital disease, especially in the brachycephalic breeds. The lesion is a functional pyloric obstruction due to hypertrophy of the pyloric sphincter.

Pylorospasm produces the same functional effects except that in these cases the pyloric sphincter is not thickened. It should be emphasised that it is clinically

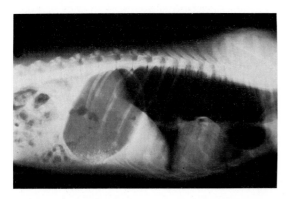

Fig. 14.2 Megaoesophagus in a 6-month-old Red Setter. The dilated oesophagus occupies the dorsal part of the thorax. The stomach is dilated with air, a finding commonly associated with megaoesophagus.

impossible to differentiate between pylorospasm and pyloric stenosis.

Unlike the previous conditions discussed, these animals will show true vomiting not related to eating. The vomiting is frequently associated with sudden activity.

Following the administration of contrast medium to a normal dog, most of the barium should have emptied from the stomach within 3 hours. In some cases, a distinct 'teat' may be seen in the contrast medium due to the hypertrophied pylorus. As a rough guide, if the stomach has not started to empty 1 hour post administration, then a delay in gastric emptying should be suspected. It should be noted that any inflammatory abdominal lesion (e.g. pancreatitis, enteritis or peritonitis) or an intestinal obstruction will delay the passage of the barium.

As pylorospasm is a functional problem, there may be no demonstrable radiographic abnormalities on both plain and contrast films. If a delay in gastric emptying is noted, it is helpful to administer metoclopramide i.v. (1 mg/kg) (Maxolon). This drug will induce gastric emptying if the delay has been caused by pylorospasm.

Treatment. Both the above conditions may respond to medical therapy with atropine or propantheline bromide and it is worth trying medical treatment before a pyloromyotomy. Ramstedt's operation is the preferred surgical treatment.

Both conditions are also seen in the older animal. When a delay in gastric emptying is detected in the adult, the possibility of a peripyloric lesion, e.g. gastric neoplasia, should be considered.

Vascular rings. Many congenital anomalies affecting the major thoracic blood vessels have been described. These cases cannot be differentiated clinically from a megaoesophagus.

One of the most fequently recorded vascular rings is a persistent right aortic arch (the aorta is on the *right* of the oesophagus). This results in the ligamentum arteriosum compressing the oesophagus against the base of the heart. Following the administration of contrast medium, radiographs of the thorax indicate that the dilation is confined to that portion of the oesophagus cranial to the base of the heart (Fig. 14.4).

The condition is treated by sectioning the ligamentum arteriosum and dilating the mediastinum surrounding the stenosed section of the oesophagus.

Cricopharyngeal achalasia. The cricopharyngeal muscle surrounds the oesophagus dorsal to the larynx. In the normal animal the muscle dilates when the animal swallows, allowing food to enter the proximal oesophagus. This does not occur in affected animals.

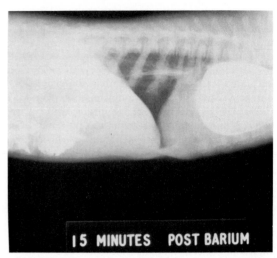

Fig. 14.4 Right-sided aortic arch in a 3-month-old Skye Terrier. Dilatation of the oesophagus is confined to the region anterior to the base of the heart.

Clinical signs are those described under pharyngeal retching. It is difficult to confirm the diagnosis without fluoroscopy to show the failure of dilation of the cricopharyngeus muscle. Spot films may show a large bolus of food retained in the posterior pharynx with a small stream of barium entering both the oesophagus and the trachea.

The condition is treated by 'cricopharyngeal myotomy' on the dorsal aspect of oesophagus (Sokolovsky 1967).

As with oesophageal dilatation the condition may develop in later life.

Differential diagnosis of persistent vomiting at weaning. Alimentary foreign bodies are unlikely to cause problems around the time of weaning. The main differentiating feature is the type of vomiting, the nature of vomitus and its relationship to eating. Using these criteria it should be possible to locate the lesion anatomically but radiology will be necessary to precisely identify the aetiology.

Persistent vomiting with no specific age incidence
1   Gastric foreign body
2   Intestinal foreign body (incomplete obstruction)
3   Oesophageal foreign body (incomplete obstruction)
4   Megaoesophagus (see above).
5   Pyloric stenosis (see above)
6   Cricopharyngeal achalasia (see above)
7   Oesophageal ulceration/stricture

8 Oesophageal diverticulum
9 Hiatus hernia
10 Gastro-oesophageal intussusception

Gastric foreign bodies. A wide variety of foreign bodies have been removed from the canine stomach ranging from razor blades to several feet of heavy link chain. Dogs tolerate gastric foreign bodies unless they are (a) are sharp, (b) obstruct the pylorus, or (c) occupy most of the stomach. Gastric foreign bodies may also move in and out of the pylorus giving a history of recurrent bouts of profuse vomiting with spontaneous remission of symptoms. Sand or gravel may cause an acute illness especially in young dogs. Chronic gastritis may result from persistent irritation of the mucosa by a rough foreign body.

The condition is best diagnosed by radiography although it should be stressed that gastric foreign bodies are a common incidental finding. Most foreign bodies are radiopaque, but contrast medium may be required to demonstrate radiolucent objects (e.g. peach stones, cloth).

Oesophageal ulceration/stricture. Ulceration of the oesophagus is uncommon in the dog. Many aetiologies have been proposed including ingestion of caustic substances and reflux of gastric acid as a sequel to an oesophageal foreign body. Several cases have been recorded following prolonged anaesthesia possibly as a result of gastric acid reflux.

Oesophageal strictures may develop as a consequence of oesophageal ulceration, but more commonly as a result of oesophageal surgery.

Both the above conditions are diagnosed by contrast radiography or endoscopy. As with many oesophageal problems, affected dogs may swallow frequently or salivate excessively.

Oesophageal diverticulum. Development of a diverticulum may be secondary to a foreign body or to a congenital weakness in the oesophageal musculature. Some cases show continuity between the oesophagus and the lung; indeed, broncho-oesophageal fistulae have been recorded. The lesion is most commonly located on the right side of the oesophagus between the base of the heart and the cardia (Pearson *et al* 1978).

Hiatus hernia. An uncommon condition in dogs. Apart from vomiting, other clinical signs noted in these cases are excessive swallowing and salivation.

As the hernia is frequently of the 'sliding' type, the lesion may be difficult to detect without the use of fluoroscopy (Gaskell *et al* 1974). The diaphragmatic defect may be obvious on surgical exploration of the abdomen.

Gastro-oesophageal intussusception. Eversion of the stomach into the oesphagus is rare in dogs. The condition has been recorded most frequently in puppies. Initially these cases present as typical oesophageal regurgitation, but with time, become markedly depressed and begin to vomit blood.

Persistent vomiting more common in the adult and aged dog
1 Uraemia (see Chapter 15)
2 Pyometra (see Chapter 16)
3 Diabetes mellitus (see Chapter 8)
4 Gastric neoplasia
5 Gastric ulceration
6 Intestinal neoplasia
7 Intestinal strictures
8 Hypertrophic gastritis
9 Oesophageal tumours
10 Masses adjacent to the alimentary canal

Gastric neoplasia. Neoplasia of the canine stomach is uncommon, gastric adenocarcinoma being the tumour

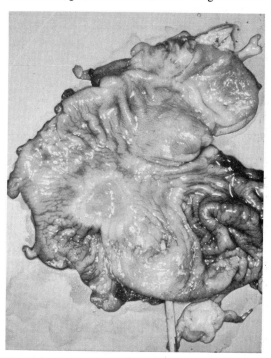

Fig. 14.5 Gastric adenocarcinoma in a 10-year-old West Highland White Terrier. A large 'punched out' ulcer is present. The normal rugal pattern is absent from the mucosa surrounding the ulcer.

Table 14.1 Radiographic changes in diseases of the stomach.

Acute gastritis
No diagnostic radiographic changes

Chronic gastritis
Rugae appear enlarged and flattened
Plaques of thickened rugae resemble intraluminal filling defect

Pyloric stenosis/pylorospasm
Delayed emptying of the stomach
Contrast projects into the sphincter giving a pyloric 'tit'
Generalised gastric enlargement

Neoplasia
Portion of the gastric lumen fails to dilate
Thickening of the stomach wall
No peristaltic movement in affected area of stomach
Persistent filling defect in the wall or lumen of the stomach

Ulceration
Outpouching of the wall beyond the lumen or crater
Rigid appearance of the wall adjacent to the crater
Mucosal folds appear abnormal

most frequently recorded. These tumours often ulcerate producing a raised, punched-out ulcer (Fig. 14.5). As a result of this, haematemesis, melaena and anaemia are often associated with the condition. A characteristic history is that the animal (usually aged) has been losing weight and vomiting for several months (Murray *et al* 1974a).

Radiographic confirmation of the diagnosis can be difficult as the lesion is rarely obvious on plain or contrast films and endoscopy may be helpful (Table 14.1).

The prognosis is poor, although surgical resection may be attempted when the lesion is discrete.

Gastric ulceration. The condition is rare in the dog although there is anecdotal evidence of an above average incidence in the Chow. The lesion has been recorded in association with many conditions (e.g. mast-cell tumours, uraemia, liver disease) and following the administration of anti-inflammatory drugs (Murray *et al* 1974b). Primary gastric ulceration, without any obvious predisposing factors, is known to occur in the dog.

Peptic ulcers may be asymptomatic although some cases will produce very similar clinical signs to gastric tumours. Even on exploratory laparotomy it may be difficult to distinguish between a primary ulcer and a neoplasm with secondary ulceration.

If the lesion is not too advanced, treatment with cimetidine (Tagamet) at 10–15 mg/kg b.i.d. may be helpful.

The use of high doses of dexamethasone as a postoperative treatment following spinal surgery for intervertebral disc protrusions has been advocated for some years. Reports have recently appeared in the literature noting a high incidence of gastro-intestinal haemorrhage which can prove fatal and should haematemesis or malaena develop in animals on this regime, corticosteroid therapy should be stopped immediately (Moore & Withrow 1982).

Intestinal neoplasia. Intestinal adenocarcinomas present as solitary or multiple annular lesions whose presence may not be suspected until ingested material impacts in the narrowed lumen producing clinical and radiographic signs of intestinal obstruction (Table 14.2). Solitary masses may be resected provided the tumour has not metastasised.

Lymphosarcoma may produce diffuse or discrete lesions (see p. 383).

Intestinal strictures. These are usually secondary to intestinal surgery although cases are seen where there is no history of surgical intervention.

Table 14.2 Radiographic changes in intestinal disease.

Obstruction
Loops of small intestine dilated with gas and fluid
Pylorus may be dilated with gas
Intestine distal to the obstruction appears empty
Conglomeration of radio dense flecks in small bowel-Gravel sign
Intestinal stasis—delayed passage of contrast medium
With linear foreign bodies, the intestine appears 'pleated'

Intussusception
Signs of intestinal obstruction (see Figs 14.6 & 14.7)
Intussuscepted segment of greater diameter than adjacent loops
Proximal end of the intussusception outlined by gas
Barium column terminates in a string through the intussusception
'Coiled watch spring' appearance (see Fig. 14.10)

Enteritis
Few detectable radiographic changes
Localised accumulations of gas in the small intestine

Discrete neoplasm (e.g. adenocarcinoma)
Signs of intestinal obstruction
Single or multiple intestinal masses

Diffuse neoplasm (e.g. Lymphosarcoma)
Flocculation and pooling of contrast media
Wide variation in intestinal diameter
Segmental narrowing of the intestinal lumen

Strictures
Signs of intestinal obstruction
Segmental narrowing of the intestinal lumen
Abnormal disposition of intestinal loops

Chronic gastritis. This problem develops as a result of hypertrophy of the gastric rugae. A variety of sequelae have been recorded including pyloric stenosis (Happe *et al* 1981) and anaemia as a result of vitamin B deficiency (Huxtable *et al* 1982). It has been postulated that gastric polyps may be an advanced form of hypertrophic gastritis.

The usual treatment is to attempt to resection of the affected gastric mucosa.

Oesophageal tumours. A rare lesion in the dog. The possibility of an oesophageal granuloma associated with *Spirocerca lupi* should be considered when the dog has been imported into this country and is presented with regurgitation and weight loss.

Contrast radiography will show a mass in the lumen of the oesophagus. Confirmation of spirocercal lesions depends upon identification of ova in the faeces.

Transient vomiting
1 Gastroenteritis
2 Travel sickness
3 Intestinal obstruction
4 Oesophageal obstruction
5 Gastric dilation/torsion
6 Pharyngeal irritation
7 Therapeutic agents

Gastroenteritis. The vomiting reflex is well developed in the dog. In the wild, both the dog and bitch feed their young by regurgitation of meat. Many normal dogs will vomit once a week.

The ease with which dogs vomit is an asset as their appetite is frequently non-selective, resulting in the ingestion of potentially injurious material. The odour of meat which is slightly 'off' has been recognised as a potent stimulator of the canine appetite. This problem will be discussed in more detail under diarrhoea.

Vomiting and diarrhoea in recently acquired young pups is very common. This is not surprising when an immature immune response is expected to cope with removal from the litter, change of environment, change of diet and stress.

Many factors have been implicated in the aetiology of canine gastroenteritis although frequently the cause cannot be determined despite obtaining a good history.

The severity of clinical signs varies from a solitary attack of vomiting to a life-threatening syndrome requiring intensive therapy.

In the majority of cases, the condition is self limiting and will clear up whatever treatment is given. Starvation for 24 hours is recognised as beneficial although each clinician advocates their own favourite treatment for this condition.

Treatment of the acutely ill case is aimed at maintaining the animals' fluid and electrolyte balance (discussed in Chapter 12).

Antiemetic drugs are summarised in Table 14.3. Metochlorpramide (Maxolon) is particularly useful as it does not induce lethargy as a side effect. It also promotes gastric emptying by relaxing the pylorus and duodenum and can be used as a premedicant when anaesthetising an emergency case which has been fed.

Travel sickness. A common problem, especially in puppies, easily treated with antiemetics.

Intestinal obstruction. A wide variety of conditions may produce clinical signs of intestinal obstruction (see Table 14.4).

Clinical signs exhibited will depend upon several factors. First, whether the obstruction is complete or incomplete. The condition of an animal with a complete obstruction (e.g. a smooth rubber ball in the duodenum), will deteriorate much more rapidly than

Table 14.3 Antiemetics.

Travel sickness antiemetics			
Acetyl promazine	Many brands	2 mg/kg	Long acting (up to 24 hours)
Promethazine	Phenergan	2 mg/kg	Long acting (up to 24 hours)
Diphenhydramine	Benadryl	4 mg/kg	Short acting (5-6 hours)
Dimenhydramine	Dramamine	8 mg/kg	Short acting (5-6 hours)
Meprobam	Mepavalon	50 mg/kg	1 hour before effects noted
Broad spectrum antiemetics			
Metoclopramide	Maxolon	0.75 mg/kg	Particularly useful
Prochlorperazine	Stemetil	0.1 mg/kg	
Chlorpromazine	Largactil	0.5 mg/kg	
Trifluorpromazine	Stelazine	0.03 mg/kg	
Trimethobenzamine	Tigan	3.0 mg/kg	

Table 14.4   Aetiology of intestinal obstruction.

Intraluminal obstruction
Radiopaque foreign bodies, e.g. stones, marbles, coal, etc.
Radiolucent foreign bodies, e.g. plastic toys, nuts, peach stones, etc.
Linear foeign bodies, e.g. tights, string, twine, etc.

Intestinal lesions producing obstruction
Intussusception
Acute enteritis
Neoplasia
Volvulus
Strictures

Obstruction although the intestinal lumen is patent
Intestinal ischaemia/infarction
Paralytic ileus

an animal with an incomplete obstruction (e.g. an intussusception). In the latter case, some fluid will pass the obstruction and be absorbed distal to the obstruction.

Second, the level at which the intestine is obstructed. As a rough guide, the higher the obstruction the more rapidly the animal's condition will deteriorate. An animal with a complete obstruction of the duodenum will vomit profusely and be moribund within a few days, whereas animals with obstruction of the distal ileum may vomit intermittently and survive for several weeks. The character of the vomitus will differ. High intestinal obstructions are associated with watery bile-stained vomitus, whereas that seen in low intestinal obstruction is almost faecal in appearance. With low obstructions, marked dilatation of the intestinal loops is present and this may be detectable on abdominal palpation. Another difference is in the type of faeces produced. High, complete obstructions are associated with absence of faeces whereas animals with low intestinal obstructions may be diarrhoeic.

Third, has the intestinal wall been perforated? Perforation is an uncommon sequel to intestinal obstruction with the exception of linear foreign bodies. These can act like a cheesewire on the intestinal wall resulting in peritonitis, abdominal pain and shock. Some metallic foreign bodies (e.g. needles) may perforate the bowel although such objects are commonly noted on survey radiographs as incidental findings.

The foreign body may be palpable. If not, well-defined radiological signs indicate the presence of an intestinal obstruction (see Table 14.2, Figs. 14.6, 14.7).

Treatment.   In some cases, the foreign body may pass into the colon without any treatment and it is good practice to take a radiograph shortly before embarking upon a laparotomy, to check the location of the foreign body. Usually, however, intestinal obstructions require therapy with three objectives.

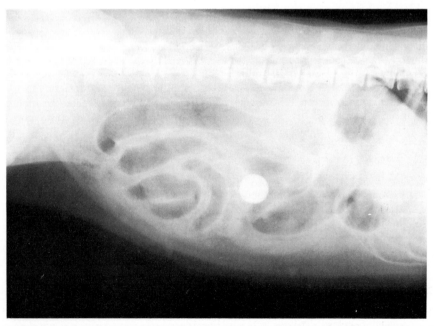

Fig. 14.6   Intestinal obstruction in a 1-year-old mongrel. The radiopaque foreign body, a glass marble, is obvious. Note the intestinal loops and the pylorus dilated with gas.

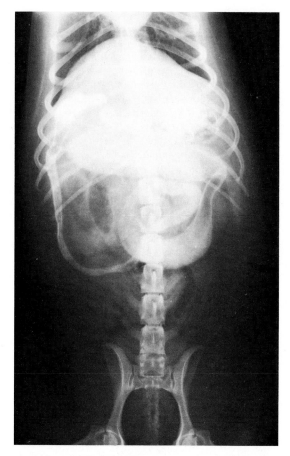

Fig. 14.7 Intestinal obstruction in a 3-year-old Collie. The radioluscent foreign body, a rubber arrow tip, is not obvious. The film was taken 2 hours after administration of barium sulphate by mouth suggesting delayed passage of contrast medium. Several dilated loops of intestine are present. The contrast medium in the caudal loop appears 'grey', suggesting dilution with fluid. Some radiodense flecks are also present in this loop.

1   To correct the animal's fluid, electrolyte and acid-base balance (see Chapter 12).
2   To administer broad-spectrum antibiotics to reduce bacterial multiplication within the gut (endotoxin shock is an important contributory factor to the severity of clinical signs).
3   To relieve the obstruction.

Clinical and radiological signs of obstruction may develop although the intestinal lumen is still patent, e.g. intestinal ischaemia/infarction. Following abdominal trauma, the dog apparently recovers but several days later begins to vomit brown, foul smelling fluid. The original trauma has damaged the mesenteric vessels resulting in ischaemia of a bowel loop. Following the administration of contrast medium, as well as the radiographic signs of obstruction, the infarcted segment appears to have a series of 'thumb prints' along the intestinal wall.

Oesophageal obstruction. Bones are by far the most common cause of oesophageal obstruction (see Fig. 14.8). The condition is commoner in Terrier type dogs

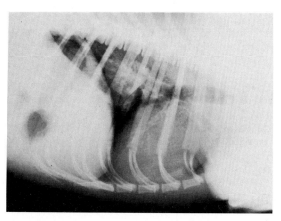

Fig. 14.8   Oesophageal foreign body in a 2-year-old Jack Russell Terrier. The flat piece of bone produced an incomplete obstruction resulting in vomiting of several months duration.

(e.g. Scotties, Westies and Bull Terriers), although all breeds may be affected (Pearson 1966). Three sites of obstruction are commonly noted; the thoracic inlet, over the base of the heart and the distal, high pressure zone between the heart and the diaphragm. Of these sites, the last has been recorded most frequently.

Clinical signs will vary depending on whether the obstruction is complete or not. If the obstruction is incomplete, the animal may survive for many months. Complete obstructions will deteriorate rapidly, exhibiting regurgitation shortly after eating, excess salivation and persistent gulping.

Although a diagnosis may often be made on history, it is always worthwhile radiographing the thorax to check for oesophageal perforation (Table 14.5) as this will influence the choice of treatment.

1   Transthoracic oesophagotomy. Good equipment and sound surgical techniques are required for this approach. If the oesophagus has perforated, this is the only method which should be used.
2   Removal per os. A wide-bore oesophagoscope and long-handled forceps are helpful when attempting to

Table 14.5   Radiographic changes in oesophageal disease.

Foreign bodies
Retention of gas, food and saliva proximal to the obstruction
Check for aspiration pneumonia
Has the oesophagus perforated? Look for
    free thoracic fluid: fissure lines between lung lobes
    mediastinitis: area around the F.B. appears fuzzy
    pneumothorax: free gas around the heart and lung lobes
    leakage: contrast media detected outside oesophagus
    pleurisy/pneumonia: loss of normal lung lucency

Megaoesophagus
Dilation of the *entire* thoracic oesophagus
Usually, dilation of cervical oesophagus as well as thoracic
Ventral depression of the trachea and PVC on lateral views
Retention of barium in the oesophagus

Vascular rings
Narrowing of the oesophagus over the base of the heart
Dilation of the oesophagus *cranial* to the stricture
Diameter of the oesophagus caudal to the heart is normal

Ulceration
Contrast media adheres to the irregular oesophageal lumen
'Smudging' of the contrast media

Stricture
Persistent segmental narrowing of the oesophageal lumen
Lumen of the narrowed segment appears irregular

Diverticulum
Oesophageal pouch usually right-sided between heart and cardia
Broncho–oesophageal fistula may be present
Advanced cases may resemble megaoesophagus

Gastro-oesophageal Intussusception
Dilation of thoracic oesophagus, especially the terminal section
Smooth intraluminal oesophageal density adjacent to cardia

remove the foreign body through the mouth. If resistance is felt when the foreign body is grasped, excessive traction should not be applied or the oesophagus will rupture.

3   Presternal oesophagotomy. Especially useful for foreign bodies located anterior to the base of the heart. Whelping forceps may be used in this approach.

4   Via the stomach. Foreign bodies in distal oesophagus may be removed via a gastrotomy incision. Again, excessive pressure should be avoided. The use of a probang to force the foreign body into the stomach should be discouraged.

Gastric dilatation and torsion. The terminology applied to this condition is very confused. Simple gastric dilatation may be defined as mild-to-moderate distension of the stomach with gas, a common problem in all breeds of dogs especially puppies and usually associated with overeating. This is rarely of clinical significance although these animals will vomit.

It is well recognised that there is an above average incidence of simple gastric dilatation and intestinal tympany in Irish Setters. Aerophagia, pyloric stenosis and defective carbohydrate metabolism have been suggested as possible aetiologies.

Acute gastrc dilatation is a life-threatening syndrome in which the viscus becomes so large that abdominal pain, impaired venous return to the heart, endotoxic and neurogenic shock and metabolic acidosis rapidly produce death (Wingfield *et al* 1974). This dilatation of the stomach is a necessary precursor to gastric torsion when the stomach rotates either clockwise or anticlockwise, producing a functional obstruction at the oesophagus and pylorus.

The problem is much commoner in large, deep-chested dogs although cases have been recorded in dogs as small as Dachshunds. Many aetiological factors have been proposed by Cornelius and Wingfield (1975). Most cases occur shortly after a large meal especially in association with postprandial exercise. Funquist and Garmer (1967) believe that the basic lesion is a dysfunction of the pyloric sphincter which allows dilatation to develop after a large meal. There is usually little problem in diagnosing gastric torsion, as the clinical signs of marked abdominal pain and distended anterior abdomen are pathognomonic; if there is any doubt as to the clinical diagnosis a radiograph will reveal the enlarged gas-filled stomach (Fig. 14.9).

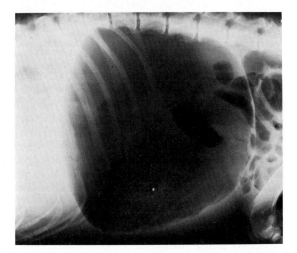

Fig. 14.9   Gastric dilation in a 3-year-old German Shepherd Dog.

Treatment. When dealing with a case of gastric torsion, there are two prime objectives; first, fluid therapy to restore the circulating blood volume and second, decompression of the stomach. The latter procedure should be carried out gradually as rapid decompression will produce a pooling of blood in the abdominal circulation causing a further drop in blood pressure. Initially, an attempt should be made to pass a stomach tube, although in some cases, even if this procedure is successful, deflation is not achieved as the stomach contents may resemble those seen in bovine 'frothy bloat'.

Other methods which may be used involve the use of a needle with a three-way tap on it, and a gastrotomy under local anaesthetic. These cases are extremely poor anaesthetic risks and the pressure should be released and the animals' fluid and electrolyte balance retored before undertaking abdominal surgery to correct the torsion.

Pharyngitis. Inflammation of the pharyngeal mucosa will result in regurgitation rather than true vomiting. It is important to determine if this inflammation has resulted from a mucosal injury, infection or as a result of a pharyngeal foreign body lodged submucosally.

Therapeutic agents. Many drugs may produce vomiting as a side effect either due to mucosal irritation e.g. salicylates and phenylbutazone, or by a central action on the chemoreceptor trigger zone, e.g. digitalis preparations.

DIARRHOEA

Diarrhoea is usually defined as an increased frequency and/or fluidity of the stool in relation to the normal for that individual. The 'normal' for any dog varies tremendously depending upon diet, temperament, training, exercise and location but it is considered normal for a dog to defaecate between one and four times daily. The quantity of faeces passed is dependant upon the diet, the size of the dog, and the consistency of faeces but as a rough guide, the daily stool weight for a Miniature Dachshund is 70 g; for a Beagle, 190 g and for a Newfoundland, 500 g (Anderson 1982).

There is surprisingly little difference between the water content of normal faeces and those from an individual with diarrhoea. The normal faecal water content is 70% whereas typical values from diarrhoeic faeces are between 80 an 83%. In a 20 kg dog, around two litres per day enters the small intestine. As 90% of this fluid has to be absorbed, it is obvious that anything interfering with this secretion and absorption will have a profound effect upon the volume excreted in the faeces.

Thus the production of normal faeces depends upon many factors:

1. Quantity, frequency and type of food.
2. Digestion of food within the alimentary canal.
3. Secretions into the alimentary canal.
4. Absorption from the alimentary canal.
5. Normal segmental and propulsive peristalsis.

Aetiology of diarrhoea

Transient diarrhoea. This group of conditions present as sudden onset diarrhoea which rarely persists for longer than a few days. Many of the cases in this group would clear up without any treatment. Conversely, this category includes the acute syndromes which may prove fatal if not treated.

Chronic diarrhoea. This classification includes the long term diarrhoeas which have persisted for months and the cases which present as recurrent diarrhoea.

Transient diarrhoea

Nutritionally induced diarrhoea
This is by far the commonest cause of diarrhoea in the dog and may be divided into three broad groups:

1. Reduced digestion or absorption of nutrients in the duodenum/jejenum
2. Passage of substrates which encourage bacterial activity in the distal small instestine
3. True dietary allergy

As a consequence of the above changes, substances are produced, e.g. organic acids, ammonia, hydrogen sulphide, amines and bacterial toxins which disturb the osmotic equilibrium of the gut and irritate the mucous membranes resulting in increased secretion into the gut. Some of these substances may block water resorption and the net effect is an increase in the water content of the faeces resulting in diarrhoea.

The first two mechanisms are closely related in that the reduced digestion or absorption of nutrients result in increased levels of undigested proteins, fats and carbohydrates in distal ileum/large intestine. These provide an excellent substrate for the growth and metabolism of micro-organisms and consequently, diarrhoea.

Reduced digestion or absorption of nutrients in the duodenum/jejenum
Most of the products of digestion are absorbed in the duodenum and the jejenum. Intestinal epithelial cells

have the highest metabolic activity of any cells in the body (there is a complete turnover of gastric epithelial cells every 2–6 days and the duodenum, every 1–2 days). This is understandable, as many substances require active, energy consuming transfer mechanisms for absorption, e.g. most monosaccharides and amino-acids.

Although a carnivore, the dog will tolerate a wide range of dietary components. Frequent changes in diet may result in reduced digestion and absorption, and diarrhoea may develop in any species, although dogs appear especially prone. The canine colon is relatively unimportant in digestion (5% of digestion in the dog is colonic compared to 35% in the horse) and as a result, the mechanisms which control bacterial growth in the colon are poorly developed. A change of diet may upset the normal balance between the colonic commensals and the pathogens, a situation exacerbated by the necessary adjustments to pancreatic secretions, e.g. in a dog on a high carbohydrate/low protein diet, these secretions will contain high levels of amylase but low levels of proteolytic enzymes. This problem is most frequently encountered when changing from a dry, complete diet, to a moist meat and biscuit diet. The faeces may be dark and evil smelling for several days.

Carbohydrate. Dogs will tolerate high levels of carbohydrate although should it form a significant part of the diet raw, uncooked starch, e.g. uncooked potatoes, flour or corn may produce diarrhoea. It is interesting to note that the misconception still exists that white bread is 'bad' for dogs. This dates back to when the bleaching agent, agene, was used, which produced epileptiform fits in dogs (Anderson 1982).

Lactose, the carbohydrate constituent of milk, is broken down by the enzymes lactase in the brush border. High levels of this enzyme are present at birth, but the amount decreases as the pup grows older, although if the dog is fed milk every day, more of the enzyme is retained. Meyer (1980) has calculated that feeding more than 1 g per kg body weight per day of lactose will produce diarrhoea in many dogs. This works out at 1 pint of milk per day to a 20 kg dog.

Batt (1979) has suggested that some dogs may be deficient in the disaccharides responsible for normal absorption and transport of specific carbohydrates across the intestinal wall. This may be one reason why some canine diarrhoeas respond to instituting a dietary regime low in carbohydrate, i.e. reducing the biscuit and meal.

Protein. In the dog, proteins of animal origin are highly digestible if fed in sensible quantities, although Meyer (1981) suggested that overcooking meat markedly reduces the digestibility of the proteins.

Raw egg whites contain a trypsin inhibiting factor (also found in unprocessed soya meal) which prevents normal digestion. This poor tolerance of milk and raw eggs shown by many dogs is particularly significant, as it is common for owners to feed a mixture of milk and raw eggs following a gastrointestinal upset.

Feeding dogs on an all-meat diet can result in watery, evil smelling faeces although faecal consistency is improved by increasing the fibre content (see p. 379). Fats of vegetable and animal origin are well tolerated and digested by dogs; thus, when investigating a recurrent diarrhoea problem, it is worth considering a change of diet as a means of therapy (see p. 386).

Passage of substrates which encourage bacterial activity in the distal small intestine
The largest numbers of gut bacteria are located in the ileum, caecum and colon. The bacteria most commonly recorded from the intestine of normal dogs are *Escherichia coli*, Lactobacilli, Streptococci and *Clostridia perfringens* (Amtsberg 1980) and the production of normal faeces depends upon a delicate balance between the commensals and the potential pathogens. Although the intestinal flora are basically established within the first two days of life, the ratio of the organisms present may be influenced by the diet, e.g. the numbers of *Closteridia perfringens* rise when a dog is fed a diet rich in meat but fall when the diet is predominantly cereal.

Increasing the numbers of Lactobacilli in the intestine is supposed to produce a more stable environment for other intestinal bacteria and this is the theoretical basis for increasing the dietary content of this organism as a treatment for acute diarrhoeas. This may be achieved by adding yoghurt or a commercial preparation containing Lactobacilli to the diet.

A well developed vomiting centre has evolved in the dog, indeed it has been estimated that it is one thousand times more sensitive than that of the cat. This provides a useful first line of defence against the effects of over eating. If however, a dog consumes more food than it can efficiently digest in a given period of time, diarrhoea may result and this is why some dogs produce more consistently normal faeces when fed several times a day rather than one large meal. If adopting this feeding regime, avoid feeding the last meal late at night as most dogs will defaecate within 5 hours of consuming a meal (Anderson 1982).

In dogs, the odour of meat which is off is a potent stimulus to eat. This preference for strong smelling, organic material is not confined to meat and the ingestion of damaged 'foodstuffs' results in a high incidence of diarrhoea in scavenging dogs.

Bacterial activity is also influenced by the fibre content of the diet. In the wild, the dog will eat the whole carcass, which results in a diet composed of highly digestible proteins and fats (skeletal muscle, liver, kidney, etc.) and material of low digestibility (skin, hair, tendon, fibres, etc.) There is little residue left in the distal ileum from the former while the fibre content in the latter stimulates peristalsis in the large intestine removing these residues.

In pets, however, the diet consists of easily digested foods with a low fibre content. Thus the residues may remain in the ileum for some time as there is little bulk to stimulate peristalsis (Morris *et al* 1971). As outlined earlier, the presence of food residues can increase bacterial activity. By adding fibre to the diet, this effect is reduced and it has been shown that faecal consistency improves if fibre is added to the diet (Ricklin & Myer 1975). A further benefit is a lower production of fatty acids.

Kendal (1982) has demonstrated that the additon of as little as 5% fibre (in the form of wheat bran) reduces faecal passage time. Owners think of bran as a laxative, but the addition of bran has little effect upon faecal weight provided this fibre comprises less than 10% of the diet. At 20%, however, faecal weight is doubled.

Dietary allergy

This is a diagnosis which is frequently made, but at the present time there has been little well-documented evidence that the condition is common in the dog. The proteins most frequently implicated are beef, wheat (gluten) and milk (casein) (Leibetseder 1982). With a true dietary allergy, the dog may exhibit skin changes as well as diarrhoea and histology of the intestinal wall reveals infiltration with plasma cells and eosinophils.

It is not clear whether the reactions to specific foods reported by owners are examples of dietary allergy, dietary intolerance or simply the effects of dietary change. It is certain, however, that the feeding of large quantities of offal is associated with an increased incidence of diarrhoea, and offal should be eliminated from the diet of a dog with recurrent diarrhoea.

If concerned about a possible dietary allergy, a useful starter diet is a mixture of meat and rice, e.g. cooked lamb, chicken or tripe, cooked rice, corn oil and a multivitamin/minerals supplement. An alternative to the above diet is a mixture of cooked rice, sunflower oil and a multivitamin/mineral supplement. This has the virtue of eliminating meat proteins and, assuming the diarrhoea clears up on this diet, indivi-

duals meats can be added one at a time to assess the effects upon the faeces.

Functional diarrhoea

It is pefectly normal for a dog to pass the occasional soft motion. For many owners, the faecal consistency of their pet is studied with morbid fascination. In most cases it is a question of convincing the owner that there is nothing wrong with the dog.

Many cases are presented with a history of passing a normal stool first thing in the morning, but the consistency becomes more fluid as the day progresses. This history is suggestive of (but by no means pathognomonic for) neural diarrhoea.

Veterinary surgeons have noted an increased incidence of digestive disturbances in giant breeds and Meyer (1980) suggested that the higher the dog's body weight then the lower its ability to cope with alimentary 'stress'.

Other forms of functional diarrhoea present when a dog is stressed, e.g. change of routine, environment, etc. Most functional diarrhoeas will respond to dietary manipulation and spasmolytics such as hyoscine butylbromide (see p. 385).

Bacteria

Bacteria certainly cause clinical problems in pups. *Escherichia coli*, Salmonella, Staphylococci and Streptococci spp. may produce severe, life-threatening diarrhoea which requires treatment with broad-spectrum antibiotics, fluids and adsorbents. In the adult, however, so-called bacterial enteritis usually results from an imbalance in the relationship between commensals and pathogens triggered off by other factors, which are most commonly dietary. The use of antibiotics in these circumstances can actually exacerbate the diarrhoea.

1 Antibiotics may themselves produce diarrhoea. Broad-spectrum antibiotics (e.g. ampicillin, oxytetracycline and chloramphenicol) at high dose rates will produce diarrhoea.
2 Antibiotics may allow super infection to develop. Antibiotics affect the dynamic relationship between colonic bacteria, allowing one form to predominate (e.g. Staphylococci or coliforms). A more serious form of super infection is the overgrowth of yeasts such as Candida spp.
3 Antibiotics may allow the development of a carrier state. There is evidence from the human that, following treatment with antibiotics, some indiviudls become chronic excretors of bacteria, especially Salmonella spp.
4 Antibiotics can induce a pseudomembranous col-

itis. This is well recognised in the human but does not appear to be a problem in dogs. The condition is associated with prolonged administration of antibiotics, the main offender being clindamycin. This drug is rarely used in veterinary medicine although it is now being prescribed for toxoplasmosis.

Thus, the use of antibiotics should be confined to those cases which are systemically ill. The object of therapy is to prevent systemic infection, *not* to sterilise the gut.

Salmonella

Studies on the prevalence of the organism have produced a wide range of incidence statistics varing from 0.6% in a 1970 West German survey to 27.6% in a 1955 survey of Florida Greyhounds. Almost all the surveys have indicated a higher incidence in young dogs and there is no doubt that young dogs are more easily infected than adults. Although many dogs appear to be Salmonella carriers, clinical salmonellosis is rare and is confined to the young animal. The dogs appear to be infected through contact with infected dogs and food-stuffs which explain the high incidence of infection in 'distribution centres' for pups. Despite this, most dogs clear Salmonella from the intestine without showing the clinical signs of vomiting, diarrhoea, fever and malaise. In young dogs with clinical salmonellosis, treatment with chloramphenicol (50 mg/kg t.i.d.) should be instituted combined with supportive fluid therapy and nursing. The organism may cause secondary problems in dogs on chemotherapy for neoplasia.

Several cases of transfer from dogs to man have been recorded and the clinician may be faced with the problem of deciding what to do with the dog excreting Salmonella in its faeces. It has been suggested that the use of antibiotics is contraindicated in Salmonella infections. In man, antibiotics do little to reduce the period of excretion of the organism and indeed may lengthen it. Also, the use of antibiotics tends to encourage the production of the carrier state. Recent work in pigs, calves, and poultry however, suggests that antibiotics may be beneficial in reducing excretion of the organism.

The possibility of a zoonosis should be brought to the owner's attention, especially if young children or elderly people reside on the premises. Should treatment be instituted, it is important to put the animal on a diet containing as few substances as possible which are likely to produce diarrhoea (i.e. low residue diet avoiding milk, liver, hearts and kidneys). It is well recognised that diarrhoea increases the number of Salmonella organisms excreted in the faeces.

Escherichia coli

Escherichia coli causes profuse, watery diarrhoea in puppies. The significance of the organism in the adult, however, is a subject of considerable controversy. The presence of large numbers of *E. coli* in the faeces may be a reflection of an alteration in the normal relationship between commensals and pathogens in the colon. In many cases of diarrhoea arising from non-bacterial factors, large numbers of *E. coli* are isolated from the faeces. Until the accurate serotyping of *E. coli*, especially the enterotoxin-secreting strains, is widespread, this controversy will continue.

Campylobacter

Although infection with campylobacter has been a familiar problem to veterinary surgeons for many years, it was not until Dekeyser *et al* (1972) applied diagnostic techniques developed in animals to human faeces that the significance of the problem in man was appreciated. Since then, the number of isolations from humans has increased dramatically to reach an incidence of around 9000 reported cases per annum (Skirrow 1981). The disease is of particular significance to the veterinary profession as reports of dog-associated campylobacter enteritis have appeared in the medical literature.

Surveys have established that campylobacter may be isolated from the faeces of around 10% of normal dogs (Hosie *et al* 1979; Holt 1980). Bruce *et al* (1980) reported that 49% of faeces sampled from *kennelled* dogs were positive for campylobacter, but in a more recent survey (1983) the same authors recorded figures in agreement with Hosie and Holt when they examined *household* dogs. There are two possible explanations for this anomaly; first, the dogs become infected after reaching the kennels (Gruffydd-Jones *et al* 1980) or secondly, some dogs may be carriers of campylobacter and only excrete the organism in their faeces under provocation, e.g. stress or conconmittant intestinal infection (Simpson & Burnie 1983).

Holt reviewed the problem in 1981 and listed five recommendations.

1 Cases of enteritis in dogs or cats which occur at the same time as human enteric disease in a household should be investigated thoroughly.
2 In the case of a positive isolation from a dog or cat, it should be ascertained that the isolate is an identical strain to that of the affected human.
3 Since the duration of excretion is unknown and the possibility exists of zoonotic spread, dogs and cats from which campylobacter have been isolated should be treated with oral tylosin at a dose of 45 mg/kg for

5 days. An alternative treatment is erythromycin at 40 mg/kg for 5 days.

4 Faecal examination for campylobacters should always be repeated in diarrhoeic animals with previous positive isolations.

5 The risk of acquiring campylobacter infections from pet animals is remote and can probably be abolished by frequent hand washing and the isolation of children from diarrhoeic dogs and cats (Skirrow 1981).

Viruses

Until the discovery of canine parvovirus (CPV) in the late 70s, it was thought that alimentary viral infections produced transient, mild vomiting and diarrhoea. This virus is covered in Chapter 13.

A coronovirus isolated by Keenan *et al* (1976) was experimentally shown to produce transient vomiting and diarrhoea. Similarly, Cartwright and Lucas (1972) described an outbreak of vomiting and diarrhoea in a kennel and demonstrated a rising titre against transmissible gastroenteritis (TGE) virus, also a coronavirus. Larson *et al* (1979) have suggested that TGE may not be pathogenic in the dog, but that this species may act as a carrier for the virus.

Rotaviruses have been isolated from diarrhoeic dogs (England & Poston 1979).

Haemorrhagic gastroenteritis (HGE)

Hill proposed the name 'canine intestinal haemorrhagic syndrome' for this disease. This is a more accurate term, both as a description of the intestinal contents and because the intestine does not show histological evidence of an inflammatory reaction.

The condition is characterised by sudden onset of vomiting and diarrhoea, rapidly progressing to severe diarrhoea which often appears to be frank blood. Although some cases are mild, most dogs with this condition are medical emergencies requiring prompt treatment. They become rapidly dehydrated and require intensive fluid therapy. The fluid imbalance develops so quickly that these animals may not exhibit the 'tenting' of a skin fold' which is seen in most dehydrated animals, even though the packed cell volume may exceed 60.

The clinical signs of HGE are very similar to those produced experimentally with bacterial endotoxin. It has been postulated that HGE may be caused by an allergic or anaphylactic response to endotoxins (the gut is a shock 'target organ' in the dog). The survey by Burrows in 1977 suggested that the condition is rare under 1 year of age with a peak incidence between 2 and 4 years. Miniature and toy breeds appear more prone prone to the disease, especially Schnauzers and Poodles.

From the above description, it is obvious that HGE may be confused with CPV infections and the necessary precautions should be observed when treating these cases.

Treatment is aimed at maintaining the circulatory blood volume using nomal saline with 1–3 mmol/kg of 8.4% sodium bicarbonate added to correct the acidosis. Intravenous antibiotics and corticosteroids are beneficial.

Intussusception

Intussusceptions are included in this section because the majority of cases present as sudden onset diarrhoea. Should the intussusception be severe enough to produce intestinal obstruction (see p. 373) then vomiting will be the main presenting sign.

The clinical signs will also depend upon the site of

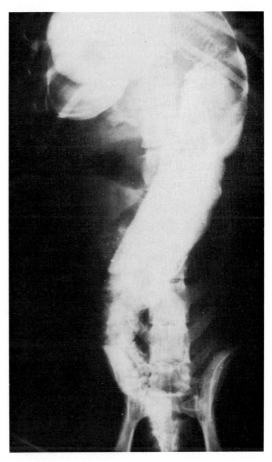

Fig. 14.10 Intussusception in a Labrador. The film was taken following administration of barium sulphate per rectum. Note the 'coiled watchspring' pattern present in the upper right corner of the film. Radiograph courtesy of the Department of Veterinary Surgery, University of Bristol.

the lesion. Most intussusceptions occur at the ileocaecal colic junction when the ileum telescopes into the colon and occasionally protrudes from the anus. These cases usually present with 'raspberry ripple' diarrhoea, so called because of the streaks of fresh blood present. Some intussusceptions, however, will occur as high as the duodenum, when vomiting is the predominant clinical sign (vomiting may develop in low intestinal intussusceptions due to incomplete intestinal obstruction).

The lesion is frequently palpable as a firm, crescentic mass. If it is not palpable then radiographic diagnosis can be difficult as a wide variety of radiological signs may be noted (see Table 14.2 and Fig. 14.10).

Treatment is by reduction of the intussuscepted segment. Frequently, this is not possible and the affected portion may have to be resected and an anastamosis performed. Routine antidiarrhoeal therapy (see below) should be instituted postoperatively to reduce the likelihood of the intussusception recurring.

Chronic diarrhoea

The first problem is to determine whether the diarrhoea is small intestinal or large intestinal in origin. From the clinical history it is usually possible to identify the site involved, although in some cases there is an overlap between the two groups of symptoms making classification difficult (Table 14.6). Note that the table refers to *chronic* diarrhoeas. In acute small intestinal diarrhoea, e.g. bacterial, a dog may pass a fluid watery stool frequently, whereas in chronic small intestinal diarrhoea, e.g. malabsorption, the dog passes a soft motion once or twice daily; compare this to chronic large intestinal lesions, e.g. colitis, where it is common for the dog to defaecate 10 times daily.

Small intestinal lesions

Small intestinal lesions showing steatorrhoea
When the clinical features indicate that the diarrhoea

originates in the small intestine, it is important to consider the appearance of the faeces. If the animal has steatorrhoea (i.e. pale, bulky, greasy, evil-smelling faeces) then the choice is narrowed to three conditions.

1 Pancreatic insufficiency
2 Malabsorption with steatorrhoea
3 Bile salt deficiency

Of the above conditions, the first is by far the commonest. All three conditions are described elsewhere.

It is important to note that steatorrhoea itself can result in diarrhoea, as perfusion of the jejenum, ileum and colon of normal dogs with fatty acids and hydroxylated fatty acids (as occurs in steatorrhoea) reduces absorption of water from the gut lumen. Hydroxylated fatty acids usually produced by intestinal bacteria, are more potent.

Small intestinal lesions showing no steatorrhoea
1 Diet induced enteropathy
2 Malabsorption
3 Parasitic
4 Partial intestinal obstruction
5 Secondary to systemic disease

Malabsorption. Malabsorption is defined as defective absorption of a dietary constituent resulting from interference with the digestive and/or absorptive phases in the processing of the molecule (Batt 1980). Thus any disease process which interferes with normal digestion or absorption can be termed a malabsorption. The basic problem can arise at four levels.

1 *Exocrine pancreatic insufficiency* (EPI) The most severe form of malabsorption resulting in impaired absorption of starch, proteins and triglycerides (p. 392).
2 *Hepatic disease* Normal absorption of triglycerides is dependent upon the formation of micelles with

Table 14.6 Differential diagnosis of small and large bowel diarrhoea.

Clinical sign	Small bowel lesions	Large bowel lesions
Weight loss	Usually present	May or may not be present
Steatorrhoea	May be present	Absent
Frequency of defaecation	Less than 3 daily	Usually exceeds 5 daily
Daily faecal output	Increased	Normal
Faecal mucus	Uncommon	Common (jelly/skin on faeces)
Tenesmus	Uncommon	Common
Faecal blood	If present—melaena	If present—fresh
Flatus/excess borborygmi	Common	Uncommon

bile salts. Thus decreased production or availability of bile salts results in malabsorption of fats.

3 *Primary deficiencies* These problems are related to the enzymes in the brush border which are responsible for the breakdown of the polysaccharides and polypeptides into a form which can be transported across the enterocyte. The best known example is a deficiency of the enzyme lactase, resulting in malabsorption of the carbohydrate lactose (p. 378).

4 *Secondary deficiencies* The disease process is interfering with the normal absorption of the basic mono- and disaccharides, oligopeptides, peptides and amino acids and lipids. If the animal is deficient in the carrier responsible for transporting a specific carbohydrate or proteins across the enterocyte, then that compound will not be absorbed.

Secondly, normal absorption of many nutrients, especially lipids, is facilitated by the enormous increase in surface area which results from the anatomical design of the villi. Any reduction in the filiform nature of the villi as a result of atrophy or damage will severely impair absorption.

Batt and Morgan (1982) have proposed a classification for these secondary deficiencies based upon estimations of serum vitamin levels.

Group 1—Low serum folate and low B12. This suggests generalised intestinal damage as folate is predominantly absorbed in the jejenum and B12 in the ileum. The condition is usually seen in older dogs and of the three groups, these are clinically the most severely affected dogs, with obvious weight loss and watery diarrhoea. Biopsies from the small intestine indicate severe villous atrophy and infiltration of the lamina propria wth chronic inflammatory cells, e.g. histiocytes, eosinophils and plasma cells. These changes suggest non-specific damage not only to the microvilli of the enterocytes but also to other organelles of these absorptive epithelial cells.

Group 2—Low folate but normal B12. These findings suggest that the jejenum is involved and these cases are less severely affected clinically than the dogs in Group 1. Villous atrophy is not a feature. Aggregates of eosinophils have been recorded in some cases.

One theory is that these changes may result from a dietary allergy and this group includes the German Shepherd Dogs with eosinophilic enteritis.

Group 3—High folate and low B12. In this group, the diarrhoea is often intermittent and the problem may be seen in young dogs. The precise aetiology is not known. It has been postulated that an immune deficiency may predispose to bacterial overgrowth in the proximal small intestine an many bacteria manufacture folate.

This bacterial overgrowth is treated with long term antibiotic therapy, e.g. tetracyclines.

Specific diseases of malabsorption. **1** Eosinophilic enteritis. This disease is characterised by focal infiltration of the mucosa with eosinophils. The affected dogs are usually less than 3 years of age and present with a chronic watery diarrhoea, steatorrhoea being uncommon. Differential white cell counts reveal between 10 and 30% of eosinophils, although the severity of eosinophilia varies from day to day and should a normal eosinophil level be recorded in a suspected case, it is worth repeating the count. The condition is more common in the German Shepherd Dog.

2 Lymphosarcoma. Invasion of the intestinal wall by lymphosarcomatous cells may result in malabsorption with diarrhoea, usually in the older dog. These animals may present with a whole range of clinical signs which depend upon the extent of the lesion within the alimentary canal, i.e. does the infiltration affect the small or large intestine or both? Further the gut lesion may be insignificant when compared with the clinical signs which may develop as a result of concomitant lymphosarcomatous infiltration in another organ, e.g. the liver. It should be emphasised that in many cases of intestinal lymphosarcoma the lesion is confined to the alimentary canal. Indeed, it may be impossible to diagnose the condition on exploratory laparotomy and intestinal biopsies are often required to establish a diagnosis. Most cases shown enlargement of the mesenteric lymph nodes, but this finding is noted in many forms of enteritis.

In a recent survey the most common presenting signs were weight loss, vomiting and diarrhoea, but a wide variety of clinical signs were recorded. Significant changes may be demonstrated on contrast radiography (see Fig. 14.11)

3 Lymphangiectasia. The term, lymphangiectasia refers to a generalised dilation of the intestinal lymphatic vessels, usually accompanied by dilation of the mucosal and sub-mucosal lymphatics.

Most dogs with lymphangiectasia present with steatorrhoea and many cases develop a protein losing enteropathy. This term is used to describe a chronic enteric disease which is characterised by an excessive loss of protein through the intestinal wall (Finco *et al* 1973; Flesja & Yri 1977). These dogs often develop ascites, oedema and hydrothorax due to the hypoproteinaemia.

There is no known treatment. Medium-chain triglycerides (MCT) have been used, as these compounds

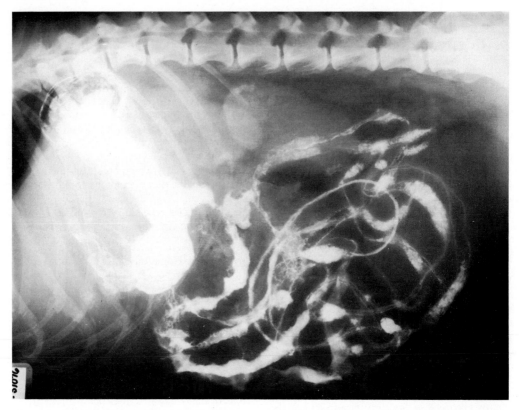

Fig. 14.11 Lymphosarcoma in a 10-year-old Labrador. There is segmental narrowing of the intestinal lumen at several points. The column of barium is irregular and narrows to a string in several places. Contrast medium has floculated.

are supposed to be absorbed directly into the portal circulation rather than through the lymphatics. However, there is evidence to suggest that if treating with MCT all other fat should be excluded from the diet, as long chain triglycerides counteract the beneficial effects of the MCT.

Putting the dog on a high protein diet will help to alleviate the hypoproteinaemia.

Parasitism. Giardia.   For many years, it was thought that Giardia were harmless commensals, but the potential of these parasites to cause disease is now clearly established. Originally they were thought to be host specific, e.g. *Giardia canis* and *G. cati*, but recent reports suggest each species may be capable of infecting more than one host, indeed Giardia cysts isolated from a human produced infections when fed to eight different species of animals (Davies & Hilber 1979).

The trophozoite form of the parasite is dorso-ventrally flattened and pear-shaped with four pairs of flagellae. The organism is attached to the duodenal epithelium by a large adhesive disc (they rarely colonise the intestinal tract lower than the jejenum).

Giardia also exists as a cyst and this is the form commonly observed in faeces and is the infective stage for another susceptible host. The cysts are oval with thick, refractible wall and it has been established in the dog that the pre-patent period between ingestion of cysts and shedding of cysts is 6–8 days (Davies & Hilber 1979).

Although most surveys have indicated that infection with Giardia is uncommon, it is now agreed that these figures are misleading as sugar and salt flotation methods render the cysts unrecognisable (the technique of choice for dignosis is zinc sulphate flotation).

Infection with Giardia may produce chronic diarrhoea in both the dog and cat and the treatment of choice is metronidazole at 25 mg/kg b.i.d. for 5 days. This regime may need to be repeated (Watson 1980).

Ascarids.   Heavy infestation with *Toxocara canis* may result in diarrhoea and checking faeces samples for *T. canis* is a valid investigation in canine diarrhoea.

Cestodes. Diagnosis is usually made on the owner's description of the segments present in the faeces although faecal examination for eggs is occasionally carried out. Should the latter investigation be necessary, then it is doubtful whether cestodes are the cause of the diarrhoea.

Trichuriasis. *Trichuris vulpis* have been included under the heading of a small intestinal parasite but, in practice, infestation by this worm will frequently present as a large intestinal diarrhoea. Clinical infection is seldom seen under 6 months of age and the condition is commoner in high density housing where the ability of *T. vulpis* eggs to remain viable in soil for several years is a major contributing factor.

Diagnosis is by identification of thick-shelled, yellowish, lemon-shaped eggs with a plug at each pole. The condition is treated with a broad spectrum anthelmintic e.g. dichlorvos or fenbendazole. Small numbers of *T. vulpis* are occasionally seen on examination of faeces samples and are of little significance.

Uncinariasis. *Uncinaria stenocephala* is found in Great Britain and like *T. vulpis* is more common in high density housing especially hound kennels. Unlike other hook worms (e.g. *Ancylostoma canium*), anaemia is not a feature of the disease (Jacobs 1978). As well as diarrhoea, foot lesions are commonly present.

Diagnosis is by identification of the eliptical, thin-shelled eggs and the condition is treated using broad spectrum anthelmintics.

Coccidiosis. As with most of the parasites discussed above, clinical outbreaks of coccidiosis are more common under conditions of high density housing. Infection is much commoner in puppies.

Diagnosis is by identification of oocysts in the faeces though more than one examination may be necessary. Treatment with nitrofurazone t.i.d. for 7 days is usually effective.

For further information on endoparasitism, see Chapter 17.

General principles of treatment of small intestinal diarrhoea

Acute diarrhoea

Diet
With the acute diarrhoeas, it is traditional to starve the dog for 24 hours. However recent work in the human has questioned the value of this therapy and many owners dislike withholding food from their pets.

To reduce the chances of malabsorption and bacterial overgrowth, the diet should contain good quality protein, e.g. lean meat, fish or cooked eggs, and not more than 25% crude fibre (Leibetseder 1982) i.e. avoid plant protein fibre or connective tissue such as tendon, fascia or cartilage.

As regards carbohydrate, avoid lactose-containing nutrients, i.e. milk and milk by-products, and the dextrinised starch of cooked cereals.

The diet should be low in fat.

Summary. *Avoid* milk and milk by-products, offal and offal by-products, biscuits and cereals (although rice is easily digested by the dog). Glucose is easily digested but the addition of excess quantities can result in an osmotic diarrhoea.

Feed lean meat, fish, cooked eggs, baby foods, cooked rice.

Anti-diarrhoeal therapy
There are two distinct peristaltic patterns recognised in the intestine:

1 Segmentation. These non-propulsive waves are associated with mixing of and absorption from chyle.
2 Propulsive. As the name suggests, these waves are responsible for mass movements *along* the intestine.

It is often assumed that hypomotility is associated with constipation and hypermotility with diarrhoea. This is not necessarily so and indeed the reverse may be true. Hypermotility may produce increased segmentation as well as increased propulsion, resulting in a net increase in total transit time and *increased* water absorption. Conversely, hypomotility may reduce segmentation giving rise to decreased water absorption. In addition, this hold up of faecal material in terminal ileum encourages bacterial fermentation, resulting in diarrhoea.

The anti-motility drugs are divided into two groups.

Opiates. These drugs increase segmentation as well as reducing propulsive peristaltic movements. They also increase water absorption and intestinal resistance. Because of these properties, the opiates are contraindicated in acute, toxogenic infections. The best know example of this group is diphenoxylate.

Anti-cholinergics. These drugs reduce gastric secretion and emptying time with a decrease in both segmental and propulsive peristalsis. There is a reduction of intestinal resistance. The most widely used drug in this group is a hyoscine derivative, of greatest benefit in the 'neural' type of diarrhoea.

Adsorbants

Kaolin, Charcoal, Bismuth compounds and Attapulgite have been used for decades in the treatment of diarrhoea. Barium sulphate is included in this group, which explains why many cases of vomiting and diarrhoea recover following a barium meal. It is now accepted that these compounds do not protect or soothe the gut but act by increasing the viscosity of the intestinal contents, although some adsorbants absorb and inactivate *E. coli* enterotoxins.

A range of compounds are now available which act by absorbing water in the distal ileum, e.g. sterculia gum.

Antibiotics

When considering therapy with antibiotics, the clinician has to choose between those which are poorly and

Table 14.7   Alimentary antibiotics.

Poorly absorbed	Partially absorbed
Neomycin	Oxytetracycline
Framycetin	Chloramphenicol
Nitrofurazone	Ampicillin
Succinylsulphathiazole	Amoxycillin
	Trimethoprim-sulphonamide

those only partially absorbed (see Table 14.7). There are three basic considerations:

1   Administering an antibiotic which is poorly absorbed would appear to be ideal. Some Gram-negative infections, however, will progress to septicaemia when systemic treatment is needed and in these circumstances an antibiotic limited to the small intestine is inadequate.
2   Parenteral dosing with an antibiotic which is effective against Gram-negative organisms and is secreted in high concentrations in bile, e.g. ampicillin or amoxycillin. With these antibiotics this route of administration will produce effective concentrations of antibiotics in both circulation and the small intestine.
3   Oral administration of an antibiotic which is absorbed such as oxytetracycline will give effective concentrations both in the small intestine and in the systemic circulation.

Anti-prostaglandin therapy

Bacterial endotoxins may stimulate secretion of fluid and electrolytes into the intestinal lumen without any apparent pathological change in the gut wall. This process is thought to be mediated via prostaglandins.

A similar mechanism has been proposed for certain food allergies. Some of the non-steroidal anti-inflammatory drugs, e.g. aspirin and indomethacin, have the ability to inhibit synthesis of prostaglandin and are helpful in many of the acute diarrhoeas.

Chronic diarrhoea

Diet

Dogs may be sensitive to a particular diet for the reasons outlined above. Thus it is always worth instituting a change in diet, bearing in mind the principles discussed earlier, especially the section on fibre and low residue diets (see p. 378). Apart from nutritional

Table 14.8   Diagnosis of intractable large intestinal diarrhoea.

Diagnostic radiographic changes	Intussusception
	Neoplasia
	Ulcerative colitis
Abnormalities on faecal examination	Bacterial
	Trichuris vulpis
Diagnostic changes on proctoscopy	Intussusception
	Neoplasia
	Ulcerative colitis
	Trichuris vulpis
Ancillary aids unhelpful	Irritable colon

reasons, a complete change of diet, e.g. switching from meat and biscuit to a dry, complete diet and vice versa may be helpful.

Increasing the numbers of Lactobacilli in the intestine is supposed to produce a more stable environment for the enteric flora and this is why the addition of live yoghurt or products containing Lactobacilli have been advocated as a treatment for chronic as well as acute diarrhoea.

With many of the conditions discussed earlier, fat absorption is impaired and the addition of a medium-chain triglyceride, such as coconut oil, is helpful, as these oils are absorbed more easily than the saturated, short-chain fatty acids found in animal fat.

Antibiotics

Oral administration of antibiotics significantly affects intestinal bacterial activity. For faecal consistency to remain normal, the delicate relationship between commensals and pathogens must be maintained. One theory is that the prolonged use of oral antibiotics induces an alteration in gut flora which can result in diarrhoea. This leads to a situation, frequently encountered in practice, where the faeces are normal while the dog is on antibiotics, but as soon as these are

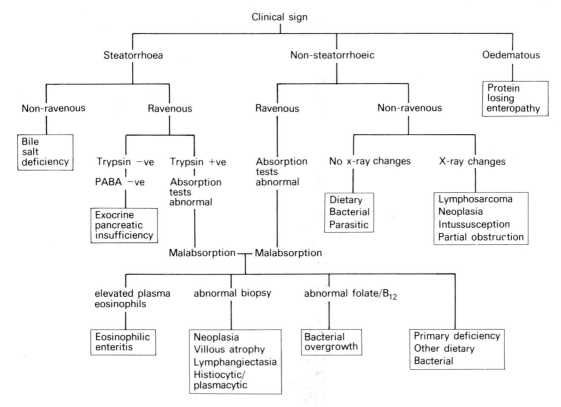

Fig. 14.12 Diagnosis of intractable small intestinal diarrhoea.

withdrawn, diarrhoea recurs. In these situations yoghurt or other sources of Lactobacilli are helpful provided antibiotic therapy is withdrawn.

Bacterial overgrowth in the proximal small intestine is a complication noted in group 3 malabsorption (p. 383). Prolonged use of oral broad spectrum antibiotics, e.g. tetracyclines, will be helpful in these cases although treatment may need to be continued for a month.

Tylosin is a macrolide antibiotic mainly active against Gram-positive, some Gram-negative, bacteria, some spirochaetes, Chlamydia and Mycoplasma. In a series of 80 cases of chronic intestinal disease (Van Kruiningen 1976), the drug produced complete recovery in some and was helpful in most of the others. With many of these dogs, however, therapy had to be administered continuously at 30 mg/kg orally. The mode of action of the drug and the reason for its undoubted efficacy in some cases is not known.

Corticosteroids
These preparations are beneficial for two reasons. Firstly, Batt (1977) has shown that corticosteroids improve absorption of carbohydrates across the small intestinal wall which is impaired in many of the conditions producing malabsorption. Secondly, the drug may reduce cellular infiltration into the gut wall. Treatment is started with high doses of prednisolone (0.75 mg/kg per day) and the dose decreased over several weeks.

Vitamins
Many forms of diarrhoea induce Vitamin B deficiency, particularly B12 and folate; indeed there is anecdotal evidence that treatment with these vitamins may produce a clinical improvement (5 mg per day of folate and 20 mg/kg/day of B12).

Pancreatic supplements
These preparations are beneficial in many cases of diarrhoea not associated with pancreatic disease and clinical improvement following the addition of pancreatic supplements to the diet is *not* diagnostic of pancreatic insufficiency.

Large intestinal lesions
The clinical signs associated with lesions of the large intestine were recorded in Table 14.6.

Colitis
For many years considerable confusion has existed regarding the terminology applied to canine colitis. Three forms of the disease are now recognised in the UK.

1   *Histiocytic ulcerative colitis (HUC)*
The basic lesion is an infiltration of the colonic sub-mucosa by histiocytes. It is probable that reports in the literature describing Boxer colitis, granulomatous colitis, and canine whipples disease are synonymous terms describing histiocytic ulcerative colitis.

Aetiology. The disease is seen almost exclusively in young Boxers although a case has been reported in the French Bulldog (Van der Gaag *et al* 1978). Some workers believe that the causal agent is a coccoid or coccobacillary organism. Beause of the specificity of the disease for the Boxer, a genetic predisposition has been suggested and it is interesting to note that the French Bulldog has the same ancestral origin as the Boxer. Several workers have postulated that the problem may be an autoimmune disease because of the histological findings.

Clinical signs. The occurrence of persistently loose faeces tinged with fresh blood and mucus in young Boxer dogs should arouse suspicion of HUC. In addition, the number of evacuations per day is greatly increased and the act of defaecation is frequently associated with tenesmus. Owners will often comment that the motions contain clear or white jelly, i.e. mucus.

80% of cases exhibit clinical signs at less than 2 years of age and the disease is uncommon in Boxers over 4 years of age. The condition is recorded more frequently in the female.

Pathology. The gross appearance of lesions varies from mucosal friability to gross ulceration, accompanied by severe haemorrhage. In advanced cases, the mucosa is replaced by granulation tissue with the development of chronic, inflammatory, fibrotic structures of the colon.

Microscopically, there is thickening of the lamina propria and the submucosa as a result of infiltration by PAS positive histiocytes, usually accompanied by plasma cells and lymphocytes.

Treatment. This will be discussed under the irritable bowel syndrome. Severely affected animals do not respond to treatment. Dogs with less advanced changes will show an initial response to treatment, but the incidence of recurrence is high and a guarded prognosis should be given in all cases.

2   *Idiopathic ulcerative colitis*
The disease is essentially the same as histiocytic ulcerative colitis except many different breeds are affected. As with the Boxer, inherited factors may play a role in the pathogenesis of the condition, e.g. Gomez and Ewing (1973) recorded the disease in 3 Basenji littermates. Most of the aetiological possibilities discussed under histiocytic ulcerative colitis could apply to this condition.

The main difference between the two problems is the microscopic appearance of the colon. A wide variety of changes have been recorded including focal mucosal ulceration, mucin cell hypertrophy, infiltration of the lamina proparia and muscularis mucosa with inflammatory cells of various types and in long-standing cases, extensive loss of the mucosa with fibrosis of the lamina propria and submucosa. Histiocytic infiltration is not recorded.

3   *Irritable colon syndrome*
This term is used to describe the dog which shows the typical clinical signs of large bowel diarrhoea under ulcerative colitis. This is the commonest form of colitis seen in the UK and is diagnosed on the clinical history and proctoscopy, as colonic biopsy and contrast radiography have proved of limited value.

Some cases will respond to dietary manipulation, the diet of choice being a low residue component, for instance meat and rice with the addition of fibre (e.g. bran and vegetables) to promote peristalsis and soften the faeces in ascending colon. Acute attacks are treated with a combination of corticosteroids and sulphasalazine. The latter drug is administered at 20 mg/kg b.i.d. for one week then the dose is gradually reduced over the next two weeks.

Recently, there have been reports of dogs developing keratitis sicca as a complication of therapy with sulphasalazine and the eyes should be checked frequently.

Colonic tumours
According to one survey (Hayden & Nielsen 1973) malignant neoplasms of the large bowel account for nearly half the alimentary tumours in the dog. Lymphosarcoma is the commonest neoplasm. Clinical signs are those of a large intestinal diarrhoea although some forms of infiltrative colonic carcinoma will produce clinical signs of a low intestinal obstruction.

Tumours of the colon are frequently palpable in the

abdomen or are noted on survey radiographs. Rectal lesions are usually detected on digital examination. Surgical removal may be attempted but the prognosis is poor when carcinomata are present because of early metastases. Polyps also occur in this region and with these lesions the prognosis is much better.

Laboratory examinations useful in diarrhoeic dogs

These have been summarised in Table 14.9. It is worth considering some of these tests in more detail.

Oral glucose tolerance test

This test is based on the premise that glucose will be absorbed across the intestinal wall to give a 'peak' blood glucose 30 minutes after oral administraton of 2 g/kg of a 12.5% solution in water. Selecting a 12.5% solution means that a considerable volume of glucose solution is necessary when investigating a large dog. The temptation to use a more concentrated solution (e.g. 40%) should be avoided, as the passage of concentrated glucose solutions through the stomach is delayed. Similarly feeding a mixture of food and glucose will delay transit into the duodenum. Thus,

the dogs should be starved for 12 hours prior to administration of glucose.

The test will also be influenced by the factors which affect serum glucose levels, e.g. insulin.

A resting sample is taken prior to the administration of glucose. In the normal dog, the concentration at 30 minutes should be in excess of 7.5 mmol/l (140 mg/100 ml) with a return to normal levels at around 2 hours. If there is impairment of carbohydrate absorption the concentration of glucose in post administration samples will vary little from the resting levels.

The advantage of this test is that estimation of blood glucose is easily performed in the practice laboratory.

Oral xylose absorption test

D-xylose is a pentose sugar which is absorbed across the small intestine both passively and actively. The advantage of the test is that there is no xylose present in normal canine serum and consequently the results are subject to fewer variables than glucose absorption. Hill *et al* (1970) reported that significant results were obtained when the xylose was mixed with meat.

Again the dog is starved prior to the test. 0.15 g/kg bodyweight of D-xylose is administered orally as a 5% solution in water or as a powder mixed with a small

Table 14.9 Summary of laboratory investigations in diarrhoeic dogs.

Test	Result	Possible diagnosis
Faeces		
Products of digestion	Muscle fibres and starch granules	EPI
Products of digestion	Fat globules	EPI, malabsorption, bile-duct occlusion
Faecal trypsin	Low levels present on serial samples	EPI
Eggs	Elliptical, thin shell, transparent	*Uncinaria stenocephela, Ancylostoma caninum*
Eggs	Lemon-shaped, yellowish, with a plug at each pole	*Trichuris vulpis*
Eggs	Oval, pitted, thick shell	*Toxocara canis*
Cysts	Oval with thick refractile wall	Giardia
Oocysts	Significant if animal shows signs of intestinal disease	Coccidiosis
Culture	Desoxycholate citrate agar	Useful for Salmonella
Culture	Blood agar, MacConkeys medium	Most enteric organisms
Culture	Anaerobic culture	Campylobacter
Blood		
Haematology	Elevated circulating eosinophils	Possible eosinophilic enteritis
Haematology	Anaemia accompanied by melaena	GI haemorrhage, e.g. ulcer, neoplasia
Oral glucose tolerance	Flat curve	Malabsorption
PABA Test	Low serum concentration at 2 hours	EPI
d-Xylose	Flat curve	Malabsorption
Serum folate	High levels plus low B12	Possible bacterial overgrowth
	Low levels	Possible malabsorption
Vitamin B_{12}	Low Levels	Possible malabsorption
Fat absorption	Serum remains clear	EPI or malabsorption
Liver function tests	Abnormal	Liver disease
Serum proteins	Less than 40 g/l total protein	Protein losing enteropathy (but many other possibilities)

quantity of meat. In the normal dog, peak levels of xylose are noted at 60 min with a gradual fall after this time as the xylose is excreted through the kidneys.

When the intestinal wall is damaged to such an extent that carbohydrate absorption is impaired, then a flat curve is obtained with a lower peak than the normal, which is noted at 2–3 hours post administration.

The procedure is more expensive and requires more specialised equipment than the glucose tolerance test.

In cases of exocrine pancreatic insufficiency absorption of D-xylose is supposed to be normal, but the author has seen cases in which a flat, abnormal curve was recorded.

This test can be combined in one procedure with the PABA Test (p. 394).

Oral fat absorption

This is a crude but useful test based on the principle that long chain fatty acids are absorbed primarily via the intestinal lymphatics.

The dog is given 3 ml/kg of corn oil, e.g. 'Mazola', orally. If fat absorption is normal, plasma taken 2 hours post administration will appear turbid and lipaemic. This indicates that the full spectrum of fat digestion is functioning, i.e. micelle formation with bile salts, breakdown by lipase, absorption across the mucosa and uptake by the lymphatics.

Should the plasma remain clear at 2 hours then this suggests a breakdown somewhere in the above cycle. This may not be due to a pathological process as the test is influenced by many variables, e.g. gastric emptying rate, and it is worthwhile repeating the fat absorption test a few days later.

Serum folate and vitamin B$_{12}$ concentrations

Bioassays are available for these estimations which are of value in differentiating the various forms of malabsorption (p. 382).

Biopsy

It is possible to take biopsies from the small intestine per os using a biopsy capsule or a paediatric fibreoptic endoscope, but the commonly used method is via an intestinal exploratory laparotomy. The most valuable sites for biopsy in the diarrhoeic dog are duodenum and proximal small intestine.

CONSTIPATION

Aetiology of constipation

1 *Functional.* Highly refined diet; megacolon (congenital or acquired).

2 *Mechanical.* Enlarged prostrate; consumption of bones, deformity of the pelvic canal as a result of a fracture; rectal diverticulum; perineal hernia; colonic strictures; peri-colonic masses, e.g. neoplasia.

Functional constipation

The problems associated with highly refined diets were discussed under dietary diarrhoea (p. 379).

Congenital megacolon. Some dogs have a congenital abnormality of the nerve supply to the colon which produces abnormal colonic peristalsis and a failure of one section to dilate. This leads to generalised colonic enlargement (megacolon) with severe constipation. Although this constipation is the main presenting sign, the owner may remark that the dog has an explosive evacuation every few days.

Acquired megacolon. Should an animal develop constipation as a result of an unrelieved mechanical obstruction, a megacolon may develop due to change in the colonic musculature.

Megacolon is easily diagnosed by abdominal palpation and survey radiographs. Establishing the aetiology of the megacolon may require further investigations with barium enemas and proctoscopy.

Mechanical constipation

Most of the conditions listed can be diagnosed by a combination of radiology and rectal palpation, although the prostate may be difficult to feel if the enlarged gland has tipped over the pelvic brim into posterior abdomen. Perineal hernias are usually palpable as a soft fluctuating mass lateral and ventral to the anus.

Treatment

In milder cases, the constipation may be relieved with oral mineral oils, e.g. liquid paraffin. More severely affected animals will require the use of enemas. In many dogs, anaesthesia may be necessary to manually remove the faecoliths (whelping forceps are useful).

Following relief of the constipation, it is important to treat the predisposing factors. Putting the dog on a high fibre diet may help to prevent recurrence of the problem.

THE PANCREAS

Exocrine diseases of the canine pancreas will be discussed in this section. Endocrine diseases have been discussed in Chapter 8.

Physiology and biochemistry

The pancreas serves two main functions. One is the production of the hormones insulin and glucagon by the islet cells and the other is the production of digestive enzymes by the zymogenic cells. These enzymes are secreted in the pancreatic juice.

Proteolytic enzymes

The pancreas secretes inactive precursors of the three proteolytic enzymes. Of these the most important is trypsinogen which is activated to trypsin by calcium ions, bile salts and intestinal enterokinase. Activation of the other two precursors, chymotrypsinogen and procarboxypeptidase depends on the presence of trypsin.

The activated enzymes act upon the complex proteins of the intestinal contents at different points of their molecules to produce polypeptides and amino acids.

Lipolytic enzymes

The enzyme lipase is responsible for hydrolysis of fats to glycerol and fatty acids, although some diglycerides and triglycerides are also produced. Normal production of bile salts by the animal is necessary for this reaction to proceed, as the bile salts emulsify the products of enzyme action to micelles which are subsequently absorbed by the small intestine.

Amylolytic enzymes

Amylase is the only enzyme secreted into pancreatic juice in its active form. The enzyme acts upon complex polysaccharides to produce carbohydrates such as dextrins, maltose and glucose. These substances are then acted upon by the intestinal disaccharidases before absorption across the gut wall.

Secretory control

Secretion of pancreatic juice is under the control of two enzymes, pancreozymin, which controls the quantity of digestive enzymes present in the juice, and secretin which controls the fluid and electrolyte components of pancreatic juice. The latter function includes the production of sodium bicarbonate which is necessary for neutralisation of the acid chyme from the stomach.

Diseases of the pancreas

Canine exocrine pancreatic disease falls into three groups:

1 Acute pancreatitis
2 Exocrine pancreatic insufficiency
3 Pancreatic neoplasia

Acute pancreatitis

The frequency of occurrence of this disease is not known with certainty. Clinical signs vary in severity from a vague malaise to peracute death. Further, there are difficulties in the diagnosis of the condition.

Two stages are noted in the development of the disease (Goodhead 1969). Firstly, some forms of pancreatic damage (e.g. obstruction of the pancreatic duct) produces interstitial oedema within the pancreas. At this stage, the only clinical sign will be a vague malaise. Should the blood supply to the pancreas be reduced, then haemorrhagic necrotic pancreatitis may develop. When this occurs, autodigestion of the pancreas begins (Interstitial trypsin inhibitors prevent this in the normal animal). The trypsin activates enzymes such as elastase, phospholipase A, kallikrein and bradykinin which produce severe systemic effects including vasodilation, increased vascular permeability, profound hypotension and shock. A positive feedback cycle occurs because pancreatic oedema results in the production of more trypsin which in turn liberates more bradykinin, etc.

The release of pancreatic enzymes into the peritoneal cavity causes a chemical peritonitis which may develop to a septic peritonitis. Considerable quantities of fluid may collect in the abdomen.

The cause of the disease is not known. The condition is much more common in obese, middle-aged bitches. It has been shown that animals on a high fat diet are more prone to the disease (Haig 1970) and that lean, working animals are more resistant (Goodhead 1971). Many other possible factors have been proposed including reflux of bile, infection, autoimmune disease, bile duct obstruction, trauma, metabolic disease and administration of glucocorticoids or adrenocorticotrophic hormones (Hardy & Johnson 1980).

Diagnosis

There is frequently a history of ingesting a large quantity of fat shortly before the onset of clinical signs. Anterior abdominal pain is frequently noted and the dog may stand with its back arched or adopt a 'praying position' with its sternum on the floor and its hindquarters elevated. Apart from abdominal pain the clinical signs most commonly recorded are anorexia, depression, dehydration and vomiting. Less commonly, affected dogs exhibit pyrexia and diarrhoea.

When presented with a case showing the above signs, the most important differential diagnosis is

Table 14.10 Differential diagnosis of acute abdominal pain.

Gastrointestinal
Acute gastroenteritis
Canine parvovirus enteritis
Haemorrhagic gastroenteritis
High intestinal obstruction
Gastric dilation/torsion
Gastrointestinal perforation

Liver
Acute hepatitis (viral, bacterial, toxic)
Cholangitis

Urinary
Acute renal disease
Urinary obstruction
Urinary rupture

Miscellaneous
Acute pancreatitis
Acute prostatitis
Splenic torsion
Testicular torsion
Metritis
Thoraco-lumbar disc protrusion

acute intestinal obstruction although other possible diagnoses should be considered (see Table 14.10).

The most reliable method for evaluating acute pancreatitis in the dog is by measuring the activity of serum lipase. Serum amylase is much less reliable as the enzyme is also elevated in renal failure, intestinal obstruction, stress and following corticosteroid therapy. Further, activity may have returned to normal 48 hours after the initial elevation. When interpreting these enzyme assays, it should be remembered that for an elevation to occur there must be enough functioning acinar tissue to permit production of these enzymes.

Other biochemical changes recorded are uraemia, increased activity of transaminases and alkaline phosphatase, hyperglycaemia, hypocalcaemia and hyperlipidaemia (Schaer 1979).

Radiography is indicated in most cases exhibiting acute abdominal pain and Gibbs *et al* (1972) reported the radiographic changes associated with acute pancreatitis. On plain films, the localised area of peritonitis may be noted as a granular, mottled density in the right cranial quadrant of the abdomen. Following the administration of contrast medium, stasis of the column of barium within a dilated, C-shaped duodenum may be observed.

Treatment
1   Correction of the animal's fluid, electrolyte and acid–base balance. These dogs may be alkalotic due to

vomiting but are more commonly acidotic as a result of shock (see Chapter 12).
2   Inhibition of further pancreatic secretion. Anticholinergic drugs such as atropine have been used to inhibit the neurogenic stimulation of pancreatic secretion, although there is now evidence to suggest that these drugs have little effect and indeed, may be contraindicated; this also applies to corticosteroids (Attix *et al* 1981). Although these dogs are usually anorexic, food should be withheld. Glucagon also reduces pancreatic secretions.
3   Control of secondary infection with antibiotics.
4   Relief of pain. Meperidine hydrochloride (pethidine) is the drug of choice administered at 10 mg/kg i.m. Morphine is contraindicated as it produces spasm of the pancreatic duct.

Exocrine pancreatic insufficiency
This title used to cover a distinct clinical entity which may develop as a result of a variety of pathological changes. Although vague, the term is used in preference to more specific descriptive terms, as confusion exists regarding the terminology applied to this disease, e.g. pancreatic hypoplasia, juvenile pancreatic atrophy, chronic pancreatitis, pancreatic fibrosis and pancreatic degenerative atrophy.

At present, there appears to be three different conditions which will produce the clinical picture associated with exocrine pancreatic insufficiency (EPI), i.e. pancreatic degenerative atrophy, pancreatic hypoplasia and chronic pancreatitis.

1   Pancreatic degenerative atrophy (PDA)
It has been postulated that dogs which develop PDA are born with a normal pancreas. At around 6 months of age, the pancreas shrinks and becomes invaded by mononuclear cells (Sateri 1975) and the condition progresses until only a few strands of normal pancreatic tissue remain (Fig. 14.13). It is not known why these changes develop although an autoimmune reaction has been postulated.

The condition is much commoner in the German Shepherd Dog and Westermack (1980) has shown that the disease is inherited via an autosomal recessive gene, although the possibility of an autosomal dominant inheritance with incomplete penetration cannot be excluded.

The dog is usually presented between 6 months and 5 years, although the majority of cases are diagnosed at 1–2 years of age. The owners main complaint is that the dog is thin but has a voracious appetite. This finding is consistent and when investigating an animal in poor condition, if the owners report that the dog leaves some food or has a selective appetite then that

Table 14.11 Aetiology of jaundice.

Category	Serum bilirubin	Urinary bilirubin
1 *Excessive breakdown of RBC* *Leptospira icterohaemorrhagiae* Incompatible blood transfusion Autoimmune haemolytic anaemia Haemobartonellosis	Unconjugated bilirubin predominates (e.g. 80% indirect 20% direct)	**1** Increased conjugated bilirubin (renal tubules can produce bilirubin from haemoglobin) **2** Increased urobilinogen
2 *Liver fails to conjugate bilirubin* Cirrhosis Neoplasms *Leptospira icterohaemorrhagiae* Infectious canine hepatitis Acute necrotising pancreatitis Myeloid leukaemia Toxic hepatitis Salmonellosis Toxoplasmosis	Van den Berg test of little significance as the ratio of direct to indirect bilirubin varies markedly	**1** Increased conjugated bilirubin **2** Increased urobilinogen
3 *Impaired excretion of bilirubin* Extrahepatic biliary obstruction Intestinal foreign body Cholestasis Cholelithiasis	Conjugated bilirubin predominates (e.g. 80% direct, 20% indirect)	**1** Increased conjugated bilirubin **2** No urobilinogen
4 *Abdominal absorption of bilirubin* Rupture of the biliary tree	Conjugated bilirubin predominates (e.g. 80% direct, 20% indirect)	**1** Increased conjugated bilirubin **2** No urobilinogen

dog does not have pancreatic insufficiency. As a result of poor absorption of fatty acids, these animals have a dry scurfy coat. A misconception has arisen that dogs with EPI exhibit watery diarrhoea; this is uncommon as the faeces usually have the consistency of porridge and are steatorrhoeic, i.e. bulky, rancid, greasy, pale and evil-smelling. A small percentage of dogs, however, will pass apparently normal faeces.

Because of malabsorption ingesta is fermented in distal ileum and colon resulting in excessive flatus and borborygmi. These changes are readily detected by the owner. A behavioural problem commonly noted is copraphagia.

Despite the gross appearance of the pancreas, diabetes mellitus is rarely recorded, indeed as a result of impaired carbohydrate absorption, the blood sugar may be subnormal (Sateri 1975). An abnormal curve may be recorded with the oral glucose tolerance test (p. 389).

Diagnosis: faecal proteolytic enzyme activity. EPI is over diagnosed because of the inaccuracies of the widely used methods for assaying the activity of the proteolytic enzymes in the faeces. Most of these tests are based on the ability of faecal proteolytic enzymes to cause hydrolysis of gelatin on radiographic film in a test tube or on petri dishes. The results obtained can be misleading for a variety of reasons.

False negatives (gelatine is not digested)
1 Pancreatic enzymes can be inactivated by the gastrointestinal microflora. This occurs when the faecal sample is not fresh or if the transit time is slow, e.g. constipation.
2 Faecal proteolytic activity varies considerably from day to day in clinically normal dogs and it is not uncommon for faeces from a normal dog to show no hydrolysis of gelatin.
3 If using x-ray film, it should not have been developed as this process hardens the gelatine.
4 The type of diet influences the quantity of proteolytic enzymes present. It is suggested that dogs fed fresh meat show higher levels of proteolytic enzymes than those fed canned meat.

False positives (gelatine is digested)
1 Bacterial proteolytic activity in the faeces may digest the gelatin masking the absence of pancreatic proteolytic enzymes.
2 Vigorous washing of the x-ray strips under the tap may wash the gelatine off.
3 If the alimentary transit time is rapid, the levels of proteolytic activity may appear artificially high.

More accurate methods for estimating faecal proteolytic activity are the azo-casein method (Hill & Kidder 1970) and the radial enzyme diffusion method (Westermarck & Sandholm 1980).

The test can be further refined by adding crude soya bean powder at 1 g/kg twice daily to the diet for two days prior to testing. Healthy dogs will show a distinct increase in faecal protease activity but dogs with E.P.I. will remain negative.

Measurement of small intestinal pancreatic activity. Several workers have described a test that indirectly measures the amount of pancreatic enzyme activity in the small intestine. The test involves the oral administration of a synthetic peptide made from N-benzoyl-tyrosine and p-amino benzoic acid (PABA), which is hydrolysed specifically by the pancreatic protease, chymotrypsin. This compound is not absorbed or degraded by any proteolytic enzyme other than chymotrypsin.

After the peptide is administered orally, it stimulates pancreatic enzyme secretion, is hydrolysed by chymotrypsin and releases free p-amino benzoic acid, which is absorbed and excreted in the urine within 6 hours of administration. It serves, therefore, as an indirect measurement of the amount of chymotrypsin activity in the small intestine.

Batt (1979) reports that an accurate diagnosis could be made simply by assaying plasma PABA 2 hours after administration of the synthetic peptide. If chymotrypsin activity in the duodenum is low (as in EPI) then PABA will not split from the protein carrier and consequently cannot be absorbed. With normal digestion, significant serum levels of PABA are recorded 2 hours post administration.

Microscopic examination of faeces in EPI. The presence of undigested proteins, carbohydrates and fats on microscopic examination of the faeces is suggestive of EPI.

Following staining with Lugol's iodine, undigested muscle fibres stain golden brown, are pointed at the ends rather than rounded and have viable cross-striations present. Note that this is influenced by the preparation of the meat and fresh meat should be fed for optimum results.

Large undigested starch granules may be present and these stain an intense blue-black colour with Lugol's iodine.

The addition of Sudan Black will stain any fat globules present in the faeces, although this finding is readily appreciable, especially if the animal is steatorrhoeic. This test can be further refined by heating the faecal smear with acetic acid. This converts the fatty acids present as water soluble soaps to insoluble free fatty acids that form fat globules.

A radioimmunoassay for serum trypsinogen is being developed which should enable an accurate diagnosis to be made on a single blood sample.

Finally, the pathological changes are usually obvious on exploratory laparotomy (Fig. 14.13).

Treatment. The most important treatment is the addition of pancreatic supplements to the diet. These should be administered at high dose rates as a considerable percentage is denatured on passage through the stomach. Further it has been suggested that human enteric coated forms should not be used as this coating may be resistant to breakdown in the canine duodenum. The administration of cimetidine 20 minutes before a meal may neutralise gastric acid and increase the quantity of enzymes reaching the duodenum.

Cases with EPI respond best to a diet which is high in protein but low in fat. If possible, it should be low residue, e.g. tripe or lean meat plus rice with a multivitamin/mineral supplement. Medium-chain triglycerides such as coconut oil are a useful addition to the diet as these substances are readily absorbed via the portal circulation. As fats tend to reduce the efficiency of pancreatic enzymes, the coconut oil is best fed separately. Supplement the food with glucose powder

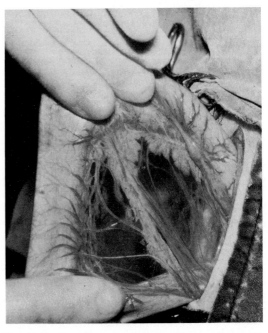

Fig. 14.13 Exocrine pancreatic insufficiency in an 11-month-old West Highland White Terrier.

as this is readily absorbed, but excessive quantities should be avoided (not more than one tablespoon per day) as this may produce osmotic diarrhoea.

The prognosis should always be guarded as reversal of the pathological changes has not been reported. Most cases will respond to treatment in that the dog's clinical condition improves, but a high percentage of owners elect euthanasia within a few months of diagnosis due to the high cost of the treatment and a lack of satisfaction at the clinical response.

2 *Chronic pancreatitis*
Uncommon in the dog. It develops when recurrent bouts of pancreatitis produce hypertrophy of the interstitial tissue with a resultant fibrosis and loss of acinar tissue.

3 *Pancreatic hypoplasia*
Again an uncommon condition in which the basic lesion is a congenital lack of pancreatic tissue. The clinical signs and treatment of the above two conditions is the same as for PDA.

Pancreatic neoplasia
Tumours may arise from the acinar tissue or from the Islets of Langerhans. The latter group present as endocrine disorders and will not be considered here.

Pancreatic tumours are uncommon. Adenocarcinomas are highly malignant and tend to metastasise early. Clinical signs are non-specific and rarely related to pancreatic dysfunction, e.g. weight loss, anorexia, vomiting and depression. Because of the anatomical proximity of the pancreas to the common bile duct, many causes are jaundiced. The presence of pancreatic carcinoma should always be suspected in middle-aged or elderly dogs where serum biochemistry has suggested an obstructive jaundice (see below) especially if a mass can be palpated in anterior abdomen. Displacement of the duodenum and pylorus may be detected radiologically but these tumours can be difficult to diagnose without exploratory laparotomy.

Prognosis is poor because the tumours metastasise early. Surgical removal may be attempted if no secondaries are seen.

LIVER DISEASE

The liver is the largest organ in the body. Its functions include:

1 Synthesis of plasma proteins (with the exception of the immunoglobulins). Many of the proteins involved in clotting are manufactured in the liver. The organ is also responsible for ammonia metabolism.
2 Regulation of carbohydrate metabolism. The liver is the most important organ involved in the maintenance of a normal blood glucose level.
3 Production and excretion of bile and bile acids.
4 Mobilisation of body fats; synthesis of cholesterol and triglycerides.
5 Breakdown and excretion of drugs, hormones and toxic substances.
6 Absorption and storage of vitamins.

Liver diseases provide the clinician with a challenge as the diagnosis and treatment of hepatic problems present considerable difficulties:

1 The liver has phenomenal powers of regeneration. It is possible to remove 75% of a dog's liver and the animal will regain normal hepatic function within 8 weeks (provided the cellular framework, biliary drainage and blood supply remain normal). This means that unless the entire liver is damaged by the disease process (e.g. infectious canine hepatitis), regeneration and degeneration will occur at the same time. Because of this rapid repair, liver function tests can only indicate the situation on the day the samples were taken.
2 There are no characteristic clinical signs associated with liver disease. Animals in acute hepatic failure may present as dull, vomiting dogs whereas the only clinical signs noted in some cases of chronic hepatic failure are dullness, weight loss and a decreased appetite. The two clinical signs classically associated with chronic liver disease (i.e. ascites and jaundice) are not invariably recorded. Even when the liver is functioning normally, ascites (e.g. abdominal neoplasia) and jaundice (e.g. ruptured bile duct) may be noted.
3 The liver is often affected as a consequence of other diseases (e.g. congestive cardiac failure, diabetes mellitus, Cushing's syndrome). The organ is also a common site for neoplastic metastases.
4 Because the liver is involved in so many aspects of metabolism there is no single laboratory test which can be used as an indicator of hepatic disease, as a pathological process does not necessarily affect all aspects of liver function to the same extent. Furthermore, the results obtained from laboratory investigations may vary markedly from one day to the next.

Clinical signs associated with liver disease

Jaundice
Jaundice is a staining of the mucous membranes, skin

Table 14.12 Differential diagnosis of abdominal fluid in the dog.

1 *Pathognomonic fluids*
Blood—neoplasia (esp. haemangiosarcoma), warfarin etc., organ rupture
Urine—ruptured bladder/urethra/ureter
Bile—rupture of the biliary tract
Chyle—rupture of the thoracic duct

2 *Serosanguineous exudate*
Acute pancreatitis
Chronic active hepatitis
Abdominal neoplasia

3 *Modified transudate*
Congestive cardiac failure
Chronic liver disease
Abdominal mass, e.g. neoplasia
Portal venous obstruction

4 *True transudate*
Massive proteinuria, e.g. membranous glomerulonephritis
Excessive faecal loss of protein, e.g. protein losing enteropathy
Reduced production of serum proteins, e.g. chronic liver disease
Mass obstructing lymphatic drainage

5 *Purulent exudate*
Gastrointestinal perforation
Ruptured pyometra

and other tissues by the yellow pigment, bilirubin. This is first noted when plasma bilirubin exceeds 35–50 μmol/l (2–3 mg/dl). An understanding of normal bile metabolism is necessary before the clinical significance of certain types of jaundice becomes apparent (Fig. 14.14).

The first stage in the production of bile is the destruction of ageing red blood cells in the spleen and reticulo-endothelial system, although some bilirubin is derived from hepatic haemoprotein and haem. The haemoglobin from these cells gives rise to a green pigment, biliverdin, which is metabolised to bilirubin. At this stage, the circulating bilirubin is loosely coupled with albumin and is termed unconjugated. It gives an indirect reading when incubated with the Van den Berg reagent. In order to be excreted in the bile, this bilirubin has to be conjugated primarily with glucuronic acid by the hepatocytes. Bilirubin glucuronide is water soluble and gives a direct reading with the Van den Berg reagent. The conjugated bilirubin passes down the bile duct into the small intestine and is further broken down by bacteria to produce stercobilinogen, the pigment responsible for the normal colour of faeces and urobilinogen which is reabsorbed and excreted through the kidneys. Thus, urobilinogen is present in urine from a normal dog. The renal threshold for bilirubin is very low in the dog and 60% of normal dogs excrete detectable amounts of bilirubin in their urine (Cornelius 1970).

The staining of jaundice is most easily detected in the sclera and gums. Wherever possible, the dog should be examined in daylight as artificial lighting (especially fluorescent strips) may simulate icterus.

One cannot correlate the levels of circulating bilirubin with the intensity of staining of mucous

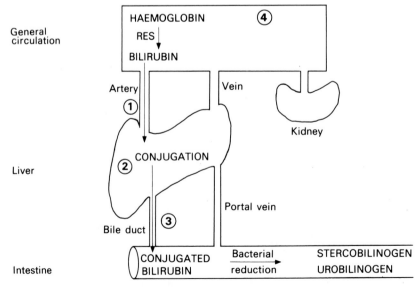

Fig. 14.14 Circulation of bile pigments. The numbers 1 to 4 refer to the categories of jaundice described in Table **14.11**.

membranes, as an animal may exhibit jaundice for several days after serum bilirubin has returned to normal. Conversely, the levels of serum bilirubin may have been elevated for several days before jaundice is obvious.

Ascites

Many cases of chronic liver disease are accompanied by ascites. A fluid thrill may be appreciable on ballottement of the abdomen. On paracentesis, the fluid obtained is a *modified* transudate with a specific gravity between 1.018 and 1.025. The colour varies from clear to yellowish/orange. Glucose is frequently present with large quantities of protein (30–40 g/l). Compare this with a *true* transudate which is clear, has a low specific gravity (below 1.010) and less than 20 g/l of protein.

Ascites may develop for several reasons.

1 The damaged liver effectively obstructs the passage of blood from the portal vein through the liver. This fibrous damage also results in the formation of functional arteriovenous anastomoses. These pathological changes produce portal hypertension and a modified transudate.
2 The liver is the main site of synthesis of albumin and other plasma proteins. Reduced production of these proteins results in decreased serum osmotic pressure and fluid leaves the circulation.
3 Increased levels of circulating aldosterone are noted due to a combination of increased production and a failure of the damaged liver to remove aldosterone from the circulation. The subsequent retention of water and sodium exacerbates the ascites.
4 The thoracic duct has difficulty clearing the large amounts of lymph produced by the damaged liver.

Although chronic liver disease is a common cause of ascites, there are many other reasons why fluid accumulates in the peritoneal cavity (Table 14.12).

Weight loss

Bile salts must be present for pancreatic enzymes to function normally. Reduced producton of these salts will result in poor digestion of food and weight loss. As was mentioned earlier, the liver plays a crucial role in the metabolism of fats, carbohydrates and proteins and any interference with these functions can lead to weight loss.

Vomiting

The causes were discussed earlier in the chapter.

Table 14.13 Summary of diagnostic tests in liver disease.

	Normal values	Acute hepatitis	Ruptured bile duct	Cirrhosis	Liver tumours	Biliary stasis	Portal shunts	Lipidosis (e.g. diabetes mellitus)
Serum or Plasma								
WBC	6–15000 ×10^6/l	Usually Increased	Increased	±Increased	±Increased	±Increased	Normal	±Increased
Total bilirubin	1.0–10.0 μmol/l	±Elevated	Elevated	±Elevated	±Elevated	Elevated	Normal	Normal
Type of bilirubin	Mostly direct	Varies	Mostly direct	Varies	Varies	Mostly direct	—	—
Alanine aminotransferase	4.8–20 iu/l	Elevated	Normal	Slight rise	Slight rise	Slight rise	Normal	Slight rise
Alkaline phosphatase	20–51 iu/l	Slight rise	Elevated	Elevated	Elevated	Marked rise	Normal	Elevated
Blood urea	3.9–6.1 mmol/l	±Elevated	±Elevated	±Elevated	±Elevated	±Elevated	Reduced	±Elevated
BSP clearance	10% at 30 mins.	Retention	Retention	Retention	Retention	Retention	Retention	Retention
Serum albumin	30–40 g/l	Normal	Normal	Usually reduced	±Reduced	Normal	±Reduced	Normal
Urine								
Urobilinogen	Present	±Elevated	Absent	±Elevated	±Elevated	Elevated	Present	Present
Conjugated bilirubin	±Present	±Elevated	Elevated	±Elevated	±Elevated	Reduced	±Present	±Present

Faecal changes

Stercobilinogen is responsible for the normal colour of faeces. Any lesion which reduces the quantity of bile reaching the duodenum (e.g. obstruction or rupture of the biliary tract) may give rise to 'chalky' faeces.

In haemolytic jaundice, the faeces are often orange as a result of over production of stercobilinogen.

Diarrhoea is commonly recorded in association with liver disease.

Haemorrhage

When liver disease has been present for many months, the clotting time may be prolonged due to impaired synthesis of prothrombin. The levels are rarely low enough to produce spontaneous haemorrhage but this point should be considered before taking a biopsy from the liver.

Hepatic encephalopathy

The liver is responsible for the conversion of ammonia, present in the systemic portal circulation, to urea. Should this function be impaired, ammonia will reach the systemic circulation producing neurological disturbances. Alternatively, the portal venous blood bypasses the liver either as a result of an acquired or a congenital portosystemic shunt. Ammonia is the most important neurotoxic substance although others have been implicated, e.g. various amino acids and amines.

Clinical signs include lethargy, aimless wandering, ataxia, blindness, head pressing and personality changes. Severe cases may develop convulsions and coma.

Diagnosis of liver disease

Serum bilirubin concentration

In the discussion on jaundice, the terms indirect (unconjugated) and direct (conjugated) bilirubin were used. The most commonly used methods of bilirubin estimation measure total serum bilirubin.

total bilirubin = direct (conjugated) + indirect (unconjugated)

Table 14.11 lists the causes of jaundice in the dog and their effect on serum bilirubin. It should be emphasised that the Van den Berg test (i.e. measurement of direct and indirect bilirubin) is only of value when there is a high percentage of one form of bilirubin present in the plasma relative to the other (e.g. 80% indirect reading bilirubin to 20% direct reading bilirubin or vice versa). The intermediate ratios (e.g. 60% direct reading to 40% indirect reading) are not significant.

Table 14.14 Sodium content of foods.

High sodium foods	Low sodium foods
Canned and processed meats	Beef and lamb
Bread and cereals	Rabbit and chicken
Kidney, heart and liver	Fresh water fish
Whole eggs	Oatmeal
Cheese	Rice and pasta
Butter and margarine	Potatoes

The following points should be noted from Table 14.11 and Fig. 14.14.

1 Excessive breakdown of RBCs is uncommon in the dog. The increase in the concentration of serum bilirubin will comprise mainly indirect reading (unconjugated) bilirubin. Conjugated bilirubin appears in the urine as the canine kidney has the ability to convert haemoglobin to conjugated bilirubin.
2 Only conjugated bilirubin will appear in the urine as the dog cannot excrete unconjugated bilirubin.
3 If bile is not reaching the small intestine (e.g. obstruction or rupture of the biliary tract), no urobilinogen will be found in the urine. Conjugated bilirubin, however, will be present in both urine and plasma. Moreover, this conjugated bilirubin will account for most of the increase in the concentration of serum bilirubin.
4 The term 'cholestasis' in Table 14.11 refers to a group of conditions which produce biliary stasis by interfering with formation or excretion of bile.

Serum alkaline phosphatase (SAP) activity

In the dog alkaline phosphatase is produced by the liver, osteoblasts, placenta, intestine and certain neoplasms. Marked elevations in activity of the enzyme indicate bile stasis, whereas with the latter conditions it is uncommon for the elevation to exceed 3 times normal. As the enzyme enters the circulation without cell damage or necrosis, it is uncommon for marked elevations to be recorded in acute or toxic hepatitis.

Serum transaminases

Alanine aminotransferase is present in the canine liver in greater quantities than in any other tissue and is virtually liver specific. Increased activity of this enzyme in serum is associated with leakage through the cell membrane either due to increased membrane permeability or necrosis and marked increases are recorded in acute conditions. Mild to moderate elevations indicate a chronic process.

Increases in aspartate aminotransferase parallels that of alanine aminotransferase, but in the dog, the enzyme is not liver specific and is released from other sources (e.g. skeletal muscle).

Gamma glutamyl transpeptidase (GGT)
This enzyme is found in the hepatobiliary tract and the kidneys but is absent from bone. Its activity has been shown to parallel that of SAP and elevations of GGT *and* SAP usually indicates bile stasis.

Serum albumin
The role of the liver in the synthesis of serum proteins was mentioned earlier. As the half life of canine albumin is 7–10 days, hypoalbuminaemia (less than 20 g/l) in liver disease indicates chronic, diffuse damage. In some cases, a rise in serum globulin concentration is noted, so although *total* serum proteins may be within normal limits, hypoalbuminaemia may be present, i.e. the albumin to globulin ration is reduced.

Bromsulphthalein (BSP) clearance
This test estimates the ability of the liver to clear foreign dyes from the circulation. The test is simple to perform and is useful indicator of impaired liver excretion. When more than 10% of the injected dye is present 30 minutes after administration, liver damage should be suspected. The test is of no value in the jaundiced animal.

Radiology in liver disease
On a lateral abdominal film of a normal dog, the ventral lobes of the liver are only just visible beyond the costal arch. The gas shadow within the stomach is aligned vertically so that the pylorus is adjacent to the ventral lobes of the liver.

Several relevant changes may be detected radiographically

1 Hepatic enlargement (Fig 14.15). The ventral lobes protrude well beyond the costal arch and are rounded. As a result of hepatic enlargement, there is posterior and dorsal displacement of the stomach, duodenum and transverse colon.

2 Reduction of liver size (see Fig. 14.16). Small changes in liver size cannot be detected radiographically, but if the organ is very small the stomach appears to be closer to the diaphragm. This change is uncommon and is usually associated with advanced cirrhosis or porto-systemic shunts.

3 Ascites. Ascites is commonly associated with liver disease. The presence of fluid reduces the detail of the viscera visible on the radiograph resulting in an overall 'ground glass' appearance with the gas in the intestinal loops easily visible.

4 Hepatic calcification. Diffuse or localised calcification of the liver may be seen in the normal dog but

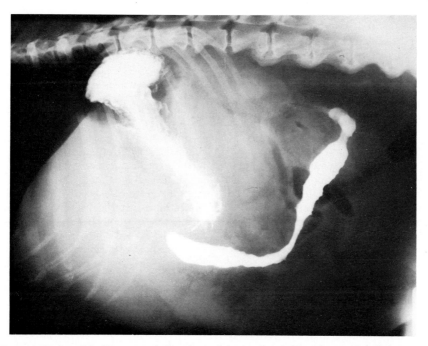

Fig. 14.15   The ventral lobes of the liver protrude from beyond the costal arch. There is posterior displacement of the plylorus and the body of the stomach.

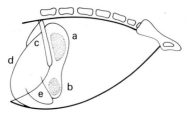

Normal liver

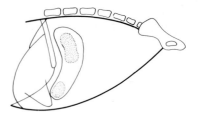

Localised hepatic enlargement
Neoplasia
Hepatic cysts
Abscess

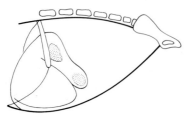

Generalised hepatic enlargement
Lipidosis e.g. D. mellitus, Cushings
Neoplasia
Hepatitis
Bile-duct obstruction
Amyloidosis

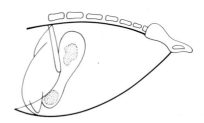

Small liver (generalised)
Cirrhosis
Porto-systemic shunt
Congenital

a. Gastric fundus b. Pylorus c. Last rib d. Diaphragm e. Liver

Fig. 14.16   Radiographic changes in liver disease.

is usually secondary to pathological change within the liver.

5   Abnormal position. When the diaphragm ruptures, the liver or part of it may enter the thoracic cavity.

Many of the above changes are more readily appreciated following the administration of barium sulphate to outline the stomach and intestine. Contrast portography is helpful in the diagnosis of portosystemic shunts and (see later section) essential if surgical correction is contemplated; 5–20 ml of a water-soluble contrast medium is injected into either the splenic or mesenteric vein and a radiograph taken as soon as the injection is completed. The same affect can be achieved by injecting contrast medium directly into the spleen.

Liver biopsy

At the beginning of the discussion on liver disease, it was emphasised that there is no one method of diagnosing the exact nature of the hepatic changes. Con-

sequently, examination of liver biopsies is a useful aid to diagnosis.

Three different methods have been described.

1   By abdominal laparotomy. More information may be obtained by direct examination of the liver than by a percutaneous approach. The disease process may not involve all lobes of the liver and the surgeon can select the site to be biopsied. The technique requires a general anaesthetic, and in animals with impaired liver function there is a greater risk of anaesthetic complications.

2   Transthoracic percutaneous biopsy (Feldman & Ettinger 1976). The biopsy needle is inserted into the thorax via the seventh intercostal space, at the level of the costochondral junction with the animal in left lateral recumbency. After entering the thorax, the needle is directed caudally through the diaphragm.

3   Abdominal percutaneous biopsy (Chapman 1965). With the dog in dorsal recumbency, the needle is inserted between the xyphoid process and the chondral portion of the last rib. The needle is advanced at an angle of 30° to the sagittal plane. This technique may be modified by inserting a finger into the abdomen via a 'keyhole incision'.

The clotting time should be determined before attempting a biopsy.

Acute liver disease

It may be difficult to differentiate between acute and chronic liver disease but the term 'acute' is used to describe a condition of sudden onset with no previous history of illness. Vomiting is usually present and the animal may or may not be jaundiced. Ascites is *not* associated with acute liver disease.

A dog may recover completely from acute liver disease, but some cases show a gradual progression to chronic hepatic failure.

Specific infections
Infectious canine hepatitis and *Leptospira icterohaemorrhagiae* have both been discussed in Chapter 13.

Toxic hepatitis
The incidence of toxic hepatitis in the dog is much lower than in large animals. One reason is that dogs are carnivores and many hepatotoxins are plant alkaloids. The ingestion of toxic chemicals is uncommon, e.g. phosporous, copper, arsenic, carbon tetrachloride and chloroform. Dogs will drink antifreeze (ethylene glycol) which may produce acute hepatic changes, although its main effect is upon the kidneys.

Many drugs are potentially hepatotoxic, e.g. phenytoin, primidone, glucocorticoids and phenobarbitone.

Acute hepatic necrosis in the dog presents as a sudden onset condition with massive necrosis of hepatocytes. Frequently, no specific aetiological agent is identified.

Ruptured bile duct/gall bladder
The condition is usually associated with abdominal injury (e.g. road traffic accident). Recovery is apparently normal following the initial trauma. Abdominal distension is noted after a period of time (which may be as long as 3 weeks) because the abdomen is filling with bile. The animal becomes jaundiced and its condition may deteriorate rapidly.

The usual site of rupture is the junction between the common bile duct and the duodenum. The treatment of choice is surgical repair.

Miscellaneous infectious agents
Bacterial hepatitis and hepatic abscesses are uncommon in the dog. Thomson and Wright (1969) recorded two cases of salmonellosis in which the hepatic changes closely resembled those seen in infectious canine hepatitis.

Toxoplasma gondii may produce necrotic foci in the liver and infection of the dog with this agent was described by Campbell *et al* (1958). Clinical signs related to the lungs and brain are frequently noted.

Chronic liver disease

Most chronic liver diseases have a history of a gradual onset, long standing problem. The usual reasons for advice being sought are weight loss, depression and intermittent gastrointestinal disturbances. The presence of ascites and jaundice is highly suggestive of chronic liver disease, but cases do occur where neither clinical sign is seen.

Cirrhosis
In both human and canine medicine, there has been confusion over the classification of cirrhosis. The current convention is that, to support a diagnosis of cirrhosis, the following criteria should be satisfied.

1   The process should involve all of the liver but not necessarily every lobule.
2   Cellular necrosis is present at some stage of the process.
3   Nodular regeneration of the liver is present.
4   The lobular architecture is distorted with diffuse fibrous bands of connective tissue.

The aetiology of cirrhosis is uncertain but several theories have been postulated including: toxic or anoxic damage, a sequel to viral infections, following chronic active hepatitis, malnutrition, autoimmune disease and a progression from hepatic lipidosis.

Both jaundice and ascites are frequently recorded in these cases although it is more common for one or the other to be present. The majority of cases are older dogs, although cirrhosis may be seen as early as 6 months of age.

Neoplasia
Hepatic neoplasms, both primary and secondary, are common in the dog. The two types of tumour most frequently seen are bile duct carcinoma and lymphosarcoma, although bile duct adenomas, hepatomas, malignant hepatomas and many other types have been recorded.

Although most hepatic neoplasms produce hepatomegaly, some tumours give rise to a shrunken liver, and the absence of hepatomegaly on clinical and radiological examination does not eliminate hepatic neoplasia as a diagnosis. Benign nodular hyperplasia is common in the dog and should not be confused with hepatic tumours.

Extrahepatic biliary obstruction

Any lesion which increases the pressure within the bile duct may produce clinical signs of obstructive jaundice. Faeces may be chalky and the intensity of the jaundice is usually greater than that seen with hepatocellular damage. The total bilirubin concentration in plasma may exceed $170\,\mu mol/l$ whereas in hepatocellular damage it rarely rises over $100\,\mu mol/l$. Pancreatic carcinomas give rise to this form of biliary obstruction although any neoplastic process in the vicinity of the bile duct may increase the intraluminal pressure. Other causes include gall stones (rare in the dog), and duodenal foreign bodies.

Portosystemic shunts

These vascular anomalies can be either acquired or congenital. The acquired forms develop as a result of generalised parenchymal damage, e.g. cirrhosis or chronic active hepatitis which in turn produces portal hypertension with opening of the collateral vessels. The congenital forms would appear to be more common than was previously suspected. A variety of anatomical abnormalities have been described, but the physiological effects are similar, i.e. blood from the portal circulation by-passes the liver and enters the systemic circulation.

The condition is seen in young pups, which exhibit a wide range of clinical signs related to hepatic encephalopathy (see earlier). In many cases, clinical signs are most obvious after a meal.

Most cases have characteristic ammonium biurate crystals present in the urine. This group of conditions are unusual in that the serum urea concentration is *lower* than normal. Excretion of BSP is delayed. Another characteristic finding is an elevated blood ammonia

Treatment. As well as the general hepatic treatments discussed later, it is helpful to attempt to control production of toxic products in the alimentary canal by administering neomycin orally. Lactulose, a synthetic disaccharide which reduces absorption of ammonia, has also been used.

Many of the congenital shunts are amenable to corrective surgery, but before considering partial ligation and occlusion of the shunt, good radiographs using contrast medium are necessary.

Chronic active hepatitis (CAH)

Many reports of this disease have appeared in the literature, but at present there is little agreement concerning the definition of the problem. Sequential biopsies should demonstrate relentless destruction of the liver parenchyma with piecemeal necrosis. Thornberg (1982) concluded that by rigidly applying the accepted criteria for diagnosis, the disease is extremely uncommon in the dog.

CAH has been described in the Bedlington Terrier, Doberman Pinscher and other breeds.

Cholangiohepatitis

It is difficult to differentiate between the various chronic liver diseases, even using laboratory tests and to reach a diagnosis of cholangiohepatitis, a biopsy is required. The condition carries a better prognosis than many of the other forms of chronic liver disease, e.g. cirrhosis, provided an early diagnosis is reached.

Chronic venous congestion

This is a common pathological change in the dog usually as a sequel to mitral endocardiosis. Enlarged, smooth, rounded ventral lobes of the liver may be palpable. On abdominal radiographs, hepatomegaly may be seen.

Hepatic lipidosis

Accumulation of fat within the liver is common in the dog and is usually secondary to dietary deficiencies or metabolic diseases such as hypothyroidism, diabetes mellitus and Cushing's syndrome. Hepatic lipidosis can alter the prognosis in these diseases, and liver function should be investigated before treatment is commenced.

Glycogen storage disease

These conditions are uncommon but may present with spectacular clinical signs. Because the animal cannot utilise the glycogen stored in the liver, frequent bouts of hypoglycaemia occur giving rise to incoordination, weakness and convulsions. Several categories of glycogen storage disease have been recorded in the dog (Bardens 1966). Treatment is by administration of sugars by mouth, corticosteroids and glucagon.

Amyloidosis

Deposition of the hyaline protein, amyloid, within the liver, is thought to be secondary to an abnormality of the immune response. Hepatomegaly occurs and the condition is diagnosed by liver biopsy. There is no treatment.

Treatment of liver disease

Diet. The diet should be formulated to supply sufficient protein to prevent endogenous protein metabolism and to help the damaged liver cells regenerate. Too much protein however will precipitate hepatic encephalopathy, although this is less likely to develop with protein of vegetable origin.

A low sodium diet will reduce water retention and consequently development of ascites (Table 14.14). Many dogs find low sodium diets unpalatable and it may be necessary to heat the food or add spices to improve acceptance.

The fat content of the diet should be low but sufficient supplied to maintain the animal's requirements for fatty acids. It is advisable to supplement the diet with the fat soluble vitamins A, D, E and K.

Ascites. Complete drainage should not be attempted as the risk of attendant complications (e.g. major haemodynamic changes, hypoproteinaemia, renal failure and peritonitis) is greater than the therapeutic benefits from a time consuming procedure. Small volume paracentesis should always be carried out for diagnostic purposes but large volume paracentesis should only be instituted when the quantity of abdominal fluid present is such that the pressure on the diaphragm results in respiratory problems.

Many diuretics are available for treatment of the ascitic dog. Frusemide is the drug of choice as it produces a diuresis in the presence of impaired liver function. There is a danger of hypokalaemia if the drug is used continuously and potassium supplementation may be necessary.

Antibiotics. A combination of penicillin and streptomycin may be safely used in hepatic disease. Tetracyclines are useful as they are concentrated in bile, although in animals with renal damage, this group of antibiotics may precipitate acute tubular failure. Ampicillin is also concentrated in bile.

REFERENCES

Alimentary

AMITSBERG G., DROCHNER W. & MEYER H. (1978) Influence of food composition on the intestinal flora of the dog. In *Nutrition of the dog and cat.* Editor, R.S. Anderson. Pergamon Press, Oxford.

ANDERSEN R.S. (1982) Personal Communication

BATT R.M. (1979) The investigation of small intestinal disease in the dog by per oral jejunal biopsy. In *Waltham Symposium No. 1—Diarrhoea in the Dog.* Pedigree Petfoods.

BATT R.M. (1980) The molecular basis of malabsorption *J. Small Anim. Pract.* **21**, 555.

BATT R.M. (1982) Role of serum folate and vitamin B12 concentrations in the differentiation of small intestinal abnormalities in the dog. *Res. Vet. Sci.* **32**, 17.

BRUCE, D., ZOCHOWSKI W. & FLEMING G.A. (1980) Campylobacter infection in cats and dogs. *Vet. Rec.* **107**, 200.

BRUCE D. & FLEMING G.A. (1983) Campylobacter isolation from household dogs. *Vet. Rec.* **112**, 16.

BURROWS C.F. (1977) Canine haemorrhagic gastroenteritis *J. Am. Anim. Hosp. Assoc.* **13**, 451.

CARTWRIGHT S. & LUCAS M. (1972) Vomiting and diarrhoea in dogs *Vet. Rec.* **91**, 571.

CORNELIUS L.M. & WINGFIELD W.E. (1975) Diseases of the stomach. In *Textbook of Veterinary Internal Medicine*, Vol 2. W.B. Saunders, Philadelphia.

COX V.S., WALLACE L.J., ANDERSON V.E. & RUSHMER R.A. (1980) Hereditary oesophageal dysfunction in the Miniature Schnauzer dog. *Am. J. Vet. Res.* **41**, 326.

DAVIES R.B. & HILBER C.P. (1979) Animal reservoirs and cross species transmission of Giardia. In *Waterborne Transmission of Giardiasis.* USEPA, Cincinnati.

DEKEYSER P., GOSSIAN-DETRAIN M., BUTZLER J.P. & STERNON J. (1972) Acute enteritis due to related vibrio in first positive stool cultures *J. Infect. Dis.* **125**, 390.

ENGLAND J.J. & POSTON R.P. (1979) Electron microscopic identification and subsequent isolation of Rotavirus from a dog with fatal neonatal diarrhoea. *Am. J. Vet. Res.* **40**, 782.

EWING G.O. & GOMEZ J.A. (1973) Canine ulcerative colitis *J. Am. Anim. hosp. Assoc.* **9**, 395.

FINCO D.R., DUNCAN J.R., SCHALL W.D., HOOPER B., CHANDLER F.W. MCKEATING K.A. (1973) Chronic enteric disease and hypoproteinaemia in 9 dogs. *J. Am. Vet. Med. Assoc.* **163**, 262.

FLESJA T. & YRI T. (1977) Protein Losing Enteropathy in the Lundehund. *J. Small Anim. Pract.* **18**, 11.

FUNQUIST B. & GARMER L. (1967) Pathogenic and therapeutic aspects of torsion of the canine stomach. *J. Small Anim. Pract.* **8**, 523.

GALTON M.M., SCATTERDAY J.E. & HARDY A.V. (1952) Salmonellosis in dogs. I, Bacteriological, Epidemiological and Clinical Considerations. *J. Infect. Dis.* **91**, 1.

GASKELL, C.J., GIBBS C. & PEARSON H. (1974) Sliding hiatus hernia with reflux oesophagitis in two dogs. *J. Small Anim. Pract.* **15**, 503.

GRUFFYD-JONES T.J., MARSTON M., WHITE E. & FRENCH A. (1980) Campylobacter infections in cats and dogs. *Vet. Rec.* **107**, 294.

HAPPE R.P., VAN DER GAAG I. & WOLVEKAMP, W. Th. C. (1981) Pyloric stenosis caused by hypertrophic gastritis in 3 dogs. *J. Small Anim. Pract.* **22**, 7.

HAYDEN D.W. & NEILSEN S.W. (1973) Canine alimentary neoplasia *Zentrabl. Veterinarmed.* **20**, 1.

HILL F.W.G., KIDDER D.E. & FREW J. (1970) A xylose absorption test for the dog. *Vet. Rec.* **87**, 250.

HOLT, P.E. (1980) Incidence of campylobacter, salmonella and shigella infections in dogs and in an industrial town. *Vet. Rec.* **107**, 254.

HOLT P.E. (1981) Role of dogs and cats in the epidemiology of human campylobacter enterocolitis. *J. Small Anim. Pract.* **22**, 681.

HOSIE B.D., NICHOLSON T.B. & HENDERSON D.B. (1979) Campylobacter infections in normal and diarrhoeic dogs *Vet. Rec.* **105**, 80.

HUXTABLE C.R., MILLS J.N., CLARK W.T. & THOMSON R. (1982) Chronic hypertrophic gastritis in a dog; successful treatment by partial gastrectomy. *J. Small Anim. Pract.* **23**, 639.

JACOBS D.E. (1978) The epidemiology of hookworm infection of dogs in the U.K. In *Veterinary Annual*, 12th Edition. John Wright, Bristol.

KENDAL P. (1982) Dietary fibre—a role in the diet of dogs? *Pedigree Digest* **9**, 5.

KEENAN K.P., JERVIS H.R., MARCHWICKI R.H. & BINN L.N. (1976) Intestinal infection of neonatal dogs with canine coronavirus 1-71: studies by virologic, histologic, histochemical and immunofluorescent techniques. *Am. J. Vet. Res.* **37**, 247.

LARSON D.J., MOREHOUSE L.G., SOLORZANO R.F. & KINDEN R. (1979) T.G.E. in neonatal puppy dogs. Experimental intestinal infection with Transmissible Gastroenteritis Virus. *Am. J. Vet. Res.* **40**, 477.

LEIBETSEDER J. (1982) Feeding animals which are ill. In *Dog and Cat Nutrition*, Edited by A. Edney. Pergamon Press.

MOORE R. & WITHROW S.J. (1982) Gastro-intestinal haemorrhage and pancreatitis associated with intervertebral disc disease in the dog. *J. Am. Vet. Med. Assoc.* **180**, 1443.

MORRIS M.L., TEETER S.M. & COLLINS D.R. (1971) The effects of the exclusive feeding on an all meat dog food. *J. Am. Vet. Med. Assoc.* **158**, 477.

MEYER H., DROCHNER W., SCHMIDT M., RIKLIN R. & THOMEE A. (1980) On the pathogenesis of alimentary disorders in dogs. In *Nutrition of the dog and cat*, Editor R.S. Anderson. Pergamon Press, Oxford.

MEYER H., SCHMITT P.J. & HECKOTTER E. (1981) Nahrstoffgehalt und verdaulichkeit von futtermittiln für hunde. *Übers. Tiernahrung* **9**, 71.

MURRAY M., ROBINSON P.B., McKEATING F.J., BAKER G.J. & LAUDER I.M. (1974a) Primary gastric neoplasia in the dog: a clinicopathological study. *Vet. Rec.* **91**, 474.

MURRAY M., ROBINSON P.B., McKEATING F.J., BAKER, G.J. & LAUDER I.M. (1974b) Peptic ulceration in the dog: a clinicopathological study. *Vet. Rec.* **91**, 441.

PEARSON H. (1966) Foreign bodies in the oesophagus. *J. Small Anim. Pract.* **11**, 403.

PEARSON H., GIBBS C. & KELLY D.F. (1978) Oesophageal diverticula in the dog. *J. Small Anim. Pract.* **19**, 341.

QUEISSAR H.G. VON (1970) Beitrag zur Salmonellose des hundes. *Dtsch. tieraerztl. Wochenschr.* **77**, 286.

RICKLIN M. & MEYER H. (1975) Untersuchungen über die beduetung von strukturstoffen in der hunderanhun. *Kleinterpraxis* **20**, 4.

ROGERS, W.A., FENNER W.R. & SHERDING R.C. (1979) Electrographic and eosophagomanometric findings in clinically normal dogs and in dogs with idiopathic megasophagus. *J. Am. Vet. Med. Assoc.* **174**, 181.

SIMPSON J.W. & BURNIE A.G. (1983) Campylobacter excretion in canine faeces. *Vet. Rec.* **112**, 46.

SKIRROW M.B. (1981) Campylobacterenteritis in dogs and cats: a 'new' zoonosis. *Vet. Res. Commun.* **5**, 13.

SOKOLVSKY V. (1967) Cricopharyngeal achalasia in a dog. *J. Am. Vet. Med. Assoc.* **150**, 281.

VAN DER GAAG I., VAN TOORENBURG J., VOORHOUT G., HAPPE R.P. & AALFS R.H.G. (1978) Histiocytic ulceration colitis in the French Bulldog. *J. Small Anim. Pract.* **19**, 283.

VAN KRUININGEN H.J. (1976) Clinical efficiency of tylosin in canine inflammatory bowel disease. *J. Am. Anim. Hosp. Assoc.* **12**, 498.

WINGFIELD W.E., CORNELIUS L.M. & DEYOUNG D.W. (1974) Pathophysiology of the gastric dilation-torsion complex in the dog. *J. Small Anim. Pract.* **15**, 735.

Pancreas

ATTIX E., STROMBECK B.R., WHEELDON E.B. & STERN J.S. (1981) Effects of anticholinergic drug and a corticosteroid on acute pancreatitis in experimental dogs. *Am. J. Vet. Res.* **42**, 1668.

BATT R.M., BUSH B.M., & PETERS T.J. (1979) A new test for the diagnosis of exocrine pancreatic insufficiency in the dog. *J. Small Anim. Pract.* **20**, 185.

GIBBS C., DENNY H.R., MINTER H.M. & PEARSON H. (1972) Radiological features of inflammatory conditions of the canine pancreas. *J. Small Anim. Pract.* **13**, 531.

GOODHEAD B. (1969) Acute pancreatitis and pancreatic blood flow. *Surg. Gynecol. Obstet.* **129**, 131.

GOODHEAD B. (1971) Importance of nutrition in the pathogenesis of experimental pancreatitis. *Arch. Surg.* **110**, 41.

HAIG B.T.H. (1970) Experimental pancreatitis intensified by a high fat diet. *Surg. Gynecol. Obstet.* **131**, 914.

HARDY R.M. & JOHNSON G.F. (1979) The Pancreas. In *Veterinary Gastroenterology*. Lea and Febinger, Philadelphia.

HILL F.W.G. & KIDDER D.E. (1970) The estimation of daily faecal trypsin levels in dogs as an indicator of gross Pancreatic Exocrine Deficiency. *J. Small. Anim. Pract.* **13**, 23.

SATERI H. (1975) Investigations of the exocrine pancreatic function in dogs suffering from chronic exocrine pancreatic insufficiency. *Acta. Vet. Scand.* suppl. 53.

SCHAER M (1979) A clinicopathological survey of acute pancreatitis in 30 dogs and 5 cats. *J. Am. Anim. Hosp. Assoc.* **15**, 681.

WESTERMACK E. (1980) The hereditary nature of canine pancreatic degenerative atrophy in the German Shepherd Dog. *Acta. Vet. Scand.* **21**, 389.

WESTERMACK E. & SANDHOLM M. (1980) Faecal hydrolase activity as determined by Radial Enzyme Diffusion: a new method for detecting pancreatic dysfunction in the dog. *Res. Vet. Sci.* **28**, 341.

Liver

BARDENS J.W. (1966) Glycogen storage disease in puppies. *Vet. Med. Small Anim. Clin.* **61**, 1174.

CAMPBELL R.S.F., MAKAY J.M.K. & VANTISS J.T. (1958) Canine toxoplasmosis. *J. Comp. Path.* **68**, 96.

CHAPMAN W.L. (1965) Liver biopsy in the dog. *J. Am. Vet. Med. Assoc.* **146**, 126.

CORNELIUS C.E. (1970) Liver function. In *Clinical Biochemistry of Domestic Animals*, Vol. I. Academic Press, New York.

FELDMAN E.C. & ETTINGER S.J. (1976) Percutaneous transthoracic liver biopsy in the dog. *J. Am. Vet. Med. Assoc.* **169,** 805.

HARDY R.M. (1975) Diseases of the liver. In *Textbook of Internal Veterinary Internal Medicine*, Vol. 2. W.B. Saunders, Philadelphia.

THOMSON H. & WRIGHT N.G. (1969) Canine salmonellosis. *J. Small Anim. Pract.* **10,** 579.

THORNBERG L.P. (1982) Chronic Active Hepatitis—What is it and does it occur in dogs? *J. Am. Anim. Hosp. Assoc.* **18,** 21.

15
Urinary System

B. M. BUSH

ANATOMY AND PHYSIOLOGY

The urinary tract consists of paired kidneys and ureters plus the bladder and urethra, and has the function of producing and eliminating urine.

The kidneys are situated retroperitoneally at the roof of the abdominal cavity on either side of the aorta and posterior vena cava. Each is bean shaped and between $2\frac{1}{2}$ and $3\frac{1}{2}$ times the length of the second lumbar vertebra. The right kidney extends forward to the level of the thirteenth rib; the left kidney is half a kidney length behind. Each is divided into an outer cortex and inner medulla, and contains approximately 400000 nephrons, the functional units for urine production (Eisenbrandt & Phemister 1979). The kidneys excrete the waste products of metabolism, maintain the amounts of water, electrolytes and other solutes at constant levels and regulate the acid–base balance of the body. In addition they secrete the hormones erythropoietin and renin, and undertake the final stage in the metabolism of vitamin D3 to its active form.

Within the nephron, ultrafiltration of blood passing through the glomerulus in the cortex produces an isotonic glomerular filtrate which enters Bowman's capsule and proceeds through the tubule. Approximately two-thirds of the filtered water, sodium and chloride is reabsorbed isotonically in the proximal tubule. Reabsorption of bicarbonate, glucose, potassium, phosphate, amino acids, proteins and uric acid plus the secretion of hydrogen and ammonium ions, and organic acids and bases, also takes place in the proximal tubule. The loop of Henle, extending deep into the medulla, acts as a countercurrent multiplier by pumping sodium chloride from the ascending limb into the interstitial tissue. Consequently a very dilute fluid enters the distal tubule. The reabsorption from here of sodium and chloride ions, and thus water, is stimulated by aldosterone from the adrenal cortex. Also, as the fluid passes along the distal tubule and collecting duct to the renal pelvis, antidiuretic hormone from the neurohypophysis increases their permeability to sodium, chloride and water thereby concentrating the urine. In both the distal tubule and collecting duct, hydrogen, ammonium and potassium ions are secreted.

Urine is conveyed through each ureter, from the renal pelvis to the bladder, by peristaltic waves. The ureters enter just in front of the bladder neck. The pear-shaped bladder is held in position in front of the pelvic bone by its lateral ligaments. As urine enters, it progressively distends anteriorly and downwards until, at a certain pressure, receptors in its walls are triggered, sending nervous impulses to both the reflex centre for micturition in the sacral spinal cord and the brain.

Simultaneous relaxation of the bladder sphincter and contraction of the detrusor muscle expels urine along the urethra. In the male the urethra comprises prostatic, membranous and penile parts; the latter passes below the os penis. It passes around the posterior border of the pelvic bone and forward to open at the tip of the penis. In the bitch the urethra is shorter and opens on an elevation from the floor of the vagina, anterior to the clitoris.

DISEASES OF THE KIDNEY

Renal disorders are among the most common diseases of the dog but, as with other organs, not all diseases or lesions of the kidney result in clinical signs.

For renal failure to occur approximately $\frac{3}{4}$ of the normal complement of nephrons must be non-functional (or fail to develop), resulting in a reduced glomerular filtration rate and the inability to remove waste products. (Nephrons once destroyed are not replaced.) This means that one complete kidney can be destroyed or removed without the development of azotaemia, the classic indicator of renal failure, and all the clinical signs which stem from it. The term azotaemia refers to the presence in the blood of an abnormally high level of *all* the products of protein catabolism including urea, creatinine, guanidine and phenolic acids and their conjugates. The term uraemia, which has been more commonly used in the past, refers only to an abnormally high blood urea level. Since the current view is that most of the clinical signs of renal failure are due to all the protein breakdown products acting in unison it is the practice to use the term azotaemia in preference to uraemia.

Nevertheless, clinical signs may arise when a *single* kidney is diseased; not signs of renal failure but those related to the cause (e.g. lumbar pain and fever arising from inflammation and infection in acute pyelo-nephritis, and cough due to secondary pulmonary metastasis of a renal neoplasm).

Renal failure is divided into acute and chronic (ARF and CRF), and it is worthwhile making the distinction in diagnosis because of the greater potential for successful reversal of acute cases. The other major syndrome is the nephrotic syndrome, character-ised by proteinuria, hypoproteinaemia and oedema.

For each of these three conditions there is a basic pattern of therapy, which may be modified according to the severity of the clinical signs, and certain specific treatments may be employed against particular aetio-logical agents. Chronic renal failure is by far the most common of the three syndromes. Wherever possible a precise diagnosis should be made because specific ther-apy may be available, and because it determines the prognosis. With conditions that are generally irrever-sible (bilateral amyloidosis or neoplasia) euthanasia may be the most humane course of action.

Primary glomerular diseases

Glomerulonephritis
In recent years glomerulonephritis (GN) has been recognised as a more important condition than pre-viously believed, although information on many as-pects is still emerging. It is a disease without obvious sex predilection, which usually occurs from middle age. However a familial GN in Doberman Pinschers appearing before one year of age has been reported (Wilcock & Patterson 1979). The primary injury is to the glomeruli. Since inflammation is not always evident, the term glomerulonephropathy may be pre-ferable to GN. Glomerular lesions are often followed by structural damage to other parts of the kidney and may result in chronic renal failure (CRF).

Glomerulonephritis in other species is associated with one of two immunological mechanisms in almost all instances (see Chapter 9). Of these by far the most commonly occurring in the dog is immune complex GN. This results from the formation of circulating antigen—antibody complexes which lodge in the glomerulus where they fix complement and initiate an inflammatory process that damages the glomerular basement membrane (GBM). The antigen may be de-rived from a virus, bacterium or parasite responsible for a long-standing infection (e.g. from *E. coli* in pyometra, or from heartworms) or from a malignant tumour (present in 40% of cases), or it may be host DNA (as in systemic lupus erythematosus). Dogs in-fected with canine adenovirus 1 (CAV-1 or infectious canine hepatitis virus) develop a focal proliferative GN, but this is only transient, disappearing with the elimination of the virus, and therefore CAV-1 is un-likely to be responsible for *progressive* glomerular dis-ease.

The second immune process is anti-GBM glomeru-lonephritis where antibodies against the GBM are formed. Naturally-occurring cases have seldom been reported in the dog.

Variation in the pathological response of the glom-erulus depends on the site of the deposition of the complexes, which is determined largely by their size, amongst other factors.

Morphologically, three major forms of canine glomerulonephritis have been described, although overlap can occur between them.

1 Membranous GN with diffuse capillary wall thick-ening and heavy leakage of protein into the urine, which may be sufficient to initiate the nephrotic syndrome. Cases of membranous GN often show a bilateral systolic murmur in the absence of valvular lesions.
2 Proliferative GN exhibits proliferation of mesangial cells with mild proteinuria, and sometimes haematuria and pyuria.
3 Exudative (or chronic) GN characterised by large fibrin deposits in the glomerular capillary walls. This may represent a natural progression from membran-ous or proliferative glomerulonephritis. Again there is proteinuria and the progressive onset of CRF. Cases can only be distinguished from chronic interstitial nephritis by certain histopathological features and immunofluorescent findings. On gross appearance the two conditions are indistinguishable ('end-stage kidneys').

The major clinical signs associated with all types of GN are:

1 Proteinuria (chiefly albuminuria) which can vary from less then 1 g/l (100 mg/100 ml) to more than 10 g/l (1 g/100 ml) (Table 15.1). Severe proteinuria is most common in membranous GN, resulting in hypoalbu-minaemia and oedema.
2 Polyuria and polydipsia. In exudative GN these signs are marked and usually form part of the

Table 15.1   Differential diagnosis of proteinuria.

Renal origin: chiefly albumin because of its small molecular size

1 MILD-MODERATE (less than 10 g/l) and not necessarily present in every case
Chronic renal failure (usually below 3 g/l and frequently below 1 g/l)
Due to: Hydronephrosis ⎫   may be no urine flow from affected kidney
           Pyonephrosis   ⎬   but will contribute to the 75% (or more)
           Nephrolithiasis ⎭   loss of nephrons
           Pyelonephritis
           Neoplasia
           Polycystic kidney
           End stage kidney: chronic interstitial nephritis, chronic amyloidosis, chronic
               (exudative) glomerulonephritis, chronic pyelonephritis and familial renal
               diseases
Early renal amyloidosis
Proliferative, and early membranous, glomerulonephritis
Glomerulosclerosis in long-standing (2 years plus) diabetes mellitus (unusual)
Physiological causes sometimes responsible: strenuous exercise, extreme heat or cold,
stress
Primary renal glycosuria and Fanconi syndrome: due to renal tubular dysfunction
Chronic passive congestion: heart or liver disease
Fever

2 SEVERE (more than 10 g/l)
                                             ⎫   Both result in nephrotic syndrome.
Membranous glomerulonephritis (advanced) ⎬   As damage progresses proportionately
Amyloidosis (advanced)   ⎭   more globulins appear

Other sources: proteinuria is usually mild
Inflammation elsewhere in urinary tract or genital tract: including discharges and pus
    (e.g. in pyometra)
Haematuria anywhere in urinary or genital tracts: since blood contains plasma proteins
Haemoglobinaemia and myoglobinaemia
Hyperproteinaemia: following the parenteral administration of plasma (renal threshold
    for plasma protein is approximately 100 g/l) or an abnormal increase in the production
    of immunoglobulins (e.g. with multiple myeloma).
Natural secretions (semen and oestral discharge)

Notes
(a) All features of nephrotic syndrome except oedema may occur with moderate proteinuria due to glomerulonephritis or amyloidosis.
(b) Commercial tests are more sensitive to albumin than to other proteins (globulin,
haemoglobin, mucoprotein) and therefore react most markedly to protein of renal origin.
(c) Protein concentrations up to 0.5 g/l often occur in normal dogs and are of little
significance. Even double this amount may be present. Usually about half of this urinary
protein is albumin.
(d) Normal protein losses in urine average 15 mg/kg/day (ranging from 0 to 30 mg/kg/
day in both males and females).
(e) Commercial tests for blood are more sensitive than those for protein and therefore a
negative result for protein does not necessarily indicate the absence of blood.
(f) 10 g/l protein in urine increases the specific gravity by 0.003.

azotaemic syndrome of CRF, whereas in membranous and proliferative GN they are usually mild and occur in the absence of azotaemia.
3 Muscle wastage and weakness.

Renal amyloidosis

Renal amyloidosis (RA) is seen mainly in middle-aged and aged dogs and may be accompanied by amyloid-osis of other organs (e.g. liver and spleen). Affected dogs frequently suffer from other diseases concurrently, especially chronic disorders, involving neoplasia or sepsis. It seems probable that amyloid is produced within the kidney by reticuloendothelial cells (and possibly other cells) in response to prolonged antigenic stimulation, and laid down as fibrils.

In the early stages, amyloid is principally deposited

around the mesangial portions of the glomerular tufts and there is slight thickening of the capillary basement membrane. Later the amyloid nodules become confluent and completely obliterate some glomeruli, resulting in a progressive loss of function in the associated tubules. Finally, it may be deposited around the tubular basement membrane and collecting ducts, and in the interstitial tissue and blood vessels.

Amyloid does not stimulate an inflammatory reaction and in general the kidney is normal sized during the early stages, but may enlarge slightly with the deposition of large amounts of amyloid, and then contract as the damaged parenchyma is replaced by fibrous tissue ('end-stage kidney').

The glomerular damage results in proteinuria which may, but not always, become so severe as to produce the nephrotic syndrome. Later the progressive destruction of functional nephrons results in the onset and signs of CRF and proteinuria is lessened. Occasionally dogs show liver or splenic enlargement due to amyloid deposition. Thrombo-embolism affecting larger blood vessels, especially the pulmonary arteries, is a more common finding and may result in sudden death. There are no features of laboratory tests *specific* to amyloidosis.

In the dog, differentiation between RA and the various forms of GN can at present be made in life only by histopathological examination following biopsy of the kidney, although in man rectal biopsy is often valuable in distinguishing cases of amyloidosis. Both diseases are progressive but whereas RA is generally irreversible and death occurs within months, cases of GN may stablise and survive two years or more (Wright *et al* 1981). Therefore biopsy techniques can be justified as a means of establishing the prognosis.

Treatment of primary glomerular diseases

It may prove possible to stop the progress of GN (and possibly even RA, though this has not been reported in dogs) by eliminating the antigen responsible for the associated disease, i.e. the infectious agent or neoplasm.

Corticosteroids, and other immunosuppressive drugs, have been widely used in man to suppress immune reactions, reduce inflammation and decrease glomerular permeability to protein in cases of glomerulonephritis. Similarly there are reports of their successful use in the dog. However they can suppress beneficial immune responses and, by stimulating gluconeogenesis, predispose to renal failure thereby increasing the mortality rate. Therefore it is recommended that if treatment with corticosteroids is attempted their effect should be assessed by monitoring the degree of proteinuria and the levels of urea, creatinine and serum proteins. In cases of amyloidosis, corticosteroid treatment usually has little beneficial effect and indeed may aggravate the condition.

Treatment with anticoagulant drugs (eg warfarin, indomethacin) has been advocated to limit the progressive deposition of fibrin in GN. Unfortunately there is as yet no procedure (such as the long-term administration of dimethylsulphoxide) which has been shown to reduce or reverse the laying down of amyloid.

Nephrotic syndrome

The nephrotic syndrome is characterised by severe proteinuria, hypoproteinaemia, hyperlipidaemia (including hypercholesterolaemia) and generalised oedema. It is associated with glomerular damage producing increased permeability to protein, which in the dog results from renal amyloidosis and glomerulonephritis, chiefly membranous glomerulonephritis.

Albumin, having a smaller molecule than globulin, is excreted in relatively greater amount producing a decreased A:G ratio. A consistent loss of 10 g/l (1 g/100 ml) urine is almost certain to give rise to oedema (Table 15.2), but it may also arise with lower concentrations. Ascites usually occurs when the total serum protein level is less than 40 g/l (4 g/100 ml) and that of serum albumin less than 20 g/l (2 g/100 ml; often considerably lower). Oedema develops gradually due to two main factors, both of which stem from the reduction in plasma proteins. One is the lower colloidal osmotic pressure of the blood and the other, and more important, is contraction of the blood volume which stimulates aldosterone secretion and increases antidiuretic hormone release (Fig. 15.1). These hormones are responsible for the retention of sodium chloride and water, thus promoting oedema, and for increased potassium loss.

The mechanism responsible for the increase in plasma lipids has not yet been identified but there is an inverse relationship with the serum albumin level. With increasing nephron destruction the blood levels of urea and creatinine rise and eventually clinical signs of CRF appear.

Treatment of the nephrotic syndrome

A high protein, low salt diet is required (Casilan) to replace the serum protein and limit retention of fluid. There is no evidence that a high protein diet increases proteinuria or adversely affects renal function. If the hypoalbuminaemia is corrected blood lipid values

Table 15.2   Differential diagnosis of oedema and ascites (after Bown 1979).

Localised
Obstruction of venous or lymphatic drainage, e.g. pressure of neoplasms, elastic bands, tight dressings, etc.; thrombo-embolism
Inflammation
Immediate-type hypersensitivity reaction

Generalised (*including ascites*)
Congestive heart failure—most commonly due to valvular endocardiosis
Chronic hepatic failure—most often due to cirrhosis
Glomerulonephritis ⎱ giving rise to the
Renal amyloidosis   ⎰ nephrotic syndrome
Protein-losing enteropathy (part of malabsorption syndrome)
Malnutrition—protein lack in diet

Other conditions which may give abdominal enlargement
Obesity (overfeeding, hypothyroidism)
Cushing's syndrome
Acromegaly in bitches
Neoplasia of abdominal organs
Pregnancy, overt pseudo-pregnancy or pyometra
Acute gastric dilation—volvulus
Accumulation of other fluids—inflammatory exudate (e.g. in peritonitis), blood, chyle, urine.

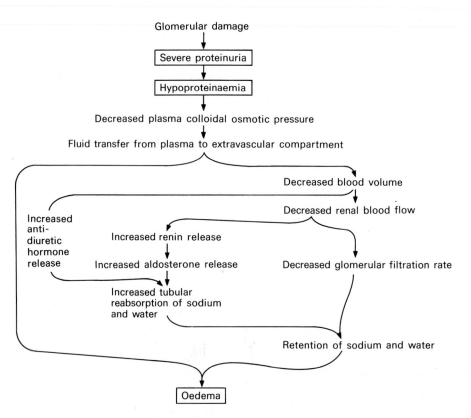

Fig. 15.1   Pathogenesis of nephrotic syndrome (After Osborne 1980).

return to normal without specific therapy. The exact amount of protein lost per day can be determined by collecting all the urine (e.g. in a metabolism cage) for 24 hours and estimating its protein content. An appropriate amount of protein food can then be given to replace it.

The low blood volume may be corrected by intravenous administration of dextran or plasma proteins, usually the former as a *salt-free* 6% or 10% dextran solution (at a dose rate of 10–20 ml/kg body weight).

Immediate relief of pain or discomfort caused by ascitic or hydrothoracic fluid can be afforded by its removal by paracentesis, but initially only 25% should be removed. However, removal of retained fluid is usually achieved with diuretics. It is recommended that spironolactone (3 mg/kg body weight twice daily) should be employed initially because it is a specific aldosterone antagonist and does not cause potassium loss. If this fails frusemide (5 mg/kg body weight once or twice a day) or ethacrynic acid (2 mg/kg body weight per day) can be used. The last-named drugs are those generally employed and during their administration potassium supplementation is advisable (e.g. potassium chloride tablets BP, one tablet per 20 kg body weight a day). All diuretics should be discontinued or their dosage reduced when the oedema is under control.

The over-hasty removal of oedema fluid (by diuretics or paracentesis) may give rise to a rapid loss of potassium, plus a rapid fall in blood volume and blood pressure producing a reduced filtration rate and the onset of renal failure. Cases of the nephrotic syndrome complicated by renal failure (i.e. with clinical signs of azotaemia) should receive a compromise between the high protein, low salt diet required by the former (see above) and the low protein, high salt diet of the latter (the precise balance depends on the severity of clinical signs), plus diuretics to control oedema, and calcium lactate, rather than sodium bicarbonate, to control acidosis.

Antibacterial agents should be given at the first sign of infection or prophylactically (e.g. after abdominal drainage).

Acute renal failure

Acute renal failure (ARF) is a condition in which there is acute suppression of renal function and consequently clinical signs appear suddenly. However speed of onset alone is not sufficient to distinguish it from chronic renal failure (CRF) since owners may miss the early signs of CRF.

The major signs of ARF are oliguria (reduced urine production, less than 7 ml/kg body weight per day) which is diagnostic of ARF, and those resulting from azotaemia. Anuria, complete cessation of urine production, is rare.

The oliguric phase lasts for up to 10 days in most cases and is then followed, in animals which survive, by a polyuric (or diuretic) phase. Oliguria causes the retention of water, protein breakdown products (azotaemia and acidosis) and potassium (hyperkalaemia). As in CRF the azotaemia is due to a lack of functional nephrons (70% or more) and a description of azotaemic signs and their development appears later under that heading.

With prompt and adequate treatment many cases of ARF will recover; if not death, or the development of CRF, may follow.

ARF may be of prerenal, postrenal or renal (intrarenal) origin.

Prerenal ARF
Prerenal ARF results from decreased perfusion of the kidneys with blood, as may occur with reduced cardiac output in heart failure, blockage of the renal blood vessels with infarcts or thrombi, or a severely depleted vascular volume following massive haemorrhage or dehydration. When the pressure in the afferent glomerular arteriole falls below 60 mmHg glomerular filtration stops and no urine is formed. The urine may show slight proteinuria and often a specific gravity above 1.025.

Treatment of cardiac failure, or the use of fluid therapy to restore the blood volume will usually reverse the condition. If the disorder to too severe or treatment too delayed, ischaemia will result in acute tubular necrosis, a renal cause of ARF.

Postrenal ARF
Postrenal ARF results from the prevention of urinary outflow, either rupture (usually of the bladder) or an obstruction which above the bladder must be bilateral (unless the unobstructed kidney is already severely diseased). Any animal showing a markedly reduced urine output should be catheterised to establish that there is no obstruction in the urethra or bladder neck, and checked radiographically for ureteral or bladder rupture and ureteral obstruction. Cases where urinary outflow from both kidneys is completely obstructed or where only one is affected but the other is non-functional will die from ARF in 4–6 days. The pathological changes characteristic of hydronephrosis therefore develop principally with unilateral obstruction where the other kidney is functional (Fig. 15.2). Complete anuria is very suggestive of obstruction.

Apart from occasional proteinuria there is no

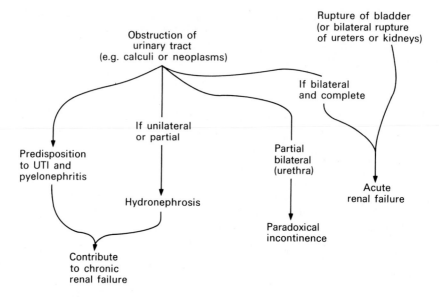

Fig. 15.2   Relationship of obstruction and rupture to renal failure.

consistent diagnostic feature of the urine. Rapid repair of rupture or removal of the obstruction is essential for recovery.

Renal ARF

In rare instances this may arise from bilateral renal rupture caused by severe abdominal trauma, but the *two major causes* of renal ARF in the dog are acute interstitial nephritis (AIN) and acute tubular necrosis (ATN). In both, the kidneys are enlarged and this may be detectable on palpation and by radiography.

1 Acute interstitial nephritis is believed to result in most cases from *Leptospira canicola* infection, mainly in dogs between 1 year and 5 years old (see Chapter 13). The kidneys show inflammatory swelling, which occludes the tubules, together with diffuse or focal cellular infiltration. The infiltrating cells include plasma cells containing antibody against the leptospirae and macrophages which phagocytose leptospiral antigen–antibody complexes and cell debris. The presence of leptospiral antibody can be demonstrated, but not that of antibodies against kidney tissue (either glomerular basement membrane or tubular epithelium). Animals rarely survive more than a few days after the onset of signs of azotaemia. Additional clinical signs usually include haematuria, proteinuria and pain in the kidney region. Not all dogs with leptospirosis develop ARF. It has been estimated that 10–40% of dogs in the USA have been infected with *Leptospira canicola* but do not develop clinical signs.

Other less common causes of acute nephritis are other bacteria (*E. coli. Proteus* spp., staphylococci) and viruses.

2 Acute tubular necrosis results from two major types of injury: nephrotoxins and ischaemia.

Commonly employed compounds known to be nephrotoxic, though to different degrees, include compounds of lead, arsenic, mercury and bismuth, amphotericin B, and the antibiotics of the polymyxin/bacitracin and aminoglycoside groups (streptomycin, neomycin, etc.), plus the less soluble sulphonamides, organic compounds such as carbon tetrachloride, chloroform, methyl alcohol, phenol, and ethylene glycol (antifreeze, which incidentally is radiopaque, a fact of diagnostic value), the analgesics phenacetin, and phenylbutazone, plus cyclophosphamide, chlorinated hydrocarbons (DDT etc.), the rat poison thallium and radiopaque contrast media. Their effects are accentuated under conditions of dehydration or reduced renal perfusion, or in the case of drugs excreted through the kidneys after pre-existing kidney damage which allows drug accumulation. They cause cellular degeneration and necrosis is mainly confined to the proximal tubules of all nephrons. Many produce other clinical signs due to toxic effects elsewhere in the body.

It is important to watch for signs of ARF when using known or potential nephrotoxins and discontinue usage immediately signs appear.

Ischaemic ARF follows a period of hypotension (e.g. complete occlusion of the renal blood supply for 45 minutes to 2 hours), as may occur in extensive surgery, severe acute haemorrhage, burns, heart failure, shock, trauma (e.g. road accidents), incompatible blood transfusion and following prolonged prerenal ARF. However, unlike the situation in man, prolonged anaesthesia and surgery on dogs that have diminished renal function does not readily provoke severe ARF, despite raised blood urea and creatinine levels (Stone *et al* 1981). Kidney pain is frequently, but not always, present. Correction of the blood volume, blood pressure and cardiac output will *not* restore normal renal function.

Variable numbers of nephrons show disruption and dissolution of the tubular basement membrane with necrosis of the tubular epithelial cells. Obstruction of tubules by casts and cell debris, and reabsorption of tubular urine through the damaged tubular epithelium, appears to be responsible for experimental ischaemic ARF, but it is still controversial as to whether this actually happens in real life.

In both types of ATN the small amount of urine contains RBCs, protein, casts, tubular cells and cell debris. The presence of oxalate crystals is a feature of ethylene glycol poisoning. Diagnosis is based principally on the history (i.e. known administration or consumption of a nephrotoxin, or known accident) and the clinical signs, supported by laboratory examination of blood and urine, radiography where necessary and even renal biopsy.

Treatment of acute renal failure

The underlying principle is to maintain the life of the patient until healing occurs. In general it is more likely that ARF will be successfully reversed than CRF, provided that the cause is removed or ameliorated and that the animal survives the uraemic crisis.

1 Oliguric stage

In the initial oliguric phase treatment differs from that of CRF mainly because of hyperkalaemia and fluid retention.

Specific therapy

Prerenal ARF. Early restoration of normal vascular volume, blood pressure and cardiac output will reverse the condition. This necessitates prompt treatment of the cardiac failure (see Chapter 1) and the correction of haemorrhage or dehydration.

Postrenal ARF. Obstructions such as calculi and neoplasms should be surgically removed wherever possible. Prostatic hypertrophy requires treatment with antiandrogenic drugs and regular catheterisation, or the use of an indwelling catheter, until urine can be passed freely. Where possible surgical repair of ureteral or bladder rupture should be undertaken.

Leptospiral ARF. To eliminate leptospirae the synergistic combination of penicillin and streptomycin should be administered for at least 7 consecutive days (suitable dose rates are 30000 iu procaine penicillin/kg body weight per day and 12 mg streptomycin/dihydrostreptomycin combined/kg body weight every 12 hours on the first day and every 24 hours subsequently).

Recovery from the acute phase carries a good prognosis since much of the available evidence suggests that CRF rarely follows. However untreated infected dogs which recover may excrete leptospirae for up to 4 years.

Nephrotoxic ARF. General treatment for oral poisoning should be instituted where appropriate (e.g. emesis and/or gastric lavage), plus any specific therapy for the particular agent (see Chapter 18).

Traumatic ARF. Severe haemorrhage may necessitate blood transfusion. Blood may be detected in the abdominal cavity on radiography and paracentesis.

Correction of fluid loss and maintenance of normal hydration (see also Chapter 12).
The degree of dehydration should be assessed by reference to the packed cell volume and clinical signs: 5% loss = slight inelasticity of skin; 7% loss = skin folds maintain their position when raised and the eye is slightly sunken; 10% loss = the same, plus dry oral mucosa; and 12–15% loss = the same, plus marked shock.

The number of the percentage deficiency multiplied by ten times the dog's body weight (in kg) indicates the fluid volume (in millilitres) of isotonic saline (if there is hyperkalaemia), or, alternatively, lactated Ringer's solution, which should be administered intravenously. To correct acidosis and hyperkalaemia part of this calculated volume should be replaced by bicarbonate and/or dextrose solution (see below). In anorexic animals a high proportion of the intravenous fluid should be 5% dextrose solution, and a mixture of two parts 5% dextrose and one part isotonic saline or lactated Ringer's solution is often advised.

In the maintenance of hydration thereafter it is important to avoid both dehydration and overhydration which, because of the difficulty in removing a fluid load, can result in pulmonary oedema (shown as dyspnoea and fluid sounds on aucultation) and cardiac failure. To achieve this balance subsequent fluid replacement should be at a rate which ensures a slight and continuous loss of the *corrected* body weight (approximately 0.5% per day), and should be checked by regular weighing. As a guide the basic fluid requirement for a medium-sized dog is around 10 ml/kg body weight per day, plus that lost in urine and vomit. Smaller dogs will require relatively more, and large dogs relatively less. Water by mouth in the oliguric phase should be restricted as there may be an increase in thirst which could result in overhydration.

In potential or established cases of ATN it is recommended that after the correction of dehydration an attempt should be made to induce diuresis by the administration of hypertonic solutions of mannitol (20%) or dextrose (10 or 20%). In potential cases (i.e. where azotaemia has *not* yet developed but it is known that a nephrotoxin has been introduced, or a severe accident sustained), the onset of ARF may be prevented by maintaining adequate renal perfusion and the normal glomerular filtration rate. In established cases of ATN, osmotic diuresis will facilitate excretion of the protein breakdown products and a reduction of azotaemia. The procedure is described at the end of this chapter.

Correction of hyperkalaemia and acidosis
The presence of hyperkalaemia (serum potassium level above 6 mmol/l) may be known from blood determination, or suspected from the existence of bradycardia, severe muscle weakness, cardiac arrhythmia or ECG findings (peaked T waves, diminished P waves, and increasing duration of the QRS complex).

It is recommended that it is treated as early as possible, certainly if the level exceeds 9 mmol/l, by administering 10% dextrose injection BP intravenously at the rate of 1 ml/kg body weight. Its effect is enhanced by adding to the solution one unit of soluble insulin for every 30 ml. Persistent cardiac arrhythmia may be treated by giving intravenous 10% calcium borogluconate solution at 0.5 ml/kg body weight. Long-term hyperkalaemia can be controlled by the oral administration of sodium polystyrene sulphonate (Resonium-A), at the rate of 2 g/kg body weight three times a day until the serum potassium level reaches 5 mmol/l.

Acidosis occurs in association with azotaemia and requires correction. Because the estimation of blood pH or bicarbonate deficit is often difficult in veterinary practice, an estimate of bicarbonate requirements can be obtained from the blood urea level.

$$\frac{\text{Blood urea level (mmol/l)} - 7}{1.6} = \text{Number of ml of 4.2\% sodium bicarbonate injection per kg body weight}$$

Half of this calculated volume should be injected during rehydration and the other half over the next 1–2 days.

Reduction of azotaemia
This may be achieved first by reducing protein catabolism, ideally by completely removing protein from the diet and if necessary administering anabolic steroids (adding dextrose to intravenous fluids is important in anorexic cases to prevent protein catabolism to obtain energy); and secondly by reducing the existing blood concentration of protein breakdown products by inducing osmotic diuresis or performing intermittent peritoneal dialysis. Both techniques are briefly described at the end of the chapter.

Treatment of secondary infection
Renal failure patients are particularly at risk from secondary infection and treatment with a non-nephrotoxic broad-spectrum antibacterial drug (e.g. amoxycillin, ampicillin, trimethoprim with sulphadiazine) should be instituted whenever sepsis is evident, or likely to follow an interference.

Avoidance of overmedication
All unnecessary medication especially with drugs requiring excretion via the kidney should be abandoned.

2 Polyuric stage
In animals which survive, polyuria follows the oliguric phase due to osmotic diuresis caused by the retention of solute and the inability of regenerating tubular cells to produce a concentrated urine. The urine remains dilute with a specific gravity usually between 1.008 and 1.012 (as in CRF). This presupposes relief of obstruction in postrenal cases and usually the onset of healing in renal cases. The polyuria may also result from osmotic diuresis induced as a therapeutic measure (see above). With the polyuria there is considerable loss of sodium. This should be replaced by providing an additional 50–75 mg of sodium chloride/kg body weight three times daily, preferably orally (ideally as enteric-coated tablets, or in the diet). Alternatively if vomiting is a problem, the urinary output can be measured and an equivalent volume of intravenous isotonic saline, or preferably lactated Ringer's solution, administered. Water intake by mouth may now be *ad libidum*, unless vomiting is present.

Acidosis should be treated by giving sodium bicarbonate, again preferably by mouth (dose: 50 mg/kg given four times daily) or intravenously (dose: 2.5 ml 4.2% sodium bicarbonate injection/kg body weight twice daily). The aim is to produce a urinary pH of 6.0–7.5, in the absence of urinary infection. Hyperkalaemia ceases to be a problem as excess potassium is excreted and the normal balance maintained.

When the kidney is able to produce a urine of specific gravity 1.025 or greater it indicates the return of renal function and is a good prognostic sign.

Other diseases leading to chronic renal failure

Both the glomerular diseases and ARF can terminate in CRF. Other diseases which can give rise to CRF are in general progressive and if unchecked most will result in the onset of CRF which is described subsequently.

Chronic interstitial nephritis

Chronic interstitial nephritis was for many years believed to be the most common cause of CRF in the dog, and there is evidence that in the UK *Leptospira canicola* infection, perhaps by immune mechanisms, can initiate the pathological changes. However, because the disease is also common in parts of the world where leptospirosis is rare there must be other aetiologies (e.g. there is evidence that CAV-1 infection can be a cause).

The kidneys are irregularly shrunken ('end-stage kidneys') with reduced cortical width and retention cysts, and they show extensive fibrosis to repair the damage inflicted by the causal agent, probably long since eliminated. This progressive scarring obliterates the glomeruli and reduces the renal blood flow, leading to the development of hypertension which in turn causes further irreversible damage. Both macroscopically and histologically these kidneys can be difficult to distinguish from end-stage kidneys resulting from other types of damage.

Hydronephrosis

Hydronephrosis is the progressive dilatation of the renal pelvis and progressive atrophy of the renal parenchyma following a complete or partial obstruction to urine flow. Such an obstruction can occur anywhere between the renal pelvis and urethral orifice and there-

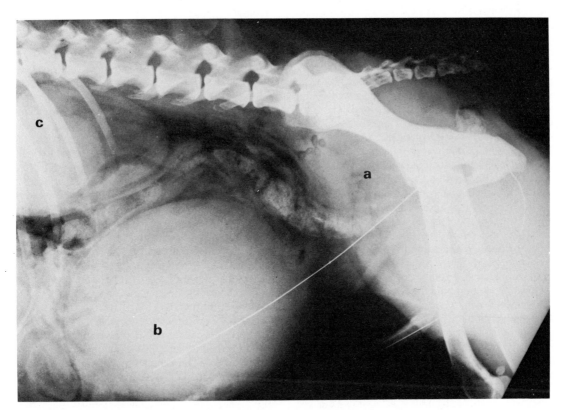

Fig. 15.3 Lateral radiograph of an 11-year-old male crossbred dog with a leiomyoma (a) dorsal to the colon and rectum. Pressure from the tumour resulted in gross distension of the bladder (b) and bilateral hydronephrosis (c). A wire stylette within a urethral catheter is clearly visible.

fore may result in either unilateral or bilateral hydronephrosis (Fig. 15.3). The most commonly encountered causes are abdominal masses (neoplastic or inflammatory) which compress the ureter(s) or urethra, and urinary calculi producing blockage anywhere in the urinary tract. Also seen are inflammatory strictures of the ureters or urethra, accidental ureteral ligation (e.g. in spaying) and ureteral involvement in fibrosis (e.g. of a healing uterine stump). In certain parts of the world, obstruction of the urinary tract with the giant kidney worm, *Dioctophyma renale*, is important. Congenital causes include urethral ectopia, abnormal development of the kidney or renal blood vessels which constrict or distort the ureters, and the congenital stenosis of ureters or urethra.

Obstruction produces back pressure on the kidney, dilating the renal pelvis and causing collapse of the renal blood vessels, which in turn causes ischaemic atrophy and necrosis of the parenchyma. The speed of these pathological changes and their severity depend on whether obstruction is complete or partial and whether it affects one or both kidneys. Complete bilateral obstruction (or unilateral obstruction when the other kidney is diseased) will result in the rapid onset of ARF culminating in death from azotaemia within a week without extensive pathological changes. With involvement of only one kidney, where the other kidney (or the major part of it) can function normally, it may take 1–2 years for clinical signs to appear (i.e. the condition may be asymptomatic for a long time). Such a unilaterally affected kidney has time to develop pronounced morphological changes, frequently becoming a large fluid-filled, thin-walled sac with a rim of atrophied parenchyma. In such cases the clinical signs first seen may be produced by the obstructive lesion (e.g. urolithiasis) and not the hydronephrosis *per se*. Alternatively they may be those of acute pyelonephritis (since obstruction predisposes to urinary tract infection, UTI); such infected hydronephrosis is referred to as pyonephrosis. With a normal opposite kidney, CRF does not develop. With a lower urinary tract obstruction hydroureter and bladder enlargement may occur.

Palpation of long-standing cases may detect renal enlargement which can be confirmed by radiography. (Exceptionally if there is no marked pressure build-up, atrophy of the kidney without enlargement results in a smaller kidney than normal.) Excretory urography will reveal the failure of the kidney (and ureter) to excrete the contrast media. Radiography may also show the cause of obstruction or this may require exploratory laparotomy. At laparotomy, fluid can often be aspirated from the pelvis, sometimes up to several litres, with the composition of normal or infected urine.

Treatment of hydronephrosis

Early removal of an obstruction, before renal changes appear, carries a good prognosis but, once present, changes are irreversible. In unilateral cases nephrectomy may be advisable if the other kidney is functioning normally but in bilateral cases the prognosis is poor. Where there are signs of CRF, appropriate therapy should be given (see p. 423) and cases complicated by infection should be treated as for pyelonephritis.

Pyelonephritis

Pyelonephritis (PN) refers to inflammation of the renal parenchyma and pelvis caused by bacterial infection. Three-quarters of cases are bilateral. It is almost always associated with a urinary tract infection (UTI) (i.e. with the passage of infected urine back up the ureters from the bladder by vesicoureteral reflux). Reflux can be demonstrated by micturating cystourethrography (see p. 438). Haematogenous bacterial spread, such as may occur in endocarditis, will result in PN *only* if the kidney has already been damaged or if there is urinary obstruction which interferes with elimination of the bacteria, and which may also produce hydronephrosis. Lymphatic spread, or direct invasion from adjacent tissues, is extremely rare.

The reflux of infected urine to the renal pelvis, and then the medulla, produces acute inflammation, and bacterial multiplication with suppuration and necrosis, which may exist as focal lesions or sometimes cause widespread nephron destruction (acute PN). Infection with CAV-1 decreases natural resistance to *E. coli* and facilitates the development of PN.

After a few weeks, especially following appropriate antibacterial therapy, resolution and healing with scar formation can occur and the kidney regains its sterile status. Alternatively the infection may remain, especially where reflux persists, resulting in chronic PN with recurrent exacerbations of the acute disease and progressive nephron destruction, and ultimately the onset of CRF. The kidneys are small and contracted ('end-stage kidneys').

The clinical signs of acute PN are firstly the signs of bacterial UTI (i.e. those of bacterial cystitis) plus the additional signs of fever—temperature of 103–105°F or more, associated with depression and anorexia—vomition, stiff gait and a tense abdomen. There is pain in the lumbar region and loins, particularly evident on prepubic palpation. In severe cases there is evidence of leucocytosis, neutrophilia and a shift to the left and the urine continues to show bacteriuria, haematuria and proteinuria. Distinguishing features from cystitis are that blood is more likely to occur throughout the urine (rather than at the end of urination) and is more likely to have been partially converted to the darker haematin. The finding of leucocyte casts (pus casts) confirms the existence of renal inflammation. Chronic PN is frequently asymptomatic unless (a) there is exacerbation with recurrence of the acute signs (i.e. fever, pain) or (b) CRF develops with azotaemic signs; but this will not occur if one kidney alone is involved. Bacteriuria is present in active cases (asymptomatic bacteriuria) but not in passive cases, and many are diagnosed only at *post mortem* examination.

Although radiography of acute cases usually shows normal-sized kidneys with a normal outline, excretory urography may show either no, or decreased amounts of, contrast media in the pelvis. There may be obvious dilatation of the renal pelvis and the ureter. Chronic cases may show the contracted irregular outline of end-stage kidneys. Exploratory laparotomy and examination of the kidneys can reveal in acute cases a very vascular capsule, whereas acute healed cases show scarring, and chronic generalised cases show both contraction and scarring. It may be possible with a fine needle to aspirate infected urine or pus from the renal pelvis.

Often it is difficult to decide whether bacteriuria is confined to the bladder or is associated with PN and although methods have been developed for use in man, diagnosis by the antibody-coated bacteria test has been shown not to be accurate in the dog, nor are bladder wash-out studies reliable.

Treatment of pyelonephritis
Cases showing bacteriuria should be treated with appropriate antibacterial drugs until the bacteria are eliminated. At least 10 days' therapy is recommended followed by reculture of the urine 1 week after its termination. With apparently successful elimination this check should be repeated at least twice more at monthly intervals. It has been found that there is increased medullary diffusion of sulphonamides, tetracyclines, and nitrofurantoin in acid urine and of gentamicin and trimethoprim in alkaline urine but that the diffusion of ampicillin is unaffected by urinary pH. The simultaneous induction of polyuria, using either salt in the diet or frusemide, is recommended. All predisposing factors to urinary obstruction should be removed (e.g. calculi, tumours and prostatic hyperplasia). In unresponsive cases, surgical removal of the affected kidney might be considered provided the other kidney appears normal (i.e. functionally, on direct inspection and, whenever possible, histologically, after biopsy).

Chronic cases showing signs of azotaemia should be treated for CRF.

Renal neoplasia
Renal neoplasia is comparatively rare in the dog. The most common primary neoplasms are renal cell carcinomas, which characteristically are large, unilateral (occasionally bilateral), and occupy one pole of a kidney. These are twice as likely to occur in male dogs, appearing from 3 years old up to extreme old age. Clinical signs which may develop include weight loss, anorexia and less commonly pyrexia and haematuria. At times overproduction of erythropoietin leads to polycythaemia. Metastasis to local lymph nodes and to the lungs is common, and they may also spread to bone.

The second most common primary neoplasms are nephroblastomas, which are most frequent in young dogs and commonly diagnosed before 1 year of age. They frequently metastasise and produce similar clinical signs to the renal cell carcinoma. Other malignant tumours occur less often; of these, transitional cell carcinomas of the renal pelvis produce obstruction and give rise to hydronephrosis.

Benign tumours are uncommon, though occasionally reported, and haemangiomas can result in considerable haematuria.

Secondary tumours, especially from the metastasis of pulmonary and mammary neoplasms, account for a considerable proportion of all renal neoplasms. Lymphosarcoma (malignant lymphoma) is seen in middle age onwards as part of generalised lymphoid leucosis (i.e. involving other organs and most lymphoid tissue).

Enlarged kidneys with an irregular outline may be detected by palpation and/or radiography. Unless both are affected (or there is a non-functional opposite kidney) signs attributable to azotaemia do not develop. Many tumours, especially benign ones, produce no signs and are only detected at necropsy although clinical signs may follow metastasis to other organs. Renal biopsy can confirm a diagnosis. Neoplastic cells rarely appear in the urine.

Treatment of renal neoplasia
Complete surgical removal of the affected kidney and its ureter is the treatment of choice where there are no metastases and the other kidney is functional. Otherwise treatment with chemotherapy or irradiation, or euthanasia, is indicated.

Renal urolithiasis
This condition is rare in the dog since the majority of uroliths form in the bladder. It may be associated with renal hypoplasia. Renal uroliths can grow to considerable size (Fig. 15.4). They may (a) not affect function, especially if unilateral, (b) if bilateral, cause sufficient

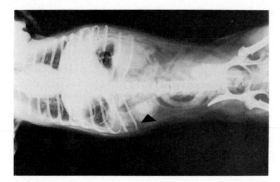

Fig. 15.4 Dorsoventral radiograph of a 9-year-old male crossbred dog with a large triple phosphate urolith in the left kidney (arrowed).

damage to produce CRF, (c) obstruct the flow and formation of urine giving hydronephrosis, and by predisposing to infection give rise to pyelonephritis, or (d) pass down the ureters, and possibly lodge there, producing severe pain.

It should be possible to demonstrate calculi radiographically and they should be surgically removed if possible (see p. 428 for causes and prevention).

Congenital renal diseases

Aplasia, hypoplasia and ectopia
If one kidney if absent or fails to develop, provided the other is functional, there will be no clinical signs (Fig. 15.5). Bilateral aplasia inevitably produces death of the newborn.

Bilateral hypoplasia if severe will provoke the early

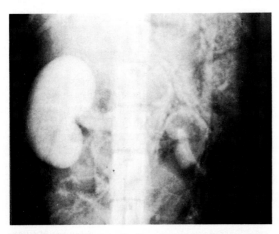

Fig. 15.5 Nephrogram of a 6-month-old Toy Poodle bitch showing hypoplasia of the right kidney. (By courtesy of Mr P.M. Webbon.)

onset of CRF. Ectopic kidneys may have insufficient drainage and are predisposed to calculi, hydronephrosis and pyelonephritis.

Polycystic kidneys
A congenital defect in the development of the renal tubules or collecting ducts gives rise to multiple cysts and progressive destruction of renal tissue (and possibly kidney enlargement) which, if bilateral, leads to CRF. If the cysts are infected this may give rise to haematuria, proteinuria, pyuria and fever with leucocytosis. The condition may be inherited (McKenna & Carpenter 1980).

Other malformations such as fusion (e.g. horseshoe kidneys) may occur. Also vascular abnormalities may occur on rare occasions.

Inherited renal diseases

Familial renal diseases
These are inherited disorders in which progressive renal damage and nephron destruction leads inexorably to the onset of CRF. The kidneys are small and irregular with evidence of glomerulosclerosis and interstitial fibrosis (end-stage kidneys). Most cases occur in animals between one and twenty-four months old; very few appear after five years old. They have been documented in certain lines of particular breeds, notably Cocker Spaniels (a condition previously referred to as renal cortical hypoplasia), Norwegian Elkhounds, Samoyeds, Doberman Pinschers, Lhasa Apsos and Shih Tzus, though similar cases have been reported in other breeds (e.g. Bedlington Terriers, Alaskan Malamutes and Keeshonds).

The diseases are not identical in all respects; for example the lesions of GN which occur in Samoyeds and Doberman Pinschers have not been described in others. In most breeds there is no sex predilection, but in Samoyeds the disease tends to be more severe, and also to have an earlier onset, in males.

Tubular defects

Hyperuricosuria. An inherent tubular defect in Dalmatians results in impaired reabsorption of filtered uric acid, in addition to the breed's reduced ability to oxidise uric acid to allantoin in the liver.

Cystinuria. The defective tubular reabsorption of cystine, and sometimes other amino acids, resulting in their excessive urinary excretion, is genetically transmitted. It has been reported in many breeds and may lead to the formation of cystine calculi (see p. 429). There is no glycosuria or hyperphosphaturia.

Primary renal glycosuria. A possibly inherited enzyme defect reduces tubular glucose reabsorption producing glycosuria in the absence of hyperglycaemia, reported most often in Norwegian Elkhounds and Basenjis. Its severity determines whether it appears with or without obvious polyuria and polydipsia.

Fanconi syndrome. A syndrome of multiple tubular reabsorptive defects resembling the idiopathic Fanconi syndrome of man has been described, involving particularly the Basenji breed (Bovée *et al* 1979a). Several cases have occurred in related individuals.

In the dog the condition is characterised by glycosuria (without hyperglycaemia), hyperphosphaturia and generalised amino aciduria (abnormally high urinary levels of many amino acids), in association with polyuria and polydipsia. Death may occur due to acute renal failure related to dehydration, acidosis and renal papillary necrosis.

Other kidney lesions

1 Many are not associated with functional impairment, e.g. spontaneous glomerular lipidosis, a distinct entity unrelated to glomerulonephritis, and solitary renal cysts which may produce an enlargement and irregular outline on radiographs. These large cysts are distinct from the multiple cysts of polycystic kidneys and the retention cysts of end-stage kidneys. If infected they may give rise to haematuria, proteinuria and pyuria.

2 Other lesions can produce severe damage. Diffuse nephrocalcinosis is associated both with hypercalcaemia (as in hyperparathyroidism, pseudohyperparathyroidism, hypervitaminosis D and certain types of malignant neoplasia; see Chapter 8) and with the hyperphosphataemia of both nutritional and renal secondary hyperparathyroidism (Schmidt *et al* 1980). The kidneys may also be damaged, on rare occasions, by the penetration of foreign bodies or (experimentally) whole body irradiation.

Chronic renal failure

This is the most common renal syndrome of the dog. Any condition in which there is progressive destruction of kidney tissue will result in CRF when approximately 75% of the nephrons have been destroyed. This implies a generalised bilateral disease or a unilateral disease where the other kidney is absent or already damaged (e.g. chronic interstitial nephritis, pyelonephritis, hydronephrosis, nephrolithiasis, glomerulonephritis, amyloidosis, neoplasia, polycystic kidneys,

familial nephropathies, or as a sequel to acute renal failure). Particular features of each of these conditions have already been described.

The end stage of many of the chronic generalised diseases (chronic PN, CIN, chronic GN, chronic amyloidosis and some familiar renal diseases) is the production of a small, irregularly contracted kidney showing capsular adhesions and retention cysts, because there has been replacement of the kidney parenchyma by fibrous tissue; the so-called 'end-stage

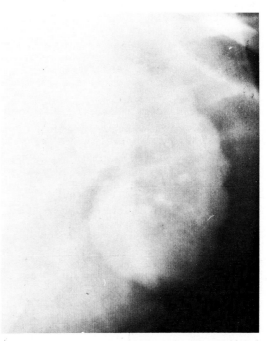

Fig. 15.6 Typical end-stage kidney of a 13-year-old male Dalmatian with chronic renal failure. This nephrogram shows the irregular outline and foci of calcification. (By courtesy of Mr P.M. Webbon.)

kidney' (Fig. 15.6). Often histopathological examination (after biopsy or at necropsy) permits differentiation of the causes, but in advanced cases it can be extremely difficult to determine whether the primary lesions occurred in the glomeruli or the interstitial tissue. In the past the blanket diagnosis of CIN has often been used.

All the vital functions of the kidney suffer with the progressive destruction of the nephrons but the most obvious clinical signs stem from the accumulation of protein breakdown products (azotaemia) as the glomerular filtration rate (GFR) of the kidney is reduced. For an individual, the product of GFR and blood urea concentration is a constant, so that a fall in one

Table 15.3   Differential diagnosis of polyuria/polydipsia.

Chronic renal failure
Due to: Hydronephrosis ⎫
           Pyonephrosis   ⎬ may be no urine flow from affected kidney but will contribute to the loss of nephrons
           Nephrolithiasis ⎭
           Neoplasia
           Polycystic kidney
           Glomerulosclerosis
           'End-stage kidney': chronic interstitial nephritis, chronic (exudative) GN, chronic PN, and some familial renal
               diseases.
Destruction of two-thirds or more of nephrons produces increased solute load on remaining nephrons resulting in osmotic
diuresis and renal insensitivity to vasopressin. CRF present when 75% of nephrons are non-functional. Polyuria/polydipsia
persists when compensated

Diabetes mellitus
Complete or partial lack of insulin results in hyperglycaemia and renal threshold is exceeded producing osmotic diuresis and
glycosuria. (Serious insulin overdosage in diabetes mellitus may also produce the same effect (Somogyi effect). The inevitable
fall in blood glucose triggers several physiological mechanisms to raise it, but in the absence of any compensatory insulin
secretion a period of hyperglycaemia results, accompanied by polyuria and polydipsia.)

Toxaemic states (chiefly pyometra)
Bacterial toxins damage renal tubules producing insensitivity to vasopressin

Hyperadrenocorticism (canine Cushing's syndrome)
Excess of glucocorticoids inhibits vasopressin release by posterior pituitary gland

Liver disease (including hepatic encephalopathy and ICH)
Due to impaired inactivation of aldosterone and cortisol, reduced conversion of urea, and hypokalaemia.

Diabetes insipidus
May be extreme polyuria/polydipsia: *no uraemia*
1 Hypothalamic-hypophyseal DI: partial or total failure to produce or release vasopressin due to damaged hypothalamus
and/or posterior pituitary gland
2 Nephrogenic DI: failure of distal and collecting tubules to respond to vasopressin

Psychogenic polydipsia
May be extreme polyuria/polydipsia: only disease condition where polydipsia precedes polyuria
Primary polydipsia probably an acquired habit in dog, though in man is associated with disorders of hypothalamic thirst
centres

Lymphocytic thyroiditis
Some end-stage cases are accompanied by polyuria/polydipsia, often of fluctuating severity, and may be distinguished by low
levels of thyroxine (T4)

Hypocalcaemia
Polyuria/polydipsia are inconsistent signs. The condition may arise due to either hypoparathyroidism (attributable to lymphocytic parathyroiditis) or hypercalcitoninism (due to medullary carcinoma of the thyroid)

Proliferative and membranous glomerulonephritis
Water is lost in association with proteinuria

Hyperviscosity syndrome
Proteinaemia (e.g. due to multiple myeloma) can result in proteinuria and consequent water loss

Acute renal failure (late stage)
Osmotic diuresis occurs due to retention of solute during oliguric phase; also damaged renal tubules are unable to concentrate
urine

Hyperthyroidism (associated with thyroid neoplasia)
Polyuria/polydipsia is a frequent sign in this rare condition; believed due to the diuretic effect of thyroid hormones

Hypercalcaemia (e.g. in primary hyperparathyroidism or pseudohyperparathyroidism)
Interference with sodium transport decreases sodium reabsorption from proximal and distal tubules. Prolonged excessive
calcium excretion results in nephrocalcinosis, impaired function of distal tubules and ultimately CRF

Hypoadrenocorticism
Decreased level of aldosterone provokes sodium loss

Acromegaly
Due mainly to hyperglycaemia resulting from overproduction of growth hormone which causes glucose intolerance and insulin
resistance. Arises in bitches from middle-age onwards, either in dioestrus or after progestagen therapy

Table 15.3—*contd.*

Primary renal glycosuria
Rare inherited defect of renal tubules limiting glucose absorption; leads to osmotic diuresis

Drug and fluid administration
Corticosteroids and diuretics stimulate polyuria and compensatory polydipsia. Overhydration with i.v. fluids will, in the normal animal, produce polyuria alone

Physiological causes (heat, exercise, dry or salty foods) and water loss secondary to other diseases (vomition and diarrhoea)
Usually polydipsia is not accompanied by polyuria as water has already been lost by other routes

Notes
(a) In all cases, except psychogenic polydipsia and intravenous overhydration, water loss precedes polydipsia. Therefore water should not be withheld as this will impose stress due to dehydration. Neither dogs that have been deprived of water, nor non-deprived dogs drink significantly *in excess* of their needs.
(b) Normal water consumption = 40–50 ml/kg body wt per day. An intake above 70 ml/kg per day can be significant and severe polydipsia exists when it exceeds 100 ml/kg body wt per day.
(c) Normal urine output = 20–40 ml/kg body wt per day (slightly more in young dogs). Definite polyuria exists when it exceeds 90 ml/kg body wt per day.
(d) Vomiting may occur after drinking very large quantities of water simply due to gastric overdistension.

results in an increase in the other. It is generally accepted that signs of azotaemia are not due to a single nitrogenous substance (e.g. urea) but to all the products of protein catabolism acting together (i.e. urea, creatinine, guanidine, phenolic acids and their conjugates, potassium and phosphates). However, the level of blood urea is often used to diagnose and to indicate the severity of renal failure (both ARF and CRF) because it is comparatively easily estimated. Fasting levels in excess of 7 mmol/l (40 mg/100 ml) are regarded as abnormal, particularly as they approach 17 mmol/l (100 mg/100 ml). However increased levels of urea may be due not only to impaired excretion but to increased production associated with high protein diets, fever, gastrointestinal haemorrhage and drugs which stimulate catabolism (e.g. corticosteroids) or inhibit anabolism (e.g. tetracyclines). Dogs with urea levels above 67 mmol/l (400 mg/100 ml) are unlikely to survive.

Creatinine estimation has been preferred because it appears to be independent of protein intake and its production from the breakdown of muscle phosphocreatine is relatively constant (i.e. less affected by the factors which influence urea production). Values below 110 μmol/l (1·25 mg/100 ml) serum can probably be considered normal (English *et al* 1980); those above 440 μmol/l (5 mg/100 ml) carry a poor prognosis. However, technically it is not so simple to estimate, and furthermore blood levels fall with muscle wasting. The current view is that neither estimation is superior. Serial determinations of the blood level of either substance and preferably both are valuable in assessing the progress of the disease. The importance of fasting values should be emphasised; after feeding there is always a rise in the level of blood urea, and also of creatinine if cooked meat has been fed. However, following the consumption of raw meat or a soft-moist food a fall in the creatinine level occurs (Watson *et al* 1981). Dehydration, up to the level of 6%, produces no appreciable increase in the blood level of either metabolite (English *et al* 1980), but in hypoadrenocorticism it is common to find a significant elevation of both.

To compensate for the reduction in total number, each surviving nephron undergoes adaptive changes, including compensatory hypertrophy, which increases its GFR, even though the GFR of the kidney as a whole is reduced. As a result of these changes renal function may be maintained for long periods though at the expense of limiting the kidney's ability to respond to physiological extremes (such as overhydration and dehydration).

A number of possible ways of detecting diminished renal function before the onset of renal failure have been investigated:

1 Monitoring the mean daily water intake, since increased urinary output begins when approximately two-thirds of the nephrons have been lost.
2 Measuring the kidney's ability to clear injected substances, or endogenous creatinine or urea, from the blood (Macdougall 1981).
3 Measuring the urine: plasma ratios for urea and creatinine; less than 10:1 is frequently found in advanced CRF but any value less than 30:1 deserves investigation (Macdougall 1981).

In addition fibrinogen–fibrin degradation products (FDP) in urine (which result from the lysis of intraglomerular fibrin deposits or the differential filtration of plasma fibrinogen and FDP through a damaged

basement membrane) may permit early glomerular damage to be detected (Steward & Macdougall 1981).
4 Measuring the level of lysozyme in the urine as an indicator of tubular damage (Biewenga *et al* 1978).

The polyuria of CRF results from the inability of the surviving nephrons to respond to vasopressin, chiefly because the increased solute load induces an osmotic diuresis (Table 15.3). This begins when more than two-thirds of the nephrons are lost. Sodium is obliged to accompany the water resulting in increased sodium loss. With defective sodium reabsorption and defective response to vasopressin the urine produced can be neither dilute nor concentrated and remains in the same range of osmolality as serum (i.e. with a specific gravity of 1.008–1.012, isothenuria). The loss of sodium produces a reduction in the extracellular fluid compartments, provoking some degree of dehydration, which further reduces the GFR and aggravates the azotaemia. Water-soluble vitamins (chiefly vitamin B) also accompany the water giving a relative vitamin deficiency.

Protein losses in the urine through the damaged nephrons may be high, depending on the cause, but protein is diluted by the large volume of water so that marked proteinuria is usually not a feature (i.e. levels are usually well below 3 g/l (300 mg/100 ml)). Proteinuria is not always present and its presence does not on its own necessarily indicate renal disease. Polyuria will of course not occur through an obstructed (e.g. hydronephrotic) kidney but its inability to function will contribute to the loss of nephrons. Oliguria may occur as a terminal event.

The stomatitis, anorexia, vomiting and diarrhoea associated with CRF are related principally to the azotaemia. The protein catabolites act directly on the brain (possibly as enzyme inhibitors) causing depression of the appetite centre and stimulation of the vomiting centre. In addition, urea is excreted through the mucosae of the alimentary tract and its subsequent decomposition produces ammonia which causes inflammation and irritation, even ulceration, and lends an ammoniacal odour to the breath. In the stomach, foci of necrosis and ulceration apparently result from anoxia caused by diffuse vascular injury compounded by increased activity of the parietal cells and the lack of the normal protective mucus barrier (Cheville 1979).

With increased capillary fragility due to azotaemia haematemesis, melaena and bleeding from the gums may be shown. There is some evidence of low grade malabsorption, including malabsorption of calcium from the small intestine.

The typical normochromic, normocytic anaemia of CRF arises principally from a depression of red bone marrow function, because of a diminution of erythropoietin production by the renal tubular epithelium. Two other factors contributing to anaemia both stem from the azotaemia, namely a reduction in RBC life-span and haemorrhagic diathesis ('uraemic bleeding') due to a qualitative platelet defect.

The blood also often shows an absolute lymphopenia following the atrophy of lymphocytic tissue and depression of lymphopoiesis.

The hypertension of CIN may give rise to cardiac hypertrophy and valvular lesions. Pericarditis associated with azotaemia is much less common in the dog than in man.

Although there is no increase in acid production, metabolic acidosis develops in the later stages of CRF due to a failure of bicarbonate reabsorption and/or reduced ammonia production resulting in less acid being excreted.

However, once present the acidosis can remain stable for long periods and patients do not become increasingly acidotic; probably because of buffer release from the skeleton which accompanies demineralisation.

As well as nitrogenous products phosphate is also derived from protein catabolism and as the GFR falls it is also found in increased concentration in the blood. This in turn causes a reciprocal decrease in the blood calcium level according to the mass law equation. The resultant hypocalcaemia is compounded by the impaired ability of the kidney cortex to carry out the final step in the metabolism of vitamin D3 to its active form, leading then to reduced intestinal absorption of calcium. This lowered blood calcium level stimulates parathyroid hyperplasia and the increased secretion of parathormone which effects the demineralisation of bone in an attempt, often successful, to return the blood calcium level to normal. Consequently in renal secondary hyperparathyroidism calcium phosphate is removed from bone and replaced by fibrous tissue (osteodystrophia fibrosa). These effects are most marked radiographically in the skull, associated with softening of the jaws, especially the mandible ('rubber jaw'), loosening of the teeth and, in younger animals, an increase in volume (facial hyperostosis) (Fig. 15.7). Very occasionally chronic stimulation of the parathyroid glands may result in their failure to respond to increasing calcium levels so that hypercalcaemia develops (Finco & Rowland 1978).

Whether there is gross parathyroid hyperplasia or not, there may be deposition of calcium salts in the soft tissues of dogs with CRF—the alimentary tract, lungs, heart, foot pads and the kidney itself—as well as an increase in SAP activity. However radiographic

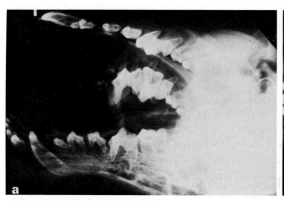 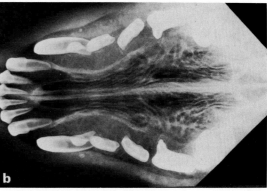

Fig. 15.7 Demineralisation of the skull produced by renal secondary hyperparathyroidism affecting a 7-month-old male crossbred dog. (a) Lateral radiograph of the upper and lower jaws; (b) ventrodorsal radiograph of the upper jaw showing lateral proliferation of fibrous connective tissue (fibrous osteodystrophy).

evidence of soft tissue calcification is rare, and there is no close correlation with the degree of mineral imbalance (Barber & Rowland 1979).

In addition to the general signs of depression and apathy which may progress to coma, attributed to the effect of the protein waste products on the brain, very occasionally dogs may show twitching and/or convulsions (so-called 'uraemic fits'). These are believed to be due, at least in part, to hypocalcaemia, and possibly calcium deposition in the brain. In young dogs with advanced renal disease these signs of uraemic encephalopathy can occur without the more typical clinical signs of CRF, and therefore this condition should be considered in the differential diagnosis of convulsions (Wolf 1980).

Increased tubular secretion of potassium usually maintains normal potassium levels in chronic renal failure although both abnormally high, and abnormally low, levels can be encountered.

Treatment of chronic renal failure

The renal damage which produces CRF is irreversible and therapy is therefore directed towards (a) arresting the progress of the underlying disease where this is possible and (b), and this is usually the most important, enabling the animal to compensate for the decreased number of nephrons. To this end, so-called conservative measures are instituted and these must be continued throughout life. However they may not always be sufficient to control the rise in the blood level of waste products (e.g. following stress or infection which increases the catabolism of protein), resulting in 'uraemic crises' with rapid deterioration in the patient's condition.

In this 'decompensated' stage additional, more intensive, therapeutic measures are necessary to achieve reduction of nitrogenous product levels and recompensation if the patient is to survive.

Conservative measures

The keystone of therapy for dogs showing clinical signs of advanced CRF is a low protein diet to minimise the production of protein breakdown products and their levels in the blood. However, it is necessary to supply simultaneously all the essential amino acids for protein synthesis (anabolism) and this is best done by providing a *small* quantity of protein of high 'biological value' (i.e. with the required amino acids in the optimum concentration so that all can be used for synthesis). Proteins of lower biological value have relative deficiencies of certain amino acids, so that more protein needs to be eaten to obtain them. This inevitably provides an excess of other amino acids which cannot be used for tissue repair or growth and so they are catabolised. Consequently high biological value proteins should be fed, of which egg is the best, followed by lean meats (e.g. beef, veal) and chicken. These should be fed at a rate of 0.7–1.3 g/kg body weight per day, depending on the severity of the azotaemia. Low biological value proteins from vegetable sources, offal, dehydrated meat and fish meal are contraindicated. Dairy products (e.g. cheese) and preparations which contain bone meal should be avoided because of their high phosphate content. There appears to be no particular reason for feeding 'white' meats.

As an alternative to animal protein a supplement of essential amino acids (Nefranutrin, Kidnamin) or their analogues (Ketoperlen) may be provided, as in man.

Doubts about the safety, as well as the efficacy, of two commercial dietary products available in the USA for dogs with CRF have been raised, related particularly to their low content of essential amino acids (Boveé *et al* 1981).

Where there is difficulty in the acceptance of low protein diets by dogs, the addition of a flavouring agent (e.g. Marmite), and feeding at blood heat and in a number of smaller meals daily, should be tried.

Adequate quantities of carbohydrates and fats should be provided to ensure that body protein is not broken down as a source of energy. Suggested calorie intake ranges from 110 kcal/kg body weight per day for a small dog to 70 kcal/kg body weight per day for large dogs. Suitable foods with no protein include butter, margarine, vegetable oils, chocolate, ice-cream, jam, honey and sugar; and those with minimal vegetable protein include rice, bread, cake, biscuits, crisps, chips and pasta products.

It has been shown that dogs with only *moderate* CRF (i.e. not having shown vomiting or anorexia and with levels of urea and creatinine less than double the upper limit of normal) can adapt to a wide range of dietary protein levels. For such animals ordinary commercial diets (i.e. with normal protein content) may well be preferable because they improve the GFR and renal plasma flow and are responsible for increased antibacterial activity in the urine which is valuable in cases of PN (Bovée *et al* 1979b; Bovée & Kronfield 1981). However, with the onset of severe clinical signs, or a marked rise in the level of protein breakdown products in the blood, a low protein diet should immediately be instituted. (Incidentally there is no evidence that high protein diets damage the kidneys of normal dogs.)

Where there is sustained anorexia or vomiting, calories can be supplied intravenously: 5% dextrose solution supplies 205 kcal/l, 10% invert sugar solution supplies 380 kcal/l and 5% dextrose solution with 5% ethanol added to it supplies 450 kcal/l. (Because of the alcohol this last-named solution should not be given to dogs with hepatic damage and, to avoid intoxication, a rate of 2 ml/kg body weight per hour should not be exceeded.)

The diet should contain an increased level of B vitamins to replace those lost through polyuria. Multivitamin injections have been recommended, particularly to provide the folic acid, cyanocobalamin and ascorbic acid needed for erythropoiesis. Salt should also be added to home-prepared diets and a dose of 50–75 mg/kg body weight three times daily is suggested, given either in the food or as tablets (preferably enteric coated). This level of salt supplementation should be introduced gradually. However in those cases with hypertension a reduction in sodium intake (i.e. salt and sodium bicarbonate) is advisable until the blood pressure is brought under control (e.g. with hypotensive drugs); then it can be increased.

Anabolic steroids can also be given to reduce protein breakdown, but in man their effect is least marked in those patients receiving a low protein diet; the diet should therefore receive priority. In male animals testosterone could be employed to produce the same effect as anabolic steroids, and such androgen therapy also replaces the stimulating effect of erythropoietin. In general, anabolic steroids administered parenterally rather than orally are preferred to reduce the risk of hepatic damage. They are contraindicated in cases of the nephrotic syndrome.

In the presence of polyuria *no restriction* in water consumption should be made as this enhances dehydration and predisposes to decompensation. The only exception to this rule is when the intake of water provokes vomition; liquid must then be supplied parenterally. Dehydration following emesis or diarrhoea should be corrected immediately. Quantities required range from 50 ml/kg body weight in 5% dehydration to 120 ml/kg body weight in 12% dehydration (see ARF for dehydration assessment). Intravenous lactated Ringer's solution (=Hartmann's solution) or 5% dextrose solution is usually advised, and its administration may need repeating. Subcutaneous administration has the disadvantage of slower absorption placing a limit on the amount that can be accommodated and therefore that can be given at one time.

Patients with CRF are unable to correct dehydration or overhydration so that as well as the former being watched for and corrected as soon as it occurs, care must be taken not to overhydrate with intravenous fluids by carefully calculating the required amount beforehand.

The acidosis of CRF will in part be corrected by the administration of lactate in lactated Ringer's solution, but it is advisable also to administer sodium bicarbonate orally at a dose rate of 50 mg/kg body weight four times daily.

Aluminium hydroxide gel orally (0.6 g/kg body weight every 8 hours) is of value in adsorbing phosphate in the gastrointestinal tract, and by its astringent and antacid effects controlling vomition and diarrhoea. In the short term, vomition can be controlled by administering chlorbutol, or preferably chlorpromazine or acetylpromazine. The last named have the advantage that they need not be given orally, and will also assist in reducing restlessness and discomfort. Demulcent mouth washes (e.g. glycerine and thymol) may help in cases of stomatitis.

Animals with renal osteodystrophy and/or impaired intestinal absorption of calcium benefit from treatment with large doses of vitamin D3 and increased calcium intake (as calcium carbonate, 100 mg/kg body weight per day). However the phosphate level should first be reduced (by the administration of aluminium hydroxide gel) until the product of the calcium and phosphate levels is less than 5.6 if measured in mmol/l (or <70 measured in mg/100 ml); otherwise the calcification of internal organs may occur. The existence of soft issue calcification *may* be revealed radiographically.

The emergency control of convulsions is probably best achieved by the intraperitoneal administration of pentobarbitone, although a reduced dose (up to 50% less) should be given because of the animal's toxaemic state. Long-term calcium borogluconate therapy (1 ml of a 10% solution/kg body weight per day) may control neurological signs. Administration of magnesium salts (e.g. Epsom salts as a purgative) is contraindicated because the kidneys have difficulty in excreting a sudden magnesium load.

Digoxin therapy for endocardiosis associated with CRF should be at a decreased (even halved) dose rate because of a reduced rate of excretion. The dosage of insulin and antibiotics which are excreted through the kidney should also be reduced, although with aminoglycoside antibiotics normal doses at lengthened intervals appear preferable (Riviere & Coppoc 1981).

In CRF the immune response of patients is impaired and there is an increased likelihood of bacterial infection. Therefore it is advisable that critically ill patients, especially those receiving interferences (e.g. peritoneal dialysis), should receive a course of a broad-spectrum antibiotic, in general ampicillin or amoxycillin or trimethoprim with sulphadiazine.

Decompensation phase
If the life of the animal is to be saved when the level of protein breakdown products suddenly increases, accompanied by a rapid decline in its clinical condition, the excess of waste products must be speedily removed. Two procedures are available, but both involve some degree of stress and should therefore be started before the animal's condition is such that it is unlikely to survive the interference. The first is to attempt osmotic diuresis which aims to stimulate solute loss through the kidney. If this does not produce the required improvement, peritoneal dialysis may be successful. These procedures are described at the end of this chapter. Usually they need to be repeated to produce an adequate response. It should be emphasised that neither procedure is capable of maintaining CRF patients permanently but both are intended to enable them to overcome periods of decompensated CRF (or ARF) even though some animals will become decompensated on several occasions. Haemodialysis

in the dog has been described (Macdougall *et al* 1977), but it is not yet a feasible routine procedure in canine practice. Renal transplantation is also a technique that has been performed on the dog but is far from being employed routinely.

One aspect of treatment not specifically described but of paramount importance is good nursing (i.e. minimising stress, keeping warm, feeding properly and ensuring the animal's comfort and well-being as far as is possible).

DISEASES OF THE URETERS

Congenital abnormalities

Ureterocoele (congenital cystic dilatation of the submucosal segment of the intravesical ureter) has been recorded on rare occasions and often produces obstruction leading to megaureter (hydroureter) and hydronephrosis. On excretory urography, the enlargement has a typical 'cobra-head' appearance. Ureteral duplication is an even rarer abnormality.

The most common congenital ureteral defect is *ureteral ectopia* with one or both ureters opening at a point other than the trigone of the bladder (i.e. into the urethra, vagina or rarely the uterus) as a result of faulty differentiation of the mesonephric and metanephric ducts in embryo. Bilateral cases account for approximately a quarter of the total. (Ectopic ureterocoele has also been recorded.)

Sometimes there may be branching of the ureters and developmental abnormalities of other parts of the urinary tract (e.g. ectopia or hypoplasia of the kidney). Hydroureter occurs in over half the cases, and in approximately 1 in 6 hydronephrosis is present.

Despite the absence of a competent uretero-vesical valve incontinence is detected in only about two-thirds of affected dogs, sometimes being intermittent or related to the animal being in a recumbent position (Holt *et al* 1982). The absence of incontinence may be due to retrograde filling of the bladder taking place, especially in males where the urethralis muscle exerts a sphincter-like action, and this could account for why fewer cases have been reported in males (less than 1 in 10). In bitches any incontinence is usually apparent from an early age, whereas in males it may appear much later in life, up to 2½ years old (Lennox 1978). The defect occurs frequently in crossbred dogs but of the pure breeds it has been seen most often in Miniature and Toy Poodles, Fox Terriers, Labrador and Golden Retrievers and Siberian Huskies. In the last three of these breeds there is evidence of a heritable tendency. Affected animals are more prone to ascending

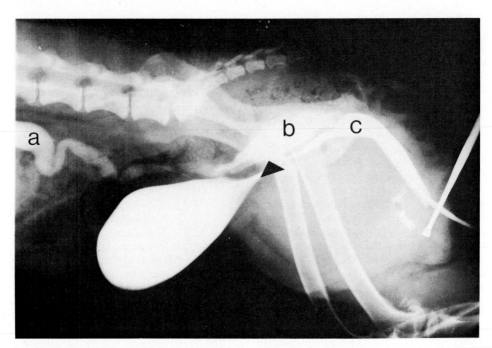

Fig. 15.8 Vagino-urethrogram of a 12-month-old Cocker Spaniel bitch showing an ectopic and dilated right ureter (a) entering the anterior vagina (b) at the point arrowed. There is evidence of stenosis between the anterior vagina and the vestibule (c). (By courtesy of Mr P.M. Webbon.)

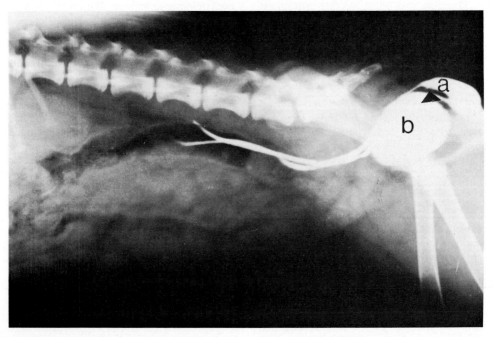

Fig. 15.9 Vagino-urethrogram of a 5-month-old Miniature Poodle bitch with bilateral uretheral ectopia. The ureters join the vagina (a) at the point arrowed, and the bladder (b) is in the pelvic cavity. (By courtesy of Mr P.M. Webbon.)

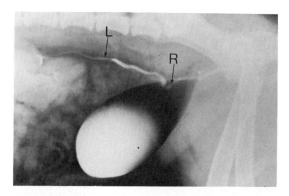

Fig. 15.10 Lateral excretory urogram of a 2½-year-old male Labrador Retriever 32 minutes after the intravenous injection of radiopaque contrast medium. The narrower left ureter (L) is clearly visible from the kidney to its entry into the bladder at the normal site. The positive contrast medium is obviously present in the bladder, which had previously been filled with air. Although the more distended ectopic right ureter (R) is not visible throughout its length, its posterior part can be seen to pass further back than the left and the medium in it is continuous with that in the urethra.

bacterial infection and reflux which may result in pyelitis or pyelonephritis.

Confirmation of the diagnosis and the site of the affected ureter(s) is best made radiographically using both excretory urography (adjusting the animals position to obtain optimum visualisation of the distal ureters), and either vagino-urethrography (vaginography) or retrograde urethrography (Figs 15.8, 15.9 and 15.10). Visualisation of the ectopic orifice is often not possible (for example bitches are often too young for vaginal endoscopy) and precisely locating the termination of the ureter(s) may not be possible in more than a quarter of cases.

Surgical treatment is necessary; the simplest is complete resection of the ureter and its associated kidney (uretero-nephrectomy), provided that the other kidney is functioning normally. Several methods of ureterovesical anastomosis (or transplantation) are available but should only be considered where the kidney drained by the affected ureter is normal, or there is bilateral ectopia or hypofunction of both kidneys. Unfortunately the translocated ureter may become stenosed, giving rise to hydroureter and HN. Occasionally vesicoureteral reflux may develop. Even in the absence of these complications the incontinence frequently does not disappear until some time after surgery, presumably because the bladder is initially overloaded and takes time to adapt to the increased volume of urine.

Obstruction

There may be interference with the passage of urine along the ureter following (a) pressure by abdominal masses including neoplasms (in or outside the ureteral wall), aberrant renal vessels and ligatures incorrectly applied during abdominal surgery, (b) internal blockage by calculi (from the renal pelvis) or blood clots, (c) kinking or twisting of the ureters due to displacement of the kidneys or bladder, and (d) congenital or acquired stenosis of the ureter (e.g. with ureterocoele or following inflammation, trauma or surgery). The effect is to produce megaureter and eventually hydronephrosis, though complete bilateral obstruction, which is rare, will result in postrenal ARF. Ureteral calculi and neoplasms are extremely rare. Abdominal pain is a sequel to trauma and the passage of calculi. Diagnosis is based on radiography (especially excretory urography). Removal of the obstruction almost always requires surgery, and treatment may also be necessary for the secondary renal damage. In many cases, provided the opposite kidney is functional, complete removal of the affected ureter and its kidney will be more successful than attempts at ureteral anastomosis.

Rupture

Rupture may follow trauma, with the passage of urine into the abdominal cavity producing a palpable soft mass in the sublumbar region. It normally takes place near the kidneys. Excretory urography shows leakage of contrast media from the ureter. Again surgical repair, or complete ureterectomy and nephrectomy, is indicated.

Vesicoureteral reflex

Most normal dogs have competent ureterovesical valves which prevent any reflux of urine to the kidney, though primary reflux (i.e. without urinary tract infection) occurs in about 10% of adult dogs and a higher proportion of younger dogs (approximately 80% at 3 months of age). In two-thirds of cases, reflux is bilateral. It was previously thought that reflux in the absence of urinary tract infection (UTI) had no deleterious effect on kidney function but recent evidence suggests otherwise. Secondary vesicoureteral reflux occurs in a proportion of animals with UTI, especially where there are factors present which encourage the persistence of the infection (i.e. obstructive lesions or defective innervation). Damage by bacterial toxins to the ureterovesical valves and to the ureters causes the cessation of normal ureteral peristalsis and the reflux of infected urine to the renal pelvis and medulla. This can result in acute pyelitis or pyelonephritis (Fig. 15.15).

Diagnosis is based on observing reflux of contrast media up the ureters during micturating cystourethrography.

Treatment should be for the underlying UTI and if necessary for CFR which may follow bilateral pyelonephritis.

BLADDER DISEASES

Anatomical abnormalities
(abnormalities of development or position)

The following are some rare congenital abnormalities which can occur: complete absence of the bladder resulting in incontinence and exstrophy of the bladder (where the ventral walls of both the abdomen and the bladder are absent so that the dorsal bladder wall substitutes for the ventral abdominal wall and the ureters discharge directly to the exterior); diverticula of the bladder body or neck, some of which represent a persistent urachus (if the urachus remains patent, urine is voided at the umbilicus) and persistent sections of secretory urachal epithelium resulting in the formation of isolated urachal cysts which may become infected.

The bladder may be displaced by prostatic enlargement (anteriorly), by uterine or vaginal prolapse (posteriorly), by adhesions formed following surgery or peritonitis (Fig. 15.11), by torsion due to trauma or tumours within the abdominal cavity, and rarely it may be involved in perineal, inguinal or abdominal hernias. There are very rare reports of prolapse of the bladder through the female urethra. These displacements can result in obstruction and pain.

Diagnosis is best made by radiography employing contrast media, and correction, where possible, requires appropriate surgical techniques. Temporary alleviation of the effects of obstruction may involve withdrawing urine from the bladder via a needle inserted through the abdominal wall.

Urinary calculi

Urolithiasis occurs in between 0.4 and 2% of the canine population. Slightly more than half of the calculi are composed mainly of phosphate (chiefly magnesium ammonium phosphate otherwise called struvite, often with some calcium phosphate, referred to as apatite). The remainder, which have as their major constituent cystine, oxalate or urate are of approxi-

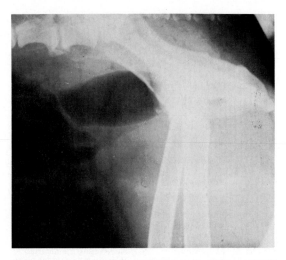

Fig. 15.11   Lateral pneumocystogram of a 5½-year-old Old English Sheepdog spayed bitch with incontinence. The bladder is displaced dorsally and appears to be misshapen, due to the formation of adhesions following ovariohysterectomy. The distortion of the bladder apparently interfered with normal sphincter action.

mately equal occurrence. Predominantly carbonate calculi rarely occur (generally in aged dogs), and cases of silica 'jack-stone' urolithiasis have been occasionally recorded in the USA, primarily in males and especially amongst German Shepherd Dogs. Most British and American reports show that overall uroliths have an equal incidence in males and females.

The majority of uroliths form in the bladder. In the bitch, 80% are composed of phosphate and the vast majority, some of which are of a considerable size, remain in the bladder. Cystine, oxalate and urate calculi occur principally in the male (Figs 15.12 and 15.13). In most affected males the calculi are found in both the bladder and the urethra and may block the latter, either behind the os penis or at the ischial arch. Calculi can arise at any age. Most are diagnosed between 4 and 6 years of age though oxalate (and carbonate) calculi are more likely to occur in older animals. A high incidence of struvite calculi in Miniature Schnauzers between 12 and 15 months old may suggest an inherited predisposition to staphylococcal infection (Klausner *et al* 1980).

Over all, the incidence of calculi appears highest in the Corgi, Dachshund, Miniature Schnauzer, Dalmatian, and Cairn Terrier and lowest in the German Shepherd Dog, Labrador Retriever and Boxer.

Infection of the urine by staphylococci is an important, if not critical, predisposing factor in the formation of phosphate calculi. The precise mechanism is unknown but is believed to be related to bacterial

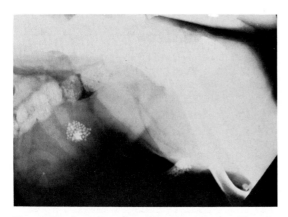

Fig. 15.12 Lateral radiograph of a 10-year-old male crossbred dog showing numerous oxalate calculi both in the bladder and in the urethra posterior to the os penis.

urease, phosphatase and coagulase production. At least three-quarters of phosphate calculi contain viable bacterial organisms; this is rare with other calculi. Struvite calculi, and possibly also calcium oxalate calculi, are more likely to form in cases of hyperparathyroidism. Cystinuria is due to an inherited renal tubular defect which predisposes to, but does not necessarily ensure, the occurrence of cystine uroliths. This appears to be especially frequent in the Irish Terrier, Bulldog, Dachshund and Bassett Hound and is common in the Corgi, Basenji and Chihuahua. Ammonium urate stones occur most frequently in the Dalmatian because it is unique in excreting most of its purines as uric acid instead of the more soluble allantoin, due to a functional deficiency in hepatic uricase activity (Yu *et al* 1971). Calculi with ammonium and uric acid components, chiefly ammonium urate calculi, frequently

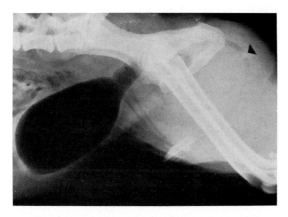

Fig. 15.13 Lateral pneumocystogram of a 7-year-old male crossbred dog revealing the presence of a cystine calculus (arrowed) in the urethra at the ischial arch.

occur in the kidney or bladder of dogs with severe liver dysfunction, which may be sufficient to produce encephalopathy, and may be the result of a congenital portosystemic shunt. Finding ammonium urate calculi in breeds other than Dalmatians is strongly suggestive of an hepatic disorder.

The non-crystalline organic matrix containing mucoproteins and mucopolysaccharides is also believed to play an important part in the formation of calculi, and the other major factors which determine whether calculi form are the concentration of the relevant salt in the urine and, to a lesser extent, the urinary pH. In general, oxalate and urate stones form in acid urine and phosphate in alkaline urine (in association with urease-producing bacteria), though phosphate stones can also occur in acid urine. Cystine stones appear equally likely to occur in slightly acid or slightly alkaline urine.

Obstruction of the male urethra produces signs of dysuria and urinary incontinence. The presence of bladder calculi in either sex can result in erosion of the wall, haematuria (especially at the end of urination) and dysuria (Table 15.4). Obstruction may lead to distension of the bladder and be followed by ARF or, if only unilateral or partial, hydronephrosis.

Bladder calculi may be palpable but, in general, diagnosis is based on finding obstruction to catheterisation and on lateral radiography, where necessary (e.g. with urate calculi) using air as a contrast medium. Phosphate and oxalate calculi are very dense and usually show clearly even when small, whereas urate stones, unless they are large or contain a high proportion of phosphate, are almost radiolucent. Cystine calculi vary in their opacity.

Treatment usually involves cystotomy, and/or urethrotomy in the male. However urethrostomy appears the better treatment in cases of male urethral blockage, creating a permanent fistula to eliminate the two common sites of obstruction from the urinary tract and allowing any small calculi from the bladder to be readily eliminated. The technique of hydropropulsion has also been advocated for removing calculi lodged in the male urethra (see p. 439). There have been reports of the fragmentation of bladder calculi by ultrasound therapy which may allow the particles to be voided naturally. Attempts at dissolving calculi by introducing chemical solutions have usually had limited success, though the use of urinary acidifiers to decrease the urinary pH (provided that the patient is not already suffering from azotaemia/acidosis) can assist in dissolving struvite calculi by increasing the solubility of struvite in the urine.

Calculi recur in between 10 and 30% of cases although no type is significantly more likely to recur

Table 15.4 Differential diagnosis of dysuria and tenesmus.

Dysuria (difficulty and pain on urination) and *stranguria* (slow, painful urination) are associated with:
Obstruction (of bladder or urethra) to the voiding of urine, e.g. calculi, neoplasm, an enlarged prostate gland or involvement of the bladder in a perineal hernia (almost invariably in males)
Inflammation of bladder or urethra (e.g. UTI)
Rupture of the bladder or urethra (rare)
Adhesion of vaginal/uterine stump to the bladder following spaying
Fracture of the os penis (rare)

Tenesmus (straining) is also associated with:
Obstruction of colon, rectum or anus (e.g. constipation, neoplasms or polyps, foreign bodies, enlarged prostate gland, anal stricture or perineal hernia)
Irritation and inflammation of colon, rectum or anus (e.g. colitis and proctitis, associated with passage of mucus and often blood, i.e. dysentery)
Parturition: normal and abnormal (dystocia)

Note. Frequency (of urination) may be associated with both dysuria and polyuria.

than another. The most important single measure to prevent recurrence is to double the water intake by adding salt to the diet or administering diuretics. It is also important to ensure the elimination of any urinary tract infection (UTI) especially in the case of phosphate calculi. In dogs with cystine and urate stones a low protein (and low purine) diet is recommended, together with the administration of sodium bicarbonate to produce an alkaline pH. In cases with oxalate stones a low intake of both protein and calcium has been advised. Cases of cystinuria may benefit from the oral administration of D-penicillamine (Cuprimine) (10 mg/kg body weight per day) to allow the excretion of a soluble cysteine–penicillamine complex, and dogs with a predisposition to urate calculi can be treated with oral allopurinol (Zyluric) (up to 30 mg/kg body weight per day for a month, then 10 mg/kg body weight per day). Provisional studies in preventing or slowing the growth of struvite calculi by administering acetohydroxamic acid (a urease-inhibitor, 25 mg/kg body weight per day) have been encouraging (Osborne *et al* 1981).

Neoplasia

Bladder neoplasms account for less than 0.5% of all tumours in the dog and over 90% are primary neoplasms. Of these, three-quarters are epithelial tumours with the two main types, carcinomas (chiefly transitional cell carcinomas) and papillomas, occurring in the ratio 4:1. The most common non-epithelial tumours are those which affect muscle tissue and connective tissue and they have an equal incidence. Bladder cancer appears to be relatively more common in Scottish Terriers, Shetland Sheepdogs and Beagles; bitches are affected more frequently. Tumours are usually found in dogs over 8 years of age (particularly

at 11 years of age, Fig. 15.14). Rhabdomyosarcomas occur most usually in dogs under eighteen months of age, particularly St Bernards, and are associated in 50% of cases with hypertrophic osteoarthropathy. Paradoxically cases of transitional cell carcinoma have developed in dogs receiving treatment with the antineoplastic drug cyclophosphamide (Weller *et al* 1979).

Secondary neoplasia of the bladder may arise by direct extension from adjacent organs (chiefly carcinoma of the prostate), implantation from the upper urinary tract, or rarely by metastasis from more distant organs (i.e. the mammary gland).

Neoplasms frequently ulcerate producing haematuria, either constantly or intermittently (Table 15.5). They may also cause dysuria (i.e. with tenesmus) and increased frequency of urination. If there is urethral or ureteral obstruction, retention of urine follows, with ARF or hydronephrosis.

Diagnosis is based on palpation of the bladder (though circumscribed tumours may simulate a calculus) and radiography, particularly after introducing contrast media into the bladder. Exploratory laparotomy is indicated in cases where other common causes of haematuria have been eliminated.

The ideal treatment is complete surgical extirpation; where this is not possible the prognosis must be poor.

Inflammatory polyps of the bladder produce identical clinical and radiographic signs to transitional cell carcinomas and can only be distinguished by histopathological examination after removal. They may predispose to cystitis (polypoid cystitis).

Cystitis

Rare cases of emphysematous cystitis (usually in association with diabetes mellitus), allergic cystitis and cystitis due to tasonemid mites have been recorded.

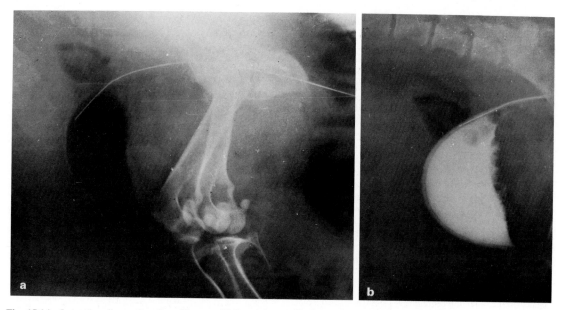

Fig. 15.14 Lateral radiographs of an 11-year-old Scottish Terrier bitch with a transitional cell carcinoma on the posterior wall of the bladder. (a) A pneumocystogram establishes an abnormal bladder shape; (b) following the intro-duction of radiopaque contrast medium the markedly irregular outline of the posterior border of the bladder indicates the position of the neoplasm.

More often cystitis is produced by trauma, calculi and neoplasia, and a sterile haemorrhagic cystitis may be a consequence of cyclophosphamide therapy. However most cases of cystitis in the dog are due to UTI with bacteria. Bacteria reach the bladder by ascending migration from the urethra, sometimes from a focus of infection in the genital tract (e.g. prostate gland or uterus). (It is believed that the bacterial organisms responsible for pyometra and prostatitis have been derived from the urethra.) The urethra is usually colonised by bacteria but defences exist to eliminate them from the bladder or prevent their multiplication there; the most important defence is the frequent and complete voiding of urine ('bladder wash out'). Consequently factors which cause retention of urine predispose to the establishment of UTI. The principal factors are blockage of the urethra (e.g. by calculi or neoplasms), neurogenic interference with normal micturition and the presence of diverticula which can harbour infected urine (Fig. 15.15). Therefore in cases of UTI, investigations should be made to discover whether such abnormalities are present. Wherever possible they should be corrected (usually by surgery); otherwise the UTI will either not be eliminated by drug therapy or soon recur.

Acute cystitis produces the clinical signs of haematuria, incontinence and frequency, plus, in severe cases, pain on bladder palpation and dysuria (with male dogs squatting to urinate). In chronic cases the bladder wall may be thickened.

Diagnosis is based on the finding of significant bacteriuria on urinalysis (i.e. more than 10^5 organisms/ml urine). However it is important to appreciate that a small number of cases of significant bacteriuria are asymptomatic and if untreated there may be reflux of infected urine up the ureters to produce pyelonephritis and, if bilateral, chronic renal failure. Consequently, the remission of clinical signs after treatment *does not* necessarily mean complete elimination of the bacterial infection.

The incidence of significant bacteriuria appears to be 1.4%. A greater proportion of bitches is affected and the incidence is higher in older animals, but there is no clear breed predilection.

The bacteria isolated in cases of UTI are those normally present in the bowel and on the skin: *E. coli* and other coliforms, *Proteus* spp., *Pseudomonas aeruginosa*, staphylococci and streptococci. In 10% of cases more than one bacterial species is present.

After performing a bacterial count or screening test to establish the existence of significant bacteriuria it is advisable to perform sensitivity testing. At least 10 days of therapy should then be given using an antibacterial drug effective *in vitro*, although a maximum of 6 days is advisable when using the relatively toxic drug polymyxin B for cases with *Pseudomonas* infection.

Table 15.5 Differential diagnosis of haematuria.

Urinary tract (any part)

Urinary calculi: may be signs of obstruction; catheterisation and radiography valuable

Severe inflammation, usually due to bacterial infection (UTI): may not be marked if (rarely) kidney alone is affected (pyonephrosis with partial obstruction, pyelonephritis); more obvious with bladder infection. Cystitis can follow cancer treatment with cyclophosphamide

Neoplasia: benign or malignant, large or small

Trauma: e.g. road accident, kick; plus kidney and bladder: vigorous palpation: bladder and urethra: catheterisation; bladder: *Capillaria plica*, very rarely

Kidney

Acute leptospirosis: finding leptospirae conclusive ⎱ early

Acute tubular necrosis; nephrotoxins or ischaemia ⎰ oliguria

Inflammation associated with proliferative glomerulonephritis

Renal infarcts: sequel to septicaemia and endocarditis

Crystalluria: less soluble sulphonamides and acid urine

Dioctophyma renale: giant kidney worm (only in imported dogs)

Idiopathic renal haemorrhage: diagnosis depends on ureteral catheterisation at laparotomy

Genital tract

Prostate gland: trauma, inflammation (prostatitis), neoplasia, hyperplasia (rarely)

Penis and prepuce: inflammation, neoplasia, trauma (e.g. mating, masturbation, licking, bite wounds)

Uterus, vagina, vulva: inflammation (metritis, vaginitis), neoplasia, trauma (mating), oestral discharge

Generalised (i.e. affecting other body systems)

Defective haemostasis—e.g. warfarin poisoning, thrombocytopenia

Severe septicaemia/toxaemia/viraemia

Chronic passive congestion

Notes

(a) Haematuria has been reported to follow violent exercise.

(b) Haemorrhage also occurs with prolapse of the male urethra or female bladder, but the lesion is obvious.

(c) Haematuria is the presence of intact RBCs in urine (derived from the urinary or genital tracts); however, if present for any length of time in this abnormal environment, especially with extremes of pH or concentration, the cells will lyse, releasing haemoglobin which will gradually be converted to dark brown acid, or alkaline, haematin. This will require distinction from haemoglobinuria (due to lead or chlorate poisoning, extensive burns, incompatible blood transfusion) and myoglobinuria (following violent exercise such as Greyhound racing).

(d) Bleeding which is most obvious at the start of urination is usually due to lesions in the urethra or genital tract. Where bleeding is most marked at the end of urination, bladder lesions are usually suspected. Blood evenly mixed with urine denotes a lesion in the kidneys, ureters, or bladder.

(e) Bleeding may not always be obvious (occult blood).

(f) Owners may be unable to distinguish between blood-stained urine, vomit and liquid faeces (dysentery) if the material is not observed being passed.

One week after the termination of treatment, urine should be re-examined to determine whether the UTI has been eliminated. If not, this procedure should be repeated with the same or another drug. Since sulphonamides, streptomycin and trimethoprim with sulphadiazine are more effective at pH 8, and penicillins, tetracycline and nitrofurantoin are more active at pH 5.5, the existing urinary pH should influence the choice of drugs. Alternatively an alkalising agent (e.g. sodium bicarbonate 50 mg/kg body weight twice daily) or an acidifying agent (e.g. sodium acid phosphate 40 mg/kg body weight per day) can be used to alter the pH, though the latter will not prove effective in the presence of a urease-producing organism. The most effective drugs (against all bacteria except *Pseudomonas*) are ampicillin, amoxycillin, trimethoprim with sulphadiazine, nalidixic acid and nitrofurantoin. Gen-

tamicin is advocated for resistant strains (Ling & Ruby 1979). Chelidonium extract and hexamine are unlikely to remove an infection. Hexamine produces an antiseptic effect only in acid urine. The supposed action of 'chelidon' tablets in the treatment of any urinary tract condition is obscure.

An increase in fluid intake (provoked by the addition of salt to the diet) and frequent urination are also recommended as aids to the elimination of bacteria. Consequently, the owner should allow the animal opportunity for frequent urination during the day.

UTI can be eliminated from 70% of dogs with one course of treatment, and only 12% fail to respond after three courses. In most of the latter cases investigation will reveal some abnormality of the urogenital tract which predisposes to the persistence of UTI.

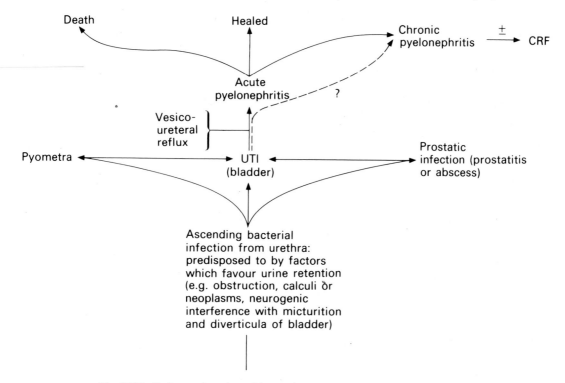

Fig. 15.15 Pathogenesis and possible consequences of urinary tract infection (UTI).

Changers in bladder tone

Primary causes

The smooth muscle of the bladder wall may be replaced by fibrous tissue (following trauma or severe inflammation) or by neoplastic tissue, producing a small firm bladder incapable of distension together with resultant incontinence (Table 15.6). Diagnosis depends on palpation and pneumocystography but treatment at this stage is unrewarding.

Secondary causes

Neurogenic

Damage to the reflex centre of micturition in the sacral region of the spinal cord (e.g. by vertebral fractures, intervertebral disc protrusion, chronic degenerative reticulomyelopathy or neoplasia) or bilateral damage to the communicating peripheral nerve fibres (principally those running in the pelvic nerves) will result in relaxation of the detrusor muscle and flaccid sphincters. There is no voluntary or reflex control of micturition and overdistension (atony) of the bladder occurs, followed by incontinence as the intravesical pressure overcomes the urethral resistance to urine flow. Lesions of the spinal cord above the reflex centre temporarily produce the same effect, but after the period of spinal shock there is spasticity of the sphincters producing urine retention and ultimately retention overflow. Then as the cord recovers (after 1–3 weeks) reflex micturition can again take place, but without voluntary control, though emptying is generally incomplete. Partial lesions of the spinal cord result in urine being passed voluntarily but in a small stream and often in short spurts with obvious straining against the pressure of a closed sphincter (reflex dyssynergia).

Lesions in the cerebral cortex remove voluntary control, and, depending on their precise position, may either facilitate or inhibit reflex micturition (i.e. produce incontinence or retention). Localising areas of increased or decreased resistance in the urethra (by a urethral pressure profile) can assist in establishing the cause of incontinence (Rosin & Barsanti 1981).

Treatment should be directed towards correction of the primary defect. Where there is lack of reflex control, manual expression of urine should be performed, although in cases with spasticity of the sphincters, catheterisation is required. Retention catheters may prove useful but tend to become dislodged or blocked

Table 15.6 Differential diagnosis of urinary incontinence.

Inflammation and incompetence, of external bladder sphincter
Can arise due to bacterial infection, presence of calculi, trauma, including surgery

Partial obstruction of urethra or bladder neck
Paradoxical incontinence (e.g. with calculi or neoplasms); therefore can be difficult to catheterise. Steady dribble of urine or sudden release with change in position

Ectopic ureters
Opening through or beyond the external bladder sphincter. Present since birth though signs may appear later, especially in males

Congenital abnormality of bladder, bladder sphincter or urethra (including urethrorectal fistula)
Rare. Present since birth

Loss of bladder muscle and replacement with neoplastic tissue or fibrous tissue
For example after trauma or severe inflammation (primary loss of bladder tone). Small indistensible bladder

Accidental fistulation between ureter and vagina
Occurs during spaying, with fairly early onset of incontinence after the operation

Uro-vagina in pseudohermaphrodites
Rare. An abnormal communication between the vagina and urethral lumen in both male and female pseudohermaphrodites allows retention of urine and subsequent leakage

Prostatic enlargement
Usually hyperplasia, sometimes squamous metaplasia, prostatitis, abscess or cyst formation, or neoplasia. In early stages causes pressure on colon/rectum but as it moves over anterior brim of the pelvis is more likely to affect urinary flow. Major cause of incontinence (and dysuria and haematuria) in male dogs beyond middle age

Endocrine imbalance
Chiefly in ovariohysterectomised dogs of any age and at varying intervals, up to several months, after operation. Responds to oestrogen (oestradiol or stilboestrol) therapy which is required life-long, though ultimately may become unresponsive.
   Also reported in a castrated male dog which responded to testosterone therapy

Displacement or distortion of bladder
Interferes with normal sphincter action. May arise with adhesions after surgery or trauma, especially adhesions of vaginal/uterine stump to the bladder after spaying. Contraction of the stump draws the bladder back into the pelvic cavity effectively shortening the urethra

Neurogenic causes
Due to damage to peripheral nerves (pelvic or pudendal), spinal cord, or brain, or even 'tight junctions' in detrusor muscle of bladder following prolonged overdistension

---

Notes
(a) Urinary incontinence is the involuntary passage of urine, producing constant or intermittent dribbling of which the animal is often unaware.
(b) Young, untrained or mentally disturbed dogs may show undesirable patterns of urination (e.g. nervous animals may urinate as part of a submissive response).
(c) Incontinence should be distinguished from polyuria where inability to retain large volumes of urine for long periods can result in it being voided on inappropriate occasions (e.g. nocturia).
(d) Persistent urachus also results in uncontrolled voiding of urine, but in this case from the umbilicus.

and predispose to urinary tract infection. Urine 'scalds' should be avoided by clipping the hair, washing the skin and applying petroleum jelly. In the short term, cases of reflex dyssenergia may respond to alpha-adrenergic blocking agents, such as phenoxy-benzamine hydrochloride (Dibenyline) (5–10 mg twice daily). Cholinergic drugs such as bethanechol chloride (Myotonine chloride) have been recommended for dogs with flaccid sphincters and loss of reflex micturition to stimulate bladder emptying (dose: 5–25 mg every eight hours); but unfortunately they have been of little benefit in most cases. Conversely anti-choli-

nergic medication, as with propantheline bromide (Pro-banthine) ($7\frac{1}{2}$–30 mg three times daily), or emepronium bromide (Cetiprin) (100–200 mg three times daily), may control cases where there is an enhanced bladder-emptying reflex resulting in sudden urination, i.e. without warning at inappropriate moments, for example following cerebellar lesions, or where no morphological change is apparent.

Paradoxical incontinence
Partial blockage of the urethra, usually by calculi, will produce overdistention of the bladder and incontin-

ence, and prolonged overdistention may result in atony. There may be constant dribbling or a sudden release of urine with any change in position. Treatment should be directed towards removal of the obstruction.

Rupture

Bladder rupture is usually due to external abdominal trauma (most often a road accident) and is the most common traumatic injury to the urinary tract. Occasionally it is the result of a puncture wound or a pelvic fracture. It may result from traumatic palpation and catheterisation, or from blockage of the urethra by a calculus. It more frequently occurs in males, and may be associated with concurrent urethral rupture. In experimental investigations the chances of survival seldom exceeded 50:50 with death occurring between one and four days later. However clinical cases are at times seen with a history of 8–9 days illness since the original trauma, and survival rates are often better. The condition produces the clinical signs of ARF but without the later polyuric phase (i.e. central nervous system depresssion, vomition, anorexia and polydipsia). There is discomfort on abdominal palpation and increasing reluctance to walk. Urine accumulates in the abdominal cavity. The body temperature and the ability or inability to urinate are *not* reliable diagnostic signs.

Diagnosis can be made on clinical signs, radiographic examination and comparision of the creatinine content of the serum and the abdominal fluid; abdominal fluid values greater than serum values in-

dicate uroperitoneum. (As with other causes of ARF there is an absolute increase in the serum levels of urea, creatinine and inorganic phosphorus.) Pneumocystograms will reveal a rupture in about 75% of cases and the injected air can often be heard escaping from the bladder. However, positive contrast cystography will demonstrate rupture in almost all cases. Before surgical repair is attempted, the metabolic abnormalities (including hyperkalaemia) should be corrected by drainage of the peritoneal fluid, institution of parenteral fluid therapy (see ARF, p. 413) and broadspectrum antibiotic therapy.

Capillaria plica infection

Although *Capillaria plica* infection of the bladder occurs in the UK, particularly in hunting dogs, the parasite is not considered of pathological importance and treatment is not usually given.

DISORDERS OF THE URETHRA

Congenital

Absence of the urethra, imperforate urethra, ectopic urethra, duplication of the urethra, hypospadias (an opening on the ventral surface of the penis or perineum) and the existence of urethrorectal fistula (resulting in urine being passed through the anus or anal sphincter as well as the urethra) have been reported (Fig. 15.16). Diagnosis is based on the history, direct inspection and, if necessary, radiography. Correction, where possible, is by surgery.

Urethritis and trauma

Inflammation of the urethra may arise in association with a UTI (see cystitis, p. 430) or with trauma inflicted by bite wounds, catheterisation, masturbation, excessive licking, obstruction with calculi, or surgery. Urethral rupture, usually at its junction with the bladder, may be a complication of pelvic fracture in a male dog (Pechman 1982). These traumatic lesions can become secondarily infected.

Patients show frequency and dysuria, often with pain and frequently haematuria. Haematuria due to localised urethral lesions is evident chiefly, or solely, at the beginning of urination and blood may drip from the urethra at other times (which should not be confused with oestral discharge).

Diagnosis may require retrograde urethrography to

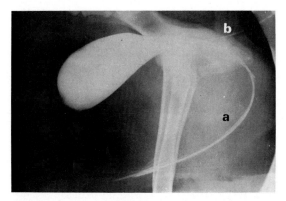

Fig. 15.16 Lateral radiograph of a 1½-year-old German Shepherd Dog with a 'urethrorectal fistula'. Radiopaque contrast medium has been introduced into the bladder through catheters inserted into both the penile urethra (a) and the abnormal channel (b) leading from the prostatic urethra to the anal sphincter. This channel represents the persistent urogenital sinus of the embryo.

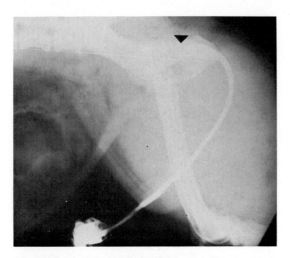

Fig. 15.17 Lateral radiograph of a 5-year-old male Labrador Retriever undergoing retrograde contrast urethrography. Radiopaque contrast medium could not be forced along the urethra beyond the point indicated. Subsequent investigation showed that the urethra was blocked at that level by a haematoma within its lumen.

discern the location and nature of the lesion. Rupture is shown by the passage of positive contrast media into the surrounding tissues.

Antibacterial therapy (parenterally, and if necessary locally) is advisable, together with surgical correction of any wounds. Masturbation may be controlled by administering oestrogen or by castration.

Obstruction

This can arise due to: (a) neoplasms, especially in bitches, and in particular those above eight years old. Squamous cell carcinomas are most frequently found, although any of the types found elsewhere in the urinary tract may occur plus transmissible venereal sarcomas; (b) calculi (see urinary calculi, p. 428); (c) prostatic enlargement; (d) stricture following previous trauma or surgery; (e) severe urethritis; or (f) a perineal hernia where there is retroflexion of the bladder and/or prostate gland (Spreull & Frankland 1980).

There may be dysuria, haematuria and the dribbling of urine and blood. Catheterisation will not always establish the site of obstruction (a catheter may for example pass certain obstructions), and excretory urography and retrograde urethrography may be of more value (Fig. 15.17). Where possible, the cause should be removed and it may be necessary to insert an indwelling catheter until normal urination is possible, otherwise ARF may follow.

Prolapse of male urethra

This rare condition appears most likely to occur in Bulldogs usually following masturbation or excessive sexual arousal, but sometimes it is associated with straining due to urethral infection or obstruction. The penile urethral mucosa protrudes beyond the orifice and drips blood. Surgical reduction or amputation is required, together with tranquillisation and if necessary the use of oestrogen therapy.

TECHNIQUES OF VALUE IN THE DIAGNOSIS AND TREATMENT OF URINARY TRACT DISORDERS

Radiography

Radiographic information should be interpreted in conjunction with the clinical signs and laboratory evidence.

Survey radiography (i.e. without contrast media)
This should precede the use of contrast media. It is best performed 2 hours after an enema, with the bladder unemptied. Radiographs can detect gross abnormalities and altered density (e.g. radiopaque calculi).

In lateral recumbency the lower kidney moves cranially, so that in left lateral recumbency there is more superimposition although less of the cranial pole of the right kidney is hidden by the ribs; in right lateral recumbency the reverse is true. A ventrodorsal radiograph is preferable to a dorsoventral view because the kidneys are nearer to the film, which produces less distortion. In the absence of fat, or when masked by fluid, no kidney outline may be visible (Webbon 1979).

Excretory urography (syn. intravenous urography, descending urography or intravenous pyelography)
Radiopaque (positive) contrast medium is injected intravenously and after filtration by the kidney, passes down the ureter into the bladder.

Rapid injection and immediate radiography is termed nephrography, which gives maximum visualisation of the kidney. With normal kidneys the immediate radiopacity is good and then progressively decreases.

Excretory urography is used (a) to detect changes in location, size, outline and excretion of the kidneys (see Table 15.7 for details); (b) to detect abnormalities of the ureters, for example, rupture (following trauma) shown by leakage of contrast media, and obstruction (calculi and neoplasms), stricture, or abnormal siting of the distal end (ectopic ureters), all of which, plus

Table 15.7 Renal changes detectable with radiography.

Increased size (left kidney usually displaces descending colon ventrally)
Neoplasia
Hydronephrosis and pyonephrosis
Cysts
Renal ARF (i.e. AIN and ATN)
Amyloidosis
Hypertrophy with contralateral renal aplasia, hypoplasia or atrophy

Decreased size
Hypoplasia
'End-stage kidney' (i.e. CIN, chronic amyloidosis, chronic GN, chronic PN, and some familiae renal diseases)

Irregular outline
Neoplasia
Hydronephrosis
Cysts
'End-stage kidney' (see above)
Abscess

Abnormal location
Ectopia
Neoplasia
Pressure from an abdominal mass

Increased density
Renal calculus
Nephrocalcinosis (generalised renal calcification)

Decreased density
Neoplasia (especially lymphosarcoma)

Reduced, or no, excretion of contrast media
Urinary obstruction: calculus, neoplasm. Results in distended renal pelvis
   (May be elsewhere in urinary tract and may produce hydronephrosis)
Reduced GFR: prerenal ARF, and 'end-stage kidney' (see above)
Obstruction to renal artery
Low concentration in conditions producing polyuria

Progressively increasing opacity with contrast media
Acute renal failure

Irregular density with contrast media
Suggests neoplasia

Contrast media outside renal capsule
Trauma with capsular rupture

For functional changes in nephrograms see Feeney *et al* (1982)

any other cause of increased pressure, can produce an increased ureteral width (megaureter); (c) for the same purposes as positive contract cystography when a catheter is difficult to pass.

Specific gravity measurements on urine samples collected after the injection of contrast media are unreliable. In general values will be increased, although previously high values (>1.040) are more likely to be decreased.

Contrast cystography (retrograde contrast cystography)
The bladder is catheterised via the urethra, drained and filled with either air (Fig. 15.18), though occasion-

ally another gas (negative contrast cystography or pneumocystography), or radiopaque contrast media (positive contrast cystography).

Often both are performed in succession, pneumocystography first. Ideally contrast media should contain 300–400 mg iodine/ml, and be given at a dose rate of 2.2 ml/kg for a 25 kg dog; more for smaller breeds (up to 4 ml/kg) and less for larger. Avoid media containing sodium salts in suspected glomerulonephritis and congestive heart failure. In general films exposed immediately, and after 5, 20 and 40 minutes, will be of maximum value in diagnosis (Feeney *et al* 1979). Multiple excretory urograms can produce, at least temporarily, a reduction in GFR.

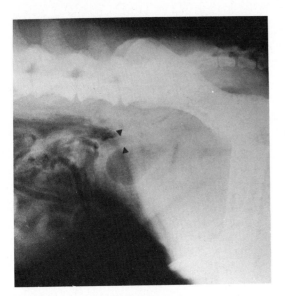

Fig. 15.18 Lateral pneumocystogram of a 2-year-old male Dalmatian taken with the animal lying on its left side. The small amount of air in the bladder has risen to the highest point, producing the erroneous impression that the bladder wall is of greatly increased thickness (as marked).

Bladder disorders which may be detected include radiolucent calculi (best seen using air as they may be obscured with dense radiopaque media), anatomical abnormalities (either congenital, e.g. diverticulum or patient urachus, or acquired, e.g. displacement or involvement in herniae), polyps, neoplasms, cystitis (with increased thickening of the bladder wall) and rupture (with leakage of contrast media).

A variant, micturating cystourethrography, is recommended for detection of vesicoureteral reflux. This involves allowing the positive contrast media to flow by gravity along a catheter into the previously emptied bladder of the anaesthetised patient and taking the radiograph as soon as spontaneous voiding occurs (i.e. when liquid flows from the urethra around the catheter).

Double contrast cystography (using both negative and positive contrast media) may clarify the appearance of suspected lesions.

Retrograde contrast urethrography

The distal end of the urethra is catheterised with a Foley catheter and its cuff inflated. Radiopaque contrast media is then injected and passes forwards. The technique is used to diagnose obstruction (e.g. calculi, enlargement of the prostate gland, congenital or acquired stricture), a diverticulum, urethrorectal fistula, periurethral abscess or neoplasm, or ectopic ureter in

a male. It is valuable where urethral damage is suspected following pelvic trauma. Reflux of the medium into the prostate gland may occur in any type of prostatic disorder (Stone *et al* 1978). Haematuria and/or UTI can arise from performing urethrography when the bladder is distended, even if only for a short period (Barsanti *et al* 1981).

Contrast vagino-urethrography (vaginography)

In the diagnosis of ectopic ureter(s) in a bitch the tip of a large Foley catheter is inserted into the vestibule and the cuff inflated. Then the radiopaque contrast medium is injected forwards. In large individuals it may be necessary to also close the vulval lips behind the cuff to prevent leakage of the contrast medium (Holt *et al* 1982). The technique is best performed in both right and left lateral recumbency, to ensure successful filling of an ectopic ureter, after first inflating the bladder with air to improve contrast in the region of the bladder neck.

Ultrasonography

Ultrasound has been found to be valuable in the diagnosis of HN, renal calculi and renal and bladder neoplasms in small animals (Cartee *et al* 1980). As well as being free from hazard to both the patient and operator, ultrasonography is better able to identify cystic structures and to distinguish dense masses within organs than is radiography, and contractile organs may be assessed without using a contrast medium. In cases of prostatic enlargement ultrasound is valuable in differentiating the possible causes.

Renal biopsy

This technique is used in the diagnosis of most renal diseases except prerenal and postrenal ARF, in which the kidneys are structurally normal and the conditions of renal abscess, pyonephrosis and hydronephrosis (although in these last-named conditions fluid can be withdrawn with a fine-gauge needle for bacterial culture and cytological examination).

Following fasting and general anaesthesia, a modified Franklin–Silvermann biopsy needle (Becton Dickinson) or Travenol 'TruCut' needle (Baxter-Travenol) is used to take a biopsy sample from the renal cortex without penetrating the renal pelvis. It can be performed through a very small opening (keyhole technique) or after laparotomy. Usually the former is preferred but the latter may be advisable in cases of suspected neoplasia so that intra-abdominal examination for evidence of neoplastic spread (invasion or metastases) can be made.

Excessive haemorrhage (e.g. from encountering arcuate vessels) is the only major complication although almost all patients show microscopic haematuria for up to 3 days afterwards. Renal biopsy has become a valuable diagnostic method though it should be pointed out that its value decreases in proportion to the length of time required to obtain a histopathological report.

Osmotic diuresis

This procedure is employed for the treatment of ATN (ARF) and the decompensated phase of CRF. The aim is to stimulate a diuresis using intravenous fluids which will also eliminate the excess of waste products in the blood. It is contraindicated in severe heart failure. Initially dehydration should be corrected with lactated Ringer's solution, and even animals without signs of dehydration should be given 40 ml/kg body weight. Then 20% dextrose solution is given at the rate of 40 ml/kg body weight; 2 ml/kg body weight per minute should be supplied for the first 15 minutes and then 1 ml/kg body weight per minute. Some authors have recommended using 20% mannitol solution but dextrose has the advantages of being cheaper and providing calories.

After weighing, the dog is catheterised to remove all residual bladder urine and the catheter is left in place to collect urine as it forms. Testing the urine with a glucose-sensitive strip will establish whether the dextrose is being eliminated. If after half the fluid has been given, urine is being produced at a rate of 1 ml or more per 10 kg body weight per minute the remainder of the fluid can be given. If not, fluid administration should cease to avoid overhydration, and frusemide should be given at a rate of 4 mg/kg body weight. If very little urine forms after 1 hour the dose of frusemide should be doubled, and if still insufficient urine forms, peritoneal dialysis is indicated as the only practicable way to reduce the high concentration of protein breakdown products.

Adequate urine production should be followed during the subsequent 24 hours by a further one or two infusions of the same volumes of lactated Ringer's solution and dextrose solution as initially employed.

The following day the dog should be weighed and its blood urea level redetermined. If it remains high, the entire procedure should be repeated. If the dog's body weight has increased, the initial administration of lactated Ringer's solution should be omitted and if it has fallen, an appropriate balancing volume of lactated Ringer's solution should be provided.

Potassium supplementation may also be required in cases of severe weakness where the blood potassium level has fallen to 3 mmol/l or less.

Intermittent peritoneal dialysis

Peritoneal dialysis is valuable in the treatment of ARF, the decompensated phase of CRF, and also in poisoning (where the toxic substance is dialysable) and over-hydration (using a fluid with a high glucose concentration). It is contraindicated in cases of peritonitis.

The principle of the technique is to use the peritoneum as a dialysing membrane. After the introduction of the dialysing fluid into the peritoneal cavity, toxic products diffuse across the peritoneum into the fluid, which can then be removed.

A site 2–3 inches behind the umbilicus and in, or a little to the right of, the midline (or alternatively in the right paralumbar fossa) is used to introduce sufficient prewarmed fluid to cause slight distension of the abdomen (400–2000 ml or more). The fluid is left *in situ* for 45–60 minutes and then removed. Commercial administration sets and peritoneal dialysis catheters are recommended as they greatly facilitate administration and, especially, removal. With the first dialysis some fluid may remain in the cavity (priming volume) but with subsequent dialysis all the fluid is recovered (i.e. the same volume is left behind each time).

Ready-sterilised commercial dialysis solutions are advocated, and the most commonly employed is an istonic solution of electrolytes containing approximately 1.4% dextrose. (When there is hyperkalaemia potassium-free solutions should be used.) Hypertonic solutions produced by the addition of more dextrose (up to 3.8%) are more efficient at removing toxic products but also withdraw larger quantities of water. Such solutions are contraindicated in the dehydrated patient, though their use can be combined with simultaneous intravenous fluid infusion.

Depending on the resultant fall in blood urea level the procedure will almost certainly need to be repeated during the same day and/or subsequent days. A soluble antibiotic should be introduced into the peritoneal cavity after each dialysis session and patients should receive increased amounts of water-soluble vitamins. Any weight loss detected by regular weighing should be made good with intravenous fluid.

Hydropropulsion

This procedure has been advocated for removing calculi lodged in the male urethra.

With the patient tranquillised or anaesthetised, digital pressure is applied through the ventral rectal wall on to the pelvic bone to occlude the urethral lumen at that point. Then through a bovine teat cannula inserted into the external urethral orifice, sterile water or saline is injected to distend the closed section of urethra (i.e. up to the point of occlusion).

Sudden removal of the cannula results in a forceful outflow of liquid often sufficient to bring calculi with it, although frequent repetition of the procedure may be required until all uroliths are removed. Alternatively, if the os penis proves an impassable obstacle the calculi can be moved back into the bladder by distending the urethra in the same manner and then suddenly releasing the pressure on the pelvic urethra.

ABBREVIATIONS IN THE TEXT

AIN: acute interstitial nephritis
ARF: acute renal failure
ATN: acute tubular necrosis
CAV-1: canine adenovirus 1 (the virus of infectious canine hepatitis)
CIN: chronic interstitial nephritis
CRF: chronic renal failure
DI: diabetes insipidus
ECG: electrocardiograph
FDP: fibrinogen–fibrin degradation products
GBM: glomerular basement membrane
GFR: glomerular filtration rate
GN: glomerulonephritis
HN: hydronephrosis
ICH: infectious canine hepatitis
IVP: intravenous pyelography
PN: pyelonephritis
RA: renal amyloidosis
SAP: serum alkaline phosphatase
UTI: urinary tract infection

Note
All the intravenous fluids mentioned in this chapter are obtainable from Travenol Laboratories Ltd., Thetford, Norfolk, with the exception of 10% calcium borogluconate solution. This may be prepared by dilution of the standard commercial 20% solution.

REFERENCES

BARBER D.L. & ROWLAND G.N. (1979) Radiographically detectable soft tissue calcification in chronic renal failure. *Vet. Radiol.* **20**, 117.

BARSANTI J.A., CROWELL W., LOSONSKY J. & TALKINGTON F.D. (1981) Complications of bladder distension during retrograde urethrography **42**, 819.

BIEWENGA W.J., GRUYS E. & GOUDSWAARD J. (1978) Quantitation of lysozyme in the urine of the dog for the diagnosis of proximal tubular damage in renal disease. *Tijdscht. Diergeneesk.* **103**, 1130.

BOVEE K.C., ABT D.A. & KRONFELD D.S. (1979a). The effects of dietary protein intake on renal function in dogs with experimentally reduced renal function. *J. Am. Anim. Hosp. Assoc.* **15**, 9.

BOVEE K.C., JOYCE T., BLAZER-YOST B., GOLDSCHMIDT M.S. & SEGAL S. (1979b) Characterisation of renal defects in dogs with a syndrome similar to the Fanconi syndrome in man. *J. Am. Vet. Med. Assoc.* **174**, 1094.

BOVEE K.C. & KRONFELD D.S. (1981) Reduction of renal hemodynamics in uremic dogs fed reduced protein diets. *J. Am. Anim. Hosp. Assoc.* **17**, 227.

BOWN P. (1979) Oedema in the dog. In *The Veterinary Annual 19th issue*, eds. C.S.G. Grunsell & F.W.G. Hill, p. 197. Scientechnica, Bristol.

CARTEE R.E., SELCER B.A. & PATTON C.S. (1980) Ultrasonographic diagnosis of renal disease in small animals. *J. Am. Vet. Med. Assoc.* **176**, 426.

CHEVILLE N.F. (1979) Uremic gastropathy in the dog. *Vet. Pathol.* **16**, 292.

EISENBRANDT D.L. & PHEMISTER R.D. (1979) Postnatal development of the canine kidney: quantitative and qualitative morphology. *Am. J. Anat.* **154**, 179.

ENGLISH P.B., FILIPPICH L.J. & THOMPSON H.L. (1980) Clinical assessment of renal function in the dog with a reduction in nephron number. *Aust. Vet. J.* **56**, 305.

FEENEY D.A., BARBER D.L. & OSBORNE C.A. (1982) The functional aspects of the nephrogram in excretory urography: a review. *Vet. Radiol.* **23**, 42.

FEENEY D.A., THRALL D.E., BARBER D.L., CULVER D.H. & LEWIS R.E. (1979) Normal canine excretory urogram: effects of dose, time, and individual dog variation. *Am. J. Vet. Res.* **40**, 1596.

FINCO D.R. & ROWLAND G.M. (1978) Hypercalcemia secondary to chronic renal failure in the dog: a report of four cases *J. Am. Vet. Med. Assoc.* **173**, 990.

HOLT P.E., GIBBS C. & PEARSON H. (1982) Canine ectopic ureter—a review of twenty-nine cases. *J. Small Anim. Pract.* **23**, 195.

KLAUSNER J.S., OSBORNE C.A., O'LEARY T.P., GEBHART R.N. & GRIFFITH D.P. (1980) Struvite urolithiasis in a litter of Miniature Schnauzer dogs. *Am. J. Vet. Res.* **41**, 712.

LENNOX J.S. (1978) A case report of unilateral ectopic ureter in a male Siberian Husky, *J. Am. Anim. Hosp. Assoc.* **14**, 331.

LING G.V. & RUBY A.L. (1979) Gentamicin for treatment of resistant urinary tract infections in dogs. *J. Am. Vet. Med. Assoc.* **175**, 480.

MACDOUGALL D.F. (1981) Assessment of renal function in the dog. *Vet. Rec.* **108**, 232.

MACDOUGALL, D.F., POWNALL R. & CRIGHTON G.W. (1977) A single catheter technique for haemodialysis in the dog. *Vet. Rec.* **100**, 200.

MCKENNA S.C. & CARPENTER J.L. (1980) Polycystic disease of the kidney and liver in the Cairn Terrier. *Vet. Pathol.* **17**, 436.

OSBORNE C.A. (1980) Glomerulonephropathy and the nephrotic syndrome. In *Current Veterinary Theory VII. Small animal practice.* ed. R.W. Kirk, p. 1053. W.B. Saunders, Philadelphia.

Osborne C.A., Klausner J.S., Krawiec D.R. & Griffith D.P. (1981) Canine struvite urolithiasis: problems and their dissolution. *J. Am. Vet. Med. Assoc.* **179**, 239.

Pechman R.D. (1982) Urinary trauma in dogs and cats: a review. *J. Am. Anim. Hosp. Assoc.* **18**, 33.

Riviere J.E. & Coppoc G.L. (1981) Dosage of antimicrobial drugs in patients with renal insufficiency. *J. Am. Vet. Med. Assoc.* **178**, 70.

Rosin A.E. & Barsanti J.A. (1981) Diagnosis of urinary incontinence in dogs: role of the urethral pressure profile. *J. Am. Vet. Med. Assoc.* **178**, 814.

Schmidt R.E., Hubbard G.B., Booker J.L. & Gleiser C.A. (1980) Dietary induction of renal mineralisation in dogs. *Can. J. Comp. Med.* **44**, 459.

Spreull J.S.A. & Frankland A.L. (1980) Transplanting the superficial gluteal muscle in the treatment of perineal hernia and flexure of the rectum in the dog. *J. Small Anim. Pract.* **21**, 265.

Steward A.P. & Macdougall D.F. (1981) Assay for fibrinogen-fibrin degradation products in canine urine. *Vet. Rec.* **109**, 179.

Stone E.A., Thrall D.E. & Barber D.L. (1978) Radiographic interpretation of prostatic disease in the dog. *J. Am. Anim. Hosp. Assoc.* **14**, 115.

Stone E.A., Rawlings C.A., Finco D.R. & Crowell W.A. (1981) Renal function after prolonged hypotensive anesthesia and surgery in dogs with reduced renal mass. *Am. J. Vet. Res.* **43**, 1675.

Webbon P.M. (1979) Radiology of the canine kidney. In *The Veterinary Annual 19th issue*, eds. C.S.G. Grunsell & F.W.G. Hill, p. 144. Scientechnica, Bristol.

Weller R.E., Wolf A.M. & Oyejide A. (1979) Transitional cell carcinoma of the bladder associated with cyclophosphamide therapy in a dog. *J. Am. Anim. Hosp. Assoc.* **15**, 733.

Wilcock B.P. & Patterson J.M. (1979) Familial glomerulonephritis in Doberman Pinscher dogs. *Can. Vet. J.* **20**, 244.

Wolf A.M. (1980) Canine uremic encephalopathy. *J. Am. Anim. Hosp. Assoc.* **16**, 735.

Wright N.G., Nash A.S., Thompson H. & Fisher E.W. (1981) Membranous nephropathy in the cat and dog. *Lab. Invest.* **45**, 275.

Yu T-F, Gutman A.B., Berger L. & Kaung C. (1971) Low uricase activity in the Dalmatian dog simulated in mongrels given oxonic acid. *Am. J. Physiol.* **220**, 973.

FURTHER READING

General

Ettinger S.J. (ed.) (1982) *Textbook of Veterinary Internal Medicine: diseases of the dog and cat.* Vol. 2, Section XIII. Diseases of the Urinary System, p. 1732. W.B. Saunders, Philadelphia.

Finco D.R., Thrall D.E. & Duncan J.R. (1979) Chapter 9, The Urinary System. In *Canine Medicine*, 4th ed. Vol. 1. Ed. Catcott, E.J. p. 419. Am. Vet. Publications, Santa Barbara.

Leaf A. & Cortan R. (1976) *Renal Pathophysiology.* Oxford University Press, New York.

Osborne C.A. (consult. ed.) (1980) In *Current Veterinary Therapy VII, Small animal practice*, ed. R.W. Kirk. Section 12: Genitourinary disorders, p. 1040. W.B. Saunders, Philadelphia.

Osborne C.A., Low D.G. & Finco D.R. (1972) *Canine and Feline Urology.* W.B. Saunders, Philadelphia.

Renal disease

Grunsell, C.S.G. & Hill F.W.G. (eds.) (1979) *The Veterinary Annual, 19th issue*, pp. 133–177, various authors. Scientechnicia, Bristol.

Morrison W.I. & Wright N.G. (1976) Immunopathological aspects of canine renal disease. *J. Small Anim. Pract.* **17**, 139.

Osborne C.A., Hammer R.F., Stevens J.B., O'Leary T.P. & Resnick J.S. (1976) Immunologic aspects of glomerular disease in the dog and cat. In *Proc. 26th Gaines Veterinary Symposium*, Columbus, Ohio, p. 15. Gaines Dog Research Center, White Plains, New York.

Diet

Osborne C.A. (1974) Dietary restriction in the treatment of primary renal failure: facts and fallacies. *J. Am. Anim. Hosp. Assoc.* **10**, 73.

Lower Urinary Tract

Burrows C.F. & Bovée K.C. (1974) Metabolic changes due to experimentally induced rupture of the canine urinary bladder. *Am. J. Vet. Res.* **35**, 1083.

Bush B.M. (1976) A review of the aetiology and consequences of urinary tract infections in the dog. *Br. Vet. J.* **132**, 632.

Osborne C.A. & Klausner J.S., (eds.) (1979) Symposium on urinary tract infections. *Vet. Clinics N. Am. Small Anim. Pract.* **9**, 585.

Pearson H. & Gibbs C. (1971) Urinary tract abnormalities in the dog. *J. Small Anim. Pract.* **12**, 67.

Radiography of the Urinary Tract

Kneller S.K. (1974) Role of the excretory urogram in the diagnosis of renal and ureteral disease. *Vet. Clinics N. Amer.* **4**, 843.

Lord P.F., Scott R.C. & Chan K.G. (1974) Intravenous urography for evaluation of renal diseases in small animals. *J. Am. Anim. Hosp. Assoc.* **10**, 139.

Park R.D. (1974) Radiographic contrast studies of the lower urinary tract. *Vet. Clinics N. Am.* **4**, 863.

16
Genital System

W. EDWARD ALLEN, DAVID E. NOAKES
AND JEAN P. RENTON

This chapter is concerned with diseases of the genital system in the dog and bitch. The main emphasis is placed on diagnosis and non-surgical treatment. Details of surgical techniques are not given and there is no reference to dystocia or its correction.

THE MALE

Clinical examination

A careful examination of the genital system of the male dog is important particularly in the puppy and also in the adult male where there is a history suggesting a genito-urinary disorder or infertility. The clinical examination is mainly dependent upon palpation and visual examination; supportive diagnostic procedures such as radiography, haematology, bacteriology and semen evaluation are useful in establishing a firm diagnosis. It is important to stress that the assay of reproductive hormones is of limited value, particularly if performed on a single sample, since there are large variations in normal values both within, and between, the individual animals.

Testes and scrotum

The scrotum of the dog is soft and thin walled. The testis is oval in shape, firm but not hard on palpation. There is considerable variation in the size of the testes in different breeds. The average dimensions are $3 \times 2 \times 1.5$ cm, with an average weight of 11 g; the testes are normally of similar size in an individual dog.

The longitudinal axis is almost horizontal in the normally descended testis with the epididymis closely attached to the dorsolateral surface. The tail of the epididymis is normally palpable as a firm, but not hard, nodule on the caudal pole of each testis. Occasionally the testes appear to be positioned in tandem, especially in the greyhound, but the normal position is readily established on palpation.

Penis and prepuce

The penis can be readily examined by digital retraction of the prepuce. The integument is smooth, pink and moist. The glans penis consists of two parts, the distal *pars longa glandis* which is 5–6 cm in length, and the thicker, proximal *bulbus glandis*. Palpation of the *os penis* is usually possible in the non-erect penis.

The prepuce should be soft, mobile and the preputial orifice large enough to allow protrusion of the non-erect penis.

Internal genitalia

The dog has no vesicular or bulbo-urethral glands, but the prostate is relatively large and well developed and is an important site of disease. The prostate gland can be palpated per rectum using the middle or index finger suitably protected with a glove or finger cot. It is bilobed and situated at the junction of the neck of the bladder and urethra. The ease of palpation depends upon (a) the length of finger, (b) the size of the dog, and (c) the condition of the prostate. Before puberty the prostate is a pelvic organ, but as the dog becomes older it increases in size and becomes more abdominal, so that after the age of 10 years it can be considered to be an abdominal organ. Even when it is enlarged because of disease it is frequently difficult to palpate, but this can be overcome by applying pressure to the posterior abdomen in order to force the gland back into the pelvic cavity. Radiography is a useful diagnostic aid. In the majority of cases considerable enlargement with forward displacement is necessary before it can be recognised. A barium enema may help to identify the enlarged prostate causing compression of the rectum, whilst a pneumocystogram or the use of other contrast material may also improve identification of the enlarged gland.

Prostatic gland biopsy has been used to identify precisely the cause of prostatic disease. Aspiration and punch biopsy has been used via the transperineal approach; the technique is difficult to perform and can result in trauma to other organs. Perhaps the most reliable method is the wedge biopsy technique, which is performed via a posterior laparotomy where the prostate can be inspected visually.

Testicular abnormalities

The testes of the dog may be the primary site of disease, *viz.* cryptorchidism, orchitis, neoplasia, or be involved secondarily *viz.* Cushing's disease (see Chapter 6). The testes have a dual function, so that disease can be demonstrated in two ways—it can affect the production of testosterone by the interstitial cells, or the generation of spermatozoa.

Cryptorchidism
The testes of the dog are intra-abdominal at birth but normally descend soon afterwards (7–10 days). In some puppies it may be possible to palpate them in the scrotum or inguinal region at 2 weeks of age, but the presence of scrotal fat makes this difficult. It should be possible to palpate the testes at 6–8 weeks of age, although it may be necessary to wait until the dog reaches puberty (5–12 months of age) before a definite diagnosis of cryptorchidism can be made; puberty occurs earlier in small breeds of dog.

A cryptorchid is an animal with one or both testes retained somewhere along the normal path of descent. Retention is usually classified as inguinal or abdominal according to whether the testis is outside or inside the deep (internal) inguinal ring. Inguinal testes usually lie cranial to the scrotum alongside the penis, whilst abdominal testes lie close to the deep inguinal ring. An ectopic testis is one which has deviated from the normal pathway of descent, usually after passing through the deep inguinal ring; ectopic testes are rare in the dog. A monorchid is an animal with only one testis. The term should not be applied to an animal with only one scrotal testis. As true monorchidism is extremely rare, an animal with only one scrotal testis must be presumed to have the second testis retained, and is thus a unilateral cryptorchid. An anorchid is an animal in which neither testis has ever developed. Anorchidism is also extremely rare, and an animal with no history of castration and no scrotal testes must be presumed to have two retained testes and is thus a bilateral cryptorchid.

Incidence
The reported incidence of cryptorchidism varies between 0.05 and 6.33%, but may be as high as 12.9% in dogs examined under 6 months of age.

Aetiology
The reason for failure of descent is obscure, but it is likely that endocrine and mechanical abnormalities are involved. Most investigators agree that the condition is inherited, so that cryptorchid dogs should not be used for breeding.

Clinical significance
There are two important conditions which are associated with retained testes. First, an increased risk of neoplasia and second, a predisposition to torsion of the spermatic cord. These will be described in greater detail below.

Abdominal testes are aspermic, so that dogs with both testes retained are sterile, but will have normal libido and secondary sex characteristics. In unilateral retention the descended testis functions normally and the dog is likely to be fertile.

Treatment
Since there is a high probability that cryptorchidism is inherited, treatment which might induce descent should be discouraged. Testosterone and human chorionic gonadotrophin (hCG) have been used to try to induce testicular descent; apparent success probably occurs in those dogs which have inguinal testes in which descent would have occurred irrespective of treatment. The technique of orchipexy has been described with little proven success.

Any retained testis should be removed surgically as soon after puberty as possible to avoid the chances of neoplasia described below.

Testicular neoplasia
Three types of testicular tumour have been described and have been classified accordingly to the main cell type involved, i.e. Sertoli cell, interstitial cell and seminomas. Neoplasia of the testes is relatively frequent and is closely related to failure of normal gonadal descent. The relative risk of Sertoli cell tumours is 23 times, and of seminomas is 16 times, greater in retained compared with descended testes. Furthermore neoplasia is twice as common in inguinal compared with abdominal testes.

Interstitial cell tumour
This is the commonest type of tumour recorded in old dogs. Frequently it causes no change in testicular size, and is rarely diagnosed: the only readily identified change is that affected testicles become hard. It rarely occurs in retained testes, is not malignant, and is generally endocrinologically inactive, although sometimes androgens are produced which result in the development of perineal tumours and prostatic hyperplasia.

Seminoma

This tumour occurs in middle aged and old dogs. The main characteristic is marked testicular enlargement which is painless and usually unilateral. Commonly it is endocrinologically inactive, although there are reports of oestradiol production; metastases occur occasionally, especially from abdominal testes.

Sertoli cell tumour

This usually occurs in middle aged and old dogs. The testis can be enlarged, firm and non-resilient, but on occasions there is no change in size. This tumour generally produces oestrogen, especially when intra-abdominal, and as a consequence there are signs of feminisation. This hormone causes gynaecomasty, pendulous sheath, penile and preputial atrophy, atrophy of the other testis if it is a unilateral lesion, prostatic enlargement (metaplasia) and bilateral symmetrical alopecia. Metastases are quite common and the dog is attractive to males.

Treatment

In all cases of testicular neoplasia the only treatment is castration. Since the condition is frequently reported in retained testes it emphasises the need to remove these gonads before the dog reaches middle age at the very latest. Frequently, and especially with Sertoli cell tumours and seminomas, both testes are involved even though there may not be obvious clinical signs.

Torsion of the spermatic cord (*testicular torsion*)

Torsion of the spermatic cord occurs rarely in the dog, but it is most frequently reported in retained or ectopic testes probably due to instability of the suspension of the gonad in allowing rotation. Torsion may also be associated with neoplastic enlargement of the testis. There does not appear to be any predisposition to side, and although the Boxer, Pekingese and Airedale Terrier have been most frequently identified with the condition, the numbers involved preclude any interpretation of a breed susceptibility.

Clinical signs

These are dependent upon the site of the affected testis. There is usually the sudden onset of pain with a reluctance to move. The dog will be anorexic, will vomit and the gait will be stiff and abnormal. If the condition occurs in a descended testis then the scrotum will be swollen, oedematous and painful. Lethargy, dysuria and abdominal pain are sometimes seen.

Treatment

Orchidectomy should be performed as soon as pos-

sible, but fatalities may occur. The degree of torsion ranges from 360° to 720°.

Orchitis

Inflammation of one or both testes and associated epididymis is not a common condition in the dog; infection can result from trauma or haematogenous spread. The raised temperature of the testis can temporarily affect spermatogenesis, but if it is allowed to remain untreated it can result in testicular degeneration.

Clinical signs usually are a stiff gait, and scrotal and testicular enlargement which is very painful and has to be differentiated from torsion of the spermatic cord. Treatment consists of systemic antibiosis.

Congenital defects

Congenital defects can be slight, involving one part of one organ, or severe, involving the whole genital system.

Aplasia of the epididymis and vas deferens

Only two cases of this condition have been described, one bilateral and the other unilateral. However it is likely to be more common and probably escapes detection at clinical examination, demonstrating the need to carefully palpate the scrotal sac and testes. If it is bilateral the dog will be sterile.

Hypospadia

This describes the abnormality where the urethra does not open at the tip of the glans penis but ventrally and posterior to the tip. The condition can be slight with opening occurring a few centimetres from the tip (glandular hypospadia) which is the most frequently reported site. However more severe forms have been described with the urethra opening at the *pars longa glandis* (penile hypospadia), at the scrotum (scrotal hypospadia) or sub-ischially (perineal hypospadia).

Glandular hypospadia requires no treatment. Successfully surgical repair at the other three sites is difficult because the urethra distal to the opening is rarely patent.

Persistent frenulum

This is a rare condition in which a narrow band of tissue extends along the ventral raphé of the penis from the preputial reflection to a point close to the penile tip. It causes ventral deviation of the protruded penis; correction is surgical.

Intersex

Intersexuality refers to a group of congenital abnormalities which are demonstrated by variations in the degree of sexual differentiation of the genital system. Although the condition is uncommon in the dog its occurrence can cause considerable dismay in breeders and disappointment for the owners of a new puppy.

The condition can be classified according to the type of gonadal tissue that is present. A true hermaphrodite has both ovarian and testicular tissue, either as a combined structure (ovotestis) or as separate gonads; externally the genitalia is atypical to both sexes. Pseudohermaphrodites may be either male or female. Male pseudohermaphrodites have testes with male and/or female internal and external genitalia. Female pseudohermaphrodites have ovaries with female and/or male internal or external genitalia. There is considerable variation in the sexual genotype and degree of differentiation of the genital system.

Diagnosis
In some cases diagnosis is straightforward, even in a young puppy, where sexing of the individual is difficult because of the position of the urogenital opening. However in others it is less obvious until the dog approaches puberty. In these cases the owner will have noted the presence of a small, poorly developed prepuce and rudimentary scrotum with no testes in what had been assumed to be a male. Conversely a supposedly normal bitch is observed to have a vulva situated more ventrally than normal with an enlarged clitoris which protrudes from the vulva and becomes traumatised when the bitch sits. Absence of oestrus and incontinence have also been reported.

Aetiology
Differentiation of the gonads occurs at the 33rd day of gestation in the dog and subsequent differentiation of the tubular genital tract is under the control of the fetal gonads. Therefore the development of intersexes occurs within the first half of gestation. The cause of the condition is generally unknown, although there is good evidence that it is genetically linked in some breeds such as the Kerry Blue, Cocker Spaniel, Dobermann and English Setter.

Intersexes can arise in puppies following the administration of hormones, especially androgens and progestagens, to the bitch during pregnancy.

Treatment
This can only be cosmetic so that the dog is more acceptable to its owner. Gonadectomy is indicated, especially if the testes are retained. Surgical reconstruction of the vulva/prepuce may be necessary and in some female pseudohermaphrodites amputation of the phallus may be indicated.

Abnormalities of the prostate gland

The prostate gland is the only accessory sex gland in the dog. Prostatic disease is quite common and should always be considered whenever a dog is presented for examination with a history of suspected urinary or intestinal disease. Perhaps one reason for the frequent occurrence of prostatic disease may be its direct blood supply from the testes via the deferential vessels which subject it to higher levels of androgens than occur in the peripheral circulation. There is some suggestion that the high rate of conversion of testosterone to dihydrotestosterone within the prostate may be important in the pathogenesis of disease.

Eight types of prostatic disease have been described: hyperplasia, metaplasia, prostatitis, prostatic tumours, cysts, abscesses, calculi and atrophy, the latter producing no clinical signs. In many cases several disease conditions occur together, particularly hyperplasia and infectious conditions. Prostatic hyperplasia is probably the commonest prostatic lesion causing symptomatic disease.

Prostatic hyperplasia and metaplasia
The prostate gland undergoes three distinct phases of activity during the life of the dog. In the young adult dog (1–5 years of age) there is normal growth, in middle age (6–10 years of age) hyperplasia occurs and in old age (11 years plus) there is senile atrophy. It has been recognised for some time that hyperplasia is a normal occurrence in middle-aged dogs and that usually there are no clinical manifestations of disease. This is because enlargement of the gland occurs outwards and therefore it is unlikely to affect the urethra, and only in severe cases does it affect the rectum. The prostate gland is normally 2.5–3 cm in diameter and it may be twice this size in cases of hyperplasia. Oestrogen-producing Sertoli cell tumours, if not removed, cause prostatic enlargement due to squamous metaplasia. A similar condition can also occur as a consequence of prolonged treatment with exogenous oestrogens, especially at high dose rates.

Clinical signs
Constipation with frequent attempts to defaecate, production of ribbon-like faeces and haematuria are commonly seen. In some cases there may be dysuria, stiffness of hind limbs and partial paraplegia. A common sequel to hyperplasia, especially in docked breeds, is the development of a perineal hernia with its attendant complications. Secondary prostatitis is a frequent sequel in which the clinical signs are intensified.

Diagnosis
This is made on the history and rectal palpation to

demonstrate an enlarged and usually painless prostate gland (there will be pain if there is a secondary prostatitis). In severe cases the gland may be palpated through the posterior abdominal wall. Catheterisation of the urethra and bladder is not impeded.

Radiography will show a large, spherical mass just cranial to the pelvic inlet.

Treatment
Cases can be treated medically with steroid hormones or surgically by castration or prostatectomy, although results from the latter technique, which is difficult, are disappointing.

Oestrogens and progestagens work indirectly by having a negative feedback effect upon the anterior pituitary gland, thus reducing testosterone production by the testes. Oestradiol benzoate at a dose rate of 1 mg per day or 5 mg per week intramuscularly or subcutaneously for 4 consecutive weeks followed by monthly treatment is effective. Alternatively ethinyl oestradiol orally at 50–100 μg/day can be used. If signs of feminisation occur, treatment should be stopped, and recommenced at half the original dose rate when signs have disappeared. Due to the likelihood of squamous metaplasia developing, castration is recommended in dogs which are not too old to undergo surgery.

Delmadinone acetate (Tardak) by intramuscular or subcutaneous injection at a dose rate of 1–3 mg/kg has proved effective, although repeated injections are necessary.

In all cases of medical treatment the size of the gland should be checked at frequent intervals after the clinical signs have disappeared so that stabilisation can be achieved.

Prostatitis
Prostatitis can be either acute or chronic, and can occur alone or associated with hyperplasia or metaplasia of the gland. The chronic form of the disease may result from partial resolution of acute prostatitis or else it may remain undiagnosed, or misdiagnosed as simple hyperplasia.

Prostatitis most frequently arises from an ascending infection from the urinary tract, although the possibility of haematogenous spread cannot be excluded. The organisms most frequently isolated are E. *coli*, Proteus spp., Pseudomonas spp., Staphylococci and Streptococci.

Acute prostatitis

Clinical signs. The condition can occur in the sexually mature dog of any age. The dog will be presented with a history of inappetence, thirst, lethargy, occasional vomiting, reluctance to move, arched back, preputial discharge, dysuria, tenesmus and haematuria. The dog will be pyrexic, and resent abdominal palpation especially towards the pelvis. Rectal palpation will show an evenly enlarged, firm and very painful prostate gland, the sulcus is usually not identifiable. This may have to be carried out under general anaesthesia.

Diagnosis. This will be made following the clinical history and initial examination. Haematological examination will reveal a leucocytosis and neutrophilia, and urine examination will show the presence of large numbers of erythrocytes and neutrophils. Bacteriological culture may demonstrate the causal organism, although it is necessary to differentiate the condition from a cystitis.

Radiography is not particularly helpful in confirming a diagnosis; it will demonstrate an enlarged prostate gland.

Treatment. High doses of antibacterial drugs are indicated for up to ten days after the clinical signs of disease have disappeared. Some attempt should be made to perform sensitivity tests on bacterial cultures obtained from urine or an ejaculate. Many antibiotics do not readily cross the lipid membrane of the prostatic epithelium, so that they do not reach adequate therapeutic levels in the gland. However some substances do, notably trimethoprim, erythromycin and possibly metronidazole.

Chronic prostatitis

Clinical signs. Recurrent haematuria, dysuria and tenesmus are typical signs. The dog will be afebrile and on rectal palpation the prostate may be slightly enlarged or small and indurated; it may or may not be painful. Some dogs show signs of recurrent anal pruritus.

Diagnosis. This will be made on the clinical history and signs; there may be a slight leucocytosis. Differentiation from cystitis or cystic calculi must be made; in some cases a concurrent cystitis may be present. Although there is frequently evidence of urinary obstruction with chronic prostatitis, because of fibrosis at the level of the prostatic urethra, the passage of the urethral catheter presents no problems.

Treatment. Treatment with the chemotherapy described above for the acute disease for a period of up to 10 days is required. If there is no response, castration or oestrogen therapy may be used.

Prostatic tumours

Prostatic neoplasia is quite common in dogs over 10 years of age, but rare in young dogs. The commonest tumour is the adenocarcinoma; squamous metaplasia is not a pre-neoplastic change.

Clinical signs

The clinical signs are similar to those described above for hyperplasia although they are usually more severe; early lesions are frequently assumed to be hyperplastic. The dog shows signs of constipation with tenesmus, haematuria, dysuria and in advanced cases partial paraplegia because of metastasis involving adjacent tissues. Secondary lesions elsewhere in the body can also result in clinical signs.

Diagnosis

This will be based upon the clinical signs but it will be necessary to exclude benign hyperplasia. Prostatic tumours should be considered when (a) the prostate is painful on palpation yet the dog shows no other signs of prostatitis, (b) the prostate is adherent to adjacent structures, (c) there is dysuria. Confirmation may be made by identifying tumour cells in the urine or urethral washings. Plain, lateral radiographs may show an enlarged gland, with irregular outline which may also be more apparent following retrograde urethrography.

A final diagnosis can only be made following the histological examination of a wedge biopsy.

Treatment

Oestrogen therapy or castration may result in temporary improvement, whilst prostatectomy might be worthwhile if metastases have not occurred. In general the prognosis is poor; in all cases the dog should be examined for the presence of secondary lesions especially in the liver, spleen, lungs and lumbar–sacral skeleton and musculature.

Prostatic cysts

These are not common. They arise either as a consequence of occlusion of the prostatic ducts, so that secretion accumulates, or from the vestiges of the Mullerian duct system; the latter condition occurs as a result of oestrogen stimulation.

Clinical signs

Small cysts do not result in clinical signs. However when they are large they cause constipation, tenesmus, haematuria and dysuria.

Diagnosis

The history is very similar to that associated with hyperplasia and can usually be differentiated from a prostatic abscess by the absence of systemic signs, especially pyrexia. Radiography, especially using contrast material in the bladder, is helpful in diagnosis since the distended bladder can readily be confused with a cyst. Rectal palpation is frequently of no value unless the cyst is very large and extends parallel to the rectum. Aspiration of fluid may be useful.

Treatment

Oestrogen therapy and castration are of no value. Simple aspiration results in temporary improvement and surgical excision is usually difficult. The best results have been obtained following the insertion of a drainage tube or marsupialisation.

Prostatic abscesses

These usually result from an untreated acute prostatitis or following treatment where chemotherapy was used for too short a period. They sometimes accompany prostatic neoplasia.

Clinical signs

These are similar to those described for hyperplasia and prostatic cysts, although the dog is frequently pyrexic. Dysuria and haematuria, especially with blood being passed at the end of urination, is almost pathognomonic. The dog frequently remains in the normal stance for urination after it is complete.

Diagnosis

This is based on the history and clinical signs; there is usually a leucocytosis. Urine samples usually show leucocytes and erythrocytes in centrifuged deposits. Rectal palpation will identify a painfully enlarged gland which is usually asymmetrical. Radiography is useful but it may be necessary to use paracentesis and aspiration as a means of differentiating the structure from a cyst. Sometimes the abscess will burst causing a peritonitis.

Treatment

Parenteral antibiotics and oestrogen therapy can be tried but they are rarely effective. Similarly aspiration and simple drainage are not often effective. Techniques of marsupialisation and the use of multiple drainage tubes have been described.

Prostatic calculi

These are rarely encountered and arise either from the gland secretions or within the urinary tract. The clinical signs are similar to those described for other diseases of the prostate gland, especially dysuria and enlargement. Radiography is invaluable in diagnosis although care must be taken to differentiate urethral calculi. Associated prostatitis can be treated with chemotherapy although complete resolution of the condition can only be achieved following surgical removal.

Prostatic atrophy

This occurs in dogs over 11 years old as a result of ageing. It produces no clinical signs.

Abnormalities of the penis and prepuce

Transmissible venereal tumour

This tumour occurs mainly on the external genitalia of both dogs and bitches. The disease is rare in Britain and is most likely to be seen in dogs in quarantine. Over the years there have been isolated reports of the disease in particular areas. It is very common worldwide, especially in tropical and subtropical climates where there are large numbers of stray and wild dogs.

The disease, which is probably of viral origin, is spread at coitus, although there are also reports of its transmission to cutaneous sites following the contamination of bites and scratches. Younger, healthier individuals tend to be more resistant to experimental transmission than older individuals.

Clinical signs

The history of a blood-stained preputial discharge should encourage the clinician to retract the prepuce so that the surface of the penis can be examined. The lesion usually appears as a pinkish-red, nodular non-encapsulated mass, measuring up to 15 mm in diameter. Rarely metastases may involve the inguinal lymph nodes.

Cutaneous lesions have been described in dogs that are in poor health. The lesions involve the skin and subcutaneous regions and consist of raised areas up to 6 cm in diameter over the back, flank, neck and limbs.

Diagnosis

This is based on the appearance of the lesion on the glans penis. When they are small the initial sign may only be the presence of a blood-stained preputial discharge, especially after mating. In the early stages there is rarely a purulent discharge, but as the disease progresses there is necrosis and ulceration of the tumour and subsequent infection. A biopsy of the tumour mass may be taken to confirm the diagnosis.

Treatment

Since the dog will develop an immunity, and provided that it is in good health, the tumour will regress spon-

taneously in about 6 months. Surgical excision and cryosurgery have proved successful.

Balanoposthitis

This describes inflammation of the penile integument and preputial lining and is quite a common condition. Young male dogs, around the age of puberty, frequently develop a preputial discharge which, apart from the inconvenience to the owner, has no effect on the dog. All entire male dogs have some degree of preputial discharge, which although it contains neutrophils is not associated with signs of inflammation. It is often difficult to decide what degree of discharge is abnormal.

Clinical signs

There is usually a history of a preputial discharge which is purulent or slightly blood-stained. The dog will frequently lick and bite the prepuce and there may be evidence of self-inflicted trauma. He may resent palpation of the prepuce and exposure of the penis. There is rarely any systemic involvement. Exposure of the glans penis shows a red and inflamed integument with small raised nodules and in severe cases there may be ulceration.

Diagnosis

This is based on the clinical signs, especially on the appearance of the glans penis and preputial lining. Bacterial culture of the discharge or preputial swabs is of limited value. There is an extensive and varied bacterial flora on the surface of the penis and preputial lining. *Staphylococcus aureus* and mycoplasmata are most frequently isolated although a large number of other bacterial species have also been isolated in mixed aerobic cultures. The isolation of Proteus spp. and Pseudomonas spp. in pure or near pure cultures may well be significant.

Treatment

In many cases, especially in the young dog, treatment is unnecessary. Broad spectrum parenteral antibiotics coupled with local application should be tried. If antiseptic washes are used care must be taken to use them at the recommended dilutions since in many cases concentrated solutions are irritant. Saline irrigation may also be tried as an alternative. Progestagens may be given in an attempt to reduce sexual self-interest.

Dog pox

This is the name given to an eruptive condition of the mucous membranes of dogs and bitches, probably caused by a canine herpes virus. The infection can occur in the colon and the recto-anal area as well as the penis of the dog and the vestibule of the bitch.

The lesions are small papules which may be present as scattered discrete eruptions or, if numerous and almost contiguous, as a moist granular mass. Individual lesions may appear haemorrhagic (although actual haemorrhage is rare) or they may glisten like vesicles (although true vesicles are unusual). In over 90% of cases the lesions are asymptomatic, but they may, however, be associated with abnormal preputial discharge and irritation (see above). The signs may be as vague as the dog turning round suddenly to nibble in a random manner at the hindquarters, hindlegs and inside of the thighs.

Treatment
When required, treatment is instillation of antibiotics into the sheath and gentle massage towards the penile root. Cautery may render the lesions less 'active' (2–5% silver nitrate washed off with saline immediately appears effective). Although venereal transmission to bitches can take place, this appears to be a relatively uncommon method of spread.

Phimosis
This is the condition where, because of an abnormally small preputial opening, the dog is unable to protrude the partially erect penis. As a consequence erection may occur within the prepuce, causing discomfort and may ultimately result in a balanoposthitis. If severe the dog may dribble urine which has accumulated in the prepuce. The condition is usually congenital and can be corrected by surgical enlargement of the preputial opening.

Paraphimosis
This occurs when the erect or partially erect penis has protruded from the prepuce, but the preputial orifice is restricted and acts as a tourniquet, thus preventing detumescence and return to the prepuce. It is most likely to be seen in young dogs and perhaps after coitus. It is sometimes difficult to differentiate this from persistent erection (priapism) which is probably due to some neurological or circulatory defect.

As well as causing embarrassment to owners it causes discomfort to the dog and if left untreated can result in severe trauma to the penis. Tranquillisers, cold compresses and attempted manual replacement may be successful. However in some cases replacement under general anaesthesia, with adequate lubrication to the glans penis, may be necessary.

If the condition is persistent it may be necessary to surgically enlarge the preputial orifice.

Hypersexuality

Young dog puppies, before the age of puberty, will frequently mount dogs of either sex or inanimate objects and show copulatory and thrusting movements. In most cases after the age of puberty and certainly when maturity is reached aberrant sexual behaviour disappears. However some dogs show evidence of hypersexuality after this time, which, if it cannot be controlled by training, requires treatment.

Hypersexuality is shown by persistent mounting of people and objects, roaming, aggression to other dogs and, especially when a bitch is in pro-oestrus or oestrus within the immediate area, territorial marking.

Treatment
The methods of treatment of hypersexuality in the male dog are contentious, with veterinarians tending to have rather fixed views. The authors make no apology for expressing theirs since in the absence of any clearly defined study it is only possible to quote clinical impressions.

In some cases firm discipline, adequate exercise and training will be sufficient. However if this fails, or there is insufficient time, hormone therapy should be implemented. Progestagens are generally effective in temporarily suppressing libido by exerting a negative feedback on the anterior pituitary, thus inhibiting gonadotrophin release and hence testosterone production from the testes. Delmadinone acetate suspension (Tardak) at a dose rate of 1.0 to 2.0 mg/kg body weight by injection is usually effective. However the response is rarely long lasting and it is usually necessary to repeat the injection every 3 to 4 weeks. Megestrol acetate (Ovarid) orally has also been used effectively.

In many cases castration will be very effective and permanent. There are some failures, but it is likely that these dogs would not respond to any other treatment. Criticisms are levelled at the procedure because it may result in obesity, lethargy and loss of male characteristics. The first can effectively be controlled by careful feeding and regular recording of body weight, the second is largely a reflection of the dog's environment, whilst the third is, in the authors' opinion, the lesser of two evils if it eliminates the undesirable facets of male behaviour. Finally, and also equally important, the dog is rendered sterile, which must reduce the likelihood of unplanned matings and unwanted puppies.

Where there is doubt that the unsocial behaviour is related to hypersexuality, then it may be desirable to determine the response of the dog to delmadinone acetate therapy before recommending castration.

Aggression towards people is rarely reduced by castration.

Infertility

The male dog is no more or less fertile than males of other domestic species. Whenever a number of bitches, particularly if they are proven, fail to conceive to a particular dog it is necessary to examine him to at least eliminate him as the cause of the problem.

It is important to obtain a reliable and detailed history of his health and the results of previous matings; the fertility of closely related males may also be useful. The dog must then be observed in the presence of a receptive bitch in oestrus and allowed to mate if he is able to do so; the importance of a quiet and undisturbed environment cannot be overemphasised for this procedure. The external and internal genitalia must be carefully examined and finally a semen sample collected and evaluated.

Normal reproductive function

The age of puberty varies from 6 to 12 months with the smaller breeds being most precocious. At two months of age puppies frequently display penile erection, and from four months onwards some male puppies will be capable of copulation but will not seek out and find a bitch in oestrus.

The age at which the first sperm-containing ejaculate is produced has been shown to be about 33 weeks in the Beagle dog. The quantity and quality of the ejaculate is very poor. A further 10–11 weeks elapse before libido and semen quality reach that observed in mature dogs. There is evidence that a dog's genotype can influence the age at which puberty occurs; line-bred collies are more precocious than out-crossed individuals.

Once spermatogenesis has commenced it will continue uninterrupted until the dog reaches old age. There is some evidence that sperm quality varies with the season of the year, but this is only slight, and there is no evidence of an effect upon fertility.

Causes of infertility

Traditionally infertility can be considered under three headings: (1) the absence of, or reduced, libido, (2) in the presence of normal libido, the inability to copulate, and (3) normal libido and ability to copulate but reduced, or complete absence of, capacity to fertilise.

Reduced or no libido

This is not usually a major problem, but since the stimulus of sexual desire is complex it can sometimes be influenced by an adverse environment, a dominant bitch rejecting forcibly the attentions of a young dog, and conditioning. It is rarely an endocrinological problem.

A suitable environment for coitus to take place is important, as young and nervous dogs are frequently distracted by extraneous noise and strange persons. Preferably the dog and bitch should have some opportunity to acquaint themselves with each other; it is unreasonable to expect a dog to immediately mate a strange bitch even though she is in standing oestrus. Kennelling dog and bitch in an adjacent run for several hours before the time of mating frequently helps in achieving success.

Some dogs show depressed libido because of the conditioning effect of owner discipline. This is particularly well demonstrated in the greyhound which, whilst he is being raced, is chastised for showing interest in a bitch, yet on retirement from the track is expected to show normal libido.

Human chorionic gonadotrophin (hCG) will stimulate the testes to produce more testosterone, but there is little evidence that it will improve libido. Induced ejaculation by digital manipulation may have some beneficial effect. Artificial insemination is not recommended but may be considered, if permitted by the Kennel Club.

Inability to copulate

Failure of erection may be due to: (1) a failure to protrude the penis either completely, as in the case of phimosis, or partially, as in the case of a persistent frenulum; (2) following normal protrusion of the penis the dog is unable to achieve intromission and complete coitus.

Disparity of size is an obvious cause, although it is surprising how readily this can be overcome. An unresponsive bitch may attract the dog but not permit intromission. Young dogs are frequently overenthusiastic; they will readily mount the bitch, who will stand, but they are unable to perform intromission. In these cases it may be necessary to assist the dog by directing the penis into the vagina. Some dogs will also be unable to copulate because of pain, discomfort or physical disability; diseases of the locomotor system and urinary system are most frequently responsible.

Reduced capacity or failure to fertilise

A history of previous unsuccessful, but apparently normal, matings to a number of proven bitches suggests a failure of fertilisation. Confirmation may be sought by the examination of the ejaculate for the presence of azoospermia, low sperm numbers or large numbers of dead or abnormal spermatozoa.

Semen collection and evaluation

Semen collection from the dog is not difficult. Artificial vaginas should not be used as they are cumbersome, and there is firm evidence that they cause the death of large numbers of spermatozoa. Collection by digital manipulation does not require any specialised equipment and the quality of the ejaculate is good; furthermore it is possible to separate the three fractions. The first fraction is clear, watery, aspermic and about 1 ml in volume; this secretion is generally assumed to arise from the urethral glands although there is a strong possibility that it may be secreted by the prostate gland. The second fraction is milky white and sperm rich and about 1–3 ml. The third fraction is clear, watery, aspermic and 5 to 30 ml; this fraction is derived from the prostate. Complete separation of all three fractions is difficult; some prostatic secretion appears to be necessary to stimulate normal sperm motility. The sperm concentration in the second fraction is usually $400–600 \times 10^3/mm^3$, with a total sperm output in each ejaculate of $100–500 \times 10^6$.

Where possible the three fractions should be collected separately. A note of volume and colour of the second fraction should be made. A small drop of this should be placed on a warm slide and the percentage of spermatozoa which are progressively motile assessed. A smear stained with eosin/nigrosin should be examined to determine the percentage of live spermatozoa and the numbers and types of morphological abnormalities. The sperm concentration in the second fraction should be determined using a haemocytometer and red blood cell pipette.

Interpretation of the results

The presence of blood or pus in the ejaculate suggests a lesion involving the urethra, bladder, prostate or epididymis. Blood is usually of prostatic origin, and is common in the third fraction of dogs over 7-years-old. A completely aspermic ejaculate is suggestive of bilateral occlusion of the ejaculatary ducts or a complete cessation of spermatogenesis. Provided that the ejaculate has been handled carefully, large numbers of dead and immotile sperm are likely to be significant in investigating an infertile dog. However, it is important, where possible, to obtain at least one more ejaculate several weeks later before a final diagnosis and decision can be made, and not all cases are clear cut.

Evaluation of defects of sperm morphology, and their clinical significance, requires the assistance of someone who is conversant with sperm structure.

Testicular biopsy

This procedure can be performed under general anaesthesia observing strict asepsis. It has the value of enabling an assessment to be made of the immediate state of spermatogenesis. Since the process of spermatogenesis takes several weeks the quality of the ejaculate is an historical reflection of the events in the seminiferous tubules. However it should not be undertaken too casually since it can result in extensive haemorrhage, haematoma formation and irritation to the dog.

Spermatogenic arrest

This condition is used to describe a condition in dogs in which sterility, associated with azoospermia, has been preceded by a history of proven fertility.

Aetiology

The cause of the condition is not known, but there is good evidence that it might be inherited since it has been shown to occur in related males. Histological examination of the testes shows evidence of degeneration with or without inflammatory changes. Although the condition may be due to a pituitary deficiency there is evidence that it might be an autoimmune disease.

History

Typically a previously fertile dog over 18 months old will have mated several proven bitches which have failed to conceive. The dog will have normal libido and be able to copulate; there will be no history of disease or ill health.

Clinical signs

The testes will be smaller than normal and flaccid, and the tails of the epididymes are reduced in size.

Diagnosis

This can be confirmed by the collection of aspermic ejaculates, *viz.* clear, watery fluid. Testicular biopsy will show that spermatogenesis is impaired or has ceased.

Treatment

Although there is a report of a spontaneous recovery after a period of sexual rest it is unlikely that the condition can be reversed. There is no evidence that hormonal therapy is of any value as a treatment.

THE BITCH

Clinical examination

Vulva

Careful, visual inspection of the vulva is indicated when the bitch has drawn attention to the organ by constant licking. In puppies, abnormal positioning due to intersexuality and congenital fusion of the vulval lips are recognised; hence young puppies when presented for vaccination need to be examined. In older animals vulvitis and perivulval dermatitis, and tumours of the vulva are seen. It is difficult to anticipate the vulval conformation which will predispose to perivulval dermatitis. Some breeds have large vulvas, e.g. Basset hounds, and some have small vulvas, e.g. greyhounds, relative to the size of bitch. Characteristic swelling of the vulva occurs during pro-oestrus and oestrus.

Vagina

Physical examination
The vestibule and posterior vagina may be examined by digital palpation where the vulval orifice is large enough to admit a finger. Most conventional auriscopes and vaginascopes only allow visual examination as far forward as the posterior vagina, and this is limited because the vagina collapses over the end of the scope. Fibreoptic instruments, after insufflation of the vagina with air, may be used to enable visual inspection of the cervix and anterior vagina. Commonly the posterior limit of the dorsal median fold of the vagina is mistaken for the external os of the cervix. The length of instrument required to reach the cervix of a bitch is usually underestimated. Radiographic examination of the vagina, after contrast medium has been introduced under pressure, is useful, but interpretation should only be attempted after the normal vagina has been studied in this way. This method will also reveal the presence of ectopic ureters, which may open into the vagina.

Vaginal smear
Material for vaginal cytology may be collected by introducing a bacteriological swab into the vestibule and subsequently rolling this on to a microscope slide, or by aspirating fluid with a pipette and smearing this onto the slide. Air dried smears may be stained with standard haematology stains, or fixed smears may be stained with trichrome stains.

Characteristically, before the onset of pro-oestrus, there is an increase in round live (nucleated) epithelial cells together with a few erythrocytes. Neutrophils are also present in small numbers at this time. As pro-oestrus progresses the number of erythrocytes increases, as do the number of epithelial cells which are dead (keratinised); these have a polygonal outline with only a small or absent nucleus. By the end of pro-oestrus there are no neutrophils in the smear. At the beginning of standing oestrus there is a diminution in

the numbers of erythrocytes, but they may remain present throughout the period of acceptance. Early in oestrus the percentage of epithelial cells which are keratinised reaches a peak (60–90%) and this is taken to indicate the optimal time for mating. Neutrophils are absent from vaginal smears until the end of oestrus, when they reappear in large numbers. There is also a reduction in the number of epithelial cells, which are now rounded and nucleated. Throughout metoestrus and anoestrus there are variable numbers of neutrophils and small and intermediate sized epithelial cells. Vaginitis is characterised by the presence of many neutrophils, although in juvenile vaginitis there is usually a preponderance of epithelial cells.

Bacteriology
A bacteriological swab may be taken from the vestibule or posterior vagina. Both these locations have a normal bacterial flora which includes β-haemolytic streptococci, coliforms and staphylococci. The significance of results of bacteriological swabbing are discussed later.

Uterus and ovaries
Abdominal palpation may reveal enlargement of the ovary (tumour) or uterus (pyometra, pregnancy, post-partum enlargement); these changes can be confirmed by plain radiography. Methods for introducing contrast medium into the non-pregnant uterus have been described but are not practical due to the difficulty encountered in trying to catheterise the bitch's cervix. Exploratory laparotomy may be necessary where disease of the reproductive tract needs to be confirmed, or when repeated failure to conceive suggests the possibility of aplasia of part of the tract.

Ovarian abnormalities

Cystic ovaries
This condition occurs most often in older maiden bitches. Clinical signs are of a persistent vaginal discharge which is first noticed after the end of an apparently normal oestrus. Unlike the discharge of pro-oestrus, which is bright red, the discharge in bitches with cystic ovaries is watery and dark red blood-stained. Bitches with cystic ovaries are not attracted to, nor seek out, the male dog, even though the male will show interest in them. The vulva is thickened, dry and pale. Cytological examination of the discharge reveals partially cornified epithelial cells and erythrocytes. Higher than normal levels of circulating plasma oestrogen are probably sustained for several weeks but never reach the peak levels found in bitches during

pro-oestrus. The bitch shows no signs of malaise. The only method of treatment is ovaro-hysterectophin. Treatment with human chorionic gonadotrophin (hCG), in an attempt to luteinise the cysts, does not appear to be successful. On removal, the ovaries are usually found to contain large cystic structures over 2 cm in size and there may be cystic glandular endometrial hyperplasia in the uterus. These ovarian cysts are different from parovarian cysts which are fluid-filled structures found lying quite close to the ovary but not part of it and having their origin in the broad ligament. Parovarian cysts do not affect fertility.

Tumours

The commonest tumour found in the ovary of the bitch is the granulosa cell tumour. Although such tumours can be found in both ovaries it is more commonly unilateral. The affected ovary is markedly enlarged and the bitch is usually present with abdominal distension; there is usually a history of anoestrus of 1–2 years' duration. The condition can occur at any age. The very enlarged ovary can be palpated as a mass in the anterior abdomen and on x-ray is seen occupying a position near to its associated kidney. Usually there is no vaginal discharge, and treatment is surgical. Primary cystadenocarcinomas can also occur.

Other types of tumours have been reported in the ovaries of bitches, but these are usually secondary to a primary lesion affecting some other parts of the body, not necessarily other regions of the reproductive tract.

Vulval abnormalities

Perivulval dermatitis

This condition is said to occur most commonly in the bitch spayed before puberty. Ulcerated lesions are found around the very small infantile vulval lips and the bitch is constantly licking at this region. There is often inflammation and necrosis of the perivulval skin, especially where folds of skin are present, as in fat bitches. Greyhounds maintained on concrete floors often have scarification and necrosis of the vulval lips which results in vaginitis. Medical treatment involves the topical use of antibiotic and corticosteroid creams, which is often resented by the bitch, and any improvement is usually only temporary. Enlargement of the very contracted vulva may be attempted by the administration of oestrogens, but the only lasting solution is radical episiostomy and vulvectomy to increase the size of the vulval orifice and remove all surrounding diseased tissue.

Occasionally there is congenital failure of the vulval lips to completely separate so that there is difficulty in urinating. Intersex dogs may have an abnormally cranial vulva and an enlarged clitoris; this is described in the previous part of the chapter dealing with the male (p. 445).

Vaginal abnormalities

Vaginal prolapse or hyperplasia of the vagina

This occurs in the bitch during late pro-oestrus and early oestrus due to hyperplasia of the vagina, which is caused by the raised circulating plasma oestrogen concentrations. The bitch is presented with a pink or red mass of tissue either visible between the lips of the vulva or protruding through the vulval lips. If protruding, it may become traumatised with consequent necrosis. If the bitch is required for breeding then the prolapsed area should be removed, since intromission by the dog is not possible when the prolapse is present.

Removal of the prolapse, which is carried out during oestrus, does not result in any subsequent difficulties at mating. In bitches that are not required for breeding, and provided there is little trauma or necrosis, no immediate treatment is necessary since the condition will be resolved when the bitch goes out of standing oestrus. Ovarohysterectomy should then be carried out.

Vaginitis

Pre-pubertal vaginitis tends to affect the larger breeds of dogs, e.g. Alsatian, Boxer and Labrador. The copious, pus-like vaginal discharge can continue for many weeks. Neither topical nor systemic use of antibiotics is of any value, in fact the former treatment may increase the amount of vaginal discharge. Some workers have suggested douching with astringent mixtures, such as 1% ferric chloride, but usually the condition quickly resolves when the bitch has her fist oestrus. Although the discharge appears to be purulent, it is composed mainly of dead epithelial cells; the cause of the condition is not known.

Vaginitis in the mature bitch can be associated with trauma at mating, or the presence of foreign bodies within the vagina. It is very irritant and the bitch frequently licks and bites the vulva and perineum. Careful inspection of the vagina is necessary to identify the presence of a foreign body, which should be removed, followed by the application of emolients and systemic antibiotics.

Outbreaks of vaginitis, as shown by abnormal vulval discharge, are also seen in breeding kennels and are frequently associated with infertility. The bacterial flora of the posterior vagina and vestibule of these bitches is the same as that of normal bitches, and includes β-haemolytic Streptococci and coliforms. The condition is usually seen on premises which have housed dogs for many years. Typically the bitches have long periods between heats and when pro-oestrus does eventually occur it appears initially to be normal, but after a few days the discharge turns from haemorrhagic to purulent; microscopic examination reveals the presence of many neutrophils with little evidence of keratinisation of epithelial cells.

The cause of the condition may be due to an increase in bacterial load in the dog's environment and/or a decreased local resistance to microorganisms in the bitch's genital tract. There may be other, unknown, predisposing factors involved. The posterior vagina and vestibule of the bitch normally have a mixed bacterial flora, but when an organism is isolated in pure culture from this area, it should probably be viewed with suspicion.

Treatment is empirical and is first aimed at reducing the number of organisms in the environment by thorough disinfection where this is possible. This is sometimes effective, but moving the dogs to new premises gives better results. Individual dogs can be treated either with an autogenous vaccine incorporating antigens of the bacteria isolated from the vaginas and faeces of the bitches, or with antibiotics. It is impossible to eliminate bacteria from the bitch's vagina, and furthermore, organisms which are normally present on the dog's penis will be introduced at coitus. Oral treatment is commenced two days before the expected first day of mating and continued for at least four days after the last mating. Ampicillin and trimethoprim are known to reach vaginal secretions in therapeutic concentrations. Vaginitis can also occur in spayed bitches. A summary of the causes of vaginal discharge and their differentiation is shown in Table 16.1.

Vaginal constriction

Difficulty in breeding in maiden bitches is sometimes attributed to constriction of the vestibulo-vaginal junction, or persistence of part of the hymen. Since there is always some constriction at this point it is sometimes difficult to establish to what degree this is abnormal. Stretching of this junction is usually possible under general anaesthesia.

Vaginal tumours

The commonest vaginal tumours are fibromata or leiomyomata, both of which usually, but not always, develop from the floor of the vagina just cranial to the urethral opening. The fibromata appear to be the canine equivalent of the human fibroid.

The owner may become aware either of distortion of the perineum between vulva and anus or, if the tumour becomes ulcerated, or a vaginal discharge or both.

Removal through an episiotomy is a relatively simple matter bearing in mind that they are submucosal *in situ*.

Uterine abnormalities

Pyometra and cystic endometrial hyperplasia

This is the commonest disease of the bitches' reproductive system. It generally occurs during metoestrus and is most frequently seen in the old and middle aged bitch. Surprisingly there are many aspects of the disease, especially related to its aetiology, which need further study. Early diagnosis often presents problems because the clinical signs can sometimes be vague, and when they are obvious can also occur in diseases unrelated to the reproductive system.

The pathological changes in the uterus have been described in great detail; these changes can be placed under four main divisions:

1 Cystic endometrial hyperplasia (CEH) is frequently seen in the uterus of the middle aged and elderly bitch; it appears to be an extension and intensification of the changes that occur in the bitch during normal metoestrus. The lesion rarely causes any clinical signs although it probably predisposes to pyometra.

2 CEH with diffuse plasma cell infiltration usually develops 40-70 days after oestrus. The only regular clinical sign is the presence of a vaginal discharge; the bitch may sometimes show slight anorexia and depression. The uterus is slightly enlarged.

3 CEH with superimposed acute endometritis, in which there is extensive neutrophil infiltration in the endometrium and in some cases the myometrium. Typically this results in the bitch showing very obvious clinical signs of disease 15–45 days after oestrus. The uterus is enlarged especially if the cervix is closed, allowing the accumulation of secretions, exudate and debris.

4 The typical histopathological signs of CEH are absent and the lesion is a chronic endometritis with lymphocyte infiltration. If the cervix is open the uterus is only slightly enlarged, but if the cervix is closed the uterus can become severely distended so that the uterine wall is very thin and liable to rupture. There is endometrial atrophy, myometrial hypertrophy and fibrosis. Typically this type of lesion occurs in the older bitch in which clinical signs appear 55–90 days after oestrus. In many cases this type of lesion results from

Table 16.1 Differential diagnosis of vaginal discharge in the bitch.

Condition	History	Gross appearance of discharge	Cytological findings*	Total blood white cell count × 10³	Condition of vulva	Comments
Pro-oestrus	Expected in 'heat'	Haemorrhagic	↑NCEC ↑RBC	7–10	Swollen	Attractive to male and frequent urination
Oestrus	Expected in 'heat'	Haemorrhagic or creamy and scant	↑CEC ↑RBC No WBC	7–10	Swollen	Attractive to male, frequent urination, allows coitus
Transmissible vaginal tumour	From outside UK	Haemorrhagic	↑RBC	7–10	—	
Vaginal ulceration	Recent trauma or mating	Haemorrhagic	↑RBC	10–12	Depends on stage of cycle	May start up to 2 weeks after mating
Cystitis	Frequent urination	Scant, usually haemorrhagic, may be purulent	↑RBC, may be ↑WBC	10–12	Normal	Restless and frequent urination (cf. oestrus)
Pyometra	Oestrus 2–8 weeks previously. Malaise & polydipsia	Purulent or blood tinged	↑WBC ↑NCEC	>15	Tumefied	Radiographic uterine shadow
Metritis	Recent parturition	Brownish red		10–12	Swollen	Severe malaise
Cystic ovaries	Continuous discharge after oestrus	Haemorrhagic	↑RBC ↑CEC (with nuclei)	10–12	Thickened	No malaise, usually old bitches
Single pup syndrome	In oestrus approx. 66 days previously, not thought to be pregnant	Brown and odorous	—	10–12	Swollen	Radiographic fetal skeleton
Juvenile vaginitis	Before first heat	Copious, thick and creamy	↑NCEC (No ↑WBC)	7–10	Normal	Refractory to antibiotics
Mummified fetuses	Around term. No straining (labour)	Thick and tarry black	—	10–40	Slightly swollen	Radiographic fetal skeletons and no malaise
Adult vaginitis	Attractive to male dogs. Licking vulva	Purulent	↑WBC	7–10	May be swollen	No malaise, may be foreign body
Subinvolution of placental sites	Whelped up to 2 months previously. Persistent discharge since	Haemorrhagic	—	7–10	Slightly swollen	No malaise and refractory to treatment
Placental separation during pregnancy	Mated within last 63 days	Haemorrhagic	↑RBC	10–12	Pink, slightly swollen	Radiographic fetal skeletons after 45 days
Normal pregnancy	Mated within last 63 days	Purulent or mucoid	↑WBC	7–10	Normal	No malaise and does not threaten pregnancy
Parturition	Mated 61–65 days previously	Greenish-black	—	7–10	Swollen and relaxed	Panting, nest making, milk production

* NCEC = non-cornified epithelial cells; RBC = red blood cells; CEC = cornified epithelial cells; WBC = white blood cells.
From Allen & Renton (1982) Br. vet. J. *138* 185–198.

a number of repeated bouts of CEH which were resolved with or without treatment.

Aetiology

It is generally accepted that there is no single causal factor for pyometra, but it is the result of a number of different effects.

Although the disease can be readily produced experimentally by the administration of progestagens at low dose rates for as little as 40 days, or at high dose rates for a much shorter period of time, it is accepted that the spontaneous development of the disease is not dependent upon abnormally elevated endogenous progesterone concentrations. There are a number of reports which have shown that bitches with pyometra do not have elevated peripheral plasma progesterone concentrations compared with clinically normal bitches at the same stage of metoestrus.

Experimentally a CEH lesion has been produced following repeated uterine biopsies during early metoestrus, possibly because trauma increased the normal metoestral response of the endometrium. Therefore if progesterone is involved in the normal pathogenesis of the condition perhaps variations in the susceptibility of the endometrium should be considered.

It is generally agreed that the commonest organism isolated from clinical cases of pyometra is E. *coli*, although Streptococci and Staphylococci are also identified. There is good evidence that the strains of E. *coli* most frequently isolated have an affinity for urinary tract epithelium and smooth muscle as well as the progesterone-dominated endometrium and myometrium. If the urinary tract organisms are involved in the pathogenesis of the condition they must gain entry to the uterus at oestrus, when the cervical canal is open. Normally one would have assumed that the oestrogen-dominated uterus would be able to eliminate such bacterial contamination, but it may be significant that in the bitch the onset of standing oestrus is associated with the early rise in plasma progesterone concentrations arising from the pre-ovulatory luteinisation of mature Graafian follicles. Such a rise in progesterone might allow these organisms to persist and to subsequently multiply.

It has long been recognised that the treatment of bitches for misalliance with oestrogen predisposes to pyometra. It may be that in these animals cervical patency persists for a longer period of time than normal, thus allowing the entry of bacteria into the uterine lumen. However it may also be due to a direct effect upon the endometrium.

Case history and clinical signs
The bitch will usually be middle aged or elderly although it must be remembered that the disease can occur in the young animal. The history will usually reveal that oestrus occurred within the last 12 weeks. Bitches that have been treated with progestagens to suppress oestrus should be considered to be at risk, as are bitches that have been treated with oestrogens for misalliance.

There is much controversy about the influence of parity, overt signs of pseudopregnancy and irregularity of inter-oestrus periods. Some authors suggest that the disease is more common in the middle aged or aged nulliparous individual, but others disagree. Similarly several authors suggest that pyometra is most frequently seen in bitches which have shown overt signs of pseudopregnancy, but the majority of bitches fall into this category. There may be a correlation between the occurrence of the disease and treatment of pseudopregnancy with steroid hormones. Irregularity of interoestrus intervals is also more common in the aged bitch, at a time when she is most prone to develop pyometra.

The severity of clinical signs will depend upon the type of endometrial lesion and the patency of the cervix.

Mild pyometra
Some bitches, especially in middle age, show vague signs of malaise during metoestrus. There may be reduced appetite, reluctance to take exercise, and the coat may appear poor. In some cases there may be a mucoid vulval discharge which persists intermittently after the end of oestrus. A similar discharge may also be present during normal pregnancy. The uterus may be enlarged on palpation and although laboratory tests and radiological examination are not conclusive, ovarohysterectomy results in the bitch returning to normal health and histopathological examination of the uterus reveals lesions typical of CEH.

Typical pyometra
There is a history of anorexia, vomiting, lethargy, abdominal distension, polydipsia and polyuria. In small bitches, the distended uterus may be palpable *per rectum* especially if the forequarters are raised. Depending on the stage of the disease, buccal and conjunctival mucous membranes may be congested or pale, and the pulse accelerated and weak. In the open case, a vaginal discharge, which may be any colour from cream to a dark, sanguinous brown, is almost pathognomonic. In some open cases, vaginal discharge may not have been noticed by the owner nor be obvious on superficial inspection, but the owner may have observed the bitch licking her vulva very often or, by manipulation of the perineal region, the clinician can observe a discharge.

The differential diagnosis of these clinical signs is given in Chapter 15, Table 15.3 (polydipsia and polyuria) and Table 16.1 (vulval discharge).

Atypical cases
In some cases appetite may be maintained, or vomiting and/or excess thirst may be absent, or there may be no obvious abdominal distension, yet the remainder of the clinical picture is characteristic.

In some animals less usual presenting signs are skeletal pain and paresis, usually of the caudal lumbar region and hind limbs. The signs are usually transient (12–72 hours) in most cases and may be due to a toxic arthritis. Usually more typical signs supervene, but if the paresis persists alone and there is no other cause, it resolves after hysterectomy.

Open versus closed

It is not a hard and fast rule that an open case is less ill than a closed case, although closed cases may at any time become open and remission of signs may follow if drainage is adequate. Very occasionally, signs of distress, pain, mild straining reminiscent of parturition or even signs of systemic collapse may accompany the transition from closed to open.

Diagnosis

Confirmation of a presumptive diagnosis of pyometra can be based upon a consideration of a large number of factors. The following may be included:

1 History and clinical signs will be consistent with such a diagnosis. Pitfalls for the unwary, however, are (a) absence of a temperature rise (well-developed cases in particular are often afebrile), and (b) a locular pyometra may resemble a 30–35-day pregnancy, and the pregnant animal may show physiological vomiting and polydipsia.

2 On examination of good radiographs the pus-filled uterus may be readily apparent. Absence of small intestine from its usual position in mid-abdomen is suggestive of uterine enlargement. A pneumoperitoneum improves contrast, but should not be performed if pyometra is suspected, because of the risk of perforating the distended uterus.

3 Haematological examination usually reveals a leucocytosis, mostly due to neutrophils with a marked 'shift to the left', but neither this nor an increased ESR are diagnostic as they may occur with any infectious inflammatory condition. However, if the case is terminal a leucocytosis will not be present. Anaemia becomes progressively apparent because of the effect of toxins on the bone marrow; low haemoglobin concentrations or PCVs are bad prognostic signs.

4 Biochemical analysis of blood reveals a slight increase in blood urea levels (up to 100 mg/100 ml) in the early stages which progressively worsens; more than 200 mg/100 ml carries a grave prognosis as it usually indicates irreversible renal damage. A high total serum protein with an exaggerated hyperglobulinaemia may also be present.

5 Urine analysis should always be carried out to assess the presence or absence of intercurrent disease such as diabetes mellitus (Chapter 8) or chronic interstitial nephritis (Chapter 15). The additional presence of either condition affects the prognosis adversely.

6 Staining a smear of the vulval discharge, or a vaginal smear taken from a swab or aspirated fluid will reveal large numbers of leucocytes.

Treatment

Treatment of choice is ovarohysterectomy and with modern anaesthetic facilities and supportive therapy (particularly fluid therapy, see Chapter 12), there is a high degree of success. Cervical catheterisation and drainage of the uterine contents through a large-bore catheter has been suggested as a form of treatment, but it is virtually impossible to see, let alone catheterise, the bitch's cervix, and in any case the contents are usually too viscid to flow readily.

Medical treatment may be required, however, either as a preoperative measure in a poor risk case or in bitches whose age and/or general condition make surgery an improper undertaking, or where the owner refuses surgery. In the poor risk case where there is evidence of bacterial proliferation (elevated temperature and severe malaise), antibacterial therapy for 12–36 hours before surgery can be most valuable, but it is always difficult to decide whether the benefit of this delay justifies postponement of surgery; each case must be judged on its merits. In the case of bitches with intercurrent disease, then it must be expected that only a small proportion will respond. Where the owner refuses surgery, he should be made aware of the probable consequences. In any case, treatment is likely to be palliative and the disease will probably reappear after the succeeding oestrus.

Ecbolics such as oxytocin are contraindicated in closed cases as the cervix may not relax and there is a risk of uterine rupture. Quinine has been recommended as a promoter of cervical opening and of uterine drainage, but despite having been well documented, regular confirmation of the results claimed has not been forthcoming. In open cases, oxytocin plus antibacterials occasionally appear to be very effective.

Various hormones have been widely used but evidence of consistently good results is lacking.

More recently some success has been reported following the use of prostaglandin $F_{2\alpha}$ at dose rates of between 0.1 and 0.25 mg/kg. This has resulted in some cases in the evacuation of the uterine contents, with an improvement in the bitches' health. Some bitches have subsequently conceived.

Segmental aplasia

Segmental aplasia of the uterus is rare. If in those parts of the uterus that are present, normal endometrial structure and function persist then uterine secretions can accumulate proximal to the aplastic section. The condition is usually asymptomatic unless the distension is excessive.

Post-partum haemorrhage

The passage of blood-stained vulva discharge is a normal occurrence after whelping, but the quantity of blood is generally small, resulting in either 'spotting' or small quantities at the end of urination, or else resulting in bloodstaining of bedding. Normally the blood-stained discharge persists for 3–4 days.

Acute haemorrhage

Occasionally a fairly copious haemorrhage occurs immediately after the expulsion of the last puppy and persists for 4–5 hours. Clinical examination of the bitch may show palor of the visible mucous membranes and rapid bounding pulse; evidence of severe blood loss can be determined by measuring the packed cell value and haemoglobin concentration.

Ecbolic drugs, such as ergometrine and oxytocin, should be given to hasten uterine involution. In severe cases it may be necessary to consider ovarohysterectomy after attempts have been made to compensate for blood loss with blood transfusions and blood volume expanders. The cause of this acute haemorrhage may be trauma to the uterus or vagina, especially if digital exploration has been performed or instruments have been used. It may also be related to premature separation of the placental attachments or in some cases interference with normal blood clotting mechanisms.

Subinvolution of placenta sites

A delay in the normal repair and regeneration of the endometrium at the sites of placental attachment can result in a slight but persistent blood-stained vulval discharge persisting for up to 2–3 months postpartum. Although it does not have a severe effect upon the bitch's health it can result in anaemia. Ecbolic drugs are of no value because the uterus is unresponsive, and antibiotic therapy is not successful. Ultimately the endometrium usually repairs and the condition resolves. In severe cases there can be perforation of the uterine wall at the margins of the placental zones and ovarohysterectomy is the only method of treatment.

Post-partum metritis

This follows prolonged parturition due to dystocia and/or retention of fetal membranes. The bitch with post-partum metritis shows severe malaise and fever (103–104°F) within 24 hours of whelping, and has a copious malodorous brown discharge from the vulva. Mastitis with a reduction in lactation often also occurs, resulting in a very discontented litter. Puppies should be removed from such bitches and hand-reared whilst the bitch is undergoing treatment. High dose systemic antibiotics should be started immediately with fluid therapy where necessary. Despite prompt treatment some bitches with this condition will die.

Retained fetal membranes

If the owner of the bitch is present at parturition, the bitch with retained fetal membranes may be presented 1–2 hours after the completion of parturition, because the owner has noted that the bitch has not expelled all the placentas. In this instance, if the bitch is relaxed, abdominal palpation may reveal the areas of the uterus where the membranes are situated, although these must be distinguished from the normal involuting uterus. In some cases the membranes have been partially expelled and on vaginal examination they may be palpated within the vagina. In this latter situation the retained placenta can be removed carefully by traction with forceps. If, however, the membranes are still retained within the uterus, stimulation of uterine contraction by the administration of oxytocin usually causes expulsion. In each instance it is always safer to give broad spectrum antibiotic treatment for several days.

Generally bitches with retained fetal membranes are presented 24–48 hours after the expulsion of the last puppy, with a persistent but perhaps intermittent green vulval discharge, the green colouration being due to the presence of the blood pigment uteroverdin. In many cases the bitch may show the typical signs, described above, of metritis. Abdominal palpation, vaginal exploration and lateral radiography will be necessary to ensure that there are no retained puppies.

Prolapsed uterus

This condition is uncommon in the bitch. Usually only one horn of the uterus is involved and this is everted into the vagina. However, in severe cases prolapse may be complete, with rupture of the broad ligament and the uterine blood vessels, resulting in sudden death. Prolapse occurs immediately after the end of parturition; the cause is excessive traction during dystocia which results in severe abdominal straining. Partial prolapse of the uterus causes the bitch to adopt an unnatural posture and shown signs of abdominal pain. If total prolapse has occurred then it is immediately obvious. A protruding prolapse rapidly becomes traumatised and necrotic. Reduction may be attempted if the uterus is undamaged. General anaesthesia is necessary and then by careful manipulation an attempt is made to replace the prolapse. In most cases, however, the uterus is so badly traumatised that amputation is the only treatment. The uterus is removed at the cervix.

Eclampsia

Eclampsia resulting from lowered blood calcium concentrations affects bitches, usually whelped 4–6 weeks, who are suckling a litter of at least three or four pups. It most commonly affects the small breeds. Symptoms vary in severity from occasional ataxia to collapse with 'fit-like' symptoms of frothing at the mouth, hyperaesthesia, whimpering and leg pedalling. The method of treatment depends on the severity of the condition. Oral administration of calcium tablets may be sufficient. More severely affected bitches require calcium borogluconate by slow intravenous injection followed by either subcutaneous injection or administration of calcium tablets over a period of several days. In all cases the puppies should be removed immediately and hand reared. Eclampsia can occur earlier and a few cases have been reported in bitches immediately prior to parturition.

Phantom pregnancy or pseudopregnancy (pseudocyesis)

There is good evidence that the majority of bitches show some signs of pseudopregnancy, but with varying severity. There is a history of the bitch being in oestrus 6–9 weeks before she is noted to have some of the signs associated with pregnancy, though she has not conceived. (In the majority of cases she has not even been mated.) The symptoms range from mammary development, with or without lactation, to making a bed and abdominal straining as if parturient.

Behavioural disturbances associated with the condition include anorexia (with normal thirst), shivering, crying, disinclination to go for walks and possessiveness over objects and territory. There is evidence that in wild dogs only dominant bitches breed, and that their puppies are nursed by other bitches in the pack. This suggests that it is normal for bitches to lactate and show maternal behaviour in the abscence of whelping. However the change in 'personality' of the bitch often worries the owner, although the anorexia is not associated with weight loss. In some cases bitches in pseudopregnancy are so aggressive towards people (whom they imagine are a threat to their expected litter) that it is unwise not to treat the condition. In the mild form tranquillisers and diuretics, to reduce milk production, may be sufficient to make the bitch comfortable, or if untreated the condition will resolve itself in 10–14 days. If signs are more severe it is necessary to use steroid hormones. There is no indication that pseudopregnancy is caused by production of abnormal amounts of progesterone. There is good evidence though that prolactin causes the lactation and probably the nervous signs. Specific anti-prolactin drugs (e.g. bromocriptine) will alleviate the condition, but since these cause vomiting in dogs they are not used in general practice. Steroid drugs (not corticosteroids) are also very effective treatments. Oestrogens *per se* can be used, e.g. oestradiol benzoate injection, or a mixture of ethinyl oestradiol and methyl testosterone is available in tablet form. Testosterone *per se*, and synthetic progestagens (e.g. megestrol acetate and proligestone) are also effective.

If the bitch is not required for breeding, ovarohysterectomy should be carried out to prevent further false (and real) pregnancies. However problems have been encountered when the operation has been carried out too soon after the treatment with steroid hormones, particularly megestrol acetate. A small number of bitches have recurrent false pregnancy following treatment, and if they are operated on just before or during the syndrome, the condition can continue to recur. It is therefore advisable not to operate until at least 6 weeks after the end of treatment. This interval may need to be longer after the use of long-acting injectable progestagens, but no information on this is available. Preferably the bitch should be spayed after an oestrus when no steroid treatment has been used to treat false pregnancy or during anoestrus. In the small number of bitches which have recurrent episodes of false pregnancy after the same heat, it may be necessary to operate during pro-oestrus, or soon after the end of heat in order to avoid the danger period. In those bitches which have false pregnancies after spaying, long-acting progestagen preparations (e.g. proligestone) should be administered when signs begin.

Control of reproductive function

Most bitches are kept as pets and are not required for breeding. The occurrence of oestrus in these circumstances is inconvenient, as it curtails normal exercise patterns and may attract male dogs. Unwanted litters only contribute to the already considerable stray dog population. Oestrus-control is therefore desirable, and there are two methods which are commonly used.

Hormonal control

The use of various progestagens to control oestrus-behaviour, presumably by their inhibitory effect on the release of gonadotrophins from the pituitary gland, has been practised for some time. At present two products are most widely used. Megestrol acetate is administered orally and may be used in a low dose regime (0.5 mg/kg daily) starting in anoestrus, to prevent the occurrence of oestrus at a particularly inconvenient time. Alternatively a larger dose (2 mg/kg daily) is administered for 8 days starting at the first signs of pro-oestrus; the signs have usually disappeared in a few days. The advantage of oral preparations is that treatment can be discontinued if side-effects occur, e.g. increased body weight. Proligestone is administered by a single injection at regular intervals at a dose rate of up to 33 mg/kg, preferably during anoestrus, although it can be given in pro-oestrus with similar responses as described for megestrol acetate. Progestagens, like progesterone can stimulate cystic glandular endometrial hyperplasia. However these effects are not as profound as those described for some of the early synthetic progestagens, e.g. medroxyprogesterone acetate.

These drugs should not be administered during oestrus since at this stage of the oestrous cycle the cervix is open and bacteria can enter the uterus. The exogenous progestagen, together with endogenous progesterone which is being produced at this time, reduce the resistance of the uterus to microorganisms, so increasing the likelihood of pyometra developing, especially if cystic hyperplasia is present. Drugs which have no adverse effect on the uterus, e.g. androgens, would be much safer for oestrous-control as they also appear to inhibit pituitary gonadotrophic function. Testosterone was formerly used to inhibit oestrus in racing Greyhound bitches, and an androgen with very few side-effects (mibolerone) is currently in use in the USA and elsewhere.

Ovarohysterectomy

In the authors' opinion this is the treatment of choice where an owner does not intend to breed from the bitch. It is more economical and reliable than constant hormone treatment, and has fewer side-effects. It also prevents pyometra, which is most common in the older non-bred bitch, and the occurrence of false pregnancies. The incidence of mammary neoplasia in ovarohysterectomised bitches is low. Spaying before puberty (first heat) is not usually carried out because of its reported association with infantile vulva and peri-vulval dermatitis. Care should be taken to ensure that a bitch is not spayed during false pregnancy. The most common side-effect of ovarohysterectomy is subsequent obesity. Owners of bitches should be advised to weigh the dog monthly and reduce food intake and increase exercise at signs of increased body weight.

Normal reproductive function

The bitch comes into oestrus at most twice a year and in some breeds only once a year. Each heat consists of a pro-oestrus of approximately 7-10 days, followed by standing oestrus which also lasts 7-10 days. The bitch then enters a luteal phase which lasts about 63 days, whether or not she is pregnant. In the pregnant bitch the corpora lutea cease to function at parturition whereas in the non-pregnant animal their function may continue a little longer. The progesterone-dominated phase is followed by a quiescent period of anoestrus which lasts for at least two months. There is confusion over the terminology used to describe events which occur after the end of oestrus. Traditionally in the bitch the period which immediately follows oestrus has been called metoestrus, and this name is applied until regression of the corpora lutea, after which the bitch enters an anoestrus with inactive ovaries. However, during this period there is remodelling of the endometrium from a secretory luteal phase to a quiescent anoestrous picture. The term metoestrus is used in other domesticated animals to describe the period of time during which the corpora lutea develop. We thus use the word metoestrus to mean something different in the bitch. Alternatively the word dioestrus can be used to describe the luteal phase which follows the end of oestrus. Neither of these words (metoestrus and dioestrus) is synonymous with the whole luteal phase of the bitch, as ovulation occurs early in oestrus and even before this time there is development of luteal tissue in unruptured follicles, with a rise in progesterone concentrations in blood. During pro-oestrus and oestrus clinical changes are demonstrated. These include behavioural changes, where a bitch during pro-oestrus will flirt, but not allow mating, and will urinate more frequently. This type of behaviour is brought about by the increased circulating levels of oestrogen produced by developing follicles. Oestrus, during which the bitch will allow coitus, is stimulated by falling oestrogen concentrations and rising progesterone values. Most ovulations occur around the first 24–48 hours of standing oestrus, although some bitches may ovulate as late as the ninth day. After ovulation progesterone levels continue to increase to peak values during the first week of metoestrus. Although over recent years much knowledge about the hormonal events of the canine oestrus cycle has been accumulated, it is still not clear how aberrations from these established patterns might affect fertility. Single or occasional blood samples for hormone (progesterone and oestrogen) assay are not informative. Daily sampling would be necessary, but cost usually makes this prohibitive. At present, most treatments for infertility are empirical as definite causes are hard to diagnose.

Abnormalities of oestrus

A bitch's first oestrus is not commonly used for breeding. On occasions this heat is prolonged, or the bitch shows signs of pro-oestrus for only a few days followed some time later by another attempt at a proper oestrus. If this behaviour is prolonged treatment should be aimed at either stimulating ovulation using 50–500 i.u. hCG if there is persistent pro-oestrus, or blocking release of gonadotrophin using progestagen (e.g. megoestrol acetate) if pro-oestrus is foreshortened and intermittent. The rationale for progestagen treatment is the assumption that inadequate gonadotrophin release will be stopped and that the next heat will be normal.

When successive periods of heat are less than 4 months apart it is possible that ovulation is not occurring. Assay of a blood sample taken 10–15 days after the end of heat is useful in diagnosis, as a low progesterone level (less than 1 ng/ml plasma) indicates no ovulations. Elevated progesterone concentrations indicate that luteinisation, and presumably ovulation, has occurred.

Since recent evidence suggests that some bitches ovulate late in oestrus, repeated services throughout the period of standing oestrus may, where possible, improve fertility.

When presented with a bitch kept as a pet, it may well be that as with all other domestic species, the cause of apparent infertility is mating at the wrong time. Most owners of pets seek advice on when to mate their bitches from breeders and mating is carried out on a particular day (e.g. 10, 12 etc.) after the beginning of pro-oestrus which is selected by the owner. Since pro-oestrus varies markedly both between breeds and within breeds, this system results in many bitches being mated at the wrong time. Some bitches kept as pets also show abnormal behaviour in that even although their vaginal cytology and blood oestrogen concentrations indicate they are ready for mating they will not stand. Some of these bitches will conceive if artificially inseminated.

Fetal resorption

The term resorption refers to the process in which the embryo or fetus dies and its fluids are resorbed. The resulting dehydrated fetus and its membranes undergo autolysis, but are eventually expelled, usually unnoticed, when the bitch's cervix opens. Resorption usually occurs between 28 and 35 days of pregnancy and a positive diagnosis of resorption can only be made when fetal units have been positively recognised at 25–30 days, but no whelps result at term. However, palpation at 28 days may occasionally demonstrate disparity in size of the units and re-examination a few days later reveals either no increase in size, or an actual decrease.

The cause of fetal resorption has not been established and may well be varied (e.g. hormonal failure to maintain pregnancy, genital tract infection or nutritional deficiency). It is usually impossible to make a positive diagnosis of the cause.

Abortion

Abortion (i.e. delivery of dead pups between 42 and 56 days) is extremely rare in the dog in the UK, although *Brucella canis* is a recognised cause in the North American continent. *B. abortus* has been reported to cause abortion in the UK, and other organisms, including viruses, may occasionally cause abortion. Some abortions go unrecognised as the bitch may eat the abortuses. If this occurs after 45 days, fetal bones may be demonstrated radiographically in the bitch's stomach.

Oestrus induction

Induced oestrus is not as fertile as spontaneous oestrus, but where delay is causing concern induction may be useful. Pregnant mare serum gonadotrophin (PMSG) may be administered in doses of 50–200 i.u. at 1–4-day intervals. The resulting pro-oestrus may be short, and mating should be allowed as soon as the bitch is receptive. Human chorionic gonadotrophin (50–200 i.u.) may be given at the time of mating to help ensure that ovulation occurs. Repeated small doses of oestrogens have also been used to stimulate ovulatory oestrus.

FURTHER READING

Cryptorchidism
Cox, J. E. and Joshua, J.O. (1979) In *Canine Medicine and Therapeutics*, p. 345. Blackwell Scientific Publications.
Cox, U.S., Wallace, L.J. & Jessen, C.R. (1978) *Teratology* **18**, 237.
Lipowitz, A.J., Schwartz, A., Wilson, G.P. & Ebert, J.W. (1973). *J. Am. Vet Med. Assoc.* **163**, 1364.
Reif, J.S. & Brodey, R.S. (1969) *J. Am. Vet. Med. Assoc.* **155**, 2005.
Willis, M.B. (1963) *J. Small Anim. Pract.* **4**, 469.

Testicular Torsion
Pearson, H. & Kelly, D.F. (1975) *Vet. Rec.* **97**, 200.

Hypospadia
ADLER, P.L. & HOBSON, H.P. (1978) *J. Am. Hosp. Assoc.* **14,** 721.

Intersex
ALLEN, W.E., DAKER, M.G. & HANCOCK, J.L. (1981) *Vet. Rec.* **109,** 468.
HARE, N.C.D. (1976) *Canadian Vet J.* **17,** 7.
JACKSON, D.A., OSBORNE, C.A., BRASNER, T.H. and JENSEN, C.R. (1978) *J. Am. Vet. Med. Assoc.* **172,** 926.

Prostate
BARSANTI, J.A., SCHOTTS, E.B., PRASSE, K. & CORNWELL, W. (1980) *J. Am. Vet. Med. Assoc.* **177,** 160.
BORTHWICK, R. & MACKENZIE, C.P. (1971) *Vet. Rec.* **89,** 374.
WEAVER, A.D. (1980) *Vet. Annual* **20,** 82.

Dog pox
JOSHUA, J.O. (1975) *Vet. Rec.* **96,** 300.

Penis
NDIRITU (1979) *Mod. Vet. Pract.* **60,** 712.

Infertility
ALLEN, W.E. & LONGSTAFF, J.A. (1982) *J. Small Anim. Pract.* **23,** 337.

ALLEN, W.E. & PATEL, J.P. (1982) *J. Small Anim. Pract.* **23,** 713.

Vaginal smears
ROSZEL, J.F. (1975) *Scope* **19,** 2.
SCHUTTE, A.P. (1967) *J. Small Anim. Pract.* **8,** 301.

Infertility and infection
ALLEN, W.E. & DAGNALL, G.J.R. (1982) *J. Small Anim. Pract.* **23,** 325.
ASCHEIM, A. (1963) *Acta. Vet. Scand.* **4,** 293.
DOW, C. (1958) *Vet. Rec.* **70,** 1102.
DOW, C. (1959) *J. Path. Bact.* **78,** 267.
DOW, C. (1960) *J. Comp. Path. Ther.* **70,** 59.
OLSON, P.N.S. & MATHER, E.C. (1978) *J. Am. Vet. Med. Assoc.* **172,** 708.
OSBALDISTON, G.W., NURU, S. & MOSIER, J.E. (1977) *J. Am. Animal Hosp. Assoc.* **8,** 93.
RENTON, J.P., DOUGLAS, T.A. & WATTS, C. (1971) *J. Small Anim. Pract.* **12,** 249.
SANDHOLM, M., VASENIUS, H. & KIVISTO, A.-K. (1975) *J. Am. Vet. Med. Assoc.* **167,** 1006.

Oestrus induction
ALLEN, W.E. (1982) *J. Small Anim. Pract.* **23,** 223.
RENTON, J.P., MUNRO, C.D., HEATHCOTE, R.H. & CARMICHAEL, S. (1981) *J. Reprod. Fertil.* **61,** 289.
WRIGHT, P.J. (1982) *Aust. Vet. J.* **59,** 123.

17

Endoparasites

W. P. BERESFORD-JONES AND D. E. JACOBS

While clinicians have long been aware of some of the veterinary problems associated with the endoparasites of the domestic dog, it is only in recent years that the full significance of these infections for small animal practice, meat production and human health has started to emerge.

The early veterinary surgeons in Great Britain attached little importance to the endoparasites of the dog, although in 1816 Richard Lawrence referred in his book *The Complete Farrier and British Sportsman* to the taenia or tapeworm, the roundworm, a third variety resembling maggots and a fourth type rather like a threadworm found principally in the rectum. He stresses how with purgatives, mercurial salts, arsenic and other metallic salts he was successful in removing tapeworms, but the dog soon became reinfected. A point he made was that worms could be fatal to puppies and that in the young and old dog they could produce fits. In 1932, the two principal kinds of worm in the dog in this country were still referred to as roundworms or *Ascarides* and tapeworms. The standard treatments at this time according to Henry Gray in *Hounds and Dogs* (ed. A. Croxton Smith) were substances such as oil of chenopodium, capsules of tetrachlorethylene or santonin followed by a purgative for the removal of roundworms and the administration of freshly powdered or grated Areca nuts, or kamala and oil of male fern (*Felix mas*) for the removal of tapeworms.

Since the publication in 1934 of Mönnig's *Veterinary Helminthology and Entomology*, knowledge has accrued steadily but it was not until the 1950s that Sprent in Australia elucidated the life-cycle of the dog ascarids, while the association between the canine coccidia and the sarcocysts of meat animals was not recognised until the mid 1970s.

This new knowledge has expanded the list of endoparasites known to occur in British dogs to a formidable length and the trend is compounded by the introduction of exotic parasites with the increasing numbers of imported animals. For the purposes of this book, the endoparasites have been grouped for easy reference into the following categories on the basis of their importance to veterinary practice: ubiquitous parasites, helminths mainly found in large kennels, parasites of public health importance, parasites of importance in meat inspection, parasites likely to occur in quarantine kennels and rare parasites and curiosities.

UBIQUITOUS PARASITES

The prevalence of a parasite in the dog population is largely dependent on factors such as climate, environment and management. *Trichuris*, for example, appears to favour a warmer climate than we can offer in the United Kingdom and heavy infections are not likely to occur except where groups of dogs share grass runs. Dietary considerations restrict the distribution of other parasites such as the tapeworms that use meat animals as intermediate hosts. Four parasites are, however, particularly common in all breeds of dogs whether urban or rural, kept as household pets, guide-dogs or in kennels for racing, breeding or hunting. These are the two ascarids *Toxocara canis* and *Toxascaris leonina*, a tapeworm, *Dipylidium caninum* and a protozoan, *Toxoplasma gondii*.

Toxocara and Toxascaris

Toxocara canis and *Toxascaris leonina* are large nematodes measuring from 7 cm up to 18 cm as adults. They are found in the small intestine. If it is required to distinguish these two nematodes, it is usually sufficient to obtain a female adult and tease the uteri apart and examine the eggs. *T. canis* shows a pitted shell, *T. leonina* a smooth shell (Fig. 17.1). The complicated life-cycle of *T. canis* is of more than academic interest because the occasional involvement of man presents a small but nonetheless important public health problem (discussed on p. 471) and because prenatal infec-

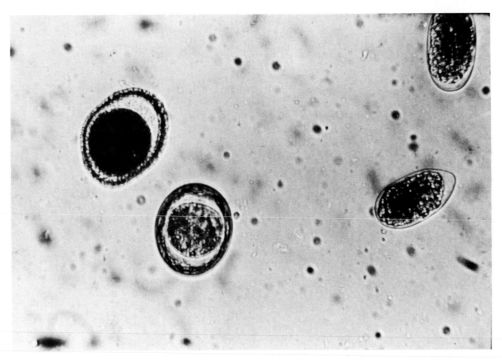

Fig. 17.1   Three types of nematode egg commonly seen in dog faeces. From left to right: *Toxocara canis, Toxascaris leonina, Uncinaria stenocephala.* Photograph by M.J. Walker.

tion with this parasite is a common cause of disease in puppies.

Clinical signs

Turner and Pegg (1977) have reported a survey of 1000 dogs in NW London, noting the following clinical signs:

Puppies up to 12 days old: noisy breathing accompanied by nasal discharge, especially when suckling, retarded growth.

Puppies 2 weeks of age: vomiting, diarrhoea, failure to grow.

Puppies 6–12 weeks of age: chronic diarrhoea often with vomiting, distended abdomen and pale almost translucent mucous membranes, together with a characteristic whining and straddle-legged posture. legged posture.

Other authors have described perforation of the intestine and/or occlusion with worms. However, most ascarid infections in dogs are seemingly without clinical effect.

Life-cycles

Perpetuation of the life-cycle of *T. canis* and the involvement of man depends on the presence of *Toxo-*

cara ova in the environment. The eggs are not immediately infective on being passed in the faeces but require a maturation period, the length of which is mainly dependent on the mean day–night temperature. In Britain, infectivity may be attained in some 2–3 weeks in midsummer but a period of months is required for eggs passed in winter, although these figures await experimental verification. During the maturation period, the faeces may be dispersed and the eggs disseminated by mechanical transfer and forces such as rain and wind. Many eggs probably have a short lifespan but some can remain viable for at least 2 years.

When ingested by a dog, the eggs hatch and the larvae migrate by way of the liver to the lungs, where a proportion will leave the bloodstream, ascend the respiratory tract and return to the small intestine where they mature. Others remain in the blood to be distributed throughout the tissues of the body as resting second stage larvae up to 0.45 mm in length. The proportion of larvae taking each of the alternative pathways is associated with the age, sex and reproductive status of the host. In young pups, virtually all will proceed to the intestine, whereas the great majority of larvae in older dogs will pass into the somatic tissues, except in bitches around the time of whelping when enteric infections may again be established. This may be associated with a partial suppression of immunity during lactation.

The next important phase of the life history of *T. canis* takes place when a bitch harbouring sedentary larvae becomes pregnant. After about the 42nd day of gestation, a proportion of the larvae become active and cross the placenta to develop in the fetus. A residual population of larvae remains in the somatic tissues and may become activated during a subsequent pregnancy. Larvae in the mammary gland may be passed to the suckling pup via the colostrum.

The life-cycle is completed when the worms in the infected pup have passed by way of the liver and lungs to the intestine, where they grow to maturity. Eggs first appear in the faeces in the third week of life, with maximum numbers occurring after a further 3–5 weeks.

As often happens in host–parasite systems, the basic life-cycle is complicated by a number of supplementary methods of dissemination and transmission. Thus, although the puppy is primarily responsible for contamination of the environment, *T. canis* eggs may be passed by a small proportion of adult dogs. Patent infections are often established in nursing bitches that ingest intestinal *T. canis* larvae expelled in the faeces of their offspring. Also, the parasite is able to take advantage of the predatory and scavenging habits of its canine hosts by infecting potential prey animals. In these cases, ingestion of the egg by rodents, or other mammalian species (including man) results in a somatic infection with sedentary larvae capable of resuming their development if eaten by a dog, fox, wolf or dingo.

In contrast, the life-cycle of *T. leonina* is rather more straightforward as there is no migration through the tissues of the final hosts (which include the cat as well as the dog), so that transplacental and transmammary passage of larvae cannot occur. Infection takes place only by ingestion of embryonated eggs or larvae that have progressed to the third stage in the tissues of prey animals that have ingested the ova. Development of *T. leonina* in the dog or cat is confined to the wall of the stomach and the lumen of the digestive tract.

Prevalence

As indicated previously, intestinal forms of *T. canis* predominate in younger dogs and the somatic forms in mature animals. Thus, in Turner and Pegg's survey of suburban pets, 30.5% of dogs under 6 months of age harboured egg-laying female worms, while only 3.6% of those over 1 year old were passing *T. canis* ova. Other surveys have shown up to 70% infection in

puppies and, as the primary route of transmission is transplacental, it can be assumed that a correspondingly high proportion of breeding bitches carry somatic larvae. While puppies frequently harbour large numbers of intestinal worms, infections in adult animals, which are more likely to occur in male dogs than bitches, usually involve relatively few egg-laying individuals.

Overall, it would appear that about 11–13% of dogs (excluding young puppies) shed *T. canis* eggs into the environment, although the figure is somewhat lower for show dogs and well-cared-for suburban pets, and rather higher in some large kennels. However, prevalence rates of 30–40% have been recorded in some city dog populations, while around 35–50% of foxes show evidence of infection.

T. leonina infections have been found in approximately 2.5% of well-cared-for dogs and 15% of dogs from some other sectors of the canine population. As prenatal infection does not occur, the highest infection rate is usually found in the 6–12 month age group.

Control

The control of ascarid infections in dogs has two main objectives:

1 The protection of the pups from the deleterious effects of infestation.
2 The reduction of the associated public health risk.

As the major part of the pup's worm burden is acquired *in utero* or via the colostrum and milk, the obvious way to control the disease is to eliminate the somatic larvae in the bitch. Recently, the oral administration of fenbendazole at a dose-rate of 50 mg/kg daily for 15–20 days before whelping and 12–18 days after parturition has been shown to prevent perinatal transmission. Hopefully, other prophylactic treatments will be developed in the near future.

Otherwise, control must of necessity be dependent on the routine treatment of lactating bitches and puppies with anthelmintics that eliminate ascarid worms from the intestine. This also serves to protect future litters by reducing the number of eggs that are shed into the environment. A single dose of anthelmintic may sometimes suppress clinical signs in pups, but multiple dosing is required to control faecal egg output. The worms in the pup are in varying stages of development and some of these are not susceptible to the effects of current anthelmintics. Ideally, pups should be treated at weekly intervals from 2 weeks of age to weaning, then fortnightly to 3 months of age and every 3–6 months thereafter, but fortnightly dosing from 3–4 weeks of age to 3 months, with further treatment at 6 months old, and when presented for booster vaccinations, might be a practical compromise. All newly acquired dogs, particularly puppies, should of course be wormed on arrival.

Anthelmintics active against the intestinal forms of both ascarid species include: piperazine, diethylcarbamazine, thenium, dichlorvos, mebendazole, pyrantel, fenbend-azole and nitroscanate.

The use of these products, however, must be accompanied by appropriate advice on management and hygiene, remembering that the long-lived eggs of *T. canis* are adhesive and resistant to disinfectants. The total elimination of eggs can only be achieved by extreme measures such as the use of a horticultural flame-gun, although vigorous scrubbing with copious volumes of hot water will substantially reduce the numbers on the concrete floors.

Dipylidium

Like *T. leonina*, *D. caninum* is a non-migratory parasite of the small intestine that can infect both dogs and cats. It can be differentiated from the large taeniid tapeworms found in these animals by the shape of the proglottids which are oval with easily visible genital pores midway along either margin. Diagnosis can be confirmed microscopically by teasing apart a gravid segment releasing the characteristic egg capsules, each containing about 20 eggs (Fig. 17.2).

Although the pathogenesis of *D. caninum* has not been studied in detail, heavy infestations may cause anal irritation, digestive disturbances and ill thrift. Such infections are also aesthetically unpleasant as the motile proglottids leave via the anus to deposit their eggs.

Further development of the tapeworm can only take place if the egg is ingested by a larval flea (or sometimes a louse). By the time the flea has emerged from its pupa for a blood meal, the metacestode is capable of establishing itself in a dog or cat. It must, however, wait for its intermediate host to be swallowed during grooming.

D. caninum is undoubtedly a common parasite in nearly all types of dog but there is little documented evidence of its prevalence. This is because the proglottids are shed erratically and are not regularly seen in faeces samples from infected dogs. Post mortem studies, however, have revealed its presence in 72% of racing Greyhounds with up to 277 tapeworms (average 41) in each animal.

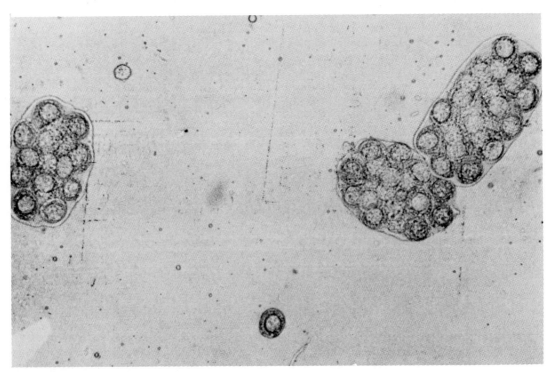

Fig. 17.2 Egg capsules from a gravid segment of *Dipylidium caninum*. Reproduced from Pegg E.J. & Shepherd R. (1966) *J. Small Anim. Pract.* **7**, 457, with permission.

Anthelmintics suitable for the treatment of *Dipylidium* infections include bunamidine, dichlorophen, nitroscanate and praziquantel. For obvious reasons, such therapy must be accompanied by vigorous steps to control the associated ectoparasitic problem.

Toxoplasma

Although *Toxoplasma gondii* was recognised as a pathogen in the early years of this century, the true identity of the organism was not established until 1970. It is now known that *T. gondii* is a coccidian parasite of the cat that can use virtually any warm-blooded animal, including man and the dog, as an intermediate host. Toxoplasmosis is of greatest significance as a zoonosis, but although dogs are frequently infected they play a minor role in the epidemiology of the human disease. The risk of *T. gondii* being transferred from canine sources to man is remote.

Clinical signs
Most *T. gondii* infections of the dog are without noticeable effect but on occasion respiratory distress, ataxia and diarrhoea may be produced. At post mortem examination, focal necrotic lesions are seen in the liver, lung and brain. Toxoplasmosis may also complicate outbreaks of distemper. It has been postulated that the immunosuppressive properties of the distemper virus may cause pre-existing subclinical Toxoplasma infections to revert from the chronic to the acute phase.

Several serological tests have been developed to detect antibodies to *T. gondii*. These include the Sabin – Feldman dye test, an indirect fluorescent antibody test and an indirect haemagglutination test. Paired samples are desirable for the diagnosis of the acute disease. At post mortem examination, a suspicion of toxoplasmosis can be confirmed by the demonstration of the parasite in tissue smears, digests or histological section.

Life-cycle
Infection of a susceptible cat gives rise to a sequence of events analogous to that seen with Eimeria in chickens. The organisms invade the epithelial cells of the small intestine and undergo several cycles of asexual division followed by gametogony, which in turn results in the formation of more than 10^{12} oocysts over a 2-week period. The intestinal infection is self limiting and the cat becomes refractory to further infection, although this immunity can wane in the absence of continued antigenic stimulation.

When a susceptible intermediate host becomes infected, the organisms invade the tissues, multiplying rapidly to form intracellular pseudocysts. These rupture, releasing numerous banana-shaped tachyzoites, approximately $6\,\mu m$ long, which become dispersed throughout the body. More cells are invaded and the process is repeated until the infection progresses after 2–3 weeks to the chronic phase. The organisms are now known as bradyzoites and divide slowly within a parasitic membrane to form the so-called tissue cyst. These may be found in any organ but are particularly common in the musculature and brain. By the time this stage is reached in the extraintestinal cycle, the host has developed an immunity and is resistant to reinfection, although the tissue cysts may persist for many months. A chronic infection may revert to the acute form if the animal is exposed to stress, immunosuppressive therapy or concurrent disease.

There are several ways in which an intermediate host may acquire infection:

1 By ingesting sporulated oocysts derived from the faeces of a cat.
2 By eating undercooked meat or the flesh of prey animals containing either pseudocysts or tissue cysts.
3 By transplacental infection, which occurs if the dam develops a parasitaemia during pregnancy.

There are fewer routes of infection for the cat as there is no prenatal transmission in this species. Also, the oocysts are of low infectivity to the definitive host, but a good mouser is constantly exposed to infection, as are cats fed uncooked meat.

Prevalence
Extrapolation of existing data suggests that approximately one-third of the world's dogs have demonstrable antibodies to *T. gondii*. Small surveys conducted in England have revealed corresponding figures of around 40%. In contrast, only 5% of Dublin dogs showed evidence of past infection.

Control
Prophylactic measures are complicated by the fact that there are several sources of infection. If all meat was fed to dogs tinned or adequately cooked, one route of transmission would be eliminated, but if there is opportunity for scavenging or hunting, these efforts would be negated. In homes where dogs and cats co-exist, the daily removal of feline faeces from the litter-tray will ensure the destruction of oocysts before sporulation. Little can be done, however, to prevent the ingestion of oocysts shed by cats outdoors. At any point in time, about 1% of a cat population may be expected to have an active intestinal infection. The

oocysts, like the eggs of Toxocara, are very resistant and can retain their viability in soil for prolonged periods.

For the treatment of acute infections, sulphonamides, such as sulphadiazine, sulphamethazine and sulphamerazine have been recommended, either alone or synergised with pyrimethamine. (It should be noted that toxicity has been reported following the use of pyrimethamine in cats.)

HELMINTHS ASSOCIATED WITH LARGE KENNELS

There are three parasites that are commonly found in animals bred or kept in large kennel establishments but which occur less frequently in other dogs. These are *Uncinaria stenocephala* (the northern or cold climate hookworm), *Trichuris vulpis* (the whipworm) and *Filaroides osleri* (a nematode found around the bifurcation of the trachea). Transmission of the two intestinal parasites is facilitated by the aggregation of large numbers of dogs sharing grass exercising runs. Knowledge of the life-cycle of *F. osleri* is incomplete, but it has been suggested that the pup acquires infection from the dam soon after birth. If this is true, it would help to explain the restricted distribution of this parasite.

Uncinaria

Most publications on the subject of hookworm disease refer to infection with the very pathogenic *Ancylostoma caninum*, but this has only been recorded in two native-born animals (both red foxes from, respectively, Argyll and SW Wales). However, *U. stenocephala* is commonly found in the United Kingdom and so the following paragraphs will refer solely to this parasite, while *A. caninum* is considered on p. 478.

The hookworms are stoutish nematodes, less than 2 cm long, that live attached to the wall of the small intestine. The two genera can only be distinguished microscopically: Ancylostoma has several pairs of 'fangs' on the ventral rim of the mouth which are lacking in Uncinaria. Both hookworms produce typical 'strongyle' eggs with those of Uncinaria (Fig. 17.1) marginally larger, although this is not a reliable diagnostic feature.

Clinical signs

U. stenocephala is generally thought to be non-pathogenic, although experimentally an infection of only 1000 larvae will cause diarrhoea. Certainly, the cold climate hookworm does not suck blood like its tropical

cousin and anaemia will result only from massive infestations. Smaller infestations are associated with a 'leakage' of protein into the gut which probably accounts for reports of 'digestive disturbances' and poor condition in infected dogs. Many Greyhound trainers believe that hookworms have an adverse effect on racing times.

Hookworm dermatitis occurs in some dogs exposed to large numbers of infective *U. stenocephala* larvae. Moderate acanthosis and hyperkeratinisation are seen on the trunk but the most severe lesions are found on the feet. The interdigital skin becomes pruritic, reddened and moist, while the hair is lost. In severe cases, the paw becomes swollen and deformities of the pads and claws may develop.

Prevalence

U. stenocephala is particularly common in Greyhounds and hunt kennels but this parasite is likely to be encountered wherever groups of dogs are exercised on grass runs. Greyhounds often acquire heavy infections within the first few weeks of life. Immunity does develop but this is a slow process, with the proportion that pass hookworm eggs in the faeces falling from some 40% in young racing dogs to 12.5% in those nearing retirement. Between 5 and 66% of sheep dogs have been shown to carry hookworm and it is possible that foxes may act as a reservoir of infection since the prevalence rate in these animals can be as high as 91% in some areas. In contrast, hookworm is rarely found in pet animals or show dogs.

Epidemiology

Although *U. stenocephala* larvae can penetrate skin (thereby provoking the pedal dermatitis described earlier) this rarely results in the establishment of an intestinal infection. Perinatal infection seldom occurs and so the primary route of infection is by ingestion.

Infective larvae can develop anywhere where there is sufficient warmth and moisture, but in kennels maintaining a good standard of hygiene indoors, the most likely source of infection is the grass exercising paddock. In this environment, the development of the egg and larva is influenced by weather conditions, producing a pattern of events reminiscent of that recorded for the trichostrongyloid parasites of ruminants. Thus, there is a regular fluctuation in the numbers of infective forms contaminating the herbage. The overwintering larvae die away in the spring or early summer to be replaced by a new generation with peak numbers occurring in the later summer or winter.

Control

Control is dependent upon hygiene, the elimination of

sources of infection (e.g. by replacing grass paddocks with concrete runs), and the use of anthelmintics. Suitable compounds include: dichlorvos, mebendazole, nitroscanate, pyrantel, thenium and fenbendazole.

Trichuris

The whipworm is easily recognised by the characteristically slender anterior portion of the body which contrasts with the substantially stouter posterior part. It grows up to 7 cm long and is found in the caecum with its head and neck buried in the mucosa, while the rest of the worm projects into the lumen.

Clinical signs
Many dogs which pass trichuroid eggs show no obvious clinical signs, but others lose condition and may be intermittently diarrhoeic, and sometimes pass dark, foul-smelling faeces. The variety of host responses to infection is possibly due to the fact that secondary invasion by potentially pathogenic intestinal microflora may follow the primary mucosal damage caused by the worm. Diagnosis can be difficult as the brown, barrel-shaped eggs (with plugs at either end) are not passed continuously in the faeces. Even if present in the faeces, they float well only in a solution with a relatively high specific gravity (e.g. sat. zinc. sulphate soln.) and may be overlooked if the customary sodium chloride is used.

Epidemiology and control
Because of the difficulties of diagnosis, there are few reliable statistics on the occurrence of this worm in the UK, but *T. vulpis* is generally found in the same groups of dogs as *U. stenocephala*. In one study, examination of racing Greyhounds at necropsy revealed that 32% were infected and it is relevant to note that only 6% of dogs from the same source had positive egg counts. The prevalence rate in pets and show dogs is, however, very low (around 1%).

The epidemiology of whipworm infections is distinct from that of the northern hookworm as the preparasitic stages of the life-cycle behave differently. The egg of *T. vulpis* does not hatch, but the larva grows to the infective stage within the tough protective shell. In the UK this process requires a period of months, as the optimum conditions for development (a mean day–night temperature of 25–30°C for 9–10 days) are rarely approached even in the height of the British summer. However the egg is very long lived and a grass paddock once contaminated will remain a potential source of infection for at least 5 years. Desiccation will kill the ova, but as drought conditions occur in-

frequently in Britain the only feasible means of reducing the risk of infection is to dig and reseed. Control is of course easier with concrete exercising areas, as regular hosing and scrubbing will prevent the accumulation of large numbers of eggs and a horticultural flame-gun can be applied if necessary.

Whipworm infections in domestic animals are notoriously difficult to treat. This is probably due to the fact that Trichuris is only distantly related to the nematode genera that usually constitute the targets for chemotherapeutic attack. In the dog, mebendazole, fenbendazole oxantel have good efficacy against *T. vulpis*, but on occasion several courses of treatment will be required to clear the infection. This is said to be because oedema at the entrance to the caecum hinders the passage of drugs (at least those that are not absorbed into the bloodstream) to the site of parasitism in that organ.

Filaroides

Filaroides osleri is a serious pathogen which poses great problems both with regard to diagnosis and treatment. The adult worms are found in clusters in nodules projecting into the trachea and bronchi, particularly around the bifurcation of the trachea. The lesions are hyperaemic, raised, elongated and/or pedunculated, varying in size from 1 mm to 2 cm. Sometimes they may partially or completely occlude a primary or secondary bronchus. The hind ends of the worms (which may be over 1 cm in length) are easily visible protruding from the nodules.

Clinical signs
Many cases are symptomless, but infection sometimes produces a severe tracheobronchitis characterised by a chronic dry cough, exacerbated by exercise, which sometimes ends with a retching action. Serious cases are emaciated and may be dyspnoeic when excited. The disease is most often seen in young animals (4–6 months old) but can also occur in young adults.

Parasitological diagnosis depends upon the demonstration of embryonated eggs or larvae in the faeces, sputum or tracheal mucus, although a negative finding does not exclude the possibility of parasitic tracheobronchitis as the ova are not produced continuously, even in heavy infections. The larvae are approximately 250 μm long with an S-shaped tail (Fig. 17.3) but care is needed to differentiate them from those of *Angiostrongylus vasorum* (see p. 480). A more reliable technique is direct visualisation of the nodules by bronchoscopy. A serological test for *F. osleri* would be of great value but none exists at the time of writing

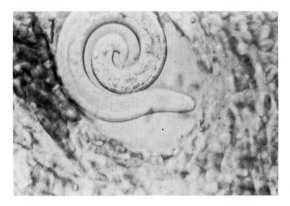

Fig. 17.3 *Filaroides osleri* larva in tracheal mucus. Photograph by P. Stevenson.

Epidemiology and control

While parasitic tracheobronchitis is diagnosed from time to time in dogs kept singly, transmission of infection is usually associated with breeding kennels. The life-cycle of *F. osleri* has not been established with certainty, but it seems likely that larvae ascending the respiratory tract of breeding bitches are transferred to the offspring by licking. It is not known whether horizontal transmission can take place in a population of weaned dogs. Although all breeds seem equally susceptible, the parasite is particularly prevalent in Greyhounds, with approximately 1 in 5 carrying infection.

At the present time, there is no treatment for parasitic tracheobronchitis that is known to be consistently effective. Surgical removal of the nodules has been recommended in the past, but there is hope that some of the newer anthelmintics will provide a simple solution to the problem. The following regimes have shown promise, but require further evaluation:

1 Oral administration of a coated tablet formulation of levamisole (Ketrax) at a rate of 7.5 mg/kg daily for 10–20 days.
2 Oral administration of thiabendazole at 32 mg/kg b.i.d. for 3 weeks, reducing the dose if the animal vomits.
3 Oral administration of fenbendazole has also given good results but at the time of writing the optimum dose rate has yet to be determined.
4 Two courses of treatment with albendazole separated by a two week interval using a dose-rate of 25 mg/kg twice daily for 5 days.

Of these anthelmintics, only fenbendazole is currently licenced for the treatment of dogs in the UK.

If modern concepts of the epidemiology of this con-

dition are correct, prophylaxis will depend on the accurate identification and treatment of symptomless carrier animals in breeding kennels.

These comments apply also to another species of Filaroides, *F. hirthi*, which is a tiny worm found in the lung parenchyma (Fig. 17.4). This is one of the few helminths that can multiply within the final host. It is found in laboratory Beagle colonies in the USA and has been suspected on occasion in the UK. It is of significance as the associated lung pathology may complicate the interpretation of toxicological studies. Respiratory problems in the USA have occasionally been associated with a third species *F. milksi* which also lives in the lung parenchyma.

PARASITES OF PUBLIC HEALTH IMPORTANCE

At an earlier period in evolutionary history, man was a potential prey animal for wolves and the ancestors of today's pets. More recently, a very close relationship has developed between man and the domestic dog. Therefore it is not surprising if some parasites of the dog involve man in their life-cycle or invade his tissues 'accidentally'. Man's involvement as a potential paratenic host in the life-cycle of *Toxocara canis* has already been described (see p. 465). There is also a tapeworm, *Echinococcus granulosus*, that utilises a wide variety of potential prey animals, but this time as intermediate hosts. In this case, man does not function very efficiently from the parasite's viewpoint as most of the intermediate forms (hydatid cysts) in human tissue are sterile and incapable of infecting a dog. Nevertheless, their presence is distressing and of considerable medical importance. The metacestode of *Taenia multiceps* (*Coenurus cerebralis*), usually found in sheep, also occurs in man, but very rarely. One adult tapeworm of pet animals is seen occasionally in man, *Dipylidium caninum*. Reference to the section on ubiquitous parasites in this chapter (see p. 466) will confirm that infection is dependent on the ingestion of a flea carrying the cysticercoid. This factor obviously limits its distribution in the human population.

Other conditions that are believed to be of little importance in the UK include human infection with *Trichuris vulpis* and cutaneous larva migrans caused by the migration of Uncinaria larvae in the skin of hypersensitive persons.

Recently some concern has been expressed about the possible role of the dog in the epidemiology of human giardiasis. This is the most frequently diagnosed form of protozoal enteritis in man in the UK. It is caused by a small pear-shaped cyst-forming flagel-

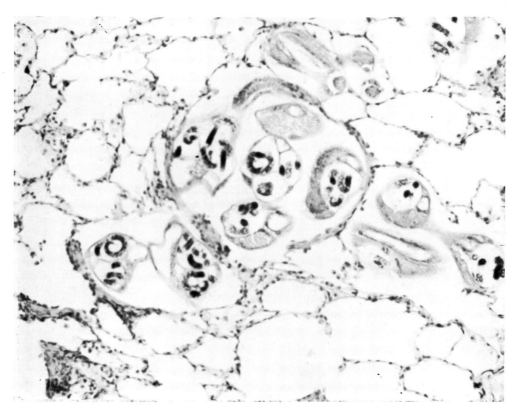

Fig. 17.4 Section of lung from a Beagle bred in the UK showing a nematode worm, probably *Filaroides hirthi*. Photograph by M.J. Walker.

late organism, *Giardia lamblia*. While it is known to occur occasionally in British dogs there is as yet no evidence to suggest canine involvement in human outbreaks. Entamoeba and Balantidium are other intestinal protozoa that have been recorded in dogs elsewhere but have no zoonotic significance in the UK.

Toxocara

Public health importance

When man ingests the embryonated ova of Toxocara, hatching takes place and, just as in any paratenic host (see p. 465), the larvae invade the tissues of the body. Fortunately, these larvae, which are rather less than 0.5 mm in length, rarely cause significant damage. However, in certain circumstances they may produce clinical disease. For example, the acquisition of an unusually large number of larvae will produce a generalised syndrome with eosinophilia, pyrexia and hepatomegaly, sometimes accompanied by encephalitis, dyspnoea or a skin reaction. Such cases usually occur in young children with a history of pica and are fortunately rare in the UK.

The second way in which trouble may occur is if just one larva by misfortune happens to settle in a particularly sensitive tissue such as the retina. When this happens the prognosis is serious as affected patients can suffer a unilateral impairment of vision. But this too is a relatively rare occurrence. For example, one medical expert, who takes a particular interest in toxocariasis, has diagnosed just one case with ocular involvement over a 5-year period. His patients are drawn from a suburban area of England housing some 300 000 people. Professor A.W. Woodruff at the Toxocaral Reference Laboratory, London, recorded 54 cases from all areas of the United Kingdom during 1977.

Professor Woodruff has also conducted a number of surveys in which selected patients suffering from various undiagnosed conditions have been tested for their reaction to the toxocaral skin test or a fluorescent antibody test. With the former test, approximately 2% of apparently healthy persons gave a positive response, whereas some 8–10% of patients with choroidoretinitis or uveitis and 7.5% of epilepsy cases were positive, suggesting that the presence of larvae in the eye or brain may be one of many factors involved in the aetiology of these conditions. More recent work in the USA using an ELISA test has compared epileptic patients whose disease was of unknown aetiology with those whose affliction had a known non-parasitic cause. An abnormally high proportion of seropositives was found in both groups indicating that toxocaral infections may be a consequence of this disease rather than a precipitating factor. The affinity of Toxocara larvae for nervous tissue led to an examination of sera from patients with paralytic poliomyelitis and it was found that 14.6% gave positive reactions, suggesting that another way in which Toxocara may cause damage is by exacerbating a pre-existing infection. Finally, Woodruff's studies, supported by those of other workers, have also led to the suspicion that Toxocara larvae may produce disease in patients susceptible to allergies, with 17–19% of patients with undiagnosed asthmatic and related conditions reacting positively to these tests.

Epidemiology and control

Man becomes infected by ingesting the sticky, embryonated eggs of Toxocara in faeces, soil or dust which have contaminated his fingers or food, and so it is necessary to define the source of this infection. It is important to remember that while all *T. canis* ova originate from the faeces of dogs and foxes, fresh faecal material is not infective to man as the eggs are not yet embryonated. If the Toxocara egg behaves like that of Ascaris, the development of the infective larva within the egg may take only 2–3 weeks in midsummer, but a period of months is required at other times of the year. During this period of weeks or months, the faecal mass will have disintegrated and dispersed. This is why there is little observed relationship between the occurrence of specific antibodies to Toxocara in children and the possession of pets.

Thus, it is important to discover to what degree our environment is contaminated by these ova. A number of investigators have conducted surveys in various parts of the United Kingdom and it is apparent that in urban areas there is a substantial reservoir of infection. For example, Toxocara eggs were found in one-quarter of a series of 800 soil samples from cities and towns throughout England, Scotland and Wales, and in 1 in 20 of 5200 soil scrapings from the London area. Not all these eggs, however, are necessarily those of *T. canis*, as the ova of *T. cati* are so similar in appearance that differentiation is impractical in this type of survey.

As might be expected, Toxocara ova are more abundant in large kennel establishments and people working in such environments would seem to be at greater risk. Two investigations conducted in the UK confirmed that such people were exposed to a greater risk than the general population, but it was found that only 2 of 34 Greyhound kennel workers and 3 of 102 dog breeders possessed significant antibody levels. It was concluded that *T. canis* infection is not readily acquired by dog handlers who maintain a reasonable standard of hygiene and this view is supported by a more recent survey of veterinarians and animal hospital employees in the USA. However, clinical cases do occur in Britain, usually in children as one cannot demand or expect a consistently high standard of hygiene in this age group. It is clearly the responsibility of the veterinary profession and the dog-owning public to make this small risk still smaller. The control measures summarised earlier in this chapter (see p. 465) will serve to reduce the public health risk as well as protect the health of the canine population. Worm control should be an integral part of all educational schemes promoting responsible pet ownership, but total elimination of Toxocara eggs from the environment involves wider issues such as the control of infection in neglected dogs, strays, foxes and cats.

Echinococcus

Echinococcus granulosus is a tapeworm that uses canine definitive hosts and a wide variety of potential prey animals, including man, as intermediate hosts. An infected dog may harbour several thousand adult worms, each of which is less than 9 mm in length and consists of only 3 or 4 proglottids. The eggs contained in the gravid segments that pass in the dog's faeces are indistinguishable from those of the other taeniid cestodes (see p. 474). The metacestode in the intermediate host is known as the hydatid cyst. This may grow up to 10 cm in diameter and typically consists of a germinal layer enclosing a fluid suspension of protoscoleces (the stage of parasite infective to the dog).

Public health importance

Most of the hydatid cysts that develop in man are found in the liver and lungs, but some develop in other organs, including the spleen, kidneys, and bone marrow. The effect is that of a space-occupying lesion in the affected organ. Rupture of the cyst (e.g. as a result of injuries sustained in a motor accident), may result in anaphylactic shock or the formation of daughter cysts. At present, the only feasible remedy for hydatidosis in man is surgical removal, but some of the newer anthelmintics give promise of a medical treatment in the near future.

Hydatid disease in man is largely confined to those areas of England, Scotland and Wales where there is frequent contact between dogs and extensively grazed sheep. During the period 1970–74, 21 people died from hydatidosis in England (this total includes some cases almost certainly contracted overseas) and 11 in Wales. This, however, is the tip of the iceberg and it has been estimated that the annual incidence rate in Powys, one of the most heavily infected areas of the United Kingdom, may be in excess of 4–5 per 10 000 inhabitants. In the same region of mid-Wales, a recent serological survey using an indirect haemagglutination test showed titres in excess of 160 in 15 of 147 volunteers, while only 14 gave no evidence of antibodies to hydatids. As a control, sera from 36 people in the Cambridge area, where hydatid disease is rare, were examined with the same test and all gave negative results.

Epidemiology

There is strong evidence to suggest that there are two strains of *E. granulosus* in the British Isles: the sheep strain (*E. granulosus granulosus*) and the horse strain (*E. granulosus equinus*); the descriptive terms refer to the preferred intermediate host of each biological form of the parasite.

The occurrence of hydatid cysts in English horses appeared to increase in the post-war years to reach a peak of between 35 and 60% in the mid-1970s. The current prevalence of infection seems to be about 10%, although this figure is greatly influenced by locality, the age structure of the population and whether or not the remains of dead cysts are included. The main source of *E.g. equinus* eggs appears to be hounds used for hunting: 11 of 21 packs were found to be infected in one survey. The increased prevalence was attributed to changes in the feeding regime in hunt kennels where more raw horse meat and offal was offered. The discovery initially caused some anxiety as rural populations, horse riders, picknickers and hunt kennel workers have apparently been exposed to a greater risk than previously. However, circumstantial evidence from Ireland suggests that *E. g. equinus* is of low infectivity for man since in that country, where the horse strain is common but the sheep strain is non-existent, human cases of hydatidosis are rarely reported. Additionally, attempts to infect non-human primates experimentally with the British horse strain of *E. granulosus* have so far been unsuccessful.

The sheep strain is undoubtedly pathogenic to man, who is infected by ingesting eggs that have originated from the faeces of dogs or foxes harbouring the adult tapeworm. Fortunately, *E. g. granulosus* is rare in town and country dogs in most areas of the UK, but prevalence rates of around 3.5% have been recorded in the Pennines and Lake District. Between 9 and 29% of farm dogs and Foxhounds in mid-Wales carry infection, as do 3–37% of foxes. Infection is also known to occur on some of the Scottish islands including Lewis, Harris and Skye.

Abattoir surveys provide a good indicator of the level of infection in an area. Thus, few sheep born and reared in eastern England show infection, whereas hydatid cysts are found in 4–5% in the north-west of England and 5–37% in Wales. Over all, 2.7% of sheep offal and 1.5% of cattle offal was partially condemned on account of hydatidosis in England and Wales during the period 1973–76. It is relevant to note that sheep from Wales are sold to all counties of England and Scotland, so that there is a risk of canine infections being established in all areas.

The areas of heaviest infestation are those where dogs are likely to scavenge sheep carcases or are fed on uncooked offal. Details of the epidemiology vary from place to place. For example, one report describes how pet dogs could acquire infection from sheep that had adopted the abnormal habit of scavenging in gardens and refuse-tips in certain towns in the mining valleys of South Wales. More often, the endemic area embraces an agricultural community where sheep are of necessity kept extensively on hilly or mountainous terrain. Under these circumstances, farm dogs are likely to find ovine casualties before even the most conscientious farmer. Dogs tend to defaecate in fields immediately adjoining farm buildings so that sheep are exposed to relatively heavy concentrations of Echinococcus eggs when the flock is gathered on lower ground for lambing or dipping.

Control

National control schemes are being practised with considerable success in Iceland, New Zealand, Cyprus and Uruguay. In New Zealand, the prevalence of infection in dogs has fallen from 3.45% at the start of the campaign in 1960 to 0.004% in 1982. In the same period the occurrence of hydatid cysts in ewes has been reduced from 57.8% to 0.21%.

In preparation for a control programme, parasitological data has to be accumulated for each district to define local epidemiological patterns and to provide a base line for assessing progress. The subsequent campaign is often based on the following principles:

1 The registration of all working, hunting and pet dogs.

2 Regular treatment of dogs with an effective anthelmintic (e.g. bunamidine, nitroscanate or prazi-quantel). The choice of drug and treatment interval depends on local circumstances but the most reliable results are achieved with praziquantel given every sixth week.

3 Routine arecoline purging to monitor progress and identify sources of infection. Regrettably examination of the purged material for the presence of adult worms is still the only reasonably accurate method of diagnosing *E. granulosus* infection in the living dog.

4 An intensive educational campaign to make dog owners aware of the risk and their responsibilities.

5 Legislation to ensure that untreated offal is not fed to dogs.

In the UK, a pilot scheme has been conducted in two Welsh valleys under the direction of the South Powys Hydatid Liaison Group. Early results have been promising and at the time of writing the feasibility of extending this project is under consideration.

PARASITES OF IMPORTANCE IN MEAT INSPECTION

It has already been noted in this chapter that many parasites of the dog exploit their predatory habits by using potential prey animals as intermediate hosts. Those exploiting man in this way were discussed above; the following paragraphs deal with those incorporating meat animals in their life-cycles.

Some parasites fall into both these categories. Echinococcus, for example, is an important zoonosis but is also a cause of considerable economic loss to the meat industry in endemic areas. In Britain, the value of offal rejected because of hydatid cysts is estimated to be in the order of £250 000 pa. Meat inspection plays an important role in safeguarding man from hydatid disease by reducing the opportunities for canine infection.

Toxocara must also be mentioned in this context as larvae passing through the liver of the pig produce 'milkspot' lesions indistinguishable from those associated with *Ascaris suum*. A recent survey showed that pigs from 14% of 1016 British herds showed serological evidence of Toxocara infection. However, fewer than 0.1% of the pigs had high antibody titres and it was concluded that Toxocara is rarely a significant factor in the production of focal interstitial hepatitis in Britain. Furthermore, this low level of infestation, coupled with the relatively short lifespan of the larvae in the pig, suggests that the consumption of pork products is an unlikely source of human toxocaral infection in the UK.

The species of Taenia harboured by the dog present only a minor hazard to man, but the occurrence of their metacestode forms in meat or offal is considered aesthetically undesirable and consequently leads to tissue condemnations. Finally, some of the sarcocysts seen macroscopically at the abattoir and microscopically in histological sections are now recognised as the intermediate stages of coccidia of the dog, cat and man. At the present time there is no evidence to suggest that the species using the dog as the final host are capable of infecting man, but new information on the biology and pathogenicity of Sarcocystis and related organisms is accumulating so rapidly that some of the views expressed in this chapter will inevitably be outdated by the time that these words appear in print.

Taenia

There are at least five species of the tapeworm genus Taenia which occur in the small intestine of dogs and foxes in temperate regions. A great deal of expertise is required to identify the adult worms although a generic diagnosis can be made quickly and easily. Taenia spp. are very considerably larger than Echinococcus; some species growing up to 3 m in length. To differentiate between Taenia and Dipylidium, it is necessary to examine individual proglottids. Those of Taenia have a single genital pore, often positioned on the opposite margins of adjacent segments. This contrasts with the double-pore pattern of Dipylidium or the single centrally placed pore of Spirometra or Diphyllobothrium (see p. 481). If a gravid segment of Taenia is crushed in a drop of water and examined microscopically the eggs, which are smaller than Toxocara ova and surrounded by the radially striated embryophore, are released individually and are not packaged in capsules.

Clinical signs and control

Diagnosis of infection in the dog depends on the chance discovery of proglottids. A more certain method of diagnosis is the arecoline purge, as used for the detection of echinococcosis. Such drastic measures are seldom necessary, however, as the adult tapeworms are of low pathogenicity. The main indications for treatment are the aesthetic requirements of the owner or the pruritus ani that may be associated with the emergence of segments from the anus. There is little public health risk associated with these worms, but as more epidemiological evidence is collected it is possible that an economic case could be made for protecting farm livestock from infection. Hydatid control programmes will also reduce the prevalence of

Taenia spp. Effective anthelmintics include: bunami-dine, dichlorophen, mebendazole, niclosamide, nitros-canate, fenbendazole and praziquantel.

Prevention of reinfection following chemotherapy involves strict dietary control, as the metacestode forms of Taenia spp. are all found in the musculature or viscera of meat animals or wild mammals. The influence that diet can have on the prevalence of the various Taenia spp. is well exemplified by a recent study comparing neighbouring kennels with different feeding regimes (Table 17.1).

Table 17.1 Influence of feeding regime on prevalence of Taenia spp. in two foxhound packs in same locality (modified from Edwards *et al* (1979) *Br. Vet. J.* **135**, 433).

Food	Pack A	Pack B
	Commercial dog food supplemented with farm livestock casualties from own farm, rabbits and hares.	Livestock carcases from local farms; offal and sheep's heads from local abattoir.
Taenia hydatigena	5.0%	46.9%
Taenia multiceps	0.6%	26.6%
Taenia ovis	1.7%	14.1%
Taenia pisiformis	6.0%	—

Life-cycles and prevalence

The Taenia spp. of the dog may be conveniently divided into three groups:

T. hydatigena and T. pisiformis

The metacestode of each of these is a cysticercus (i.e. a bladder worm with one inverted scolex) found in the peritoneal cavity of the intermediate hosts, which include the sheep, ox and pig in the former case and the rabbit and hare in the latter. The metacestode of *T. hydatigena* is known as *C. tenuicollis* in meat inspection and is a fluid-filled cyst of up to 7–8 cm diameter found free or adhering to the omentum, mesentery or other serosal surface. *T. pisiformis* infections often have the appearance of a bunch of grapes on the omentum and mesentery.

The intermediate host is infected by eating herbage contaminated with Taenia eggs. An adult tapeworm may persist in the dog for several years and 50 000–100 000 eggs may be passed each day. The eggs from a single faecal deposit have been observed to spread irregularly over an area of 20 000 m² within 10 days.

The oncospheres are immediately infective and may survive for several months under winter conditions but exposure to hot dry conditions will quickly kill them. Following infection, the oncosphere hatches out, passes by way of the hepatic portal system to the liver and migrates through the parenchyma to reach the abdominal cavity. In doing so, haemorrhagic and fibrotic tracts are formed and if considerable numbers of parasites are involved an acute disease syndrome reminiscent of fascioliasis may result.

There are very few reliable figures for the prevalence of Taenia spp. in the definitive host in the UK, but *T. pisiformis* has been recorded in 10% of Foxhounds in mid-Wales and 3–25% of farm dogs in various areas. Corresponding figures for *T. hydatigena* are 49% and 0 (East Anglia) to 55% (mid-Wales), respectively. A recent survey in Dyfed showed that 40% of the lambs in that area were infected with *C. tenuicollis*.

T. ovis

The dog–sheep/goat life-cycle of *T. ovis* is very similar to the better-known man-ox cycle of *T. saginata*. The cysticerci measure up to 6 mm and are found in the striated musculature. The prevalence of *T. ovis* in British dogs is generally low, as is the level of infection in the intermediate host. Infection levels of up to 14% have, however, been recorded in some groups of dogs in Wales.

This parasite has, however, been the cause of substantial economic loss to some meat-exporting countries. For example, 12.5% of Australian shipments of boneless mutton to the USA, valued at over $1½ million, were rejected during the first half of 1968 because of *T. ovis*. Consequently, an experimental vaccine has been produced using antigens collected during the *in vitro* incubation of activated oncospheres. Early results suggest that lambs can be protected from infection in this way but further evaluation is required before the commercial value of this approach can be assessed.

T. multiceps and T. serialis

The characteristic shared by this pair of tapeworms is the development of a coenurus in the intermediate host (i.e. a bladderworm with multiple inverted scolices). That of *T. serialis* is found in the intermuscular connective tissue of the rabbit and that of *T. multiceps* (which is also known as *Multiceps multiceps*) in the brain of the sheep. In the latter case the metacestode, termed *C. cerebralis*, may produce an intracranial space-occupying lesion up to 5 cm in diameter which in turn may result in behavioural changes such as the classical 'gid' or impairment of the surefootedness so necessary in mountainous terrain.

A survey in mid-Wales (B.M. Williams, pers. comm.) showed that cases of 'gid' had occurred on 80% of 610 farms with average losses of 3% of the lamb flock. At a local slaughterhouse, 58 of 1000 heads from apparently normal lambs contained coenuri. Approximately 1 in 10 farm dogs and hounds in the area harboured *T. multiceps*, but only 1 of 360 foxes was infected. The prevalence of *T. serialis* in British dogs is generally below 5%.

Sarcocystis and other intestinal coccidia

The dog is the definitive host of at least ten species of coccidia. One of these, *Hammondia heydorni*, is closely related to Toxoplasma, but the veterinary and public health implications of this parasite are at present unclear.

The remaining coccidial species belong to two ge-nera: Isospora and Sarcocystis (Fig. 17.5). Unfortunately there is confusion regarding the nomenclature of this group of parasites. Some workers maintain that the Isospora species of the dog should be assigned to a new genus named 'Levineia' or 'Cystoisospora' on the grounds that the canine species use facultative or obligatory intermediate hosts whereas most Isospora spp. have a direct life-cycle. Rodents are able to act as intermediate host in the laboratory but it is not known which animals perform this role in nature. The intestinal forms of Sarcocystis were previously thought to be Isospora spp. but it is now known that the life-cycles of these parasites are fundamentally different, as will become apparent below, and so there is no doubt as to their true generic name. There is, however, disagreement over the species names. One school of thought advocates descriptive names, *S. bovicanis*, for example, being a species using cattle as intermediate host and the dog as final host. Others insist on the

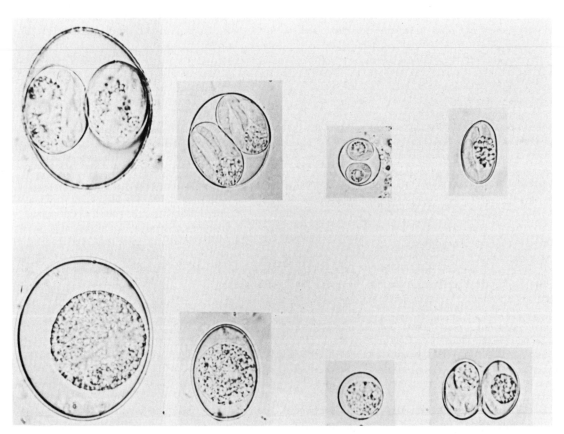

Fig. 17.5 Coccidial oocysts and sporocysts from the faeces of the dog. From left to right: *Isospora canis, I. ohioensis, Hammondia heydorni, Sarcocystis cruzi*; to scale, the oocyst of *I. canis* measures approx. 38 × 30 μm. Reproduced from Rommel (1975) Neue Erkenntnisse zur Biologie der Kolkzidien, Toxoplasmen, Sarkosporidien und Besnoitien. *Berl. Münch. tierärztl Wschr.* **88,** 112, with permission.

strict application of the International Laws of Nomenclature, which in this case gives the name *S. cruzi* precedence.

Clinical signs

Some parasitologists doubt reports of the pathogenicity of the canine coccidia as many attempts to reproduce the disease experimentally have failed. There have been descriptions, however, of epidemic outbreaks of diarrhoea in kennels associated with high faecal isosporan oocyst counts. Sulpha drugs or nitrofurazone are recommended in such cases.

Life-cycle

A dog becomes infected with Sarcocystis when it consumes the flesh of an animal harbouring the tissue-cysts of an appropriate species of the parasite. The definitive host seems unable to produce a protective immunity to Sarcocystis spp. and so reinfection is possible. The bradyzoites released from the tissue-cyst invade the lamina propria of the small intestine. In this site, they immediately undergo gametogony forming oocysts which sporulate and are subsequently released slowly over an extended period of time. The oocyst wall is very fragile and so faecal examinations usually reveal free sporocysts in very low numbers.

When sporocysts contaminating herbage are ingested by the intermediate host, the sporozoites that are released invade the body and undergo schizogony in the endothelial cells of blood vessels. This is followed by the formation of tissue-cysts in the musculature. The cysts are much larger and more elaborate than those of Toxoplasma; they are divided into compartments and vary in size from a few millimetres to several centimetres. A further phase of asexual multiplication involving cells termed metrocytes occurs within the cyst, and finally gives rise to the infective form, the bradyzoite.

Prevalence

A high proportion of meat animals harbour macroscopic or microscopic sarcocysts in their musculature. It has become apparent in recent years that the sarcocysts seen at the abattoir belong to a variety of species, with some using the dog and fox as definitive hosts while others use the cat or man. Intensive work is in progress to define the morphology and biological characteristics of each species, but at the time of writing the situation is confused and it is not possible to assess the relative frequency of occurrence of each.

Sarcocystis spp. oocysts or sporocysts have been recovered from the faeces of 36.5% of sheepdogs and 17.0% of foxes in North Wales and 24.0% of Greyhounds in South-east England. The species recovered were *S. cruzi*, *S. ovicanis* and *S. miescheriana* which infect cattle, sheep and pigs respectively. Experimentally, *S. cruzi* and *S. ovicanis* are extremely pathogenic to their intermediate hosts. The period of multiplication in the vascular endothelium is associated with an acute febrile disease with anaemia, abortion and even death. Several suspected field outbreaks have been reported in cattle in North America, but the true incidence of this condition is unknown. There are also two species of Sarcocystis, not as yet isolated from British dogs, that infect the horse.

PARASITES LIKELY TO OCCUR IN QUARANTINE KENNELS

Dogs entering the United Kingdom and the Republic of Ireland are subject to the *Rabies (Importation of Dogs, Cats and Other Mammals) Order (1974) (Amendment) Order (1977)*. This involves restriction to a licensed quarantine kennel for a period of 6 months, during which time the animals are under veterinary supervision. Although there is no regulation relating to the control of endoparasites in imported dogs, it is obviously desirable that exotic infections should be detected and treated.

There is little published information on the number of imported animals that harbour exotic parasitisms. Routine faecal examination of 320 dogs from all parts of the world kept at one quarantine kennel in South-east England over a 4-year period, demonstrated the presence of hookworms in 35 (of which 19 originated from the USA and Carribean, with 7 from Africa). No attempt was made to distinguish the ova of Uncinaria and Ancylostoma but many of the infections were undoubtedly of the latter genus. Ascarids were found in 15 dogs (10 from the USA) and Trichuris in 5 (3 from the USA).

Not all parasites can be detected by faecal examination. *Dirofilaria immitis*, a filarial nematode, is the cause of heartworm disease which presents particular problems to the veterinary surgeon both with respect to diagnosis and treatment. Canine dirofilariasis is considered to be one of the most important conditions seen in small animal practice in the USA and is found from time to time in quarantine dogs. Disease causing intracellular protozoan parasites occurring in warmer climates include *Babesia canis*, found in erythrocytes, and Leishmania spp. in macrophages.

Dirofilaria

D. immitis is generally considered to be a parasite of tropical and subtropical regions, confined to these areas by the high temperatures required for completion of larval development in the intermediate host, the mosquito. Twenty years ago heartworm disease in the USA appeared to be widespread at serious disease-producing levels only within 50–70 miles of the Atlantic and Gulf coasts south of New Jersey with only one enzootic centre outside this region (in Minnesota). Since that time a rapidly increasing number of severe clinical cases have been recorded throughout the northern states of the USA and in some parts of Canada. A similar trend has been observed in Australia where heartworm has spread southwards along the eastern coastal strip into Victoria, but the endemic foci in southern Europe do not seem to be expanding.

The reason for this extension of the enzootic zone is unknown but is possibly connected with the greatly increased mobility of the human population, with pets moving into and out of endemic areas with their owners. Whether or not new strains of the parasite have evolved that are better adapted to more temperate climates is still a matter of speculation.

Whatever the reason, the spread of *D. immitis* into much cooler areas raises the question of whether the disease could become established in the UK. Several species of mosquito capable of acting as intermediate hosts do occur in this country but population densities are mostly lower than in the new endemic areas of the USA. Also the summer temperatures tend to be rather cooler and so, hopefully, the chances of transmission of infection from dog to dog taking place here are small. But in view of the seriousness of the disease and the number of dogs which are imported from endemic areas (3 a month from the Bahamas alone), the veterinary profession should be aware of the possibility.

Clinical signs

Affected dogs are often presented because of loss of exercise tolerance, sometimes associated with a shallow cough. Advanced cases may show weakness, haemoglobinuria and other signs of chronic right-sided cardiac insufficiency. Large numbers of worms in the posterior vena cava occasionally produce an acute syndrome with haemoglobinuria, jaundice and collapse.

Life-cycle and diagnosis

The adult worms grow to a length of 12–30 cm in the right ventricle and pulmonary artery. The females produce embryonic larvae known as microfilariae which circulate in the peripheral blood. More than 70 species of mosquito can act as intermediate hosts and disseminators of the infection.

The microfilariae, which are present in about 85% of heartworm-infected dogs, are easily detected by examining the sediment formed when 1 ml of freshly drawn blood and 10 ml of 2% formalin are mixed and centrifuged. A drop of 1% aqueous methylene blue assists microscopy. This is known as the modified Knott's technique. The microfilariae of *D. immitis* can be distinguished from those of the non-pathogenic *Dipetalonema reconditum* (see p. 480) as they are longer (more than 300 μm), have a tapered head and a straight tail. The numbers of microfilariae are not, however, always related to the severity of the disease and other aids to diagnosis such as biochemistry and radiology may be required to monitor the degree of organ damage and response to treatment.

The prepatent period of *D. immitis* averages $6\frac{1}{2}$ months, so infections acquired immediately prior to importation may not show clinically during the quarantine period.

Control

A non-infected dog entering an endemic area may be protected by the daily administration of diethylcarbamazine. This prophylactic treatment should continue for 80 days after exposure to infective mosquitoes has ceased.

Treatment to infected dogs can be hazardous and is divided into three phases:

1 Symptomatic therapy to improve the condition of the animal as much as possible before administering the necessary toxic drugs.
2 Elimination of the adult worms by giving thiacetarsamide or levamisole. The patient must be hospitalised and appropriate action taken if signs of toxicity appear.
3 Elimination of the circulating microfilariae with multiple doses of levamisole or dithiazanine.

Ancylostoma

Three species of *Ancylostoma* occur in the dog: *A. braziliense*, *A. ceylanicum* and *A. caninum* (the latter is the most common and the most pathogenic). All are found in the warmer regions of the globe. *A. caninum* is an avid blood-sucker producing anaemia. Transmission occurs by ingestion of third stage larvae, by skin penetration or via the colostrum and milk. As with Toxocara, the somatic larvae are extremely difficult to kill and so puppies born to imported bitches may be at risk. Infected animals build up a protective immunity and a successful vaccine has been developed although this is no longer available commercially. The anthelmintics listed as active against Uncinaria (see p. 468) are also effective against Ancylostoma.

Babesia

Canine babesiosis, also known as canine piroplasmosis or infectious haemoglobinuria, is a febrile disease characterised by progressive anaemia and jaundice. The acute form is usually fatal if untreated but chronic cases do occur. In endemic areas, such as southern Europe and parts of the USA, Latin America and Asia, many dogs are protected by premunity (i.e. they remain immune while possessing a low level parasitaemia). The intermediate hosts include a number of ticks. The most important of these is *Rhipicephalus sanguineus* which has been reported on rare occasions in the United Kingdom but generally requires a much hotter climate. It can, however, thrive in warm buildings and is often introduced into quarantine kennels where it can become a considerable nuisance. Prompt eradication is necessary under these circumstances to eliminate any possibility of the disease being transmitted to susceptible animals. Clinical cases can be confirmed by the demonstration of the large paired intraerythrocytic pyriform organisims in stained blood smears. Treatment with quinuronium sulphate or berenil aceturate has been recommended.

Leishmania

Canine visceral leishmaniasis can remain clinically inapparent for long periods of time and can thereby occur in dogs long after they have been released from quarantine. Several such cases have been diagnosed in the UK. Clinical signs are non-specific and leishmaniasis should be considered in the differential diagnosis of any imported dog showing chronic illness characterised by wasting, lymphadenopathy, skin lesions or diarrhoea. *Post mortem* examination will in addition reveal an enlarged spleen and multifocal granulomatous lesions in many organs. Leishmania spp. are intracellular protozoan parasites, closely related to the trypanosomes, that are transmitted by the bites of certain sandflies. Endemic zones encompass many of the warmer regions of the world including southern Europe and the Middle East. The organism can be demonstrated in smears made from *post mortem* lesions or biopsy material taken from lymph nodes or bone marrow. When stained with colophonium-Giemsa, the organisms can be seen in the cytoplasm of macrophages (Fig. 17.6). Extreme care is needed when handling suspect tissues. Antimonials are used

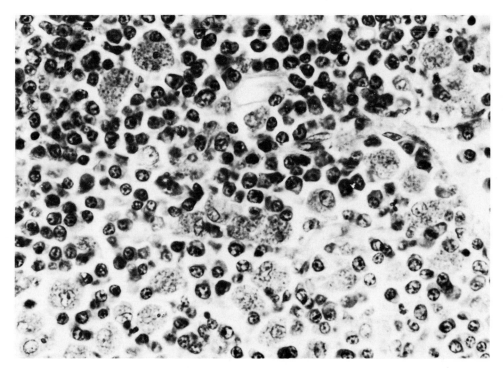

Fig. 17.6 Photomicrograph of lymph node cortex of dog suffering from leishmaniasis showing parasitised macrophages and plasma cells. Reproduced from Longstaffe *et al* (1983) *J. Small Anim. Pract.* **24**, 23, with permission.

for chemotherapy but treatment is difficult and perhaps undesirable outside of endemic areas as this parasite does pose a zoonotic hazard.

RARE PARASITES AND CURIOSITIES

As well as the infections of major interest described in the preceding sections of this chapter, there are many other parasites that can infect the dog. Some are endemic in the fox population but cannot maintain their life-cycles in a domestic environment. Others may be of considerable importance in other parts of the world but are only recognised occasionally in dogs imported into the British Isles. Two parasites that fall into neither of these categories, Angiostrongylus and Dipetalonema, are of sufficient clinical significance to warrant brief descriptions.

Angiostrongylus

A. vasorum is a metastrongyloid nematode found in the right ventricle and pulmonary artery (Fig. 17.7). It

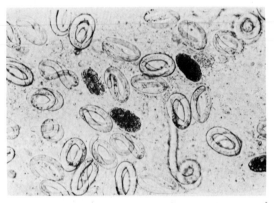

Fig. 17.7 *Angiostrongylus vasorum* larvae and eggs in tracheal mucus. Reproduced from Jacobs D.E. & Prole J.H.B. (1975) *Vet. Rec.* **96**, 180, with permission.

is 1–2 cm in length but only 0.2 mm wide. The eggs are carried to the lungs where they lodge in the capillaries. The larvae hatch, ascend the respiratory tree and can be found in large numbers in the faeces. Care is necessary to differentiate between the larvae of *A. vasorum* and *F. osleri* as each has an S-shaped tail. Those of the former species are, however, longer and more slender with a 'button' at the anterior extremity (Fig. 17.8). Dogs acquire infection by ingesting the intermediate hosts which include slugs and snails of various genera.

Infections are seen in Greyhounds and other breeds in Ireland, Cornwall and, rarely, elsewhere in Britain. Affected dogs lose condition and racing form, and later develop large subcutaneous swellings and an as-

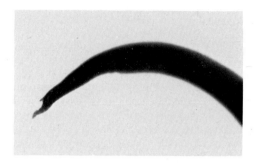

Fig. 17.8 *Angiostrongylus vasorum* Larva from faecal preparation stained with cotton blue to show structure of the tail. Photograph by P. Stevenson.

sociated deficiency in the blood clotting mechanisms. The condition responds to levamisole administered subcutaneously on three consecutive days at a dose rate of 10 mg/kg.

Dipetalonema

This non-pathogenic parasite lives under the skin and in fibrous tissue. Its significance in veterinary practice is that it gives rise to circulating microfilariae that could be mistaken for those of the canine heartworm. In wet blood smears, however, the microfilariae of Dipetalonema differ from those of Dirofilaria in that they show progressive movement, while in a Knott's preparation (see. p. 478) they are shorter (less than 300 μm), have a blunt head and a forward-curving ('button-hook') tail. Five per cent of British and Irish Greyhounds are infected with an unidentified species of this worm which is transmitted by the flea (Fig. 17.9).

Parasites of the fox

Capillaria aerophila is found in the trachea and bronchi of dogs in some large kennel establishments. The eggs, which are passed in the faeces, are double plugged and easily confused with those of Trichuris, but they are slightly smaller, have a greenish tinge and a rougher surface. *Capillaria plica* occurs in the bladder and kidney calices, with the eggs being passed during micturition. It is usually associated with hunt Terriers, Foxhounds and Beagle packs, but is of little pathogenic significance. More damaging is *Crenosoma vulpis*, a parasite of the bronchi and bronchioles which is recognised by the cuticular rings around the anterior of the body, but it is rarely reported in British dogs.

The dietary restrictions imposed on the domestic dog protect it from other parasites of the fox. Thus, several trematode species may be acquired by the consumption of raw fish containing cercariae and a tape-

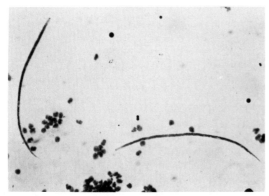

Fig. 17.9 Microfilariae from a British Greyhound (Knott's preparation). The species of *Dipetalonema* found in the British Isles lacks the button-hook tail typical of *D. reconditum*. Photograph by P. Stevenson.

worm from the ingestion of wild vertebrates harbouring the metacestode of *Mesocestoides lineatus*.

Exotic parasites

1 *Spirocerca lupi*, a spiruroid parasite of widespread occurrence in the tropics, is found in the oesophagus where it produces nodules that may become neoplastic.

2 Physaloptera and Gnathostoma, are spiruroid parasites of the stomach found in the Far East and certain other regions.

3 *Strongyloides stercoralis* occurs sporadically in the small intestine worldwide, but has not been reported from the UK. The dog may act as a reservoir for human infection but generally canine strains are of low pathogenicity to man.

4 *Dioctophyma renale*, the largest nematode of domestic animals, is found in the kidney and occurs in many temperate countries, but not in the UK.

5 Thelazia spp., another spiruroid, is found in the conjunctival sac: one species occurs in the Far East, another in California and neighbouring states.

6 *Diphyllobothrium latum* and Spirometra spp. are both pseudophyllidean cestodes and both are of importance as zoonoses. The former is found in temperate and subarctic regions while various species of the latter are found in North America, Asia and Australia.

FURTHER READING

The facts and figures quoted in this chapter originate from sources so numerous that it is not possible to acknowledge the authors individually. The following titles will lead the reader to more detailed accounts of many of the topics covered.

General
KELLY J.D. (1977) *Canine Parasitology*. University of Sydney Post-graduate Foundation in Veterinary Science, Review No. 17. (An excellent 110-page paperback with copious illustrations and comprehensive bibliography.)

Selected References
BARLOUGH, J.E. (1979) Canine giardiasis: a review. *J. small Anim. Pract.* **20**, 613.
CARLISLE C.H. (1980) Heart worm disease in dogs with particular reference to a protocol for treatment. In *Veterinary Annual*, 20th edn., p. 135, Eds. C.S.G. Grunsell & F.W.G. Hill. John Wright, Bristol.
CLARKSON, M.J. (1978) Hydatid disease in Wales: 2. Eradication. *Vet. Rec.* **102**, 259.
CLAYTON H.M. (1983) The management and treatment of respiratory nematode infections in small animals. In *Veterinary Annual*, 23rd edn, p. 254. Eds. C.S.G. Grunsell & F.W.G. Hill. John Wright, Bristol.
CLAYTON H.M. & LINDSAY F.E.F. (1979) *Filaroides osleri* infection in the dog. *J. small Anim, Pract.* **20**, 773.
DUBEY J.P. (1977) Toxoplasma, Hammondia, Besnoitia, Sarcocystis and other tissue cyst-forming coccidia of man and animals. In *Parasitic Protozoa* Vol. III, p. 101, Ed. J.P. Kreier. Academic Press, New York.
DÜWEL D. & STRASSER H. (1978) Versuche zur Geburt helminthen-freier Hundewelpen durch Fenbendazol-Behandlung. *Dtsch. Tierärztl. Wschr.* **85**, 239.
EDWARDS G.T. (1982) Observations on the epidemiology of equine hydatidosis in Britain. *Vet. Rec.* **110**, 511.
GEORGI J.R., GEORGI M.E., FAHNESTOCK G.R. & THEODORIDES V.J. (1979) Transmission and control of *Filaroides hirthi* lungworm infection in dogs. *Am. J. Vet. Res.* **40**, 829.
JACOBS D.E. (1978) The epidemiology of hookworm infection in dogs in the UK. In *Veterinary Annual*, 18th edn., p. 220, Eds. C.S.G. Grunsell & F.W.G. Hill. John Wright, Bristol.
JACOBS D.E., PEGG E.J. & STEVENSON P. (1977). Helminths of British dogs: *Toxocara canis*—a veterinary perspective. *J. small Anim. Pract.* **18**, 79.
LLOYD S., AMERASINGHE P.H. & SOULSBY E.J.L. (1983) Periparturient immunosuppression in the bitch and its influence on infection with *Toxocara caris. J. small Anim. Pract.* **24**, 237.
LONGSTAFFE J.A., JEFFERIES A.R., KELLY D.F., BEDFORD P.G.C., HERRTAGE M.E. & DARKE P.G.C. (1983) Leishmaniasis in imported dogs in the United Kingdom; a potential human health hazard. *J. small Anim. Pract.* **24**, 23.
MAHAFFEY M.B., LOSONSKY J.M., PRESTWOOD A.K., MAHAFFEY E.A. & LEWIS R.E. (1981) Experimental Canine Angiostrongylosis: II: Radiographic Manifestations. *J. Am. Anim. Hosp. Assoc.* **17**, 499.
PRESTWOOD A.K., GREENE C.E., MAHAFFEY E.A. & BURGESS D.E. (1981) Experimental Canine Angiostrongylosis: I. Pathologic Manifestations. *J. Am. Anim. Hosp. Assoc.* **17**, 491.
TURNER W.T. & PEGG E.J. (1977) A survey of patent nematode infestations in dogs. *Vet. Rec.* **100**, 284.
WALTERS T.M.H. (1978) Hydatid disease in Wales: 1. Epidemiology. *Vet. Rec.* **102**, 257.

18
Poisoning

M. L. CLARKE

Every species has certain characteristics which render it either more or less liable to poisoning. In the dog the traits which incline it towards being poisoned are its greed, its scavenging habits, its complete lack of discrimination in what it eats and its hunting instincts; those which count against it being poisoned, or which mitigate the outcome of any poisoning that occurs, are, first its fairly adequate detoxication mechanisms and, second the readiness with which it vomits.

It is difficult to get any figures with regard to the frequency of poisoning. In a small animal practice in the south of England it was estimated that about one case in a thousand might have been due to poisoning. Figures from Switzerland suggest that one dog in 2500 is poisoned at some time in its life, with 20% of the cases having a fatal outcome.

The number of cases of poisoning due to any particular poison will vary from one country to another depending upon which toxicants are in common use. There are no recent figures for the UK. In several countries from which figures are available strychnine was found to be the commonest source of poisoning until approximately a decade ago. Recent figures indicate that, in some areas, the trend has changed to pesticides. In the Los Angeles area, of 289 cases of poisoning in dogs and cats 27% were due to N-methyl carbamate, 15% to organophosphorus insecticides, 19% to anticoagulant rodenticides, 5% to Vacor (a rodenticide effective against warfarin-resistant rats) and metaldehyde, and 4% to chlorinated hydrocarbon insecticides and arsenical ant poisons. In the Mexico City area, however, of 49 dogs presenting clinical signs of poisoning, strychnine was found in 21. In Israel fluoracetamide baits have been a more common cause of death than strychnine and in the UK several reports of fatalities due to paraquat baits have been recorded.

DIAGNOSIS OF POISONING

The diagnosis of poisoning is not easy and cannot be made from a single observation. A final conclusion can be reached only from the assessment of four types of evidence: clinical, circumstantial, pathological and analytical. To these some authorities add a fifth: experimental (i.e. the evidence obtained by administering some of the suspect material to another animal). With this the author disagrees for two reasons. First, such evidence may be most misleading. For the experiment to be of any value the material would have to be fed to members of the same species as that suspected of having been poisoned. A dog may be fed indefinitely on food preserved with benzoic acid, of which a single meal would kill a cat, and, as experiments with one animal are valueless, a significant number would have to be used. It is obviously undesirable, both for humane and economic reasons, to sacrifice a dozen dogs because one member of the species is suspected of having been poisoned. Second, such a procedure would rank as a vivisection experiment, and in the United Kingdom could only be performed by someone holding a Home Office licence. Any veterinary surgeon carrying out unauthorised experiments of this kind would find himself in serious trouble with the law.

Clinical evidence is provided by the veterinary surgeon's own observations, or by interrogation of the dog's owner, who alone is likely to have seen the initial signs.

To diagnose poisoning from the clinical signs alone is no easy task, as there is no sign that is pathognomonic of intoxication nor any syndrome produced by a poisonous substance that cannot be duplicated by some other cause. In addition, the signs produced by any poison in any given species are not constant, but vary considerably from one case to the next. For few poisons have we enough records to give any idea of the frequency with which the various signs of poisoning occur, but figures are available for poisoning in dogs by lead and by thallium.

In the case of lead, 87% of dogs poisoned showed gastrointestinal signs, 76% nervous signs. In the former category are included vomiting (78%), anorexia (62%), abdominal pain (55%) and diarrhoea

(42%). In the latter category are hysteria (33%), convulsions (30%) and other nervous signs such as hyperaesthesia, behaviour changes, ataxia and whining (67%). It is noteworthy that there is no single sign that occurred in every case. With thallium, vomiting occurred in 82% of cases, cutaneous alterations in 71%, depression in 62%, anorexia in 53%, nervous disorders in 47%, diarrhoea in 44%, dyspnoea in 44%, conjunctivitis in 41% and dehydration in 24%. Once again, there is no constant feature; it is interesting that cutaneous changes, usually regarded as characteristic of thallium poisoning, occurred in fewer than three-quarters of the cases.

With commonly occurring poisons like lead and thallium it is possible to build up a picture like this from the records of many cases, but with unusual poisons it is impossible, as our knowledge is based on the records of only a few, or at the worst of only a single case. For example, the writer knows of only one case of acrolein poisoning in the dog and two of poisoning by laburnum. In circumstances like this, difficulty arises from the fact that at times quite atypical clinical signs occur. For example, a man is recorded as having died quietly in his sleep after a massive dose of strychnine, while a girl had violent convulsions after an overdose of phenobarbitone. Had these been the only cases recorded, quite erroneous pictures of the syndromes caused by these compounds would have been perpetuated in the literature.

Thus, the symptomatic or clinical evidence can at best produce only a tentative diagnosis of poisoning. Nevertheless, this first diagnosis may be of great value in enabling symptomatic treatment to be initiated and in starting enquiries as to the availability of a particular poison. As an aid to this diagnosis the more common clinical signs have been listed in Table 18.1 together with the toxicants reported as having given rise to them. It must be emphasised that this list must be treated with very considerable reserve. It should be regarded more as an *aide-memoire* than as a key to differential diagnosis.

It must be realised that there is considerable difference in the probability that any clinical sign is due to any particular toxicant. For example, convulsions will almost certainly be seen in poisoning due to strychnine or fluoroacetate, will probably be seen in poisoning due to metaldehyde or DDT, and may be seen in poisoning caused by chloralose (alphachloralose) or nicotine. Sometimes closer observations may serve to distinguish between different toxic agents. The convulsions due to strychnine and to metaldehyde are greatly exacerbated by external stimuli, those due to organochlorine compounds are potentiated to a lesser extent and those due to fluoroacetate are unaffected.

Circumstantial evidence is also provided by interrogation of the owner and from the veterinary surgeon's own observations. The aim is to find out to what poisonous substance or substances the dog could have had access. What food has it had? If possible, samples of anything the animal has eaten should be taken and refrigerated for possible future analysis. Has there been any change in the diet? Could the children have given it anything unusual? Has there been any painting or plumbing done in the house recently? Have any pesticides been used? To what outside area has the dog access? a garden? a farm? woodland? open country? Some pesticides, no longer on the market, may remain as a potential source of poisoning until a shed or greenhouse is cleared out.

Whatever the answers, a personal search is often much more fruitful than extensive cross-examination. The owner may deny the presence of anything harmful in the house, whereas personal investigation reveals several possible toxicants.

In the case of proprietary preparations of unknown composition, by far the best procedure is to telephone the manufacturers. They will usually be extremely helpful in supplying details of any possible toxic compounds which their products may contain.

An assessment of the clinical and circumstantial evidence should have provided a tentative diagnosis. The pathological evidence will help to confirm or refute this. Of course, it will only be available if treatment has failed, or when the dog has been found dead, in which case the autopsy will be of extreme importance.

Pathological evidence can come from two sources: the macroscopic examination made by the clinician himself, and the detailed histopathology carried out at a specialist's laboratory. Consideration of the latter is outside the scope of this chapter.

On opening the body the first thing to notice is any unusual odour. This may become more apparent when the stomach itself is opened. Cyanide poisoning is indicated by the smell of bitter almonds (evanescent and difficult to detect); phenol by the smell of carbolic; phosphorus and zinc phosphide by an odour not unlike that of garlic; metaldehyde by the formalin-like smell of acetaldehyde. Any unusual object in the stomach should be noted and removed for future examination. Twigs or tablets should give a clue to poisoning by plants or drugs. The shell of an egg or the remains of a bird or rodent is often found in cases of strychnine and of calves or lambs in paraquat poisoning.

Table 18.2 lists some of the more common lesions to be found in different organs. It must be emphasised that, as with the clinical signs, there may be considerable variation in the severity of the lesions caused by

Table 18.1 The more common clinical signs of poisoning and their toxicants.

Clinical signs	Toxic agents	Clinical signs	Toxic agents
Abdominal pain	Anticoagulant rodenticides, arsenic, carbamates, chlorate, death-cap, fluoroacetate, fly agaric, lead, mercury (inorganic), organophosphorus insecticides, paraquat, phenol, phosphorus, thallium, zinc phosphide		wood, reserpine, thallium, theobromine
		Dilated pupils	Barbiturates, cyanide, mistletoe, snakebite, strychnine
Anorexia	Aflatoxins, calciferol, chlorate, chlorophenoxy herbicides, fly agaric, lead, mercury (organic and inorganic), paraquat, phenol, Philodendron, redwood, thallium, triazine herbicides, zinc phosphide	Dyspnoea	Acrolein, anticoagulant rodenticides, antu, carbamates, carbon monoxide, chlorate, cyanide, Dieffenbachia, fly agaric, nicotine, organophosphorus insecticides, paraquat, thallium, triazine herbicides
Blindness	Carbon monoxide, lead, mercury (organic), metaldehyde, organochlorine insecticides, salt	Excitement	Caffeine, cannabis, chloralose (alphachloralose), cyanide, fluoroacetate, lead, organochlorine insecticides, reserpine, snakebite, strychnine
Cardiac arrhythmia	Oleander, redwood, toad venom	Haematuria	Chlorate, ethylene glycol
Collapse	Acrolein, anticoagulant rodenticides, arsenic, nicotine, redwood, snakebite, theobromine, toad venom	Incoordination	Antu, arsenic, barbiturates, carbamates, chloral hydrate, chloralose (alphachloralose), chlorophenoxy herbicides, ethylene glycol, garbage, laburnum, mercury (organic and inorganic), metaldehyde, mistletoe, nicotine, organochlorine and organophosphorus insecticides, phenol, red squill, salt, snakebite
Coma	Arsenic, barbiturates, carbamates, carbon monoxide, chloral hydrate, chloralose (alphachloralose), chlorophenoxy herbicides, cyanide, ethylene glycol, fluoroacetate, fly agaric, metaldehyde, organochlorine and organophosphorus insecticides, phenol, phosphorus, zinc phosphide		
		Jaundice	Aflatoxins, paraquat, phenol, phosphorus
Constipation	Calciferol, lead	Muscle tremors	Carbamates, cyanide, hexachlorophane, lead, metaldehyde, organophosphorus insecticides, penitrem A, reserpine (shivering), snakebite, triazine herbicides
Convulsions	Caffeine, carbamates, chlorophenoxy herbicides, crimidine, cyanide, ethylene glycol, fluoroacetate, garbage, laburnum, lead, metaldehyde, nicotine, organochlorine and organophosphorus insecticides, phenol, phosphorus, red squill, strychnine, thallium, zinc phosphide	Paralysis	Fly agaric, lead, mistletoe, organophosphorus insecticides, salt
		Salivation	Antu, arsenic, benzalkonium chloride, cannabis, carbamates, chloralose (alphachloralose), Dieffenbachia, dumb cane, fly agaric, metaldehyde, mistletoe, nicotine, organochlorine and organophosphorus insecticides, Philodendron, phosphorus, strychnine, toad venom
Cyanosis	Acrolein, antu, carbamates, metaldehyde, organophosphorus insecticides, paraquat		
Depression and weakness	Aflatoxins, anticoagulant rodenticides, arsenic, barbiturates, benzalkonium chloride, cannabis, carbon monoxide, chloral hydrate, chloralose (alphachloralose), chlorate, chlorophenoxy herbicides, Dieffenbachia, ethylene glycol, garbage, lead, nicotine, paraquat, phenol, Philodendron, reserpine, snakebite, triazine herbicides, zinc phosphide	Sudden death	Arsenic, carbon monoxide, cyanide, strychnine
		Vomiting	Aflatoxins, antu, arsenic, benzalkonium chloride, carbamates, chlorophenoxy herbicides, death-cap, Dieffenbachia, ethylene glycol, fluoroacetate, garbage, laburnum, lead, mercury (inorganic), metaldehyde, nicotine, oleander, organochlorine and organophosphorus insecticides, paraquat, phenol, Philodendron, phosphorus, red squill, reserpine, thallium, theobromine, zinc phosphide
Diarrhoea	Aflatoxins, antu, arsenic, benzalkonium chloride, calciferol, carbamates, death-cap, Dieffenbachia, fly agaric, garbage, lead, mercury (inorganic), nicotine, oleander, organophosphorus insecticides, Philodendron, red-		

Table 18.2 The more common lesions found in various organs and the toxicants.

Organ	Lesion	Toxic agent
Skin	Alopecia, hyperkeratosis	Thallium
Mucous membranes	Pink	Carbon monoxide
	Cyanotic	Fluoroacetate
	Pallid	Anticoagulant rodenticides
	Congested	Dumb cane, thallium, toad venom
General	Widespread haemorrhages	Aflatoxins, anticoagulant rodenticides
	Petechiae	Organochlorine insecticides
Blood	Cherry red	Carbon monoxide, cyanide
	Chocolate brown	Chlorate, nitrite
	Unclotted	Anticoagulant rodenticides, cyanide
Heart	Hydropericardium	Antu
	Petechiae	Arsenic, lead, organochlorine and organophosphorus insecticides, triazine herbicides
Lungs	Congestion	Arsenic, cyanide, metaldehyde, organochlorine insecticides, paraquat
	Oedema	Antu, zinc phosphide
Liver	Congestion	Aflatoxins, arsenic, chlorate, fluoroacetate, metaldehyde, paraquat, thallium, triazine herbicides
	Jaundice	Aflatoxins, anticoagulant rodenticides, phosphorus, thallium
	Degenerative changes	Chlorophenoxy herbicides, phenol
	Fatty degeneration	Phosphorus
Kidneys	Congestion	Antu, arsenic, chlorate, fluoroacetate, metaldehyde, triazine herbicides
	Degenerative changes	Chlorophenoxy herbicides, mercury (inorganic)
	Calcium oxalate crystals	Ethylene glycol
Stomach	Bitter almond smell	Cyanide
	Carbolic smell	Phenol
	Formalin smell	Metaldehyde
	Garlic smell	Phosphorus, zinc phosphide
	Gastritis	Ethylene glycol, laburnum, mercury (inorganic), phosphorus, zinc phosphide
	Haemorrhagic gastritis	Arsenic, chlorophenoxy herbicides, thallium
	Petechiae	Metaldehyde
	Remains of rat or bird	Paraquat, strychnine
	Contents fluorescent	Phosphorus
Intestines	Enteritis	Phosphorus, mercury (inorganic)
	Haemorrhagic enteritis	Aflatoxins, arsenic, thallium
	Petechiae	Chlorophenoxy herbicides, metaldehyde

any one poison, and that many toxicants, particularly those of vegetable origin, cause no visible lesions at all.

Finally, there is the question of chemical or analytical evidence. It might be thought that, as this is capable of giving a definite answer in many cases, it could be a matter of routine to have it carried out on every occasion; but there are several difficulties. In the first place, laboratories willing to undertake this work are not easy to find. Secondly, toxicological analysis has nowadays become an extremely expensive business. Modern analytical techniques require complicated apparatus, and in order to get a reasonable return on capital outlay, high fees have to be charged.

It is quite impracticable to ask an analyst to make a 'search for poisons'. This might take weeks, the cost would be prohibitive, and in the end the result might be completely negative. If the clinician cannot make a diagnosis the laboratory is unlikely to be able to supply one. Its role is purely confirmatory. If the veterinary surgeon thinks that he has a case of metaldehyde or strychnine or organophosphate poisoning, he should ask the analyst to test for that compound or class of compound and nothing else. Only in this way can the cost of an analysis be kept to a reasonable figure. Finally, a good laboratory has a heavy case load. It is difficult for it to produce a rapid answer in cases where this is needed, as with suspected lead poisoning, in order to initiate treatment.

Samples should never be sent to a laboratory without prior warning. The first step is to telephone and ask them if they can undertake the case and, if so, what samples they need, and how these should be preserved, packed and despatched. They should be warned of any particular urgency, and whether legal action is probable; in the latter case, samples should be taken in the presence of a witness and sealed in such a way that tampering with the samples is impossible. A full report of the case, including clinical signs, post mortem findings and details of all medicines given in treatment, together with instructions concerning the analysis to be carried out, should accompany the sample.

The samples usually needed for analysis are liver, kidney, stomach contents, intestinal contents, blood and urine. In view of prohibitive postal charges plastic containers are probably the most satisfactory form of packaging, in spite of the fact that they are permeable to certain substances and may confuse subsequent chemical analysis. Preservatives are best avoided, but if one has to be added it is advisable to use alcohol, which is of little significance in veterinary toxicology. A specimen of the same alcohol should be included with the samples as a control.

TREATMENT OF POISONING

Any case of poisoning should be regarded as an emergency and treatment should be initiated as quickly as possible. This proceeds along three lines.

The first aim is to prevent the absorption of any further poison. Any suspect material, half-eaten food and so on should be removed and kept for subsequent examination and possible analysis. This also applies to vomit. Any skin contamination should be washed off with running water (e.g. a hose). There is some disagreement about using soap or detergent as it may increase absorption. Probably the best compromise is to use a hose in the case of water-soluble materials such as made-up solutions of garden chemicals, but in the case of oily materials such as paint or tar to remove as much as possible by rubbing with rags or kitchen paper, then cover the area with cooking oil, again

remove with rags or paper, then wash well with warm water and detergent.

To remove material that has been ingested but not yet absorbed it is best to give an emetic, except when the animal is comatose or in convulsions, or in cases of poisoning by petrol, paraffin or corrosive liquids. Apomorphine, 0.1 mg/kg may be given subcutaneously, but if it is not available, salt and water (two teaspoonsfuls in a cup of warm water), mustard and water (in the same proportion), or washing soda (a crystal placed on the back of the tongue) are readily available substitutes. Speed is the all-essential factor; there is little point in administering an emetic more than 4 hours after the poison has been ingested.

Gastric lavage may be performed instead of, or subsequent to, an emetic. Wash out the stomach with water or saline until all solid material has been removed, or the smell of the suspected poison (e.g. phenol) has gone. Some activated charcoal may be left in the stomach. A saline purgative may be given to remove material which has passed into the gut.

The second type of treatment comprises supportive and symptomatic therapy, aimed at reinforcing the body's own defences until the toxicant is metabolised, neutralised or eliminated. Clinical conditions are treated with appropriate agents. Convulsions may be controlled with pentobarbitone sodium, 20 mg/kg intravenously if possible, if not, intraperitoneally. Coma may be treated with an analeptic such as nikethamide, 20 mg/kg subcutaneously, but its use is better avoided if possible as it may precipitate convulsions. Cardiac arrhythmia may be reduced with propranolol, 0.5 mg/kg intravenously. Dehydration may need parenteral administration of glucose saline or compound sodium lactate BP. Hypothermia (as from chloralose) needs hot blankets or a warm hot water bottle, hyperthermia (as from pentachlorophenol or dinitro-orthocresol) calls for cold water or ice.

The final line of treatment is the use of the specific antidote, if there is one. This can be employed only when the identity of the poison has been established. Details are given later in this chapter under individual toxicants. Examples are: sodium calcium edetate for lead, dimercaprol for arsenic and mercury, pyridoxine for crimidine, atropine and pralidoxime for the organophosphates and antivenin for snakebite.

DOMESTIC HAZARDS

Acrolein
Acrolein is an unsaturated aldehyde produced by the oxidation of glycerin when fat is overheated. It is a compound of considerable toxicity; it was used as a

chemical warfare agent in World War I. A concentration of 1 part/10^6 becomes intolerable in 5 minutes.

A poodle shut up in a small kitchen with a chip-pan of overheated fat showed swollen tonsils, blood from the nostrils and elevated temperature. Next day the signs were dyspnoea, cyanosis, a rapid pulse and congested eyes. Collapse and death followed.

Carbon monoxide
Carbon monoxide poisoning usually arises when a dog is shut up in a room with either a leaking coal-gas appliance or with a stove burning propane gas, oil, or solid fuel in an inadequate supply of air. Coal-gas poisoning is becoming less common with the advent of 'natural gas' which contains no carbon monoxide, but poisoning due to incomplete combustion and bad ventilation is on the increase due to the popularity of central heating; probably most cases occur at night when the dog is shut up near the boiler with the draught reduced and all the windows shut. Poisoning has also arisen in caravans with propane heaters and in cars with defective exhausts.

The toxic effect of a gas is approximately proportional to the product of the concentration of the gas and the time of exposure (Haber's law). In the case of carbon monoxide, a dog exhibits signs of poisoning when the concentration of carboxyhaemoglobin in the blood reaches 30%. This occurs after an exposure of 1 hour to a concentration of 1200 parts/10^6 or of 2 hours at half this concentration. The clinical signs are weakness, dyspnoea and coma; often the animal is found dead. Blindness and deafness may occur; the latter is sometimes slow to clear and may become permanent. It is due to anoxia of the brain. The mucous membranes are pink and the blood cherry red.

Immediate treatment consists of removing the animal to the open air. Often this will suffice; otherwise oxygen, preferably with 5% of carbon dioxide, should be administered. Carbon monoxide can be detected and estimated in the blood by chemical and spectrophotometric methods.

Cyanide
Cyanide, usually the potassium salt, is still sometimes used for destroying wasps' nests, and tins of it stored in garden sheds have given rise to poisoning, as has sodium cyanide from a lorry which had shed its load. Poisoning is so rapid that the animal is usually found dead. The lethal dose in the dog is about 2 mg/kg. Clinical signs include excitement, muscle tremors, dyspnoea, dilatation of the pupils, convulsions, coma and death. On opening the stomach the bitter almond smell of HCN may be noticed. The blood is bright cherry red and coagulates slowly. There may be

congestion and haemorrhage of the lungs and stomach. Treatment is by the injection of sodium nitrite and sodium thiosulphate. A suggested dosage is 0.1 ml/kg of a solution made by mixing one volume of a 20% solution of the former with three volumes of a 20% solution of the latter.

Detergents and disinfectants
Detergents and disinfectants, used at the recommended dilution, are usually harmless, but a 1% solution of benzalkonium chloride can cause moist erythematous purulent lesions of the paws if walked in, and salivation, vomiting and depression if ingested.

Young puppies are much more susceptible than adult dogs to intoxication with hexachlorophane. A puppy with acute dermatitis, bathed daily for a week in 3% hexachlorophane emulsion developed severe muscle tremors and was destroyed. Oedematous changes were noted in the CNS. Death of a suckling puppy also followed washing the mammae of the dam in 3% hexachlorophane solution.

Recently, cases of dermatitis have been reported following the use of dry powder carpet cleaner.

Ethylene glycol
Ethylene glycol is used extensively as an antifreeze. Dogs, attracted by the sweet taste, are usually poisoned by drinking the water drained from a car radiator. The lethal dose is about 8 ml/kg.

The toxicity of ethylene glycol is due partly to its depressant action on the CNS, but chiefly to the toxic action of its metabolites, particularly oxalic acid. The initial syndrome, which may become apparent within an hour or two and includes vomiting, depression, weakness and incoordination, is probably due to the first of these factors. There may be apparent recovery after a few hours, but the clinical signs will recur and become more acute, including haematuria or anuria, thirst, convulsions and coma followed by death. This second phase is due to the oxalic acid. With large doses there may be no remission of clinical signs and death may occur within 24 hours. Calcium oxalate crystals are found in the brain and kidney tubules at post mortem examination.

Treatment aims to prevent the oxidation of glycol to oxalic acid by offering ethanol as an alternative substrate, thus 'swamping' the enzyme alcohol dehydrogenase which catalyses the reaction. This is achieved by the i.v. injection of 20% ethanol (5.5 ml/kg) and 5% sodium bicarbonate solution (8.8 ml/kg) every 6 hours for 2 or 3 days. This should be combined with the oral administration of activated charcoal at a level of 5 g/kg. Convulsions may be controlled with pentobarbitone sodium. Intravenous calcium borogluconate is also useful. If the ethanol–bicarbonate treatment can be initiated within 4 hours recovery is likely.

Phenol

Phenol poisoning is much less common in the dog than in the cat or pig but can arise from ill-advised medication or gross contamination with tar or creosote. Clinical signs are vomiting, depression, anorexia, abdominal pain, incoordination, anaemia, jaundice and, in serious cases, convulsions, coma and death. *Post mortem* lesions are congestion and haemorrhages, particularly of the liver, which may show centrilobular necrosis. The smell of carbolic may be obvious. Treatment is by the administration of an emetic or gastric lavage, with the latter being continued until there is no longer a smell of phenol. White of egg or milk may be left in the stomach. Intravenous glucose-saline hastens the elimination of phenol. Any material spilled on the body should be removed by washing with soapy water or methylated spirit.

DRUGS

Poisoning by drugs occurs in two ways: either the drug is administered to the dog or the dog helps itself.

There are several reasons for iatrogenic poisoning. The most common is probably overdosage. This may occur from normal human error, or, in the case of a newly-introduced drug, from lack of appreciation of its toxicity. Oestradiol cypionate given intramuscularly in small doses (0.2 mg/kg) to bitches has recently been shown to produce a depressive effect on bone marrow with leucopenia and thrombocytopenia and 0.75–1 mg/kg may be fatal. Another common cause of poisoning is individual idiosyncrasy, which can occur with any drug if, given at an accepted level, it causes untoward clinical signs. There are numerous examples on record. A course of phenylbutazone, well below the toleration level, has caused haemorrhage and renal degeneration in a Dachshund. Phenytoin at the recommended dose has caused anorexia, vomiting, hepatitis and death in a Collie; its toxicity may be increased by the simultaneous administration of chloramphenicol. A normal dose of nalidixic acid has caused lethargy and depression in a Great Dane. A minute portion of a 25 mg tablet of acepromazine caused deep unconsciousness, lasting several hours, in a 6-month-old Labrador puppy. It is difficult to estimate the frequency of such hypersensitivity as there are so few records. It has, however, been noted that diethylthiambutene caused tetanic spasms in 25 out of 667 dogs (3.7% of cases).

Quite different situations arise when an owner doses his dog without veterinary advice. These usually follow the administration of a drug intended for human consumption. First, the dose is usually far too large; a tablet meant for a man may contain ten times the dose for a dog. Numerous small animals have been poisoned by a vegetable laxative tablet. Second, there may be a difference in species susceptibility between man and the dog, with the drug being much more toxic to the dog. This is true of the monoamine oxidase inhibitors, which have an antidepressant action in man, but in the dog produce incoordination, convulsions, and haemolytic anaemia. Again, the benzodiazepines, which are used as tranquillisers in man, may give rise to excitement and aggression in a dog. A dog, treated by the owner with a bovine selenium preparation died following convulsions. Widespread degenerative lesions indicative of chronic selenium poisoning were found at *post mortem.*

By far the most common cause of poisoning is due to the dog (or, more often, the puppy) finding a packet of tablets intended for its owner and eating it, consuming at one sitting the quantity intended to last a man for a month. This type of accident has become even more common since plastic containers have replaced glass ones. People are notoriously careless about failing to keep medicines out of the reach of children and animals but, even with reasonable care, accidents can happen. A dog has been poisoned by Easton's tablets knocked off the mantelpiece by the cat.

Numerous examples could be quoted. A puppy which had eaten 2.5 g of thyroid tablets became blind and dyspnoeic, and died. Another puppy which had eaten 75 mg of amitriptyline became unconscious but recovered after injection of bemegride. Three grams of caffeine eaten by a small dog, and a packet of caffeine tablets eaten by a puppy caused excitement, rapid pulse and convulsions. In spite of administration of barbiturate both animals died. Ingestion of 50 migraine tablets containing both ergotamine and caffeine also caused death. Another migraine preparation, Bellergal, containing atropine, ergotamine and phenobarbitone caused a retriever to remain incoordinate for 3 days. A terrier which had eaten 450 mg of the tranquilliser hydroxyzine and which exhibited excitement and aggression with rapid pulse and respiration, recovered after injection of diethylthiambutene. A puppy which had consumed a packet of marihuana (cannabis) cigarettes showed salivation, weakness and alternate unconsciousness and hyperaesthesia, but recovered in a few hours, while another, which had eaten 180 mg of phenelzine, died. A month's supply of 'the pill', however, had no apparent effect.

These examples serve to show the great variety of

compounds available to a dog in a modern drug-orientated society, and the frequency with which accidents can have a fatal outcome. Poisoning of this type poses a number of problems. The first of these is the identity of the poison. The owner may know definitely that the unconscious puppy has eaten the packet of tranquillisers, but may have no idea of the name of the drug, and the label, if still extant, may only state 'Mrs Smith, as directed', which is of no help with regard to treatment. Contact with the doctor who prescribed the tablets or the chemist who dispensed them may produce some information, although this may be withheld on the ground of professional ethics. Even if they do disclose the identity of the drug they may not be able to help in the matter of treatment, and it may be that the substance is one used only in human medicine and with which the veterinary surgeon is not familiar. In this case there are two possible lines of action. The first, as has already been suggested, is to approach the manufacturer. If this is unsuccessful, the best thing to do is to look up the drug in The Extra Pharmacopoeia. This admirable work gives toxic effects and suggests possible treatments for most available drugs, and although directed towards human poisoning this can usually be interpreted in a veterinary context. All university and reference libraries, and many pharmacists, will have a copy. Failing this, the only procedure is to treat the case symptomatically as suggested above.

ENVENOMATION

Bees and wasps

Dogs are frequently stung by these insects, whose venom contains amines, peptides and enzymes, the several actions of which are as yet imperfectly understood. Most cases are trivial and may be treated with a topical application of an antihistamine or a 1:4 dilution of the papain solution sold as a meat tenderiser.

Multiple stings may be more serious. A dozen or so may result in no more than a stiffness and a slightly elevated temperature, but upwards of a thousand, due to a swarm settling on the animal, may result in death preceded by vomiting and diarrhoea. Multiple stings should be treated with an injection of an antihistamine and with corticosteroids. If visible the stings may be removed.

In man the most frequent cause of death following bee or wasp stings is allergy. In a sensitised person this may follow even a single sting, with the victim collapsing and dying within a few minutes of anaphylactic shock. The condition is rare in the dog, but has been recorded.

Snakes

The common adder (*Vipera berus*) is the only venomous snake found in Britain. The other two indigenous species, the grass snake (*Natrix natrix*) and the smooth snake (*Coronella austriaca*) are quite harmless. Dogs are frequently bitten as they blunder into snakes or attempt to play with them. The bite is considerably more dangerous to the dog than it is to man owing to the dog's smaller size and to the fact that it is usually bitten on the head or neck while a man is usually bitten on a limb. Bites frequently occur on sunny days in spring, when the snake has come out of hibernation and is basking in the sunshine. The author has known a case as early as 10 February.

There is great variation in the severity of the poisoning, as the expression of venom from the glands, and hence the amount injected, is a voluntary action entirely under the snake's control. The reptile instinctively conserves its venom, which is the means by which it obtains its food. A bite inflicted on a dog is a defence action only, as a snake cannot regard the animal as a potential meal.

The signs of poisoning include excitement followed by depression, muscular tremors, incoordination, dilatation of the pupils, collapse and death. There is considerable swelling in the neighbourhood of the bite, where the fang marks may often be seen, particularly if the skin is shaved. When bitten, the dog should be carried to where veterinary help is available; exercise should be avoided as it tends to spread the venom.

The only worthwhile treatment is injection of the correct antivenin; one covering all European vipers is available in this country. The manufacturer's instructions should be followed but it must be remembered that these usually refer to a human victim, and that the dog needs a larger, not a smaller, dose of antiserum than a man. Supportive therapy consists of corticosteroids and antibiotics, but not antihistamines or permanganate. If the dog has been bitten on a limb, a tourniquet to delay the spread of the venom may be helpful as a first aid measure. Cutting the area of the bite and applying suction will do little good and can only serve to distress the animal.

In the case of a dangerous snake such as a cobra or a rattlesnake the same line of treatment should be followed, although the urgency is greater. Once again, the effects of a bite are quite unpredictable. Of two dogs bitten one after the other by a mamba (*Dendroaspis angusticeps*), the first exhibited no signs of poisoning, the second died almost at once.

Toads

All toads secrete a complex venom from glands in the skin. This contains numerous toxic factors including cardioactive steroids such as bufotoxin, indole derivatives such as bufotenine and serotonine and catecholamines such as adrenaline and noradrenaline. Luckily the species found in Great Britain, of which *Bufo vulgaris*, the common toad, is the most plentiful, are far less dangerous than many exotic species.

Poisoning occurs from a dog biting or mouthing a toad. Within a few minutes the animal appears distressed, retches continually and exhibits hypersalivation with masses of ropey saliva hanging from its jaws. With the common toad often no other signs occur, and the dog recovers without treatment, but if part of the toad has been eaten, or in the case of a more dangerous species, these clinical signs may be followed by prostration, cardiac arrhythmia, collapse and possibly death.

Treatment consists of washing out the mouth with much water (e.g. a hose) and intravenous injections of 1.0–2.0 mg of atropine to control the salivation and 0.5 mg/kg of propranolol to deal with the effect on the heart. Convulsions may be controlled with pentobarbitone sodium. Corticosteroids may also be used.

FOOD

In this connection, 'food' denotes some substance fed to the animal; it does not include unwholesome materials which it scavenges for itself.

Food poisoning may arise from one of four causes: the food may be inherently toxic; it may have had some toxic substance added to it either deliberately or inadvertently; it may have become contaminated during processing, transport or storage; or it may have become infected with some fungus or bacillus.

Few substances fed to dogs are potentially poisonous in themselves. An exception is chocolate which contains about 0.25% of theobromine. Poisoning can only arise from gross overeating but Dachshunds which had eaten about 300 g died suddenly, an adult Springer Spaniel died 12 hours after eating 250 g household cocoa, while dogs fed food (under wartime conditions) containing 0.2% of theobromine showed vomiting, diarrhoea, thirst and collapse, followed by death. The classic example of poisoning due to a substance deliberately added to food was the canine hysteria produced by agene (nitrogen trichloride) at one time used as an 'improver' in flour. A much more common addition is salt. This normally causes no trouble as the dog either refuses the food or promptly vomits. Puppies, however, can show incoordination, pain in the lumbar region, and paralysis of the hindlegs after eating such substances as salt fish or meat pickled in brine. Recovery is usually complete, although the

paralysis may be slow to clear. Salt poisoning can also arise when a dog drinks sea water, particularly in hot weather. The clinical signs are incoordination, paralysis, convulsions and blindness. Such cases often have a fatal outcome. Fresh water should be given as soon as possible. If the animal is unable to drink, water may be given forcibly by stomach tube, or isotonic glucose injected intraperitoneally.

Incidentally, potassium chloride, which is used as a fertiliser, produces quite a different syndrome: unconsciousness, subnormal temperature, imperceptible pulse, flaccid limbs and bluish mucous membranes.

Food poisoning may also occur when horse-meat fed to a dog contains the euthanasia agent used to destroy the animal. Both barbiturates and chloral hydrate have caused drowsiness, incoordination, coma and, in some cases, death. The drug can usually be found in the urine of the poisoned dog. Fatalities have also arisen from the consumption of the meat of a horse poisoned with fluoroacetate from a rubbish dump, after the carcase had been sold to local pet shops. The feeding of the ears of cattle which had been implanted with stilboestrol has caused anoestrus and fetal deaths in breeding bitches.

Food can, of course, become contaminated with pesticides and other poisonous substances in numerous ways: in manufacture, in transit, in storage and in the home. For example, dogs have been fatally poisoned after their feed has become accidentally contaminated with organochlorine pesticides in the process of milling, and in one incident 80 dogs died after eating poultry meat contaminated with fluoroacetate. Chemical analysis can usually put the matter beyond doubt, but as has already been pointed out, unless the analyst can be told the nature of the poison suspected, a quick answer is almost impossible. If local contamination can be ruled out, and the food was purchased in the original container, the manufacturer may be willing to have a rapid analysis made. Pending the result of this, symptomatic and supportive therapy should be maintained.

In addition to contamination with chemical substances, food can also become infected with fungi or bacteria. The dog appears to be particularly susceptible to aflatoxin B_1, produced by *Aspergillus flavus*, administered orally or parenterally. The first signs of poisoning are dullness, anorexia and loss of weight. These are followed by gastrointestinal disturbances, ascites and death. The lesions include widespread haemorrhages and necrosis of the liver and gall bladder as well as pancreas, kidneys, thymus, heart and adrenal glands. The acute LD_{50} of aflatoxin B_1 in the dog is about 1 mg/kg, but clinical signs can be produced by feeding 0.05–0.1 parts/10^6 in the food for 5 months. In an outbreak of aflatoxicosis in Kenya aflatoxin levels of 1000–3000 μg/kg were found in commercially prepared dog food and aflatoxin B_1 was detected in the liver and kidneys of many affected dogs. There is no specific treatment. In recent years poisoning of dogs with mycotoxins has been reported from several countries. Two dogs developed severe muscular tremors and generalised seizures after eating mouldy cream cheese, and an adult Boxer became ataxic and showed mydriasis and convulsions following ingestion of mouldy walnuts. *Penicillium crustosum* and its toxin penitrem A were isolated from the cheese and walnuts. Haemorrhages and liver lesions have also been produced experimentally in dogs injected intraperitoneally with penicillic acid, a mycotoxin produced by several species of Penicillium and Aspergillus, and rubratoxin B, produced by *Penicillium rubrum*, which gives rise also to degenerative changes in the renal tubular epithelium. Experimental nephrosis has also been induced following administration of ochratoxin A (produced by *A. ochraceus* and *P. viridicatum*) and citrinin (produced by *P. palitans*). A combination of both toxins has resulted in lesions of lymphoid tissue ulceration of the intestinal mucous membrane. There is no specific treatment. Recently toxic myopathy in a Sheltie has been reported, resulting from contamination of dry dog food with monensin, a food conversion supplement prepared from *Streptomyces cinnamonensis*. A milling company produced dog food as well as cattle and poultry rations.

Botulism in dogs is rare, but has been recorded. The chief signs are stiffness, paralysis and regurgitation of food. Treatment is by injection of polyvalent botulinum antiserum. Recovery may take up to a month, and some animals die. There are no characteristic lesions.

A condition known in America as 'garbage poisoning' and characterised by malaise, vomiting, diarrhoea, depression, incoordination and convulsions is probably caused by staphylococcal enterotoxin acquired by eating putrid material found when scavenging.

PESTICIDES

Herbicides

Arsenical herbicides

Although sodium arsenite, the traditional homicidal weedkiller, is seldom used nowadays, organic compounds of arsenic such as cacodylic acid and disodium methanearsonate (DSMA) are sometimes employed for special purposes. They are far less toxic than in-

organic arsenic, but clinical signs and treatment are the same (see Arsenic, p. 497).

Bipyridyl herbicides

Diquat (Reglone) and paraquat (Gramoxone; Weedol, which also contains diquat dibromide) are contact herbicides which rapidly destroy vegetation and are used for such purposes as stubble clearing, potato haulm destruction and clearing weeds between bushes. They are rapidly inactivated by contact with soil and were originally thought to be comparatively harmless. They are now known to be among the most dangerous poisons in use. The acute LD_{50} for dogs is 100–200 mg/kg for diquat and 25–50 mg/kg for paraquat. For prolonged feeding the 'no effect' levels in the diet are 50 and 35 parts/10^6 respectively.

Poisoning may occur from drinking from vessels containing solutions of the herbicide, from eating carcases deliberately baited with it to kill foxes, from malicious administration or from access to treated herbage. The first sign of illness, usually apparent after 24 hours, is vomiting. This is followed by anorexia, lethargy and dyspnoea which becomes progressively worse until it forms the dominant feature. Cyanosis, jaundice, abdominal pain and ulceration of the tongue have also been recorded. Death may occur in from 1 to 10 days. At necropsy the lungs are purple-red and congested, with petechial haemorrhages, the liver is enlarged and congested.

Treatment is usually ineffective, although, recently, administration of cyanocobalamin has been suggested. Parenteral antibiotic, corticosteroid and fluid therapy has proved successful in a cat. In human cases Fuller's Earth or Bentonite, given by mouth, has been recommended to deactivate any unabsorbed herbicide. Both diquat and paraquat may be detected in stomach contents, urine, liver and kidneys.

The chlorophenoxy acids (2,4-D; 2,4,5-T; MCPA; etc.) are selective weedkillers extensively used for removing weeds from lawns. They are sold under various trade names, which are usually mixtures. They are of fairly low toxicity and if used correctly are unlikely to cause poisoning. The dog, however, is more susceptible than most other species, having an LD_{50} for 2,4-D of about 100 mg/kg, and cases of poisoning have arisen from animals drinking solutions prepared for horticultural use and left unattended, or from ditches sprayed with the herbicide. Death may be delayed for several days. There is some cumulative effect. Signs of poisoning are anorexia, depression, vomiting and incoordination, followed by convulsions and coma. *Post mortem* lesions include haemorrhagic gastritis and degenerative changes of liver and kidneys. There is no specific antidote. Treatment is by induction of emesis, gastric lavage and supportive therapy. The chlorophenoxy acids may be detected in stomach contents and urine.

Sodium chlorate is strongly phytotoxic to all green plants, and as it is cheap and readily available it finds considerable use as a total weedkiller. It is used either in the solid state or in solution. Dogs eating the solid material usually vomit and show no further ill effects. Concentrated solutions are refused, but an animal may drink enough of a 2% solution to absorb a lethal dose. Poisoning may arise from drinking from the gutters after city streets have been sprayed to clear them of weeds. The lethal dose in the dog is approximately 2 g/kg.

The toxic effect of chlorate is mainly due to tissue anoxia caused by the conversion of haemoglobin to methaemoglobin, but the compound also acts as an irritant poison. Signs of poisoning are depression, anorexia, abdominal pain and haematuria. Sometimes blood-stained faeces may be passed. The mucous membranes are at first cyanosed, but later brown. Mild cases may show only pharyngitis, renal irritation and tenderness over the loins, with no methaemoglobinaemia. *Post mortem* lesions are characterised by the brown colour of methaemoglobin. Liver, kidney and spleen are congested.

Except in mild cases, the prognosis is not favourable. For treatment, the stomach may be washed out with 1% sodium thiosulphate solution. Two per cent methylene blue solution may be injected intravenously at a level of 10 mg/kg and repeated if necessary. Milk or other demulcents may be given.

Chlorate may be detected in tissue, plasma or urine. In the latter it may be found up to 24 hours after ingestion.

The triazine herbicides (atrazine, simazine, etc.) are used for clearing weeds from garden paths. Although rather more toxic than the chlorophenoxy acids, poisoning is unlikely if they are correctly used. They may cause anorexia, depression, dyspnoea and muscle spasms. Lesions consist of congested liver and kidney and petechiae on the epicardium. Treatment is as for the chlorophenoxy acids. Metabolites of the triazines may be detected in the urine.

Insecticides

The traditional insecticides of vegetable origin, such as derris and pyrethrum, seldom, if ever, cause poisoning in domestic animals. Even nicotine, which is extremely toxic, the lethal dose in the dog being about 2.0-3.0 mg/kg, does not cause poisoning when used as an insecticide, although it has been known to do so when puppies have eaten cigarettes or cigar ends. The signs of poisoning are vomiting, diarrhoea, depression and salivation, followed by incoordination, dyspnoea, convulsions and collapse. Treatment should be by gastric lavage with dilute potassium permanganate solution and careful use of stimulants.

During the last 30 years many synthetic organic compounds have come into use as insecticides. The three main classes are the organochlorine compounds, the organophosphorus compounds and the carbamates.

Organochlorine compounds

The organochlorine insecticides, or chlorinated hydrocarbons, came into use during World War II. They include DDT (dicophane), gamma-HCH (gamma-BHC; gammexane, lindane), aldrin, dieldrin, chlordane, endrin, heptachlor, camphechlor and numerous others. They vary considerably in toxicity and are very stable compounds and resistant to biodegradation. Poisoning can arise from contamination of food and from careless use, particularly of gamma-HCH and DDT, for destruction of ectoparasites.

The first signs of poisoning are usually restlessness and hypersensitivity, salivation, vomiting and incoordination. These may be followed by convulsions, blindness, coma and death. The first 24 hours is the critical period. If the animal survives this it will probably recover, although it may remain dull and incoordinate for 4 or 5 days. *Post mortem* findings are not typical, but may show congestion of the lungs and widespread small haemorrhages. Treatment should be by gastric lavage, and intravenous or intraperitoneal injection of pentobarbitone sodium, 20 mg/kg, to control the convulsions. Calcium borogluconate is also useful.

Organochlorine compounds can be detected in blood or viscera.

Organophosphorus compounds

The organophosphorus insecticides form a large group of compounds developed from World War II nerve gases. Nearly 100 of them have been described. Among the better known are: azinphosmethyl (Gusathion), carbophenothion (Trithion), chlorfenvinphos (Birlane), chlorpyrifos (Dursban), crotoxyphos (Ciodrin), crufomate (Ruelene), demeton-S-methyl (Metasystox), diazinon (Basudin), dichlorvos (Nuvan, Vapona), dimethoate (Rogor), dioxathion (Delnav), disulfoton (Disyston), fenchlorphos (Nankor), fenthion (Tiguvon), fonofos (Dyfonate), malathion (Malathion), mevinphos (Phosdrin), parathion (Bladan), phorate (Thimet), phosalone (Zolone), phosmet (Imidan), phosphamidon (Dimecron) and trichlorphon (Neguvon, Dipterex).

Toxicity varies widely. The newer organophosphorus compounds are much less toxic than the older ones, having been synthesised with a view to producing a compound highly toxic to insects but not to mammals. They are all less persistent than the organochlorine compounds.

Poisoning usually arises from the dog drinking from a vessel of made-up solution, but may also occur from chewing a plant which has been sprayed.

In spite of their differences in toxicity, the organophosphorus compounds all act in the same way by inhibiting the action of cholinesterase and thus allowing acetylcholine to accumulate. The signs are thus those of overstimulation of the parasympathetic nervous system, and include salivation, abdominal pain, vomiting, diarrhoea, incoordination, muscle tremors, dyspnoea, cyanosis, convulsions, coma and death. Not all cases will exhibit every clinical sign and the order in which these appear may depend upon the particular compound ingested.

Treatment follows two lines. First, the administration of atropine to counter some of the effects of the acetylcholine accumulation. A solution of 0.15% of the sulphate in physiological saline should be given at a rate of 0.25 mg/kg, repeating as necessary, judging the effect by the alleviation of hypersalivation and the onset of mydriasis. A quarter of the dose is given intravenously and the rest intramuscularly or subcutaneously. Second, the slow intravenous injection of pralidoxime (2-PAM) in dilute solution at a level of 40 mg/kg. This serves to reactivate the phosphorylated enzyme, but must be injected as soon as possible before irreversible inactivation has taken place.

There are no characteristic *post mortem* lesions.

Some of the organophosphorus compounds are unstable and difficult to detect by chemical analysis, but diagnosis may often be confirmed by the estimation of whole-blood cholinesterase, although this may not correspond with the severity of the poisoning; but if it is below 25% of the normal range there is likelihood of poisoning.

Carbamates

Carbamates resemble organophosphorus compounds in that they are inhibitors of cholinesterase, but the reaction differs in being one of carbamylation, not phosphorylation, and also in being readily reversible. Carbamates are used as fungicides, insecticides and molluscicides. Well-known examples are carbaryl (Sevin), methiocarb (Draza) and pirimicarb (Pirimor). Like the organophosphorus compounds they vary widely in toxicity; aldicarb (Temik) is as

poisonous as strychnine and carbaryl is practically harmless.

Being cholinesterase inhibitors, they give rise to the same clinical signs as the organophosphorus compounds, and poisoning by them is treated in the same way with atropine. Pralidoxime should not be used, as it is incapable of reactivating the carbamylated enzyme, and may even exacerbate the condition.

As the carbamate–cholinesterase complex is unstable, blood samples for analysis should be refrigerated at once and dealt with as quickly as possible.

Molluscicides

Metaldehyde

Metaldehyde is used as a slug-killer either mixed with bran or as a proprietary preparation; the latter is available in both pellet and liquid form. The substance seems to be extremely attractive to dogs, and cases of poisoning are common. The acute oral LD_{50} for dogs is 600–1000 mg/kg.

Signs of poisoning are salivation, vomiting, hyperaesthesia, incoordination and convulsions, with increased heart and respiration rate. Tremors, rigidity and blindness have also been noted. Delayed death from liver damage may occur. *Post mortem* examination shows hyperaemia of lungs, liver and kidneys, with petechial haemorrhages of the gastrointestinal tract. The stomach contents (and vomit) may have the formalin-like smell of acetaldehyde.

Treatment aims at controlling the convulsions by the injection, intravenously or intraperitoneally, of pentobarbitone sodium, 20 mg/kg. Alternatively, acepromazine, 0.5 mg/kg intramuscularly, may be used. The stomach may be washed out with dilute sodium bicarbonate solution. Calcium borogluconate or glucose-saline may be given intravenously. Chlorprothixene (3 mg/kg) followed by vitamins B_{12} and C has also been recommended.

Metaldehyde poisoning may be confirmed by the detection of acetaldehyde in the stomach contents.

Methiocarb

Methiocarb (Mesurol, Draza) is also used as a molluscicide. It is a carbamate and acts as an inhibitor of cholinesterase (see above).

Rodenticides

Antu

Antu is not often used nowadays. It is extremely toxic to dogs; the lethal dose is 30 mg/kg. It is more toxic to older dogs than to younger ones, and more effective on a full stomach than an empty one. Clinical signs are vomiting, salivation, incoordination, dyspnoea and diarrhoea. Death is due to anoxia caused by accumulation of fluid in the lungs. *Post mortem* lesions include pulmonary oedema, hydrothorax and hydropericardium. There is no specific treatment; apomorphine and atropine may be helpful in the early stages.

Calciferol

Calciferol (vitamin D_2, Sorexa CR) has recently come into use as a rodenticide. It acts by causing calcification of the arteries. Signs of poisoning are anorexia, depression, diarrhoea or constipation, spinal arching, polydipsia and polyuria. Suggested treatment is a diet with a high fluid intake, high salt and low calcium. Sunlight should be avoided.

Calciferol is sometimes used in admixture with warfarin.

Chloralose

Chloralose (alphachloralose) is used particularly against mice. It has both stimulant and depressant properties, but the latter usually predominate. Signs of poisoning are dullness, incoordination, hypothermia and coma, sometimes preceded by excitement. For treatment it is usually sufficient to remove the animal to a warm environment. If the coma is deep or prolonged an analeptic such as nikethamide may be given, but its use is best avoided as it may precipitate the opposite syndrome. Sedatives should never be given. Fatal cases are very rare. The lethal dose in the dog is about 600 mg/kg.

Crimidine

Crimidine (Castrix) is widely used in Europe. It acts by antagonising pyridoxine, producing violent convulsions, which may be controlled by a barbiturate. An effective antidote is pyridoxine given intravenously at a level of 20 mg/kg.

Fluoroacetate and fluoroacetamide

These substances are used as rodenticides in many parts of the world. They are extremely toxic to all species, with the lethal dose in the dog being about 0.10 mg/kg, and frequently give rise to secondary poisoning. Fluoroacetate is converted in the body to fluorocitrate which blocks the citric acid cycles. Clinical signs are vomiting, abdominal pain, excitement, wild running and barking, convulsions (which are not triggered by external stimuli) coma and death. *Post mortem* lesions include cyanosis of the mucous membranes and congested liver and kidneys. There is

no effective antidote, but convulsions may be controlled with minimal doses of barbiturate.

Phosphorus

Yellow phosphorus is still occasionally met with as a rodenticide. Poisoning has also been caused by phosphorus incendiary bombs used by terrorists. Clinical signs are vomiting, abdominal pain, salivation, jaundice, convulsions, coma and death. *Post mortem* lesions are gastroenteritis and fatty degeneration of the liver. On opening the stomach a garlic-like smell may be noticed. The vomit and stomach contents may glow in the dark. Treatment consists of giving an emetic and gastric lavage with 0.5% copper sulphate solution.

Red squill

This is probably the safest rodenticide known, as domestic animals usually refuse to eat it and, if they do, promptly vomit. Unfortunately, its use in the UK is prohibited. The lethal dose in the dog is about 150 mg/kg. Signs of poisoning are vomiting, hyperaesthesia, incoordination and convulsions. There is no specific antidote, but dogs usually recover. *Post mortem* lesions are those of gastroenteritis.

Reserpine

Reserpine (Betakil) is an alkaloid of the tropical shrub *Rauvolfia serpentina*, and is used in human medicine as a hypotensive. It has sedative and depressant properties, which are responsible for its rodenticidal action. Signs of poisoning are diarrhoea, vomiting and shivering, followed by sedation and respiratory depression, although excitement is sometimes seen. There are no characteristic *post mortem* lesions. For treatment, an emetic should be given, followed by nikethamide, subcutaneously, 20 mg/kg. The lethal dose of reserpine in the dog is about 10 mg/kg.

Strychnine

Strychnine is controlled in the UK and its use as a rodenticide is forbidden. In many countries, however, it is freely available, and where this is so it is usually the most frequent cause of poisoning in dogs. In Great Britain, cases arise from the eating of poisoned carcases put down illicitly for foxes, or from secondary poisoning. The lethal dose of strychnine is about 0.75 mg/kg.

The first signs of poisoning, which usually occur within half an hour, are excitement, apprehension, stiffness and salivation. Then violent tetanic spasms commence; these become more severe and frequent, possibly being initiated by external stimuli, until the animal dies of cerebral anoxia in the throes of a convulsion. Death usually takes place within a few hours.

The onset of rigor mortis is rapid. There are no characteristic *post mortem* lesions, but the remains of rats or birds may often be found in the stomach.

Treatment aims at controlling the convulsions by the intravenous or intraperitoneal injection of pentobarbitone sodium 20 mg/kg. There is some disagreement as to the value of apomorphine. It certainly removes much unabsorbed strychnine, but it may exacerbate the convulsions. However, diazepam (2 mg/kg intravenously) followed by apomorphine has been recommended. Once anaesthesia has been established the stomach may be washed out with tannic acid (1%) or potassium permanganate, 1:1000.

If the animal survives for 24 hours the prognosis is good, as strychnine is rapidly eliminated from the body and has no lasting ill-effects.

The alkaloid may be detected in stomach contents, liver, kidney or urine.

Thallium

Thallium is an extremely toxic substance; the lethal dose in the dog is less than 20 mg/kg. Poisoning may be acute, subacute or chronic. The clinical signs are vomiting, haemorrhagic diarrhoea, anorexia, abdominal pain, convulsions and dyspnoea. There is reddening of the oral mucous membranes, followed by cutaneous changes such as alopecia and hyperkeratosis. *Post mortem* lesions include haemorrhagic gastroenteritis and fatty degeneration of the liver. For treatment, an emetic may be given within a few hours of the consumption of the poison. This may be followed by diphenylthiocarbazone (50 mg/kg) or prussian blue (0.15 mg/kg), both drugs given orally three times daily with supportive therapy, but the prognosis is not favourable. Thallium may be detected in urine and viscera.

Warfarin

Warfarin is the most common of a series of rodenticides which act by inhibiting the production of prothrombin, thus interfering with the clotting mechanism. They also damage the capillaries, causing widespread internal haemorrhage. Other members of the class are coumachlor (Tomorin), coumatetralyl (Racumin) and difenacoum (Neosorexa), which resemble warfarin in being hydroxycoumarins, and diphacinone (Diphacin), chlorophacinone (Drat) and pindone (Pival), which are indandione derivatives. All are of about the same toxicity, and resemble warfarin in their mode of action. As rodenticides they are more effective if taken in repeated small doses than in a single larger dose. A dog would be killed by a single dose of 50 mg/kg, but a daily dose of 1.0 mg/kg might cause death in about a week. Secondary poisoning may occur but is unlikely to be caused by the ingestion of a single poisoned rodent. A massive dose causes death very rapidly, but usually there is an interval of several days before the onset of signs.

The clinical signs are pallor of the mucous membranes, subnormal temperature, increased rate of respiration, abdominal pain, lameness, dyspnoea and collapse. There may be bloody vomit and faeces and pregnant bitches may abort. The necropsy shows widespread haemorrhages, and jaundice may be present.

During treatment, restraint and handling should be minimal; a sedative should be given if necessary. Phytomenadione (vitamin K_1) should be injected intravenously or intramuscularly, at a level of 10-30 mg. This may be repeated on two subsequent days. In severe cases whole blood may be administered, 20 ml/kg, half rapidly, half at a rate of 20 drops a minute. The citrated blood is made by mixing 100 ml of a solution containing 2 g of sodium citrate and 12.5 g of glucose with 300 ml of arterial whole blood (see Chapter 12).

Metabolites of warfarin may be identified in the urine for up to 10 days.

Zinc phosphide

Zinc phosphide is one of the older rodenticides, but is still available in parts of the USA. The lethal dose in the dog is about 40 mg/kg. Unlike most poisons it is more effective on a full stomach. Clinical signs are vomiting, anorexia, depression and abdominal pain. Convulsions and coma sometimes precede death. There is no specific antidote, but gastric lavage may be effective if initiated in time. Gastritis and oedema of the lungs are found *post mortem*. The garlic-like smell of phosphine may be detected on opening the stomach.

POISONOUS PLANTS

Plant poisoning is normally associated with farm stock, not with small animals, but due to the dog's predilection for chewing anything it can find, a number of cases are on record. Those cited below are in the literature, or are known to the author, but it should be realised that poisoning can occur from chewing any toxic plant to which the dog may have access. In this connection it must be noted that a number of species grown as house plants are well known to be poisonous in their land of origin, although their toxicity is not appreciated here.

Plant poisoning may usually be diagnosed from the history of the case, the dog having been seen to eat or chew the plant, or from recognisable pieces of the plant in the vomit. In all cases of suspected plant poisoning (except from Dieffenbachia spp.) an emetic should be given as quickly as possible, even if the dog has already vomited. Poison is extracted but slowly from vegetable material, and the longer any of the latter remains in the stomach the more chance there is of a fatal dose being absorbed. It is noteworthy, however, that a lethal dose of, say, a highly toxic alkaloid can be absorbed from the mucous membrane of the mouth without any of the plant having been actually swallowed.

Both *Amanita muscaria* (fly agaric) and *A. phalloides* (death cap) have caused poisoning. The former gives rise to dullness, salivation, anorexia, aggression, abdominal pain, diarrhoea, dyspnoea, contraction of the pupils and posterior paralysis, sometimes followed by coma. Treatment is by subcutaneous injection of atropine, 0.05 mg/kg. Recovery may be expected. Poisoning by *A. phalloides*, on the other hand, is usually fatal. Signs of poisoning are not apparent for 12 hours or so after the fungus has been eaten. These usually consist of vomiting and diarrhoea, with blood in the vomit and faeces, and intense abdominal pain. Death may not occur for several days and is usually preceded by coma. A specific antiserum has been prepared but is unlikely to be available. Otherwise treatment is by emetic or gastric lavage and supportive therapy.

The berries of mistletoe (*Viscum album*) have caused death in a puppy 50 hours after ingestion. The clinical signs were incoordination, posterior paralysis, hyperaesthesia, salivation, dilatation of the pupils and polyuria. Berries of the black nightshade (*Solanum nigrum*) are said to have caused incontinence and a garlic smell in the breath, although these signs are not usually symptomatic of poisoning by this plant in other species.

Laburnum (*Laburnum anagyroides*) poisoning is well known in most species of domestic animal, as well as in children. In one case, of only two recorded in the dog, a Terrier died within an hour of chewing a branch cut from a tree 3 months previously. It vomited and exhibited incoordination and mild convulsions. The chewing of yew twigs has also caused vomiting, with rapid recovery. In America, a Labrador puppy, having eaten leaves of chokecherry (*Prunus virginiana*), which contains a cyanogenetic glycoside, was found prostrate, gasping and thrashing about, and died shortly afterwards; its stomach was full of the leaves.

A case of anaemia with Heinz body formation in a puppy, with a predilection for eating raw onions, was soon reversed when a meat and biscuit diet was given.

Among the house plants that have caused poisoning are dumb cane (Dieffenbachia spp.), Philodendron spp. and oleander (*Nerium oleander*). The leaves of Dieffenbachia contain bundles of fine crystals of calcium oxalate and possibly also a toxic protein. On being bitten these cause intense pain in the mouth, salivation, oedema of the buccal mucous membrane, paralysis of the tongue and dysphagia. Treatment is by washing out the mouth with dilute bicarbonate solution, injection of pethidine to relieve the pain and corticosteroids. Recovery is usually complete but may take several days, during which time parenteral feeding may be required. Oleander is becoming increasingly popular as a house plant. No case of poisoning in a dog has yet been reported in the UK, but cases have occurred in warmer localities where the plant flourishes. Signs of poisoning are continued vomiting, diarrhoea and cardiac arrhythmia. Treatment is with atropine and propranolol.

Dogs have died after having been bedded on the shavings of African redwood (*Mansonia altissima*). The material gives rise to ulcers on the mouth and paws, causes anorexia, diarrhoea and prostration, and exerts a digitalis-like action on the heart.

Although the incidents cannot be considered as plant poisoning, it is noteworthy that complete obstruction of the bowel has been caused when dogs have swallowed such objects as horse chestnuts and pieces of sweet corn cob. Similarly the 'burrs' of burdock can cause granular stomatitis. Small papules, which grow and become ulcerated, develop on the tongue. These may be treated by curettage under general anaesthesia.

TOXIC METALS

Arsenic

Arsenic poisoning is much less common than it used to be due to the decreasing use of this substance; its place has been taken by less toxic and more effective compounds. It is still, however, used as a rodenticide, a wood preservative and a defoliant, while lead arsenate is used for spraying fruit trees. Poisoning usually arises from careless disposal of the material. Malicious poisoning is also known. Percutaneous absorption can arise if animals walk through foliage that has been sprayed with a defoliant.

The lethal dose of arsenic trioxide is about 100 mg/kg. Sodium arsenite, which is soluble, is about ten times as poisonous; organic compounds of arsenic are considerably less toxic.

In the USA the arsenic content of 32 commercial pet foods was found to vary from 0.02–1.55 parts/10⁶. A mean 0.48 parts/10⁶ was present in dry food, 0.28 parts/10⁶ in canned and 0.21 parts 10/⁶ in semi-moist food.

The clinical signs of arsenical poisoning are vomiting, salivation, weakness, incoordination, abdominal pain and profuse haemorrhagic diarrhoea, followed by collapse and death. With large doses death occurs rapidly, but with smaller quantities the animal may survive for 2 or 3 days. Chronic poisoning is rare; at least it is rarely diagnosed.

The *post mortem* examination shows reddening and swelling of the whole length of the gastrointestinal tract, particularly the stomach. The contents are fluid and evil smelling, and may contain blood. There is usually inflammation of liver, kidneys and lungs.

If treatment can be initiated very soon after the arsenic has been taken, apomorphine may be given, and gastric lavage carried out, but if signs of arsenical poisoning have appeared such procedures are contraindicated. The specific antidote is dimercaprol (BAL), but its value is limited. It is given intramuscularly in a 5% solution in 10% benzyl benzoate in arachis oil at a rate of 3 mg/kg four times daily until recovery. If dimercaprol is not available one of the older remedies may be tried. For example, 20% sodium thiosulphate may be injected intravenously at a level of 20 mg/kg; twice this quantity should be given by mouth if practicable. As supportive therapy glucose-saline solution or Ringer-lactate (compound sodium lactate injection BP) may be given to replace loss of fluid. Vitamin B complex is also useful. After vomiting has ceased, care must be taken in the administration of solid food.

Arsenic may be detected by analysis in all parts of the body, including the hair. The latter is useful in cases of suspected chronic poisoning.

Copper

In a recent study of the offspring from five matings of Bedlington Terriers affected with copper toxicosis the high hepatic copper concentrations in this condition were found to follow an autosomal recessive pattern of inheritance. Selective breeding by test matings is advocated to reduce the prevalence of copper toxicosis.

Lead

Lead poisoning in dogs, particularly in puppies, is comparatively common. This is due to their indiscriminate eating habits and their tendency to chew anything they encounter whether edible or not. Paint is by far the most common source of lead poisoning, particularly old and flaking paint which contains a high proportion of lead. In addition to chewing furniture and skirting boards, animals may inhale lead-laden dust from household decorating activities such as the removal of old paint with a sander. As well as paint,

putty, red lead, linoleum and metallic lead objects can cause poisoning.

The acute lethal dose of lead in the dog is probably of the order of 1.0 g/kg, but lead is a cumulative poison. In five weeks, 8.0 mg/kg a day may be fatal, 2.5 mg/kg a day in five months. In 38 brands of American commercial pet food the lead content was 0.025–5 parts/10^6. The amounts (in parts/10^6) in dry, canned and semi-moist foods were 1.28, 1.399 and 2 respectively.

Clinical signs of poisoning may be gastrointestinal or nervous; either or both types of condition may be present, although a combination of the two is the most common picture. Gastrointestinal signs seem to predominate in older dogs. The syndrome includes anorexia, vomiting and abdominal pain, with diarrhoea or constipation, while the nervous signs are depression or excitement, hyperaesthesia, muscular spasms, convulsions, paralysis and blindness. Arching of the neck, champing of the jaws and lateral recumbency with running movements are sometimes seen.

Diagnosis is best confirmed by estimation of the lead level in the blood. This is normally about 0.1 parts/10^6. Values over 0.6 parts/10^6 are diagnostic for lead poisoning, and even 0.35 parts/10^6 is significant if taken together with the clinical signs. A urine level of 0.75 parts/10^6 is suggestive of poisoning, but is less satisfactory than blood as it is very variable. It may increase tenfold after Ca-EDTA therapy. Stomach contents, liver and kidney normally contain about 1.0 part/10^6, but may contain 10–100 times as much in cases of poisoning. Another diagnostic criterion is the basophilic stippling of the red blood cells. If this is present, it is good evidence of lead poisoning, but if it is absent it does not mean that the condition may not be present.

Post mortem lesions vary and are not characteristic.

The specific treatment is by the chelating agent sodium calcium edetate (Ca-EDTA). The 'injection of sodium calcium edetate B.Vet.C.' is a 25% solution, and should be diluted before use at the rate of one volume of the solution to five volumes of normal saline. This gives a solution containing about 4% of Ca-EDTA. The recommended daily dose of 75 mg/kg represents about 2 ml/kg of this solution. This should be given by slow intravenous injection in divided doses, four times a day for 3 or 4 days. Some authorities recommend the subcutaneous injection of a more dilute solution, 10 mg/ml, or the B.Vet.C. solution diluted 25 times.

The specific Ca-EDTA therapy should be accompanied by supportive treatment: pentobarbitone sodium to control convulsions, glucose-saline if the animal is dehydrated, and magnesium sulphate to remove any unabsorbed lead such as the insoluble lead sulphate.

Mercury

Mercury poisoning in the dog is rare, but cases have arisen from poisoning of food from mercurial fungicides, from eating the flesh of pigs and chickens poisoned by mercury-dressed corn and from inhalation of vapour during illicit smelting. Mercury contamination of industrial effluents is converted into soluble methylmercury in rivers and eventually taken up by sea fish from which tinned food is preserved, a potential source of poisoning. Signs of poisoning are gastroenteritis, anorexia, incoordination and blindness. Stomatitis and nephritis may be seen in cases of poisoning by inorganic mercury, but not in those due to organic mercurials, where nervous symptoms are more likely to occur. Mercury may be found in liver, kidney, urine and, particularly, the brain.

Post mortem lesions may include gastroenteritis and nephritis, but not usually after poisoning by organic compounds.

Treatment is by dimercaprol, as for arsenical poisoning.

ACKNOWLEDGEMENT

This chapter was originally written by the late Professor E.G.C. Clarke in the first edition of this book, and has been up-dated by his wife, Mrs M.L. Clarke.

FURTHER READING

Aronson A.L. (1972) Chemical poisonings in small animal practice. *Vet. Clinics N. Am.* **2**, 379.

Buck W.B., Osweiler G.D. & van Gelder G.A. (1976) *Clinical and Diagnostic Veterinary Toxicology.* 2nd edn. Kendall Hunt, Dubuque, Iowa.

Clarke E.G.C. (1973) Lead poisoning in small animals. *J. Small Anim. Pract.* **14**, 183.

Clarke M.L., Harvey D.G. & Humphreys D.J. (1981) *Veterinary Toxicology*, 2nd Edn. Baillière Tindall, London.

Darke P.G.G., Gibbs C., Kelly D.F., Morgan D.G., Pearson H. & Weaver B.M.Q. (1977) Acute respiratory distress in the dog associated with paraquat poisoning. *Vet. Rec.* **100**, 275.

Darke P.G.G., Roberts T.A., Smart J.L. & Bradshaw P.R. (1976) Suspected botulism in Foxhounds. *Vet. Rec.* **99**, 98.

Harris W.F. (1975) Clinical toxicities of dogs. *Vet. Clinics N. Am.* **5**, 605.

Hatch R.C. (1977) Veterinary toxicology. In *Veterinary Pharmacology and Therapeutics*, eds. M.L. Jones, N.H. Booth & L.E. McDonald, p. 1121. Iowa State University Press, Ames, Iowa.

Kelly D.F., Morgan D.G., Darke P.G.G., Gibbs C., Pearson H. & Weaver B.M.Q. (1978) Pathology of acute respiratory distress in the dog associated with paraquat poisoning. *J. Comp. Path.* **88**, 275.

Oehme F.W. (1975) Veterinary toxicology. In *Toxicology: The Basic Science of Poisons*, eds. L.J. Casarett & J. Doull, p. 701. Macmillan, London.

Radeleef R.D. (1970) *Veterinary Toxicology*, 2nd edn. Lea & Febiger, Philadelphia.

Worthing C.R. (1979) *The Pesticide Manual*, 6th edn. The British Crop Protection Council, London.

Zook B.C., Carpenter, J.L. & Leeds E.B. (1969) Lead poisoning in dogs. *J. Am. Vet. Med. Assoc.* **155**, 1329.

Zook B.C. & Gilmore C.E. (1967) Thallium poisoning in dogs. *J. Am. Vet. Med. Assoc.* **151**, 206.

19
Behavioural Problems

V. L. VOITH

INTRODUCTION

The veterinarian is the first person to whom the public turns regarding their animal's behaviour. The veterinarian therefore must be prepared to give initial advice regarding behavioural problems. Sometimes it is sufficient to provide a simple answer to a question why the animal is acting as it does, an explanation to the owner that s/he is reinforcing the behaviour, or advice on how to extinguish the behaviour. At other times, more complicated counterconditioning and desensitising programmes are required. Occasionally, drug therapy, hormonal manipulation, castration, or other surgical procedures might be indicated. The practitioner may elect to refer the owner to a behavioural specialist, however, the veterinarian usually must make the first differential diagnosis.

Fortunately, many behaviour problems can now be corrected by pooling knowledge from ethology, psychology, and medicine. This, of course, assumes that the owners are willing and able to devote some energy to eliminating the problem. Happily, many owners are only too willing to do so.

Most owners are as distraught about having their pet destroyed because of a behaviour problem as they would be if it was euthanised because of disease or injury. It seems unfair to destroy a healthy animal that is a good companion most of the time, but that has a behavioural trait that is intolerable for the remainder. Although the owners do not know what could be done about the problem, they usually feel that something should be possible.

In a series of 100 behaviour problems information was collected to ascertain owner's attitudes towards their pets (Voith 1981a). Sixty-two per cent of the cases involved dogs and 38% involved cats. The problems covered the range of behaviours commonly presented to behaviourists. The majority of dog problems involved aggression towards people; second, some form of destructive behaviour; and third, elimination in the house. The most common reason cats were presented was because they were not using the

litterbox, and, second, because they were aggressive towards other cats. The duration of the problems ranged from several months to several years. None was of short duration. Ninety-nine per cent of the clients indicated that they considered the problem either serious or very serious. The majority of people who brought in a pet also had other animals and were living with other people. Fifty-two per cent of the dog owners had either another dog or a cat. Only four of the dog owners had never had a dog before.

Towards the end of the interview, the clients were asked why they had kept the animal this long despite the behaviour problem. The owners usually gave between one and three responses, which fell into ten categories (Table 19.1). Overwhelmingly, the first response (55% of both dog and cat owners) was a term of affection. The second most common first response (16% of both dog and cat owners) was a humanitarian reason, such as 'No one else would take the animal. I feel that people have a responsibility to a pet.' The third largest category of first responses was simply the statement that getting rid of the animal was not a consideration. There were no statistical differences between any of the ten first responses of dog and cat owners. Except for one category, there were no correlations between type of response and number of people in the household or whether the person had other pets. However, two clients (one cat and one dog owner) answered that they could not live without the animal and these were individuals living alone without

Table 19.1 Responses to question of why behaviour problem dog was kept.

Statement of affection	Thought problem was curable
Humanitarian reason	Monetary value
Not a consideration	Cannot live without dog
Referred to dog as a person	Dog couldn't live without person
Positive attributes outweighed negative	Protective value

other pets in the household. This should not be construed as implying that all people living alone with no other pets answered as such. A social worker (on the staff at the Veterinary Hospital, University of Pennsylvania) has also observed a correlation between extreme dependency on an animal and solitary living situations (Quackenbush 1981).

More dog owners than cat owners (45% vs. 34%) referred to the pet as a person sometime during the interview. Perhaps because dogs have a wider range of and/or more easily recognised facial and postural expressions, people identify more with dogs than with cats. Sixty per cent of both dog and cat owners endured some sort of social ridicule from their friends for seeking behavioural consultation to solve the problem of their pets.

Owners quite clearly can recognise their attachment to the pet and at the same time acknowledge that the animal is causing them inconvenience, financial or social expenses, or emotional pain. People with problem pets can be as attached to them as persons are attached to animals without misbehaviours.

People become very attached to companion animals and indicate this in a variety of ways. Over 700 people (32% men and 68% women) filled out all or part of an 81 item questionnaire available to any person entering the veterinary hospital of the University of Pennsylvania throughout the year 1981 (Voith 1983a). Ninety-eight per cent of respondents considered their dog a member of the family. Ninety-seven per cent indicated they talked to their dogs frequently (once a day or more), and 45% talked to their dog at least once a month about events important to them. Ninety-nine per cent thought they were aware of their dog's moods and 98% believed that the dog was aware of the owner's moods. Fifty-six per cent of the owners allowed the dog to sleep on the bed with a human member of the family and most owners shared their food with their pet. At mealtimes sixty-four per cent gave tidbits from the table to their dogs and 86% shared snacks with their dogs at other than mealtimes. Most owners (68%) indicated that they spent more than an hour each day talking to, playing with, exercising, training or caring for their dog. Fifty-six per cent celebrated their dog's birthday; 9% had paintings of their dogs, and 91% had photographs. Clearly, people can be very attached to their pet dogs. Owners of problem pets are no exception.

CLASSIFICATION OF BEHAVIOUR PROBLEMS

Behavioural problems can be classified in a variety of ways. It is helpful to classify each problem according

Table 19.2   Classification of behaviour problems.

Normal
Species-typical
Learned
Abnormal
Pathophysiological
genetic
acquired
Experiential
early experience
phobias
psychosomatic

to three classification systems: normal to abnormal (Table 19.2), descriptive, and functional (Voith 1979a; Borchelt & Voith 1982).

Normal behaviours include both species-typical behaviours and learned behaviours. Species-typical behaviours are those that are generally thought of as 'instinctive' such as maternal behaviour sequences, intermale aggression, territorial behaviours, etc. Most of these are adaptive or beneficial to the animal either in an immediate or evolutionary perspective. Most learned behaviours are also normal and beneficial from the animal's perspective (a view not always held by the owner).

Like normal behaviours, abnormal behaviours can be genetic or acquired. Abnormal behaviours are not characteristic of the species nor beneficial to the animal in either an immediate or evolutionary perspective. Flank sucking (Fig. 19.1), cataplectic narcolepsy, and some forms of epilepsy are genetically determined behaviours which can be considered abnormal. Disease processes, particularly neurological, endocrine, and urogenital disorders, can also result in abnormal behaviours. Sometimes learning can lead to abnormal behaviours, such as phobias and psychosomatic manifestations, which are disruptive and detrimental to the animal. Adverse early experiences can also result in pervasive, abnormal behaviours.

Behaviours can also be classified according to a description of the problem, such as aggression, elimination problems involving urination and defaecation, fearful behaviour and overactivity.

The description of a behaviour problem does not offer a complete diagnosis. For example, just as polyuria may be a sign of a variety of different medical disorders, eliminating in the house may be a sign of potentially different behavioural motivations. The dog may be defaecating in the house because of disease, inappropriate housebreaking, separation anxiety, a fear response, or lack of opportunity to eliminate in an appropriate place.

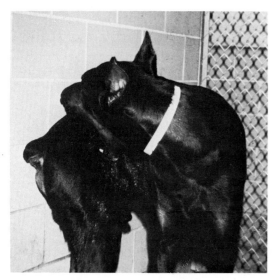

Fig. 19.1   A Doberman engaging in flank sucking, an abnormal behaviour.

An accurate description of the behaviour and the context in which the animal performs the behaviour, as well as the animal's physiological state, is what allows one to make a functional classification. For example, a mother dog that is only aggressive to other dogs and people when she is near her puppies would be classified as demonstrating parental or maternal aggressive behaviour. A dog which physically resists being pushed over, growls with a vertical retraction of the lip and stares at the owner with its ears forward, would tentatively be classified as manifesting dominant aggressive behaviour.

The more accurately a problem can be classified, the greater the probability of an accurate prognosis and subsequent successful therapeutic regime.

FACTORS THAT INFLUENCE BEHAVIOUR

The behaviour of an animal is a product of the animal's interaction with the environment. Behaviour is influenced by genetics, early experience, and learning as well as immediate internal and external stimuli. An example with which veterinarians are readily familiar is intermale aggression. Some breeds and individuals are more predisposed than others to fight. Environmental factors, such as the presence or absence of a bitch in oestrus, may influence whether a dog fights another male. Previous learning experiences such as the outcome of a previous fight and reinforcement or

punishment by an owner will also influence a dog's readiness to fight another. Androgens tend to facilitate intermale aggression and progestins tend to suppress it. Intermale fighting has a genetic basis, but whether or not the animal engages in the fight is influenced by a multitude of stimuli and experiences (Fig. 19.2).

Effects of early experience

The early experience of an individual is the environment in which it spends the first few weeks or months of life or repeated exposure to specific situations or circumstances during that time interval. The effects of early experience on behaviours tend to be pervasive and profound. Deprivation or aversive early experiences rarely result in a single, abnormal behavioural response but, rather, alter the future emotional baseline of the animal.

In a series of studies done at McGill University, puppies were raised alone or in pairs in cages with opaque sides. Littermates were raised in homes or normal laboratory conditions. At 9 months of age, all the puppies were kept in a normal laboratory setting. In test situations the dogs that had been raised in restricted environments tended to exhibit neophobic responses in novel environments, hyperactive behaviour, were less interested in social interactions with other dogs, had difficulty with learning simple problems, and persisted in repeating errors and self-injurious behaviours. For example, the dogs raised in restricted environments took five times as long to learn to avoid a mobile toy car that delivered a shock. In fact, these dogs frequently ran into the electric toy. During the course of the experiments, one of the puppies repeatedly bumped its head on a permanently fixed water pipe in its pen. These animals appeared not to be able to learn how to manipulate or interact with objects in their environment (Melzack 1954; Melzack & Thompson 1956; Melzack & Scott 1957).

Several people have reported that dogs that are not handled before 14 weeks of age are thereafter always suspicious of humans. In general, these dogs remain timid and more like wild animals than domestic ones. Dogs that are not exposed to a variety of environmental situations generally remain apprehensive in novel situations as adults (Scott & Fuller 1965; Whitney 1971). The apprehensiveness and hyperactivity of such dogs not only makes them undesirable pets but also raises the question of how suitable they are for physiological, medical, or behavioural research.

Scott and Fuller (1965) concluded that puppies need little daily interaction with people to prevent appre-

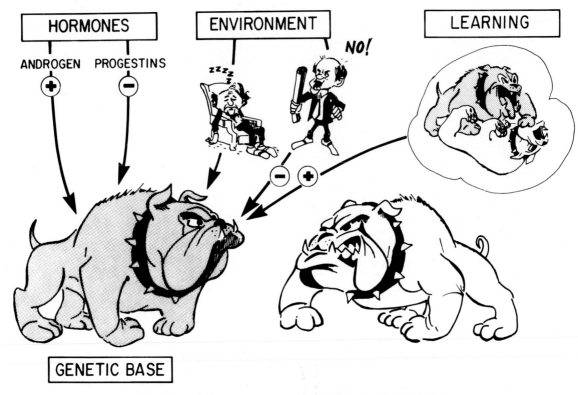

INTERMALE AGGRESSION IN DOGS

Fig. 19.2 Intermale aggression in dogs is a genetically based behaviour, the expression of which is influenced by numerous internal and external variables (from Voith 1979a). With permission from the editor of *California Veterinarian*.

hensiveness in adulthood. To minimise the probability of developing neophobia or timidity in novel situations, puppies should be taken on progressively further journeys from their kennel area. They need exposure to a wider range of environments than simply where they live.

The results of isolation studies have led some veterinarians to recommend that orphan animals not be raised for fear that a puppy will likely develop into an abnormal individual and will show the above mentioned behaviour abnormalities. Whilst it is important to be aware of the devastating effects that isolation and deprivation during the first several months of life can have on an animal, it is not valid to extrapolate that information verbatim to a home setting where there can be active interaction with an orphan. If an orphan animal is not allowed to interact with other dogs, it is possible that they may not be a willing breeder later in life (Beach 1968). However, reproduction is usually not of concern to most pet owners. Interacting with the orphan and exposing it to novel stimuli and situations will prevent it from developing the hyperactivity, neophobia, and other undesirable behaviours that can result from deprivation or isolation. A small survey (Voith, unpubl. obs.) of 16 dog breeders who had raised orphan puppies, in litters or singly, indicated that all the animals developed normally and exhibited behaviours within the range of normal behaviours of adult dogs.

Owners of orphan puppies should be encouraged to pick them up, handle, and in general move them about. In addition to stimulating the puppies to urinate and defaecate by wiping the urogenital and rectal area with a moist piece of cotton, it would probably be beneficial for the animals to receive some tactile stimulation on their face and body as is provided by the bitch. As a puppy gets older, it should be played with and, whenever possible, exposed to other dogs of the same age. Above all, the orphan should not simply be fed and then left alone or the owner may indeed end up performing his/her own isolation or deprivation study.

Learning

Learning can be defined as a change in the behaviour of an animal as a result of previous experience. Even though many problem behaviours involve species-typical behaviours such as trying to maintain contact with a social member of the group, intermale aggression and elimination behaviours, learning plays a role in the development and maintenance of these behaviours. Frequently excessive barking, scratching at the door, overactivity, phobias, and some forms of aggression are learned behaviours that have often paid off for the animal. In order to assess the part learning may be playing in the animal's behaviour and to utilise learning principles to treat behaviour problems, one must be familiar with some principles of learning.

Habituation

Habituation is one of the simplest forms of learning. It is the loss or reduction of the performance of an instinctive behavioural response as the result of repeated exposure to an eliciting stimulus that is without consequence to the animal. The classical example is that of a young bird's response to moving stimuli overhead. Any movement overhead, be it a duck, hawk, or leaf floating by, causes a young quail to run for cover. Eventually the bird loses its escape response to repeatedly seen stimuli that are of no consequence, such as the drifting leaf, bird, or goose flying overhead. However, the chick does not habituate readily to the form of a hawk flying overhead. This is partially because the chick is more predisposed to flee from such a shape and because there is less frequent exposure to hawks.

Most dogs readily habituate to novel stimuli. For example, initially a puppy might be frightened of a large box or a room that has rearranged furniture. Simply repeated or continued exposure to these stimuli leads to a decrease in the initial apprehensive behaviour.

Classical conditioning

In classical conditioning, a neutral stimulus is paired with an unconditioned stimulus (UCS) which evokes an unconditioned response (UCR). The taste of food (UCS) will evoke salivation (UCR) (Fig. 19.3). If the sound of a metronome or bell (neutral stimulus) is paired with the taste of food (UCS), eventually the sound will evoke salivation. The sound is then called a conditioned stimulus (CS) and the evoked salivation response a conditioned response (CR) (Fig. 19.4). The letdown of milk in dairy cows in response to the banging of milking equipment or music is another example of a classical conditioning phenomena.

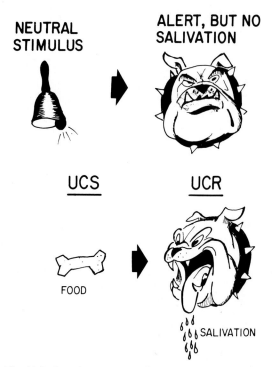

Fig. 19.3 In reference to a salivatory response, a neutral stimulus is a stimulus which does not normally (or naturally) evoke salivation. Food is an unconditioned stimulus (UCS) that naturally revokes the unconditioned response (UCR) of salivation.

An interesting experiment that leads to speculation that neutral stimuli consistently paired with a disease response might be able to subsequently evoke the disease response is as follows: guinea-pigs that were sensitised to a particular antigen were placed in a specific room and exposed to the antigen (UCS). The guinea-pigs manifested an asthmatic attack (UCR). After several such episodes, merely placing the sensitised guinea-pigs in that room resulted in an asthmatic attack—without exposure to the antigen. The room or the placement of the guinea-pig in the room had become a conditioned stimulus that resulted in the conditioned response of an asthmatic attack. The investigators also demonstrated that the sound of a ringing bell could become a conditioned stimulus that would evoke the conditioned response of an asthmatic attack (Otterberg *et al* 1958).

Instrumental conditioning

When a behaviour is followed by a positive or negative event the subsequent performance of that behaviour may change. If a puppy is repeatedly scolded for jumping onto furniture, the frequency of jumping onto

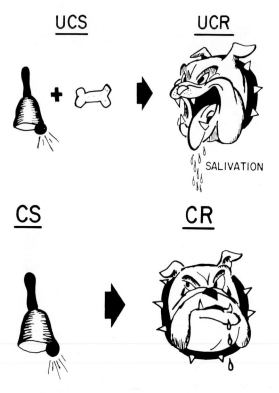

Fig. 19.4 When a neutral stimulus (bell) is paired with the UCS (bone) and the UCR (salivation), eventually the neutral stimulus becomes a conditioned stimulus (CS) and evokes a conditioned response (CR) (salivation). The CR is not perfectly identical to UCR.

furniture is reduced. If a dog is frequently fed after the opening of a refrigerator door, it may begin running to the kitchen whenever the refrigerator is opened.

A reinforcement is a stimulus or event that increases the future probability of the performance of a behaviour. A positive reinforcement is a stimulus or event which follows the response of an animal and increases the probability of that response reoccurring. It is, in effect, a reward. Positive reinforcements are most effective when they occur 0.5 seconds after the response. Behaviours that are quickly followed by positive reinforcements tend to be repeated.

An aversive event or stimulus can also increase the frequency of the performance of a behaviour. The animal may perform a behaviour to avoid or escape such stimuli. Aversive stimuli that increase the performance of a behaviour are called negative reinforcements.

A punishment is a stimulus or event that occurs after a behavioural response and leads to the decrease in the frequency of performance of that behaviour.

Punishment is usually an aversive stimulus. Punishment decreases a performance of behaviour and reinforcement increases the frequency of behaviour.

A response that has been acquired as a consequence of reinforcement will eventually extinguish if the animal is no longer reinforced. For example, if a dog had learned to gain access to the house by barking or scratching at the door, the response could be extinguished if the owner no longer let the animal inside when it barked or scratched. The more valuable a reinforcement is, the longer it will take to extinguish the learned behaviour. For dogs, which are social animals, being reunited with the owner is a powerful reinforcement. Therefore, it may take a long time to extinguish a response of scratching on the door for admittance.

If a dog is rewarded immediately and every time it engages in a particular behaviour, it will acquire that response quickly; delayed and intermittent reinforcements will prolong the acquisition of a response. However, if all rewards are ceased, animals that have been reinforced on a delay or intermittent schedule will persist in the behaviour much longer than an animal that has been immediately and continuously rewarded (Table 19.3). Intermittent reinforcements result in persistent responses (Fig. 19.5). Many behaviours of animals that owners find undesirable have been intermittently reinforced. Sometimes the dog who barks or scratches on the door gains entry and sometimes it does not. The dog may be admitted immediately or not at all. The more variable the intermittent schedule of reinforcement, the more persistent will be the response. When an owner decides to extinguish a response that has been intermittently reinforced s/he should be prepared for a long wait. Unfortunately, many owners stop too soon. Owners should also be prepared for a temporary increase in frequency and intensity of the behaviour when they begin ignoring the dog. When extinction is employed, animals often initially increase the intensity and frequency of its response. Extinction, by itself, may take a very long time. However, there are a variety of techniques, such

Table 19.3 Schedules of reinforcement.

Optimal for rate of acquisition of a response	Optimal for prolonging extinction of a learned response
Immediate	Delayed

Continuous	Intermittent
	    Variable ratio
	    Variable interval

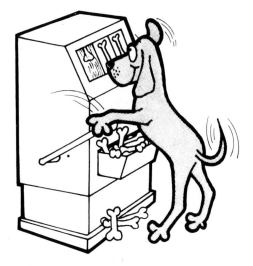

Fig. 19.5 Intermittent schedules of reinforcement produce very persistent behaviours (Voith 1979b). With permission from the editor of *Modern Veterinary Practice*.

as punishment and counterconditioning, that can be employed simultaneously to facilitate extinction.

Generalisation

Generalisation is the phenomenon or process by which a response to specific stimuli is elicited by similar stimuli. When animals acquire a response to a particular stimulus, they also acquire responses to similar stimuli. The more similar the stimuli are to the original stimulus the more similar the responses are to the original response. For example, a dog may have learned that scratching at the back door allows it access to the house. If, one day, the dog finds itself at the front of the house, it may also scratch at the front door to get in. The stimulus of a door, when the dog is isolated outside of the house, evokes the behaviour of scratching at the door. The dog may not scratch at the front door as hard as or as long as it does at the back door, but it is still likely to scratch at the front door. A dog that responds to the approach of an owner's car is likely to respond to the approach of a car of a similar model. A dog that has learned to sit when its owner says sit will often respond similarly to that voice command by another person. An animal that has learned to be afraid of men with beards may also be somewhat afraid of a man with a moustache. The more similar stimuli are to the initial stimulus, the closer the responses to these other stimuli resemble the original response.

The generalisation of stimuli and responses allows a clinician to identify stimuli along a gradient that evoke undesirable behaviours. While it often is impos-

sible to work with an animal when it is presented with the full intensity of an eliciting stimulus, it usually is possible to countercondition, desensitise, or extinguish responses to similar stimuli which elicit weaker responses. The new, acceptable response to the weaker stimuli should then generalise to more intense stimuli and allow the clinician to gradually expose the dog to the full intensity of the stimulus (Fig. 19.6).

Behaviour modification

Behaviour modification is the application of learning principles to treat problem behaviours. It generally utilises positive reinforcement, desensitisation, and counterconditioning rather than punishment.

Systematic desensitisation is a technique used to break down anxieties and fears in a piecemeal fashion. It involves repeatedly exposing the animal to a very weak fear-eliciting stimulus without evoking a fear response. It is done by repeatedly exposing the individual to a stimulus that resembles the fear-eliciting stimulus and gradually metamorphising or changing the presented stimulus into the original stimulus. The change should occur so slowly that fears and anxieties are not provoked.

Counterconditioning is a method of ameliorating undesirable behaviours by conditioning the animal, both by classical and instrumental conditioning, to engage in responses which are incompatible with the undesirable response. Counterconditioning is frequently used in conjunction with systematic desensitisation.

Spontaneous recovery

After an animal has been desensitised or counterconditioned to a specific stimulus, if a long period of time lapses between the training procedures and the occurrence of a real incident, the dog may again react in an undesirable way when the original stimulus is presented. In order to prevent 'spontaneous recovery' from occurring, the dog should be periodically exposed to some form of the stimulus after treatment. For example, if a dog that has been treated for fear of people does not usually come into contact with people, the owner should definitely plan such exposures. Otherwise the animal may revert to its original fearful response to unfamiliar people. If an animal has been desensitised to thunderstorms, it should be periodically exposed to stereo recordings or sounds of thunderstorms.

Constraints on learning

While it may appear that one can teach an animal to do anything, that is, of course, not true. There are constraints concerning what an animal can learn.

a

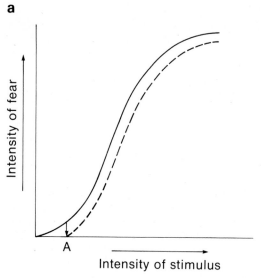

b

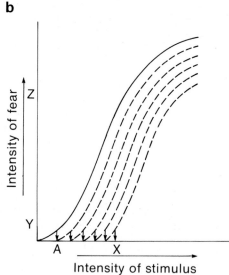

Fig. 19.6 Theoretical representations of desensitisation procedure. (a) As the intensity of an aversive stimulus, such as the onset of a thunderstorm or approach of a person, increases, the intensity of the fear also increases as indicated in the response curve prior to desensitisation (—). Following desensitisation at a stimulus level A, the animal's fears may be reduced to zero (---). This desensitisation may also result in reduction of fear at all higher levels of intensity of the aversive stimulus, as indicated by the new response curve. (b) Several successive desensitisation sessions given to an animal may result in successively lower response curves. Thus, a stimulus at point X will evoke a fear reaction of level Y after five desensitisation sessions compared with a response at point Z prior to any desensitisation (Voith & Hart 1978). From *Canine Neurology*, 3rd edn., Hoerlien (ed.), W.B. Saunders, Philadelphia, with permission.

There are genetic limitations as to what can be learned and there are species differences (Thorndike 1898; Breland & Breland 1961; Seligman 1970). Not all behaviour problems can be eliminated by utilising learning principles.

BEHAVIOURAL THERAPY

Because a behaviour can be influenced by a multitude of variables, it is logical to assume that there are a number of ways of intervening in order to change a behaviour and that people with different backgrounds could intervene successfully. However it is also logical to deduce that the greater one's knowledge in the area of animal behaviour, the better the individual should be in diagnosing the problem designing therapeutic procedures. A wider range of techniques should be available to that individual.

There are three major ways of intervening to treat a behaviour problem (Table 19.4). One is to manipulate the environment to change the probability of a problem occurring; the second is to alter the physiology of the animal either by a surgical procedure or drug therapy; and third, by utilising behaviour modification techniques or learning principles. For exam-

ple, if the dog is only aggressive to male dogs when a bitch is in oestrus, manipulating the environment by prohibiting access to oestrus females or prohibiting access to other male dogs will prevent the problem. Male dogs can also be trained to engage in nonaggressive behaviours when faced with another male dog. Housebreaking problems are generally treated by manipulating the environment in such a way that the dog learns where to eliminate and will inhibit itself in other circumstances. Castration or progestin therapy can suppress intermale aggression and urine marking behaviour by male dogs. A dog that urine marks in specific circumstances can also be counterconditioned to perform competing behaviour in those situations.

Sometimes intervening in one way will suffice, other times it is more helpful to utilise two or three of these avenues. The treatment methods of choice depend on

Table 19.4. Major ways to change behaviour.

Environmental manipulation
Physiological intervention
Pharmacological
Surgical
Behaviour modification

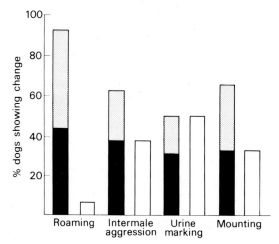

Fig. 19.7 Behavioural changes following castration of adult male dogs. Percentage of dogs experiencing rapid decline (solid sections), gradual decline (shaded sections), or no change (blank sections) in roaming, aggressive interactions with other males (intermale aggression), urine markings in the house, and mounting of other animals or people, after castration. Modified from Hopkins *et al* (1976).

the probability of it working, owner's preferences, potential side-effects, and specific constraints imposed by the owner or dog.

Physiological intervention

Effects of castration

Veterinarians and husbandrymen have employed castration for centuries to alter the behaviour of male animals. The procedure is an effective way to reduce typically masculine behaviour traits in dogs. A retrospective study of 42 dogs, which had been castrated between 0.67 and 12.0 years of age, indicated that within six months following surgery, 50–70% of the dogs decreased mounting people or animals, urine marking in the house, and intermale aggressive behaviour. Roaming behaviour declined by about 90% (Fig. 19.7; Hopkins *et al* 1976). Approximately half of the dogs showed a decline in these behaviours within two weeks and the rest within six months following surgery. The age of the dog at the time of castration did not appear to influence the effects of the surgical procedure. Several owners commented that their dogs appeared calmer after castration but there was no indication that any of the dogs became abnormally inactive or lethargic. All the owners expressed positive comments concerning effects of the castration. Dogs which underwent surgery because of hyperactivity did not reduce their activity level following surgery, nor did dogs who were protective of their property show any decrease in their protective behaviour.

There is a wide degree of variation in the impairment of copulatory behaviour of male animals following surgery. Laboratory experiments have shown that some dogs retain copulatory behaviour for years post-castration (Beach 1970). Studies with Beagles indicate that persistence in copulatory behaviour is independent of pre-castration sexual experience (Hart 1968). However, all dogs that continue to copulate following castration do show some impairment of sexual activity. Detriments in performance include longer latencies before mounting or cessation of mounting, more pelvic thrusting prior to intromission, a shorter length of time in lock, and fewer copulations per session.

The persistence of sexual or typically masculine behaviours is probably not due to sustained serum testosterone levels following castration or to circulating adrenal androgens. The concentration of plasma testosterone drops to nearly non-detectable levels within six hours post castration (Resko 1970; Resko & Phoenix 1972) and neutered animals that have also been adrenalectomised still persist in sexual activities (Warren & Aronson 1956).

It is not clear what the relationship is between testosterone and dominance aggression of dogs directed toward people. Clinically, male dogs are presented for dominance aggression overwhelmingly more often than are females (Voith 1979a, 1981a; Line & Voith 1983; Borchelt 1983). These dogs usually do not begin exhibiting aggression until sometime after reaching puberty. Since most typically masculine behaviour traits are effected by castration and dominance aggression is a typically masculine behaviour trait, it is logical to assume that castration may effect this behaviour. However, unlike the other behaviours affected by castration, persistence of this trait may be influenced by the length of time the dog has engaged in the behaviour prior to castration. It is my clinical impression that castration does suppress the expression of dominance aggression towards people and that the procedure is more likely to be effective in younger male dogs.

A study comparing the behaviour of three 3-month-old puppies castrated at forty days with the behaviour of three intact male litter mates reported that castration did not influence aggressive behaviours or the dominant status of the individuals with each other during play, competition for bones, or sexual responsiveness; nor did castration impair the dogs' ability to compete for receptive oestrus females. Size appeared to be a more important influencing factor than the presence of testosterone (LeBœuf 1970).

The effects of psychotropic drugs on behaviour

Veterinarians frequently administer drugs as a means of restraining or subduing animals. These drugs are usually general and selective central nervous system depressants such as the barbiturates, benzodiazepines, and phenothiazines. These hypnotic, sedative, and tranquilizing drugs decrease general activity level, suppress excitement, calm anxious individuals, produce drowsiness, and promote sleep. Sometimes this class of drugs also act as antiepileptic agents, muscle relaxants, anti-anxiety drugs, and anaesthetics.

The benzodiazepines such as diazepam and chlordiazepoxide (Valium and Librium) are commonly used to reduce anxiety in people. Their success would suggest that they are likely candidates for treatment of anxieties in dogs and cats; however, the benzodiazepines are not general depressants and can sometimes cause excitement. Not infrequently owners report that their dogs become more restless, agitated, or aggressive following the use of diazepam or chlordiazepoxide. Lapras (1977) also noted that diazepam was 'capable of increasing excitability and worrying ... dogs'. However high levels of diazepam (0.5–2.2 mg/kg per os) have been found to reduce a dog's phobic reaction to thunderstorms (Voith 1983b).

The phenothiazine drugs are used for sedative effects and to treat severe psychiatric illnesses in people. In animals, these drugs generally are termed tranquillisers and are used to treat anxiety. However, although an animal's learned responses and motor abilities can be depressed with phenothiazines, the animal can still be quickly aroused when it receives a painful stimulus. Unconditioned responses, such as response to pain, are not suppressed by phenothiazines. Phenothiazines may suppress a dog's learned fear response of an approaching veterinary surgeon, but the animal will react when it experiences pain. Sudden aggressiveness in dogs has been reported following the use of acepromazine maleate (Waechter 1982).

Phenothiazines potentiate seizure activity and are contraindicated in epileptic animals. The phenothiazines probably should not be used in animals manifesting false pregnancies because phenothiazines are dopamine agonists and dopamine is a prolactin inhibiting factor.

Lapras (1977) treated 138 animals over a period of three years with the psychotropic drugs, trimeprimine and medifozamine. He reported that behaviours indicative of anxiety and depression were relieved with the use of these drugs and noted few intolerances other than that of occasional sleepiness. The essence of his paper was that there is a potential usefulness of psychotropic drugs for the treatment of behavioural problems in animals. Psychotropic drugs do open up a potential resource for the treatment of behavioural disorders in animals; however, it should be remembered that these drugs are marketed for people and their effects can vary greatly between species. Veterinarians should familiarise themselves thoroughly with information available on psychotropic drugs before prescribing them to animals. Current human therapy books (such as the *Physicians Desk Reference*) should be consulted. Information can also be sought from the drug companies that market the product. The products may have been tested on dogs prior to marketing for people. The owners should be informed if a drug is not marketed for animals and be made aware that it is essentially an experimental drug in such situations. When prescribing such drugs, it would be best to warn the owner to watch for side effects and remain with the dog for 24 hours when first administering the drug.

To limit the use of drugs to the few tranquillisers and hormones marketed for use in animals potentially reduces the possibility of successful treatment of several serious behavioural problems in animals. However, if psychotropic drugs are used, it should be done cautiously.

Amitriptyline hydrochloride is an antianxiety/antidepressant medication marketed for humans, but in my experience, it can suppress separation anxiety responses in dogs. If the behaviour problem is mild, the drug therapy will work without concurrent behavioural modification techniques. If the behaviour problem is very severe, behaviour modification techniques may need to be supplemented with some drug therapy. Amitriptyline has been found to be effective for separation anxiety at doses of 2–4 mg/kg per os administered an hour prior to departure. This initial dose can be used for two weeks, then the medication should be progressively decreased over several weeks. Amitriptyline and imipramime also decrease the tone of smooth muscle in the bladder and could be used to treat selective enuresis problems. They *would not* be effective in suppressive enuresis related to hypoestrogenism.

Potential side-effects of amitriptyline in people are anticholinergic responses such as blurred vision, a dry mouth, constipation, urinary retention, cardiac arrhythmias, tachycardia, orthostatic hypotension, general weakness, muscle tremors, and occasionally, manic episodes.

Methylphenidate and amphetamines have been used to treat naturally occurring hyperkinetic dogs (Corson *et al* 1976) (see p. 520).

Amphetamine overdose in dogs results in an increase in activity level, elevated heart and respiratory rate, and increased oxygen consumption. At higher doses, the animal may become anorexic, engage in nonsensical repetitive motions such as circling or running backwards, hyperthermia, and convulsions. Amphetamine poisoning has been reported to be treatable with 0.1–1.0 mg/kg of acetylpromazine maleate intramuscularly, immersion in cold water, and if necessary, barbiturate anaesthesia (Stowe *et al* 1976).

Amphetamine is also used in diagnosis and treatment of narcolepsy in dogs. This syndrome is adequately covered in numerous neurology texts pertaining to companion animals.

Effects of progestins on behaviour

Typically masculine behaviour traits such as roaming, intermale aggression, urine marking, mounting, and dominance aggression directed toward people, exhibited by intact or castrated dogs can be reduced with the treatment of synthetic progestins. Interestingly progestins will also reduce these behaviours when exhibited by a female.

Repository medroxyprogesterone acetate at 10–20 mg/kg/IM or SQ can suppress masculine behaviour traits of castrated dogs for several weeks or months. Intact males should respond similarly. The response to the drug is variable and it is difficult to retrieve once administered. Evans (1978) reported that 69.1% of 55 intact male dogs reduced or stopped engaging in roaming, mounting, or urine marking in the house when treated with megestrol acetate at 1–4 mg/kg per os daily for one week, followed by 0.1–1.0 mg/kg for two weeks. Two months after cessation of medication, 66.6% of the dogs were reported to have maintained their improved behaviour. When the author (VLV) uses megestrol acetate to treat typically masculine behaviours, she prescribes 1.0–2.0 mg/kg per os daily for two weeks followed by progressive reduction over 2–6 more weeks. However, unless the owners simultaneously engage in behaviour modification or training procedures, the undesirable behaviours often return as the drug is withdrawn.

Progestin therapy should be stopped periodically. The variables influencing the behaviour may have changed and the dog may no longer be motivated to engage in the undesirable behaviour. Periodically stopping the medication may also reduce the possibility of inducing side-effects with the drug.

If it is anticipated that progestin therapy will be used for more than one month, it would be wise to obtain a complete blood count and serum chemistry profile prior to treatment and periodically assess these parameters during the course of therapy. Admittedly, most of these measures will only detect late changes that are occurring in the physiology of the dog, but it is one method of monitoring possible aversive side-

effects. An advantage to the use of oral medication is that if side-effects are observed, the medication can be stopped, whereas repository injections are not easily retracted. Side-effects of progestin therapy are often reversible if medication is stopped early in the course of pathological response.

The progestins can cause an increase in appetite and mammary gland hyperplasia. Recent studies and reviews of the literature (Eigenmann & Venker-van Haagen 1981; Eigenmann & Eigenmann 1981; Eigenmann 1981) have reported that in the dog synthetic progestins and naturally elevated progesterone levels such as those that occur after oestrus, can cause hyperglycaemia, elevated insulin and growth hormone levels, acromegaly, glucose intolerance/diabetes mellitus, polyphagia, polyurea, and polydipsia unaccompanied by hyperglycaemia, lower packed-cell volume, reduced exercise tolerance, thickening of the gall bladder epithelium with possible sequelae of jaundice, development of mammary gland nodules, and in the intact female, chronic hyperplastic endometrium–pyometra complex. The older the dog the greater the risk of inducing glucose intolerance/diabetes mellitus. Because prolonged administration of progestins has been incriminated in pyometra–hyperplastic-endometrium complexes in dogs, the author does not use progestins for behavioural therapy in intact females. Progestins also suppress spermatogenesis, although sperm production and libido should return after progestin therapy is stopped.

Clearly the use of progestins should not be taken lightly. The use of the drug, the possible side-effects, the alternative therapies available, and the possibility of immediate euthanasia must all be weighed by the practitioner and owner. The use of progestin therapy should be based on appropriate diagnosis and not used simply in the hope it will change any behaviour that an animal engages in. It should be remembered that masculine behaviour traits are most likely to be influenced by progestin therapy. For example, whereas urine marking may be suppressed by progestins, lack of housebreaking will not be affected.

The progestins also have an antianxiety or tranquillising effect and may be effective in ameliorating anxiety-related behaviours. However, other antianxiety drugs with lower probabilities of producing side-effects should also be considered.

HISTORY-TAKING AND INTERVIEWING TECHNIQUES

If a behaviour problem has been longstanding or the owner's question complex, a few minutes of history-taking and a short answer will not suffice. A considerable amount of information is often needed to make a diagnosis and to structure a therapeutic regime which fits that particular owner and dog. To do justice to a problem, time must be set aside to collect information and learn something about the daily activities of the owner and dog.

The styles of history-taking and interviewing technique vary among individuals. What is essential, in either an office or home visit, is to collect enough information from the history and by observing the owner and animal to make a diagnosis, and to transmit enough information to the owner that s/he is able to work with the problem. Home visits have the advantage of being able to see the animal and owner in the usual environment where problem behaviour occurs. The clinician can also personally assess the physical layout of the environment for aids in treating the problem. In a large office, where an animal is allowed to wander about, one can also see typical interactions between the owner and animal and how the owner responds to behaviours of the animal. Behavioural therapists vary in the number of times they see a particular case. Some find it beneficial to see the client, either at home or in the office, several times in order to personally assess the degree of improvement and to directly help the owner further shape the behaviour of the animal. Other therapists believe they are able to monitor the situation by telephone after a visit. A great deal of personal expertise and art is involved in collecting the information and dispensing the treatment procedures. Whether at home or in the office, a critical amount of information is needed.

A relaxed friendly attitude on the part of the clinician is even more important during a behaviour interview than during an office examination regarding a medical problem. Owners often feel guilty when their animals have a serious behavioural problem, particularly when they believe that their method of raising the dog may have contributed to its possible destruction. If the clinician appears judgmental the client is unlikely to reveal a complete description of events, some of which may be helpful in understanding the situation.

Although a structured interview would be the most efficient way of collecting information, it is usually an unproductive way to begin. The owner does not initially see the purpose of such questions and feels frustrated if the interview is structured too rigidly.

After the owners have described what they consider to be the major problem and what they feel is important about it, the owner should be asked to relate in detail the last three incidents, detailing who was present, in which room the behaviour occurred, what happened within the few minutes preceding and immediately after the behaviour occurred. The purpose of this questioning is to determine if there are specific stimuli that evoke the behaviour and if the dog is being reinforced in some way for performing the behaviour. The owner is likely to remember the sequence of events of the last several incidents in great detail. After those incidents have been described they should be asked to relate events in a chronological order; when the behaviour began, what sort of stimuli were involved at the initial precipitation of the behaviour, etc., until the owners have listed everything that they remember.

By now, an experienced clinician has an idea of the nature of the problem and may begin asking questions to confirm the tentative diagnosis. The owner may not have volunteered some information because they did not believe it to be related to the problem. For example, if the stimuli which evoke growling and biting are reaching for the dog, hugging or petting the dog, and trying to take objects from it, the dog may be exhibiting dominance aggression. This alerts the clinician to ask about other situations that are often indicative of dominant characteristics, such as what happens if the owner grabs the dog by the neck or the muzzle, pulls on its neck, lifts it, pushes it over, or scolds it. The owner may reveal that some of these activities evoke a lift of the lip, growl, or other threat. These responses would support a diagnosis of dominance aggression.

During the interview, the owners should be encouraged to answer with actual descriptions of behaviours and not explain the dog's behaviour in terms of 'happy, aggressive, angry, etc'. If these terms are used the owner should be asked to describe what the animal did or looked like that made them attribute that description. The owner should be able to relate what they observed rather than their interpretations of the behaviours.

After obtaining detailed descriptions of the behaviour problem incidents, the owner should be asked for a description of a typical day in the life of the dog, giving the sequence of events in which the owners interact with the dog. Do they immediately take the dog out upon wakening? Does it eliminate outside? Do they find that it has eliminated in the house overnight? Where is the dog when they eat breakfast and how does it behave? When do they feed the dog? Who feeds it? When they leave for work does the dog show signs of distress or apprehensiveness—does it pace, salivate, etc.? When they return from work do they find it has eliminated, destroyed objects, are the neighbours complaining about howling behaviour? How does the dog greet the returning owner? What is the owner's response? This segment of the interview, which may take 10-15 minutes, usually proves invaluable. It shows the times of the day the behaviour may be occurring, how much attention and exercise the dog is getting, and other immediate factors that may relate to the behaviour problem. The author also use this information to structure the treatment programme to fit the owner's schedule.

It is important, of course, to find out how many people live in the household, how many other animals there are, how each of these individuals interact with the pet that has the problem and what the dog's response is to them, what kind of training it has received, and its early history.

Towards the end of the interview, possible treatments are explored to determine what the owners have already tried, what their attitudes are towards keeping the dog despite the behaviour problem, if they have considered euthanasia and what their views on euthanasia are, etc. For example, some cases of aggression may have a poor prognosis and are exceedingly risky to treat, particularly if children are in the household.

Throughout the behavioural interview, it is important to watch the dog, owner, and their interactions. It is also valuable to observe how the dog reacts to outside noises or stimuli or new persons coming into the room or vicinity. The clinician is often able to see both behaviours of the animal that are indicative of the problem and those of the owner which may facilitate the problem. Such observations not only help in the diagnosis of the problem but also serve as an opportunity to discuss the behaviour and how the owner responds to it. The clinician can explain or demonstrate alternative and appropriate ways for the client to interact with the dog at that time.

A clinician should not feel pressured to offer an immediate prognosis and treatment plan if s/he is unsure what the diagnosis is or the best method to approach a problem. It is better to consider the matter and for the interim, advise and instruct the owner how to teach the dog to sit-stay or other simple procedures, because these techniques frequently are incorporated in subsequent behaviour modification programmes. Subsequent instructions can then be posted to the owner, or a subsequent meeting or telephone conversation can go over the prognosis and the treatment procedures. The short delay thus created in developing a specific programme is usually well accepted.

FEARS AND PHOBIAS

The underlying treatment of a fear or phobia is to experience the fear eliciting stimulus without being afraid. This can be achieved in a variety of ways although the underlying element of treatment is al-

ways the same. Desensitisation and counterconditioning are the traditional methods of treating fears and phobias in animals (Tuber *et al* 1974, 1982). Flooding or response prevention is commonly used to treat fear responses of people and may have some application in treating dogs (Young 1982). Desensitisation and counterconditioning involve gradually exposing the animal, without eliciting a fearful response, to the fear eliciting stimulus. Flooding employs almost the opposite tactic and involves exposing the animal to a sufficiently intense stimulus to elicit a fearful response, but the fear eliciting stimulus is *not removed* until the animal has stopped responding fearfully or at least has begun to habituate. Thus, by the end of the treatment session, the animal is experiencing the fear eliciting stimulus in a non-fearful state. It is theoretically possible that removal of the animal or the fearful stimulus while the animal is still engaging in the fearful response perpetuates the response. The animal associates the fearful response with the termination of the stimulus. If a clinician utilises flooding as a treatment procedure, s/he should be prepared for potentially very long sessions.

Noise phobias

A phobic reaction is a fear response that is out of proportion to the real threat of the stimulus. Some dogs are so frightened of thunderstorms that they will leap through glass windows or doors in an attempt to escape the noise. Dogs have jumped out of windows in high rise buildings, broken their jaws trying to manipulate latches on doors, destroyed household furniture and collapsed in flaccid paralysis for the duration of the storm. They can inflict serious injury upon themselves as well as their environment in futile attempts to escape.

Desensitisation and counterconditioning techniques have been used successfully to treat thunderstorm phobias of dogs and the paradigm provides a good model for treatment of other fears. Dogs react to the approach, intensity and dissipation of thunderstorms along an intensity gradient. When the storm is at a distance, the dog begins exhibiting mild signs of anxiety such as pacing, salivating, or muscle tremors. As the storm increases in intensity, the dog's responses increase. As the storm dissipates, the responses dissipate. While the dog may be reacting to a variety of stimuli involved with the storm, noise is clearly one of the more powerful components.

A real thunderstorm has too rapid an onset and is too intense to utilise within a therapy session. However, if a facsimile can be produced and its intensity controlled, the dog can be desensitised and counter-conditioned to the artificial storm with the anticipation that the new responses will generalise to the real thunderstorm. In order for this programme treatment to work, the artificial stimulus has to be of sufficient quality to generate a fear response. In addition to excellent stereo equipment and recordings, it is sometimes necessary to darken the room, increase the base component of the sound, and add flashing strobe lights to elicit a fear response. As soon as it is determined that the artificial situation is effective in eliciting a response, the equipment should be immediately turned off.

The actual treatment sessions involve rewarding the dog with a delicious food reward for remaining quiet as the artificial storm is produced and gradually increased and decreased in intensity: in effect creating a mini-storm. The situation should be controlled so that it does not evoke a fear response. As long as the dog remains calm, it receives food rewards. If the dog appears nervous, it does not get any food rewards nor should the clinician or owner pet or speak to the dog in attempts to relieve the anxiety. These actions may act as reinforcement for the anxiety. If a mild response has been elicited the animal may quickly habituate and, after it does so, it should get a food reward. If the dog does not habituate, the volume of the recording should be reduced until the dog is again relaxed. The clinician should wait a while before again resuming dispensing food rewards. Later the volume should again be increased but more slowly so as not to evoke a fear response. Sessions generally last 20–30 minutes and are repeated over a course of several days until the owner is taught the rudiments of the techniques — particularly when to reward and withhold reinforcements. Gradually the dog is put on intermittent schedules of reinforcement. Sometimes the dog must tolerate 2–3 thunderclaps before receiving a reward and several minutes must lapse between rewards. The procedure should be practised in several locations and, of course, eventually in the owner's home. After the dog is tolerating loud recordings, it may be beneficial to softly play the recordings at low levels at time unassociated with therapy sessions.

It is unlikely that the dog's reactions to the recordings will generalise perfectly to real storm situations. The dog will probably never enjoy thunderstorms. However, its new response to the recordings should generalise sufficiently to real storms that it will not engage in phobic reactions. After the dog has been desensitised and counterconditioned it should periodically be exposed to the recordings between thunderstorm seasons to prevent spontaneous recovery of the phobia from occurring.

If a real thunderstorm occurs between treatment sessions, the owner should not reinforce the dog's fearful behaviour by talking to it soothingly, hugging or petting it. If necessary, the owners should restrain the dog so it does not injure itself or the environment and if possible, the dog should be heavily tranquillised prior to the onset of the storm. The drug found most effective in attenuating fear responses of thunderstorms is diazepam dosed at 0.25–0.50 mg/kg per os.

Fear responses to people

The facial and body expressions of fearful dogs are well known to veterinarians and have been described by several authors (Schenkel 1947; Fox 1971). The fearful dog lowers its head, retracts its ears, tucks its tail between its legs, and may lie down or roll over on its side (Fig. 19.8). It may also draw its mouth back into a horizontal grin and avoid direct eye contact. Dogs generally try to avoid fearful stimuli, but if cornered or ambivalent about the situation, the fearful dog may bite. Fear-induced aggression is one of the more common causes of aggressive behaviour of dogs towards people. Dogs, like people, can experience several emotions simultaneously or, to word it less anthropomorphically, appear to be motivated to perform two or more behaviours simultaneously. A dog may be afraid of someone but also motivated to protect its puppies or territory. The dog may exhibit a composite of fearful and offensively aggressive signals or rapidly alternate the two signals.

If it is determined that a dog is afraid of people, a hierarchy of stimuli that elicit the responses needs to be determined; the physical appearance and movement of the people, situations or locations, etc. If counterconditioning and desensitisation are employed, the stimuli must be arranged according to a hierarchy and gradually presented to the dog while it is in a non-fearful state. For example, a dog may be more afraid of men than women, more afraid of bearded men than clean shaven men (Fig. 19.9). Distance is also a variable. The dog may not be afraid of a person at 5.7 m, but begins showing anxiety at 6 m and is overtly afraid at 5.1 m. The dog may not be afraid of a person standing still, but if s/he reaches towards the dog, the dog exhibits fear. The dog may be afraid of specific parts of its body being touched or reached for. It may take 10 or 15 minutes to obtain a list of stimuli and determine the gradient of intensity of these stimuli that will evoke fearful behaviour but only after these stimuli are identified can the desensitisation and counterconditioning procedures be implemented.

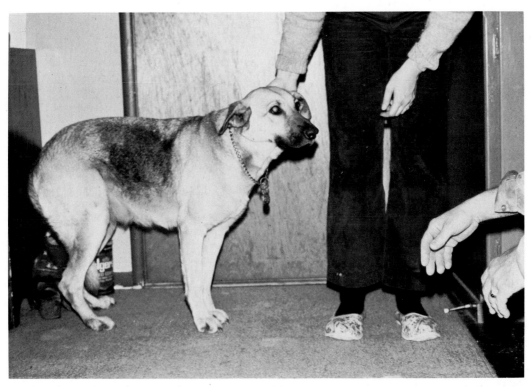

Fig. 19.8   This German Shepherd Dog's facial expression and body posture indicate that she is afraid of the people reaching towards her.

Prior to initiating the desensitisation and counter-conditioning sessions, the owners should practice sit-stays with the dog. The dog should learn to anticipate a delicious food tidbit with sitting or lying still and a neutral or non-fearful motivational state. When the actual sessions begin, the dog receives tidbits for remaining in a quiet, non-fearful state while weak fear eliciting stimuli are presented. As long as the stimuli do not evoke fear the dog is rewarded with food tidbits as well as petting and praise.

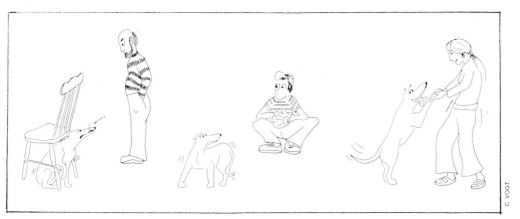

Fig. 19.9   Dogs that are afraid, and consequently aggressive, often react with varying intensities of fear to different groups of people. This dog is most afraid of men, less afraid of boys, and not afraid of women. Delineation of such a hierarchy of fear inducing stimuli is necessary before embarking on a desensitisation programme (Voith, 1979c). With permission from the editors of *Modern Veterinary Practice*.

If a dog has indicated that it is more afraid of men than women, more afraid of a person reaching out than not, more afraid if it is in a corner than in the centre of the room, the desensitisation and counter-conditioning session might begin outdoors or in the centre of a large room with a woman at a distance with her arms beside her. The woman moves closer to the dog. If the dog does not demonstrate any signs of apprehension—lowers ears, quivers or moves backwards, etc.—the dog is rewarded. The person then takes another step forward. The woman might then add a moving stimulus, such as raising and lowering her arm, reaching toward the dog, or wiggling her hand. The dog is rewarded if it tolerates these actions. Gradually the woman moves closer and closer until she can extend her hand over the head of the dog. About this time, food tidbits can be shown to the dog and transferred to the approacher's hand who then slowly gives the tidbits to the dog. The woman may carefully begin almost or actually petting and touching various parts of the dog's body. A tidbit is paired with tolerating these advances.

At the slightest indication of apprehension, the tidbit is withheld and the person stops increasing the intensity of the stimulus complex. If this happens, one can wait to see if the dog habituates and as soon as the ears again come forward or the body again straightens into a taller position, the dog gets a tidbit. If it appears that the dog is not going to habituate, the person should back up. However, the dog does not immediately get a reinforcement when it resumes its non-fearful state because one does not want to inadvertently reward the fearful behaviour that was just exhibited. Instead, the approacher should make a modified movement towards the dog. If the dog tolerates this abbreviated increase in intensity of stimulus, the dog gets a reward.

Not only do visual and auditory stimuli, location, distance from the dog, and arm movements evoke fearful responses, but the length of time these stimuli are presented also functions as a variable in eliciting a response. A dog may tolerate a fearful stimulus for a short while, but eventually become apprehensive. It is often best to keep the treatment sessions relatively short—15–20 minutes, particularly if the 'approaching' person is close to the dog.

Factors that must be taken into consideration vary for each case. Staring at the dog, tones of voice, rapid movement *away from the dog* as well as towards the dog may elicit responses. It is important to determine as many eliciting stimuli as possible and gradually introduce them to the dog.

Between therapy sessions, the owner should try to avoid situations or people that might elicit a fearful response. For example, if one is trying to desensitise and countercondition a dog's fearful response to judges in a show ring, the dog should not be exposed to this situation until it is predicted that it will not react apprehensively. Every time the dog engages in a fear response between therapy sessions, the treatment process is retarded. If, between sessions, an owner, inadvertently or by necessity, exposes the dog to people in a situation that evokes a fear response, the owner should restrain, but otherwise ignore, the dog. The owner should refrain from talking soothingly or petting the dog in an attempt to relieve its anxiety because the dog may interpret these behaviours as reinforcements. If the dog habituates to the stimulus and assumes a calm appearance, then the dog should be praised and petted.

Punishment, of course, is contraindicated in treating fearful behaviours including fear-induced aggression. It is ridiculous to believe that punishing a dog for being afraid of a thunderstorm will alleviate its fearful response to the thunderstorm. Likewise, punishing a dog who elicits fear-induced aggression does not treat the underlying cause of the aggressive problem. While it is possible that an intimidating person may inhibit or suppress an aggressive response of a fearful dog, the dog is still afraid of people and is likely to demonstrate aggression at another time or to another individual. Neutering (castration or spaying) is not effective in ameliorating fearful behaviours, including fear-induced aggression.

Theoretically, drugs may be helpful as an aid in treating fearful behaviours. The drugs that are reported to alleviate anxieties and fears of people and of experimental animals are the benzodiazapines and phenothiazines. Such drugs may be helpful between sessions if the dog is exposed to fearful stimuli. It is debatable whether or not to use drugs in conjunction with desensitisation procedures because of the phenomenon known as drug-dependent learning. An animal can learn to engage in a specific behaviour while under the influence of a drug, but when the drug is withdrawn the animal will no longer engage in that learned behaviour. The animal only exhibits the behaviour under the influence of the drug.

Every case involving fears or phobias has its own idiosyncrasies and these must be determined to develop a treatment plan. Once the stimuli are identified and gradients established, the author finds it helpful to give individually designed handouts to the owners which they can follow (Fig. 19.10). A systematic checklist helps the owners proceed at an appropriate rate and provides information concerning the problems with the programme. The most common mistake of owners is that they proceed too fast and precipitate

Date	Location	Approacher	Distance	Dog's Reaction
16·3-83	outdoors	Jane Doe	10 ft	good
	"	"	9 ft	"
	"	"	8 ft	"

Fig. 19.10 Example of handout provided to owner for practice sessions involving desensitisation and counterconditioning of a fearful dog (Voith 1976).

mistakes. If they evoke a severe fear response, it is an indication that the programme is being implemented inappropriately. Desensitisation and counterconditioning procedures must proceed slowly to be effective.

Separation anxiety

Dogs are social creatures and sometimes howl, whine, dig, chew, pace, pant, salivate, eliminate, or become anorexic when they are separated from their owners. Eventually the responses of the dogs generalise from the actual time of separation to predeparture behaviours of the owner. A dog may begin showing signs as the owners engage in behaviours that routinely predict a departure—such as straightening magazines, putting the dishes away, locking the windows, going to the coat closet, or putting on specific shoes or trousers. Like other anxieties or fears, the key to treatment is to experience the situation without being afraid. The stimuli that elicit the anxiety are predeparture be-

haviours of the owner, the actual departure, and an interval of time after departure.

Dogs with separation anxiety often have histories of abruptly being left alone for long periods of time after months or years of constant human companionship. Typically the dog had either accompanied the owner everywhere or someone was always present at home. Some dogs have histories of repeated and frequent abandonment; they were strays in the street, kept in humane shelters, or had been frequently kennelled for several week intervals.

Dogs presented for this syndrome usually engage in exaggerated and prolonged greeting responses when reunited with their owners and rarely separate themselves from the owners while at home. The dog follows the owner from room to room, frequently crawls onto the owner's lap or leans against the owner. Occasionally, these dogs demonstrate aggression as the owner tries to depart. Whereas the complaint of the owner is that the dog refuses to let the owner leave, the specific stimulus that elicits the aggression is usually the owner trying to restrain the dog in an attempt to prevent the dog from accompanying him/her. The dog is not actually trying to prevent the owner leaving, but is resisting the restraint being employed to prevent it from accompanying the owner. A detailed history reveals that these dogs also are aggressive toward the owners in other circumstances which are compatible with dominance aggression. Two syndromes, dominance aggression and separation anxiety, need to be investigated.

Interestingly, many dogs that cannot be left alone at home for five minutes can be safely left alone in a car for any length of time. Most people have gradually 'trained' or accustomed their dog to tolerate staying alone in the car. Even after the dog has demonstrated tolerance of long separations it is periodically left alone in the car for short intervals such as the time it takes to post a letter, pay a petrol station attendant, or do a quick bit of shopping. Whereas, initially the departures of an owner from a car are short—usually only a few minutes—and gradually the owner extends the absence, departures from a house are usually initially very long—often 4, 8, or 10 hours—and most subsequent absences are long.

The key feature of a therapeutic programme is many short departures of variable lengths that gradually allow the dog to experience longer, atraumatic separations from the owner. The initial departures should be so short that the dog does not engage in any of the undesirable responses. This may mean one or two minute departures. Gradually the departures become longer, but not in steady progression. For example, a typical series of departures may be 2, 1, 3, 5, 1, 10, 5, 5, 15 minutes etc. (Fig. 19.11).

In addition to the gradual departures, ancillary treatment measures can be employed. Novel cues such as a radio, a loud ticking clock or other obvious cues, can be paired with the short practise departures to facilitate an association of the cue with a 'safe' or short departure—much the same way that dogs learn that departures from cars are 'safe'. The 'safe' departures are gradually made longer. After the dog has experienced several long 'safe' departures, the cue can be dropped out. The owner should not present the cue to the dog for longer intervals than have been gradually practised or the value of the cue as a safety signal will be lost. Obviously the owner should not initially pair the cue with all day departures.

The owners should try to prevent the dog from engaging in the misbehaviours between the practice departures. Until the dog can be left alone for extended periods of time, the owners might take the dog with them, hire a dog sitter or put the dog in a commercial kennel. Confinement systems at home, such as a crate, are not always an appropriate method of managing separation anxiety problems. When left alone in a crate some dogs injure themselves trying to escape. If crates are used, the dog should gradually become accustomed to the cage in the presence and then in the absence of the owner. The idea is not to permanently manage the problem with confinement, but eventually leave the dog free while the owner is away.

Most distress at being left alone is usually confined to an interval of time surrounding the owner's departure. If a dog can be conditioned to tolerate a 90 minute departure, it will usually tolerate departures for many hours. It is important to do practice departures at different times of day and on weekends as well as on weekdays. If departures are only done during daylight hours and then the owner leaves the dog for a long interval at night, the dog may not consider this a 'safe' departure and may react with distress.

Gradual and periodic separations when dog and owner are home helps decrease the dependence of the dog on the owner. For example, the dog can be taught to stay as the owner leaves the room for progressively longer periods of time. Eventually the dog may be required to sleep on the floor or outside the owner's bedroom instead of on the owner's bed. The owners can discourage the dog from sitting on their laps and plastering itself against them.

In cases where dogs are so distraught at the time of departure that the owner cannot leave them even for a few minutes, it is helpful to countercondition the animal to predeparture cues. The dog can be taught to associate quiet, relaxed behaviour (such as sit-stays) with delicious food rewards, and predeparture cues such as the owner putting on his/her shoes, walking to the door, rattling car keys. Eventually the owner actually departs for several minutes with the dog quietly remaining in a sit-stay.

Sometimes it is beneficial to utilise antianxiety drugs such as amitriptyline (2 mg/kg per os), or megestrol acetate (1.0–2.0 mg/kg per os) in conjunction with behaviour modification techniques. Theoretically, the benzodiazapines such as diazepam (Valium) and chlordiazepoxide (Librium) might be helpful. These drugs are frequently used for anxiety responses in people. However, some owners have reported that their dogs become more active after receiving benzodiazapines. None of these drugs are marketed for behavioural therapy of animals in the United States. If a clinician decides to use a drug s/he should familiarise her/himself with all possible side-effects and explain to the owner the experimental nature and potential side-effects of the use of the drug. Of course, the dog should first receive a physical examination to determine if there are any contraindications. If a clinician pre-

Date	Time	Departure (min)	Remarks	Obedience*	Exercise**
1		5			
2		5			
3		10			
4		5			
5		10			
6		5			
7		10			
8		10			
9		5			
10		15			
11		5			
12		15			
13		10			
14		5			
15		20			
16		5			
17		15			
18		10			
19		30			
20		10			
21		5			
22		5			
23		10			
24		30			
25		5			

*Check if you practiced routine obedience procedures that day

**Check if you exercised dog that day

Fig. 19.11 An example of a schedule that could be used as a guideline for graduated departures designed to alleviate separation anxiety (Voith 1975).

scribes a drug for separation anxiety, it is wise to first have the owners give the drug while they are home all day to observe the responses of the dog to the drug. If there are no undesirable effects, the drug should be given an hour before the owner's departure. Occasionally, mild separation anxiety responses can be ameliorated with short-term drug therapy without concurrent behaviour modification techniques. However, severe separation anxiety reactions usually necessitate behavioural intervention.

One of the greatest services a practitioner could offer an owner of a new puppy is to advise them to leave the puppy alone for gradually longer periods of time and thereafter periodically leave it alone for a few hours each week. This should prevent the development of a separation anxiety syndrome.

It should be remembered that dogs can howl, dig, chew and/or eliminate for reasons other than separation anxiety, and that a differential diagnosis must be made when a dog is presented with these signs. The reason the dog is engaging in a specific behaviour must be determined in order to prescribe the most beneficial treatment.

The key features associated with separation anxiety are that the dog engages in behaviours in a relatively short period of time after separation from the owner, shows signs of extreme attachment by following the owner from room to room, engages in overexuberant, prolonged greetings when the owner returns, demonstrates predeparture anxieties such as pacing, salivating, or trembling as the owner prepares to depart and usually does not eat when the owner is gone. Treatment necessitates treating the dog's anxiety related to separation from the owner.

ELIMINATION BEHAVIOUR PROBLEMS

The major differentials for elimination problems in the house are disease, housebreaking, marking behaviour, submissive urination, excitement urination, fear-induced elimination, separation anxiety, and simply lack of opportunity to eliminate in an appropriate place. Disease aetiologies should, of course, be differentiated by clinical signs, obtaining a good history and necessary laboratory tests.

Housebreaking

If a dog is presented for both urinating and defaecating in the house, the most likely behavioural aetiologies are lack of appropriate housebreaking, not taking the dog out frequently enough, or separation anxiety behaviours. If a dog is not well housebroken, the elimination behaviour is usually not related to the absence or presence of the owner, but is related to the length of time since the dog last had access to an appropriate place to eliminate. The problem is unlikely to be a separation anxiety problem if the dog eliminates after the owner has been gone for several hours. In housebreaking problems a large amount of urine is usually voided, not a small amount such as occurs with cystitis or marking behaviour. An unhousebroken animal may also show a preference for one or two locations in the house. Males and females are equally likely to develop a preference for eliminating in the house.

Housebreaking techniques involve frequent access outside or an appropriate location, supervising the dog carefully while inside or confining it in a small space when it cannot be watched, managing its feeding and water schedule or training the dog to eliminate on papers. If paper training is utilised, the owners can put plastic under the paper in the location where the dog is eliminating in the house, gradually reduce the amount of paper and then remove it and the plastic. The essential features of housebreaking are establishing a preference for eliminating outside and developing an inhibition of eliminating inside.

If the dog is caught in the act of eliminating, punishment may be appropriate. However, punishment after the dog has eliminated is not an effective way to solve the problem. Many people report that they have trained their dog to become housebroken by disciplining it whenever they find it has eliminated in the house; however, they also utilised other techniques. It actually is the other techniques that housebreak the dog, not the punishment. It may be true that upon the owner's return the dog 'looks guilty' (assumes a submissive posture and expression) only if it has eliminated in the house. However, this does not mean that the dog associates the forthcoming punishment with the fact that it eliminated previously. What the dog does associate is that simultaneous presence of excrement and return of owner is followed by punishment. If the owner returns and there are no excretory products in the house, only one of the stimuli is present (the returning owner) and the dog does not react with a submissive expression. But, if there is urine or faeces in the house, both stimuli are present and the dog anticipates punishment. A recent case history illustrated this. An owner housebroke his Boston Terrier by spanking and rubbing her nose in the excrement when he found the dog had done something wrong. The dog became housebroken and was perfectly well housebroken for seven years. The owner had also used other housebreaking methods but had not attributed the success to these methods. The owner then got another dog, a Boston Terrier puppy, which was not housebroken. The character of the stools and the urine volume of the puppy could be differentiated from that of the adult dog. However whenever the owner returned and the puppy had eliminated in the house, the adult dog greeted the owner looking guilty.

Urine marking

If the owner complains of small amounts of urine and the dog is a 12–18-month-old male who lifts its leg, the dog is probably urine marking. This behaviour is usually unrelated to the presence of the owner, although it may occur in specific circumstances such as when someone comes to the door or the owner returns. Urine marking is highly likely to be suppressed by castration or progestin therapy. However the beneficial effects of the progestins may only last while the dog is on the drug therapy. Consistent punishment immediately associated with every onset of the behaviour, may also suppress the expression of this behaviour. However, punishment is usually not effective if the dog also urinates in the owner's absence. When certain environmental events are associated with urine marking, such as the entrance of a visitor, the dog can be conditioned to sit-stay or engage in a play behaviour in these circumstances, rather than urine mark. While there is some indication that dominant wolves urine mark more than submissive wolves, all members in the pack may urine mark (Peters & Mech 1975). There does not appear to be a strong correlation between urine marking and dominance status in dogs.

Occasionally dogs may use faeces to mark. Some dogs defaecate on the top of bushes or fence posts, and Beagles have been described as standing on their forelegs and defaecating on high vertical objects (Hart 1969). However, defaecation is not frequently associated with marking behaviour of house dogs.

Submissive/greeting urination

The dog who greets a person by squatting and urinating may be doing so as a part of a greeting and submissive urination behavioural sequence. This behaviour, often accompanied by rolling onto its side, ears back, and tail down, often occurs when someone enters the house, approaches or reaches for the dog. It is usually manifested by puppies and, if the owner does nothing, the dog usually outgrows it. Punishment may only exacerbate or aggravate the situation. Petting or pleasantly talking to the dog as it urinates might be interpreted as a reinforcement by the animal. The situation can usually be treated by ignoring the behaviour or redirecting greeting behaviour into another activity such as chasing a ball or playing with a toy. If the problem persists, counterconditioning may be necessary. The stimuli that elicit the behaviour need to be identified, such as type of person, body posture, and locations that elicit the behaviour, and then the dog is reinforced for standing rather than squatting when these stimuli are presented.

Excitement urination

A related situation is the dog who urinates in a standing as well as squatting posture whenever it is excited. Exciting stimuli may be greeting situations, play or noises. This dog should neither be punished for the behaviour nor reinforced with petting and conversation by the owner. The problem can be treated by identifying the stimuli that elicit the behaviour and conditioning the animal to be calm in the presence of the stimuli.

Fear-elicited elimination problems

Occasionally, dogs urinate and defaecate because of fear. For example, it is not unusual for dogs afraid of thunderstorms to eliminate when a storm occurs. The solution to this problem is to identify the fear eliciting stimuli and treat the fear response.

Separation anxiety

Dogs may urinate and/or defaecate as a consequence of separation from the owner. The key features associated with separation anxiety are that the dog engages in behaviours in a relatively short period of time after separation from the owner, shows signs of extreme attachment by following the owner from room to room, engages in overexuberant, prolonged greetings when the owner returns, demonstrates predeparture anxieties such as pacing, salivating, or trembling as the owner prepares to depart and usually does not eat when the owner is gone. Treatment necessitates treating the dog's anxiety related to separation from the owner (see pp. 515–518).

OVERACTIVITY

Overactivity or hyperactivity is a common complaint of many dog owners. There are numerous possible aetiologies: exuberant play, reinforcement, normal physiological predisposition (such as has been selected for in some hunting breeds) and physiological disorders. Hyperthyroidism has been associated with overactivity and states of agitation; however, most animals exhibiting hyperthyroidism also show signs of weight loss, cardiac abnormalities and other physiological disturbances. Hyperkinesis is a rare activity disorder that responds to pharmacological treatment with some central nervous system stimulants such as amphetamine.

Play and reinforcement

Most dogs are active because they are playful and/or intermittently reinforced for the active behaviour. It is guaranteed to get attention. The owner interacts with the dog, chases it, etc., and maybe even tries to discipline it—which the dog often turns into fun. Play and overexuberant behaviours related to play are very common in dogs under 2 years of age.

The appropriate therapeutic approaches to this problem are to redirect the play and activity into an appropriate channel before the animal initiates the misbehaviour, stop all possible reinforcement of the behaviour, and perhaps counterconditioning and punishment. For example, if the owner can predict that the dog will 'go crazy' and run throughout the house when the owner returns, the owner should initiate a vigorous acceptable method of play before the dog begins 'going crazy'. Inappropriate responses should be extinguished, that is, not reinforced. The owner is to ignore the dog when it becomes 'crazy'. The circumstances and stimuli that elicit the exuberant behaviours (such as someone coming to the door or running past the yard) could be identified and counterconditioned; that is, the dog conditioned to engage in a behaviour that is incompatible with the overactivity, such as sitting or lying down. This requires that the dog learns to inhibit itself in unexciting circumstances first. Sometimes punishment is a helpful adjunctive method.

If the dog is highly motivated to play or is a hunting dog bred for a high activity level, punishment and/or conditioning the dog to inhibit itself will not suffice. These animals must be allowed to play and redirect their energies in an acceptable manner for the owners. Long walks, playing fetch, running or jogging with the owner should reduce the activity level of these dogs. Only if the owner has allowed the dog appropriate play and activity outlets should the owner employ extinction, counterconditioning and/or punishment.

Hyperkinesis

Corson *et al* (1976, 1980) have described hyperkinetic dogs as showing signs of overactivity, increased heart rate, increased respiratory rate, increased oxygen consumption, and inability to tolerate restraint. The dogs demonstrate the intolerance by thrashing, biting and chewing and clawing at the restraining apparatus until it is demolished or the animal becomes exhausted. Tranquillisers such as chloropromazine and meprobamate usually do not affect these dog's behaviour; however, some will respond to pharmacological treatment with amphetamines or methylphenidate (Corson *et al* 1976).

Therapeutic dosages varied among individuals. Methylphenidate (2–4 mg/kg per os) was reported as

reducing hyperactivity, but not as being effective as amphetamines. Hyperkinetic behaviour was reduced by the oral administration of 0.2–1.3 mg/kg dextroamphetamine or 1.0–4.0 mg/kg levoamphetamine.

A physiological hyperkinetic dog usually responds to a therapeutic dose of dextro- or levoamphetamine within two hours of oral administration. The dogs stopped panting, the heart rates decreased, and the dogs tolerated restraint. Corson *et al* also noted that amphetamines would reduce the aggressive behaviour of some hyperkinetic dogs. Interestingly, the dextro- and levoisomers were equally potent at 0.2–1.3 mg/kg per os in suppressing the aggressive behaviour.

To determine a therapeutic dose and/or arrive at a diagnosis of hyperkinesis, it is wise to hospitalise the animal and first obtain an activity baseline using an objective behavioural measure such as number of seconds it remains still or number of metres it travels per unit of time. Then the lowest dose recorded to be effective could be administered to the dog. The animal's behaviour and physiological responses should be evaluated 1–2 hours post administration of the medicine. If there was no response, the animal could be treated again in 24 hours at an increased increment of 0.2 mg/kg dextroamphetamine or 0.5 mg/kg levoamphetamine. The dosage should be slowly increased until the dog either decreases its activity level or increases it. The latter would indicate that the dog may not be hyperkinetic or that the therapeutic window of the drug was missed. It is important to increase the dosage slowly because hyperkinetic dogs, as well as normal dogs, can be overdosed with amphetamines, resulting in an increase in activity, abnormal behaviours, and amphetamine poisoning (see p. 508).

Remember, however, that most animals that are presented for overactivity are not physiologically hyperkinetic but behave that way because they have been reinforced for their active behaviour.

AGGRESSION

Aggression is the most common behavioural problem of dogs presented to behavioural therapists. To maximise the probability of successful treatment, it is important to correctly diagnose why the dog is demonstrating the aggressive behaviour. The therapeutic procedures are designed to reduce the probability of aggression; sometimes the probability can be reduced nearly to zero, but there is never any guarantee that the dog will never bite or injure anyone in the future. Before a clinician begins working with an aggression case, the owners should realise the risks involved and be fully aware that they are responsible for the behaviour of the dog during and after therapy.

Behaviourists do not uniformly agree how to define aggression. The term is usually applied to behaviours which appear to an observer to lead to the damage or destruction of some goal entity (Moyer 1968). Behaviours that signal an intent to inflict damage are also considered aggressive behaviours—such as snarling, lifting of the lip, snapping, threatening barks and growling. Predatory behaviour is not usually traditionally classified as aggression by most behaviourists. The postures and behavioural sequences of a dog while catching prey are quite different from the animal's behaviours when engaging in other types of aggression.

Aggressive encounters may involve competition over a resource or opportunity to enhance an animal's genetic representation (production or survival of offspring or relatives). Sometimes the resource the animal is defending is readily identifiable, such as food, shelter, or territory. Other times the resource or the benefit is not immediately apparent but the animal is able to collect a payoff later on. Aggressive encounters are used in the establishment and maintenance of dominance hierarchies and dominant animals usually have first access to resources. For example, in wolf packs the dominant members are usually the animals that most frequently breed and produce offspring.

Not all displays of aggression are related to dominance. A dog may utilise threats to protect or defend itself or its territory or offspring. There are a multitude of reasons for a dog manifesting aggression and not all forms of aggression can be treated identically. It is important to be familiar with natural manifestations of aggression in order to differentiate them from pathophysiological behaviours.

Most aggressive behaviours of dogs are performed for adaptive reasons—from the perspective of the dog. However, normal species-typical behaviours of canids are not necessarily desirable qualities in a pet, nor does the fact that they are normal behaviours minimise the dangers in keeping such a dog.

Moyer (1968) developed a classification system for aggressive behaviours that was primarily based upon the stimulus situation which elicited the aggression. He also tried to take into account that experience, physiology, and genetic variability affected the expression of aggression. His classifications were: predatory, intermale, fear-induced, irritable, territorial defence, maternal, and instrumental. This basic classification system has been followed by most veterinarians (Houpt 1979; Voith 1980). This schema forces one to identify the stimuli, physiological state and circumstances associated with the aggressive behaviour.

Consequently one can tentatively make a functional or motivational classification of the aggressive behaviour. Then, a rational course of therapy is possible. A synergism of knowledge of species-typical behaviour patterns, facial and body expressions of dogs, learning principles, behavioural modification techniques, physiology and pharmacology will maximise a clinician's ability to functionally classify, offer an accurate prognosis, and develop a successful treatment plan.

Intermale aggression

Intermale aggression provides a good model depicting the numerous variables that can influence the expression of a behaviour (Fig. 19.2) as well as the major therapeutic avenues of change (environmental changes, physiological manipulation, and behaviour modification techniques). While it is true that fighting does include ritualised behaviours and that canids have evolved submissive signals that often deter offensive attacks, it is not true that dogs will not seriously injure each other or kill another in a fight. It is also a fallacy that wild animals in their natural environments never inflict serious injury or kill each other; they do. Advising an owner to let two male dogs 'fight it out' could have serious consequences.

There are two major circumstances of intermale fighting problems: the male dog that challenges strange male dogs and the male dog that threatens another living in the same household. Owners of single aggressive male dogs often attempt to cope with the problem by avoiding other dogs. However, this is usually impossible to achieve realistically; besides this approach also reduces social contact among people. When this male dog does see another, he charges aggressively toward it, often dragging the owner behind, and causing general havoc if not injury to all in his path. Sometimes, if the owner tries to restrain the dog, the dog redirects the aggression to the owner. This type of dog can usually be successfully controlled using behaviour modification techniques; however, castration and/or a temporary course of progestin therapy may facilitate treatment. While training can help control intermale aggression within a household, castration and/or progestin therapy have a greater likelihood of ameliorating the behaviour.

Castration will suppress intermale aggression in many dogs. A retrospective survey of 8 adult male dogs presented for castration reported that intermale aggression ceased or was markedly reduced in 5 of the cases (Hopkins *et al* 1976; Fig. 19.7). Dunbar (1979) reported that aggression between two male dogs was more likely to be reduced if both animals were castrated rather than just one. To maximise the probability that castration will reduce aggression within a household, both male dogs, regardless of who is the aggressor, should be castrated.

Synthetic progestogens will reduce aggression in some castrated as well as intact male dogs. Progestins suppress LH and testosterone production as well as spermatogenesis. The drug clearly has properties in addition to androgen suppression. Progestins can be effective in suppressing typically masculine behaviours, such as intermale aggression, even when castration is not. The drugs are particularly helpful in lowering the motivation for aggression while a dog is being taught to tolerate the approach of other males and to remain with his owner rather than fight. The dosage regime should be adjusted to suit the particular individual.

Occasionally stimuli in the environment, such as an oestrous bitch, can be identified and avoided. Avoiding the stimuli does not correct the problem but simply prevents it from occurring.

Prohibiting free access of males to each other within a household may be the best solution to domestic intermale fighting. Drug therapy and castration do not always work nor are they acceptable to some owners. Although dogs may be trained to tolerate each other *in the owner's presence* they are likely to resume fighting when the owner is gone. If the dogs are constantly vying, fights may periodically erupt even in the owner's presence. It is difficult for most owners to constantly be aware of the interactions of two dogs living together. How successful even a very 'dominant' and experienced owner is in maintaining peace is largely dependent on the intensity of rivalry between the dogs; it is often easier and safer to control the access of the dogs to each other. Even if this environmental approach is taken, the dogs should still be trained to inhibit their aggressive tendencies toward each other and periodically be exposed to each other in controlled situations.

Training techniques are highly successful in allowing an owner to safely walk a pugnacious male dog and are helpful in controlling dogs within a household. Castration and temporary progestin therapy may be beneficial adjunctive measures.

I have found the following schedule of procedures useful for owners of the single dogs. Variations of this technique can be used for dogs within households.

First the owner spends about a week teaching the dog to sit and stay on command. After the dog is performing well and has come to anticipate a very palatable food reward for his behaviour, the owner enlists the aid of a friend with a friendly dog, preferably one that is known to be liked by the owner's male dog. The owners arrange a rendezvous. With the male dog on a lead the owner waits at a designated location. When the other dog and handler come into view, the male dog is told to sit and when he does, he is given a delicious tidbit. The dog must remain sitting while the other dog and handler turn around and disappear from view. As they turn, the male dog receives another tidbit if he remains seated and does not exhibit any aggressive signs. The owner then allows the dog to get up and walk around. When the other handler and dog again come into view, the male dog is again rewarded for sitting, and must remain sitting as the other dog and person approach closer before stopping. The male dog receives a tidbit for tolerating this approach. When the other dog and handler turn and leave, the male is again rewarded for remaining quiet. This sequence is repeated until the other dog and handler are able to approach quite closely and eventually pass the male dog without eliciting any signs. *After* the dog has demonstrated his ability to sit in an unaggressive manner as a friendly, familiar dog passes him at various speeds, different dogs and handlers are enlisted to participate (Fig. 19.12). Sometimes it is helpful if the owner conditions the male dog to wear a muzzle prior to practising these sequences. Muzzles are available

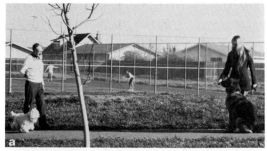
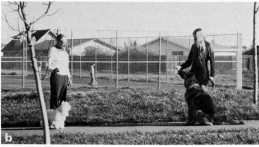

Fig. 19.12 During the final stages of treating intermale aggression, the dog is rewarded for sitting quietly while another male dog approaches closer and closer.

that fit snugly and yet allow the dog to have a tidbit. Eventually the procedures should be done without a muzzle.

If the male shows any signs of aggression during these approaches, he does not get a reward. The particular step of the procedure that elicited the aggression is repeated until the male shows no aggressive signs. Whether or not scolding or punishment is appropriate depends on whether fear is contributing to the dog's aggressive behaviour. Ideally, the procedures should be done so slowly that little or no aggression is ever evoked. If the owner or clinician sense the dog is becoming uneasy, the dogs should not be brought any closer together, and that particular step should be repeated until the male easily tolerates the other dog at that distance.

It may take several sessions until the male appears comfortable tolerating another dog to approach within six feet and then walk past. The closer the dogs are, the more careful the owners must be. It is also important to know that *distance and time can interact* in precipitating an aggressive behaviour. The male dog may tolerate an approach to six feet; however, if the other dog stays there too long, the male dog may no longer inhibit his aggressive tendencies and will attack. Initially the approaching handler and dog should not remain near the male dog for very long. Time is a variable which also needs to be gradually increased at progressively closer distances.

If fear is not a component of the intermale aggressive behaviour (surprisingly it often is), *and* if the dog is not aggressive in any way toward the owner, punishment might be added to this therapeutic procedure. Generally a non-painful punishment is preferred if the dog demonstrates aggression, because pain sometimes elicits aggression. The owner might grab the dog's head and muzzle and scold him severely until he exhibits a submissive look.

There are numerous variations of this procedure that can be designed to treat the problem. The underlying principle should be to reward the dog for an alternative, unaggressive behaviour in the presence of other male dogs. If the dog is not afraid of other male dogs and the dog is not dominant or aggressive towards the owner, a non-painful punishment for aggressive behaviours may be instigated in the practice situations. However, the basis of the programme is rewarding appropriate behaviour.

These techniques can be expanded upon when teaching dogs within a home to tolerate each other. Such dogs should also learn to tolerate people petting the other dog and the other dog approaching people to be petted. All circumstances that are likely to lead

to an aggressive display should be identified and the dogs conditioned to remain quiet and unaggressive.

Interfemale aggression

Aggressive behaviour of one female dog toward another generally occurs among dogs within the same home environment. It frequently occurs in competitive or arousing situations such as feeding time, when the owner returns home, or when a visitor enters. The onset of this behaviour generally occurs when one of the dogs is between 1 and 3 years of age. Spaying is only likely to affect this problem if the aggression is related to the oestrous cycle, which is usually not the case. Generally this aggressive behaviour is independent of oestrous cycles and consequently spaying has no effect. Since interfemale aggression is not a typically masculine trait, progestin therapy is unlikely to have an effect.

In my experience to date, the only effective approach to this problem is to condition the dogs to inhibit themselves or engage in alternative behaviours in situations that are likely to lead to aggressive encounters. The eliciting stimuli must be correctly identified and then counterconditioning procedures implemented. Usually these dogs should be kept separated in unsupervised situations because occasionally such dogs have killed another when the owners were not present. Aggression among animals is not all ritualized behaviours; serious injuries and deaths do occur. Even after the dogs have been conditioned to inhibit themselves in specific circumstances, it probably continues to be a good idea to keep them separated in the absence of the owner.

Fear-induced aggression

Fear-induced aggression can occur at any age and be exhibited by either male or female dogs. Neutering is not effective in eliminating fear-induced aggression. Therapy involves desensitisation and counterconditioning procedures, extinction, and the avoidance of punishment. Fear-induced aggression is treated as described in the section discussing fears of people (pp. 512–515). Dogs that are afraid of other dogs can be treated with the same procedures.

Theoretically, antianxiety drugs might be helpful in treating this problem. Occasionally the author prescribes such drugs for between therapy sessions, but they are rarely used during therapy sessions.

Bilateral amygdalectomies (Andersson & Olsson 1965) have been reported to eliminate fear-induced aggressive behaviours in dogs, but not other types of aggressive behaviours. Side-effects of this procedure were loss of housebreaking and loss of memory of other learned behaviours.

Pain-induced aggression

Aggression is a protective mechanism. It is not unreasonable to expect a dog to react to pain with a threat or aggressive behaviour. A dog that is clearly submissive to the people with whom it lives may inhibit its aggressive reaction to a pain-induced stimulus longer than a dog who is relatively dominant. However, there is a threshold of response for every animal. Panosteitis, otitis, anal saculitis, etc. may eventually elicit a growl or a snap from the gentlest dog.

Pain or disease aetiology should be suspected when there is a relatively sudden onset of aggression, particularly related to touching specific areas of the body. The appropriate therapy is to treat the underlying cause of pain and to avoid eliciting the pain if at all possible. If an aggressive response is repeatedly evoked, it is possible that the dog will become conditioned to elicit aggression whenever reached for, and aggression may persist after the aetiology of the pain is gone.

If it is impossible to avoid touching a painful area, measures can be taken to reduce the probability that the dog will learn to react aggressively while it has the painful disorder. The dog should learn not to anticipate pain each time the owner approaches it. The owner should frequently touch, pet, and manipulate parts of the animal's body which are not painful and subsequently reward the dog when it does not display aggression. If this is done, the patient will not anticipate a painful encounter each time the owner approaches. The dog will associate most approaches and touching by the owner with pleasant experiences rather than painful ones.

If the owner must manipulate a painful area, the manipulation should be done as gently as possible and the dog generously rewarded when it does not respond aggressively. The patient can also be gradually trained to tolerate treatment of a painful area. If an otitis condition needs to be treated, the owner can frequently approach the dog with the medication in hand and given the dog a tidbit for simply allowing the approach. Then the dog is rewarded for allowing the owner to touch areas of the body such as the neck and shoulder with the tube of medication. The owner gradually moves towards the head, rewarding the dog for tolerating touches closer and closer to the ear. Gradually the owner moves to the site of pain and

very gently touches and medicates the area. If it is necessary to restrain the dog to do so, the dog should be restrained. Care should be taken to avoid eliciting pain. If the dog tolerates the entire procedure without a threatening display, it should get several wonderful tidbits and much petting and praise. If it does act aggressively, it does not get a tidbit or reward but the ear is medicated anyway. Then the owner touches distal areas and rewards the dog for tolerating at least some manipulation.

In summary, the owner should frequently touch the dog in a region far enough away from the painful locus that the dog does not react and the dog should be rewarded for letting itself be touched and manipulated. Then the owner gradually touches the dog closer to the painful area. Finally, the owner gently touches the painful area and rewards the dog for tolerating manipulation. Gradually the owner increases the manipulation necessary to the level which allows the owner to treat or manage the disease process. Of course, the owner generously rewards the dog for tolerating the pain. Even if the owner can manipulate the painful area, the dog should be rewarded for tolerating touch and manipulation of non-painful areas. This is done so that the dog does not anticipate pain every time a person reaches toward it. After the pathology is corrected, it may be beneficial for the owner to continue for a short while, approaching, touching, and manipulating the area and rewarding the dog for not displaying aggression.

Pain is acknowledged as a stimulus which can evoke aggression and anxiety. Therefore, physical punishment involving pain can be expected to cause anxiety and sometimes aggression. Punishment involving pain is definitely contraindicated when trying to treat pain-induced or fear-induced aggression.

Learned aggression

One example of a learned aggression is that alluded to above—a sequel of pain-induced aggression. After the aetiology of the painful disorder is gone, aggression may persist because the dog has come to anticipate being hurt whenever the owner reaches towards it. The therapeutic approach to this problem is essentially the same as that designed to reduce the probability of evoking pain-induced aggression or treating fear-induced aggression. The stimuli that evoke the aggression are identified and presented along a gradient as the dog is rewarded for non-aggressive behaviours. The rewards should be generous and the procedure implemented slowly so as not to evoke an undesirable response.

Some aggression is maintained by positive reinforcements from the owner. Not infrequently owners unwittingly reward a dog for being aggressive. The owner may recognise that the dog is apprehensive when a visitor comes to the door or that the dog is 'upset' when a strange dog approaches. As the dog growls and barks at the approaching figure, the owner strokes the dog and soothingly tells the dog that everything is all right. The soothing voice and petting are immediate, positive reinforcements paired with the threatening behaviour. The dog may, in fact, be comforted, but it is also being immediately reinforced for its aggressive behaviour. Extinction and counterconditioning can be stimultaneously employed to eliminate such reinforced behaviours. That is: stop reinforcing the undesirable behaviour, and teach the dog to perform a response incompatible with the aggressive response. Punishment is to be avoided if pain or submission is part of the aggressive response.

Both male and female dogs can learn to be aggressive and neutering will not suppress learned aggressive behaviours.

Territorial aggression

Territory is frequently defined as an area that an animal will defend. What a dog considers its territory may be a specific location within the owner's property, a boundary that exceeds the owner's property, the house of the owner, and/or the yard of the owner. It is not abnormal for a dog to act aggressively in order to prevent or try to prevent strange dogs or people from entering its territory.

Males as well as females can be territorial and neutering has no effect on this behaviour (Hopkins *et al* 1976). The behaviour usually develops around 6-9 months of age.

Owners often play a part in influencing the degree to which their dogs develop territorial aggression. Some owners actively encourage the dog to bark whenever it hears something and praise it for aggressive behaviours. Other owners unwittingly reward the dog's aggressive stances with soothing petting and talk.

Training or counterconditioning, restraint, and supervision are the methods available to control territorial aggression. A dog can learn to assume non-threatening behaviours when its territory is approached. Depending on the dog's predisposition, the presence of the owner may be necessary to assure that the dog inhibits its aggressive behaviour. The neutral or friendly behaviour reinforced during training sessions may not generalise to times when the owner is absent. Therefore, when the owner is not present, precautions may still have to be taken to prevent the dog from harming someone.

Dogs highly predisposed to guarding and territorial aggressive behaviours will probably recognise a truly threatening situation and act aggressively. It is the author's belief that most dogs can discriminate between an inappropriate entrance or approach of a stranger and more normal, unthreatening entrances. Since the types of approaches the dog has been counterconditioned to accept are normative approaches, these dogs are still likely to act aggressively when something out of the ordinary happens.

Parental aggression

Wolves, as well as many other canids, live in social groups and several members of the community may participate in rearing the offspring. Members of the pack hunt, bring back or regurgitate game and act as 'wet nurses' as well as providing shelter, warmth and protection to the litter (Rabb, Ginsburg & Andrews 1962; Rabb, Woolpy & Ginsburg 1967; Ryden 1975; Klinghammer 1979). A mother dog, as well as other adult dogs in the household, may act aggressively to protect puppies from perceived potential harm, even if these dogs have never before exhibited aggression to people or other animals. The owners of dogs exhibiting parental aggression should take precautions not to evoke or reinforce the aggression. If the behaviour poses a serious problem and/or the owner must manipulate the bitch or her puppies, counterconditioning utilising positive reinforcement of non-aggressive behaviours to ameliorate the aggression.

False pregnancy

Oestrous cycles of canid bitches in groups tend to be synchronised. If only one bitch has offspring, which often happens in a wolf pack, the other females may experience false pregnancies that coincide with the real pregnancy. Barren female wolves and coyotes can then nurse the puppies of the breeding female. Pseudocyesis, or false pregnancy, is probably a normal consequence of the oestrous cycle of a sterile mated or unmated bitch.

The physical signs of false pregnancy in dogs are a distended abdomen, an engorged uterus, the development of mammary glands and/or lactation. Behavioural components include nervousness, 'mothering' and protectiveness of 'surrogate' puppies, nesting behaviour and guarding of nest sites. A bitch may show one or any combination of physical or behavioural signs. These behaviours often have a sudden onset in an intact bitch 6–8 weeks post oestrus. Physical changes may or may not accompany behavioural changes. Occasionally, if a bitch, usually with a history of pseudocyesis, is spayed in early metoestrus, she will immediately develop signs of false pregnancy.

Dogs exhibiting aggression as a component of false pregnancy can be treated as though they actually do have a litter of pups, and the owners should take precautions to avoid situations that evoke the aggression. The dog will gradually stop exhibiting these behaviours in 4–6 weeks. If she is spayed well into dioestrus, she will not exhibit these behaviours again. If the aggression poses a problem which can not be avoided, the stimuli that evoke the behaviour should be identified and the dog's responses counterconditioned.

Drug therapy for the treatment of pseudocyesis is controversial. Several texts mention oestrogens, testosterone or progestins as being effective in terminating physical and behavioural signs of false pregnancy. The efficacy of these treatments is presently being questioned by endocrinologists. If the condition is treated early, megestrol acetate, 2 mg/kg per os for 5–7 days, administered immediately after the onset of false pregnancy, is reportedly effective 80% of the time in shortening or terminating the false pregnancy cycle. Bromocriptine is a dopamine agonist used to treat hypergalactia in people. Dopamine is a prolactin inhibiting factor. Prolactin has been identified as inducing or facilitating maternal or parental behaviour in many birds and is suspected to do so in mammals. Increasing amounts of dopamine available should decrease prolactin and subsequent milk secretion and maternal behaviours. An appropriate dosage of bromocriptine for this problem in dogs has not yet been determined. A side-effect of bromocriptine administration is emesis.

Drugs, such as the phenothiazines and butyrophenones, which inhibit or antagonise dopamine are contraindicated for treatment of pseudocyesis. These drugs may result in an increase in prolactin release and therefore enhance the pseudocyesis phenomena.

Dominance aggression

One of the most common reasons dogs are presented to behaviour therapists is for aggression towards the owner. While the owner presents the case as unprovoked aggressive attacks, a detailed history usually reveals specific stimuli or circumstances that are involved in eliciting the reaction. These stimuli and circumstances support the hypothesis that the dog is demonstrating aggression related to its dominance of the owner.

The typical signalment of a dominant aggressive dog is a purebred, intact, 2-year-old male, although females and mixed breeds are occasionally presented for this problem. Dominance aggression is one of the few behaviour problems that is seen more frequently in purebred dogs than in mixed breeds. Perhaps qualities that are selected for in show rings are too similar to dominance gestures (tail up, head very erect, tall stance). The individuals that do well in show rings are frequently inbred, hence concentrating the gene pool of these potentially dominant traits.

Dominance aggression may be manifested to all or only some of the people in the household. The dog may not be aggressive to strangers. It is often very friendly toward and may solicit attention from people to whom it is periodically aggressive.

The circumstances in which the dog demonstrates aggression are related to access to 'critical resources' and in response to what it interprets as dominant signals by a person. Critical resources are items that maximise the probability of survival and reproductive success of an individual. Such items are food, water, shelter and access to a favourite person or mate. These dogs frequently guard food or stolen items. Dominant dogs may, however, exchange objects with the owner during play without exhibiting aggression. Play occurs in a different context than a dominance conflict. Occasionally a dog which is dominant will interpose itself between a 'favourite person' and another individual. First access at a passageway is another situation in which a dominant dog sometimes signals aggression. A dog presented for this syndrome frequently growls when it is disturbed on the bed or on a chair. Sometimes merely walking near him wherever he is resting will elicit an aggressive response.

Stimuli that often trigger aggression are petting, grooming, pushing down on the dog, pulling on the dog, trying to make it lie down, restraining it, putting on or taking off a collar or a lead. Tactile pressure is a frequent dominant gesture in canid communication. Dominant dogs put their necks or forefeet over or on the neck or back, or grab the muzzle of individuals lower in the hierarchy. Dominant dogs often respond to being stared at with aggression. Subordinate dogs will passively submit to such signals; however, a dog that is vying for a dominant place will object if a person (whom the dog is trying to dominate), engages in a behaviour similar to those that signal dominance among canids. A dominant dog may also frequently display non-aggressive dominant signals to the owner such as standing over the owner, staring at the owner, pressing its chin down against the owner's shoulder or head, etc.

At first the aggression may be mild and intermittent. Eventually the dog becomes aggressive in more situations, more frequently, and with greater intensity. The dog that tends to be dominant usually resists punishment or threats by escalating its aggression.

The species-typical signals, facial, body and vocal expressions have been described in detail in texts such as Schenkel (1947) and Fox (1971).

Signs of aggression can be a snarl, a lift of the lip, a growl or bark, a snap, an inhibited bite or a bite that actually inflicts injury. If the eliciting stimulus is presented slowly the dog may give warning signals, otherwise it may immediately bite.

In the management and treatment of dominance aggression problems, the goals are to avoid injury to people and to eventually allow the person to engage in the activities that previously elicited aggression.

Theoretically, a physical confrontation can reverse or stop a dominance challenge. However, this will only work if the person is able to win. The size and motivation of the dog and the degree of intimidation the person feels can easily prohibit an individual from winning a physical confrontation. It is far easier for a stranger to intimidate a dog than an owner who has previously lost hundreds or thousands of minor challenges. When such an owner begins to utilise discipline, the aggression usually rapidly and dramatically escalates, and the person may be bitten. Reversal of the dominance hierarchy must be done safely.

Treatment of this problem involves changing the daily behavioural interactions between the owner and dog. Often detailed behavioural modification programmes, castration and progestin therapy can facilitate the reversal of the hierarchy.

Since this behaviour is primarily a masculine behaviour trait it is logical to assume that castration might affect dominance aggression, and in male dogs this is often the case.

Although behavioural effects of castration may not be manifested for several months following surgery (Hopkins *et al* 1976), progestins, which tend to suppress typically masculine behaviours, can affect dominance aggression within days. Spayed females manifesting dominance aggression are as likely to respond to progestin therapy as are males. An initial dose is 2.0 mg/kg per os megestrol acetate daily or 10 mg/kg IM or SQ of medroxyprogesterone acetate. The megestrol acetate is reduced by half every two weeks and discontinued by 8 weeks. Repository injections of medroxyprogesterone acetate would be administered as needed. The side-effects of progestin therapy must be explained to the owner (see p. 509). Prolonged progestin therapy in intact bitches, elderly or obese animals is not advisable. Oral administration of progrestins is thought to permit better regulation of the drug than does repository injection.

The behavioural techniques used in reversing dominance aggression can be complex and must accommodate the individual situation. Clinicians that wish to develop this expertise are referred to more in depth articles (Voith 1981c,d; Voith & Borchelt 1982). Unless the practising veterinarian has developed an expertise in behavioural therapy, the client and dog are best referred to an animal behavioural therapist for the behavioural treatment techniques.

For safety's sake, most dominance hierarchies should be reversed subtly and slowly. The dog can first be taught to sit or lay down for progressively longer periods of time. Within a few days the rule 'nothing in life is free' is instituted. For the dog to gain access to anything it wants, it must first sit or lie down. It must assume a moderately submissive posture before it goes out, comes in, gets fed, gets petted, etc. As time progresses the owner adds extra requests that the dog must submit to before obtaining what it wants. The dog may have to tolerate its muzzle being held, accept pressure on its neck for a moment before it is let outside, etc. The owner gradually uses stronger dominance signals, without exceeding the threshold that triggers aggression. For example, if it has been determined that petting the dog four times elicits aggression, initially the owner should only pet the dog two or three times. Over a period of weeks, the owner accustoms the dog to being petted progressively longer and harder, having his muzzle held more firmly, being pushed over and restrained in lateral recumbency, and being pulled by the neck. The dog must also tolerate being stared at without growling back. It may be necessary to condition the dog to tolerate wearing a muzzle before instigating some of these techniques. Gradually the owner requests the dog to assume submissive roles in the situations that it previously demonstrated aggression.

Electroconvulsive therapy (ECT) has been reported to ameliorate aggressive behaviour in dogs (Redding & Walker 1976). The type of aggressive behaviour that appeared to be affected was dominance aggression towards human members of the family. Remission of the aggressive behaviour lasted a few months to several years and some dogs were successfully retreated. Owners reported that the dog appeared confused and did not seem to recognise them for 2–4 weeks. The dogs also required rehousebreaking. Perhaps, while the dog was experiencing a memory loss, a new social hierarchy was established in which the dog was subordinate.

Treating a long-standing dominance aggression problem involves a commitment of diligence and time from both owner and clinician, and should not be taken lightly. Treatment of these cases often only results in the aggression being reduced, but not completely eliminated (Line 1983). People who have children should be advised not to keep a dominant aggressive dog or, at least, to keep the dog and child separated until the child is old enough to understand how to carefully interact with the dog.

Aggression towards infants is unlikely to be dominance-related. Dominance struggles occur between individuals in a group that are competing for resources or a specific status. It is difficult to imagine how a baby could transmit signals interpreted as a dominance threat to dogs. Dogs, however, may bite and kill a baby because they respond to the small infant as a prey object. Most of the cases with which the author is familiar of dogs killing an infant have occurred within a few hours of the infant's arrival into the house when the dog was either left alone with the child or not adequately supervised. At least one of the dogs had a history of killing numerous small animals. The author is not aware of any cases of dogs killing babies after the two had had months of continuous, close, amicable social contact.

Redirected aggression

When an animal is in conflict (that is, motivated to perform two behaviours simultaneously, or prevented from engaging in a highly motivated behaviour) the animal may redirect one of the behaviours to another target. For example, a restrained dog threatening another dog may turn and bite the owner. Sometimes a dog will redirect aggression to another dog. Redirected aggression is a normal behaviour, manifested by many species including man. Interestingly, in all cases of redirected aggression involving dogs that the author has investigated, the dogs have only redirected aggression to a subordinate. When presented with a redirected aggression problem, the clinician should also explore the dominance relationship between the dog and the person bitten. In addition to treating the immediate, inciting stimulus of an aggressive bout, dominance aggression related to the owner also has to be considered.

Aggression over food

Usually, dogs that are aggressive concerning their food are also dominant to the individual they are threatening. However, sometimes a dog that is sub-missive to a person in all other circumstances may growl related to food. Mech (1970) describes subordinate wolves growling and threatening a dominant individual if the latter tries to take food away. Possession sometimes is 9/10 of the law. If aggression over food is part of a dominance complex, the dominance hierarchy should be reversed. Aggression over food, unrelated to dominance, may respond to a counter-conditioning procedure whereby the dog is conditioned to relinquish non-food objects, then gradually more palatable food items. Whether or not punishment should also be used depends on the individual case.

Punishment-elicited aggression

Pain has long been recognised as an aggression-eliciting stimulus. If painful punishment is used, anxiety and aggression are always possible sequelae. Sometimes punishment is a convenient and appropriate approach to stopping a behaviour, however if it involves pain it must be carefully modulated. Punishment is, of course, contraindicated in fear and anxiety situations (see section on punishment).

Predation

Predatory behaviour of animals is not generally classified as aggressive behaviour. However, predation is occasionally presented to the clinician as aggression. The targets of predation are frequently small animals such as birds, rabbits, and squirrels. Some breeds and individuals are more predisposed to predatory activities than are other dogs. Sometimes dogs, particularly when facilitated by others, will chase and kill livestock and, occasionally, predation becomes part of an attack sequence directed towards a human being. The latter cases usually involve groups of dogs (Borchelt *et al* 1983).

Initiating causes that have eventually led to predation of humans have been redirected predatory sequences and territorial or defensive aggression that progressed to bodily injury of the person and subsequent predation. Hunger does not appear to be a strong motivating factor in these incidents. Most of the dogs in such cases have had histories of threatening people prior to the predatory incidents. Histories of dogs that kill infants and small children (3 years old and younger) do not always reveal previous aggression to human adults, but reveal previous predation of small animals or use as hunting dogs.

Small running objects, particularly if they are fleeing, tend to elicit chasing behaviour. Chasing, stalking, and sometimes biting, of children or small mammals, as they run past a dog, might be related to predatory behaviour.

The most effective way to control predation is to prohibit the dog's access to the target animal. This means adequate fencing and leash control or good verbal command over the dog is necessary. Predatory sequences appear to be facilitated by other dogs and even a well trained dog is less likely to respond to an owner's command if it is running with other dogs. A dog that does not chase moving objects in the owner's presence may do so when the owner is absent.

Punishment in the form of an electric shock, delivered by a remote control electric shock collar, is often used on hunting dogs to train them not to chase the wrong game. For such punishment to be effective, however, the shock collar must be used appropriately. It should be paired with the onset of the chase behaviour, be of adequate strength to disrupt the behaviour without inducing subsequent apprehensiveness, should cease as soon as the dog stops chasing the target, and should be used every time the dog begins to chase the forbidden object. Shock collars can be misused and it is possible to produce a neurotic or phobic animal. Pain also has the possibility of evoking aggressive behaviour. Shock collars and other punishment methods are less likely to work if dogs are facilitated by other dogs in a chase sequence.

The 'Garcia effect' has been used with mixed results as an effort to stop coyotes from preying on sheep. Nausea and vomiting are induced with apomorphine and/or lithium chloride after the coyotes have eaten sheep meat. Theoretically, this should produce an aversion to eating sheep and therefore stop predation. However, dogs rarely eat livestock brought down in a predatory chase sequence. Even among wild and feral canines the predatory sequence *per se* is far enough removed from the ingestion phase that the 'Garcia effect' is unlikely to prevent hunting sequences, even though it might prevent the animal from eating the prey. It is doubtful that the 'Garcia effect' would inhibit dogs from killing small mammals or birds.

Aggression related to pathophysiological disorders

Laboratory experiments involving stimulation and lesioning of regions of the brain can produce a variety of aggressive behaviours. It is not unreasonable to assume that some clinical cases might involve brain disorders that result in aggression.

Ablative lesions usually have to be bilateral to induce behavioural changes. Therefore, if a space occupying lesion is suspected, it is more likely to be along the midline of the central nervous system. Irritative lesions which can result in seizure activity may be unilateral.

Meierhenry and Lui (1978) reported a correlation between sudden personality changes involving unprovoked vicious attacks by dogs towards people and cardiac abnormalities and neuronal changes indicative of cerebral hypoxia. It was theorised that the cardiac conduction system lesions resulted in cerebral hypoxia and the subsequent behavioural changes.

Theoretically, spontaneous electrical discharges in the brain could result in aggressive behaviours similar to aggression elicited by electrical stimulation. The literature regarding psychomotor seizures and aggression in people is inconclusive. Whether or not aggression can be a form of epilepsy is controversial. Many investigators believe epilepsy rarely, if ever, can be incriminated as a direct cause of well coordinated aggressive sequences in people.

The following criteria would support a diagnosis of seizure activity involving aggression.

1 The aggression does not fit a description of a normal species-typical behaviour or an adaptive learned behaviour.
2 Other concurrent neurological or pathophysiological signs such as an abnormal EEG, grand mal seizures, etc.
3 Epileptogenic drugs, such a phenothiazines, are able to elicit the aggressive behaviour.
4 Antiepileptic drugs can suppress the behaviour.

An interesting case that meets many of the above diagnostic criteria involved an intact, male Lhasa Apso that would growl and attack the air around himself, whirling in circles, when presented with food (Fig. 19.13). This behaviour would last for a few minutes, then the dog would resume eating and again begin whirling, growling and barking. The dog never injured himself, but if someone's arm or hand had been put in the path of the dog's attack, the dog undoubtedly would have bitten it. Throwing a blanket over the dog could also elicit this circling, swirling, aggressive behaviour. Oral administration of 5–10 mg of diazepam (Valium), an antiepileptic drug, allowed the dog to eat without engaging in the aggressive sequence. An intravenous injection of chlorpromazine (Largactil, Thorazine) immediately elicited the aggressive behaviour in the absence of food or a blanket. Perhaps the stimuli that triggered the seizure activity did so because they increased the excitement level of the dog. Perhaps the food directly activated neural excitation of the olfac-

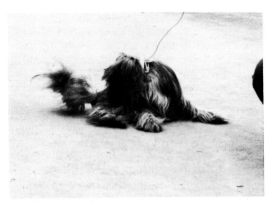

Fig. 19.13 Presentation of food, being covered with a blanket, and intravenous chloropromazine evoked an aggressive response in this Lhasa Apso. The dog would growl, snap, and 'attack' the area around him. He never bit himself.

tory system (which is intricately related to the limbic system) and thus precipitated the aggressive bout. Similar food-elicited aggressive behaviours have been described in a variety of dogs, including mixed breeds.

Behavioural disturbances might result from biochemical disturbances as well as abnormal electrical discharges. Corson *et al* (1976) reported that aggressive behaviour in some dogs was suppressed with oral administration of 0.2–1.3 mg/kg per os dextro- or levoamphetamine. The type of aggressive behaviour that responded to the amphetamines was not described in detail. The results were dramatic and took effect within two hours. Under the influence of the drug, the dogs solicit petting and are able to interact with people and other dogs in a friendly manner. After several treatments, one dog, which was also physiologically hyperkinetic, was able to retain an unaggressive attitude in an unmedicated state; another dog reverted to his aggressive behaviour after 3–4 hours.

Infectious diseases involving the nervous system should always be considered as a possible cause of aggressive behaviour. Rabies is a viral disease that is widely recognised as causing behavioural abnormalities including aggression. Inflammation resulting from any infectious agent or process may be sufficiently irritating to cause aggression, particularly if the limbic system is involved.

Summary

While much can be done with behaviour modification, physiological intervention and environmental manipulation to reduce aggressive behaviour of dogs, no guarantee can ever be made that a dog will never again demonstrate aggressive behaviour. It should always be made clear to the client that the treatment of species-typical, learned or pathophysiological aggression is aimed at reducing the probability of recurring aggression and is not a guaranteed elimination of all possible future aggressive behaviour.

Aggression related to brain disorders is not always predictable and not all pathophysiological disorders will respond to therapeutic intervention. If long periods of time normally elapse between episodes, it is difficult to ascertain if a therapeutic approach is effective. Owners should always be cautioned concerning the risks of trying to treat such dogs.

PATHOPHYSIOLOGICAL BEHAVIOURAL DISORDERS

The behaviour of an animal and its organic substrate, particularly the brain, are intertwined and inseparable. Bizarre, unusual, or abnormal behaviour (not species-typical or adaptive learned behaviour) of an animal may reflect an organic pathological disorder. Some behavioural problems of dogs can be related to known physiological abnormalities. Others can only be classified as functional disorders because, as yet, no underlying physical abnormalities have been found. Some disorders appear to be genetic in that they present in specific breeds, for example, flank sucking in Doberman Pinschers (Fig. 19.1).

There is a paucity of information correlating organic disorders and abnormal behaviours in animals. Portions of this section are composed, therefore, of extrapolation from what is known about people and projections as to the incidence of similar disorders in animals.

In man, correlations are known to exist between specific behaviours and the experience of certain sensations, states of consciousness, or emotions. If one attaches feelings or emotions to animals that are known to occur in people, one is accused of anthropomorphism. It is true we may not be able to prove what animals are perceiving, but rather than assume that animals do not experience similar sensations to man, why not assume that, under the same circumstances, they are indeed experiencing similar sensory and emotional feelings?

Epilepsies or seizures are clinical events usually associated with a measurable electrical disturbance of the brain. The signs are disturbances of movement, feeling and/or consciousness. We are most familiar with motor seizures in animals, however, other types of seizures such as sensory and psychomotor probably also occur.

Hallucinations are the perception of visual, auditory, gustatory, olfactory, mechanical or tactile sensations in the absence of an external eliciting stimulus. Hallucinations may be the result of epileptic seizures, electrical stimulation of the brain or biochemical alterations. Dreams are considered by some to be a normal occurring hallucinogenic experience.

Hormones, neurohormones, and neurotransmitters all influence behaviour. A normal range of hormonal levels must be maintained for appropriate behavioural expression. For example, hyperthyroidism or thyrotoxicosis is associated with agitated states or nervousness. A deficiency of thyroid hormone early in life results in cretinism and mental retardation. Central nervous system catecholamine abnormalities or disturbances result in hyperkinesis, narcolepsy, depression or manic behaviours. Testosterone is important for the expression of male sexual behaviours in most male animals. Oestrogen is necessary for receptive sexual behaviour in the female. The above are just a few examples of the relationships between hormones and behaviour. If there is an alteration or an abnormality occurring in the hormonal status of an animal, behavioural disturbances or abnormalities can result.

Metabolic disturbances such as hypoglycaemia, hyperammonaemia, uraemia, effects of starvation, and heavy metal poisoning (most commonly lead) can cause unusual behaviour or seizure activity.

Experimental stimulation of regions of an animal's brain can elicit behaviours such as predation, sleep, grooming, and aggression. Electrical stimulation of areas of the brain can also result in animals that show extreme fear reactions. In the light of this evidence it would seem reasonable to assume some behavioural problems in animals could be the result of abnormal brain activity.

If a pathological alteration occurs, either electrically or chemically, particularly in the limbic or hypothalamic regions, perhaps an animal can experience emotions such as aggression or rage and act in a rather coordinated manner with stimuli in the environment. It is also possible that some extreme phobias exhibited by some animals may be related to abnormal brain activity in the limbic or hypothalamic areas.

Psychomotor seizures

Seizure activities which involve sensory perception, emotions, and relatively coordinated behaviour patterns are classified as psychomotor seizures. During the seizures, which usually last only a few minutes, the victim appears to respond in a limited fashion to the environment and is capable of carrying out coordinated motor acts. Human patients report experiencing intense emotions, usually of fear and anxiety, and may react with undirected rage, flailing out to resist restraint.

Occasionally, people who experience psychomotor seizures will engage in behaviours such as undressing in public, driving somewhere, or putting dishes in the clothes dryer. When they return to the normal state of consciousness they do not remember anything. These people are able to interact with their environment to a certain extent and appear to be perceiving and reacting to some stimuli in the environment which direct their behaviours.

Sensory seizures

Spontaneous electrical discharges in the motor areas of the brain result in motor convulsions. Stimulation of sensory areas evokes sensations. People experiencing sensory seizures report feelings of numbness, tingling, and movement as well as auditory, vertiginous, visual, olfactory and gustatory experiences. Visual seizures usually, but not always, have epigenic foci in the occipital lobes. The visual sensations reported are: dimming of vision, seeing spots, flashes of light, and dancing or twirling objects. Auditory seizures are reported as buzzing, ringing, hissing, or machine-like sounds. Olfactory and gustatory seizures are usually described as horrible smells and unpleasant tastes. Visceral sensory seizures are described as nausea and epigastric sensations which are unaccompanied by motor activity of viscera. Sensory epilepsy does exist in people and probably also occurs in dogs. Dogs have been reported to exhibit signs of anxiety prior to motor seizures, which may indicate the occurrence of a sensory experience (Holliday *et al* 1970).

Unfortunately, in the dog, unless seizure activity in the hypothalamus, limbic system or temporal lobe spreads to the dorsal cortex, conventional canine EEG recordings are unlikely to reflect any abnormalities. A dog can have epileptic foci in these structures and demonstrate a normal EEG.

Occasionally, a dog that has been exhibiting bizarre behaviours may respond favourably to antiepileptic medication. Precautions to consider when treating an aggressive dog with epileptic medication are discussed in greater depth in the section on aggression.

It is possible for seizure activity to be instrumentally reinforced or classically conditioned. The confounding and contributory influences of learning must always be considered when unusual behaviours are demonstrated. In such cases the animal's response may be only partially suppressed with antiepileptic medication and the learned components of the behaviours remain. If learning is thought to be a probable contributing factor to the animal's behaviour, extinction and counterconditioning will have to be employed as well as medication.

Visceral sensory and motor seizures

Seizure activity may involve visceral motor areas of the brain as well as sensory and somatomotor regions. Breitschwerdt *et al* (1979) reported that several dogs which persistently vomited or had diarrhoea, for which no gastroenteric aetiology could be found, had abnormal EEGs. The manifestation of gastroenteric disorders stopped when the dogs were treated with antiepileptic medication of phenytoin and/or phenobarbital. Since these drugs can also have a direct effect on the gastrointestinal system it is still unclear if the dogs did have visceral motor and sensory epilepsy.

Uncinate fits

Persons afflicted with seizure activity in the uncinate cortex experience disagreeable odours and sometimes tastes, frequently exhibit movements of chewing and lip smacking, and report having epigastric sensations. Not uncommonly dogs engage in mouth smacking, flicking of the tongue in and out, and chewing movements that appear to the owner as though the dog were tasting something unpleasant. Identical movements can be elicited with a bitter tasting substance such as ophthalmic atropine. This lipsmacking syndrome in dogs may be similar to uncinate fits that occur in people. Unfortunately, conventional canine EEGs are unlikely to show any abnormalities because of the location of the uncinate cortex. A diagnosis of epilepsy would be supported if the behaviour could be elicited by epileptogenic drugs or suppressed with antiepileptic medication.

Trance-like behaviour

Occasionally, dogs are observed to assume rigid stances, appear to stare transfixed at the floor or into space, and are seemingly unaware of their environment (Fig. 19.14). Dogs exhibiting this behaviour do not appear to be suffering any discomfort nor are they impaired by the episode. These behaviours appear similar to what are described as petit mal seizures in people. Such persons experience a transient short lapse into unconsciousness without loss of muscle tone and exhibit paroxysmal 3/sec spike and wave EEG patterns. The victim is unaware of his/her behaviour.

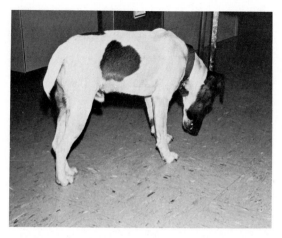

Fig. 19.14   A 3-year-old male Fox Terrier that occasionally 'stared' transfixed at the floor. This dog did not exhibit a 3/sec spike and wave EEG pattern.

Although dogs appear to demonstrate behaviour that corresponds to petit mal seizures, characteristic EEG recordings of 3/sec spike and wave patterns have not been documented in the dog or correlated with this behaviour. An experimental study has demonstrated 3/sec spikes and wave sequences in EEGs of kittens (Guerrero-Figueroa *et al* 1963); perhaps the neural substrate for such activity is also present in the dog. The cause of short 'trance-like' behaviour could be 'floating objects' in the animal's visual field that are apparent to the dog when it looks at a uniformly coloured and smooth surface, visual seizures or hallucinations, petit mal seizures and/or a learned behaviour for which the dog has been reinforced.

An ophthalmic examination, EEG recordings, and response to antiepileptic medication can be used in attempting to arrive at a diagnosis of 'trance-like behaviour'. Unless the dog appears distressed or is being injured during these attacks, treatment is probably unnecessary. If it appears that the episodes are a result of learned behaviour, appropriate behaviour modification techniques could be instigated.

Flank sucking

Flank sucking has to date only been described in Doberman Pinschers (Fig. 19.1). These dogs grasp their flank with their mouths and may remain that way for hours. The dog can be either lying down or standing. Excitement frequently precipitates this behaviour. Despite persistent and obsessive grasping of their flanks, injuries are rare. Occasionally these dogs also engage in behaviour which can be described as snapping and biting at imaginary flies. The aetiology of this syndrome is unknown and an effective treatment has not yet been found.

Fly biting and attacking the ground

A variety of breeds, as well as mixed breeds, have been described leaping and biting at 'imaginary objects' in the air or on the ground (Fig. 19.15). The exact aetiology is not known. Possible causes are visual defects (which might be seen upon an ophthalmic examination), seizure activity, hallucinations, (which may or may not be the result of seizures in the visceral sensory cortex), or behaviour acquired as a result of reinforcement from the owner.

Flashes of light, scotomata, or spots in the visual field of people have been associated with abnormal electrical activity of the occipital lobe. Correlations have been observed between 'hallucinogenic' spots in the visual field, abnormal EEGs of the occipital area and sensitivity or allergic reactions of the central nervous system to specific foods (Dees 1954).

In dogs, abnormal EEGs and/or response to anti-epileptic drugs would support sensory epilepsy. Should drug therapy be unsuccessful, a systematic deletion and addition of foods can be tried to determine if hypersensitivity to foods is a cause of this disorder.

Drugs used to control hallucinations in people are not approved for animals, but with consent from the owner, such drugs might be tried. Drugs that fall into this classification are the phenothiazines, butyrophenones, and the dibenzodiazepines. It should be remembered that phenothiazines and butyrophenones will facilitate seizure activity whereas benzodiazepines suppress it.

If the behaviour seems to be associated with specific stimuli, such as the entry of the owner into the room, behaviour modification can be employed. The dog can be taught a competing response, such as sit-stay, to perform in situations which predictably precipitate the compulsive behaviour. The dog is then rewarded with a delicious morsel of food for the approved behaviour. Extinction is another approach. Whenever the dog engages in the behaviour, the owner should either ignore the dog or turn and walk away, leaving the dog alone.

It is possible that there could be neurological and learned components to such behaviours, in which case both medication and behaviour modification would be necessary. Of course an ophthalmic examination should always be done to determine if there are observable visual defects.

Psychosomatic disorders

Psychosomatics can be defined as the interrelationship between learning, emotions and manifestation of disease. Psychosomatic medicine encompasses the effects of physiological variables on behaviour and the effects of social and psychological events on disease. Psychological factors can affect the time course, severity, and precipitation of diseases. In humans, disorders such as asthma, heart disease, peptic ulcers, gastrointestinal disorders, and neurodermatitis frequently are the result of psychosomatics. Dogs, which are social crea-

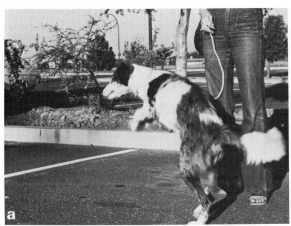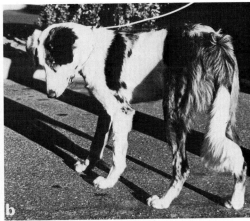

Fig. 19.15 This female Australian Shepherd Dog leapt and stared at 'imaginary objects'. When she was treated with internal and external variables (from Voith 1979). With permission from the editor of *California Veterinarian*.

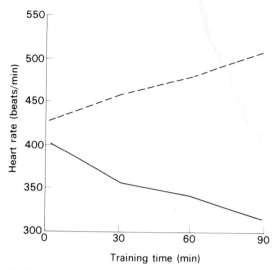

Fig. 19.16 Rats can be conditioned to increase or decrease heart rate independently from changes in rate of gastro-intestinal peristalsis (reward fast heartbeat, dotted line, reward slow heart beat, solid line) (DiCara 1970).

tures, subjected to the same environment and stresses as people may possibly manifest psychosomatic disease.

The learned asthma experiment with guinea pigs (p. 503) is an example of a psychosomatic phenomenon. Conditioning of the visceral, smooth muscle and autonomic nervous system is not, however, confined to classical conditioning. These systems can also be instrumentally or operantly conditioned (Fig. 19.16) (Di Cara 1970). Rats have been conditioned to increase or decrease their heart rate independent of gastro-intestinal changes and motility, and alter intestinal motility independent of a change in heart rate. Utilising either positive or negative reinforcement, animals have also demonstrated the ability to change blood pressure, control blood vessel diameter, and rate of urine formation (Miller 1969). Dogs which vomit usually receive immediate attention from their owner. Often this attention is one of concern accompanied by a caring voice and tactile stimulation. A dog which is lame is often reinforced with attention. Whereas the original cause or aetiology of such disorders may be due to a physiological disturbance, because the behaviours are followed by positive reinforcements, the behaviour may persist after the original aetiology is gone. Persistent manifestation of a disease after the original and complicating physical aetiologies have been removed can be the result of either classical or instrumental conditioning. In such cases extinction and/or counterconditioning must be employed to

eradicate the remnant manifestations of the disease.

Dramatic examples of conditioning body systems to react in an abnormal way are probably rare. More frequent forms of psychosomatic disorders that occur in animals are probably related to daily stress. Emotional stress has a cumulative effect and influences the onset of disease, recovery from an illness or surgical procedure, incidence and rapidity of death. Most of these correlations have been compiled in human medicine, but the same phenomena undoubtedly also occur in veterinary medicine.

REPRODUCTIVE BEHAVIOUR

Normal reproductive behaviour

A bitch is in behavioural oestrus 1–3 times a year. Her receptivity corresponds to elevated oestrogen levels and is termed 'oestrus' or 'standing heat'. Although she may only accept the male over a 3–5-day interval, the female dog attracts males for several days before becoming sexually receptive. Pheromones, excreted in the urine, are the probable mechanism by which male dogs are attracted to females. Anal sac excretions of bitches on heat do not appear to be a sexual attractant (Doty & Dunbar 1974).

The presence of an oestrus bitch frequently evokes fights between males. When a female in a household or neighbourhood is in heat, there may be fighting among previously amiable male dogs.

A sexually active male and receptive female may engage in courtship behaviour prior to copulation. The dogs may sniff each other's noses, followed by investigation of the female's hindquarters by the male. The male then usually attempts to mount. The female may, however, bound away for a short distance. The two dogs may then engage in chasing behaviour consisting of short dashes and play soliciting behaviours such as crouching on elbows, pawing, and barking. Eventually the female stands and copulation takes place.

A receptive female may present her rearquarters to a male, and elevate and cock her tail to one side. The male mounts from the rear, grasps the female around the flanks with his front legs, and begins pelvic thrusting. The penis becomes erect and when partial intromission has been achieved, pelvic thrusting increases in intensity until complete intromission. The male then tightens his hold on the female, lowers his tail, rapidly steps alternatingly with his hindlegs and engages in intense pelvic thrusting. This intense reaction lasts about 15–30 seconds and is accompanied by the ejaculation of the sperm. The female either throws the male off or the male dismounts shortly after the intense ejaculatory response. However, the dogs remain locked together for 10–30 minutes.

Problems related to breeding behaviour

Ideally, both male and female should be acclimatised to the breeding area. However it is more important that the male be comfortable and familiar with the territory than it is for the female. Although erection and ejaculation are primarily spinal reflexes, these behaviours can be cortically inhibited.

An inexperienced male may initially mount the female from the front or side before assuming the proper position. Novice males also spend more time engaged in pelvic thrusting and may mount a female several times before completing copulation. Such behaviours are exaggerated in males raised without contact with other dogs. As the male gains experience, however, he usually becomes a more effective breeder.

If the first few times an inexperienced dog tries to service a bitch, he encounters a female that is not in standing heat or a female with an aggressive temperament, he may become subsequently reluctant to mate, or he may develop an aversion to a particular female or colour of female. Care should be taken to have a novice male breed females that are definitely in standing heat and preferably females known to be unaggressive.

Males can be taught to serve females expediently thus saving many hours of observation time and avoids the need to put the dogs together unobserved for long intervals such as overnight. A specific area should be chosen as a breeding area and a standard routine followed in order that the male comes to expect and to mate a receptive oestrus female every time he is brought to the designated area.

Ovariectomised female dogs can be brought into standing heat for 14 days following two administrations of 1 mg oestradiol cypionate, subcutaneously or intramuscularly, 48 hours apart. The training female should be spayed to prevent the possibility of reproductive tract pathologies developing as a consequence of hormonal manipulation. Because of the risk of drug-induced bone marrow suppression, the bitches should not be kept on hormonal treatment for long periods of time and they should be periodically haematologically monitored.

To train the stud dog, first acclimatise him to the breeding area. Then daily or every other day a routine sequence of procedures should be followed until the dog becomes conditioned to anticipating the breeding activities. The male is first placed in the chamber followed by the known receptive female. After the male has mated her the female is removed and then the male. Initially it may be necessary to leave the dogs together for several hours before breeding occurs. When this sequence has been repeated several times, the male usually begins to anticipate being placed in the test area and mates the female within a few minutes.

A virgin bitch that is in full oestrus (as determined by vaginal smears) may continue to evade a male dog. Holding her head and supporting her thorax to keep her standing will allow the male to mate her. The female may subsequently stand for breeding procedures.

If a male or oestrus female ignores the other, it does not necessarily mean that either animal has lost all libido. Partner preferences do exist among dogs as does specific discrimination against particular individuals or groups of individuals that resemble each other. Although a dog may reject one individual he or she may readily respond to another.

REFERENCES

ANDERSSON B. & OLSSON K. (1965) Effects of bilateral amygdaloid lesions in nervous dogs. *J. Small Anim. Pract.* **6**, 301.

ARNOLD L.E., KIRILCUK V., CORSON S.A. & CORSON E. (1973) Levoamphetamine and dextroamphetamine: differential effect on aggression and hyperkinesis in children and dogs. *Am. J. Psychiatry* **130**(2), 165.

BEACH F.A. (1968) Coital Behavior in dogs. III. Effects of early isolation on mating in males. *Behavior* **30**, 217.

BEACH F.A. (1970) Coital behavior in dogs. VI. Long-term effects of castration upon mating in the male. *J. Comp. Physiol. Psychol.* **70**, 1.

BORCHELT P.L. (1983) Aggressive Behavior of Dogs Kept as Companion Animals: Classification and Influence of Sex, Reproductive Status, and Breed. *Appl. Anim. Etiol.* **10**, 45–61.

BORCHELT P.L., LOCKWOOD R., BECK A. & VOITH V.L. (1983) Attacks by packs of dogs involving predation on human beings. *Public Health Rep.* **98**(1), 57–66.

BORCHELT P.L. & VOITH V.L. (1982) Classification of animal behavior problems. *Vet. Clin. North Am.* (*Small Anim. Pract.*) **12**, 511–85.

BRELAND K. & BRELAND M. (1961) The misbehavior of organisms. *Am. Psychol.* **16**, 681.

BREITSCHWERDT E.B., BREAZILE J.E. & BROADHURST J.J. (1979) Clinical and electroencephalographic findings associated with 10 cases of suspected limbic epilepsy in the dog. *J. Am. Anim. Hosp. Assoc.* **15**, 35–50.

CORSON S.A., CORSON E.O., ARNOLD L.E. & KNAPP W. (1976) Animal models of violence and hyperkinesis. Interaction of psychopharmacologic and psychosocial therapy in behavior modification. In *Animal Models in Human*

Psychology, eds. G. Serban & A. Kling. Plenum Press, New York.

CORSON S.A *et al* (1980) Interaction of genetics and separation in canine hyperkinesis and in differential responses to amphetamine. *PAV. J. Biol. Sci.* **15**(1), 5–11.

DEES S.C. (1954) Neurologic allergy in childhood. *Vet. Clin. North Am.* **1**, 1017.

DICARA L.V. (1970) Learning in the autonomic nervous system. *Sci. Am.* **222**(1), 30.

DOTY R.L. & DUNBAR I.F. (1974) Attraction of beagles to conspecific urine, vaginal, and anal sac secretion odors. *Physiol. Behav.* **12**, 825.

DUNBAR I.F. (1979) *Presented at Ann. Am. Vet. Ethol. Soc. Meeting*, Seattle, Washington.

EIGENMANN J.E. (1981) Diabetes Mellitus in elderly female dogs: recent findings on pathogenesis and clinical implication. *J. Am. Anim. Hosp. Assoc.* **17**, 805–12.

EIGENMANN J.E. & EIGENMANN R.Y. (1981) Influence of medroxyprogesterone acetate (Provera) on plasma growth hormone levels and on carbohydrate metabolism I and II. *Acta Endocrinol.* **98**, 599–62, 602–8.

EIGENMANN J.E. & VENKER-VAN HAAGEN A.J. (1981) Progestagen-induced and spontaneous canine acromegaly due to reversible growth hormone over production: Clinical picture and pathogenesis. *J. Am. Anim. Hosp. Assoc.* **17**, 813–22.

EVANS J.M. (1978) Current thoughts concerning hypersexuality in dogs, with particular reference to the role of progestogens. *Proc. Refresher Course for Veterinarians No. 37, Post-Graduate Committee in Veterinary Science.* University Press, Sydney.

FOX M.W. (1971) *Behavior of Wolves, Dogs and Related Canids*. Harper & Row, New York.

FREEMAN D.G., ELLIOT E. & KLING J.A. (1961) Critical period in social development of dogs. *Science* **133**, 1016.

FULLER J.L. & Clark L.D. (1966) Genetic and treatment factors modifying the postisolation syndrome in dogs. *J. Comp. Physiol. Psychol.* **61**, 251.

GOODMAN L.S. & GILMAN A. (1975) *The Pharmacological Basic of Therapeutics*, 5th edn. Macmillan, New York.

GUERRERO-FIGUEROA R., BARROS A., DEBABBIAN VERSTER F. & HEATH R.G. (1963) Experimental 'Petit Mal' in kittens. *Arch. Neurol.* **9**, 297–306.

HART B.L. (1968) Role of prior sexual experience in the effects of castration and sexual behavior of male dogs. *J. Comp. Physiol. Psychol.* **66**, 719.

HART B.L. (1969) Unusual defecation behaviors in the male dog. *Commun. Behav. Biol.* **41**, 237–8.

HOLLIDAY T.A., CUNNINGHAM J.G. & GUTNICK M.J. (1970) Comparative clinical and electroencephalographic studies of canine epilepsy. *Epilepsia* **II**, 281.

HOPKINS S.G., SCHUBERT T.A. & HART B.L. (1976) Castration of adult male dogs: Effects of roaming, aggression, urine marking, and mounting. *J. Am. Vet. Med. Assoc.* **168**, 1108.

HOUPT K.A. (1979) Behaviour: Aggression in dogs. *The Compendium in Cont. Ed. for the Small Anim. Pract.* **3**, 123–8.

KLINGHAMMER E. (1979) Social Behavior of Wolves, lecture at University of Pennsylvania, Philadelphia.

LAPRAS M. (1977) Modern Psychotrope Therapy in the Dog. *Proceedings of the 6th World Congress, World Small Animal Vet. Assoc. Post. Acad. onder wiis Publikatie No. 8.*

LEBŒUF B.J. (1970) Copulatory and aggressive behavior in the prepuberally castrated dog. *Horm. Behav.* **1**, 127.

LINE S. (1983) Review of Dominance Agression. *Amer. Soc. Vet. Ethology Newsletter* **6**, 3–5.

MECH L.D. (1970) *The Wolf: Ecology and Behavior of an Endangered Species*. The Natural History Press, Garden City, N.Y.

MEIERHENRY E.F. & LUI S. (1978) Atrioventricular bundle degeneration associated with sudden death in the dog. *J. Am. Vet. Med. Assoc.* **172**, 1418.

MELZACK R. (1954) The genesis of emotional behavior: an experimental study of the dog. *J. Comp. Physiol. Psychol.* **46**, 166.

MELZACK R. & SCOTT T.H. (1957) The effects of early experience on the response to pain. *J. Comp. Physiol. Psychol.* **50**, 155.

MELZACK R. & THOMPSON W.R. (1956) Effects of early experience on social behavior. *Canad. J. Psychol.* **10**, 82.

MILLER N.E. (1969) Learning of visceral and glandular responses. *Science* **161**, 434–45.

MOYER K.E. (1968) Kinds of aggression and their physiological basis. *Commun. Behav. Biol. Part. A.* **2**, 65.

OTTERBERG P. *et al* (1958) Learned asthma in the guinea pig. *Psychosom. Med.* **20**, 395.

PETERS R. & MECH L.D. (1975) Scent-marking in wolves. *Am. Sci.* **63**, 628–47.

QUACKENBUSH J.E. (1981) Pets, Owners, Problems, and the Veterinarian: Applied Social Work in a Veterinary Teaching Hospital. *The Compendium on Continuing Education* **3**(9), 764–70.

RABB G.B., GINSBURG B.E. & ANDREWS S. (1962) Comparative studies of *Canid* behavior, IV, abstract 207, *Am. Zool.* **2**, 440.

RABB G.B., WOOLPY J.H. & GINSBURG B.E. (1967) Social relationships in a group of captive wolves. *Am. Zool.* **7**, 305–11.

REDDING R.W. & WALKER T.L. (1976) Electroconvulsive therapy to control aggression in dogs. *Mod. Vet. Pract.* **57**, 595.

RESKO J.A. (1970) Androgens in systemic plasma of male guinea pigs during development and after castration in adulthood. *Endocrinology* **86**, 1444.

RESKO J.A. & PHOENIX C.H. (1972) Sexual behavior and testosterone concentrations in the plasma of the rhesus monkey before and after castration. *Endocrinology* **86**, 499.

RIMM D.C. & MASTERS J.C. (1974) *Behavior Therapy Techniques and Empirical Findings*. Academic Press, New York.

RYDEN, H. (1975) *God's Dog*. Coward, McCann and Geoghegan, N.Y.

SCHENKEL R. (1947) Ausdrucks—studien an wolfen. *Behavior* **1**, 81–129.

SCOTT J.P. & FULLER J.L. (1965) *Genetics and the Social Behavior of the Dog*. University of Chicago Press, Chicago.

SELIGMAN M.E.P. (1970) Phobias and preparedness. *Behav. Ther.* **2**, 307–20.

SELIGMAN M.E.P. (1971) On the generality of the laws of learning. *Psych. Rev.* **77**, 406–418.

STOWE C.M. *et al* (1976) Amphetamine poisoning in dogs. *J. Am. Vet. Med. Assoc.* **168**, 504.

THOMPSON W.R. & HERON W. (1954) The effects of restricting early experience on the problem solving capacity of dogs. *Canad. J. Psychol.* **8**, 17.

THORNDIKE E.L. (1898) Animal intelligence, an experimental

study of the associative process in animals. *Psychol. Rev. Mono.* **2**, 109.

TUBER D.S., HOTHERSALL D. & PETERS M.F. (1982) Treatment of fears and phobias. *Vet. Clin. North Am. (Small Anim. Pract.)* **12**, 607.

TUBER D.S. HOTHERSALL D. & VOITH V.L. (1974) Animal clinical psychology: a modest proposal. *Am. Psychol.* **29**, 762.

TURNER W.A. (1973) *Epilepsy, a study of the idiopathic disease.* Raven Press, New York.

VOITH V.L. (1975) Destructive behaviour in the owners absence. Parts I and II. *Canine Pract.* **2**(3), 11; **2**(4), 8.

VOITH V.L. (1976) Fear-induced aggressive behaviour. Parts I and II. *Canine Pract.* **3**(5), 14; **3**(6), 14.

VOITH V.L. and HART B.L. (1978) Principles of Behavior. In B.F. Hoerlein (ed.) *Canine Neurology*, 3rd Ed. W.B. Saunders Co., Philadelphia.

VOITH V.L. (1979a) Clinical Animal Behaviour. *Calif. Veterinarian*, June, 21–25.

VOITH V.L. (1979b) Learning principles and behavioral problems. *Mod. Vet. Prac.* **60**(7), 553–5.

VOITH V.L. (1979c) Treatment of fear reactions: canine aggression. *Mod. Vet. Prac.* **60**(11), 903–5.

VOITH V.L. (1980) Diagnosis and treatment of aggression behaviour problems in dogs. *AAAH 47th Annual Proceedings*, 35–8.

VOITH V.L. (1981a) The attachment of owners to pets despite behavior problems of the animal. Proceedings of Thamatology Foundation Symposium. *Vet. Med. Pract: Pet Loss and Human Emotion.*

VOITH V.L. (1981b) You, too, can teach a cat tricks. *Mod. Vet. Pract.* 639–42.

VOITH V.L. (1981c) Diagnosing dominance aggression. *Mod. Vet. Pract.* **62**, 639–42.

VOITH V.L. (1981d) The treatment of dominance aggression toward people. *Mod. Vet. Pract.* **62**, 149–152.

VOITH V.L. & BORCHELT P.L. (1982) Diagnosis and Treatment of Dominance Aggression in Dogs. In V.L. Voith and P.L. Borchelt (eds.), *Vet. Clin. North Am. (Small Anim. Pract.)* **12**(4), 655–63.

VOITH V.L. (1983a) Human-Animal Relationships. In R. Anderson (ed). *Proceedings of 1st Nordic Veterinary Medical Symposium.* Pergamon Press, Oxford.

VOITH V.L. (1983b) Possible pharmacological approaches to treating behavioural problems in animals. *Proceedings of 1st Nordic Veterinary Medical Symposium.* Pergamon Press, Oxford.

WAECHTER R.A. (1982) Unusual reaction to acepromazine maleate in the dog. *J. Am. Vet. Med. Assoc.* **180**(1), 73–4.

WARREN R.P. & ARONSON L.R. (1956) Sexual behavior in castrated adrenalectomized hamsters maintained on DCA. *Endocrinology* **58**, 293.

WHITNEY L.F. (1971) *Dog Psychology: The basis of dog training.* C.C. Thomas, Springfield, Ill.

YOUNG M.S. (1982) Treatment of fear-induced aggression in dogs. *Vet. Clin. North Am. (Small Anim. Pract.)* **12**(4), 645–53.

20
Canine Nutrition and Disease

A. T. B. EDNEY

Compared with cats, dogs are relatively robust nutritionally. Most canids, foxes in particular, manage to thrive in relatively unpromising circumstances when food supplies are uncertain. As small- to medium-sized mammals go, domesticated dogs are relatively long lived, many surviving well beyond 10 years. However nutrition-related canine problems do arise in small animal veterinary practice. These may be a result of faulty feeding practices, but also include a wide range of illnesses where nutritional adjustments play a role in their management but are not the actual cause of the condition. Both groups will be explored in this chapter as they are of practical importance to clinicians in general practice.

Faulty feeding can arise out of providing excesses or as absolute or relative shortages of essential nutrients. The majority of cases seen which come into the category of faulty feeding are where too much food is provided rather than the deficiency diseases which are well documented in other works. Canine obesity is a direct result of maintaining an individual in positive energy balance by providing more energy than it needs, so that the excess is stored as body fat. The result is the commonest form of malnutrition seen in veterinary practice.

Pancreatic failure is an example of a condition coming into the second group because dietary adjustment is normally needed in the management of such cases, although the condition is not normally caused by any feeding practices. Although the division of the conditions covered in this chapter into two groups is somewhat arbitrary, it is useful to help to explain to the owner what is being done and why. Misunderstandings often arise when a dog's diet is changed, if the reasons for such action are not made clear. Owners readily assume that if the food they are giving their animal has been changed, then that food must be the cause of the illness, even though a new diet may be prescribed for sound medical reasons.

The purpose of this chapter is to compile a guide for veterinarians attending cases which have come into either of the two groups described and to list some general guidelines for feeding dogs which are ill. This approach is taken in preference to listing all the obscure conditions which are possible but are rarely seen in clinical practice.

CONDITIONS ASSOCIATED WITH FAULTY FEEDING

Many problems arise from faulty nutrition in dogs, but deficiencies and excesses of single nutrients are not usually encountered in isolation. Apart from an overall excess of calorie intake leading to obesity, what usually occurs is a collection of signs relating to a number of irregularities in the diet. Clinical illness relating to deficiencies is usually accompanied by some degree of inappetence which in turn compounds the problems which already exist.

Canine obesity

Far and away the commonest form of malnutrition in dogs is obesity. Dogs are said to be obese when there is an accumulation of body fat sufficient to cause some impairment of body function. Obesity is always a result of positive energy balance where the dog's calorie intake exceeds its requirements. The resulting excess is stored as body fat, mainly in the subcutaneous areas. Once the obese state has been reached it can usually be maintained without over eating, so when presented for clinical examination, obese dogs may not be eating very much more than otherwise comparable individuals.

Dogs tend to be opportunist feeders, engorging themselves on available supplies all the time they continue to be provided. Some breeds tend to be more greedy than others. Hounds, many gundogs, particularly Labradors, Boxers and many Terriers, tend to be more voracious than others, e.g. toy breeds or most Setters. However much depends on what feeding habits have been allowed to develop.

A number of surveys have indicated that overt obesity is present in 28–34% of the canine population in the UK (Mason 1970; Anderson 1973), and elsewhere in Europe the proportion of the canine population judged to be obese may be even more (Steininger 1981). However, these data are based on limited numbers and a more extensive survey is clearly needed. There is also some evidence that obese owners tend to keep obese dogs, probably because of over-generous traditions of hospitality in the household. Dogs from such households are particularly difficult to treat and are the ones most likely to require hospitalisation to achieve a satisfactory outcome in the management of the case.

Obese dogs are seldom presented to veterinarians because of their obesity. Each case is usually brought for veterinary attention for the results of obesity. Canine obesity is frequently associated with many of the complications seen in human medicine. Circulatory difficulties, particularly cardiopulmonary congestion, with some joint damage, are frequent sequelae to canine obesity. It is, however, difficult to separate cause and effect in trying to establish what contribution being grossly overweight makes to the malfunctioning of the circulatory or locomotor systems, particularly as debility from such complications leads to further inactivity with reduced energy output, thus tending to exacerbate the obese state. Infertility, lowered resistance in infectious disease, increased surgical and anaesthetic risk as well as poor heat tolerance due to an increased level of insulation, have all been found to be associated with canine obesity. Feldman (1980) reports the development of hepatomegaly, reduced expiratory reserve volume, decreased chest wall compliance, alveolar hypoventilation and tracheal collapse in obese dogs. These conditions eventually lead to cyanosis and heart failure.

The neutering of male and female dogs increases the likelihood of obesity developing unless dietary measures are taken to prevent it. Not only does neutering alter the life style of castrated or spayed animals, it is likely that some metabolic pathways are modified; for example the utilisation of amino acids to build muscle protein under the influence of testosterone and the effect of an increase in circulating follicle stimulating hormone on the deposition of body fat in spayed bitches are significant changes which follow neutering (Anderson & Lewis 1980). However, body fat can only come from food and owners need to exercise sufficient control over the food intake to prevent the development of obesity in their dogs. Clinicians carrying out neutering operations need to give clear feeding guidance to owners when spaying or castrating their dogs.

Management of canine obesity

As owners do not usually bring their dogs to veterinarians because of the development of obesity, but more often to remedy its complications, it is often difficult to convince owners of the threat to their dog's health and the need to take firm action.

Each case should be examined carefully to determine the extent of any of the usual complications of obesity and to discover if any condition is present, such as a heart valve lesion, which could influence treatment or recovery. The owner must then be counselled fully and an explanation given regarding what is wrong with the dog, and what must be done to put it right. Some estimate of how long the treatment will take is needed, as well as an understanding of the need to maintain a disciplined feeding and exercise regime for the rest of the animal's days. Anything less than all this and disappointing results are likely, in which case everyone's time is wasted and the dog's health prejudiced further.

As obesity results from a positive balance in the dog's energy metabolism, its resolution can only be brought about by establishing and maintaining a negative energy balance until sufficient body fat has been mobilised to restore the animal to its optimum bodyweight. This can be achieved by allowing the dog less calories than it is using. Calorie restriction may be partial or total, that is deprivation of all food. It is possible to increase energy output as well by forced exercise, but this is only advised in the greatest moderation. It is safer to allow the dog to increase its own level of activity as it becomes less bulky on its prescribed diet. Most clinicians prescribe modest but strict calorie restriction accompanied by some voluntary increase in activity as the dog becomes fitter. Forced exercise at any stage of obesity treatment is likely to be positively harmful particularly if there are any cardiorespiratory signs evident.

Calorie restriction is often more effective if it is not too severe, as owner compliance is usually better than with more demanding regimes. Starvation or semi-starvation are not normally well accepted by owners. Non-compliance with instructions can waste a good deal of time and effort and may not be discovered for several weeks. Hospitalisation is necessary for any starvation therapy.

The objective of the treatment regime recommended is to find the level of food allowance which will just effect a progressive loss of body weight. It has been found that trying to adjust the dog's existing diet to bring about weight reduction is less effective than prescribing a new diet for the dog.

Having discussed the case with the owner and insisted on complete co-operation of all who come into contact with the dog, the following procedure should be adopted.

1 Weigh the dog carefully and record the result. A reasonably accurate and reliable set of scales is needed. Weighing the owner plus dog on bathroom scales and subtracting the weight of the owner gives a rough indication of the dog's bodyweight, but is not accurate enough for effective monitoring of weight control procedures.

2 Estimate the weight that the dog should be. This can be done by reference to the weights of the usual breeds and types of dog, or if the animal is a crossbred, a target weight of 15% less than the weight the dog is presented at can be used as a starting point.

3 Estimate the energy needs of the dog at the target weight. A diet which allows 60% of the calories needed for a dog of the target weight is the initial allowance.

4 In addition to setting a target bodyweight (say −15%), a date for achieving this should be set. This would normally be 12 weeks after treatment begins.

5 Insist that the dog has only the diet prescribed and nothing else at all except drinking water.

6 The dog should be examined every week at the same time of day and carefully weighed on the same scales in the same place. The bodyweight is then carefully recorded.

7 Every week there is no appreciable bodyweight reduction, the total amount of food prescribed is decreased by 20% until there is.

8 If a simple graph of the dog's bodyweight is kept against time, this will show the point at which negative energy balance is achieved and will help to motivate the owner. Even quite good progress may not be evident for several weeks except as an indication on a graph. Once a steady weight loss occurs the line of the graph can be projected forwards to show the owner that with sustained application of the dietary regime, the target weight can be achieved within a reasonable time.

9 If the owner can be persuaded to keep a diary of everything the dog does, it can help considerably. This serves to reinforce the discipline of dietary control and to record any voluntary increase in the dog's own activity.

10 Once the target weight has been achieved, it is necessary to prescribe a maintenance diet to stabilise the dog at an acceptable bodyweight. This rarely needs to be more than an additional 15% of the calories needed to effect a bodyweight reduction.

11 Follow-up examinations should be carried out 1, 3 and 6 months after treatment has finished to ensure that the maintenance diet is sufficient to prevent further weight loss or is not being abused so that relapses occur.

Table 20.1 shows the theoretical calorie needs of dogs of normal bodyweight and the 60% calorie allowance given to obese subjects (after Edney 1972).

The gross calorie content of any dog food can be calculated from a proximate analysis assuming 1g of protein yields 4 kcal, 1g of carbohydrate, 3.5 kcal and 1g of fat, 9 kcal. As a rule of thumb canned wet foods normally yield 75–100 kcal/100 g, those with cereal will have the higher figure. Dog biscuit and other dry foods with a moisture level of <10% usually contain 350/400 kcal/100 g. Some commercially available canned diets have material such as bran added to reduce the digestibility and thus decrease the amount of available calories.

Many owners find the giving of additional 'treats' to the dog, especially last thing at night, a difficult practice to abandon. As these are usually calorie-dense foods such as chocolate, they frequently represent the difference between success and failure. Rather than trying to prohibit this supplementary feeding the simple expedient of cutting up small cubes of the dog's dietary allowance and substituting this for the 'treat' has been shown to be an effective strategy (Edney & Hughes 1980).

Total starvation, to the extent of depriving the dog entirely of nutrients, except water and a vitamin/mineral supplement, is practised effectively by some workers. In man this has proved effective enough, although some deaths have occurred after apparently successful treatment. Bodyweight losses of the order of 23% after 5 weeks can be achieved (Lewis 1977) apparently without ill effect as ketosis does not seem to follow starvation in dogs (de Brunjie 1983). No problems of refeeding have so far been reported. With otherwise healthy animals starvation may be a useful alternative although disproportionate losses from lean body mass such as those which occur in man could present additional complications. In any case hospitalisation and constant surveillance are needed to enforce the regime and the obvious cost of such measures is an additional point which must be considered before embarking on this approach. Field work has shown that simple disciplined calorie restriction is an effective treatment for canine obesity and hospitalisation is only needed where owner co-operation is inadequate or the dog's scavenging activity is difficult to control.

Overnutrition of growing giant dogs

A problem occasionally encountered in veterinary practice is the overnutrition of growing dogs of the giant breeds, especially Great Danes. This is usually

Table 20.1 The calculated calorie requirement and amount to be prescribed to obese dogs based on an estimated optimum bodyweight (after Edney 1972).

Estimated optimum bodyweight of dog		Approximate daily energy requirement (NRC 1974) kcal	Daily energy intake recommended to begin weight reduction (kcal)
lb	kg		
10	4.5	400	250
20	9.0	700	400
30	13.5	950	550
40	18.0	1150	700
50	23.0	1400	800
60	27.0	1550	950
70	32.0	1750	1000
80	36.0	1900	1200
90	41.0	2100	1300
100	45.5	2300	1500

the result of attempts to force puppies beyond their normal growth capacity. *Ad libitum* feeding of a calorie-dense highly palatable food has been shown to produce many skeletal problems in Great Danes when compared with litter mates allowed only two-thirds the amount of food (Hedhammar *et al* 1974). The high rate of bodyweight increase and deposition of bone is believed to outstrip the dog's capacity to lay down properly structured bone.

The popular belief that giant breeds of dog need proportionately very large amounts of calcium is probably responsible for the development of hypercalcitonism which impairs remodelling of bone during rapid growth and interferes with the absorption of zinc and magnesium (Hedhammar 1980).

Hypervitaminosis A

Excess vitamin A intake leading to toxicosis occasionally occurs in dogs as a result of the overzealous administration of cod liver oil or other supplements containing high levels of fat soluble vitamins. The effects of hypervitaminosis A are cumulative because of storage in the liver. The condition is usually seen in puppies where owners still maintain a belief that 'more is better' with vitamin supplementation. The cortex of the long bones becomes thin and the epiphyseal cartilage narrow. Exostoses occur at the point of tendon attachments. There is considerable joint pain and puppies are eventually unable to stand. Characteristically the affected individuals resent handling of their extremities. Remodelling of bone becomes irregular and appetite deteriorates, leading to complete anorexia. This is usually accompanied by gingivitis, when severe tooth loss is extensive.

Hypervitaminosis D

Dogs which live in normal conditions are believed not to need a dietary source of vitamin D. Although the absorption of calcium from the gut is enhanced by available vitamin D, its main action is to maintain normal plasma calcium concentrations. So where mineral intake is critically low, the dog is especially vulnerable to the ill effects of additional vitamin D, as plasma levels are eventually maintained by the demineralisation of bone. Thus an owner's efforts at 'building strong bones' by supplementing an inadequate diet with a rich source of vitamin D such as cod or halibut liver oil, can easily provoke the reverse of the effect intended. Vitamin D toxicosis leads to high serum calcium and phosphorus levels, which in turn result in extensive soft tissue calcification. Bone lesions normally only occur if there is an excess of vitamin A as well.

Doses of 25 000–50 000 iu of vitamin D are sufficient to raise the serum Ca and P levels enough to cause soft tissue calcification. As with vitamin A toxicosis, the effects of over supply of vitamin D are cumulative, as both vitamins are stored in the liver. Eventually renal lesions occur with hypervitaminosis D, resulting in uraemia and eventually death.

The early signs of hypervitaminosis A or D are likely to be reversible if a normal unsupplemented diet is eaten. That is where the effects of inappetence are not so profound as to prevent the dog from taking in enough nutrients to remain healthy.

Hypervitaminosis E

Although all fat soluble vitamins are toxic in excess, in the normal course of events toxicosis due to vitamin

E is unlikely to occur. Ten times the recommended level (NRC 1974) has been fed to growing puppies without ill effects being observed (Burger 1982).

Inanition

The feeding behaviour of dogs is very different from cats, although both species seem to be able to withstand food deprivation in accidental circumstances very well, provided sufficient water is available to drink. However, dogs are less able to conserve water by concentrating their urine to the extent cats do readily. Dogs also differ in that as a general rule they do not normally starve themselves in the presence of wholesome food and seem to be less subject to the effects on their feeding behaviour of environmental stresses such as boarding or hospitalisation, although both may lead to a measure of inappetence. Young puppies and other individuals with a high demand for nutrients may suffer from undernutrition simply because they are unable to accommodate enough of an energy-dilute food. An increase in the number of meals offered helps to overcome some of the shortfall, but in most cases a more calorie-dense food is needed. Bitches which are heavily pregnant, where the gravid uterus occupies so much abdominal space that the capacity of the mother's stomach becomes progressively less, need to be fed more frequently. Problems with general underfeeding are fairly common where bitches are rearing large litters. Owners often judge the effectiveness of their bitches feeding regime only by looking at the puppies being reared. What frequently happens however is that the demands of a growing litter (which itself may collectively weigh as much as their mother), are such that at least three times the bitch's maintenance requirements are needed at the peak of lactation. When this is not provided the bitch will draw on her own body reserves to feed her puppies. A dramatic loss of both body fat and lean body mass can occur quite rapidly in such cases. If a bitch is eating readily there is no need for her to lose bodyweight during lactation.

The opposite effect of too dilute a food, where a dog is replete and cannot physically accommodate more, can occur with energy-rich foods. In which case, the dog can become satiated with an excess of calories before some essential nutrients have been eaten. This is not a frequent problem with dogs as they mostly have a tendency to overeat when the opportunities to do so are presented. However, the demands of growing dogs are more critical and a diet which, on the face of it, may have adequate amounts of essential nutrients present, in more practical terms, may be unbalanced

when expressed as concentration per 400 kcal Burger (1982). Only by expressing nutrient content in this way can meaningful comparisons be made; 400 kcal represents about 100 g of most wet diets.

Proteins

For practical purposes 22% of metabolisable energy (ME) as protein is needed to cover all stages of a dog's life (NRC 1974); that is 22 g of protein per 400 kcal. This is achieved with most prepared foods.

The effects of protein-calorie deficiency are dependent upon the limiting amino acid present, but in general body protein breakdown occurs as the animal goes into negative nitrogen balance. Wasting of lean body mass is the usual feature of protein-calorie deficiency. Where such wasting occurs, even though apparently adequate amounts of food may be being eaten, the protein calorie content of the dog's diet should be estimated from the proximate analysis as a first step. If this is less than 22% then adjustments in the proportion of the protein component are needed. If the percentage calories from protein appears adequate, it is more likely that the amino acid make-up is inadequate and additional sources of essential amino acids are needed. Even so analysis is not all. It may be necessary to investigate the digestibility of the proteins in the diet fed and to examine the amino acid profile. The following are known to be essential amino acids for dogs: threonine, valine, methionine, isoleucine, leucine, phenylalanine, histidine, tryptophan, lysine. Although animal-derived proteins generally have these amino acids present in greater abundance and in a more balanced form, vegetable proteins can be a valuable source of much of them. In this case there is usually a shortfall of lysine as the limiting amino acid, which can usually be made up from animal sources. It is possible, but not very practical, to feed a dog adequately entirely on vegetable material.

Undermineralisation

Calcium
Inadequate provision of minerals has serious consequences in growing puppies and results in severe osteodystrophy. The commonest cause of canine osteodystrophy is an over reliance on muscle meat as the main component of the diet, without any mineral additions. Not only does the skeleton become undermineralised, with characteristic thin cortices, poor bone density and spontaneous fractures, but Hendrik-

son (1968) has shown that severe periodontal disease results from feeding a diet grossly imbalanced in its ratio of calcium: phosphorus (0.12:1.20). Alveolar bone becomes progressively eroded, leading to considerable tooth loss. Subsequent work showed that these signs could be avoided if the calcium content of the diet was raised from 0.12% to 0.6%. Where insufficient available calcium is present, excessive bone resorption occurs as a result of nutritional hyperparathyroidism. Jaw bones are often the first to show signs of demineralisation, this may be followed by vertebral compression and spontaneous fractures of long bones. Tetanic convulsions ultimately occur, eventually leading to death from cardiac arrest.

Phosphorus

As phosphorus is found in most cellular material a straightforward phosphorus deficiency is not likely to be encountered in the normal course of events. It is only when the calcium:phosphorus ratio is grossly imbalanced to favour calcium, of the order of 20:1 or more, that rickets is likely to occur in growing dogs (see p. 544).

Zinc

Mineral deficiencies other than calcium or phosphorus are relatively rarely seen in dogs with the possible exception of zinc. Even when otherwise adequate amounts of zinc are present in a diet, high levels of calcium may interfere with zinc absorption. A diet containing 3.3 mg of zinc/100 g and 1.1% calcium (dry matter) has been shown to produce signs of skin and hair lesions, especially keratitis (NRC 1974). Less specific signs of anorexia, conjunctivitis and emaciation also occur. Additional zinc in the diet eliminates all these signs, provided the dog can continue eating.

Copper

Although straightforward copper deficiency is unlikely to occur in canine veterinary practice, a curious condition of copper toxicity occurs in some Bedlington Terriers. Affected individuals are unable to dispose of copper effectively, so toxic levels build up in the liver, leading to hepatitis and eventual cirrhosis, where analysis shows that copper levels reach < 10 mg/g dry weight of liver tissue (Owen & McCall 1983). Restricting the copper intake of affected Bedlingtons is the only course open to the owner, although stimulation of biliary secretions with relatively high fat intakes may help increase copper excretion, as this is mainly by way of bile. Copper intake can be restricted by avoiding the feeding of liver or any mineral supplements containing copper.

Iron deficiency and anaemia (see Chapter 11)

Vitamins

The days when vitamins were looked upon as 'cure-alls' may not yet have passed. Many owners and some breeders still regard vitamins as having restorative powers beyond the therapeutic effects of making good deficiencies. Problems relating to injudicious supplementation, largely with fat soluble vitamins, outweigh deficiency diseases by a wide margin. However, clinical cases of inadequate vitamin intake do occur, usually in growing puppies.

Vitamin A

Unlike cats, dogs are not limited in their use of carotenoid precursors, so the vitamin A present in vegetable material is available to them as β-carotene from which active vitamin A is derived. Cats as well as having a greater need for vitamin A are unable to use β-carotene in this way.

Growing puppies may need up to 1000 iu of vitamin A per 400 kcal of their diet. Adults can continue to thrive on about half this amount. When puppies are deficient they rapidly grow weak and deformed. Eye changes develop, characteristic signs of xerophthalmia are readily seen to accompany conjunctivitis. Eventually corneal opacity and ulceration cause irreversible changes leading to blindness which may be hastened by retinal dysplasia in severe cases. Bone remodelling becomes disorganised, leading to degenerative nerve changes particularly involving the eighth cranial nerve leading to deafness. Similar changes occur with the optic nerve. Epithelial degeneration occurs in the respiratory system, leading to encrustation of the nares and a chronic nasal discharge. Epithelial degeneration also occurs in the seminiferous tubules and endometrium leading to infertility. Similar changes may occur in the pancreas and salivary glands causing serious digestive disturbances due to inadequate secretion.

It is usually worth examining the vitamin A status of dog breeding establishments where poor results are evident. Either males or females may be infertile, or both. A low grade endometritis may be detected, bitches may fail to come into oestrus, or abort. Any puppies carried to term are likely to be born deformed or show stunted growth.

Any food which has been subjected to temperatures greater than 125°C for long periods should be suspected as inadequate unless supplemented, as vitamin A is made unavailable by overheating.

Vitamin D

Dogs are able to form their own vitamin D from lipid compounds in the skin under the influence of ultraviolet light. Changes subsequently occur in the liver and kidneys to convert vitamin D into an available form (NRC 1974). Deficiencies are therefore rare and the level of availability is only usually critical when calcium and phosphorus intakes are low. The combination of these circumstances leads to rickets (see p. 543).

Vitamin E

As with vitamin D, deficiencies of vitamin E are not usually seen in domestic dogs. But as in other species high levels of polyunsaturated fatty acids (PUFA) increase the need for the anti-oxidant effect of vitamin E. The ratio of vitamin E:PUFA (as mg:g) needs to be 0.5 or more in favour of vitamin E to prevent signs of illness due to cellular changes (NRC 1974).

Signs of inadequate vitamin E intake include myodegeneration leading to skeletal muscular dystrophy and possibly testicular and endometrial degenerative changes. Such individuals show low levels of circulating tocopherol concentration (<5 parts 10^6). Although the estimation of tocopherol status may present practical difficulties, it is a useful strategy in kennels where infertility is evident.

Vitamin B1—thiamin

One of the few straightforward deficiencies encountered in small animal veterinary practice is a lack of available vitamin B_1, or thiamin, in the diet. The reason for this is that thiamin is both thermolabile and can be inactivated by the enzyme thiaminase. The situation is complicated by the fact that thiamin is a co-enzyme which plays an integral part in carbohydrate metabolism. A high fat/low carbohydrate diet tends to spare the need for thiamin. Conversely diets with a high percentage of carbohydrate, like various dry meals/biscuits, need more thiamin to complete the metabolic processes involved. Core temperatures within the food during processing in excess of 100°C reduce the amount of thiamin available with time. Thiamin is progressively inactivated by heating, not, as is widely believed, suddenly destroyed at a particular temperature. Most manufactured foods are supplemented before processing to compensate for any subsequent losses.

Where food is cooked by owners, loss of thiamin will occur unless the diet is supplemented with a rich source of vitamin B such as Brewer's Yeast. The thiaminase present in raw fish also destroys thiamin, but as most fish is fed cooked and therefore the thiaminase is inactivated, there is not usually clinical illness.

The clinical manifestations of thiamin deficiency begin with anorexia, which is likely to compound the problem so that other deficiencies result if no action is

taken to rectify the matter. Unsteadiness of gait, postural abnormalities accompanied by a loss of muscle tone and reflexes, especially in the hind limbs, are seen. There is a degeneration of the myelin sheath of the peripheral nerves and eventually of the spinal cord. Death follows from cardiac failure (NRC 1974).

Injections of 500–1000 μg of thiamin rapidly reverse clinical signs, unless cardiac or neurological damage is advanced. Once any deficiency of thiamin has been corrected, it is vital that the intake is maintained permanently by feeding an adequate diet, because, as with all water soluble vitamin deficiencies, there is no storage of thiamin in body tissues.

Vitamin B6—pyridoxine

Occasionally a clinical case of vitamin B6 or pyridoxine deficiency is presented in canine veterinary practice. In puppies non-specific signs of depression, anorexia and subsequent retarded growth occur. This is accompanied by a microcytic hypochromic anaemia, eventually followed by death as a result of severe epileptiform convulsions (NRC 1974). However the provision of only 5 μg/kg/day is enough to prevent signs developing in growing dogs.

Niacin—nicotinic acid

The classic picture of 'black-tongue' in dogs, that is severe inflammation with ulceration of the mouth and thick cords of saliva, which may be bloodstained, running continuously from the mouth, accompanied by an offensive smell, is rarely seen now. The exceptional occurrence is in occasional working dogs fed almost entirely on cereal grains. Signs resembling human pellagra progress to a bloodstained diarrhoea and necrotic lesions of the large and small intestines. Malabsorption results from extensive damage to intestinal villi. Dehydration and death eventually follow; 250 μg/kg/day are sufficient to reverse early signs and prevent recurrence.

Biotin

For practical purposes all the biotin needs of dogs can be derived from their own gut flora. Deficiencies can occur however when there is prolonged antibiotic therapy or if large quantities of raw egg white are fed. Avidin present in egg white inactivates biotin so that signs of deficiency follow. Dogs develop a dry scaly skin with dull, brittle hair; eventually there is hyperkeratosis, pruritus and ulceration of the skin (Glättli *et al* 1973). Avidin is however readily destroyed by heat so where eggs are fed cooked, biotin deficiency is not likely to occur.

Biotin supplementation is however indicated after prolonged antibiotic therapy. Levels of 2.2 μg/kg/day are said to prevent the signs of deficiency appearing in adult dogs and 4.4 μg/kg/day in puppies (NRC 1974).

Vitamin C

Although it is well known that dogs, in common with most mammals, are independent of any need for dietary vitamin C, many claims have been made for its role in preventing conditions such as hip dysplasia. However, there is very little credible evidence to support any belief that such conditions can be influenced by even high doses of vitamin C. However, a disease similar to human infantile scurvy (Moeller–Barlow's disease) is said to respond to vitamin C therapy, although positive evidence of low circulating levels of vitamin C is so far wanting (see p. 146).

Carbohydrate

Until recently it was generally held that dogs did not have a dietary requirement for carbohydrate in their diet, provided enough nutrients were available for energy needs from other nutrients. Recent work has suggested however that a high fat/carbohydrate free diet may be insufficient to maintain gestation and survival of growing puppies (Romsos *et al* 1981). Further work is needed to substantiate such claims. In practical terms however any latent deficiency is not likely to become manifest, as the great majority of pregnant and lactating bitches have some form of cereal mixer in their diet. It is certainly advisable to continue to supply some energy from carbohydrate sources at this time.

Essential fatty acids

The needs for essential fatty acids (EFAs) can be met for dogs by providing 1% of the dietary dry matter as linoleic acid (Burger 1982). Unlike cats, dogs have the enzyme system to elongate the short chain fatty acids so a dietary source of arachidonic acid is not needed and dietary fat of animal origin is not essential as it probably is in cats.

EFA deficient dogs show keratinisation of the skin evident in scurfiness, with dull dry, brittle coats which respond to the administration of corn oil or other rich source of EFAs.

THE DIETARY MANAGEMENT OF CANINE DISEASE

The management of canine conditions where the fault lies in the provision of too much or not enough of particular available nutrients is relatively straightforward. Once the cause has been determined it can usually be rectified.

The rationale for such remedial action is usually clear, although the procedure may be lengthy and tedious. The adoption of a feeding regime based on foods designed and manufactured for the purpose intended, will resolve most nutritional problems. This is provided the dog will eat enough of the food and changes are still reversible. The dietary management of canine disease which is not actually caused by faulty feeding, but has a dietary component in its management is a science which has not attracted much detailed investigation when compared with more basic studies. Much of the available advice is extrapolated from experience in other species.

GENERAL GUIDELINES FOR FEEDING DOGS WITH POOR APPETITES

Unlike most cats, dogs are less effected by environmental factors and rarely starve themselves in the presence of wholesome food; however most illnesses are associated with some degree of inappetence. Such individuals can usually be encouraged to eat by applying the following guidelines.

1 Feed small amounts on a 'little and often basis', rather than large meals at infrequent intervals.

2 Dispose of all food not eaten after 15–20 minutes.

3 Feed wet foods to improve palatability. Canned foods can be made wetter by adding around 50–100 ml of water to each meal.

4 Offer food at around 37–38°C, but not higher than 40°C. Palatability is improved with food temperatures up to about 'blood heat', that is the temperature live prey would normally be. Warming food also releases a number of odours making it more attractive to dogs. The improvement in palatability declines rapidly above 40°C.

5 Feed at the time of day the dog is accustomed to, at its usual location, preferably with its own utensils, provided by the dog's usual attendant. Although dogs are generally much less sensitive to environmental influences on feeding behaviour than cats, a dog used to being fed in the morning may well have a completely different attitude to food provided in the late afternoon or evening.

6 Even when a special diet is indicated, the food may be flavoured by small amounts of the dog's favourite foods.

7 Feed in a group situation if this is possible, unless there is good reason not to. Most animals eat more in a competitive environment. Although there is much less control over what is actually eaten, it may provoke an otherwise reluctant individual to begin eating.

8 Whilst bland easily digested foods may be indicated, particularly with alimentary disturbances with vomiting or diarrhoea, food with a more obvious odour may help stimulate an interest in eating in an otherwise reluctant feeder.

Some owners may simply fail to provide enough calories. Dogs are less likely to supplement their diet by hunting or scavenging, although this may mask potential nutritional inadequacy for a time in some individuals.

A dog's energy needs may vary from between 150 kcal/kg to 50 kcal/kg daily. The least demanding is the basic maintenance of a large inactive adult dog, much more taxing are the needs of lactating bitches rearing a large litter and the extreme needs of dogs doing very hard work in a cold environment. In these circumstances four or more times the normal maintenance energy level may be needed. Such an individual may find it impossible to accommodate its daily needs at one meal, so three or even more meals may be necessary every day, to the extent of feeding during the night.

FOOD-INDUCED ALLERGY

The commonest manifestations of food related allergy in dogs are gastrointestinal disturbances and skin changes. Occasionally a severe anaphylactic reaction can occur which can even be life-threatening. Allergic skin responses may take several hours to develop, up to half a day or more. Alimentary disturbances may occur after similar periods resulting in vomiting and diarrhoea which may continue for 2–3 days even after the allergen has been removed from the diet.

Inflammatory skin responses may be complicated by self-inflicted injury and superimposed infection and the basic nature of the lesion may be masked. Symptomatic treatment is likely to be unrewarding if the allergen is still present in the diet. The main difficulties when food-induced allergy is suspected is the identification of the allergen and convincing the owner that the fault lies with the animal not the food. Each case must be investigated methodically as the putative allergen must be eliminated from the diet permanently. Test feeding requires a sustained effort on the part of the investigator as well as the owner. It may be necessary to hospitalise the dog to make sure that the controlled introduction of potential allergens is not prejudiced by 'unauthorised' feeding and to prevent hunting or scavenging food which will nullify attempts at identifying the dietary component causing the allergic response.

The dog must be taken off the diet it is being fed and put onto a single source of protein such as cooked fish, chicken or rabbit with boiled drinking water as the only supplement allowed. This feeding regime should continue for 5 days. If the signs do not recede this may be due to intercurrent infection or continued self-inflicted injury, if either of these is the case, further treatment will be needed. Persistence of the clinical signs may also be because the protein source selected is the actual allergen or failing that the condition is not a food-induced allergy at all. If the signs recede on the basal test diet, possible allergens may be introduced one at a time, allowing up to five days on each to see if the clinical signs return. If they do the allergen can be confirmed by removing, then re-introducing it. It is best to start the challenge procedure with the most common food allergens, these are cow's milk (casein being the usual allergen), beef, fish and wheat gluten.

Although food-induced allergies account for only a small percentage of all allergies, dogs are more likely to be allergic to wheat protein (gluten) than cats. To date attempts at hyposensitisation have not been rewarding (Walton 1977). Multiple sensitivities are less usual than in man, although some dogs may be allergic to cow's milk and some meats as well. Where this does occur lesions may return if only one of these allergens is introduced into the diet.

Only small amounts of a dietary allergen are usually needed to trigger an allergic response and one of the principal problems is convincing owners that any known allergen must be totally excluded for the rest of the animal's life. In EEC countries it will be of help after 1984 as manufacturers will be required to do what most in the United Kingdom have done for some time, that is declare lists of ingredients on packs of prepared foods. This is a valuable guide in the selection of foods to exclude particular components. Where more detailed information is needed manufacturers may be asked directly.

DIABETES MELLITUS

As with other mammalian species diabetic dogs show hyperglycaemia with a persistent glycosuria when fasted. Dogs are usually good subjects for insulin therapy when diabetic, provided the owner is sensible and motivated to co-operate fully. Once fluid balance disturbances have been corrected, the dietary regime should be stabilised. It is most important to keep energy intake and output as unchanged as is practicable. Prepared foods have a definite advantage in this respect where there is effective quality control and foods are relatively unchanging. Dogs normally stabilise their own energy output, but it may be necessary to confine more active individuals. Foods containing simple sugars, as are sometimes used in semi-moist foods as humectants, are best avoided as they may provoke hyperglycaemic peaks in diabetic animals. Contrary to a widely held belief there is no indication for withholding all carbohydrate from a diabetic animal's diet. Up to 40% of the total calories provided may be as carbohydrate without causing additional hyperglycaemia. Dogs fed on canned meat and biscuit on a 50:50 volume:volume basis would receive about 35–45% of their energy as carbohydrate, which is a reasonable proportion for most diabetics. Dividing the food allowance into several meals spread out evenly during the day may help a brittle case accommodate. This can best be done by allowing half the total energy allowance in the middle of the day and dividing the remainder equally between the morning and evening meals (Leibetseder 1982). So prepared foods containing wheat, rice or potato may be quite suitable for feeding to diabetic dogs. There is evidence that high fibre diets actually decrease the amount of insulin which needs to be administered to human diabetics, but it is not known whether this effect occurs in dogs.

CHRONIC DIARRHOEA/ MALABSORPTION

Diarrhoea is a clinical sign manifest as an increase in fluidity and frequency of defaecation and not a disease in itself. Dietary adjustment may be part of the process of investigation (see Food-induced allergy) or the actual treatment of cases.

The inability of an individual's gut to digest or absorb any part of the diet is likely to lead to diarrhoea in some degree.

Exocrine pancreatic failure is more common in dogs than cats. German Shepherd Dogs account for the majority of cases, making up 75% of cases presented (Darke 1977; Leibetseder 1982).

Dogs with normal pancreatic function are able to tolerate high levels of dietary fat; up to 40% in the diet is satisfactory provided other nutrients are present in proportion (NRC 1974). Fat restriction is needed where there is a lack of pancreatic enzymes.

Some individuals may show an intolerance to certain dietary components for reasons which remain obscure. Clearly such foods need to be excluded from the dog's diet, either completely or in amounts which can be digested. Many dogs are unable to tolerate liver in any form for example, although they may safely eat, say, kidney or heart. Liver from pigs is usually more difficult to digest as it is more fibrous than lamb's liver.

Soy protein, as textured vegetable protein (TVP) is normally found to be useful in dog nutrition, however some dogs produce very loose faeces when fed TVP-containing foods. Such dogs are often digestively sensitive to many meats as well and often thrive on canned mixtures of fish and cereal which contain no TVP or meat. Some individuals have insufficient lactase in their gut to be able to digest lactose. The result is twofold as undigested lactose in the small intestine allows lactose-fermenting bacteria to proliferate, causing a considerable amount of local inflammation. This, combined with the osmotic effect of a large molecule polysaccharide in the gut, results in very wet profuse diarrhoea all the time the dog is allowed access to milk. Lactose intolerance becomes evident when the supplies of lactase are exhausted. It is advisable therefore to withhold all forms of milk from cases of diarrhoea for a period of 2–3 days. Most cases of lactose intolerance will then resolve spontaneously. The majority of dogs are able to accommodate up to 3 g of lactose per 400 kcal daily (see p. 378). Resolution will also occur in those dogs which are allergic to casein. It is worth making up a test feed with casein but without lactose to differentiate between the conditions as this will be needed to determine the future diet of the individual.

The general treatment of chronic diarrhoea is otherwise based on withholding solid food for a period of 24 hours and providing only drinking water or an electrolyte solution by mouth. Food of a bland easily digested type may be introduced in small amounts on a 'little and often' basis providing the total food needs are spread over at least 3–4 meals each day. When diarrhoea persists agents which absorb fluid and harden faeces such as kaolin and chalk mixtures may be administered; in addition dehydrated potato powder fed dry or mixed in with prepared foods, helps to give some structure to the faeces. Live yoghurt is occasionally very effective in resolving otherwise intractable cases of diarrhoea where the aetiology is bacterial.

CHRONIC RENAL FAILURE

When a dog's kidneys are no longer able to effectively eliminate the end products of protein metabolism, uraemia results due to the accumulation of potentially toxic material in all the individual tissues. Protein restriction is usually needed to control the effects of uraemia. The objective is to try to supply enough protein to meet the dog's amino acid needs and not go beyond that, so far as it is practical to do so. Adequate energy supplies from non-protein sources are needed to reduce the amount of protein contributing to uraemia. Bovee (1977) has shown that around 75% of the total kidney mass has to become inoperative before the signs of renal failure begin to develop. In addition to protein restriction water soluble vitamins, as well as calcium, are lost by way of the damaged kidney so a vitamin/mineral supplement is usually indicated, especially where there is diarrhoea, as intestinal absorption is likely to be affected as well.

Although there is general agreement that some protein restriction is needed for dogs with chronic renal failure, the extent of the restriction is the subject of much debate.

Inevitably some measure of compromise is needed. If less protein is provided than is actually required for maintenance purposes, there is a breakdown of the dog's lean body mass. This contributes to uraemia as well as weakening the dog. On the other hand any excesses have to be deaminated and also contribute to uraemia.

A further complication arises from most normal dog's dislike of low protein diets. It is easy to lose sight of the fact that only food which is eaten has any nutritive value. Dogs with renal failure usually have some degree of inappetence which tends to compound the problem of controlling dietary protein intake. Fortunately the need to supply the most useful proteins for the dog, and thus reduce the amount of waste material, means that proteins of high biological value are needed. This in turn has palatability advantages as in general, the better 'quality' the proteins are in terms of amino acid profile, the more palatable the diet is likely to be.

The total amount of protein actually offered to each dog with renal failure is for the veterinarian in charge of the case to judge. A useful starting point is to feed 1.3 g/kg bodyweight daily. The effect on the uraemic state of the dog can be monitored by determinations of the circulating urea levels and assessing the state of the dog's nitrogen balance.

It is usually clear when the dog is in negative nitrogen balance as there is usually a progressive loss of lean body mass, although the dog may be eating reasonable quantities of food. A reasonably positive nitrogen balance should be aimed for where the amount of protein in excess of requirements is reasonably generous, this will be reflected in the circulating urea levels. When feeding dogs with severe uraemia, however, a protein intake of 0.66 g/kg bodyweight daily is advised (Osborne 1974).

Feeding dogs with chronic renal failure requires continuous supervision. Urinary protein losses are difficult to assess without collecting 24 hour urine samples; not usually a practical measure in general veterinary practice. As a rule of thumb, however, one lightly boiled hen's egg can be added to the diet for every 100 mg protein per dl urine. The effect of this can then be monitored by examining fasting, blood, urea levels, assessing lean body mass and the general clinical state. Although this approach is empirical and rather crude, it is normally effective in practice.

GASTRIC DILATION AND TORSION

A life-threatening and sudden accumulation of gas in the stomach of certain types of dog is one of the genuine emergencies of veterinary practice. The dogs affected are usually the large deep chested varieties such as Irish Wolfhounds, Great Danes, as well as Bloodhounds, Borzois, German Shepherd Dogs and St Bernards. A number of Irish Setters, Basset Hounds, Boxers and Bull Terriers are also affected.

A good deal of the gas which collects in the dog's stomach is analytically very similar to atmospheric air. It is assumed that aerophagia is a major factor in the development of the condition. The condition rarely occurs in fussy feeders.

The distress experienced by dogs with acute gastric dilation is rapidly worsened to a state of shock when torsion supervenes. When the stomach twists, circulatory collapse can occur as a result of the obstruction of blood vessels supplying the gut.

It is clear that a number of factors need to coincide to precipitate an episode of gastric dilation/torsion, some of these may be nutritional. Van Kruiningen *et al* (1974), in an extensive review of the subject, identified aerophagia following excited greedy feeding with a readily fermentable substrate in the stomach of susceptible types of dog as being amongst the usual circumstances accompanying the condition. Because of these pointers towards the cause of gastric dilation/torsion it is possible to frame some guidelines to prevent a recurrence or even avoiding primary cases in potentially susceptible animals.

Dogs should be fed smaller, frequent meals rather than large single allocations of the day's food supply. Exercise and excitement at and around feeding times should be kept to a minimum.

These measures present profound difficulties in breeding kennels with large numbers of dogs, but if a sensible attitude is maintained, much can be achieved with sympathetic staff. Foods should be fed wet, preferably as canned foods made wetter by the addition of 100–200 ml water per kg of food. Any biscuit fed should be presoaked. Aerophagia can be further reduced if the dog is fed with its head in an elevated position.

FEEDING AGED DOGS

Old age is not a specific condition in any species, but there are some trends which may help feeding aged dogs. However, practically all conditions usually associated with ageing can occur much earlier in life.

As a dog ages its organoleptic senses dull and food may become less attractive simply because of the reduced capacity to appreciate flavours and odours. Degenerative changes in the mouth such as periodontal disease and dental deposits may lead to discomfort or simply physical difficulty in eating.

The dog's gut may be chronically inflamed leading to vomiting of undigested or partially digested food, often quite some time after meals. The processes of digestion and assimilation may be functioning so inefficiently that the dog is unable to accommodate normal sized meals. Quite often the motility of the gut is reduced to the extent that constipation becomes a serious problem.

Renal, liver and cardiac failure are relatively common conditions of aged dogs. These subjects are covered elsewhere. Where there is a normal food intake without any difficulties of digestion or absorption, obesity can follow where the dog's activity has reduced but it is still eating the same amount of food as when it had the behaviour of a younger animal.

The following are general guidelines for feeding old dogs. Care needs to be taken to assess each case individually as what might be suitable for one may be contraindicated in another individual:

1 Feed small amounts frequently rather than large single allocations of food especially where there is malabsorption.

2 Make food attractive by warming to blood heat and providing food with a clearly recognisable odour and flavour.

3 Feed reasonably non-abrasive and less hard foods where there is gingivitis or dental disease which cannot be eliminated surgically.

4 Restrict protein intake where there is evidence of renal failure. Possibly supplement with salt, vitamins/minerals, additional high biological value protein.

5 Restrict salt intake where there is sodium retention associated with cardiac insufficiency.

6 Feed bulking agents such as bran mixed in with the diet where gut motility has resulted in constipation.

7 Restrict calorie intake where adiposity has resulted in a positive energy state following reduced levels of the dog's activity.

REFERENCES

ANDERSON R.S. (1973) Obesity in the Dog and Cat. *Vet. Ann.* **14,** 182–6.

ANDERSON G.L. & LEWIS L.D. (1980) Obesity. In *Current Veterinary Therapy* Vol. VII, edited by R.W. Kirk, pp. 1034–1039. W.B. Saunders, Philadelphia.

BOVEE K.C. (1977) Diet and Kidney Failure. *Proceedings of the Kal Kan Symposium for the Treatment of Dog and Cat Diseases*, pp. 25–8. Ohio State University.

BURGER I.H. (1982) A Simplified Guide to Nutritional Needs. In *Dog and Cat Nutrition*, edited by A.T.B. Edney, pp. 13–31. Pergamon, Oxford.

DARKE P.G.G. (1977) Pancreatic Dysfunction. In *Diarrhoea in the Dog*, edited by A.T.B. Edney, 1st Waltham Symposium, pp. 27–8.

DE BRUNJIE J.J. (1983) Some Effects of Starvation in the Dog. In *Proceedings of 1983 Voorjaarsdagen, Netherlands Small Animal Veterinary Association*, pp. 170–4.

EDNEY A.T.B. (1972) Current Trends in Small Animal Nutrition. In *Vet. Ann.* **13,** 194–9.

EDNEY A.T.B. & HUGHES I.B. (1980) Practical Experience in the Dietary Control of Obesity in Dogs. *Pedigree Digest.* **8,** (2), 10–11.

FELDMAN E.C. (1980) Influence of Non-Cardiac Disease on the Heart. In *Current Veterinary Therapy*, edited by R.W. Kirk, pp. 340–7. W.B. Saunders, Philadelphia.

GLÄTTLI H.R., SCHATZMANN H. & ZINTZEN H. (1973) Dietary Measures and Essential Substances in the Treatment of Skin Diseases in Dogs. *Kleintierpraxis* **18,** 203–10.

HEDHAMMAR Å.A., WU E., KROOK L., SCHRYVER H.F., DELAHUNTA A., WHALEN J.P., KALLFELZ F.A., NUNEZ E.A., HINTZ H.F., SHEFFY B.E. & RYAN G.D. (1974) Overnutrition and Skeletal Disease. An Experimental Study in Growing Great Dane Dogs. *Cornell Veterinarian* **64,** Supplt. 2, 1–159.

HEDHAMMAR Å.A. (1980) Over-Nutrition in Large Breeds of Dogs. In *Over and Under-Nutrition*, edited by A.T.B. Edney, 2nd Waltham Symposium, pp. 30–3.

HENDRIKSON P.Å. (1968) Periodontal Disease and Calcium Deficiency. An Experimental Study in the Dog. *Acta. Odont. Scand.* **26,** Supplt. 50, 1–132.

LEIBETSEDER J. (1982) Feeding Animals Which are Ill. In *Dog and Cat Nutrition*, edited by A.T.B. Edney, pp. 85–96. Pergamon, Oxford.

LEWIS, L.D. (1977) Obesity in the Dog. In *Proceedings of 1st Kal Kan Symposium for the Treatment of Dog and Cat Diseases*, Ohio State University, pp. 19–24.

MASON E. (1970) Obesity in Pet Dogs. *Vet. Rec.* **86,** 612–16.

NRC (1974) *Nutrient Requirements of Dogs*, Report No. 8, National Academy of Sciences, Washington.

OSBORNE C.A. (1974) Dietary Restriction in the Treatment of Primary Renal Failure; Facts and Fallacies. *J. Am. Anim. Hosp. Assoc.* **10,** 73–7.

OWEN C.A. & MCCALL J.T. (1983) Identification of the Carrier State of the Bedlington Terrier Copper Disease. *Am. J. Vet. Res.* **44,** 694–6.

ROMSOS D.R., PALMER H.J., MUIRURI K.L. & BENNINK M.R.

(1981) Influence of a Low Carbohydrate Diet on Performance of Pregnant and Lactating Dogs. *J. Nutr.* **111,** (4),
678–89.

STEININGER E. (1981) Obesity in Dogs. *Weiner Tierärtzliche
Monatsschrift* **68,** 122–30.

VAN KRUNININGEN H.J., GREGOIRE K. & MENTON D.J.
(1974) Acute Gastric Dilation; A Review of Comparative
Aspects by Species and a Study of Dogs and Monkeys. *J.
Am. Anim. Hosp. Assoc.* **10,** 294–324.

WALTON G.S. (1977) Allergic Responses to Ingested Allergens. In *Current Veterinary Therapy* **VI,** edited by R.W.
Kirk, pp. 576–9. W.B. Saunders, Philadelphia.

Glossary

Trade name	Description	Manufacturer
Acthar	ACTH gel	Armour
Actrapid MC	Insulin, neutral soluble	Novo Laboratories Ltd
Adalat	Nifedipine	Bayer
Alugan	Bromocyclen	Merck
Alupent	Orciprenaline	Boehringer
Amerlex TF4	RIA measurement of free T4	Amersham Int.
Aminofusin L600	Parenteral supplement	BDH Pharm.
Aminoplex	Parenteral amino acid supplement	Geistlich
Amipaque	Metrizamide	Nyegaard
Apresoline	Hydralazine	CIBA
Arquel	Melcofenamic acid	Parke Davis
Benadryl	Diphenhydramine hydrochloride	Parke Davis
Betsolan drops	Betamethasone sodium phosphate	Glaxo
Bisolvon	Bromhexine	Boehringer
Biricanyl	Terbutaline	Astra
Capoten	Captopril	Squibb
Casilan	High protein low fat diet	Glaxo
Catapres inj.	Clonidine	Boehringer
Cetiprin	Emepronium bromide	Kabivitrum
Conray 60	Meglumine iothalamate	May & Baker
Cordilox	Verapamil	Abbott
DDAVP	Desmopressin	Ferring
Daranide	Dichlorphenamide	Merck
Depo-medrone	Methylprednisolone acetate	Upjohn
Dextrostix	Diagnostic test sticks	Ames
Diabinese	Chlorothiazide	Pfizer
Diamox	Acetazolamide	Lederle
Dibenylene	Phenoxybenzamine hydrochloride	SKF
Dramamine	Dimenhydramine	Searle
Eltroxin	Thyroxine	Glaxo
Endemine	Diazoxide	Allen & Hanbury
Epanutin	Phenytoin	Parke Davis
Eurax	Crotomiton lotion	Ciba Geigy
Felocell	Live FPV vaccine	SKF
Florinef	Fludrocortisone acetate	Squibb
Fungassay	Dermatophyte test medium	C. Vet Ltd.

Glucagon injection	Glucagon	Eli Lilly
Haemaccel	Urea crosslinked gelatin	Hoechst
Harleco apparatus	Plasma bicarbonate measurement	American Hosp. Supply Co.
Healan-Vet	Sodium hyaluranate	Pharmacia
Hydrocortone	Cortisol	Merck
Inderal	Propranolol	ICI
Intralipid	Parenteral fat supplement	KabiVitrum
Isoptoplain	Hydroxypropyl methylcellulose (hypromellose)	Alcon
Keto-diastix	Diagnostic test sticks	Ames
Ketoperlen	Amino acid supplement	Pfrimmer
Ketrax	Oral levamisole	ICI
Kidnamin	Amino acid supplement	KabiVitrum
Lanoxin	Digoxin	Wellcome
Largactil	Chlorpromazine hydrochloride	May Baker
Librium	Chlordiazepoxide	Roche
Lipiodol	Contrast material	May & Baker
Liquifilm	Polyvinyl alcohol	Allergan
Lysodren	Mitotane, *op'* DDD	Bristol-Myers
Macrodex	Dextran 70	Pharmacia
Maxalon	Metoclopramide	Beechams
Mepavlon	Meprobamate	ICI
Mucodyne	Carbocisteine	Berk
Mydriacyl	Tropicamide	Alcon
Myocrisin	Sodium aurothiomalate	May & Baker
Myodil	Iodo-phenylundecyclate	Glaxo
Myotonine chloride	Bethanechol chloride	Glenwood
	Acetohydroxamanic acid	Sigma London Chemical Co. Ltd
Numotac	Isoetharine	Riker
Ophthaine	Proparacaine hydrochloride	Squibb
Oradexon injection	Dexamethasone	Organon
Ovarid	Megestrol acetate	Glaxo
Panalog	Steroid/antibiotic/fungal cream	Squibb
Percorten M	Deoxycortone pivilate	Ciba
Pevidine medicated wash	Povidine-iodine	Berk
Phenergan	Promethazine hydrochloride	May & Baker
Pitressin	Vasopressin-tannate-in-oil	Parke Davis
Ponstan	Mefanamic acid	Parke Davis
Pro-Banthine	Propontheline bromide	Searle
Quellada	BHC-shampoo	Stafford Miller
Reflotest-glucose	Diagnostic test sticks	BCL Labs
Resonium-A	Sodium polystyrene sulphonate	Winthrop Labs
Rheumacrodex	Dextran-40	Pharmacia
Rythmodan	Disopyramide	Roussel

Saventrine	Isoprenaline	Pharmax
Solganol	Sodium auriothioglucose	Schering
Solu-Cortef	Cortisol sodium succinate	Upjohn
Somatotropin	Growth hormone	Koch-Light Laboratories Ltd
Stelazine	Trifluoperazine hydrochloride	SKF
Stemetil	Prochloperazine mesylate	May & Baker
Synalar lotion	Fluocinolone	ICI
Syncathen	Tetracosactrin	Ciba
Synthamin 7S	Amino acid supplement	Travenol
Syntopressin	Lysine vasopressin nasal spray	Sandoz
Tagamet	Cimetidine	SKF
Tardak	Delmadinone acetate	Syntex
Thrombo-Wellcotest	Fibrin test	Wellcome
Thytropar	Thyroid stimulating hormone	Armour
Tosmilen	Demecarium bromide	Astra/Sinclair
Unopettes	Blood counting system	Becton-Dickinson
Vacutainer	Blood vacuum tubes	Becton-Dickinson
Valium	Diazepam	Roche
Vamin fructose		KabiVitrum
Ventolin	Phenylephrine, ephedrine or salbutanol	A&H
Vetsovate	Betamethasone valerate 0.05%	Glaxo
Xylocard	Lignocaine	Astra
Zyluric	Oral allopurinol	Wellcome

INDEX

Page numbers suffixed by 't' indicates tabulated material, and by 'f' indicates figures.